Neurological Aspects of Substance Abuse

Neurological Aspects of Substance Abuse

Second Edition

John C. M. Brust, M.D.

Professor of Clinical Neurology, Columbia University College of Physicians and Surgeons; Director, Department of Neurology, Harlem Hospital Center, New York, New York

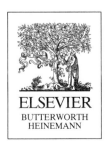

ELSEVIER
BUTTERWORTH
HEINEMANN

ELSEVIER
BUTTERWORTH
HEINEMANN

RM
316
.B78
2004

170 S. Independence Mall W.
300 E. Philadelphia, PA 19106-3399

NEUROLOGICAL ASPECTS OF SUBSTANCE ABUSE   ISBN 0-7506-7313-3

NOTICE

Medicine is an ever-changing field. Standard safety precautions must be followed but as new research and clinical experience broaden our knowledge, changes in treatment and drug therapy may become necessary or appropriate. Readers are advised to check the most current product information provided by the manufacturer of each drug to be administered to verify the recommended dose, the method and duration of administration, and contraindications. It is the responsibility of the treating physician, relying on experience and knowledge of the patient, to determine dosages and the best treatment for each individual patient. Neither the Publisher nor the author assumes any liability for any injury and/or damage to persons or property arising from this publication.

The Publisher

Library of Congress Cataloging-in-Publication Data

Brust, John C. M. (John Calvin M.), 1936-
  Neurological aspects of substance abuse/John C. M. Brust–2nd ed.
    p. ; cm.
  Includes bibliographical references and index.
  ISBN 0-7506-7313-3
   1. Psychopharmacology. 2. Substance abuse–Complications. I. Title.
   [DNLM: 1. Neurologic Manifestations. 2. Substance-Related
  Disorders–physiopathology. 3. Nervous System–drug effects. WM 270 B912n 2004]
  RM316.B78 2004
  616.86–dc22

                                                        2003065533

Editor: Susan F. Pioli
Editorial Assistant: Joan Ryan
Publishing Services Manager: Joan Sinclair
Project Manager: Mary Stermel

Printed in the United States of America

Last digit is the print number: 9   8   7   6   5   4   3   2   1

As before, for Meridee, Mary, Frederick, and James

Contents

Preface for First Edition

Reminiscent of "The Sorcerer's Apprentice," we are awash in a deluge of redundant medical texts. Nevertheless, my colleague Dr. Lewis P. Rowland persuaded me that neurologists would welcome a book on drug abuse. If you disagree, blame him. If you agree with the premise but don't like the product, blame me.

The title has been carefully considered, for it is my view that most biomedical aspects of drug abuse are in fact neurological. Accordingly, the text addresses pharmacology and animal studies, overdose and withdrawal, medical and neurological complications, fetal effects, and pharmacotherapy. Historical background and epidemiology are also considered, partly because the subject is often quite entertaining, and partly because contradictory and bizarre societal attitudes toward particular substances are better understood in an historical context.

Some of this material has appeared in a chapter on drug dependence I wrote for Joynt's *Clinical Neurology*, and I thank the publishers at Harper & Row for letting me occasionally plagiarize my own sentences without fear of copyright infringement. I also thank Dr. Robert Joynt for inviting me to write that chapter, without which I doubt I would have had the fortitude to proceed with the present text.

Other thanks are due to Nancy Megley, formerly at Butterworth, for early encouragement; Christopher Davis, also formerly at Butterworth, whose cheerful patience remained unflagging as one promised delivery date after another receded into the future; Susan Pioli, currently at Butterworth, who brought the final product to the finish line; Sandra Sands, Janet Rivera, and Jeffrey Green for indispensable assistance with the manuscript; Dr. Edward B. Healton and Ellen Giesow of the Columbia P&S Dean's office at Harlem Hospital Center, for support tangible and intangible; and—even though his suggestion effectively demolished 52 consecutive weekends—Dr. Lewis P. Rowland.

John C.M. Brust, M.D.
New York, New York

Preface

The observation in Ecclesiastes that there is nothing new under the sun might apply to public attitudes toward substance abuse and addiction; as the decades roll by, the March of Folly otherwise known as America's War on Drugs continues apace. Amidst political posturing, media distortions, and corporate turpitude, however, enough is new on the neurobiological and clinical fronts to justify a second edition of this text.

In no particular order, questions addressed in the present volume include: Is there a pharmacological common denominator for all addictive drugs? What is the extended amygdala? Is sensitization the switch that turns on addiction? Does ethanol bind to neurotransmitter receptors? How many Americans currently use illicit drugs? How many American 21-year-olds are binge drinkers? What are blunts? What are bidis? What do nitrites have to do with AIDS? What ever happened to the "crack babies"? What percent of United States federal antidrug expenditures is for education and treatment? What is bad about Stadol? What is bad about Oxy-Contin? How do endocannabinoids act? Why was it so difficult for the FDA to ban ephedra products? What drugs turn up at "raves"? What is "whack"? How many people worldwide will the tobacco industry kill over the next three decades? Does angel dust cause schizophrenia? What is "doing a shotgun"? What effect on U.S. illicit drug consumption has defoliation of the South American continent had? What effect on international drug trafficking has the War in Afghanistan had? Does marijuana cause lasting cognitive impairment? Does cocaine? Does "Ecstasy"? Does tobacco? What is a grimmie? What is "candyflipping"? What is post-hallucinogen perceptual disorder? Why would someone drink toner cartridge cleaner? Does ethanol cause strokes or prevent them? Does ethanol cause dementia or prevent it? What is "U4Euh"? Does heroin maintenance therapy make sense? How does kava affect eye movements? What is DARPP-32? Does therapeutic ibogaine have a future? What are the "date-rape" drugs? Who didn't inhale?

A number of people deserve thanks for advice, encouragement, or simply forbearance, but some merit special mention. My secretary, Shirley E. Myers-Jones, working as she does with a word processor illiterate, was a good deal more involved with the text than secretaries these days expect to be. Susan Pioli of Elsevier once again cheerfully nudged the book to completion as one missed deadline succeeded another. Finally, Columbia University's former Chairman of Neurology, Dr. Lewis P. Rowland, continues to visit us regularly at Harlem Hospital Center, as does his successor, Dr. Timothy A. Pedley. Without their support, out-of-job-title projects like "Neurological Aspects of Substance Abuse" would not be possible.

John C.M. Brust, M.D.
New York, New York

Chapter 1
Questions and Definitions

Giving up smoking is easy. I've done it hundreds of times.
—Mark Twain

Just say no.
—Nancy Reagan

I didn't inhale.
—William Jefferson Clinton

What Do We Mean by *Dependence*, *Addiction*, and *Abuse*?

In 1964, the World Health Organization (WHO) Expert Committee on Addiction-Producing Drugs recommended that the terms *drug addiction* and *drug habituation* be replaced by *drug dependence,* defined as:

> a state of psychic or physical dependence, or both, on a drug, arising in a person following administration of that drug on a periodic or continuous basis. The characteristics of such a state will vary with the agent involved ... for example, dependence of morphine type, of barbiturate type, of amphetamine type, etc.[1]

Psychic dependence is "... a feeling of satisfaction and a psychic drive that requires periodic or continuous administration of the drug to produce pleasure or avoid discomfort." Physical dependence is "... an adaptive state that manifests itself by intense physical disturbances when the administration of the drug is suspended or when its action is affected by administration of a specific antagonist." Psychic dependence thus induces "psychic" symptoms and compulsive drug-seeking behavior. Physical dependence induces "physical" symptoms and objective signs. Psychic and physical dependence can occur independently or together, and only mind–brain dualists need concern themselves over the *voluntary* or *nonorganic* aspects of the former and the *involuntary* or *organic* aspects of the latter.

These definitions were subsequently subjected to a fair amount of tinkering. For example, in 1982, a WHO memorandum suggested replacing *physical dependence* with *neuroadaptive state* and explicitly distinguished dependence from *drug-related disability.*[2] The American Psychiatric Association's Diagnostic and Statistical Manual (DSM-IV), moreover, has its own set of criteria for dependence and abuse (Tables 1–1, 1–2).[3] Nevertheless, the original definitions of physical and psychic dependence have remained in general usage.

Addiction is psychic dependence. An *addict* is someone whose psychic dependence—with or without physical dependence—has made drug procurement a daily preoccupation. Addiction used to be equated with physical dependence; it was believed

Table 1–1. DSM-IV Criteria for Substance Dependence

A maladaptive pattern of substance use, leading to clinically significant impairment or distress, as manifested by three (or more) of the following, occurring at any time in the same 12-month period:
1. Tolerance, as defined by either of the following:
   (a) need for markedly increased amounts of the substance to achieve intoxication or desired effect
   (b) markedly diminished effect with continued use of the same amount of the substance
2. Withdrawal, as manifested by either of the following:
   (a) the characteristic withdrawal syndrome for the substance
   (b) the same (or a closely related) substance is taken to relieve or avoid withdrawal symptoms
3. The substance is often taken in larger amounts or over a longer period than was intended
4. There is a persistent desire or unsuccessful efforts to cut down or control substance use
5. A great deal of time is spent in activities necessary to obtain the substance (e.g., visiting multiple doctors or driving long distances), use the substance (e.g., chain-smoking), or recover from its effects
6. Important social, occupational, or recreational activities are given up or reduced because of substance use
7. The substance use is continued despite knowledge of having a persistent or recurrent physical or psychological problem that is likely to have been caused or exacerbated by the substance (e.g., current cocaine use despite recognition of cocaine-induced depression, or continued drinking despite recognition that an ulcer was made worse by alcohol consumption)

Specify if:
With Physiological Dependence: evidence of tolerance or withdrawal (i.e., either Item 1 or 2 is present)
Without Physiological Dependence: no evidence of tolerance or withdrawal (i.e., neither Item 1 nor 2 is present)

Source: Modified from Diagnostic and Statistical Manual of Mental Disorders, 4th edition. Washington, DC: American Psychiatric Association, 1994, with permission of the publisher.

that prolonged exposure of neurons to a drug led to adaptive responses, which in turn led to craving, which in turn led to drug-seeking. Such a sequence of events would occur whether the drug was self-administered (by an animal or human) or passively administered (by an investigator or nurse). In fact, many patients who receive morphine passively for pain have prominent withdrawal symptoms yet little or no craving for the drug. Conversely, abstinent tobacco smokers often have intense craving without observable physical signs. Conditioning and learning are crucial to the development of addiction[4]—as emphasized by the U.S. Surgeon General, when in 1988 he pronounced tobacco an addictive drug.[5]

The term *drug abuse* is a social judgment. One might be considered a drug abuser for using an illegal substance (e.g., heroin or cocaine), for using a legal substance in amounts that others consider excessive (e.g., ethanol), or for using a legal substance in any amount (e.g., tobacco). Pharmacologists often use the term *abuse liability* to signify a drug's potential for inducing addictive behavior; indeed, that concept is the basis of Drug Enforcement

Table 1–2. DSM-IV Criteria for Substance Abuse

A. A maladaptive pattern of substance use leading to clinically significant impairment or distress, as manifested by one (or more) of the following, occurring within a 12-month period
   1. Recurrent substance use resulting in a failure to fulfill major role obligations at work, school, or home (e.g., repeated absences or poor work performance related to substance use; substance-related absences, suspensions, or expulsions from school; neglect of children or household)
   2. Recurrent substance use in situations in which it is physically hazardous (e.g., driving an automobile or operating a machine when impaired by substance use)
   3. Recurrent substance-related legal problems (e.g., arrests for substance-related disorderly conduct)
   4. Continued substance use despite having persistent or recurrent social or interpersonal problems caused or exacerbated by the effects of the substance (e.g., arguments with spouse about consequences of intoxication, physical fights)
B. The symptoms have never met the criteria for Substance Dependence for this class of substance

Source: Modified from Diagnostic and Statistical Manual of Mental Disorders, 4th edition. Washington, DC: American Psychiatric Association, 1994, with permission of the publisher.

Administration (DEA) drug scheduling under the 1970 Controlled Substances Act (Table 1–3). In clinical practice, however, abuse is not the same as addiction. Even one-time use of a drug is abuse if it causes harm to oneself—for example, cocaine—or to others—for example, ethanol. Conversely, although by the above-mentioned definition caffeine is an addicting drug, its legality and lack of perceived harmfulness allow coffee drinkers to pass their days free of social stigma. As we shall see, in the United States neither addiction liability nor physical harm has much bearing on a drug's legal status.

Table 1–3. Federal Schedules of Controlled Drugs, 2003

	Opioids	Stimulants	Sedatives/Hypnotics	Other

Schedule I	Benzylmorphine
	Dihydromorphinone
	Heroin
	Ketobemidone
	Levormoamide
	Morphine-
	  methylsufanate
	Nicocodeine
	Nicomorphine
	Racemoramide
		Cathinone
		N-methylamphetamine
		3,4-Methylenedioxy-
		  methamphetamine
		MDMA
		Ecstasy
		Phenylpropanolamine
		4-methylaminorex
		4-bromo-3, 4-dimethoxy-
		  phenylethylamine
			Methaqualone
			Quaalude
				Bufotenine
				Ibogaine
				Lysergic acid
				  diethylamide
				LSD
				Marijuana
				Mescaline
				Peyote
				Phencyclidine
				PCP
				Psilocybin

Schedule II	Alfentanil *Alfenta* Codeine Fentanyl *Sublimaze* Hydromorphine *Dilaudid* Levorphanol *Levo-Dromeram* Methadylacetate (LAAM) Meperidine *Demerol* Methadone Morphine Oxycodone *OxyContin* *Perocet* *Percodan* Oxymorphone *Numorphan* Pantopon Sufentanil *Sufenta*	Amphetamines Cocaine Dextroamphetamine *Dexedrine* Methamphetamine *Desoxyn* Methylphenidate *Ritalin* Phenmetrazine *Fastin* *Preludin*	Amobarbital *Amytal* Glutehimide *Doriden* Pentobarbital *Nembutal* Secobarbital *Seconal*	
Schedule III	Buprenorphine *Buprenex* *Subutex* Buprenorphine + Naloxone *Suboxone* Codeine compounds *Tylenol #3* *Tussionex*	Benzphetamine *Ditrex* Phendimetrazine *Plegine*	Butabarbital *Butisol* Butalbital *Fiorecet* *Fiorinal* Methyprylon *Noludar* Gamma- hydroxybutyrate *Xyrem*	Dronabinol *Marinol* Testosterone

Continued

Table 1–3. *Continued*

	Opioids	**Stimulants**	**Sedatives/Hypnotics**	**Other**
Schedule IV	Propoxyphene	Diethylpropion	Alprazolam	
	Darvon	*Tenuate*	*Xanax*	
	Darvocet	Phentermine	Chloral betaine	
	Pentazocine	*Fastin*	Chloral hydrate	
	Talwin	Modafinil	*Noctec*	
		Provigil	Chlordiazepoxide	
			Librium	
			Clonazepam	
			Klonopin	
			Clorazepate	
			Tranxene	
			Diazepam	
			Valium	
			Estazolam	
			Prosom	
			Ethchlorvynol	
			Placidyl	
			Ethinamate	
			Flurazepam	
			Dalmane	
			Halazepam	
			Paxipam	
			Lorazepam	
			Ativan	
			Mazindol	
			Sanorex	
			Mephobarbital	
			Mebaral	
			Meprobamate	
			Equanil	
			Methohexital	
			Brevital Sodium	
			Methylphenobarbital	
			Midazolam	
			Versed	
			Oxazepam	
			Serax	
			Paraldehyde	
			Paral	
			Phenobarbital	
			Luminal	
			Prazepam	
			Centrax	
			Temazepam	
			Restoril	
			Triazolam	
			Halcion	
			Zaleplon	
			Sonata	
			Zolpidem	
			Ambien	

Continued

Table 1–3. *Continued*

	Opioids	Stimulants	Sedatives/Hypnotics	Other
Schedule V	Opium preparations *Donnagel PG* *Kaopectalin PG*	1-Deoxyephedrine *Vicks Inhaler*	Chlordiazepoxide *Librax*	

Schedule I: High potential for abuse, no accepted medical use
Schedule II: High potential for abuse, currently accepted medical use
Schedule III: Accepted medical use, lower potential for abuse than Schedule I and II drugs
Schedule IV: Lower potential for abuse than Schedule III drugs
Schedule V: Lowest abuse potential of the controlled substances; includes over-the-counter antitussives and antidiarrheals

What Is *Tolerance* and What Does It Have to Do with Physical Dependence and Addiction?

Tolerance is "... an adaptive state characterized by diminished response to the same quantity of drug or by the fact that a larger dose is required to produce the same degree of pharmacodynamic effect."[1] There are several kinds of tolerance. Metabolic, dispositional, or pharmacokinetic tolerance results from increased metabolism and decreased availability of the drug at its locus of action. Cellular or pharmacodynamic tolerance, on the other hand, is a reduced response despite unchanging drug concentrations and availability; it signifies an adaptive change in the brain.[6]

Different from pharmacokinetic and pharmacodynamic tolerance are behavioral and environmental tolerance. Behavioral tolerance is a reduced response consequent to a drug's negative effect on reward-seeking or punishment-avoiding behavior.[7] For example, rats intoxicated with ethanol and performing equilibratory tasks develop tolerance to the drug's ataxic effects faster than rats not being tested.[6] Environmental tolerance is the result of a drug being administered in a setting of familiar cues.[8] It could be considered an atypical pavlovian response. Pavlov observed classical conditioning in dogs receiving morphine injections (the unconditioned stimulus); after enough trials, the appearance of the technician (the conditioned stimulus) was sufficient to produce morphine-like effects of salivation, vomiting, and sleep.[9] By contrast, animals receiving morphine "in the context of pre-drug cues" may be *less* sensitive to its analgesic, thermic, locomotor, sedating, and even lethal effects than animals tested in an unfamiliar setting.[8,10] This particular conditioned response— environmental tolerance—seems to result from an *anticipatory compensation*, which attenuates the drug's effect, perhaps by causing environmentally cued changes in drug disposition.[11]

The interrelationships between tolerance, physical dependence, and drug-seeking behavior are complex.[12] In animals, tolerance and physical dependence for psychoactive addicting agents tend to develop and persist together, and inhibitors of protein synthesis block both.[13] On the other hand, in humans, marijuana and lysergic acid diethylamide (LSD)-like drugs produce striking tolerance, yet marijuana causes few symptoms of physical dependence, and with hallucinogens withdrawal symptoms do not occur. With opioids, which produce predictable, severe withdrawal symptoms and signs, tolerance is much more marked for psychic and analgesic effects than for smooth muscle actions. Withdrawal from amphetamine and cocaine causes depression, hunger, and intense craving but few objective signs, and although tolerance develops to the euphoric effects of these psychostimulants, there seems to be *reverse tolerance (sensitization)* to psychosis, abnormal movements, and seizures. Whether tolerance is required for physical dependence is unclear, and it is possible that an explanation of either phenomenon—in terms of, say, enzyme regulation, receptor change, or functional hypertrophy of alternate pathways—will shed little light on addiction per se.

What Is the Significance of Sensitization?

As noted, with repeated drug administration some effects decrease (tolerance) yet others increase ("sensitization," "reverse tolerance"). This phenomenon, perhaps comparable to electrophysiological kindling, is particularly evident with psychostimulants. Chronic cocaine users, for example, develop increasingly severe psychosis and abnormal movements, and their seizure thresholds decrease. In animals repeated intermittent administration of cocaine or amphetamine results in a progressive increase in the ability of the drugs to produce locomotor hyperactivity or stereotyped behavior and facilitates the acquisition of drug-seeking behavior.[14–17]

Considerable current research is focused on sensitization, in the hope that understanding its biology might explain why occasional recreational drug use switches to psychic dependence (addiction).[18–20] Conditioning to environmental stimuli associated with a drug plays a significant role in sensitization, but the extent of its contribution is disputed; sensitization is not simply pavlovian conditioning.[21,22] It should be noted, moreover, that some workers, while acknowledging sensitization to locomotor response in animals and to psychosis in humans, do not believe sensitization plays a major role in reinforcement.[23]

What Then, Is the Neurobiological Basis of Addiction?

To explain addiction and reward in neurobiological terms would be a profound achievement, with ramifications far exceeding the problem of substance abuse. Accordingly, over the past decade major-league scientists have entered the field in increasing numbers, producing an exhilarating if voluminously daunting literature. Their achievements—including the anatomy of the reward circuit, neurotransmitters, signal transduction pathways, and genetics—are summarized in Chapter 2 as well as in chapters on individual agents.

How Many Americans Use or Abuse Drugs?

Modern drug abuse prevalence in the United States is crudely estimated by examining data from diverse sources. These include (1) acute medical interventions—for example, reports of hepatitis or acquired immunodeficiency syndrome (AIDS) and statistics from the Drug Abuse Warning Network (DAWN), a federally operated system that monitors emergency rooms, hospital inpatient services,

medical examiner offices, and crisis centers; (2) treatment programs, including the National Institute of Drug Abuse's Client Oriented Data Acquisition Process (CODAP); (3) law enforcement agencies; and (4) household, school, and college surveys.

Monitoring the Future (a long-term research project of the University of Michigan) and the National Household Survey on Drug Abuse (NHSDA, conducted by the Substance Abuse and Mental Health Services Administration of the Department of Health and Human Services) identified declines in the use of many illicit drugs—including marijuana, hallucinogens, cocaine, amphetamines, heroin, barbiturates, and tranquilizers—between the mid-1980s and the mid-1990s.[24,25] During the late 1990s, however, illicit drug use rose. In 2001, 15.9 million Americans aged 12 years or older (7.1% of the population) had used an illicit drug during the prior month.[25] Of those current illicit drug users, 76% used marijuana and 44% (7 million people) used other illicit drugs either alone or with marijuana. Of those 7 million people, 4.8 million (2.1% of the population) used "psychotherapeutic drugs" ("prescription-type drugs"—pain relievers, tranquilizers, stimulants, and sedatives), 1.7 million (0.7% of the population) used cocaine (including alkaloidal "crack"), 1.3 million (0.6%) used hallucinogens, 8.1 million (3.6%) used methylenedioxymethamphetamine (MDMA, "Ecstasy"), and 123,000 (0.1%) used heroin (Table 1–4).[25]

Rates of current illicit drug use varied substantially with age, peaking among 18-to 20-year olds

Table 1–4. Percentage of Americans Aged 12 Years or Over Using Illicit Drugs During the Past Month

	1999	2000	2001
Any drug	6.3	6.3	7.1
Marijuana	4.7	4.8	5.4
Psychotherapeutic	1.8	1.7	2.1
Cocaine	0.7	0.5	0.7
Hallucinogen	0.4	0.4	0.6
Heroin	0.1	0.1	0.1

Source: Substance Abuse and Mental Health Services Administration. Results from the 2001 National Household Survey on Drug Abuse: Vol I. Summary of National Findings. Rockville, MD: Office of Applied Studies, NHSDA Series H-17, DHHS Publication No. SMA 02-3758, 2002.

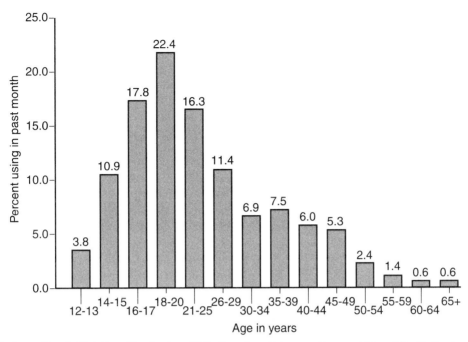

Figure 1–1. Past Month Illicit Drug Use, by Age: 2001. (Data from Substance Abuse and Mental Health Services Administration. Results from the 2001 National Household Survey on Drug Abuse: Volume I. Summary of National Findings. Rockville, MD: Office of Applied Studies, NHSDA Series H-17, DHHS Publication No. SMA 02-3758, 2002.)

and declining steadily thereafter (Figure 1–1). Young adults showed increases in most categories of illicit drug use between 2000 and 2001, continuing upward trends that began in the early-to-mid-1990s (Table 1-5). (Of special note is that although the prevalence of "Ecstasy" use fell slightly from 2000 to 2001, between 1991 and 2001 it rose among 19-to 20 year old Americans from 0.6% to 11.0%.[24])

NHSDA categorized ethanol use as either current (at least one drink during the past 30 days), binge use (5 or more drinks on the same occasion at least once during the past 30 days), and heavy use (5 or more drinks on the same occasion on at least 5 different days during the past 30 days).[25] Nearly half (48.3%) of Americans aged 12 years or older were current drinkers during 2001, up from 46.6% during 2000. One-fifth (20.5%) of Americans aged 12 years or older were binge drinkers, and 5.7% (12.9 million people) were heavy drinkers. Current use was 2.6% at age 12 years, peaked at 67.5% at age 21 years (binge 48.2%, heavy 17.8%), declined to 55.2% at age 45 to 49 years (binge 19.1%, heavy 5.4%), and fell to 35% after age 65 years (binge 5.8%, heavy 1.4%) (Figure 1–2). Current, binge, and heavy drinking were significantly more prevalent among college students than among others aged 18 to 22 years. Underage current drinkers (age 12 to 20 years) varied among ethnic groups (Figure 1–3).

Table 1–5. Percentage of Americans Aged 19–28 Years Using Illicit Drugs During the Past Month, 2001

	2001	Change from 2000 to 2001
Any illicit drug	18.8	+0.7
Any illicit drug other than marijuana	7.0	+0.6
Marijuana	16.7	+0.6
LSD	0.7	0
MDMA (Ecstasy)	1.8	−0.1
Cocaine	2.2	+0.6
Heroin	0.3	+0.1
Amphetamines	2.4	+0.1
Barbiturates	1.7	+0.3
Tranquilizers	2.1	+0.3
Inhalants	0.4	−0.1

Source: Johnston LD, O'Malley M, Bachman JG. Monitoring the Future: National Survey Results on Drug Use, 1975–2001. Bethesda, MD: NIH Publication No. 02-5107, NIDA, 2002.

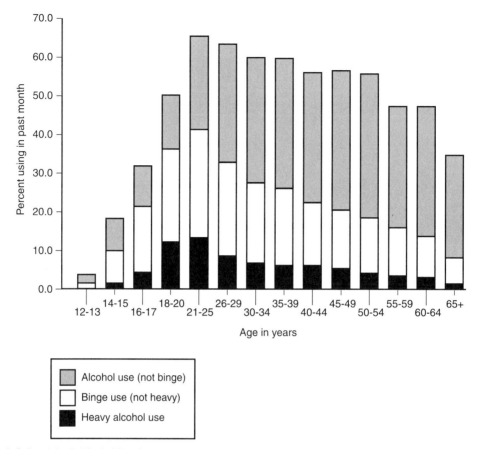

Figure 1–2. Past Month Alcohol Use, by Age: 2001. (Data from Substance Abuse and Mental Health Services Administration. Results from the 2001 National Household Survey on Drug Abuse: Volume I. Summary of National Findings. Rockville, MD: Office of Applied Studies, NHSDA Series H-17, DHHS Publication No. SMA 02-3758, 2002.)

Addressing tobacco, NHSDA found that 29.5% of Americans aged 12 years or older (66.5 million people) smoked tobacco products; 24.9% smoked cigarettes, 5.4% smoked cigars, 3.2% used smokeless tobacco, and 1.0% smoked tobacco in pipes.[25] Tobacco use was most prevalent among young adults aged 18 to 25 years (Figure 1–4). The prevalence of cigarette use among children aged 12 to 17 years fell from 14.9% in 1999 to 13% in 2001 (Figure 1–5). Among all Americans aged 12 years or older, the prevalence of cigarette use varied with ethnicity (Figure 1–6).

NHSDA estimated that during 2001, 16.6 million Americans aged 12 years or older (7.3% of the total population) met DSM-IV criteria for dependence on or abuse of either ethanol or illicit drugs (Table 1–6)[25] Among the total number of Americans who used heroin, 50% were considered dependent on it or

abusers of it. Among cocaine users the figure was 24.9%. Among marijuana users the figure was 16.5%. These figures represented substantial increases from the previous year. During 2000 the number of Americans dependent on or abusing ethanol, illicit drugs, or both was 14.5 million (6.5% of the population). From 2000 to 2001 the percentage of the population with dependence on or abuse of illicit drugs increased from 1.9% to 2.5%. Ethanol dependence or abuse increased from 5.4% to 5.9%.

In contrast to these mostly upward trends, a Monitoring the Future study of 8th, 10th, and 12th graders during 2002 found decreased prevalence rates, compared with 2001, for use of marijuana, Ecstasy, LSD, ethanol, and cigarette smoking. Crack cocaine use, however, increased among 10th graders, and sedative use increased among 12th graders. Heroin use among all three groups remained stable.[26]

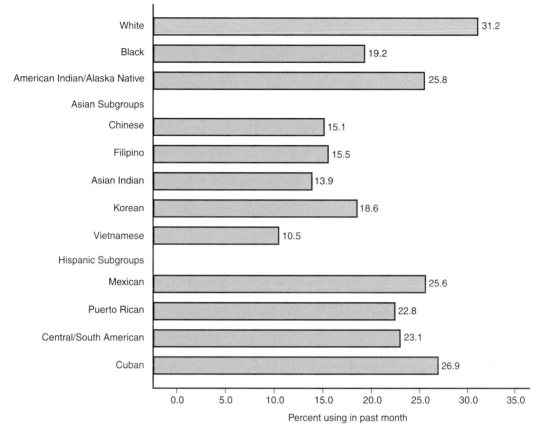

Figure 1–3. Past Month Alcohol Use among Youths Aged 12 to 20 Years, by Race/Ethnicity: 2000–2001 Annual Averages. (Data from Substance Abuse and Mental Health Services Administration. Results from the 2001 National Household Survey on Drug Abuse: Volume I. Summary of National Findings. Rockville, MD: Office of Applied Studies, NHSDA Series H-17, DHHS Publication No. SMA 02-3758, 2002.)

A study addressing injection drug use among adolescent boys found that reported prevalence rates were significantly higher when an audio computer-assisted self-interviewing instrument replaced a participating interviewer. This observation suggests that Monitoring the Future and NHSDA underestimate prevalence rates.[27]

Is There Such a Thing as an *Addictive Personality*?

Although among their disparate properties all addicting drugs have a common neuropharmacological effect—namely, facilitation of firing by dopaminergic neurons in the midbrain ventral tegmental area and release of dopamine into the nucleus accumbens (see Chapter 2)—the answer to this question remains no. Animal drug preferences vary between species and strains, but when a highly addictive drug such as cocaine is made available, most animals self-administer it.[28] Similarly, sudden availability of a drug can produce epidemics of human abuse—for example, methamphetamine in Japan in the 1940s and cocaine in the United States in the 1980s. It is of course significant that even when highly reinforcing drugs are plentiful, some animals do not self-administer them, and that among humans who do, most are not compulsive daily users. Drug availability, in other words, does not by itself predict drug addiction. That does not mean, however, that either addicted humans or addicted rats have an *addictive personality*.

Objective psychological testing has repeatedly failed to define a personality profile or psychopathological state specific to drug addiction in general

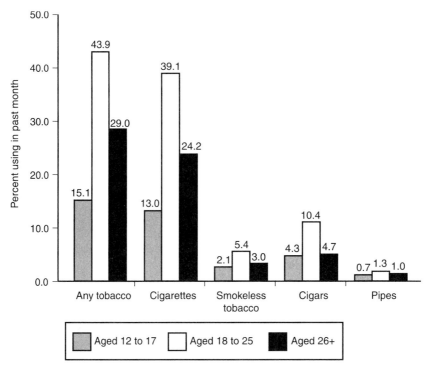

Figure 1–4. Past Month Tobacco Use among Persons Aged 12 Years or Older: 2001. (Data from Substance Abuse and Mental Health Services Administration. Results from the 2001 National Household Survey on Drug Abuse: Volume I. Summary of National Findings. Rockville, MD: Office of Applied Studies, NHSDA Series H-17, DHHS Publication No. SMA 02-3758, 2002.)

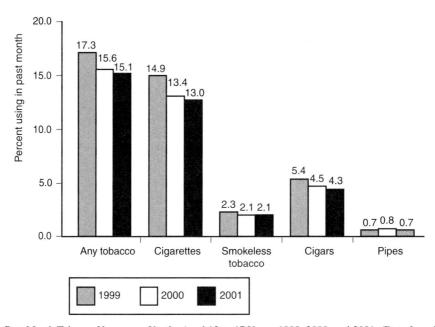

Figure 1–5. Past Month Tobacco Use among Youths Aged 12 to 17 Years: 1999, 2000, and 2001. (Data from Substance Abuse and Mental Health Services Administration. Results from the 2001 National Household Survey on Drug Abuse: Volume I. Summary of National Findings. Rockville, MD: Office of Applied Studies, NHSDA Series H-17, DHHS Publication No. SMA 02-3758, 2002.)

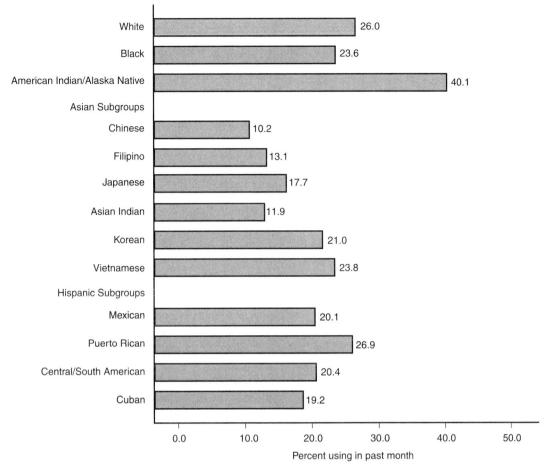

Figure 1–6. Past Month Cigarette Use among Persons Aged 12 Years or Older, by Race/Ethnicity: 2000–2001 Annual Averages. (Data from Substance Abuse and Mental Health Services Administration. Results from the 2001 National Household Survey on Drug Abuse: Volume I. Summary of National Findings. Rockville, MD: Office of Applied Studies, NHSDA Series H-17, DHHS Publication No. SMA 02-3758, 2002.)

Table 1–6. Number of Americans Aged 12 Years or Older Meeting DSM-IV Criteria for Substance Dependence or Abuse: 2001

Both ethanol and illicit drugs	2.4 million
Illicit drugs but not ethanol	3.2 million
Ethanol but not illicit drugs	11 million
Heroin	200,000
Cocaine	1 million
Marijuana	3.5 million

Source: Substance Abuse and Mental Health Services Administration. Results from the 2001 National Household Survey on Drug Abuse: Vol I. Summary of National Findings. Rockville, MD: Office of Applied Studies, NHSDA Series H-17, DHHS Publication No. SMA 02-3758, 2002.

or to abuse of any one substance.[29–42] To be sure, among drug abusers a variety of psychopathologies are over-represented. Anxiety, emotional immaturity, antisocial personality, or depression can lead to drug use in the first place, and many addicts—for example, cocaine users with depression—are self-medicating psychiatric symptoms.[43–50] Novelty-seeking may be especially over-represented, and animals showing a greater locomotor response to a novel environment are reportedly more likely to engage in drug self-administration behavior.[51,52] (Interestingly, such animals also have enhanced dopamine release in the nucleus accumbens in response to novelty, amphetamine, or cocaine.)[15] Some workers report that the majority of drug-abusing or drug-dependent individuals have an additional psychiatric diagnosis.[53] In a study of drug-abusing adolescents, 82% had an Axis I disorder, and three-fourths of these had more than one disorder; 61% had mood disorders, 54% conduct disorder, and 43% anxiety disorder.[54] In another study of adolescents, 71% had conduct disorder, 31% major depression, and 14% both.[55] In that study, depression was considered more often the consequence of drug abuse than its cause, but it can be difficult to tell whether psychopathology precedes or follows drug use. Drug abusers, moreover, tend to be attitudinally and emotionally "different from the average person in society" to the degree that their particular drugs "meet with severe disapproval."[6] Again, such linkage need not imply the existence of an addictive personality, for prior delinquency in itself is conducive to obtaining an illicit drug.[56] As an example, marijuana may or may not serve as a "gateway" drug to more dangerous agents, but if so the reason may simply be that marijuana's illegality brings users in contact with purveyors of cocaine or heroin. Moreover, the prevalence of drug abuse in minority "ghettos" (or, for that matter, in suburban white "ghettos") might reflect reinforcing properties of a drug abuser's lifestyle, offering excitement and risks to those either bored in sterile surroundings or denied normal opportunities for self-fulfillment.

In addition to such operant aspects, drug abuse has pavlovian features. Animals exposed to environmental stimuli previously associated with a drug demonstrate drug-seeking behavior.[57] Their human counterparts are successfully detoxified addicts who relapse into drug-seeking on returning to their old neighborhoods.[58] Conversely, patients made physically dependent on morphine while hospitalized usually do not crave the drug on discharge[59,60] and the great majority of U.S. servicemen addicted to heroin during the Vietnam War did not crave the drug when they returned home.[61]

As already noted, animals exposed to drug-associated surroundings may even display signs of drug intoxication in the absence of drug administration. Their human counterparts are parenteral drug abusers who obtain subjective drug effects after unwittingly self-injecting saline ("needle freaks").

Finally, Siegel[62] suggests that drug "intoxication" is a basic drive in both humans and animals, independent of psychological makeup and no more repressible than eating, drinking, or sex.

How Are Drugs Identified in Body Fluids and Tissues?

A technical discussion of drug detection is beyond the scope of this text. Different testing systems exist for identifying drugs in urine, which is more often analyzed than blood.[63–67] Testing of hair can detect drug use days to months earlier, and detection in meconium can identify fetal exposure.[68–70] Although ethanol itself cannot be measured in hair or meconium, its fatty acid ethyl esters can be identified in meconium, and the nicotine metabolite cotinine can be measured in neonatal hair.[71] Many emergency rooms use thin-layer chromatography, which requires 3 to 4 hours to perform and is insensitive when only small doses of a drug have been taken (especially cocaine and phencyclidine). More sensitive and therefore suitable for screening are immunoassays, which include enzyme immunoassay, radioimmunoassay, fluorescence polarization immunoassay, and latex agglutination inhibition assay. Of these, the qualitative or semiquantitative enzyme immunoassay known as enzyme multiplied immunoassay technique (EMIT) is widely available and inexpensive. With thin-layer chromatography, enzyme immunoassay, radioimmunoassay, and fluorescence polarization immunoassay, positive results for cocaine and marijuana are highly predictive. For amphetamines and opioids, positive results are less specific. Most toxicology laboratories confirm any positive screened sample with gas chromatography/mass spectrometry (GC/MS), which is more expensive, more time-consuming, more sensitive, and more specific.[72] GC/MS is required for confirmation by the U.S. Armed Forces and by federal regulations for workplace testing. Even GC/MS can be misleading, however. For example, benzphetamine (Didrex) and selegiline (Eldepryl) are metabolized to amphetamine and methamphetamine, and poppy seeds contain morphine.[73] Other confirmatory techniques include high-performance liquid chromatography and gas-liquid chromatography (Table 1–7).[66,72]

Drug abuse screening has problems in addition to sensitivity and specificity. Persistence of a drug or its metabolite in the urine varies widely

Table 1–7. Cut-Off Points (in Nanograms per Milliliter) of Different Drugs of Abuse by Different Analytical Techniques

Drug Group	Immunoassay		Chromatography	
	Enzyme Immunoassay	**Radioimmunoassay**	**Thin-Layer Chromatography**	**Gas Chromatography/ Mass Spectrometry**
Cannabinoids	20–100	100	25	1–15
Cocaine	300	300	2000	5
Phencyclidine	75	25	500	5
Dextroamphetamine	300	1000	500	10
Morphine/heroin	300	300	500	5

Source: Schwartz JG, Zollars PR, Okorodudu AO, et al. Accuracy of common drug screen tests. Am J Emerg Med 1991; 9:166.

among agents and users. For example, urine can be positive for cannabinoids several days after single casual use of marijuana, and in heavy chronic cocaine users, the major metabolite benzoyl-ecgonine is detectable for several weeks. Unless observed, users may substitute "clean" urines (or apple juice) or adulterate urine with water, sodium chloride, vinegar, ammonia, sodium hypochlorite, or soap.[66] "Chain of custody"—the accountability of a specimen from its production to its analysis—must be tightly controlled, and equipment and technique must be continually monitored.[74] These issues are of obvious importance in forensic cases and—along with the problems of invasion of privacy and cost-effectiveness—in the debate over workplace screening.

What About Treatment?

A drug abuser might be treated for overdose, for withdrawal, for medical or neurological complications, or for addiction itself. Each of these areas is covered in this book, but selectively and, perforce, sometimes superficially. General principles of management in poisoning or overdose are discussed in other texts,[75] and such controversies as whether gastric emptying does more harm than good after ingestion of a poison[76] are outside the bounds of space, time, and my own experience. Similarly, although I address some specific chronic therapies—methadone for heroin abusers, antidepressants for cocaine abusers, disulfiram for alcoholics, nicotine gum for tobacco abusers—readers seeking broad coverage of the treatment of addiction are advised to look elsewhere.[77–79]

Two points are worth emphasizing, however. First, drug addiction is a chronic, not an acute, illness. Short-term interventions such as detoxification are therefore bound to fail. (One review remarked, "Imagine this same strategy applied to the treatment of hypertension."[80]) Second, unimodal approaches are unlikely to work. For one thing, drug abusers do not usually limit themselves to one agent. A familiar scene is the emergency room patient simultaneously intoxicated with multiple drugs or intoxicated with one agent while withdrawing from another.[81] Heroin addicts frequently

Table 1–8. Components of Comprehensive Addiction Treatment

Core elements
    Intake processing and/or assessment
    Treatment plan
    Pharmacotherapy
    Behavioral therapy and counseling
    Substance use monitoring
    Self-help and peer support groups
    Clinical and case management
    Continuing care
Associated services
    Mental health services
    Medical services
    Educational services
    AIDS/HIV services
    Legal services
    Financial services
    Housing and/or transportation services
    Family services
    Childcare services
    Vocational services

Source: Leshner I. Science-based views on drug addiction and its treatment. JAMA 1999; 282:1314.

become successfully maintained on methadone and then become alcoholic or addicted to cocaine. Biological, psychological, or socioeconomic approaches to drug abuse are not mutually exclusive, and drug abuse treatment involves (or should involve) them all (Table 1–8).[82–84]

What About Prevention?

In 2002 President George W. Bush unveiled a $19 billion national anti-drug strategy for the United States. Eighty-seven percent of the budget was targeted at interdiction and law enforcement; 13% was for education and treatment. Interdiction included resumption of American counternarcotics flights over Colombia and Peru and the claim (citing, among a number of terrorist organizations, the Afghan Taliban) that the War on Drugs was part of the War on Terrorism.[85,86]

Supply, not demand, is thus the principal target of governmental anti-drug policies, reflecting the widely held view that illicit drug use should be criminalized, not medicalized. According to 47 national surveys between 1978 and 1997, most Americans consider drug abuse a moral issue and favor a continuation of existing anti-drug policies even though they acknowledge that the War on Drugs has so far been a failure.[87]

One consequence of the disproportionate focus on supply rather than demand has been a skyrocketing prison population. In 1972, after 50 years of a stable incarceration rate, 200,000 Americans were in state and federal prisons; today 1.3 million are, and nearly two-thirds have a history of substance abuse. Draconian laws in a number of states (e.g., "3 strikes and you're out," disproportionate mandatory sentencing for possession of "crack" cocaine vs. cocaine hydrochloride) have resulted in life sentences for possession. The cost of "warehousing" drug offenders is twice that of treating them, and a RAND Corporation study concluded that for every dollar spent on treatment, US$7 are saved in other services (e.g., reduced crime, increased productivity, fewer emergency room visits).[88–90] In the meantime, as noted above, during the past decade the prevalence of illicit drug use has increased.

Politics is "the art of the possible," and the March of Folly resulting from the criminalization of drug addiction has not only been a bipartisan effort in the United States but is the basis of drug policy in many other countries as well. For example, the United Kingdom spends 75% of its anti-drug budget on law enforcement and interdiction (with interception of as little as 5% to 10% of smuggled drugs).[91] Supply reduction and demand reduction are of course not mutually exclusive, and recognition of drug addiction as a neuropsychiatric disease with obsessive-compulsive features does not mean that law enforcement is irrelevant. Indeed, the U.S. federal government has paid lip service to a "balanced strategy" since the Nixon administration.[92] The balance, however, has consistently been lopsided.

What About *Legalization*?

Legalization is a social, not a medical issue, with many ramifications. For example, economists do not agree whether consumption depends on drug prices or how much tax revenue could be anticipated if drugs were legally marketed.[93] From a medical standpoint, however, the harm a drug does—to a user or to society—has obvious bearing on its legal status. A few points are worth considering in this regard:

1. Nearly every society since recorded history has countenanced the use of one or more mind-altering drugs.
2. Some mind-altering drugs are more harmful than others.
3. Attempts to stamp out abuse of particular drugs by declaring them illegal have been spectacularly unsuccessful.
4. When drugs are freely available, however, more people use them.
5. The two biggest killer drugs in the United States are legal.

A decade ago the crack cocaine epidemic generated a contentious debate over drug legalization, with proponents comparing governmental policies to American Prohibition of alcohol during the 1920s.[94–97] Today, although over a million Americans still currently use cocaine, the most vocal debate has shifted toward legalization (or decriminalization) of marijuana (which, it might be noted, was entirely legal in the United States when ethanol was not).

Whatever drug policy the United States adopts, it is not going to be the first society in recorded history to eliminate the use of mind-altering substances. The question, then, short of outright legalization, is whether society should accept a certain level of drug abuse (as it does with ethanol and tobacco) or whether it should attempt to eliminate the use of those drugs it has declared illegal, knowing that that goal cannot succeed. The prohibition of alcohol 70 years ago and the War on Drugs as currently conducted illustrate not only the futility but also the danger of overzealous law-enforcement. As the editors of the *New England Journal of Medicine* put it, "All we can do is try to keep the number of drug-dependent people to a minimum without destroying the fabric of society in our efforts to do so."[90] In the meantime physicians, and in particular neurologists and psychiatrists, whether or not they favor legalization or decriminalization, should participate in the debate, reminding politicians that substance abuse is a disease of the brain, not a moral weakness.[98–99]

References

1. Eddy NB, Halbach H, Isbell H, Seevers MH. Drug dependence: its significance and characteristics. Bull WHO 1965; 32:721.
2. Edwards G, Arif A, Hodgson R. Nomenclature and classification of drug and alcohol-related problems: a shortened version of a WHO memorandum. Br J Addict 1982; 77:3.
3. Diagnostic and Statistical Manual of Mental Disorders, 4th edition (DSM-IV). Washington, DC: American Psychiatric Association, 1994.
4. Stolerman I. Drugs of abuse: behavioural principles, methods and terms. Trends Pharmacol Sci 1992; 13:170.
5. Department of Health and Human Services. The Health Consequences of Smoking. A Report of the Surgeon General. Washington, DC: DHHS Publication No. (CDC) 88-8406, US Government Printing Office, 1988.
6. O'Brien CP. Drug addiction and drug abuse. In: Hardman JG, Limbird LE, eds. Goodman and Gilman's The Pharmacological Basis of Therapeutics, 10th edition. New York: McGraw-Hill, 2001; 621.
7. Dews PB. Behavioral tolerance. In: Krasnegor NA, ed. Behavioral Tolerance: Research and Treatment Implications. Washington, DC: National Institute on Drug Abuse, DHEW Publication No. (ADM) 78-551, US Government Printing Office, 1977; 18.
8. Siegel S, MacRae J. Environmental specificity of tolerance. Trends Neurosci 1984; 7:140.
9. Pavlov IP. Conditioned Reflexes (Anrep GV, trans.). Oxford: Oxford University Press, 1927.
10. Siegel S, Hinson RE, Krank MD, McCully J. Heroin "overdose" death: contribution of drug-associated environmental cues. Science 1982; 216:436.
11. Goudie AJ, Griffiths JW. Environmental specificity of tolerance. Trends Neurosci 1984; 7:310.
12. Dewey WL. Various factors which affect the rate of development of tolerance and physical dependence to abused drugs. NIDA Res Monogr 1984; 54:39.
13. Snyder SH. Receptors, neurotransmitters, and drug responses. N Engl J Med 1979; 300:465.
14. Genova L, Berke J, Hyman SE. Molecular adaptations to psychostimulants in striatal neurons: toward a pathophysiology of addiction. Neurobiol Dis 1997; 4:239.
15. Vezina P, Lorrain DS, Arnold GM, et al. Sensitization of midbrain dopamine neuron reactivity promotes the pursuit of amphetamine. J Neurosci 2002; 22:4654.
16. Nestler EJ. Neurobiology. Total recall–the memory of addiction. Science 2001; 292:2266.
17. Everitt BJ, Wolf ME. Psychomotor stimulant addiction: a neural systems perspective. J Neurosci 2002; 22:3312.
18. Tzschentke TM, Schmidt WJ. Functional heterogeneity of the rat medial prefrontal cortex: effects of discrete subarea-specific lesions on drug-induced conditioned place preference and behavioral sensitization. Eur J Neurosci 1999; 11:4099.
19. Vanderschuren LJ, Kalivas PW. Alterations in dopaminergic and glutamatergic transmission in the induction and expression of behavioral sensitization: a critical review of preclinical studies. Psychopharmacology 2000; 151:99.
20. Carlzon WA, Nestler EJ. Elevated levels of GluR1 in the midbrain: a trigger for sensitization to drugs of abuse? Trends Neurosci 2002; 25:610.
21. Robinson TE, Browman KE, Crombag HS, et al. Modulation of the induction or expression of psychostimulant sensitization by the circumstances surrounding drug administration. Neurosci Biobehav Rev 1998; 22:347.
22. Beninger RJ, Miller R. Dopamine D1-like receptors and reward-related incentive learning. Neurosci Biobehav Rev 1998; 22:335.
23. DiChiara G, Tanda G, Bassareo V, et al. Drug addiction as a disorder of associative learning. Role of nucleus accumbens shell/extended amygdala dopamine. Ann N Y Acad Sci 1999; 877:461.
24. Johnston LD, O'Malley M, Bachman JG. Monitoring the Future: National Survey Results on Drug Use, 1975–2001. Bethesda, MD: NIH Publication No. 02-5107, NIDA, 2002.
25. Substance Abuse and Mental Health Services Administration. Results from the 2001 National Household Survey on Drug Abuse: Volume I. Summary of National Findings. Rockville, MD: Office of Applied Studies, NHSDA Series H-17, DHHS Publication No. SMA 02-3758, 2002.
26. HHS News. 2002 Monitoring the Future survey shows decrease in use of marijuana, club drugs, cigarettes and tobacco. http:\\www.nida.nih.gov/

27. Turner CF, Ku L, Rogers SM, et al. Adolescent sexual behavior, drug use, and violence: increased reporting with computer survey technology. Science 1998; 280:867.

28. Dole VP. Addictive behavior. Sci Am 1980; 243:138.

29. Hill HE, Haertzen CA, Davis H. An MMPI factor analysis study of alcoholics, narcotic addicts and criminals. Q J Stud Alcohol 1962; 23:411.

30. Monroe JJ, Ross WF, Berzins J. The decline of the addict as "psychopath": implications for community care. Int J Addict 1971; 6:601.

31. Mott J. The psychological basis of drug dependence: the intellectual and personality characteristics of opiate users. Br J Addict 1972; 67:89.

32. Dole VP. Narcotic addiction, physical dependence, and relapse. N Engl J Med 1972; 286:988.

33. Overall JE. MMPI personality patterns of alcoholics and narcotic addicts. Q J Stud Alcohol 1973; 34:104.

34. Feldstein S, Chesler P, Fink M. Psychological differentiation and the response of opiate addicts to pharmacological treatment. Br J Addict 1973; 68:151.

35. Robins LN, Helzer JE, Davis DH. Narcotic use in southeast Asia and afterward: an interview of 898 Vietnam returners. Arch Gen Psychiatry 1975; 32:955.

36. Craig RJ. Personality characteristics of heroin addicts: review of empirical research 1976–1979. Int J Addict 1982; 17:227.

37. Sutker PB, Moan CE, Goist KC, Allain AN. MMPI subtypes and antisocial behaviors in adolescent alcohol and drug abusers. Drug Alcohol Depend 1984; 13:235.

38. O'Malley PM, Bachman JG, Johnson LD. Period, age, and cohort effects on substance use among American youth, 1976-1982. Am J Public Health 1984; 74:682.

39. O'Mahony P, Smith E. Some personality characteristics of imprisoned heroin addicts. Drug Alcohol Depend 1984; 13:255.

40. Khantzian EJ. The self-medication hypothesis of addictive disorders: focus on heroin and cocaine dependence. Am J Psychiatry 1985; 142:1259.

41. O'Connor L, Berry JW. The drug-of-choice phenomenon: why addicts start using their preferred drug. J Psychoactive Drugs 1990; 22:305.

42. Campbell BK, Stark MJ. Psychopathology and personality characteristics in different forms of substance abuse. Int J Addict 1990; 25:1467.

43. Pope HC. Drug abuse and psychopathology. N Engl J Med 1979; 301:1341.

44. McLellan AT, Woody GE, O'Brien CP. Development of psychiatric illness in drug abusers. Possible role of drug preference. N Engl J Med 1979; 301:1310.

45. Sutker PB, Archer RP, Allain AN. Psychopathology of drug abusers: sex and ethnic considerations. Int J Addict 1980; 15:605.

46. Rounsaville BJ, Novelly RA, Kleber HD. Neuropsychological impairment in opiate addicts: risk factors. Ann N Y Acad Sci 1981; 362:79.

47. Weller MP, Ang PC, Zachary A, Latimer-Sayer DT. Substance abuse in schizophrenia. Lancet 1984; I:573.

48. Marlatt GA, Baer JS, Donovan DM, Kivlahan DR. Addictive behaviors: etiology and treatment. Annu Rev Psychol 1988; 39:223.

49. Butcher JN. Personality factors in drug addiction. NIDA Res Monogr 1988; 89:87.

50. Hesselbrock V, Meyer R, Hesselbrock M. Psychopathology and addictive disorders. The specific case of antisocial personality disorder. In: O'Brien CP, Jaffe JH, eds. Addictive States. Res Publ Assoc Res Nerv Ment Dis 1992; 70:179.

51. Pierre PJ, Vezina P. Predisposition to self-administer amphetamine: the contribution of response to novelty and prior exposure to the drug. Psychopharmacology 1997; 129:277.

52. Marinelli M, White FJ. Enhanced vulnerability to cocaine self-administration is associated with elevated impulse activity of midbrain dopamine neurons. J Neurosci 2000; 20:8876.

53. Weinberg NZ, Rahdert E, Colliver JD, et al. Adolescent substance abuse: a review of the past 10 years. J Am Acad Child Adolesc Psychiatry 1998; 37:25.

54. Stowell RJA, Estroff TW. Psychiatric disorders in substance-abusing adolescent inpatients: a pilot study. J Am Acad Child Adolesc Psychiatry 1992; 31:1036.

55. Bukstein OG, Glancy LJ, Kaminer Y. Patterns of affective comorbidity in a clinical population of dually diagnosed adolescent substance abusers. J Am Acad Child Adolesc Psychiatry 1992; 31:1041.

56. Robins LN, Murphy GE. Drug use in a normal population of young Negro men. Am J Public Health 1967; 57:1580.

57. Siegel S. Drug anticipation and the treatment of dependence. NIDA Res Monogr 1988; 84:1.

58. Wikler A. Interaction of physical dependence and classical and operant conditioning in the genesis of relapse. Res Publ Assoc Res Nerv Ment Dis 1968; 46:280.

59. Dole VP. Narcotic addiction, physical dependence, and relapse. N Engl J Med 1972; 286:988.

60. Foley K. The treatment of cancer pain. N Engl J Med 1985; 313:84.

61. O'Brien CP, Nace EP, Mintz J, et al. Follow-up of Vietnam veterans. 1. Relapse to drug use after Vietnam service. Drug Alcohol Depend 1980; 5:333.

62. Siegel RK. Intoxication. Life in Pursuit of Artificial Paradise. New York: EP Dutton, 1989.

63. Hawks RL, Chiang CN, eds. Urine Testing for Drugs of Abuse. Rockville, MD: NIDA Res Monogr 1986:73.

64. Gold MS, Dackis CA. Role of the laboratory in the evaluation of suspected drug abuse. J Clin Psychiatry 1986; 47(Suppl):17.

65. Schwartz RH. Urine testing in the detection of drugs of abuse. Arch Intern Med 1988; 148:2407.

66. Schwartz JG, Zollars PR, Okorodudu AO, et al. Accuracy of common drug screen tests. Am J Emerg Med 1991; 9:166.

67. Osterloh JD, Snyder JW: Laboratory principles and techniques to evaluate the poisoned or overdosed patient.

In Goldfrank LR, Flomenbaum NE, Lewin NA, et al, eds. Goldfrank's Toxicologic Emergencies, 6th edition. Stamford, CT: Appleton & Lange, 1998:63.

68. Nakahara Y, Takahashi K, Shimamine M, Takeda Y. Hair analysis for drug abuse. I. Determination of methamphetamine and amphetamine in hair by stable isotope dilution gas chromatography/mass spectrometry method. J Forensic Sci 1991; 36:70.

69. Moore C, Negrusz A, Lewis D. Determination of drugs of abuse in meconium. J Chromatogr Biomed Sci Appl 1998; 713:137.

70. Gaillard Y, Pepin G. Evidence of polydrug use using hair analysis: a fatal case involving heroin, cocaine, cannabis, chloroform, thiopental, and ketamine. J Forensic Sci 1998; 43:435.

71. Koren G, Chan D, Klein J, et al. Estimation of fetal exposure to drugs of abuse, environmental tobacco smoke, and ethanol. Ther Drug Monitor 2002; 24:23.

72. Moeller MR, Kraemer T. Drug of abuse monitoring in blood for control of driving under the influence of drugs. Ther Drug Monitor 2002; 24:210.

73. Kwong TC, Shearer D. Substances that give false-positive results by both initial and confirmatory testing. Obstet Gynecol Clin North Am 1998; 25:59.

74. Wilson JF, Williams J, Walker G, et al. Performance of techniques used to detect drugs of abuse in urine: study based on external quality assessment. Clin Chem 1991; 37:442.

75. Goldfrank LR, Flomenbaum NE, Lewin NA. Principles of managing the poisoned or overdosed patient: an overview. In: Goldfrank LR, Flomenbaum NE, Lewin NA, et al, eds. Goldfrank's Toxicologic Emergencies, 6th edition. Stamford, CT: Appleton & Lange, 1998:31.

76. Kulig K. Initial management of ingestions of toxic substances. N Engl J Med 1992; 326:1677.

77. Lowinson JH, Ruiz P, Millman RB, Langrod JG. Substance Abuse: A Comprehensive Textbook, 2nd edition. Baltimore, MD: Williams & Wilkins, 1992.

78. Graham AW, Schultz TK, Mayo-Smith MF, et al, eds. Principles of Addiction Medicine, 3rd edition. Chevy Chase, MD: American Society of Addiction Medicine, 2003.

79. National Institute on Drug Abuse. Principles of Drug Addiction Treatment. Bethesda, MD: NIH Publication No. 99-4180, 1999.

80. McLellan AT, Lewis DC, O'Brien CP, et al. Drug dependence, a chronic medical illness. JAMA 2000; 284:1689.

81. Khantzian EJ, McKenna GJ. Acute toxic and withdrawal reactions associated with drug use and abuse. Ann Intern Med 1979; 90:361.

82. McLellan AT, O'Brien CP, Metzger D. How effective is substance abuse treatment-compared to what? In: O'Brien CP, Jaffe JH, eds. Addictive States. Res Publ Assoc Res Nerv Ment Dis 1992; 70:231.

83. Gerstein DR. The effectiveness of drug treatment. In: O'Brien CP, Jaffe JH, eds. Addictive States. Res Publ Assoc Res Nerv Ment Dis 1992; 70:253.

84. Leshner I. Science-based views of drug addiction and its treatment. JAMA 1999; 282:1314.

85. Marquis C. Bush's $19 billion antidrug plan focuses on law enforcement and treatment. NY Times, February 13, 2002.

86. Jones AN. Strong views, pro and con, on ads linking drug use to terrorism. NY Times, April 2, 2002.

87. Blendon RJ, Young JT. The public and the war on illicit drugs. JAMA 1998; 279:827.

88. Orenstein P. Staying clean. NY Times Magazine, February 10, 2002.

89. Butterfield F. Number of people in state prisons declines slightly. NY Times, August 13, 2001.

90. Angell M, Kassirer JP. Alcohol and other drugs–toward a more rational and consistent policy. N Engl J Med 1994; 331:537.

91. Working Party of the Royal College of Psychiatrists and the Royal College of Physicians. Drugs: Dilemmas and Choices. London: Gaskill, 2000.

92. Acker CJ. Creating the American Junkie: Addiction Research in the Classic Era of Narcotic Control. Baltimore, MD: Johns Hopkins University Press, 2002.

93. Grossman M, Chaloupha FJ, Shim K. Illegal drug use and public policy. Health Affairs 2002; 21:134.

94. Nadelmann EA. Drug prohibition in the United States: costs, consequences, and alternatives. Science 1989; 245:939.

95. Goldstein A, Kalant H. Drug policy: striking the right balance. Science 1990; 249:1513.

96. Jarvik ME. The drug dilemma: manipulating the demand. Science 1990; 250:387.

97. Schwartz RH. Legalization of drugs of abuse and the pediatrician. Am J Dis Child 1991; 145:1153.

98. Cami J, Farré M: Drug addiction. N Engl J Med 2003; 349:975.

99. Vastag B. Addiction poorly understood by clinicians. Experts say attitudes, lack of knowledge hinder treatment. JAMA 2003; 290:1299.

Chapter 2
The Neurobiology of Addiction

My case is a species of madness, only that it is a derangement of the Volition, and not of the intellectual faculties.
—Samuel Taylor Coleridge

The Role of Sensitization

The neurobiological basis of addiction—defined as "the loss of control over drug use, or the compulsive seeking and taking of drugs despite adverse consequences"—remains poorly understood.[1a] Neither tolerance nor physical dependence are essential features of chronic drug seeking behavior, which can re-emerge after months or years of abstinence upon exposure either to drug-associated cues (e.g., drug-taking paraphernalia, familiar environments), to stress, or to the drug itself.[2,3] This phenomenon—protracted or relapsing craving—has obvious analogies to long-term memory and seems to represent the essence of addiction.[4,5] During the past decade it has been studied in terms of "sensitization"—defined as "enhanced drug responsiveness with repeated exposure to a constant dose."[1] In contrast to tolerance, which is most readily produced by continuous or frequent administration of low doses of a drug, sensitization is most readily produced by intermittent administration of high doses.[6] In some animal models sensitization appears after several days of drug abstinence but not after shorter intervals of abstinence.[7] Evidence exists that acquisition of sensitization and maintenance of sensitization involve separate anatomical structures. Once sensitization has been induced, animals may remain hypersensitive for months or years to the psychomotor or rewarding effects of subsequent drug exposure.[7a]

Tolerance probably contributes to the escalation of drug use during the development of an addiction, and physical dependence probably contributes to the dysphoria and somatic symptoms that lead to high rates of relapse during early withdrawal. Sensitization may be what makes addiction a chronic—often lifelong—relapsing disorder, and as such it involves long-term plasticity and "extremely stable changes in the brain."[1]

Studies with animals, focusing on this plasticity, shed light not only on the anatomical structures and neurotransmitter systems involved in addiction, but also on intracellular signal transduction pathways and transcriptional mechanisms.

Animal Models

There are a variety of animal models for studying addicting drugs.[8–12] In drug discrimination studies, animals learn to tell one drug from another (or from saline) for a reward; generalization from one drug to another implies similar mechanisms of action.[9,13,14] Moreover, many investigators believe that the ability of a drug to act as a discriminative stimulus in animals reflects its subjective rewarding properties in humans—euphorigenic or otherwise. Nearly all drugs that are addicting to humans have discriminative stimulus effects in animals.[8]

Other models more specifically reveal how "reinforcing" or "rewarding" a drug is. In conditioned place preference (CPP) models, drug and saline injections are paired with different environments, for example, one of two compartments in a cage; an animal's later preference for one or another environment indicates that the drug associated with it was rewarding.[2] Some drugs, rather than producing CPP, produce conditioned place aversion (CPA).[15–17]

A large number of psychostimulants with dopamine D_2 agonist activity—including cocaine, amphetamine, methylphenidate, bupropion, apomorphine, and bromocriptine—produce CPP. So do morphine, heroin, and other μ-opioid receptor agonists. Mu-receptor antagonists produce CPA. Delta-opioid receptor agonists are less likely to produce CPP than μ-agonists, and κ-agonists more often produce CPA than CPP. Nicotine-induced CPP shifts to CPA with increasing dosage. Nicotine antagonists and muscarinic antagonists produce neither CPP nor CPA. With ethanol and sedatives findings have been inconsistent; ethanol produced both CPP and CPA, diazepam and lorazepam produced CPP, phenobarbital and pentobarbital produced CPA, and γ-hydroxybutyrate produced CPP. The glutamatergic antagonist phencyclidine produced either CPP or CPA or had no effect. Delta-9-tetrahydrocannabinol produced CPP at low doses and CPA at high doses. LSD produced CPP, as did glue thinner vapors.[17]

Numerous studies have involved drugs in combination—the ability of one agent to block the production of CPP by another. For example, amphetamine-induced CPP was attenuated by both D_1 and D_2 dopamine receptor antagonists, whereas cocaine-induced CPP was blocked by D_1 antagonism but not by D_2 antagonism. Both amphetamine- and cocaine-induced CPP were blocked by naloxone. D_1 antagonists blocked morphine-induced CPP. D_2 antagonists blocked morphine-induced CPP in some studies and were without effect in others. Psychostimulant-induced CPP is little influenced by serotonin agonists or antagonists, whereas morphine-induced CPP is consistently blocked by $5HT_3$ antagonists. Others have studied CPP in particular settings, for example after intracranial drug injection, after brain lesions, in different animal strains, in genetically engineered animals, and in relation to dosage, tolerance, and sensitization.[17]

In other models, drugs are assessed for their ability to lower the threshold for self-stimulation through electrodes implanted in *reward areas*, which include the pathway from the midbrain ventral tegmental area (VTA) through the medial forebrain bundle to the nucleus accumbens (NA).[18]

In self-administration models, animals ingest drugs or self-inject them, either systemically or into various parts of the brain, especially reward areas.[3–5,19] In these models, when self-injection of a particular drug increases the rate of responding on subsequent occasions, the animal's response is defined as an operant and delivery of the drug as a reinforcer.[20] Different schedules of reinforcement are used, based on whether the reinforcer follows a given number of responses (ratio schedules) or whether it follows a response after a given period of time has elapsed (interval schedules). In ratio schedules, the number of responses required to produce an injection may be constant (fixed ratio), increase over time (progressive ratio), or vary irregularly from injection to injection (variable ratio). With progressive ratio schedules, the response requirement at which responding declines or ceases is called the breakpoint.

Drug-seeking behavior has two phases: acquisition and maintenance. Fixed ratio testing measures acquisition: how rapidly an animal learns to self-administer a drug. Progressive ratio testing measures maintenance: how reinforcing a drug continues to be once addiction is established. The addiction liability of a drug is usually defined in terms of acquisition. By such criteria, cocaine is more addicting than heroin, for after 5 days of testing, 70% of animals learn to self-administer cocaine, whereas only 30% self-administer heroin. Ethanol is much less addicting than either.[21]

When an animal has been pharmacologically pretreated (for example, with a dopamine antagonist), subsequent increased rate of drug self-administration is usually taken to indicate decreased reinforcing efficacy; increased administration is compensatory. Such an interpretation has been challenged, however, and discrepancies between fixed ratio and progressive ratio results have called into question the reliability of rate of drug intake as an indicator of drug reinforcement.[22] Self-administration studies are further complicated by the direct effects of the drugs themselves. For example, increasing rates of cocaine self-administration could be secondary to increased locomotor activity rather than a result of cocaine's reinforcing properties per se, and decreasing rates of responding might ensue when enough drug has been delivered to be behaviorally disruptive. Such confounding effects vary with the particular schedule of reinforcement selected.

Self-administration studies reveal that animals self-administer most drugs abused by humans, including ethanol, opioids, amphetamine, cocaine, barbiturates, benzodiazepines, phencyclidine, and nicotine. They do not self-administer hallucinogens such as LSD. They do self-administer some drugs not abused by humans, including apomorphine, ketocyclazocine, and procaine. Results with cannabinoids, caffeine, and 3,4-methylenedioxymethamphetamine (MDMA, "Ecstasy") are conflicting.[23]

Striking differences exist in the manner in which animals self-administer "rewarding" drugs. For example, with amphetamine, periodic self-administration tends to alternate with periodic self-imposed abstinence; saline substitution for amphetamine is followed by a few hours of self-administration and then cessation. With morphine, self-administration is done in gradually higher daily doses that prevent both toxicity and signs of withdrawal; with saline substitution, the animal continues to self-administer for weeks.[22–26] Perhaps analogously, human parenteral amphetamine abusers tend to "burn out" after a few years; with opioids, physical and psychic dependence can persist for decades.[27,28]

The Neuroanatomy of Reward

The Reward Circuit

As noted, a reinforcer is an event that increases the likelihood of a response. Reward is defined similarly, with the added implication of affective pleasure.[29] In 1954, Olds and Milner, studying rats, reported that electrical stimulation of certain parts of the brain, particularly the septal area, was positively reinforcing: animals repeatedly pressed levers to stimulate themselves.[30] Further investigation revealed that stimulation of many other areas—motor, sensory, and associational—was rewarding. The most sensitive sites were along the medial forebrain bundle (MFB), especially at the level of the lateral hypothalamus and the VTA. The MFB was considered therefore a final common pathway of the reward circuit, its principal component consisting of rostrally projecting dopaminergic fibers from neurons in the VTA to forebrain areas that include the NA, limbic cortex, and amygdala.[31] Its function was seen as "converting emotion into motivated action" by filtering signals from the limbic system that ultimately produce motor acts via extrapyramidal output.[29] Lesions in the system lead to decrease in the locomotor activity ordinarily induced by a novel environment, reduction in the distraction usually associated with irrelevant information, difficulty in certain learning tasks, and perseveration.[29,32]

The reward circuit is considered the anatomical and physiological substrate not only for drug addiction but also for reward associated with eating, drinking, and sex.[33] Such a system obviously must consist of more than rostrally projecting dopaminergic fibers. In fact, more than 50 fiber systems traverse the MFB, and electrophysiological studies reveal that the great majority of MFB fibers that mediate the reward of electrical self-stimulation project in a caudal direction.[31] Some of these fibers project to the VTA, where dopaminergic neurons, with thresholds too high to be directly activated by electrical stimulation, can be indirectly activated transynaptically. Other directly activated MFB fibers project further caudally to the pedunculopontine and other tegmental nuclei of the upper brainstem, which in turn send cholinergic projections to the VTA.[34] It is possible, but unproven, that these ascending cholinergic fibers participate in the "first stage" of activation during MFB electrical stimulation.

Thus, the reward circuit is much more than a rostrally projecting dopaminergic cable. Furthermore, the precise role this complex circuitry plays in addiction remains to be clarified. Several theories have been proposed.[35] Hedonic theories of addiction hold that mesocorticolimbic systems mediate the pleasure of addictive drugs and the anhedonia of withdrawal. In other words, dopaminergic cell firing directly produces the subjective responses to a drug reward.[36] Learning theories of addiction hold that sensitized mechanisms of stimulus–response learning and reward prediction result in ingrained drug-taking habits. In other words, mesocorticolimbic dopaminergic projections, rather than directly producing subjective pleasure, fire to cues that predict reward.[4,37–39,39a] Incentive-sensitization theories of addiction propose that drugs sensitize mesocorti-colimbic "substrates of incentive salience." In other words, an addict might "want" drugs dispropor-tionately to "liking" them.[35,40–42,42a]

Component Structures of the Reward Circuit

Ventral Tegmental Area

The VTA contains dopaminergic neurons, which project via the MFB to the NA, olfactory tubercle, frontal cortex, amygdala, and septal areas. Activity of these dopaminergic neurons is modulated by numer-ous neurotransmitter inputs.[43] Somato-dendritically released dopamine produces inhibitory feedback via D_2 dopamine autoreceptors, and inhibition is further provided by GABAergic neurons within the VTA. Additional inhibitory and excitatory con-trol comes from serotonergic, noradrenergic, cholinergic, GABAergic, glutamatergic, and pep-tidergic afferents which originate in cortical, thala-mic, brainstem, and other limbic areas, and which synapse onto either the dopaminergic cell bodies or the local GABAergic interneurons. By inhibiting GABAergic interneurons (via μ- and δ-receptors, but not κ-receptors), opioids indirectly increase firing of the dopaminergic neurons.[44] Mu- and δ-opioid agonists are self-administered into the VTA. Cocaine and amphetamine are not.[45–47] Administra-tion of nicotinic cholinergic agonists into the VTA is rewarding, presumably by activation of excitatory nicotinic receptors on dopaminergic neurons.[48]

Nucleus Accumbens

The NA consists of three parts: the shell, the core, and the rostral pole, which in rodents are anatomi-cally and pharmacologically distinct.[49–52] In humans the NA is anatomically more continuous with the striatum and is often referred to as the ventral stria-tum. Most important from the standpoint of drug abuse is the shell; acute systemic administration of all drugs that are reinforcing in animals increases extracellular levels of dopamine in this structure.[53] Glutamatergic afferents to the NA come from the medial prefrontal cortex, amygdala, and hippocam-pus, and electrical stimulation of each of these areas is rewarding. Inhibitory control is principally pro-vided by GABAergic and cholinergic interneurons

and by post-synaptic μ- and δ-opioid receptors. Each of the NA's efferent projections originates from GABAergic medium spiny neurons.[53a] One pathway projects back to the VTA, forming a direct VTA–NA–VTA feedback loop. Another synapses in the ventral pallidum (VP), which in turn projects to the VTA, forming an indirect VTA–NA–VP–VTA feedback loop[1,45] (Figures 2–1, 2–2). GABAergic NA neurons that project directly to the VTA contain dynorphin and substance P; GABAergic NA neurons that project to the VTA indirectly via the VP contain enkephalin.[53b] Other projections are to the midbrain pedunculopontine nucleus, the dorsomedial thalamus, and the preop-tic and lateral hypothalamus. Areas receiving lesser projections include the septum, the amygdala, and the nucleus basalis of Meynert.

Dopaminergic input to the NA is from the VTA, and addictive drugs with different molecu-lar mechanisms of action facilitate the release of dopamine from VTA neurons projecting to the VTA.[53c] As in the striatum (which receives dopaminergic afferents from the substantia nigra pars compacta), dopamine D_1 receptor expression in the NA is correlated with expression of sub-stance P, whereas D_2 receptor expression is corre-lated with expression of enkephalin.[54] D_1 and D_2 receptors do not co-localize, but D_3 receptors (which correlate with substance P expression) are found in subsets of D_1- and D_2-expressing neu-rons.[55] It has been long-debated whether dopamine receptors in the striatum and the NA are excitatory or inhibitory. They are both, depending on the state of the neuron.[56] GABAergic medium spiny neurons of the NA and the striatum move between two membrane states, termed up-state or down-state. Down-state neurons are hyperpolarized, but when they receive temporally convergent excitatory synaptic input (e.g., from the hippocampus to the NA), they depolarize to the up-state, close to the threshold for spike generation. Within the NA are functionally related microzones of highly corre-lated state transitions.[57] Dopamine D_1-receptor activation suppresses transition from down-state to up-state, but once a neuron has achieved up-state, D_1-receptor activation enhances spike generation, probably by augmenting L-type Ca^{2+} currents and indirectly increasing glutamate AMPA- and NMDA-mediated excitatory post-synaptic potentials (EPSPs). D_1 receptor stimulation thus selectively

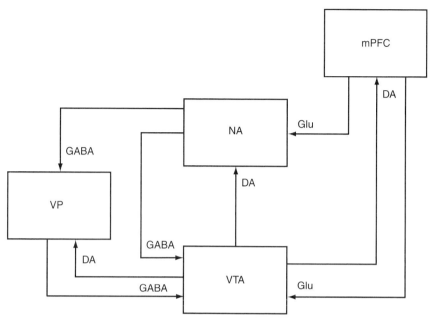

Figure 2–1. Principal components of the reward circuit. VTA: ventral tegmental area; NA: nucleus accumbens; mPFC: medial prefrontal cortex; VP: ventral pallidum; DA: dopamine; Glu: glutamate; GABA: γ-aminobutyric acid. (Modified from McBride WJ, Murphy JM, Ikemoto S. Localization of brain reinforcement mechanisms: intracranial self-administration and intracranial place-conditioning studies. Behav Brain Res 1999; 101:129.)

activates neuronal ensembles receiving highly convergent excitatory input and thereby increases signal-to-noise ratio.[56] Such state-dependent modulation of target cells by dopamine probably explains paradoxical reports that dopamine receptors can be both excitatory and inhibitory at the same time and probably accounts for conflicting descriptions of responses to drugs.

GABAergic medium spiny neurons in the NA express μ- and δ-opiate receptors and are inhibited by morphine. Mu- and δ-, but not κ-, opioid agonists are self-administered into the NA, and this effect is independent of dopamine, persisting even after VTA efferents to the NA have been blocked.[58–60] Amphetamine and cocaine are also self-administered into the NA, and this response is dopamine-dependent.[45] (Early reports that cocaine was not self-administered into the NA are probably explained by inadequate dosage or by injection into the core rather than the shell.[45]) Phencyclidine (PCP) self-administration into the NA is dopamine-independent; PCP probably blocks glutamatergic excitation of medium spiny neurons.[61] The net effect of opioid, psychostimulant, and PCP self-administration

thus appears to be inhibition of GABAergic spiny neuron efferents. (That electrical stimulation of the NA is rewarding in animals is presumably because elements of the NA other than the medium spiny neurons are preferentially activated.[31])

Medial Prefrontal Cortex

The medial prefrontal cortex (mPFC) receives dopaminergic afferents from the VTA and sends glutamatergic efferents to the VTA, the NA, and other areas. Animals self-administer cocaine into the mPFC. Animals also self-administer PCP into the mPFC, and such injections result in increased dopamine turnover in the NA.[31,61,62] Surprisingly, animals do not self-administer amphetamine into the mPFC.[63,63a] Injection of opioids into the mPFC is also not rewarding.[64] The mPFC is not a homogeneous structure, however, and lesions of different areas produce different conditioned place preference and sensitization responses to cocaine, amphetamine, and morphine. Within the mPFC the anterior cingulate cortex appears to play a significant role in pavlovian conditioning.[65]

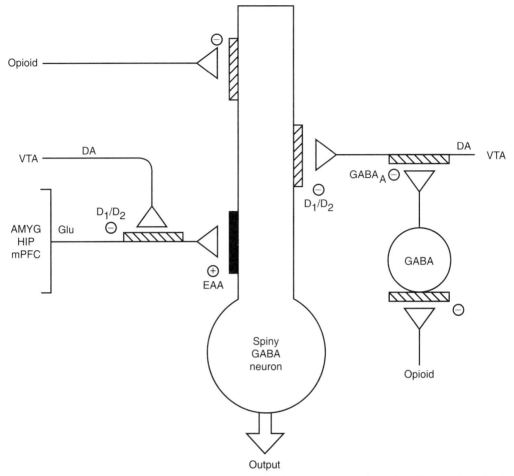

Figure 2–2. Interactions within the nucleus accumbens (NA). Reinforcement occurs when spiny GABAergic projecting neurons are inhibited. Activating dopaminergic receptors on these GABAergic neurons reduces their firing rate and initiates reinforcement. Activating dopaminergic receptors on glutamatergic inputs to the NA produces additional indirect inhibition of GABAergic output. Opioids produce reinforcement by directly inhibiting the GABAergic projecting neurons. They also produce reinforcement by inhibiting GABAergic interneurons in the VTA, thereby disinhibiting VTA dopaminergic neurons and enhancing dopamine release in the NA. VTA: ventral tegmental area; AMYG: amygdala; HIP: hippocampus; mPFC: medial prefrontal cortex; Glu: glutamate; GABA: γ-aminobutyric acid; DA: dopamine; EAA: excitatory amino acid receptor; D_1/D_2: dopamine receptor. Hatched receptors are inhibitory; black receptors are excitatory. (Modified from McBride WJ, Murphy JM, Ikemoto S. Localization of brain reinforcement mechanisms: intracranial self-administration and intracranial place-conditioning studies. Behav Brain Res 1999; 101:129.)

Ventral Pallidum

As noted, the ventral pallidum (VP) receives a major inhibitory GABAergic projection from the NA and in turn projects back to the VTA and to other limbic, thalamic, and midbrain areas, including the dorsomedial nucleus of the thalamus, which in turn is reciprocally related to the prefrontal cortex.[65a] In addition to modulating dopaminergic output from the VTA, the VP also conveys information from the NA to neural systems involved in motor response—i.e., drug-seeking behavior. The VP is necessary for drug-induced hyperactivity. Animals self-stimulate the VP electrically, and they self-administer amphetamine and cocaine into it.[60,66] Agents that directly or indirectly inhibit GABAergic medium spiny neurons in the NA disinhibit the VP and activate reinforcement.[45,66a]

Together the NA and VP can be viewed as components of a "ventral striatal-pallidal system" analogous to the dorsal striatal-pallidal system (putamen, caudate, and globus pallidus). Adjacent to each other and composed of parallel cortico-striatal-pallidal-thalamic-cortical projections, each is basically a cortical-subcortical re-entrant circuit.[65a] Related principally to the motor and supplementary motor cortices, the dorsal system is involved in motor planning. Related principally to prefrontal and limbic areas, the ventral system is involved in emotion and reward.

Dorsal Striatum

In contrast to the NA (ventral striatum), the principal afferents of which are from limbic structures and the mPFC, the caudate and putamen (dorsal striatum) receive afferents from sensorimotor and associative cerebral cortex. Through recurrent synaptic relays in the midbrain (including dopaminergic projections from the substantia nigra) the ventral striatum communicates with the dorsal striatum, and this pathway is probably involved in the late stages of addiction. The dorsal striatum is considered "a brain center for habit formation."[66b] Striatal synaptic plasticity may be necessary for the progression of drug use to addiction, a kind of habit not unlike obsessive-compulsive disorder and Tourette syndrome (which also involve dorsal striatal circuits).

Amygdala

The amygdala contains three major nuclei. The corticomedial nucleus receives largely olfactory afferents and projects to the ventromedial nuclei of the hypothalamus. The basolateral nucleus receives afferent information from all sensory modalities and relays this information to the central nucleus, which has two major efferent projections. The stria terminalis projects to the hypothalamus, the bed nucleus of the stria terminalis, and the NA. The ventral amygdalofugal pathway projects to the brainstem, the thalamus, the cingulate gyrus, and the orbitofrontal cortex. The amygdala plays a major role in reward and learning; autonomic expression of emotional states is mediated by connections of the amygdala to the hypothalamus whereas conscious emotional feeling is mediated by connections to the cingulate and the prefrontal cortex.[67]

The central nucleus of the amygdala (CeA) shares cytoarchitectural and circuitry similarities with the NA shell and the bed nucleus of the stria terminalis, suggesting that these structures— collectively termed the "extended amygdala"— form a common anatomical substrate for the "limbic–motor interface," or, more particularly, for acute drug reward and compulsive drug use and, possibly, for negative effects of compulsive drug administration on reward function.[53a,62,67a,68] All three components of the extended amygdala receive major dopaminergic input from the VTA and major glutamatergic input from the amygdala's basolateral nucleus.[69] They also receive efferents from the hippocampus and send major efferents to the VP and the hypothalamus. Microinjection of various neurotransmitter agonists and antagonists into the CeA alters responses to a variety of drugs, including ethanol, cocaine, morphine, nicotine, and tetrahydrocannabinol. Lesions of the CeA abolish the potentiative effects of psychostimulants on responding with conditioned reinforcement. Similar effects follow NA shell lesions, consistent with functional commonality between the CeA and NA. Some manipulations of the CeA and NA shell, however, do not produce identical effects. For example, lesions of the CeA abolish aversive pavlovian conditioning; lesions of NA shell do not. The extended amygdala is thus not functionally homogeneous, and some anatomists restrict the term "extended amygdala" to the CeA and bed nucleus of the stria terminalis.[65a]

Hypothalamus

The preoptic and basolateral areas of the hypothalamus receive direct input from the NA shell and are directly interconnected with the amygdala, the hippocampus, and other limbic structures. Animals self-administer morphine into the lateral hypothalamus, and other studies using more selective ligands suggest that δ-opiate receptors, rather than μ- or κ-receptors, are more important in hypothalamic reward.[45,60,70,71]

Hippocampus

The hippocampus, which is crucial to declarative memory and learning, sends direct glutamatergic projections to the NA. This excitatory input is modulated within the NA by inhibitory presynaptic input from local cholinergic neurons and within the hippocampus by input from prefrontal and entorhinal cortices, amygdala, and thalamus. Animals self-administer morphine into the hippocampus, especially the CA3 region, which is rich in opioid receptors. The hippocampus does not appear to affect psychostimulant reward.[60]

Pedunculopontine Tegmental Nucleus

The pedunculopontine tegmental nucleus (PPTN) contains cholinergic and glutamatergic neurons. GABAergic inhibitory projections from the basal ganglia, the NA, and the VP synapse largely on noncholinergic cells. Output from the PPTN is both rostral and caudal, with major cholinergic projections to the substantia nigra, thalamus, lateral hypothalamus, and amygdala. Other projections include the VTA, posterior pons, medulla, cerebellum, and spinal cord. The PPTN thus appears to serve as a further interface between limbic/motivational information and complex motor response. Lesions of PPTN raise the threshold for opioid and psychostimulant reinforcement.[60,72,73]

The Habenula and the Fasciculus Retroflexus

The major input to the habenular nuclei (medial and lateral) is the stria medullaris, which contains projections from the septal area (largely cholinergic), the diagonal band of Broca, the NA, the hypothalamus, the frontal cortex, the globus pallidus (largely GABAergic), the raphe nuclei, the periaqueductal gray of the midbrain, the VTA, and the substantia nigra (SN). Input from the VTA and the SN is dopaminergic. Efferent projections from the habenula pass through the fasciculus retroflexus to the interpeduncular nucleus, the VTA, the raphe nuclei, the SN, and several nuclei of the thalamus and the hypothalamus. Not surprisingly, in view of its extensive limbic connectivity, lesions of the habenula produce alterations in electrical self-stimulation. The habenula and the fasciculus retroflexus seem particularly vulnerable to damage

inflicted by repeated psychostimulant administration[74] (see Chapter 4).

Other Areas

Other areas likely involved with reward include the midbrain periaqueductal gray (PAG), the septal area, and the serotonergic raphe system. Animals self-administer morphine into the PAG, and septal lesions lower the threshold for cocaine reinforcement.[60,75]

Reward Circuitry and Memory

Viewed as a manifestation of learning, drug reinforcement involves separable memory systems and their anatomical substrates.[76] At least three forms of memory play a role in drug reinforcement. Incentive learning (classical pavlovian conditioning, which has autonomic, behavioral activating, and stimulus-orienting components) produces either reinforcing or aversive responses and depends on conditioned cues, either external (i.e., environment) or internal (i.e., the subjective effect produced by a drug). This form of memory is unconscious ("implicit") and requires the amygdala. It presumably contributes to drug craving.[77] Habit learning (instrumental conditioning) refers to repetitive motor responses (e.g., barpress to self-administer a drug) performed in the presence of drug-related stimuli (again, external or internal). Also unconscious, habit learning requires the caudate/putamen.[78] Being unconscious, incentive and habit learning produce behaviors that require post-hoc explanations. These are provided by declarative memory, which assesses drug-related information (including environmental setting and affective states) at a conscious cognitive level. Some workers view the NA shell as preferentially involved with incentive learning and the NA core as preferentially involved with habit learning.[79] The hippocampus plays an essential role in conscious declarative memory. Although different drugs share anatomical substrates, they do not interact with these memory systems in identical fashion.[76]

Neurotransmitter Systems and Reward

The complexity of reward is reflected in a voluminous and often contradictory literature addressing the effects of particular neurotransmitters and neuromodulators on behavioral responses to reinforcing drugs. The following is a highly selective sample.

Neurotransmitters and Neuromodulators

Dopamine

As noted, whether dopamine depolarizes or hyperpolarizes target neurons depends on the membrane state of the target neurons. Dopamine affects postsynaptic membrane potentials indirectly through G-protein and second messenger systems (see later). Although they have opposing effects on these second messenger systems, D_2-like dopamine receptors (which include D_2, D_3, and D_4 subtypes) and D_1-like dopamine receptors (which include D_1 and D_5 subtypes) each mediate direct reinforcing effects, and they do so independently of one another.[80,81] Studies in humans using positron emission tomography (PET) and a D_2-receptor ligand ($[^{11}C]$raclopride) found that the perceived rewarding effects of psychostimulants correlated with the rapidity of D_2-receptor activation.[78] In non-drug-abusing humans who received psychostimulants, those who described the effects as pleasant had (by PET measurement) lower levels of D_2 receptors than those who described the effects as unpleasant, suggesting an optimal range for D_2-receptor stimulation to be perceived as reinforcing: too little might be insufficient but too much might be aversive.[82]

Animals self-administer both D_1- and D_2-selective agonists, and D_1, D_2, and D_3 antagonists all attenuate the rewarding effects of psychostimulant drugs.[83–87] D_2 agonists selective for autoreceptors (which, as a negative feedback mechanism, inhibit dopamine release) are not self-administered. Studies using D_3-receptor agonists and antagonists implicate a role for D_3 receptors in drug addiction.[88–92] Studies addressing the effects of the preferential D_4 antagonist clozapine on cocaine reinforcement have been conflicting, probably because clozapine affects other receptors. Mesocorticolimbic dopamine neurons have higher densities of D_3 and D_4 receptors than do nigrostriatal dopamine neurons.[93] Knockout mice lacking D_4 receptors are supersensitive to the locomotor stimulatory effects of cocaine,

methamphetamine, and ethanol (considered an animal counterpart to euphoria).[94]

Studies addressing the effects of dopamine D_1 and D_2 agonists and antagonists on opioid reinforcement have also been inconsistent, probably because opioid reinforcement is both dopamine-dependent at the level of the VTA and dopamine-independent at the level of the NA.[95–97] Similarly conflicting findings emerge from studies involving ethanol and sedative reinforcement, yet it is worth keeping in mind that, as noted above, acute administration of all reinforcing drugs increases extracellular levels of dopamine in the shell of the NA.[62] Conversely, during withdrawal from reinforcing drugs, extracellular dopamine is decreased in the NA (reflecting decreased firing rates, not the number of spontaneously active neurons).[98] Similarly reflecting adaptive change, withdrawal from psychostimulants, opioids, ethanol, δ-9-tetrahydrocannabinol, and nicotine is associated with an elevated threshold to intracranial brain self-stimulation.[53,62]

Serotonin

Most of the 14 known 5HT receptor subtypes are metabotropic, activating G-protein-linked signaling pathways, but the $5HT_3$ receptor is ionotropic, with a ligand-gated ion channel. The variety of 5HT receptors makes it difficult to study the effects of serotonin on reward. In animals, raising brain serotonin levels with a tryptophan-enriched diet decreased psychostimulant self-administration, and administering a serotonin uptake inhibitor (fluoxetine) decreased self-administration of psychostimulants, heroin, and ethanol.[99–102] Such observations could indicate either a decrease in reward (i.e., reduced motivation to administer the drug) or an increase in reward (i.e., a lesser dose required to achieve the desired affect). Favoring reduction in brain reward are observations that raising serotonin levels lowers the breakpoint on progressive ratio scheduled self-administration studies and that a $5HT_1$ autoreceptor agonist (which would reduce serotonergic activity) produced a conditioned place preference.[103,104] Acutely opioids, via μ-receptors, disinhibit brainstem serotonergic neurons by suppressing inhibitory GABAergic projections onto them. Chronic morphine induces upregulation of GABAergic input, resulting in decreased serotonergic activity during opioid withdrawal.[104a] One study showed that stimulation of $5HT_{1B}$ receptors enhanced the reinforcing effects of cocaine.[105] Other studies found that $5HT_3$ antagonists prevented stimulation of mesolimbic dopaminergic transmission by opioids and reduced ethanol intake in animals.[106–108] Most data, however, favor an overall inhibitory effect of serotonin on drug reward. Studies with 5HT receptor subtypes have to date failed to indicate subtype specificity in such inhibitory effects.

Glutamate

Receptors for the excitatory amino acid neurotransmitter glutamate are of three major subtypes. Ionotropic glutamate receptors, which directly gate ion channels, consist of those that bind *N*-methyl-D-aspartate (NMDA) and those that do not. The latter in turn are subdivided into those that bind either alpha-amino-3-hydroxy-5-methyl-4-isoxazole propionate (AMPA) or kainate. AMPA and kainate receptors regulate a channel permeable to Na^+ and K^+. NMDA receptors regulate a channel permeable to Na^+, K^+, and Ca^{2+}. NMDA receptors have binding sites for glycine, which facilitates activation of the receptor by glutamate, opening the channel, and for phencyclidine and dizocilpine (MK801), which noncompetitively block the channel. The third type of glutamate receptor, metabotropic receptors, indirectly gate ion channels by activating second messenger systems.[109]

Drugs that block NMDA receptors are rewarding; PCP and dizocilpine produce place preference in animals and are self-administered by them.[110,111] Independently of dopamine, PCP and dizocilpine are self-administered into the NA.[112] Studies addressing the effects of NMDA blockers on other rewarding drugs are less consistent.[113,114] A potential confounder is that NMDA antagonists nonspecifically disrupt some types of learning.[115]

The role of glutamate neurotransmission in tolerance and sensitization is complex. NMDA antagonists can prevent both tolerance and sensitization to psychostimulants and to opioids; such seemingly opposing effects are reminiscent of the obligate role of NMDA receptors in both long-term potentiation (LTP) and long-term depression (LTD).[116–118] In LTP, activation of AMPA receptors, which are permeable to sodium ions, produces a

depolarization that in turn activates NMDA receptors, which are permeable to calcium ions. The result is influx of calcium and activation of various kinases (in particular calcium/calmodulin) and their signaling pathways. Activation of these signaling pathways causes phosphorylation of AMPA receptors as well as recruitment of previously inactive AMPA receptors to the post-synaptic cell membrane. The result is increased response of post-synaptic neurons to glutamate. Altered gene expression (see later) probably produces an even longer lasting increase in synaptic efficacy.[56,119,120]

One investigator declared that "drug addiction should be viewed as a form of glutamate-dependent plasticity."[121] Others, noting *enhancement* of psychostimulant sensitization by NMDA antagonists, have emphasized the complexity of interactions between the drugs being studied.[122] For example, NMDA antagonists prevent the cellular events (increased D_1-receptor sensitivity, decreased D_2-autoreceptor sensitivity) associated with psychostimulant sensitization, yet they produce these cellular changes when given alone.[123] Microinjection of psychostimulants into the VTA initiates sensitization, but microinjection into the NA is necessary to sustain sensitization, and this "transfer" of sensitization from the VTA to the NA, likely reflecting a change in the firing rate or pattern of VTA/NA dopaminergic neurons, requires local glutamatergic input and probably involves AMPA and metabotropic as well as NMDA receptors.[116] Lesion studies suggest a crucial role in the development of sensitization for glutamatergic projections from the ventral mPFC, which synapse onto both dopaminergic and non-dopaminergic cells in the VTA.[124] By contrast, lesions of the dorsal mPFC, which sends glutamatergic projections to the NA, prevent the expression of sensitization.[125] Precisely how glutamate and dopamine (which have receptors on the same projecting GABAergic inhibitory medium spiny neurons of the NA) interact at the cellular level to produce sensitization is unclear and controversial.[116,126]

Ethanol inhibits NMDA receptors, and in drug discrimination studies animals substitute glutamate antagonists for ethanol.[127] Both NMDA antagonists and L-nitroarginine, a nitric acid synthase inhibitor, block the development of tolerance for ethanol, suggesting that tolerance involves LTP or LTD.[128]

Gamma-Aminobutyric Acid

Gamma-aminobutyric acid (GABA) receptors, which mediate inhibitory synaptic actions, are of two major types. The GABA$_A$ receptor is an ionotropic receptor that gates a Cl$^-$ channel. The GABA$_B$ receptor is a metabotropic receptor that acts through G proteins and second messenger systems; among its effects is activation of an inhibitory K$^+$ channel.[109] Ethanol, barbiturates, and benzodiazepines facilitate GABA$_A$ receptors. In animals a GABA$_A$ agonist increased oral intake of ethanol and a GABA$_A$ antagonist decreased it, but as with other self-administration studies, these did not conclusively demonstrate whether the agonists or the antagonists actually increased or decreased reward.[129] Microinjection of GABA$_A$ antagonists into the central nucleus of the amygdala also reduces ethanol self-administration.[130,131] Studies using the GABA$_B$ agonist baclofen suggest that GABA$_B$ receptors are not involved in ethanol reward.[60]

Stimulation of the benzodiazepine site is rewarding; animals self-administer benzodiazepines and most (but not all) studies have shown conditioned place preference for benzodiazepines.[132,133] Benzodiazepine agonists interfered with place preference for amphetamine but not for morphine,[134] and they reduced cocaine self-administration.[135]

Acetylcholine

Studies on the role of acetylcholine in reward have involved the cholinergic agonist nicotine. Place preference studies with nicotine are conflicting, suggesting that its rewarding properties are weak.[136] Consistent with this view, nicotine self-administration in animals is less predictable than that of cocaine or amphetamine.[137] Nicotine withdrawal can be precipitated by opioid antagonists.[138]

Opioids

Opioid μ- and δ-agonists are rewarding, and they also enhance psychostimulant reward. Morphine, heroin, and the partial agonist buprenorphine reduce cocaine self-administration (interpreted as increasing reward) and enhance cocaine conditioned place preference.[139,140] Opioid antagonists interfere with psychostimulant place preference and attenuate the rewarding properties of ethanol.[141,142]

In contrast to μ- and δ-opioid receptors, κ-receptors do not mediate drug reward.[143] In fact, κ-opioid receptor activation in humans produces dysphoria.[144] The κ-receptor agonist, dynorphin, becomes functionally activated during chronic cocaine administration and attenuates cocaine reward, probably by inhibiting dopamine release in the NA via presynaptic κ-receptors.[145]

Glucocorticoids

In animals and humans, stress can trigger the transition from occasional to compulsive drug use. The locomotor response of a rat to novelty (a mild stress) predicts the amount of psychostimulant the animal will subsequently self-administer.[146] A mediator of this behavioral response to stress may be glucocorticoids. In rats receiving either cocaine or morphine, adrenalectomy resulted in reduced extracellular dopamine levels in the NA shell, an effect reversed by giving corticosterone (the major glucocorticoid in the rat).[147] The mechanism by which corticosterone stimulates the activity of VTA dopaminergic neurons is uncertain. Possibilities include increased dopamine synthesis by facilitation of tyrosine hydroxylase, decreased dopamine metabolism by inhibition of monoamine oxidase, decreased dopamine re-uptake, or increased response of dopamine receptors to dopamine.[148]

Molecular Mechanisms

When voluntary administration of a drug leads to further drug intake, reinforcement has occurred. As noted, the major challenge to neurobiologists studying substance abuse is to understand why occasional, controlled drug use progresses to compulsive, uncontrolled drug use, i.e., addiction. Animals with limited access to cocaine (e.g., 1 hour of access per session) maintain low and stable intake, whereas animals with 6-hour sessions gradually escalate intake over days. Dose–response curves in these animals suggests an elevated "hedonic set point"—an attempt to maintain a higher state of intoxication rather than a compensatory response to drug tolerance.[149,150] Mechanisms for such transformation are being sought at the molecular level.

Receptors and Intracellular Signaling

Dopamine Receptors, G-Proteins, and Cyclic AMP

Dopamine D_2-like receptors (including D_2, D_3, and D_4 subtypes), opioid μ- and δ-receptors, and cannabinoid receptors are all coupled to G-proteins of the G_i and G_o type (Table 2–1). These G-proteins inhibit adenylyl cyclase and cAMP formation. Cyclic-AMP-dependent protein kinases are thereby deactivated, with decreased phosphorylation of their target proteins, including enzymes, ion channels, and other receptors. G_i and G_o also directly activate inwardly rectifying potassium channels, an inhibitory effect.[7a] Reduced protein kinase A activity results in reduced phosphorylation of sodium channels, further lowering neuronal excitability.[81]

By contrast, D_1-like dopamine receptors (including D_1 and D_5 subtypes) are coupled to the stimulatory G-protein G_s, which stimulates cAMP formation and the second messenger protein phosphorylation system.

These opposing actions would predict that if D_2-like receptors (as well as μ- and δ-receptors and cannabinoid receptors) mediate reinforcement, D_1-like receptors do not. D_1 receptors stimulation however *is* reinforcing, even in the presence of D_2 receptor antagonism.[151] This seeming paradox is unexplained. One proposed mechanism is that the two pathways operate in separate neuronal populations. Another is that the opposing effects on the cAMP pathway have different temporal properties; for example, sustained D_1-mediated increase in cAMP activity could augment the effect of a subsequent transient D_2-mediated decrease in cAMP activity.[81]

Pertussis toxin inactivates G_i and G_o proteins, and cholera toxin activates G_s proteins. Local instillation of these toxins into the NA produces behavioral evidence of reduced reinforcement to either cocaine or heroin, suggesting that acute elevation of cAMP antagonizes drug reinforcement.[81,152]

DARPP-32

In similar studies involving a further step in the signal transduction pathway, local infusion into the NA of an inhibitor of cAMP-dependent protein kinase facilitated cocaine reinforcement, whereas infusion of a protein kinase activator reduced cocaine reinforcement.[153] It appears, therefore, that drug reinforcement is related to reduced phosphorylation by cAMP-dependent protein kinases of particular protein substrates. Of special interest is *dopamine- and cAMP-regulated phosphoprotein* (DARPP-32), which is a target for cAMP-dependent protein kinase A. DARPP-32 is regionally distributed with high levels in striatal and mesolimbic areas; it is present in dopaminoceptive GABAergic medium spiny neurons of the NA but not in dopaminergic neurons of the VTA. DARPP-32 is modulated by reinforcing drugs.[154,155]

Activated PKA phosphorylates DARPP-32 in response to D_1-receptor activation and dephosphorylates it in response to D_2-receptor activation.

Table 2–1. Acute Actions of Some Drugs of Abuse

Drug	Action	Receptor Signaling Mechanism
Opioids	Agonist at μ-, δ- and κ-opioid receptors	G_i
Cocaine	Indirect agonist at dopamine receptors by inhibiting dopamine transporters	G_i and G_s
Amphetamine	Indirect agonist at dopamine receptors by stimulating dopamine release	G_i and G_s
Ethanol	Facilitates $GABA_A$ receptor function and inhibits NMDA receptor function	Ligand-gated channels
Nicotine	Agonist at nicotinic acetylcholine receptors	Ligand-gated channels
Cannabinoids	Agonist at CB_1 and CB_2 cannabinoid receptors	G_i
Phencyclidine (PCP)	Antagonist at NMDA glutamate receptors	Ligand-gated channels
Hallucinogens	Partial agonist at $5-HT_{2A}$ serotonin receptors	G_q
Inhalants	Unknown	

Source: Modified from Nestler EJ. Molecular basis of long-term plasticity underlying addiction. Nat Rev Neurosci 2001; 2:119–128.

When phosphorylated on threonine-34, DARPP-32 inhibits protein phosphatase-1 (PP-1). As a result, target proteins of PP-1 remain phosphorylated. These target proteins include ion channels and transcription factors (for example, *cyclic AMP response element-binding protein* [CREB]). Other phosphatases (for example, calcineurin) can remove the threonine-34 phosphate groups from DARPP-32, thereby blocking DARPP-32 inhibition of PP-1 and counteracting the effects of PKA. DARPP-32 is thus considered a "molecular switch" which balances the opposing actions of PKA and calcineurin. Knockout mice lacking DARPP-32 have increased motor sensitization to chronic cocaine administration, suggesting that PKA's activation of DARPP-32, and DARPP-32's inhibition of PP-1, dampens the effects of chronic cocaine use—i.e., compensatory negative feedback.[156,157]

CART

Another source of current investigation is *cocaine-and amphetamine-regulated transcript* (CART), mRNA of which is increased in rat NA after acute administration of cocaine or amphetamine. CART is present in many areas of the central nervous system, including the olfactory bulbs, cerebral cortex, thalamus, hypothalamus, retina, and basolateral amygdala. (It is not present in the VTA.) It is tentatively associated with a number of physiological functions, including feeding behavior, stress response, sensory processing, central autonomic processing, and reward/reinforcement.[158] CART peptide (or smaller fragments) are present in GABA-containing axon terminals, consistent with a neurotransmitter or neuromodulatory role. Intracerebroventricular injection of antisera to CART attenuates cocaine-induced increases in locomotor activity.[159,160]

Adaptations, Withdrawal, and Sensitization

Neurotransmitter Adaptations

Chronic administration of different reinforcing drugs results in adaptive changes in the VTA and the NA. During early withdrawal from psychostimulants, opioids, or ethanol, both basal and drug-induced dopamine release in the NA are decreased,

plausibly reflected in tolerance and the dysphoria of acute abstinence.[81,161] There is often a brief period following acute withdrawal during which human addicts do not seek drugs, a reinforcement opposing state. In animals during this period there is elevation in the threshold for electrical brain stimulation.[162] Later, however, basal dopamine release is normal, and drug-induced dopamine release is increased.[163] At this point morphine injections into the VTA or amphetamine injections into the NA reinstate drug-seeking behavior in animals with previous drug self-administration experience.[164] Such injections also enhance conditioned pavlovian reinforcement produced by environmental stimuli associated with prior drug use.[165] Increased dopamine release is thus reflected in increased locomotor response and reinforcing effects of the drugs, i.e., sensitization, possibly the basis for human compulsive drug taking during relapse. The mechanism for increased dopamine release is uncertain, however, and studies are not entirely consistent. Some report early subsensitivity of D_2 autoreceptors in the VTA, caused by their chronic overstimulation, and leading to decreased levels of G_i and G_o proteins in dopaminergic neurons.[166] The result would be increased firing of these neurons. Other studies describe persistent reductions in dopamine transporters in the NA during drug withdrawal.[167] Still others report increased tyrosine hydroxylase levels and increased dopamine synthesis in the VTA.[168]

In sensitized animals dopamine D_2 agonists markedly reinstate drug-seeking behavior, but D_1 agonists do not. In fact, some studies suggest that D_1 agonists suppress cocaine craving.[81] It is unclear why D_1 agonists are reinforcing in other settings.

Possibly playing a role in increased dopamine release and sensitization are adaptations in glutamate AMPA receptors on VTA dopaminergic neurons. One study found enhanced responsiveness of these neurons to AMPA glutamate receptor stimulation, perhaps reflecting increased expression of specific AMPA receptor subunits in VTA neurons. In fact, transgenic mice with overexpression of specific AMPA receptor subunits in the VTA became sensitized to the reinforcing effects of morphine.[169–171] On the other hand, some studies describe decreased rather than increased spontaneous activity of VTA neurons during these same time periods, suggesting that chronic adaptations in VTA neurons and dopamine release in the NA cannot fully explain drug sensitization.[81,172]

G-Protein and cAMP Adaptations

Chronic drug administration (psychostimulants, morphine, and ethanol) produces functional D_1-receptor supersensitivity in the NA which is not accompanied by changes in the receptors themselves but rather is associated with decreased levels of G_i and G_o proteins and increased levels of adenylyl cyclase and cAMP-dependent protein kinases.[173,174] When caused by cholera toxin infusion into the NA, up-regulation of the cAMP system produces increased locomotor responses to psychostimulants, i.e., behavioral sensitization.[175] Up-regulation of the cAMP system following chronic drug administration appears to be a homeostatic compensatory adaptation to drug-induced inhibition of cAMP activity and could contribute to tolerance, aversive withdrawal symptoms, and sensitization.[81,176] Consistent with such a common mechanism are observations that psychostimulants, opioids, and other reinforcing drugs elicit cross-sensitization, i.e., early exposure to one drug produces sensitization to others.[176,177]

CREB and IEGs

Drug exposure alters gene expression, likely contributing to both short-term and long-term adaptive changes in the brain. Studies involving short-term adaptive changes have focused on two families of transcription factors, namely cAMP response element-binding protein (CREB) and the products of the immediate early genes (IEG) such as c-*fos* and c-*jun*.[53a] CREB protein, upon being phosphorylated by cAMP- or calcium-dependent protein kinases, binds to specific DNA sequences—cAMP response elements (CREs)—and regulates transcription. c-*Fos*, c-*Jun*, and similar IEG protein products bind to specific DNA sequences referred to as activating protein-1 (AP-1) binding sites.[178]

Up-regulation of the cAMP pathway by reinforcing drugs activates CREB. Inasmuch as opioids, cocaine, ethanol, and other addictive drugs are more likely acutely to inhibit the cAMP pathway, this up-regulation probably represents a compensatory homeostatic response.[179] Overexpression of CREB

in a subset of inhibitory GABAergic dynorphin-containing medium spiny neurons in the NA results in increased inhibitory feedback onto dopaminergic nerve endings projecting to the NA from the VTA.[180,181] Overexpression of CREB in the NA and the VTA likely contributes to the dysphoria of early opioid withdrawal, and overexpression of CREB in the locus ceruleus and the periaqueductal gray likely contributes to the symptoms and signs of physical dependence and withdrawal.[182–184] Up-regulation of cAMP and CREB lasts only a few days or a week after drug withdrawal, however, and so cannot account for long-term sensitization and craving.[185]

c-*Fos* is induced by opioids and psychostimulants within a few hours of drug administration, but the induction wears off within several hours because of instability of the protein and its mRNA.[185–188] Several other members of the Fos family, referred to as acute fos-related antigens (FRAs) are induced over a longer period, but their induction is also transient, resolving within 12 hours.[185,189,190] By contrast, isoforms of ΔFosB, referred to as chronic FRAs, are induced only slightly by acute drug exposure, yet their stability allows them to accumulate with repeated drug administration.[191] The accumulation of ΔFosB might underlie relatively long-lived sensitization to drugs of abuse.[192] Induction of ΔFosB selectively in the NA of mice markedly increases the sensitivity to the locomotor activating and rewarding responses to cocaine and to morphine.[193,194] ΔFosB knockout mice lose sensitization to repeated cocaine administration.[195] ΔFosB might contribute to sensitization by inducing particular subunits of the glutamate AMPA receptor, resulting in "enduring changes in the responses of the brain to drugs of abuse."[53b,196]

ΔFosB does undergo proteolysis, and its intracellular levels revert to normal within a month or two. While it might be the basis of sensitization within that time, it cannot be the direct basis of sensitization lasting months, years, or a lifetime. Perhaps ΔFosB causes changes in the brain which themselves become permanent.[197]

Another transcription factor, nuclear factor-κB (NF-κB), is induced in the NA by cocaine acutely in mice overexpressing ΔFosB and chronically in wild-type mice. These findings suggest that NF–κB is a target for ΔFosB and that NF-κβ signaling pathways play a role in long-term adaptation of NA neurons to cocaine.[198]

Structural Adaptations

Repeated administration of opioids decreases the size and caliber of dendrites and soma of dopaminergic neurons in the VTA. By contrast, repeated administration of cocaine or amphetamine increases the number of dendritic branches and spines in medium spiny neurons of the NA and pyramidal cells of the medial prefrontal cortex (mPFC), both of which receive dopaminergic input.[199] These changes, which persist for at least a month, might represent a neural substrate for long-lasting sensitization reflected in behavioral responses to these drugs. Chronic exposure to opioids also inhibits neurogenesis in the hippocampus of adult rats.[200] Repeated cocaine or morphine administration causes decreased levels of neurofilament proteins in VTA neurons.[201]

Neurotrophic factors might be involved in these changes in neural structure and neurogenesis. Chronic administration of cocaine or opioids causes altered cellular responses to brain-derived neurotrophic factor (BDNF), glial-derived neurotrophic factor (GDNF), and other neurotrophic factor systems.[202] Chronic cocaine administration raises levels of cyclin-dependent kinase 5 (Cdk5) within the NA, and local inhibition of Cdk5 prevents cocaine-induced increases in dendritic spine density. Cocaine-induced upregulation of Cdk5 is mediated through ΔFosB, and the structural changes that result persist long after the ΔFosB signal has dissipated.[203]

Drosophila Genes

The role of altered gene expression in behavioral responses to drugs has been studied in the fruitfly *Drosophila*, which undergoes a dose-dependent behavioral change on exposure to cocaine: low doses produce intensive grooming with little locomotion, moderate doses produce increased locomotion and rotation, and high doses produce tremor and paralysis.[204] Repeated exposure results in sensitization to locomotor and stereotypic responses, which, similar to that seen in rodents, is dependent on monoamine transporters and D_1-like dopamine receptors.[205] In *Drosophila*, genes involved in circadian rhythmicity play a role in cocaine sensitization; knockout flies lacking the period, clock, cycle, or doubletime genes have a normal initial cocaine response but do not develop sensitization, and flies that do not sensitize owing to absence of these genes do not demonstrate the induction of tyrosine decarboxylase normally seen after cocaine exposure.[206]

G-Proteins, GRKs, and Tolerance

Tolerance—reduced drug effect after repeated exposure—is of several kinds. With opioids, cellular (pharmacodynamic) tolerance is plausibly related to desensitization of G-protein coupled opioid receptors. Such desensitization has been attributed to reduced receptor number, in turn resulting from either reduced transcription/translation or receptor internalization.[207–209] A proposed mechanism for increased internalization is up-regulation of G-protein-receptor kinases (GRKs), which phosphorylate agonist-bound forms of receptors, leading to their internalization. Also probably contributing to opioid tolerance is down-regulation of G_i protein alpha subunits, which are necessary for coupling G-proteins and their opioid receptors.[210,211] Further contributing to opioid tolerance could be opioid-induced changes in ion channels; for example, the inwardly rectifying K^+ channel is acutely activated by opioids.[212] Finally, in addition to their inhibitory effects (via G_i signaling, inhibition of adenylyl cyclase, activation of K^+ channels, and inhibition of Ca^{2+} channels), opioids can activate adenylyl cyclase via other G-proteins in some cell types, and evidence exists that these excitatory effects of opioids become up-regulated after chronic opioid administration, opposing the inhibitory effects, and contributing to tolerance.[213]

Other Neurophysiological Aspects of Withdrawal

Drug withdrawal is associated with an aversive mental state—dysphoria, anxiety, irritability—and controversy exists over the degree to which such symptoms contribute to reinforcement (in this case negative reinforcement) and drug-seeking.[81] There are also somatic physical signs—e.g., tremor, autonomic changes—which vary considerably from drug to drug, reflecting different anatomical circuits. Somatic withdrawal symptoms probably play little if any role in motivating drug use, but like the motivationally significant adaptive changes produced in the reward circuit by chronic drug use, they represent adaptive responses.[62] Molecular adaptations in the cAMP second-messenger system of the locus ceruleus (LC) during chronic opioid administration results in increased activity of LC neurons during opioid withdrawal,[81,214,215] although to what degree this overactivity contributes to opioid withdrawal somatic symptoms is controversial.[215,216] Adaptive changes in the midbrain periaqueductal gray matter also likely contribute to opioid abstinence somatic symptoms. Also contributory is the hypothalamic–pituitary–adrenal axis, which is activated during chronic administration of reinforcing drugs.[217] Extracellular corticotropin releasing factor (CRF) is increased in limbic structures during withdrawal from cocaine, ethanol, and δ-9-tetrahydrocannabinol,[218,219] and intracerebroventricular administration of a CRF antagonist in rats dependent on cocaine, nicotine, or ethanol reversed behavioral signs of withdrawal, as did injection of a CRF antagonist into the central nucleus of the amygdala in animals withdrawing from either ethanol or opioids.[220] (After months of abstinence from ethanol, rodents display a decreased release of CRF, and CRF receptors are up-regulated. Like the plasticity observed in other drug-exposed neurotransmitter/neuromodulator systems, such adaptation might signify "new physiological set points outside the normal range," referred to as "allostasis" or "homeostasis through change."[221] As noted above, corticosteroids also modulate positive reinforcement.[148])

Addiction and the Genome

Epidemiological studies (including family, twin, and adoption) show that 40% to 60% of a person's risk for addiction, whether to cocaine, opioids, sedatives, cannabis, or ethanol, is genetic. There appear to be risk factors for particular classes of drugs as well as for substance abuse in general.[222–224] In some cases different subjective responses to drugs might depend on individual variation in particular metabolizing enzymes or brain transporter and receptor systems.[225] Unlike hereditary disorders that are explained by mutations of a single gene, however, addiction liability appears to be polygenetically inherited, and whereas monogenetically inherited disorders (e.g., Huntington's disease) are rare, polygenetically inherited disorders (e.g.,

hypertension, schizophrenia, and addiction liability) are common.[226] Disease occurs when various genes—perhaps dozens—are present in particular allelic combinations and when this particular genetic pattern interacts with environmental factors, including infectious agents and social milieu. Phenotypes are therefore quantitatively rather than dichotomously distributed, and psychic and behavioral effects of addictive drugs are graded.

To locate different genes contributing to addiction liability, animal studies have employed strategies that identify quantitative trait loci. A quantitative trait locus (QTL) is a chromosomal region that can be shown by genetic mapping to contribute to phenotypic differences. Each QTL confers only a small degree of total risk, but taken together several or many QTLs that affect a trait (e.g., response to a drug) account for most or all of the genetic contribution to the risk of developing the phenotype in question.

Mapping methods involve inbred strains of rodents in which same-sex animals are for practical purposes the same as monozygotic twins. Crossing two such strains produces an F_1 generation that is heterozygous at all genes that differ in the parents. Crossing F_1 animals to obtain an F_2 or backcrossing an F_1 to one of the parenteral inbreeds produces a generation that segregates genetically. Many individual animals are then examined, and the quantitative phenotypic trait expressed (e.g., drug preference) is correlated with specific marker alleles. If the frequency of a particular marker allele statistically correlates with the frequency of a particular trait, then a nearby (linked) gene likely affects the trait. The strategy identifies a neighborhood for the gene in question—the QTL—and the probability that a gene actually exists within a particular region is often expressed as the "logarithm of the odds of linkage," or "LOD score." Thus, the gene in question is mapped but not identified.

By the late 1990s more than 50 chromosomal regions (QTLs) had been identified as contributing to different responses to ethanol, morphine, cocaine, amphetamine, and nitrous oxide.[226,227] Responses include severe versus mild ethanol- and barbiturate-withdrawal seizures, ethanol-conditioned taste aversion, ethanol preference, cocaine seizures, and morphine preference. Cross-breeding a strain of ethanol-preferring mice with a strain of ethanol-avoiding mice allowed in ethanol-preferring offspring the identification of homozygous marker alleles that had been present in the ethanol-preferring parents; these alleles were absent in ethanol-avoiding offspring. QTLs for these alleles were mapped to chromosomes 1, 2, 4, and 9, and although, as noted, QTLs do not define the genes themselves, the QTL on chromosome 9 contains two plausible candidate genes, namely Drd2, which codes for the dopamine D_2 receptor, and Htr1b, which codes for the $5HT_{1B}$ receptor.[228] QTLs for morphine preference were mapped to chromosomes 6 and 10, and the region on chromosome 10 contains a candidate gene, Oprm, which codes for the μ-opioid receptor.[226]

Genetic influences on drug response can also be studied using mutant mice that under- or over-express specific genes. Knockout strategies have produced mice completely lacking $5HT_{1B}$ receptors; these animals consume twice as much ethanol as controls and are overly responsive to cocaine. Dopamine-D_4-receptor-deficient mice have enhanced sensitivity to methamphetamine, cocaine, and ethanol.

QTL map resolution is coarse (typically 10–30 centimorgans), and different strategies are employed to enhance it. Sufficient resolution (e.g., to a fraction of a centimorgan) could make possible positional cloning and identification of gene products. Increasingly sophisticated statistical techniques are used to clarify unique and common effects of QTLs on particular traits. Microarrays (DNA chips) are allowing thousands of cDNAs, reverse-transcribed from transcripts, to screen mRNAs from drug-exposed and control animals.[226] Finally, the influence of the Human Genome Project on drug abuse research and, eventually, clinical management, will undoubtedly be profound.

References

1. Nestler EJ. Molecular basis of long-term plasticity underlying addiction. Nat Rev Neurosci 2001; 2:119.
1a. Nestler EJ, Malenka RC. The addicted brain. Sci Am 2004; 290:78.
2. Shaham Y, Erb S, Stewart J. Stress-induced relapse to heroin and cocaine seeking in rats: a review. Brain Res Rev 2000; 33:13.
3. Robinson TE, Browman KE, Crombag HS, et al. Modulation of the induction or expression of psychostimulant sensitization by the circumstances surrounding drug administration. Neurosci Biobehav Rev 1998; 22:347.
4. Berke JD, Hyman SE. Addiction, dopamine, and the molecular mechanism of memory. Neuron 2000; 25:515.
5. Nestler EJ. Common molecular and cellular substrates of addiction and memory. Neurobiol Learning Memory 2002; 78:637.
6. Kuribara H. Effects of interdose interval on ambulatory sensitization to methamphetamine, cocaine and morphine in mice. Eur J Pharmacol 1996; 316:1.
7. Jung BJ, Dawson R, Sealey SA, et al. Endogenous GABA release is reduced in the striatum of cocaine-sensitized rats. Synapse 1999; 34:10.
7a. Genova L, Berke J, Hyman SE: Molecular adaptations to psychostimulants in striatal neurons: toward a pathophysiology of addiction. Neurobiol Dis 1997; 4:239.
8. Stolerman I. Drugs of abuse: behavioral principles, methods and terms. Trends Pharmacol Sci 1992; 13:170.
9. Geary N. Cocaine: animal research studies. In: Spitz HI, Rosecan JS, eds. Cocaine Abuse: New Direction in Treatment and Research. New York: Brunner/Mazel, 1987:19.
10. Koob GF, Vaccarino FJ, Amalric M, Serdlow NR. Neural substrates for cocaine and opiate reinforcement. In: Fisher S, Raskin A, Uhlenhuth EH, eds. Cocaine: Clinical and Biobehavioral Aspects. New York: Oxford University Press, 1987:80.
11. Wise RA, Rompre P-P. Brain dopamine and reward. Annu Rev Psychol 1989; 40:191.
12. Singh J, Desiraju T. Differential effects of opioid peptides administered intracerebrally in loci of self-stimulation reward of lateral hypothalamus and ventral tegmental area–substantia nigra. NIDA Res Monogr 1988; 87:180.
13. Colpaert FC, Janssen PAJ. Factors regulating drug cue sensitivity: limits of discriminability and the role of a progressively decreasing training dose in cocaine–saline discrimination. Neuropharmacology 1982; 21:1187.
14. Woods JH, Winger GD, France CP. Reinforcing and discriminative stimulus effects of cocaine: analysis of pharmacological mechanisms. In: Fisher S, Raskin A, Uhlehuth EH, eds. Cocaine: Clinical and Biobehavioral Aspects. New York: Oxford University Press, 1987:21.
15. Bardo MT, Rowlett JK, Harris MJ. Conditioned place preference using opiate and stimulant drugs: a meta-analysis. Neurosci Biobehav Rev 1995; 19:39.
16. Calcagnetti DJ, Keck BJ, Quatrella LA, Schechter MD. Blockade of cocaine-induced conditioned place preference: relevance to cocaine abuse therapeutics. Life Sci 1995; 56:475.
17. Tzschentke TM. Measuring reward with the conditioned place preference paradigm: a comprehensive review of drug effects, recent progress and new issues. Prog Neurobiol 1998; 56:613.
18. Kornetsky C, Bain G. Neuronal basis for hedonic effects of cocaine and opiates. In: Fisher S, Raskin A, Uhlenhuth EH, eds. Cocaine: Clinical and Biobehavioral Aspects. New York: Oxford University Press, 1987:66.

19. Johanson CE. Assessment of the dependence potential of cocaine in animals. NIDA Res Monogr 1984; 50:54.

20. Spealman RD, Goldberg SR. Drug self-administration by laboratory animals: control by schedules of reinforcement. Annu Rev Pharmacol Toxicol 1978; 18:313.

21. Bozarth MA. New perspectives on cocaine addiction: recent findings from animal research. Can J Physiol Pharmacol 1989; 67:1158.

22. Arnold JM, Roberts DCS. A critique of fixed and progressive ratio schedules used to examine the neural substrates of drug reinforcement. Pharmacol Biochem Behav 1997; 57:441.

23. Iwamoto E, Martin W. A critique of drug self-administration as a method for predicting abuse potential of drugs. NIDA Res Monogr 1988; 81:457.

24. Johanson CE, Balster RL, Bonese K. Self-administration of psychomotor stimulant drugs: the effects of unlimited access. Pharmacol Biochem Behav 1976; 4:45.

25. Woolverton WL, Balster RL. Reinforcing properties of some local anesthetics in rhesus monkeys. Pharmacol Biochem Behav 1979; 11:661.

26. Downs DA, Harrigan SE, Wiley JN, et al. Continuous stimulant self-administration in rhesus monkeys. Res Commun Psychol Psychiat Behav 1979; 4:39.

27. Kramer JG, Fischman VS, Littlefield DC. Amphetamine abuse: patterns and effects of high doses taken intravenously. JAMA 1967; 201:305.

28. Vaillant G. A 20-year follow-up of New York narcotic addicts. Arch Gen Psychiatry 1973; 29:237.

29. Koob GF. Drugs of abuse: anatomy, pharmacology and function of reward pathways. Trends Pharmacol Sci 1992; 13:177.

30. Olds J, Milner P. Positive reinforcement produced by electrical stimulation of septal area and other regions of rat brain. J Comp Physiol Psychol 1954; 47:419.

31. Wise RA. Drug-activation of brain reward pathways. Drug Alcohol Dep 1998; 51:13.

32. LeMoal M, Simon H. Mesocorticolimbic dopaminergic network: functional and regulatory roles. Physiol Rev 1991; 71:155.

33. White FJ. A behavioral/systems approach to the neuroscience of drug addiction. J Neurosci 2002; 22:3303.

34. Yeomans JS, Mathur A, Tampakeras M. Rewarding brain stimulation: role of tegmental cholinergic neurons that activate dopamine neurons. Behav Neurosci 1993; 107:1077.

35. Kelley AE, Berridge KC. The neuroscience of natural rewards: relevance to addictive drugs. J Neurosci 2002; 22:3306.

36. Koob GF, LeMoal M. Drug addiction, dysregulation of reward and allostasis. Neuropsychopharmacology 2001; 24:97.

37. Waelti P, Dickinson A, Schultz W. Dopamine responses comply with basic assumptions of formal learning theory. Nature 2001; 412:43.

38. Fiorillo CD, Tobler PN, Schultz W. Discrete coding of reward probability and uncertainty by dopamine neurons. Science 2003; 299:1898.

39. Shizgal P, Arvanitogiannis A. Gambling on dopamine. Science 2003; 299:1856.

39a. Richmond BJ, Liu Z, Shidara M. Predicting future rewards. Science 2003; 301:179.

40. Schultz W. Dopamine neurons and their role in reward mechanisms. Curr Opin Neurobiol 1997; 7:191.

41. Hyman SE, Malenka RC. Addiction and the brain: the neurobiology of compulsion and its persistence. Nat Rev Neurosci 2001; 2:695.

42. Spanagel R, Weiss F. The dopamine hypothesis of reward: past and current status. Trends Neurosci 1999; 22:521.

42a. Robinson TE, Berridge KC. Addiction. Annu Rev Psychol 2003; 54:25.

43. Kalivas PW. Neurotransmitter regulation of dopamine neurons in the ventral tegmental area. Brain Res Rev 1993; 18:75.

44. Johnson SW, North RA. Opioids excite dopamine neurons by hyperpolarization of local interneurons. J Neurosci 1992; 12:483.

45. McBride WJ, Murphy JM, Ikemoto S. Localization of brain reinforcement mechanisms: intracranial self-administration and intracranial place-conditioning studies. Behav Brain Res 1999; 101:129.

46. Devine DP, Leone P, Pocock D, Wise R. Differential involvement of ventral tegmental mu, delta, and kappa opioid receptors in modulation of basal mesolimbic dopamine release: in vivo microdialysis studies. J Pharmacol Exp Ther 1993; 226:1236.

47. Devine DP, Wise RA. Self-administration of morphine, DAMGO, and DPDPE into the ventral tegmental area of rats. J Neurosci 1994; 14:1978.

48. Museo E, Wise RA. Place preference conditioning with ventral tegmental injections of cytosine. Life Sci 1994; 55:1179.

49. Pennartz CMA, Groenewegen HJ, Lopes da Silva FH. The nucleus accumbens as a complex of functionally distinct neuronal ensembles: an integration of behavioral, electrophysiological and anatomical data. Prog Neurobiol 1994; 42:719.

50. Zahm DS, Brog JS. On the significance of subterritories in the "accumbens" part of the rat ventral striatum. Neuroscience 1992; 50:751.

51. Zahm DS. Functional-anatomical implications of the nucleus accumbens core and shell subterritories. Ann N Y Acad Sci 1999; 877;113.

52. Haber SN, McFarland NR. The concept of the ventral striatum in non-human primates. Ann N Y Acad Sci 1999; 877:33.

53. Pontieri FE, Tanda G, DiChiara G. Intravenous cocaine, morphine, and amphetamine preferentially increase extracellular dopamine in the "shell" as compared with the "core" of the rat nucleus accumbens. Proc Natl Acad Sci USA 1995; 92: 12304.

53a. Harlan RE, Garcia MM. Drugs of abuse and immediate-early genes in the forebrain. Mol Neurobiol 1998; 16:221.

53b. Kelz MB, Chen J, Carlezon WA, et al. Expression of the transcription factor ΔfosB in the brain controls sensitivity to cocaine. Nature 1999; 401:272.

53c. Saal D, Dong Y, Bonci A, et al. Drugs of abuse and stress trigger a common synaptic adaptation in dopamine neurons. Neuron 2003; 37:549.

54. Lu XY, Ghasemzadah MB, Kalivas PW. Expression of D1 receptor, D2 receptor, substance P and enkephalin messenger RNAs in the neurons projecting from the nucleus accumbens. Neuroscience 1998; 82:767.

55. LeMoine C, Bloch B. Expression of the D3 dopamine receptor in peptidergic neurons of the nucleus accumbens: comparison with the D1 and D2 dopamine receptors. Neuroscience 1996; 73:131.

56. Nicola SM, Surmeier DJ, Malenka RC. Dopaminergic modulation of neuronal excitability in the striatum and nucleus accumbens. Annu Rev Neurosci 2000; 23:186.

57. Stern EA, Jaeger D, Wilson CJ. Membrane potential synchrony of simultaneously recorded striatal spiny neurons in vivo. Nature 1998; 394:475.

58. Gracy KN, Svingos AL, Pickel VM. Dual ultrastructural localization of mu-opioid receptors and NMDA-type glutamate receptors in the shell of the rat nucleus accumbens. J Neurosci 1997; 17:4839.

59. Jiang ZG, North RA. Pre- and postsynaptic inhibition by opioids in rat striatum. J Neurosci 1992; 12:356.

60. Bardo MT. Neuropharmacological mechanisms of drug reward: beyond dopamine in the nucleus accumbens. Crit Rev Neurobiol 1998; 12:37.

61. Carlezon WA, Wise RA. Rewarding actions of phencyclidine and related drugs in nucleus accumbens shell and frontal cortex. J Neurosci 1996; 16:3112.

62. Koob GF, Sanna PP, Bloom FE. Neuroscience of addiction. Neuron 1998; 21:467.

63. Carr GD, White NM. Anatomical dissociation of amphetamine's rewarding and aversive effects: an intracranial microinjection study. Psychopharmacology 1986; 89:340.

63a. Tzschentke TM. The medial prefrontal cortex as part of the brain reward system. Amino Acids 2000; 19:211.

64. Bals-Kubik R, Ableitner A, Herz A, Shippenberg TS. Neuroanatomical sites mediating the motivational effects of opioids as mapped by the conditioned place preference paradigm in rats. J Pharmacol Exp Ther 1993; 264:489.

65. Tzschentke TM, Schmidt WJ. Functional heterogeneity of the rat medial frontal cortex: effects of discrete subarea-specific lesions on drug-induced conditioned place preference and behavioral sensitization. Eur J Neurosci 1999; 11:4099.

65a. Heimer L. A new anatomical framework for neuropsychiatric disorders and drug abuse. Am J Psychiatry 2003; 160:1726.

66. Johnson PI, Stellar JR, Paul AD. Regional reward differences within the ventral pallidum are revealed by microinjections of a mu opiate receptor agonist. Neuropharmacology 1993; 32:1305.

66a. Napier TC, Mitrovic I. Opioid modulation of ventral pallidal inputs. Ann N Y Acad Sci 1999; 876:176.

66b. Gerdeman GL, Partridge JG, Lupica CR, et al. It could be habit forming: drugs of abuse and synaptic plasticity. Trends Neurosci 2003; 26:184.

67. Iverson S, Kupfermann I, Kandel ER. Emotional states and feelings. In: Kandel ER, Schwartz JH, Jessell TM, eds. Principles of Neural Science, 4th edition. New York: McGraw-Hill, 2000:992.

67a. Koob GF. The role of striatopallidal and extended amygdala systems in drug addiction. Ann N Y Acad Sci 1999; 877:445.

68. Everitt BJ, Parkinson JA, Olmstead MC, et al. Associative processes in addiction and reward. The role of amygdala–ventral striatal subsystems. Ann N Y Acad Sci 1999; 877:412.

69. Everitt BJ, Morris KA, O'Brien A, Robbins TW. The basolateral amygdala–ventral striatal system and conditioned place preference: further evidence of limbic striatal interactions underlying reward-related processes. Neuroscience 1991; 42:1.

70. David V, Cazala P. Differentiation of intracranial morphine self-administration behavior among five brain regions in mice. Pharmacol Biochem Behav 1994; 48:625.

71. Agmo A, Gomez M. Conditioned place preference produced by infusion of metenkephalin into the medial preoptic area. Brain Res 1991; 550:343.

72. Inglis WL, Winn P. The pedunculopontine tegmental nucleus: where the striatum meets the reticular formation. Prog Neurobiol 1995; 47:1.

73. Corrigall WA, Coen KM, Adamson KL, Chow BL. Manipulations of mu-opioid and nicotine cholinergic receptors in the pontine tegmental region after cocaine self-administration in rats. Psychopharmacology 1999; 145:412.

74. Ellison G, Irwin S, Keys A, et al. The neurotoxic affects of continuous cocaine and amphetamine in habenula: implications for the substrates of psychosis. NIDA Res Monogr 1996; 163:117.

75. Gong W, Neill DB, Justice JB. Increased sensitivity to cocaine place-preference conditioning by septal lesions in rats. Brain Res 1995; 683:221.

76. White NM. Addictive drugs as reinforcers: multiple partial actions on memory systems. Addiction 1996; 91:921.

77. Horacz JL, Mash DC, Sircar R. A multi-component learning model of drug abuse. Drug taking and craving may involve separate brain circuits underlying instrumental and classical conditioning, respectively. Ann N Y Acad Sci 1999; 877:811.

78. Volkow ND, Fowler JS, Wang G-J. Role of dopamine in drug reinforcement and addiction in humans: results from imaging studies. Behav Pharmacol 2002; 13:355.

79. DiChiara G, Tanda G, Bassareo V, et al. Drug addiction as a disorder of associative learning. Role of nucleus

accumbens shell/extended amygdala dopamine. Ann N Y Acad Sci 1999; 877:461.

80. Beninger RJ, Miller R. Dopamine D1-like receptors and reward-related incentive learning. Neurosci Biobehav Rev 1998; 22:335.

81. Self DW, Nestler EJ. Molecular mechanisms of drug reinforcement and addiction. Annu Rev Neurosci 1995; 18:463.

82. Volkow ND, Wang G-J, Fowler JS, et al. Prediction of reinforcing responses to psychostimulants in humans by brain dopamine D2 receptor levels. Am J Psychiatry 1999; 156:1440.

83. Koob GF, LeMoal M. Drug abuse: hedonic homeostatic dysregulation. Science 1997; 278:5.

84. Epping-Jordan MP, Markou A, Koob GF. The dopamine D1 receptor antagonist SCH23390 injected into the dorsolateral bed nucleus of the stria terminalis decreased cocaine reward in the rat. Brain Res 1998; 784:105.

85. Woolverton WL. Effects of a D1 and a D2 dopamine antagonist on the self-administration of cocaine and piribedil by rhesus monkeys. Pharmacol Biochem Behav 1986; 24:531.

86. Self DW, Stein L. The D1 agonists SKF82958 and SKF77434 are self-administered by rats. Brain Res 1992; 582:349.

87. Caine SB, Koob GF. Effects of dopamine D1 and a D2 antagonists on cocaine self-administration under different schedules of reinforcement in the rat. J Pharmacol Exp Ther 1994; 270:209.

88. Pilla M, Perachon S, Sautel F, et al. Selective inhibition of cocaine-seeking behavior by a partial dopamine D3 receptor agonist. Nature 1999; 400:371.

89. Caine SB, Koob GF. Modulation of cocaine self-administration in the rat through dopamine D3 receptors. Science 1993; 260:1814.

90. Caine SB, Koob GF, Parsons LH, et al. D3 receptor test in vitro predicts decreased cocaine self-administration in rats. Neuroreport 1997; 8:2373.

91. Staley JK, Mash DC. Adaptive increase in D3 dopamine receptors in the brain reward circuits of human cocaine fatalities. J Neurosci 1996; 16:6100.

92. Duaux E. Homozygosity at the dopamine D3 receptor gene is associated with opioid dependence. Mol Psychiatry 1998; 3:333.

93. Gardner EL, Ashby CR. Heterogeneity of the mesotelencephalic dopamine fibers: physiology and pharmacology. Neurosci Biobehav Rev 2000; 24:115.

94. Rubinstein M, Phillips TJ, Bunzow JR, et al. Mice lacking dopamine D4 receptors are supersensitive to ethanol, cocaine, and methamphetamine. Cell 1997; 90:991.

95. Nader K, Bechara A, Roberts DCS, et al. Neuroleptics block high- but not low-dose heroin place preferences: further evidence for a two-system model of motivation. Behav Neurosci 1994; 108:1128.

96. DiChiara G. The role of dopamine in drug abuse viewed from the perspective of its role in motivation. Drug Alcohol Depend 1995; 38:95.

97a. Shippenberg TS, Herz A. Motivational effects of opioids: influence of D1 versus D2 receptor antagonists. Eur J Pharmacol 1988; 151:233.

98. Diana M, Pristis M, Carboni S, et al. Profound decrement of mesolimbic dopaminergic neuronal activity during ethanol withdrawal syndrome in rats: electrophysiological and biochemical evidence. Proc Natl Acad Sci USA 1993; 90:7966.

99. Carroll ME, Loc ST, Asencio M, et al. Intravenous cocaine self-administration in rats is reduced by dietary L-tryptophan. Psychopharmacology 1990; 100:293.

100. Peltier R, Schenk S. Effects of serotonergic manipulations on cocaine self-administration in rats. Psychopharmacology 1993; 110:390.

101. Lyness WH, Smith FL. Influence of dopaminergic and serotonergic neurons on intravenous ethanol self-administration in the rat. Pharmacol Biochem Behav 1992; 42:187.

102. Higgins GA, Wang Y, Sellers EM. Preliminary findings with the indirect 5-HT agonist dexfenfluramine on heroin discrimination and self-administration in rats. Pharmacol Biochem Behav 1993; 45:963.

103. McGregor A, Lacosta S, Roberts DCS. L-tryptophan decreases the breaking point under a progressive ratio schedule of intravenous cocaine reinforcement in the rat. Pharmacol Biochem Behav 1993; 44:651.

104. Papp M, Willner P. 8-OH-DPAT-induced place preference and place aversion: effects of PCPA and dopamine antagonists. Psychopharmacology 1991; 103:99.

104a. Jolas T, Nestler EJ, Aghajanian GK. Chronic morphine increases GABA tone on serotonergic neurons of the dorsal raphe nucleus: association with an upregulation of the cyclic AMP pathway. Neuroscience 2000; 95:433.

105. Parsons LH, Weiss F, Koob GF. Serotonin 1B receptor stimulation enhances cocaine reinforcement. J Neurosci 1998; 18:10078.

106. Carboni EE, Acquas R, Frau R, DiChiara G. Differential inhibitory effects of a $5HT_3$ antagonist on drug-induced stimulation of dopamine release. Eur J Pharmacol 1989; 10:1179.

107. Grant KA: The role of $5HT_3$ receptors in drug dependence. Drug Alcohol Depend 1995; 38:155.

108. LeMarquand D, Pihl RO, Benkelfat C. Serotonin and alcohol intake, abuse, and dependence: findings of animal studies. Biol Psychiatry 1994; 36:326.

109. Kandel ER, Siegelbaum SA. Synaptic integration. In: Kandel ER, Schwartz JH, Jessell TM, eds. Principles of Neural Science, 4th edition. New York: McGraw-Hill, 2000:212.

110. Layer RT, Kaddis FG, Wallace LJ. The NMDA receptor antagonist MK-801 elicits conditioned place preference in rats. Pharmacol Biochem Behav 1993; 44:245.

111. Carroll ME, Carmona GN, Rodefer JS. Phencyclidine (PCP) self-administration and withdrawal in rhesus

monkeys: effects of buprenorphine and dizocilpine (MK801) pretreatment. Pharmacol Biochem Behav 1994; 48:723.

112. Carlezon WA, Wise RA. Rats self-administer the noncompetitive NMDA receptor antagonists phencyclidine (PCP) and MK-801 directly into the nucleus accumbens. Soc Neurosci Abstr 1993; 19:830.

113. Kim HS, Jang CG, Park WK. Inhibition by MK801 of morphine-induced conditioned place preference and postsynaptic dopamine receptor supersensitivity in mice. Pharmacol Biochem Behav 1996; 55:11.

114. Schenk S, Valadez A, McNamara C, et al. Development and expression of sensitization to cocaine's reinforcing properties: role of NMDA receptors. Psychopharmacology 1993; 111:332.

115. Trujillo KA, Akil H. Excitatory amino acids and drugs of abuse: a role for N-methyl-D-aspartate receptors in drug tolerance, sensitization and physical dependence. Drug Alcohol Depend 1995; 38:139.

116. Wolf ME. The role of excitatory amino acids in behavioral sensitization to psychomotor stimulants. Prog Neurobiol 1998; 54:679.

117. Trujillo KA, Akil H. Excitatory amino acids and drugs of abuse: role for N-methyl-D-aspartate receptors in drug tolerance, sensitization, and physical dependence. Drug Alcohol Depend 1995; 38:139.

118. Bhargava HN. Diversity of agents that modify opioid tolerance, physical dependence, abstinence syndrome, and self-administrative behavior. Pharmacol Rev 1994; 46:293.

119. Nestler EJ. Total recall–the memory of addiction. Science 2001; 292:2266.

120. Kandel ER. Genes, synapses, and long-term memory. J Cell Physiol 1997; 173:12.

121. Wolf ME. NMDA receptors and behavioral sensitization: beyond dizocilpine. Trends Pharmacosci 1999; 20:188.

122. Tzschentke TM, Schmidt WJ. Does the noncompetitive NMDA receptor antagonist dizocilpine (MK801) really block behavioral sensitization associated with repeated drug administration? Trends Pharmacosci 1998; 19:447.

123. Jake-Matthews C, Jolly DC, Queen AL, et al. The competitive NMDA receptor antagonist CGS 19755 blocks the development of sensitization of the locomotor and dopamine activating effects of amphetamine. Soc Neurosci Abstr 1997; 23:1092.

124. Tong Z-Y, Overton PG, Clark D. Stimulation of the prefrontal cortex in the rat induces patterns of activity in midbrain dopaminergic neurons which resemble natural burst events. Synapse 1996; 22:195.

125. Pierce RC, Hicks J, Reeder D, et al. Bilateral ibotenic acid lesions of the dorsal prefrontal cortex block the expression of behavioral sensitization to cocaine. Soc Neurosci Abstr 1996; 22:930.

126. Pierce RC, Kalivas PW. A circuitry model of the expression of behavioral sensitization to amphetamine-like psychostimulants. Brain Res Rev 1997; 25:192.

127. Tabakoff B, Hoffman PL. Alcohol addiction: an enigma among us. Neuron 1996; 16:909.

128. Koob GF, Roberts AJ. Brain reward circuits in alcoholism. CNS Spectrums 1999; 4:2.

129. Boyle AE, Segal R, Smith BR, Amit Z. Bidirectional effects of GABAergic agonists and antagonists on maintenance of voluntary ethanol intake in rats. Pharmacol Biochem Behav 1993; 46:179.

130. Hyttia P, Koob GF. $GABA_A$ receptor antagonism in the extended amygdala decreases ethanol self-administration in rats. Eur J Pharmacol 1995; 283:151.

131. Roberts AJ, Cole M, Koob GF. Intraamygdala muscimol decreases operant ethanol self-administration in dependent rats. Alcohol Clin Exp Res 1996; 20:1289.

132. Woods JH, Katz JL, Winger G. Abuse liability of benzodiazepines. Pharmacol Rev 1987; 39:251.

133. DiScala G, Oberling P, Rocha B, Sandner G. Conditioned place preference induced by RO 166028, a benzodiazepine receptor partial agonist. Pharmacol Biochem Behav 1992; 41:859.

134. Pettit HO, Batsell WR, Mueller K. Triazolam attenuates amphetamine but not morphine conditioned place preference. Psychopharmacology 1989; 98:483.

135. Goeders NE, McNulty MA, Guerin GF. Effects of alprazolam on intravenous cocaine self-administration in rats. Pharmacol Biochem Behav 1993; 44:471.

136. Calcagnetti DK, Schechter MD. Nicotine place preference using the biased method of conditioning. Prog Neuro-Psychopharmacol Biol Psychiat 1994; 18:925.

137. Donny EC, Caggiula AR, Knopf S, Brown C. Nicotine self-administration. Psychopharmacology 1995; 122:390.

138. Dani JA, Heinemann S. Molecular and cellular aspects of nicotine abuse. Neuron 1996; 16:905.

139. Winger G, Skjoldager P, Woods JH. Effects of buprenorphine and other opioid agonists and antagonists on alfentanil- and cocaine-reinforced responding in rhesus monkeys. J Pharmacol Exp Ther 1992; 261:311.

140. Masukawa Y, Suzuki T, Misawa M. Differential modification of the rewarding effects of methamphetamine and cocaine by opioids and antihistamines. Psychopharmacology 1993; 111:139.

141. Trujillo KA, Belluzzi JD, Stein L. Naloxone blockade of amphetamine place preference conditioning. Psychopharmacology 1991; 104:265.

142. Samson HH, Doyle TF. Oral ethanol self-administration in the rat: effect of naloxone. Pharmacol Biochem Behav 1985; 22:91.

143. Negus SS, Henriksen SJ, Mattox A, et al. Effect of antagonists selective for mu, delta, and kappa opioid receptors on the reinforcing effects of heroin in rats. J Pharmacol Exp Ther 1993; 265:1245.

144. Schlaepfer TE, Strain EC, Greenberg BD, et al. Site of opioid action in the human brain: mu and kappa agonists' subjective and cerebral blood flow effects. Am J Psychiatry 1998; 155:470.

145. Hyman SE. Addiction to cocaine and amphetamine. Neuron 1996; 16:901.

146. Exner E, Clark D. Behavior in the novel environment predicts responsiveness to D-amphetamine in the rat: a multivariate approach. Behav Pharmacol 1993; 4:47.

147. Barrot M, Marinelli M, Abrous DN, et al. The dopaminergic hyper-responsiveness of the shell of the nucleus accumbens is hormone-dependent. Eur J Neurosci 2000; 12:973.

148. Piazza PV, LeMoal M. Pathophysiological basis of vulnerability to drug abuse; role of an interaction between stress, glucocorticoids, and dopaminergic neurons. Annu Rev Pharmacol Toxicol 1996; 36:359.

149. Ahmed SH, Koob GF. Transition from moderate to excessive drug intake: change in hedonic set point. Science 1998; 282:298.

150. Weiss F, Ciccocioppo R, Parsons LH, et al. Compulsive drug-seeking behavior and relapse. Neuroadaptation, stress, and conditioning factors. Ann N Y Acad Sci 2001; 937:1.

151. Self DW, Lam DM, Kossuth SR, Stein L. Effects of D1- and D2-selective antagonists on SKF 82958 self-administration. NIDA Res Monogr 1993; 132:230.

152. Self DW, Terwilliger RZ, Nestler E, Stein L. Inactivation of G_i and G_o proteins in nucleus accumbens reduces both cocaine and heroin reinforcement. J Neurosci 1994; 14:6239.

153. Self DW, Chi S, Nestler EJ. Modulation of cocaine self-administration by cyclic AMP analogues in the nucleus accumbens. Soc Neurosci Abstr 1993; 19:1858.

154. Caporaso GL, Bibb JA, Snyder GL. Drugs of abuse modulate the phosphorylation of ARPP-21, a cyclic AMP-regulated phosphoprotein enriched in the basal ganglia. Neuropharmacology 2000; 39:1637.

155. Hemmings HC, Walaas SI, Ouimet CC, Greengard P. Dopaminergic regulation of protein phosphorylation in the striatum: DARPP-32. Trends Neurosci 1987; 10:377.

156. Fienberg AA, Greengard P. The DARPP-32 knockout mouse. Brain Res Rev 2000; 31:313.

157. Gupta A, Tsai L-H. A kinase to dampen the effects of cocaine? Science 2001; 292:236.

158. Kubar MJ, Dall Vechia SE. CART peptides: novel addiction- and feeding-related peptides. Trends Neurosci 1999; 22:316.

159. Koylu EO, Couceyro PR, Lambert PD, Kuhar MJ. Cocaine- and amphetamine-regulated transcript peptide immunohistochemical localization in the rat brain. J Comp Neurol 1998; 391:115.

160. Adams LD, Gong W, Vechia SD, et al. CART: from gene to function. Brain Res 1999; 848:137.

161. Rosetti ZL, Hmaidan Y, Gessa GL. Marked inhibition of mesolimbic dopamine release: a common feature of ethanol, morphine, cocaine, and amphetamine abstinence in rats. Eur J Pharmacol 1992; 221:227.

162. Markou A, Koob GF. Postcocaine anhedonia. An animal model of cocaine withdrawal. Neuropsychopharmacology 1991; 4:17.

163. Kalivas PW, Duffy P. Time course of extracellular dopamine and behavioral sensitization to cocaine. 1. Dopamine axon terminals. J Neurosci 1993; 13:266.

164. Stewart J, Wise RA. Reinstatement of heroin self-administration habits: morphine prompts and naltroxone discourages renewed responding after extinction. Psychopharmacology 1992; 108:79.

165. Kelley AE, Delfs JM. Dopamine and conditioned reinforcement. 1. Differential effects of amphetamine microinjections into striatal subregions. Psychopharmacology 1991; 103:187.

166. Wolf ME, White FJ, Nassar R, et al. Differential development of autoreceptor subsensitivity and enhanced dopamine release during amphetamine sensitization. J Pharmacol Exp Ther 1993; 264:249.

167. Cerruti C, Pilotte NS, Uhl G, Kuhar MJ. Reduction in dopamine transporter mRNA after cessation of repeated cocaine administration. Mol Brain Res 1994; 22:132.

168. Sorg BA, Chen S-Y, Kalivas PW. Time course of tyrosine hydroxylase expression after behavioral sensitization to cocaine. J Pharmacol Exp Ther 1993; 226:424.

169. White FJ, Hu X-T, Zhang X-F, Wolf ME. Repeated administration of cocaine or amphetamine alters neuronal responses to glutamate in the mesoaccumbens dopamine system. J Pharmacol Exp Ther 1995; 273:445.

170. Fitzgerald LW, Ortiz J, Hamedani AG, Nestler EJ. Regulation of glutamate receptor subunit expression by drugs of abuse and stress: common adaptations among cross-sensitizing agents. J Neurosci 1996; 16:274.

171. Carlezon WA, Boundy VA, Haile CN, et al. Sensitization to morphine induced by viral-mediated gene transfer. Science 1997; 227:812.

172. Ackerman JM, White FJ. Decreased activity of rat A10 dopamine neurons following withdrawal from repeated cocaine. Eur J Pharmacol 1992; 218:171.

173. Henry DJ, White FJ. Repeated cocaine administration causes persistent enhancement of D1 dopamine sensitivity within the rat nucleus accumbens. J Pharmacol Exp Ther 1991; 258:882.

174. Terwilliger RZ, Beitner-Johnson D, Sevarino KA, et al. A general role for adaptations in G-proteins and the cyclic-AMP system in mediating the chronic actions of morphine and cocaine on neuronal function. Brain Res 1991; 548:100.

175. Cunningham ST, Kelley AE. Hyperactivity and sensitization to psychostimulants following cholera toxin infusion into the nucleus accumbens. J Neurosci 1993; 13:2342.

176. Nestler EJ. Molecular mechanisms of opiate and cocaine addiction. Curr Opin Neurobiol 1997; 7:713.

177. Cunningham ST, Kelley AE. Evidence for opiate-dopamine cross-sensitization in the nucleus accumbens: studies of conditioned reward. Brain Res Bull 1992; 29:675.

178. Torres G, Horowitz JM. Drugs of abuse and brain gene expression. Psychosom Med 1999; 61:630.

179. Shaw-Lutchman TZ, Impey S, Storm D, et al. Regulation of CRE-mediated transcription in mouse brain by amphetamine. Synapse 2003; 48:10.

180. Steiner H, Gerfen CR. Dynorphin opioid inhibition of cocaine-induced, D_1 dopamine receptor-mediated immediate-early gene expression in the striatum. J Comp Neurol 1995; 353:200.

181. Cole RL, Konradi C, Douglass J, Hyman SE. Neuronal adaptation to amphetamine and dopamine: molecular mechanisms of dynorphin gene regulation in rat striatum. Neuron 1995; 14:813.

182. Lane-Ladd SB, Pineda J, Boundy V, et al. CREB in the locus coeruleus: biochemical, physiological, and behavioral evidence for a role in opiate dependence. J Neurosci 1997; 17:7890.

183. Shaw-Lutchman TZ, Barrot M, Wallace T, et al. Regional and cellular mapping of cAMP response element-mediated transcription during naltrexone-precipitated morphine withdrawal. J Neurosci 2002; 22:3663.

184. Maldonado R, Blendy JA, Tzavara E, et al: Reduction of morphine abstinence in mice with a mutation in the gene encoding CREB. Science 1996; 273:657.

185. Nestler EJ, Aghajanian GK. Molecular and cellular basis of addiction. Science 1997; 278:58.

186. Nguyen TV, Kosofsky BE, Birnbaum R, et al. Differential expression of c-Fos and Zif268 in rat striatum after haloperidol, clozapine, and amphetamine. Proc Natl Acad Sci USA 1992; 89:4270.

187. Liu J, Nickolenko J, Sharp FR. Morphine induction of Fos in striatum is mediated by NMDA and D1 dopamine receptors. Soc Neurosci Abstr 1993; 19:1022.

188. Moratella R, Elibol B, Vallejo M, Graybiel AM. Network-level changes in expression of inducible Fos-Jun proteins in the striatum during chronic cocaine treatment and withdrawal. Neuron 1996; 17:147.

189. Hope BT, Kosofsky B, Hyman SE, Nestler EJ. Regulation of IEG expression and AP-1 binding by chronic cocaine in the rat nucleus accumbens. Proc Natl Acad Sci USA 1992; 89:5764.

190. Hope BT, Nye HE, Kelz MB, et al. Induction of long-standing AP-1 complex composed of altered Fos-like proteins in brain by chronic cocaine and other chronic treatments. Neuron 1994; 13:1235.

191. Chen J, Kelz MB, Hope BT, et al. Chronic Fos-related antigens: stable variants of ΔFosB induced in brain by chronic treatments. J Neurosci 1997; 17:4933.

192. Merlo-Pich E, Pagliusi SR, Tessari M, et al. Common neural substrates for the addictive properties of nicotine and cocaine. Science 1997; 275:83.

193. Kelz MB, Nestler EJ. ΔFosB: a molecular switch underlying long-term neural plasticity. Curr Opin Neurol 2000; 13:715.

194. Colby CR, Whisler K, Steffen C, et al. Striatal cell type-specific overexpression of Delta-FosB enhances incentive for cocaine. J Neurosci 2003; 23:2488.

195. Hiroi N, Brown J, Haile C, et al. FosB mutant mice: loss of chronic cocaine induction of Fos-related proteins and abnormality in locomotor and reinforcing responses to cocaine. Proc Natl Acad Sci USA 1997; 94:10397.

196. Carlezon WA, Nestler EJ. Elevated levels of GluR1 in the midbrain: a trigger for sensitization to drugs of abuse? Trend Neurosci 2002; 25:610.

197. Nestler EJ. Molecular basis of long-term plasticity underlying addiction. Nat Rev Neurosci 2001; 2:119.

198. Ang E, Chen AE, Zagouras P, Magna H, et al. Induction of nuclear factor-kappa B in nucleus accumbens by chronic cocaine-administration. J Neurochem 2001; 79:221.

199. Robinson TE, Kolb B. Alterations in the morphology of dendrites and dendritic spines in the nucleus accumbens and prefrontal cortex following repeated treatment with amphetamine or cocaine. Eur J Neurosci 1999; 11:1598.

200. Eisch AJ, Barrot M, Schad LA, et al. Opiates inhibit neurogenesis in the adult rat hippocampus. Proc Natl Acad Sci USA 2000; 97:7579.

201. Beitner-Johnson D, Guitart X, Nestler EJ. Neurofilament proteins and the mesolimbic dopamine system: common regulation by chronic morphine and chronic cocaine in the rat ventral tegmental area. J Neurosci 1992; 12:2165.

202. Messer CJ, Eisch AJ, Carlezon WA, et al. Role of GDNF in biochemical and behavioral adaptations to drugs of abuse. Neuron 2000; 26:247.

203. Bibb JA, Chen J, Taylor JR, et al. Effects of chronic exposure to cocaine are regulated by the neuronal protein Cdk5. Nature 2001; 410:376.

204. Wolf ME. Cocaine addiction: clues from *Drosophila* on drugs. Curr Biol 1999; 9:R770.

205. McClung C, Hirsh J. Stereotypic behavioral responses to free-base cocaine and the development of behavioral sensitization in *Drosophila*. Curr Biol 1998; 8:109.

206. Andretic R, Chaney S, Hirsh J. Circadian genes are required for cocaine sensitization in *Drosophila*. Science 1999; 285:1066.

207. Pak YS, Kouvelas A, Scheideler MA, et al. Agonist-induced functional desensitization of the mu-opioid receptor is mediated by loss of membrane receptors rather than uncoupling from G protein. Mol Pharmacol 1996; 50:1214.

208. Freedman NJ, Lefkowitz RJ. Desensitization of G protein-coupled receptors. Recent Prog Horm Res 1996; 51:319.

209. Zhang L, Yu Y, Mackin S, et al. Differential mu opiate receptor phosphorylation and desensitization induced by agonists and phorbol esters. J Biol Chem 1996; 271:1144.

210. Sim LJ, Selley DE, Dworkin SI, Childers SR. Effects of chronic morphine administration on micro opioid receptor-stimulated [^{35}S]GTPgammaS autoradiography in rat brain. J Neurosci 1996; 16:268.

211. Gold SJ, Ni YG, Dohlman H, Nestler EJ. Regulators of G protein signaling: region-specific expression of nine subtypes in rat brain. J Neurosci 1997; 17:8024.

212. Kovoor A, Henry DJ, Chavkin C. Agonist-induced desensitization of the mu opioid receptor-coupled potassium channel (GIRK1). J Biol Chem 1995; 270:589.

213. Smart D, Lambert DG. The stimulatory effects of opioids and their possible role in the development of tolerance. Trends Pharmacol Sci 1996; 17:264

214. Nestler EJ. Under siege: the brain on opiates. Neuron 1996; 16:897.

215. Koob GF, Maldonado R, Stinus L. Neural substrates of opiate withdrawal. Trends Neurosci 1992; 15:186.

216. Christie MJ, Williams JT, Osborne PB, Bellchambers CE. Where is the locus in opioid withdrawal? Trends Neurosci 1997; 18:134.

217. Kreek MJ, Koob GF. Drug dependence: stress and dysregulation of brain reward pathways. Drug Alcohol Depend 1998; 51:23.

218. Merlo-Pich E, Lorang M, Yeganeh M, et al. Increase of extracellular corticotropin-releasing factor-like immunoreactivity levels in the amygdala of awake rats during restraint stress and ethanol withdrawal as measured by microdialysis. J Neurosci 1995; 15:5439.

219. Rodriguez de Fonseca F, Carrera MRA, Navarro M, et al. Activation of corticotropin-releasing factor in the limbic system during cannabinoid withdrawal. Science 1997; 276:2050.

220. Koob GF. Drug addiction; the yin and yang of hedonic homeostasis. Neuron 1996; 16:893.

221. Goldman D, Barr CS. Restoring the addicted brain. N Engl J Med 2002; 347:843.

222. Merikangas KR, Stolar M, Stevens DE, et al. Familial transmission of substance use disorders. Arch Gen Psychiatry 1998; 55:973.

223. Kendler KS, Karkowski LM, Neale MC, et al. Illicit psychoactive substance use, heavy use, abuse, and dependence in a U.S. population-based sample of male twins. Arch Gen Psychiatry 2000; 57:261.

224. Tsuang MT, Lyons MJ, Meyer JM, et al. Co-occurrence of abuse of different drugs in men. The role of drug-specific and shared vulnerabilities. Arch Gen Psychiatry 1998; 55:967.

225. Nestler EJ, Landsman D. Learning about addiction from the genome. Nature 2001; 409:834.

226. Crabbe JC, Phillips TJ, Buck KJ. Identifying genes for alcohol and drug sensitivity: recent progress and future directions. Trends Neurosci 1999; 22:173.

227. Kubar MJ, Joyce A, Dominguez G. Genes in drug abuse. Drug Alcohol Dep 2001; 62:157.

228. Tarantino LM, McClearn GE, Rodriguez LA, et al. Confirmation of quantitative trait loci for alcohol preference in mice. Alcohol Clin Exp Res 1998; 22:1099.

Chapter 3
Opioids

Thou only givest these gifts to man, and thou hast the keys of Paradise, O just, subtle, and mighty opium.
—Thomas De Quincey

Everything one does in life, even love, occurs in an express train racing towards death. To smoke opium is to get out of the train while it is still moving.
—Jean Cocteau

Junk is not … a means to increased enjoyment of life. Junk is not a kick. It is a way of life.
—William Burroughs

Persons addicted to morphia are inveterate liars.
—William Osler

Opium is derived from seed capsules of the poppy, *Papaver somniferum*, indigenous to the Middle East and Southeast Asia. The dried juice (gum opium) contains more than 20 alkaloids, including morphine and codeine.[1] Today there are also commercially available semisynthetic and synthetic opioids, including agonists, antagonists, and mixed agonist-antagonists (Table 3–1).

Pharmacology and Animal Studies

Opioid Receptors and Endorphins

Some investigators use the term *opiate* for morphine-like drugs derived directly or indirectly from opium and *opioid* for drugs with morphine-like actions but quite different chemical structures. To avoid confusion, only opioid is used here, referring to both agonists and antagonists, whether or not they structurally resemble morphine. Similarly misleading is the term *narcotic*, which not only fails to describe why opioids are usually taken (medically or illicitly), but also when used by law enforcement agencies refers to cocaine and marijuana as well.

Some agonist-antagonists (e.g., buprenorphine and nalbuphine) are *partial agonists*, having agonist effects when given alone or in the presence of small doses of strong agonists but antagonizing the effects of large doses. Other agonist-antagonists (e.g., nalorphine and cyclazocine) have agonist effects at low doses but dysphoric psychotomimetic effects at high doses and antagonize the effects of either low or high doses of pure agonists.[2] Such complex properties have been better understood since the discovery in 1973 of stereospecific opioid receptors in mammalian brain and the subsequent identification of endogenous opioid peptides (endorphins).[3–6] High concentrations of opioid receptors and endorphins in particular regions of the central and peripheral nervous system correlate with opioid effects, including euphoria, addiction, nausea, analgesia, sedation,

Table 3–1. Opioids Currently or Recently Available in the United States

Agonist
Powdered opium
Tincture of opium (laudanum)
Camphorated tincture of opium (paregoric)
Purified opium alkaloids (Pantopon)
Morphine (Morphine Sulfate Injection;
    MS Contin; Oramorph)
Heroin (legally available only for investigational use)
Methadone (Dolophine)
Fentanyl (Sublimaze; in Innovar; Duragesic Patch)
Sufentanil (Sufenta)
Alfentanil (Alfenta)
Oxymorphone (Numorphan)
Hydromorphone (Dilaudid)
Codeine
Dihydrocodeine (Synalgos)
Oxycodone (Oxy-Contin, and in mixtures, e.g., Percodan,
    Percocet, Tylox)
Hydrocodone (in mixtures, e.g., Hycodan, Lortab, Lorcet,
    Tussionex, Vicodin)
Levorphanol (Levo-Dromoran)
Meperidine (pethidine; Demerol, Pethadol)
Alphaprodine (Nisentil)
Propoxyphene (Darvon, and in Darvocet, Wygesic)
Diphenoxylate (in Lomotil)
Etorphine (for animal use)
Apomorphine

Antagonist
Naloxone (Narcan)
Naltrexone (Trexan)
Nalmefene (Revex)

Mixed Agonist-Antagonist
Pentazocine (Talwin, Talwin Nx, and in Talacen)
Butorphanol (Stadol)
Buprenorphine (Buprenex)
Nalbuphine (Nubain)
Cyclazocine (for investigational use only)
Propiram (for investigational use only)
Profadel (for investigational use only)
Meptazinol (for investigational use only)
Dezocine (for investigational use only)

Table 3–2. Correlation of Opioid Effects with Regional Opioid Receptors

Analgesia	Spinal cord, midbrain periaqueductal gray matter, limbic structures
Emotion	Limbic structures, locus ceruleus
Sedation	Midbrain reticular formation, cerebral cortex
Memory, learning	Hippocampus
Miosis	Midbrain
Hypothermia	Hypothalamic preoptic nucleus
Respiratory depression	Brainstem respiratory centers
Cough suppression	Medulla

Source: References 7–9, 35.

Table 3–3. Receptor Specificities of Natural and Synthetic Opioids

Mu
Beta-endorphin
Morphine
Levorphanol
Fentanyl
[Met]enkephalyl-Arg-Arg-Val-NH$_2$
[D-Ala^2-NMePhe^4, Gly-ol]enkephalin (DAMGO)
[Met]enkephalyl-Arg-Arg-Val-Gly-Arg-Pro-Glu-Trp-
    Trp-Met-Asp-Tyr-Gln (BAM 18)
[Met]enkephalyl-Arg-Phe-Tyr-D-Arg-Phe-Lys-NH$_2$
D-Phe-Cys-Tyr-D-Trp-Orn-Thr-Pen-Thr-NH^2 (CTOP)

Delta
[Leu]enkephalin
[Met]enkephalin
Beta-endorphin
[D-Ala^2-D-Leu^5]enkephalin (DADLE)
[D-Pen^2-D-Pen^5]enkephalin (DPDPE)

Kappa
Dynorphin A (1–17)
Dynorphin B
Alpha-neo-beta-neoendorphin
Dynorphin A (1–18)
[D-Pro^{18}]dynorphin A (1–11)
U-69, 593
PD 117302
Ketocyclazocine
Pentazocine
Butorphanol
Nalbuphine
Nalorphine

Source: References 7–9.

miosis, respiratory depression, cough suppression, appetite stimulation, constipation, bradycardia, hypotension, temperature regulation, immunological responses, and seizures.

In addition to their different anatomical distributions, endogenous opioids have different receptor affinities, although they are not receptor-specific (Tables 3–2, 3–3).[7–9] Beta-endorphin arises, with adrenocorticotropic hormone (ACTH), from a precursor molecule, pro-opiomelanocortin. It is at highest concentration in the pars intermedia and pars distalis of the pituitary, the arcuate nucleus of the hypothalamus, the locus ceruleus, limbic areas, and the midbrain and has higher affinity for μ- than for δ-receptors.[9,10] Methionine-enkephalin and leucine-enkephalin, derived from pro-enkephalin, are more widely distributed in the brain and spinal cord. They are especially concentrated in the hypothalamus, the amygdala, and other limbic areas and in brain stem and spinal cord areas involved with pain (e.g., the midbrain periaqueductal gray matter, the spinal trigeminal nucleus, and laminae I and II or the dorsal horn); enkephalins are also released, with catecholamines, from the adrenal medulla. They are more bound to δ- than to μ-receptors.[8,9] The dynorphins, derived from pro-dynorphin, contain the leucine-enkephalin amino acid sequence at one end yet have affinity for κ-receptors, in the case of dynorphin A and B to a greater extent than for μ- and δ-receptors.[8,11] Also widely distributed in the central nervous system (CNS), dynorphins share brain areas with the enkephalins, yet within these areas they often occupy different neuronal groups.

In addition to these well-studied endorphins, the brain contains numerous fragments of pro-opiomelanocortin, pro-enkephalin, and pro-dynorphin, the functional significance of which is uncertain. "Endomorphins" are endogenous ligands containing only four amino acids yet highly selective for μ receptors.[11a] Even more obscure is the physiological role in mammalian brain of endogenous morphine, codeine, and 6-acetylmorphine, synthesized in liver (using the same steps as in the opium poppy) and transported across the blood–brain barrier as a presumed peripheral-to-central hormone.[12] Finally, a 91-amino acid peptide from the pituitary, β-lipotropin, also derived from pro-opiomelanocortin, has a sequence at residues 61 to 65 identical to methionine-enkephalin and at 61 to 91 identical to β-endorphin, yet β-lipotropin has no opioid activity itself.[13]

A receptor partly homologous with the δ-receptor has little affinity for opioids but binds strongly to a ligand known as orphanin FQ/nociceptin (OFQ/N).[14] Widely distributed in the CNS, OFQ/N reverses opioid analgesia through actions on opioid-sensitive pain-modulating regions of the brainstem (including the midbrain periaqueductal grey matter and the medullary nucleus raphe magnus). At the level of the spinal cord OFQ/N can produce either hyperalgesia or analgesia depending on the state of the animal.[15] It does not cause respiratory depression.[11a] Possibly relevant to drug dependence, OFQ/N receptors are abundant in reward circuit areas, and OFQ/N delivered into the ventral tegmental area (VTA) increases γ-aminobutyric acid (GABA) levels in the (VTA) and reduces dopamine levels in the nucleus accumbens (NA). Although studies are not entirely consistent, OFQ/N, unlike opioid antagonists, appears to attenuate morphine's rewarding properties without inducing aversion and without suppressing food intake.[16,17]

Skin of the amphibian *Phyllomedusa* contains two classes of heptapeptides, namely, dermorphins, which are selective for μ-receptors, and deltorphins, which are selective for δ-receptors. Interestingly, substitution of a single amino acid confers strong μ-receptor affinity in deltorphins without any decrease in δ-receptor affinity. This feature has aroused much research interest in deltorphins.[18]

Although highly homologous with one another, genes encoding the three opioid receptors are present on different chromosomes, suggesting that their divergence was not recent in evolutionary history.[19]

A peptide, Phe-Met-Arg-Phe-NH2 (FMRF-amide), originally identified in molluscs, is present in mammalian CNS, where it exerts anti-opioid effects. Its physiological importance is uncertain, but speculation includes a possible role in tolerance and dependence.[20] Rats receiving intrathecal injections of cerebrospinal fluid (CSF) from morphine-tolerant rats develop immediate tolerance to morphine effects, and an FMRF-amide–like peptide precipitates signs of opioid withdrawal.[21]

Receptor Distribution, Function, and Subtypes

Opioid μ-receptors are widely distributed in the CNS; δ-receptors are restricted largely to the forebrain; and κ-receptors are found in limbic and other diencephalic areas, brainstem, and spinal cord.[22–24] Distribution of receptors and their endogenous ligands within the mesocorticolimbic reward system is shown in Table 3–4. Receptors vary in their affinities for exogenous opioids. For example, the

Table 3–4. Opioid-Receptor and Peptide Distribution

Region	Receptors			Peptides		
	μ	δ	κ	POMC	Pro-Enk	Pro-Dyn
VTA	++	0	+	++	++	+
NA	++++	++++	++++	+	+++	++
VP	+	+	+	0	++++	+++
LH	+	0	++	+++	++	+++
AMYG (lateral)	++++	+++	+++	++	+++	+
MPF	+++	++	++	0	++	+
PAG	+	0	++	++++	+++	+
PPN	++++	+++	+++	0	+++	0

++++, very dense; +++, dense; ++, moderate; +, low; 0, undetectable.

Abbreviations: POMC, pro-opiomelanocortin; Pro-Enk, pro-enkephalin; Pro-Dyn, pro-dynorphin; VTA, ventral tegmental area; NA, nucleus accumbens; VP, ventral pallidum; LH, lateral hypothalamus; AMYG, amygdala; MPF, medial prefrontal cortex; PAG, periaqueductal gray; PPN, pedunculopontine nucleus.

Source: Shippenberg TS, Elmer GI. The neurobiology of opiate reinforcement. Crit Rev Neurobiol 1998; 12:267. Reprinted with permission.

μ-receptor has highest affinity for morphine, levorphanol, and fentanyl, and synthetic analogs have been developed with selective agonism for μ-, δ-, and κ-receptors.[9,25] There are also receptor-selective antagonists. Receptors are not functionally specific. For example, μ-, δ-, and κ-receptors each participate in analgesia, but μ-receptors play the major role.[8] Mu-receptor knockout mice have exaggerated nociceptive responses and are unaffected by morphine.[26]

Evidence supports the existence of receptor subtypes (μ_1, μ_2, μ_3, δ_1, δ_2, κ_{1-4}), with dissociable effects (e.g., analgesia vs. respiratory depression), but the molecular basis of such differences is uncertain.[2,10,19,27,28] Possibly they are the result of heterodimerization of various opioid receptors. Alternatively, different cellular responses to particular agonists for the same receptor could be the result of recruitment of molecules to form distinctive "signaling complexes" with the receptor.[29] Interestingly, in knockout mice lacking the first exon of the μ-receptor gene morphine is pharmacologically inactive yet its metabolite, morphine-6-beta-glucuronide (M6G), as well as heroin and the heroin metabolite 6-acetylmorphine, continue to be analgesic.[30] μ_2-receptors affect pain and respiration equally; μ_1-receptors are more specifically analgesic.[2] μ_1-receptors bind morphine and the enkephalins with equal affinity; μ_2-receptors bind morphine more avidly than the enkephalins. Naloxone antagonizes both μ_1- and μ_2-receptors; naloxonazine selectively antagonizes μ_3-receptors,

thereby blocking analgesia, prolactin release, acetylcholine turnover, and hypothermia but not respiratory depression, growth hormone release, bradycardia, sedation, inhibition of electrically stimulated guinea pig ileum, or dopamine turnover.[27,28] Similarly selective agents have been developed to study δ- and κ-receptors. For example, naltrindole antagonizes δ_1- and δ_2-receptors, BNTX antagonizes only δ_1-receptors, and naltriben antagonizes only δ_2-receptors.

Although δ-receptors may contribute, μ-receptors are the principal mediators of opioid euphoria and reinforcement. Animals self-administer morphine (which is more μ-specific than any endorphin) systemically and directly into the VTA, the NA, the lateral hypothalamus, the amygdala, and the hippocampus, and genetic manipulation in mice to increase μ-receptor density enhances morphine's efficacy as a reinforcer.[31] Knockout mice lacking μ-receptors show no morphine-induced place preference.[32] Animals also self-administer δ-receptor agonists into the VTA and the NA, and either δ_1- or δ_2-receptor agonists induce place preference. By contrast, κ-receptor agonists are not self-administered either systemically or into the VTA or the NA, and they produce aversion for an environment associated with their administration.[10] Mixed opioid agonist-antagonists are also aversive in most studies, probably due to their κ-agonist effects and their μ-antagonist effects; reports of self-administration are probably explained by μ-agonism at certain doses.[10]

The non-selective opioid antagonist naloxone maintains negative reinforced behavior in non-opioid-dependent animals, suggesting the existence of a tonically active endogenous opioid reward pathway, disruption of which produces aversion.[10]

Sigma-receptors have affinity for mixed agonist-antagonists such as cyclazocine as well as for phencyclidine. Their effects are not blocked by naloxone, and they are not classified as opioid receptors.[33] Additional opioid receptors or receptor subtypes mediate inhibition of smooth muscle contraction, hypothermia or hyperthermia, and proconvulsant or anticonvulsant effects.[34] Such diversity explains the complex actions of particular opioids. For example, the effects of nalorphine result from competitive antagonism at μ-receptors, partial agonism at κ-receptors, and agonism at ζ-receptors. Some opioid effects are not understood in terms of any combination of receptors, for example, why morphine produces sedation in some subjects but not others.[2]

The existence of multiple opioid receptor types also helps to explain different abstinence syndromes, for example, of morphine, cyclazocine, and nalbuphine. A partial agonist such as nalbuphine relieves abstinence symptoms in subjects no longer receiving morphine by occupying vacant receptor sites but precipitates abstinence in subjects fully dependent on morphine by replacing a weak agonist for a strong one. A mixed agonist-antagonist such as cyclazocine precipitates abstinence in subjects dependent on drugs occupying receptor types for which it is a competitive antagonist but does not precipitate abstinence when both it and the drug of dependence are agonists for the same receptors. It and the dependent drug are then cross-tolerant.[2]

The different actions of different opioids are exemplified in the hippocampus, which has μ- and δ-receptors and enkephalins as well as κ-receptors and dynorphins. Enkephalins increase the excitatory responses of hippocampal pyramidal cells in the CA1 region by presynaptically inhibiting GABAergic inhibitory interneurons. By this action enkephalins facilitate long-term potentiation (LTP), critical for learning and memory. They are also, by the same mechanism, epileptogenic. Dynorphins, by contrast, inhibit excitatory glutamatergic neurotransmission at perforant path terminals in the hippocampal dentate gyrus. By this action dynorphins inhibit LTP, learning, and epileptogenesis. Opioids thus provide a fine-tuning of hippocampal excitability.[35,35a]

Opposing actions of μ- and κ-receptors are seen in other regions as well. Although κ-receptor agonists are weakly analgesic, they reverse the analgesic actions of μ-receptor agonists at the level of the spinal cord and the brainstem. Kappa-receptor agonists, which themselves lack reinforcing effects (and in humans produce dysphoria), block the reinforcing effects of morphine in both self-administration and conditioned place preference models, and they suppress morphine tolerance.[36]

Opioids and Pain Control

Opioid-related pain control has at least two anatomical and functional components. The first is concerned with pain perception threshold. Beta-endorphin, the enkephalins, and the dynorphins are each present in high concentration in the midbrain periaqueductal gray matter, electrical stimulation of which causes naloxone-reversible analgesia. Analgesia also follows injection of morphine into this area. The periaqueductal gray matter is part of a descending system that ultimately inhibits nociceptive impulses in the dorsal horn of the spinal cord. It probably contributes to analgesia associated with placebo; acupuncture; transcutaneous nerve stimulation; fear; and other stresses such as fighting, sexual arousal, food deprivation, or temperature changes; each of these analgesic effects is reversible with naloxone.[11a,37,38] The responsible descending pathways are anatomically and pharmacologically complex, with important relays in the nucleus raphe magnus of the medulla and involvement of serotonin, norepinephrine, dopamine, acetylcholine, histamine, somatostatin, thyroid-releasing hormone, neurotensin, and cholecystokinin.

The second component of pain control involves psychological response. Morphine-induced analgesia depends as much on relief of the anxiety and tension that accompany pain as on elevation of pain perception threshold. This action involves limbic structures; in functional imaging studies of healthy volunteers experiencing sustained pain, there was release of endogenous μ-receptor agonists in thalamus, amygdala, insula and prefrontal cortex.[39] Pain is separable into at least two types. *Phasic* (sudden, sharp) pain is mediated by the lateral spinothalamic tract and relays mainly to the sensory cortex. *Tonic* (persistent) pain is mediated by a more medial system and relays mainly to limbic areas. Opioids appear to affect tonic pain at the limbic rather than the spinal level. Interestingly, although phasic pain shows considerable tolerance to opioid analgesia, tonic pain does not.[40]

Reinforcement and Dependence

As noted, μ- and δ-receptor agonists are self-administered directly into the VTA and the NA, demonstrating the critical role of the mesocorticolimbic reward system on opioid positive reinforcement. Opioids increase firing of the VTA dopaminergic cells by inhibiting local inhibitory GABAergic interneurons within the VTA. Reinforcement from NA self-administration, however, is independent of VTA dopaminergic neurons and seems to involve direct inhibitory actions on GABAergic projecting neurons within the NA (see Chapter 2). Dopamine D_1 antagonists, D_2 antagonists, and mixed D_1/D_2 antagonists do not attenuate heroin self-administration in rats, and 6-hydroxydopamine (6-OHDA) lesions of the NA (which selectively destroy dopaminergic nerve endings) decreased cocaine self-administration without affecting heroin self-administration. On the other hand, dopamine D_1 antagonists and 6-OHDA lesions of the NA do prevent heroin-induced conditioned place preference. It is possible that dopamine is involved in the acquisition of opioid self-administration, being necessary for "salience attribution" and the acquisition of conditioned responses, but not in maintenance of opioid self-administration once it is established.[10] Also uncertain are the relative roles of the NA shell and the NA core.[41]

The ventral pallidum (VP), considered a region necessary for the motor expression of limbic-generated reward seeking (see Chapter 2), receives GABAergic and opioid projections from the NA, glutamatergic projections from the prefrontal cortex and the basolateral nucleus of the amygdala, and dopaminergic projections from the substantia nigra and the VTA. Opioid transmission in the VP tends to attenuate GABA and dopamine influences while potentiating the efficacy of glutamate. The overall effect is to "diminish the influence of reinforcement (VTA and NA) in the transduction of cognition (prefrontal cortex) and affect (amygdala) into behavior".[42]

The anatomy of opioid reward is widely distributed. For example, local injection of an opioid antagonist into the bed nucleus of the stria terminalis and lesions of the pedunculopontine tegmental nucleus of the brainstem each reduce the rewarding effects of opioids.[16,43]

Kappa-receptor agonists decrease extracellular dopamine levels in the NA by activating inhibitory κ-receptors on dopaminergic nerve endings.[44] Like other reinforcing drugs, ethanol, nicotine, and cannabis increase dopamine levels in the NA, and these increases are blocked by naloxone or naltrexone. It thus appears that the rewarding properties of a number of drugs are mediated by opioid systems.[45–47]

There are no known exogenous or endogenous opioids that are strongly analgesic without producing physical dependence. (Interestingly, the association of analgesia and abuse potential is seen with a number of non-opioid drugs as well, including anticholinergics, alpha-2 adrenergic agonists, dopamine D_2 agonists, cannabinoids, and adenosine antagonists [e.g., caffeine].[48]) On the other hand, the μ_1-antagonist naloxonazine reduces morphine analgesia in rats without preventing the development of physical dependence, and the δ_2-receptor antagonist naltrindole-5′-isothiocyanate attenuates heroin self-administration but not antinociception.[49] Such dissociability of analgesia and physical dependence has spurred search for more selective agonists.

Reward seeking and physical dependence are also dissociable. Rats self-administer morphine directly into the VTA at intervals too long to produce signs of physical dependence,[50] and in place preference and intravenous self-administration models, rats demonstrate heroin seeking for weeks after receiving doses too small to produce physical dependence.[51,52] Conversely, chronic infusion of methionine-enkephalin, β-endorphin, or morphine into rodent periaqueductal gray matter causes signs of physical dependence following naloxone challenge, but infusion into the VTA does not.[28,50] Animals do not self-administer morphine into the periaqueductal gray matter, and opioids passively injected into the periaqueductal gray matter inhibit rather than facilitate brain stimulation reward.[7] Knockout mice lacking dopamine D_2-receptors do not develop reinforcing responses to opioids, yet they do demonstrate opioid physical dependence, providing evidence that dopaminergic mechanisms are involved in opioid reward, whereas non-dopaminergic mechanisms underlie physical dependence.[53,54] Of course the desire to relieve withdrawal symptoms can contribute to drug-seeking behavior, but the relative roles of reward and abstinence are disputed, for opioids and for other drugs.[55]

Can there be physical dependence on endogenously released endorphins? Such is suggested by naloxone's ability to precipitate typical opioid withdrawal in physically stressed mice.[56] In humans strenuous physical exercise causes elevated plasma levels of β-endorphin.[38] A child with recurrent apnea and elevated CSF β-endorphin had signs suggesting opioid withdrawal following treatment with naltrexone.[57]

Is drug-seeking behavior, tolerance, or physical dependence associated with changes in endorphin concentration or in the number or sensitivity of opioid receptors? Chronic, but not acute, administration of μ-receptor agonists causes down-regulation of μ-receptors, and the non-specific opioid antagonist naltrexone produces up-regulation of opioid systems.[38] Rats receiving chronic morphine do have increased levels of brain enkephalinase and decreased levels of pituitary and brain β-endorphin and enkephalin.[58] Plasma β-endorphin levels are reduced in heroin-dependent humans and increase during withdrawal.[59] Heroin-dependent humans also have a rise in CSF β-endorphin during withdrawal; CSF methionine-enkephalin levels rise when acupuncture is additionally given.[60] Heroin users lack a normal circadian rhythm of secretion of the pro-opiomelanocortin-derived peptides, ACTH, β-lipotropin, and β-endorphin.[61] CSF endorphin levels are often abnormally high in humans receiving long-term methadone, and heroin users, in whom levels are quite variable, tend to respond best to methadone maintenance treatment when pretreatment levels are either abnormally low or high.[62] Although these reports imply that perturbations of endorphins or their receptors do contribute to symptoms and signs in opioid abusers, they hardly produce a consistent picture.

Interactions with Other Neurotransmitters and Neuromodulators

Other systems affected by opioids include norepinephrine, serotonin, acetylcholine, adenosine, glutamate, GABA, nitric oxide, and cholecystokinin (Table 3–5).[63–67] As usual, studies are conflicting. Particular attention has focused on norepinephrine. Neurons of the locus ceruleus have high concentrations of opioid receptors and fire in response to

Table 3–5. Opioid Interactions with Non-Dopaminergic Neurotransmitter and Signaling Systems

Norepinephrine[68–70]

Clonidine decreases symptoms of opioid withdrawal and on discontinuation produces similar symptoms itself

Animals self-administer clonidine

Serotonin[10,73,74,84]

Serotonin accelerates development of tolerance to morphine

Chemical destruction of serotonergic neurons decreases morphine tolerance and lessens signs of dependence

Acetylcholine[63]

Opioid withdrawal in dependent rats is exacerbated by cholinergic agonists and relieved by antagonists

In nonopioid-dependent dogs, carbachol injected into the midbrain periaqueductal gray matter causes signs indistinguishable from opioid withdrawal

Adenosine[38,64,84]

Adenosine and drugs acting at the adenosine A_1 receptor suppress, in vitro, naloxone-precipitated withdrawal contractions in opioid-dependent guinea pig ilium and, in vivo, morphine withdrawal signs in mice

Alkylxanthines (theophylline, caffeine), which block adenosine function, antagonize morphine analgesia and precipitate signs suggesting opioid withdrawal

Glutamate[38,65]

MK-801, which antagonizes N-methyl-D-aspartate (NMDA) receptors, in rats attenuates the development of tolerance to morphine analgesia as well as morphine physical dependence

Direct injection of glutamate into the locus ceruleus precipitates withdrawal in morphine-dependent rats

Injection of the non-NMDA antagonist CNQX into the locus ceruleus or amygdala attenuates naloxone-precipitated withdrawal

Acamprosate, which antagonizes NMDA receptors, suppresses morphine-induced sensitization of locomotor activity

Cannabinoids[38]

CB_1-receptor antagonists or deletion of the CB_2 receptor prevents acquisition of morphine self-administration

Gamma-aminobutyric acid (GABA)[38,84]

μ-receptor agonists inhibit GABAergic neurons in the VTA

Benzodiazepines attenuate tolerance to morphine analgesia and suppress withdrawal signs precipitated by naloxone in morphine-dependent animals

Continued

Table 3–5. *continued*

Nitric oxide[84]

Nitric oxide synthase (NOS) inhibitors attenuate the development of tolerance to morphine

Chronic administration of μ- and κ-receptor agonists increases NOS activity

Thyrotropin-releasing hormone (TRH)[84]

TRH antagonizes the sedative and hypothermic actions, but not the analgesic actions, of morphine. It prevents the development of tolerance to morphine analgesia and inhibits naloxone-precipitated withdrawal

Alpha-calcitonin gene-related peptide (αCGRP)[85]

Knockout mice (–/–) for αCGRP display marked reduction in heroin withdrawal signs

Substance P[86]

Morphine reward and physical dependence are reduced in substance P receptor knockout mice

Cholecystokinin[66]

The analgesic effect of morphine applied to rat spinal cord is abolished by spinal cord release of the neuropeptide cholecystokinin. Such antianalgesia might play a role in opioid tolerance

Chronic morphine up-regulates cholecystokinin receptors in the supraoptic nuclei of the hypothalamus

A cholecystokinin antagonist decreases withdrawal signs in morphine-dependent rats

---

painful stimuli, an effect blocked by exogenous or endogenous opioids. Locus ceruleus cells also have norepinephrine receptors, and α_2-adrenergic agonists such as clonidine decrease cell firing. Naloxone reverses the depressant effect of opioids but not of clonidine; piperoxan, an α_2-adrenergic antagonist, reverses clonidine inhibition and in nonhuman primates causes behavior resembling opioid abstinence and attributable to noradrenergic hyperactivity. Similar effects follow electrical stimulation of the locus ceruleus and are reversible with either opioids or clonidine. Tolerance develops to suppression of locus ceruleus neurons by exogenous opioids.[67] In humans, clonidine produces analgesia, miosis, sedation, and respiratory depression, and sudden discontinuation causes symptoms resembling opioid withdrawal, with increased plasma levels of 3-methoxy-4-hydroxyphenylglycol (MHPG). Clonidine, moreover, decreases abstinence symptoms and elevated MHPG levels following

opioid withdrawal in humans.[68] Rats and monkeys self-administer clonidine.[69,70] Whether these observations mean that the locus ceruleus is a principal substrate of opioid withdrawal signs is controversial, however. Withdrawal excitability of midbrain periaqueductal gray neurons is also attenuated by α_2-adrenergic agonists,[71] and β-receptor activation of the bed nucleus of the stria terminalis, which receives adrenergic projections from the brainstem medulla rather than the locus ceruleus, is necessary for the expression of opioid withdrawal signs.[72]

Interactions of opioids with serotonin (5-HT) are complicated by the large number of 5-HT receptors. In rats the 5-HT uptake inhibitor dexfenfluramine suppresses heroin self-administration; the receptor subtypes involved are likely 5-HT_1 and 5-HT_2.[10,73] The 5-HT_2 antagonist ritanserin, however, attenuates morphine-induced place preference, as does the 5-HT_3 antagonist ondansetron.[10] Morphine increases 5-HT release in the NA; the mechanism is probably inhibition of inhibitory GABAergic neurons in the dorsal raphe nucleus of the brainstem.[74]

Opioids and Intracellular Signaling

Whatever the effects of opioids on dopamine and other neurotransmitters, they are indirect and do not explain how opioids ultimately act. Opioids induce membrane hyperpolarization and neuronal inhibition.[75] Opioid receptors are members of the seven transmembrane G-protein-coupled receptor family.[10,76] Acting through G_i/G_o membrane proteins, opioids decrease adenylyl cyclase and cAMP production. Their inhibitory effects on neuronal excitability are probably the result of inhibition of excitatory calcium conductances and facilitation of inhibitory inwardly rectifying potassium currents. They also regulate mitogen-activated protein (MAP) kinases, consistent with a role in growth and differentiation and in immune response. Not surprisingly, however, opioid actions are not straightforward. At least nine isoforms of adenylyl cyclase exist, and depending on the experimental design, opioids can stimulate rather than inhibit some of them. Similarly, κ-receptor agonists under certain circumstances can stimulate rather than inhibit L-type calcium channels.[29] By and large, however, μ-, δ-, and κ-receptors have common molecular actions—that is, they decrease adenylyl cyclase and cAMP production, they inhibit calcium currents, and they facilitate potassium currents. The effects of μ-, δ-, and κ-receptor agonism are opposed because in brain regions where they coexist they act on different types of neurons—for example, μ-receptors might attenuate inhibitory GABAergic neurotransmission and κ-receptors might attenuate excitatory glutamatergic neurotransmission.[36]

In neuroblastoma/glioma cell cultures possessing opioid receptors, tolerance develops to opioid-induced reduction of adenylyl cyclase levels, and upon withdrawal there is rebound increase in cAMP levels above predrug levels.[77] Injection into the VTA or the NA of pertussis toxin, which inactivates G_i and G_o proteins, antagonizes morphine self-administration.[78] Agonist-induced desensitization and down-regulation of receptors is the consquence of agonist-induced receptor phosphorylation. β-arrestin then binds to the phosphorylated receptor, competing with G-protein. The β-arrestin-bound receptor can then be internalized, dephosphorylated, and recycled to the membrane.[29,79–81]

Receptor genes are regulated by activation of transcription factors such as cAMP response element binding protein (CREB). Studies with mice implicate CREB in tolerance and physical dependence; when the gene encoding CREB is mutated, there is considerable attenuation of morphine withdrawal signs.[82] Knockout mice lacking β-arrestin-2 (which binds G-protein-coupled receptors after their phosphorylation) do not develop tolerance to morphine analgesia, although they still become physically dependent.[83]

Genetics

Twin studies show that heroin use carries a heritability of 0.54 but shares very little genetic vulnerability with other abused drugs.[87] Inbred mouse strains demonstrate marked differences in morphine sensitivity and preference.[88] The molecular basis of these genetic influences is unknown.

Genes for major opioid receptors and ligands have been identified and cloned (Table 3–6). In each, polymorphisms have been identified and attempts have been made to correlate particular polymorphisms with pharmacological properties. For example, a polymorphism in the μ-receptor gene is associated with a threefold increase in its binding

Table 3–6. Chromosomal Localizations of Human Opioid System Genes

Gene	Location
μ-opioid receptor	6q24-25
δ-opioid receptor	8q11.2
κ-opioid receptor	1p34.3-36.1
Pro-opiomelanocortin	2p23.3
Enkephalin	8q23-q24
Dynorphin	20p12-pter

Source: Laforge KS, et al. Eur J Pharmacol 2000; 410:249.

to β-endorphin. Studies have also tried to correlate polymorphisms with susceptibility to opioid addiction. For example, several studies reported an association of specific alleles of the μ-receptor gene and opioid dependence (as well as dependence on ethanol and other drugs). Most reports, however, are either conflicting or negative.[89] Animal and human studies have similarly failed to implicate alterations in dopamine receptors or transporters, serotonin receptors or transporters, GABA receptors, or cannabinoid receptors.[90] In one report the TaqIA(1) allele of the dopamine D_2 receptor, controversially associated with alcoholism and other addictive behaviors, was associated in heroin addicts with poor response to methadone maintenance therapy.[91] An association was also described between heroin addiction and a particular polymorphism of the gene for catechol-*O*-methyltransferase (COMT).[92]

A neuronal cytochrome enzyme, CYP2D6, is necessary for the transformation of codeine, oxycodone, and hydrocodone into morphine, oxymorphone, and hydromorphone, and individuals homozygous or heterozygous for defective alleles of this gene are less responsive to these analgesics. They also might be less susceptible to dependence on these oral opioids.[93]

Historical Background and Epidemiology

The poppy has been harvested for its opioid content for more than 6000 years. Appearing in ancient Assyrian and Egyptian art, it was used for analgesia; whether early use was also recreational is unknown.[5,94] During the 5th century BCE Herodotus, visiting the Massaget people north of the Caspian

Sea, described their custom of inhaling smoke from burnt poppy heads in order to induce euphoria.[95] Opium was imported into Europe by the crusaders, and its use was widespread by the middle of the 16th century; Paracelsus is said to have formulated laudanum (tincture of opium often containing other ingredients such as saffron, cloves, and cinnamon), and 18th-century physicians recognized its dependence potential.[1,96] By the 19th century, opium was popular in many countries as a euphoriant.[97,98] In 1839, the British successfully waged the "Opium War" with China to preserve its profitable opium trade, and in Europe during this time laudanum was readily available; celebrated users include Thomas De Quincey and Samuel Taylor Coleridge. (Such self-styled "opium eaters" were actually "opium drinkers.")

During and after the Civil War, opioid use became increasingly popular in the United States. Morphine was easily obtained with or without a prescription, and opium was present in over-the-counter remedies such as "Dover's Powder," "Godfrey's Cordial," "Darby's Carminative," and "Mrs. Winslow's Soothing Syrup." The invention of the hypodermic needle led to injectable morphine and more rapid and powerful effects than could be achieved with oral preparations. Opium continued to be legally imported, morphine was legally manufactured from it, and opium poppies were legally grown.[99] The number of Americans addicted to opioids by the end of the 19th century is controversial—estimates range from 200,000 to more than 1 million (4% of the population). Most were white, middle-class, middle-aged women taking either opium in patent medicines or injectable morphine.[100] (A possible explanation for female preponderance is that they were not welcome in saloons.) In the 1890s, heroin was introduced as a "nonaddictive" opioid for treating morphine dependence and as an over-the-counter antitussive.[101,102]

A notable addict of this period was the surgeon, William Halsted, who successfully "cured" a debilitating addiction to cocaine by switching to morphine; maintaining himself on 180 mg daily, he remained professionally productive—and to his colleagues and friends mentally and physically sound—for more than three decades.[103] During this time, it was a common medical practice to try to convert alcoholics to morphine.

The first steps toward opioid prohibition in the United States were racially motivated: Chinese immigrant laborers had brought with them the custom of smoking opium in "dens," and during the 1880s, many localities banned them and restricted the preparations of opium for smoking. The result was a widespread switch to morphine.[99] In 1914, the Harrison Narcotics Act curtailed a physician's right to give opioids to addicts, banned their non-medical availability, and regulated their manufacture and distribution. Whether the Harrison Act led to a decrease in opioid addiction depends on which figures one accepts for the number of addicts before its passage. In 1918, the number of current American opioid addicts was estimated at 238,000. At least 12,000 received daily morphine from legal dispensing clinics set up by local health departments. In 1924, however, the U.S. Treasury Department closed down these clinics, and thereafter opioid addiction became a crime.[104] (In 1952, the U.S. Supreme Court ruled that imprisonment for merely being an addict represented "cruel and unusual punishment" and was therefore unconstitutional. "Purchase" and "possession" are still punishable, however, making it rather difficult for someone to be addicted to illicit opioids without breaking the law.[99])

During the 1930s, most opioid abusers smoked opium; only 13% injected heroin, and only 17% were black.[105] Following World War II, epidemics of heroin use occurred in black communities, for example, Chicago in the late 1940s, affecting largely non-delinquent adolescents. During the 1950s, heroin-related deaths rose steadily in New York City—from 50 in 1950 to 311 in 1961—with blacks representing more than half. By the mid-1960s, minority use became widespread, especially among unemployed young men who had often been criminally active before they used drugs. In 1972, the number of heroin users in the United States was estimated at more than 600,000, over half of whom were in New York City.[106] In the late 1980s, it was estimated that heroin had been used at least once by more than 2 million Americans—including 1.3% of high school seniors.[107,108]

In the early 1970s, when Turkey was reducing its opium crop (estimated at about 80 metric tons in the 1960s), the purity of street heroin averaged about 3% to 5%. A few years later, with rising opium production in Iran, Afghanistan, and Pakistan, New York City street heroin purity rose to 17%.[109] During this period heroin of high purity ("China White," "China Cat") was also imported from the "Golden Triangle" of Southeast Asia (the juncture of borders of Thailand, Laos, and Myanmar). In New York City in 1991, the purity of street heroin was typically 40% to 45%, and the price had fallen sharply.[110] By the mid-1990s heroin from the Middle East and Southeast Asia was being displaced by importation of even more potent heroin from South America and Mexico.[111,112] During the 1990s, as the price of heroin on the street fell from US$220,000 to US$60,000 per kilogram, the number of regular users in the U.S. rose from 600,000 to nearly 1 million. By 2003 most of the heroin sold east of the Mississippi was high-grade "Colombian white," often with purity exceeding 90%. Heroin sold west of the Mississippi was mostly "Mexican brown," usually of lesser purity (and, when of particularly low grade, referred to as "black tar" or "Mexican mud.") The American heroin market is roughly divided into three ethnically controlled regions, with Mexicans operating out of Southern California, Nigerians out of Chicago, and Dominicans (fronting for Colombians) out of New York. Smaller Chinese gangs continue to function in New York and San Francisco.[113,114]

Accompanying these economic shifts were changing patterns of use.[115] Older inner city addicts increasingly switched from injecting heroin to snorting or smoking it.[116] At the same time, heroin use became epidemic in middle-class suburban and rural communities, and the percentage of users who injected it steadily increased.[117,118] The doubling of heroin consumption during the 1990s especially affected young adults and adolescents.[119]

In 1998, 3.5% of 198,000 Long Island students interviewed in the 7th through 12th grades admitted to using heroin, and 1% were regular heavy users.[120] According to the federal government's National Household Survey on Drug Abuse, the number of 18- to 25-year olds who had used heroin in the past month rose from 26,000 in 2000 to 67,000 in 2001.[114] Deaths from overdose increased concomitantly.[121,122]

In 1996 the cost of heroin addiction in the United States was an estimated US$21.9 billion (productivity loss US$11.5 billion, criminal activities US$5.2 billion, medical care US$5.0 billion, social welfare US$0.1 billion).[123]

A resurgence of heroin use also struck Europe during the 1990s, with Afghanistan a principal supplier.[124] In 2000, under the Taliban regime, poppy cultivation in Afghanistan was banned, and during the next year Afghan opium production fell from over 4000 tons (70% of the opium produced in the world) to 82 tons (largely from poppies grown in that part of the country under the control of the opposition Northern Alliance).[125] Processing and trafficking were not banned, however, and so huge stockpiles allowed heroin prices to remain stable in Britain, Germany, and other European countries. Although the Afghan government that followed the Taliban in 2002 banned poppy cultivation, as well as processing and trafficking, the ban proved unenforceable.[126] By 2003 opium production in Afghanistan had increased 19-fold and was the major source of the world's heroin.[126a]

Relevant to attempts by law enforcement agencies to stamp out heroin use by curtailing opium supply abroad is the fact that the amount of heroin imported annually into the United States is derived from less than 2% of world opium production, an amount that would require fewer than 25 square miles of poppy cultivation.[104] Countries like Myanmar and Afghanistan produce many times the opium needed for the entire U.S. heroin market. The manufacture of heroin is quite simple, and only a small percentage of what is smuggled into the United States is blocked.[127]

Often unappreciated is the fact that the majority of heroin users do not take it daily. Most experiment with it for months before obvious dependence develops and repeatedly discontinue use—often for more than a year—after becoming physically dependent.[128,129] Naloxone challenge reveals that many applicants to methadone maintenance programs are not physically dependent on opioids.[130] In fact, estimates of the prevalence of intermittent or "controlled" heroin users ("chippers," "joy poppers") in the United States have been as high as 4 million.[131] In contrast to psychostimulant abusers, who often "burn out" and cease use after several years, heroin users are more likely to maintain stable use patterns for many years. In a follow-up study of male heroin addicts who had received compulsory drug treatment 33 years earlier, 40.5% reported past-year heroin use.[132] The relationship between opioid use and crime is complex, yet urban crime rates do rise and fall with heroin retail price.[133,134] Inner city heroin users engage in almost daily crimes (not including drug trafficking or use), largely thefts, check forgery, and prostitution. Criminal activity frequently precedes heroin use, however,[135] and drug-related violent crime, including homicide, most often involves users and dealers.[106,128]

Preparations

Heroin (diacetylmorphine) crosses the blood–brain barrier faster than morphine and is then metabolized to 6-acetylmorphine (which has opioid activity) and morphine. Three milligrams of heroin are equivalent to 10 mg of morphine (Figure 3–1).[1] Experienced users cannot tell heroin from morphine when they are given subcutaneously but are often able to do so when they are given intravenously.[136] It is uncertain if heroin's more rapid effect confers greater dependence liability. (That possibility—along with efficacy, side effects, and potential for street diversion—is relevant to the debate over the comparative merits of heroin and morphine in treating cancer pain.[137] Further complicating the controversy are observations in rats that heroin and 6-acetylmorphine are each more rewarding than morphine[138] and in mice and rats that heroin has direct CNS receptor specificities not shared by morphine.[139])

The major metabolites of morphine are morphine-3-glucuronide (M3G) and morphine-6-glucuronide (M6G). Following a low dose (3–12 mg) of heroin, morphine is detectable in urine for one to one-and-a-half days.[139a] M6G is a μ-receptor agonist and probably contributes to analgesia and respiratory depression. M3G in animals antagonizes morphine- and M6G-induced analgesia and respiratory depression; it might therefore play a role in the development of tolerance. Animal and human studies suggest that M3G may also be responsible for the non-opioid-mediated hyperalgesia/allodynia and seizures/myoclonus seen after very high doses of morphine or heroin.[140]

Illicit heroin—"horse," "crank," "jive," "smack," "junk," "skag," "dope," "shill," "H," "white stuff," "Lady Jane," "boy," "lemonade" (poor-grade heroin), "dynamite" (high-grade heroin) "China White," "China Cat," "Mexican black tar," "Colombian White," "scramble" (heavily adulterated heroin)—was traditionally sold in glassine envelopes ("bags") containing about 90 mg of white powder, with heroin concentrations ranging from zero to over 90%. (Until the late 1980s, most bags contained 5–10 mg heroin.) New York City samples frequently contain quinine, originally added in the 1930s for its antimalarial properties and retained because it produces vasodilation, which some users believe enhances the "high," and also, from the dealer's standpoint, because its bitter taste disguises the true content of heroin present.[141] (On the West Coast, quinine is infrequently present in heroin preparations.) Other pharmacologically active adulterants include, variably, diazepam, lidocaine, procaine, ephedrine, theophylline, caffeine, diphenhydramine, thioridazine, tripolidine, phenylpropanolanine, thiamine, nicotinamide, aminopyrine, acetaminophen, hydroxyzine, amitriptyline, methylparaben, aspirin, and strychnine. Inert adulterants include mannitol, starch, lactose, cellulose, sodium chloride, dextrose, and even on occasion curry powder, Vim, or Ajax.[115,142,143] The rapidly rising numbers of heroin users in the United States and Europe has resulted in an increasingly diverse clientele, including urban professionals, suburban teenagers, and denizens of the inner city. The response of traffickers has been "microbranding"—selling vials (or, for injection, gelcaps) color-coded to indicate amount, purity, and price.[113]

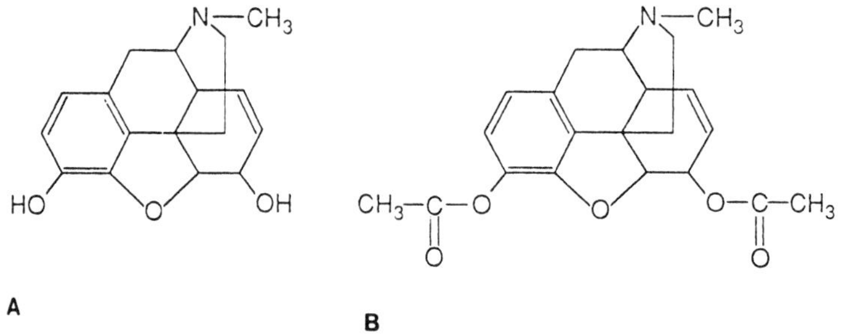

Figure 3–1. Morphine (**A**) and Heroin (**B**).

Dissolved in unsterile water in a bottle cap or spoon and heated with a match, heroin is drawn into an eye dropper or syringe through cotton (purportedly to filter out impurities) and injected either intravenously ("mainlining") or subcutaneously ("skinpopping"). Smokers, "sniffers," or "snorters" are less likely than parenteral users to become compulsive daily users, although some do become severely addicted without ever injecting heroin.[144,145] An additional advantage of nonparenteral use is that overdose is unlikely. (Worldwide, a growing number of heroin users "chase the dragon"; the drug is placed on tinfoil and heated from beneath and the vapor produced is then "chased" and inhaled through a straw or tube.[146] The popularity of this technique seems to have resulted from the ready availability of impure "brown heroin," which is difficult to dissolve for injection.[147,148])

Other practices include snorting or smoking dried gum opium and drinking teas made from opium or from poppy seeds.[149] Opium, which cannot be injected, has been smoked or eaten in China, Southeast Asia, and the Indian subcontinent for millennia. Attempts by Asian governments to eradicate opium use have resulted in widespread replacement by heroin and a rapid spread of human immunodeficiency virus (HIV) infection. The increasing popularity of opium use in North America has been linked to Asian refugees, particularly Laotian.[150]

"Shotgunning" refers to the practice of inhaling smoke and then exhaling it into another person's mouth.[151]

Acute Effects

Effects at Intended Doses

Heroin or morphine causes drowsiness, difficulty concentrating, and euphoria, although sometimes there is fear or anxiety, especially in nondependent, pain-free normal subjects (Table 3–7). (Psychotomimetic effects and visual hallucinations can occur after morphine or heroin administration, but are much more often associated with mixed agonist-antagonists such as pentazocine.[152]) Analgesia is more to deep burning pain than to pinprick; both threshold of pain perception and the ability to tolerate pain are increased. Nausea and vomiting occur less often in dependent than naive subjects

Table 3–7. Acute Effects of Heroin

"Rush"
Euphoria or dysphoria, "drive"
Drowsiness, "nodding"
Analgesia
Nausea and vomiting
Miosis
Dryness of the mouth
Pruritus
Sweating
Suppression of the cough reflex
Respiratory depression
Hypothermia
Postural hypotension
Constipation
Biliary tract spasm
Reduced gastric acid secretion
Urinary retention
Suppression of rapid eye movement sleep

but can be severe in daily users, who, far from being bothered, refer to the symptoms as "a good sick."[153] Miosis may be so marked ("pinpoint") that the light reflex—which opioids do not interrupt—is difficult to discern. (Opioid-induced miosis is usually attributed to disinhibition of pupilloconstrictor neurons in the Edinger–Westphal nucleus. However, locally instilled conjunctival naloxone reportedly produced pupillary dilation in opioid-dependent subjects but not in controls.[154]) Other acute effects include dryness of the mouth, pruritus, sweating, suppression of the cough reflex, respiratory depression, hypothermia, postural hypotension, constipation (resulting from gastrointestinal hypertonicity and decreased propulsion), reduced gastric acid secretion, biliary tract spasm, and urinary retention. There is electroencephalographic slowing as in natural sleep, but the time spent in the rapid eye movement (REM) phase is decreased.[155] With high doses, the electroencephalogram may have irritative features, and rarely multifocal myoclonus or seizures occur.[136,156–158] There is increased production of antidiuretic hormone (ADH), prolactin, and calcitonin and reduced secretion of ACTH, luteinizing hormone, and growth hormone.[1,104,159–162] Libido is decreased, although early in the course of dependence potency may be enhanced.[163,164] The insulin response to glucose is reduced, and platelet and coagulation alterations resemble those found in diabetics.[165–167]

Parenteral heroin produces a "rush" ("kick," "thrill," "hit," "flash"), an ecstatic feeling lasting about a minute and often compared to orgasm but usually referred to the abdomen and accompanied by itching and flushing of the skin. The user may then "go on the nod," experiencing a dream-like, pleasant drowsiness and alternately dozing and suddenly awakening; skeletal muscle tension may be decreased only in the neck and face, so the subject seems asleep on his feet. (A "rosette of cigarette burns on the chest" is an almost pathognomonic sign of "nodding.") Alternatively, there may be "drive," with increased psychomotor activity and garrulous boastfulness ("soap-boxing").

Marked tolerance develops to euphoria, analgesia, and respiratory depression; doses of 500 mg morphine daily have been achieved in only 10 days, and addicts have received 5000 mg morphine without serious consequence. There is less tolerance to smooth muscle effects (e.g., constipation and miosis).[104,168,169] Tolerant users tend to be dysphoric, depressed, hypochondriacal, irritable, and socially withdrawn most of the time except briefly after each injection, and there is greater tolerance to "drive" than to "nodding."[170]

Overdose

Overdose causes coma with pinpoint but reactive pupils and respiratory depression or apnea.[171–173] Anoxic brain damage, however, can produce large, unreactive pupils. Fatal overdose has followed not only parenteral administration (including penile injection[174]) but from non-injecting routes including inhalation, nasal snorting, and swallowing.[175] Suicide was accomplished by sniffing heroin.[176]

Treatment of overdose begins with attention to apnea or shock (Table 3–8). Because opioids depress brainstem carbon dioxide sensitivity, oxygen use should be carefully monitored in patients dependent on hypoxic respiratory drive.[1] Hypotension usually responds quickly to correction of hypoxia and administration of fluids (which, because heroin pulmonary edema may be present, should be given cautiously); vasopressors or plasma expanders are rarely needed.[171]

For patients with respiratory depression, naloxone is given in an initial dose of 2 mg intravenously.[172] If signs are not promptly reversed, boluses of 2–4 mg

Table 3–8. Treatment of Opioid Overdose

Ventilatory support
If hypotension does not respond promptly to ventilation, IV fluids (pressors rarely needed)
Consider prophylactic intubation
If respiratory depression, naloxone, 2 mg IV, IM, or SC, and then 2 mg to 4 mg repeated as needed up to 20 mg. If no respiratory depression, naloxone, 0.4 mg to 0.8 mg IV, IM, or SC, and if no response, 2 mg repeated as needed
Hospitalization and close observation, with additional naloxone as needed
Consider overdose with other drugs, especially cocaine and ethanol

Source: Nelson LS. Opioids. In: Goldfrank LR, Flomenbaum NE, Levin NA, et al., eds. Toxicologic Emergencies, 6th edition. Stamford, CT: Appleton & Lange, 1998; 975.

are repeated up to a total dose of 20 mg. High doses may be required for propoxyphene, pentazocine, diphenoxylate, nalbuphine, butorphanol, or buprenorphine overdose, but failure to respond to 20 mg should make one consider alternative diagnoses, superimposed anoxic-ischemic brain damage, or additional drugs. Patients who lack adequate veins and are not hypotensive can be given naloxone intramuscularly or subcutaneously. Patients with depressed sensorium but normal respirations should initially receive smaller doses to avoid "overshoot" and precipitation of withdrawal signs; 0.4–0.8 mg naloxone is given and if there is no response, 2 mg doses are repeated every 2–3 minutes. Maximal effect occurs 2–3 minutes after intravenous naloxone but only about 15 minutes after intramuscular or subcutaneous administration. In some centers, because of frequent vomiting, routine endotracheal intubation is performed before giving naloxone. Although too much naloxone can precipitate opioid withdrawal symptoms, naloxone is shorter-acting than most opioids, and unobserved patients can slip back into coma and apnea. Close observation is required for at least 24 hours with morphine or heroin and for 72 hours with methadone or propoxyphene, and it may be necessary during that time to give naloxone either in 5 mg hourly boluses or by prolonged infusion. (Naloxone infusion can be established at an hourly rate of two-thirds whatever dose reversed respiratory depression; the rate can then be titrated to the reappearance of respiratory depression or the emergence of withdrawal signs.) Anecdotal reports describe seizures, cardiac arrhythmia, and severe agitation as rare complications of conventional naloxone doses.[173]

Nalmefene, a long-acting opioid antagonist, does not restore normal ventilation as rapidly as naloxone, and it can produce unintended prolonged withdrawal symptoms.[173,177]

A common feature (10% to 15%) of opioid overdose is noncardiogenic pulmonary edema, either present at the outset or appearing during the first 24 hours of hospitalization. It can follow either parenteral or intranasal heroin, and its cause is unclear. Possibilities include anaphylaxis, hypoxia, and vascular damage secondary to street adulterants, especially quinine.[178] Aspiration further complicates the picture. Treatment is with positive pressure ventilation and oxygen, not digitalis, diuretics, or morphine.[1,172] Naloxone reportedly can precipitate non-cardiogenic pulmonary edema by reversing opioid-induced vasodilation and venous pooling, with increased venous return to the lungs. Some workers believe naloxone should therefore be avoided in overdose patients who are hemodynamically stable.[179]

When heroin is combined with parenteral cocaine or amphetamine ("speedball"), paranoid psychosis can predominate or become unmasked by naloxone.[180] Heroin is also smoked with "crack" cocaine or phencyclidine.[181] (In self-administration studies with animals, heroin combined with cocaine is more rewarding than either drug alone, and the combination produces synergistic elevations of extracellular dopamine in the nucleus accumbens.[182,183]) Opioids taken with barbiturates, benzodiazepines, antidepressants, or ethanol produce atypical signs including coma unresponsive to naloxone.[184–187] Conversely, naloxone has reportedly reversed signs of ethanol intoxication, perhaps by inhibiting GABA, and so a response may not be opioid-specific (see Chapter 12).[188] Also sometimes added to heroin are marijuana and scopolamine ("polo," "super buick," "homicide").[189,190]

Dependence and Withdrawal

Acute and Protracted Abstinence

Accompanying opioid tolerance are psychic and physical dependence and withdrawal symptoms and signs (Table 3–9).[104,191,192] Four to 6 hours after

Table 3–9. Symptoms and Signs of Opioid Withdrawal

Drug craving
Irritability, anxiety
Lacrimation
Rhinorrhea
Sweating
Yawning
Myalgia
Mydriasis
Piloerection
Anorexia, nausea, and vomiting
Diarrhea
Hot flashes
Fever
Tachypnea
Productive coughing
Tachycardia
Hypertension
Abdominal cramps
Muscle spasms
Erection, orgasm

the last heroin dose, drug craving begins. At 8 to 12 hours, irritability and anxiety become marked, and there is weakness, lacrimation, rhinorrhea, sweating, and yawning, often followed by several hours of restless, tossing sleep from which the addict awakens feeling worse than ever, with achiness, mydriasis, piloerection ("cold turkey"), severe anorexia, nausea, vomiting, abdominal cramps and tenderness, hyperactive bowel sounds, diarrhea, violent yawning, hot flashes, fever, tachycardia, hypertension, and sweating alternating with chills. Pain in the back and limbs accompanies muscle spasms and kicking movements ("kicking the habit"). Erection or ejaculation occur in men and orgasm or menorrhagia in women. The respiratory response to carbon dioxide is exaggerated, with increased respiratory rate. Hypersecretion of bronchial mucous glands produces clear sputum and rales or rhonchi relieved by coughing. There is increased urinary excretion of epinephrine and 17-hydroxycorticosteroids and often leukocytosis. Dehydration and ketosis can rarely lead to cardiovascular collapse, but in contrast to ethanol or barbiturate abstinence, opioid withdrawal does not cause seizures (except perhaps in newborns), hallucinations, or delirium tremens and is hardly ever life-threatening. In fact, the syndrome is often compared to a bad case of "the 'flu," and its unpleasantness does not fully explain the degree of drug craving. Symptoms peak at 24 to 72 hours with morphine and heroin and usually last 7 to 10 days, but full recovery takes longer—sometimes much longer.

Protracted abstinence is two-phased, with mild behavioral abnormalities and increased pulse, blood pressure, temperature, and carbon dioxide sensitivity lasting several weeks, followed by several months of pulse, blood pressure, temperature, carbon dioxide sensitivity, and pupillary size below predependence levels. During this time, there is increased urinary epinephrine excretion, an elevated cold pressor response, increased response of the autonomic nervous system to nociceptive stimuli, and continued abnormalities of REM sleep.[192]

Protracted abstinence is observed in animals. Monkeys display signs of acute abstinence for up to several months after withdrawal from morphine, and rats have electroencephalographic abnormalities, "wet-dog" shakes, fever, hypermetabolism, increased water intake, and drug-seeking behavior for up to a year.[193,194] Protracted abstinence may be related to dopamine receptors. Striatal dopamine D_2 receptors in rats demonstrated abnormally increased binding during morphine dependence and abnormally decreased binding during protracted abstinence.[195] The degree to which protracted abstinence contributes to persistent drug craving in humans is uncertain but has obvious implications for treatment.

Former opioid addicts have persistent decreased pain sensitivity, a phenomenon not affected by administration of naltrexone. The cause is probably up-regulation of non-opioid pain suppression systems.[196]

Methadone's action lasts 24 to 36 hours, and there is a similar abstinence syndrome, beginning 8 to 24 hours after the last dose and peaking at 3 to 8 days; the most severe symptoms last up to 3 weeks (Figure 3–2).[197] Rifampin, phenytoin, carbamazepine, and barbiturates (but not valproate) accelerate methadone metabolism and precipitate withdrawal symptoms in patients receiving maintenance therapy.[198–200] By unclear mechanisms, metyrapone also precipitates opioid abstinence.[201]

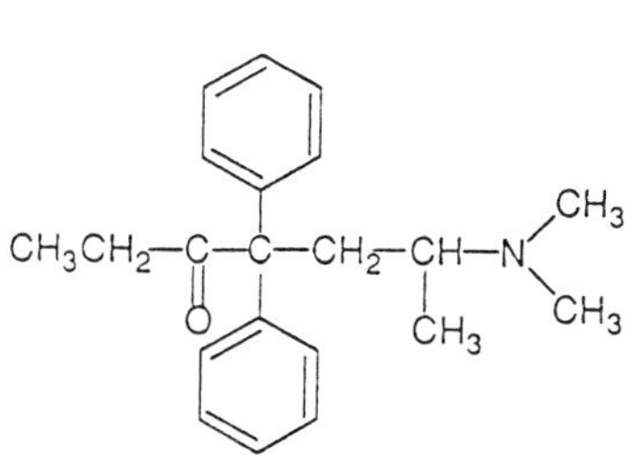

Animal studies suggest that both tolerance and physical dependence can develop after a single opioid dose.[202] The matter is controversial, however; as noted earlier, there are animal models in which widely spaced low doses of opioids produce reward seeking without evidence of tolerance or physical dependence. Human subjects receiving morphine several times daily for 2 weeks develop mild abstinence symptoms when it is stopped. Naloxone precipitates severe abstinence symptoms after only 2 days of morphine and mild symptoms if given within 24 hours of a single dose of morphine or within a week of a single dose of methadone—at a time when acute effects of the opioid are no longer measurable.[203–205] The severity of the abstinence syndrome is dose-dependent up to about 500 mg morphine daily.

Treatment of Withdrawal

Opioid abstinence symptoms are usually relieved by oral methadone, 20 mg once or twice in the first 24 hours, with subsequent tapering titrated to symptoms.[171] Patients already receiving high doses of methadone as maintenance therapy may require more. About one-fourth of each previous day's dose prevents recurrence. (It is a violation of U.S. federal law, however, to give opioids to relieve abstinence symptoms except as "emergency" therapy for inpatients or in federally approved drug-treatment programs.[206]) A British study found that oral heroin also effectively prevented opioid withdrawal symptoms, but frequent doses throughout the day were required, and the mean daily heroin dose (55 mg) was significantly higher than the equivalent mean daily methadone dose (36 mg).[207]

Restrictions on the use of opioids to treat opioid withdrawal in ambulatory patients has stimulated a search for effective non-opioid therapies.[197] In contrast to methadone, clonidine suppresses autonomically mediated symptoms and signs of abstinence without occupying opioid receptors. Its efficacy is probably related to inhibitory action on the locus ceruleus, but additional mechanisms are

Figure 3–2. Methadone.

also possible; in both heroin addicts and controls, clonidine raised plasma β-endorphin levels. Used in conjunction with methadone, clonidine reduces the time required for detoxification from long-term methadone.[68] In patients detoxified from heroin or methadone, clonidine caused a significant reduction in withdrawal symptoms and signs compared with methadone itself or placebo.[208] Comparable success has been claimed with lofexidine, a similar drug. In some patients, clonidine suppresses objective autonomic signs of morphine withdrawal but not subjective discomfort or craving.[209] Postural hypotension, a common side effect with clonidine, is less often encountered with lofexidine.[210] Clonidine abuse, with psychic dependence, was reported in two patients receiving methadone maintenance treatment.[211]

The more specific alpha$_2$-adrenergic agent, guanfacine, in one study relieved autonomic symptoms (e.g., lacrimation, sweating, hot flashes, orgasm) more than psychological (anxiety), neuromuscular (achiness, tremor), or gastrointestinal (abdominal cramps, diarrhea) symptoms, and craving persisted.[212] In another study, all symptoms except "sleep disturbances" were relieved in over 80% of patients.[213] In a randomized controlled trial, guanfacine was superior to clonidine but inferior to methadone.[214]

Clonidine/naltrexone and lofexidine/naltrexone combinations have been given to achieve simultaneous opioid withdrawal and initiation of antagonist maintenance.[215–218] Large doses of these agents can produce rapid and comfortable detoxification in only 4 days. Another approach to acute detoxification involves substituting buprenorphine (2–8 mg sublingually daily) for heroin or methadone. After a month, it is abruptly stopped, and a high dose (35 mg) of naloxone is given; the resulting abstinence syndrome is usually mild and well tolerated.[218,219] Buprenorphine substitution has also been followed by 1-day detoxification with combined naltrexone/clonidine.[217]

"Ultra-rapid" detoxification refers to the direct transition in an ambulatory setting from heroin or methadone to oral naltrexone after deep sedation with a benzodiazepine and symptomatic support with clonidine and ondansetron or octreatide (for nausea and vomiting).[220,221] Controversial at best, the procedure has been condemned as unnecessary and potentially dangerous. A 1998 review of nine published studies revealed that only two followed patients for more than a week, and both of these reported high rates of relapse.[222] In one, withdrawal symptoms were still present 24 hours after detoxification, and 80% of patients relapsed during a 6-month follow-up.[223] In 1999 ultra-rapid detoxification was associated with several fatalities in a single clinic in New Jersey.[224]

The alkaloid ibogaine is anecdotally reported to block signs of opioid withdrawal and to produce sustained relief of craving.[225] Controlled studies have not been reported.

Similarly anecdotal are reports that the non-opioid antitussive dextromethorphan relieves withdrawal signs and craving in heroin addicts; a suggested mechanism is the drug's antagonism at glutamate N-methyl-D-aspartate (NMDA) receptors.[226] (Interesting in this respect is that methadone, unlike morphine, is also an NMDA receptor antagonist.[227])

As might have been predicted from studies with endorphins, acupuncture can relieve abstinence symptoms.[228] In animals, transcutaneous cranial stimulation potentiated analgesia and attenuated opioid abstinence signs.[229]

Neonatal Withdrawal and Fetal Effects

In newborns of opioid-dependent mothers, withdrawal signs can be severe or even fatal (Table 3–10). With heroin exposure they usually begin within 24 hours of delivery. Screaming is

Table 3–10. Neonatal Opioid Withdrawal

Irritability
Tremor, jitteriness
Increased muscle tone and tendon reflexes
Screaming
Sneezing
Yawning
Lacrimation
Sweating
Skin pallor or mottling
Fever
Tachypnea and respiratory distress
Tachycardia
Vomiting
Diarrhea
Myoclonus, seizures (?)

high-pitched and protracted, diarrhea is explosive, and there is vomiting and poor feeding yet frantic thumb or fist sucking. Myoclonus or seizures, which can be difficult to tell from severe jitteriness, probably occur in 1% to 4% of heroin-exposed babies, most often at 1 to 2 weeks of age.[230,231] Mortality is as high as 90% without treatment, and signs resemble those associated with neonatal hypoglycemia, hypocalcemia, intracranial hemorrhage, meningitis, or sepsis, any of which could coexist.[232–234] Withdrawal signs are especially severe in newborns of mothers taking heroin plus cocaine.[235] Disordered sleep and respiration can persist for weeks or months.

Sudden withdrawal from opioids during pregnancy carries a high risk of premature labor, fetal distress, meconium aspiration, and fetal death.[236,237] Gradual withdrawal with methadone or other agents is impractical when—as it is not unusual—the mother's first appearance at a health care facility is after labor has begun. Even if slow detoxification is accomplished earlier in pregnancy, abstinence through term is unlikely. Methadone maintenance causes its own neonatal withdrawal syndrome. Signs appear on the second or third day of life, are more protracted, and, according to some but not all workers, more severe than with heroin; seizures reportedly occur in 5% to 20% of such infants.[230,231,234,238,239]

Recommended treatment includes barbiturates, benzodiazepines, phenothiazines, methadone, and paregoric (camphorated tincture of opium, with an ethanol concentration of 45%).[232,240] On the basis of a single prospective randomized trial comparing opioids with sedatives[241]—as well as theoretical considerations of cross-tolerance—the Center for Substance Abuse Treatment in 1992 recommended oral paregoric as the treatment of choice.[231] A Cochrane review in 2002 also concluded that opioid therapy was preferable to sedative therapy in treating neonatal opioid withdrawal. In fact, phenobarbital was no more effective than general supportive treatment.[241a] At the time of this report a study was under way to determine the efficacy of phenobarbital added to an opioid. In the meantime, intravenous phenobarbital is appropriately used for intractable withdrawal seizures.

Such infants are often of low birth weight and small for gestational age.[242] The Moro reflex is hyperactive and persists well beyond the usual 20 weeks.[243] Respiratory distress syndrome is common, and the frequency of sudden infant death is more than 5 times that of non-opioid-exposed infants.[244,245] Later in life, there is hyperactivity, disturbed sleep, or impaired cognition.[245,246] Small birth weight and behavioral abnormalities follow intrauterine opioid exposure in animals.[247,248] Rats exposed in utero to morphine had decreased density of neurons and reduced axonal branching and dendritic arborization, whereas rats exposed in utero to naloxone had increased neuronal density and process length.[249] In mice, on the other hand, fetal exposure to methadone produced small-for-date offspring but no abnormalities of brain development.[250] Physiological evidence of impaired hippocampal cholinergic function was observed in mice prenatally exposed to heroin.[251] Both animal and human mothers and offspring have demonstrated chromosomal aberrations.[252–254]

Some of these reports are problematic. Several studies of such children during the first few years of life found no long-term developmental or cognitive sequelae.[255] However, because mothers tend to underreport drug use during pregnancy, differences between users and nonusers could be masked. Studies claiming abnormalities have not always addressed the quality of prenatal care, including the use of other drugs, ethanol, or tobacco, or factors such as maternal psychopathology or low intelligence.[242,256–259] A controlled study did show "low average and mildly retarded intellectual performance" in preschool children of mothers taking heroin or methadone during pregnancy, but correlation was with inadequate prenatal care, "prenatal risk score," and home environment, not with maternal opioid use per se.[260] Other follow-up studies of opioid-exposed infants have been inconsistent regarding abnormalities of attention, communication skills, tone, or motor coordination.[261] Compared to controls, one-month-old infants exposed prenatally to opioids had delays in auditory evoked responses.[261a]

Medical and Neurological Complications

Violence, Overdose, and Sudden Death

Before the acquired immune deficiency syndrome (AIDS) epidemic, the average case fatality rate of heroin addicts in both the United States and Europe was 1% to 2% per year.[262–265] During the late 1960s, heroin-related fatalities were the most common cause of death among New York City men aged 15 to 35 years. Of these, 40% resulted from violence, especially homicide. Slightly more than half followed overdose or acute adverse reaction to the opioid or an adulterant. Wide variations in the content of street heroin make overdose a continued risk. Subjects dying within 3 hours of injection have higher blood morphine levels than those dying later, and there is strong correlation between the clinical diagnosis of overdose and brain morphine concentrations.[266] The frequency of sudden death in a community correlates positively with the amount of heroin in street packages and inversely with prices.[267–270]

Heroin "body packers" or "mules" swallow or insert in body orifices drug-containing condoms to smuggle or to avoid detection by police.[271,272,272a] Opioid intoxication, intestinal obstruction, and sudden death occur, and attempted endoscopic removal can cause packet rupture.[273] In one case, blood concentration of morphine was 120 mg/L and that of 6-acetylmorphine 184 mg/L.[274] Fatal asphyxiation followed an attempt to swallow a packet of heroin.[275] Increasingly, drugs are smuggled into U.S. airports by this method; in New York a 12-year-old boy traveling from Nigeria was founded to have swallowed 87 condoms filled with heroin.[276] Couriers have also been found dead near international airports, their abdomens ripped open to salvage the heroin inside.[277]

In 1985, a striking rise in the number of fatal heroin overdoses in New Mexico was attributed to the availability of Mexican "black tar" heroin, which is difficult to dilute to sublethal levels.[278]

Table 3–11. Noninfectious Medical Complications of Heroin Use

---

"Nonoverdose sudden death"
  Pulmonary edema
  Asthma
  Quinine cardiotoxicity
Thrombophlebitis, pulmonary embolism
Pulmonary hypertension
Hepatotoxicity
Intestinal pseudo-obstruction
Myalgia/periarthritis
Nephropathy
  Immune
  Amyloid
Decreased glucose tolerance
Thrombocytopenia

In some patients, coma and death are difficult to explain on the basis of true overdose (Table 3–11). The needle may be found in the vein, implying sudden death. Pulmonary edema is frequently present, and even in the absence of other drugs or anoxic-ischemic brain damage, coma may not respond to naloxone.[267] Death has followed very small amounts of heroin or even oral methadone,[279] and blood or even brain opioid levels are sometimes no higher than found in heroin users who die from other causes. Opioids alone can cause pulmonary edema (as noted more than a century ago by Osler);[280] other adulterants damage pulmonary capillaries; and quinine causes cardiac conduction abnormalities, peripheral vasodilation, and ventricular fibrillation. Quinine-related cardiotoxicity has been reported in heroin users.[281] Most patients who die following acute administration of heroin have significant blood levels of ethanol or benzodiazepines.[173] Heroin and ethanol are also individually associated with cardiac arrhythmia, and synergism between heroin, ethanol, and quinine could underlie sudden heroin death.[267,270,281–283] Hypersensitivity reaction or asthma secondary to histamine release is also possible.[178,263,267,284] Inhaled heroin can trigger status asthmaticus, sometimes fatally.[285] Valsalva maneuvers during heroin inhalation can cause pneumomediastinum.[286]

Sudden death occurred following intravenous "speedball" injection; autopsy revealed a broken hypodermic needle which had embolized to the right heart ventricle.[287]

Miscellaneous Organ Damage

Additional medical complications in heroin users include thrombophlebitis and pulmonary emboli;[285] pulmonary hypertension from talc microemboli;[286] hepatotoxicity;[287] chronic abdominal pain and intestinal pseudo-obstruction;[288] and a syndrome of fever, myalgia, and periarthritis.[289] Heroin nephropathy, probably an immunological disorder (perhaps related to adulterants rather than to heroin per se), can cause neurological disease, including uremia, malignant hypertension, hypertensive encephalopathy, and hemorrhagic stroke.[290,291] Renal damage could also be secondary to amyloidosis or to the immune complex glomerulonephritis of bacterial endocarditis.[292] Altered pulmonary function is common in heroin users, and, as noted, heroin inhalation has precipitated fatal asthma.[284,293] Heroin users have decreased glucose tolerance.[294] Thrombocytopenia is associated with antiplatelet antibodies.[295]

Infection

Hepatitis

Before the AIDS epidemic, infection accounted for about 5% of New York City heroin deaths (Table 3–12). Especially common is viral hepatitis. In a 1989 survey of New York City parenteral drug abusers, 86% had serological evidence of hepatitis B infection,[296] and among parenteral drug abusers in the Netherlands, 74% were seropositive for hepatitis C.[297] Of 110 Spanish heroin addicts with acute hepatitis, 63 had hepatitis B and 35 hepatitis C; nearly half of those with hepatitis B also had hepatitis D. All the patients with hepatitis C and 75% of those with hepatitis D developed chronic liver disease.[298] In the early 1980s, an epidemic of hepatitis A in Portland, Oregon, was linked to intravenous drug abuse.[299] In 2000, an outbreak of hepatitis B affected 60 parenteral drug users in Washington State, and three co-infected with hepatitis D died.[300]

By 2001 nearly 4 million people in the United States had chronic hepatitis virus C (HCV) infection.[301] Drug use accounted for up to 50% of these chronic infections and nearly two-thirds of newly acquired cases. Of the one-and-a-half million Americans who inject drugs, 80% to 95% are infected with HCV.[302,303] Cirrhosis develops in up to 20% of people with chronic HCV-infection causing 8,000 to 10,000 deaths in the United States annually and accounting for nearly 10% of deaths in New York City patients receiving methadone maintenance therapy.[301,304] It is predicted that within several years, deaths from HCV infection will surpass AIDS-related deaths among such patients.[304]

Treatment approaches in HCV-infected active drug users are controversial. In 1997 the National Institutes of Health recommended withholding pharmacotherapy—alpha interferon plus ribavirin—until illicit drug use was stopped for at least 6 months.[301] Reasons included the likelihood of non-compliance, the high prevalence among such patients of co-morbid psychiatric conditions considered contraindications to interferon therapy, coexisting ethanol abuse, and availability of needles. Needless to say, such policy has not gone unchallenged.[304a,304b]

Bacteria, Fungi, Malaria

Bacterial infections in parenteral drug abusers affect almost any organ and often involve exotic organisms. Skin poppers develop local abscesses, cellulitis, and pyomyositis, and parenteral abusers of any type are at continued risk for sepsis, pneumonia, and a host of direct or blood-borne infections.[305]

Endocarditis is common, affecting in equal frequency the mitral, aortic, and tricuspid valves and most often caused by *Staphylococcus aureus*, which street-purchased antibiotics render resistant to methicillin or oxacillin.[263,306–308] The source of the organism appears to be neither the drug itself nor the injection paraphernalia but rather carriage in the nose.[309] Other organisms include *Pseudomonas* (which may be harbored in areas of heart valve fibrosis caused by street heroin additives)[310] and *Candida* (which may necessitate surgical valve replacement)[311] as well as unusual organisms such as *Neisseria subflava, Wangiella,* and *Gemella morbillorum.*[312–314]

Table 3–12. Non-HIV Infectious Complications of Heroin Abuse

Hepatitis
Skin abscesses, cellulitis
Pyomyositis
Fasciitis
Pneumonia
Sepsis
Infected venous pseudoaneurysm
Enophthalmitis
Chorioretinitis
Episcleritis
Arthritis, including pyogenic sacroiliitis and
    sternocosto-chondritis
Osteomyelitis, including vertebral
Endocarditis
Malaria
Tick-borne relapsing fever
Tetanus
Botulism
Candidiasis, including cardiac and disseminated
Nocardiosis
Mucormycosis
Tuberculosis

A malaria epidemic among heroin users in California was traced to a Vietnam veteran.[315] Similar cases in Spain were traced to a traveler from Africa.[316]

During a single summer, four heroin users were admitted to the same hospital in Seville, Spain, with tick-borne relapsing fever (*Borrelia*).[317]

In 2000, 35 heroin users in the UK and Ireland died from gas gangrene and sepsis caused by *Clostridium novyi*. All were intramuscular injectors who mixed heroin with citric acid, favoring survival of the anaerobic organism.[318]

A heroin skin popper developed local anthrax with septic shock and meningitis.[319]

Nosocomial outbreaks of *Pseudomonas pickettii* and *Serratia marcescens* bacteremia were traced to contamination of hospital supplies of fentanyl, which had been illicitly used by hospital workers.[320,321]

Nervous System Complications of Infections

Such infections directly or indirectly affect the nervous system. Infectious hepatitis or cirrhosis causes encephalopathy and if clotting is deranged predisposes to traumatic or even spontaneous intracranial hemorrhage.

Vertebral osteomyelitis causes back or neck pain, radiculopathy, and sometimes cord compression.[322–324] Cervical infection is especially common among addicts who inject into the jugular vein.[325] Symptoms frequently precede diagnosis by several weeks. Early in the course, plain cervical radiographs are often normal; computed tomography (CT) and magnetic resonance imaging are more sensitive. In one series, *Staphylococcus aureus* was grown in 10 of 14 cases.[326] Others have reported a preponderance of gram-negative organisms, especially *Pseudomonas*.[327–329] Subacute tetraplegia in an intravenous heroin user was the result of an intramedullary spinal cord abscess caused by *Staphylococcus aureus*.[330] Paraparesis in another intravenous heroin user was the result of spondylodiscitis and epidural abscess caused by *Candida albicans*.[331]

Endocarditis causes intraparenchymal or extraparenchymal abscess of the brain or spinal cord, meningitis, cerebral infarction, diffuse vasculitis, and subarachnoid hemorrhage from rupture of a septic ("mycotic") aneurysm.[332–335] Subtle or insidiously progressive neurological or systemic symptoms, such as headache, fever, syncope, hemiparesis, or aphasia, are common with mycotic aneurysms; sudden onset suggesting subarachnoid hemorrhage is less frequent than with saccular aneurysms, and CSF white cell pleocytosis can precede rupture. Although mycotic aneurysms sometimes disappear with antimicrobial therapy, they also persist, enlarge, or burst. At Harlem Hospital and St. Luke's–Roosevelt Hospital in New York City, 28 cerebral mycotic aneurysms were identified in 17 patients; five patients had aneurysmal rupture during or following appropriate antimicrobial therapy, and of 20 aneurysms followed angiographically, 10 became smaller or disappeared whereas 10 remained unchanged or enlarged, one with fatal rupture (Table 3–13).[336] Such unpredictability argues for prompt angiographic detection and preemptive surgery in patients with endocarditis and unexplained neurological symptoms. Mycotic aneurysms in heroin users have occurred on the carotid, subclavian, and pulmonary arteries.[337–339]

Tetanus

Tetanus, usually severe, is especially common in skin poppers with multiple skin abscesses, making it nearly impossible to identify the lesion that harbors *Clostridium tetani*.[340] Quinine, which

Table 3–13. Mycotic Aneurysm Behavior in Relation to Antibiotic Therapy

Behavior During Therapy	No. of Aneurysms
Bled before treatment, early excision	4
Bled before treatment, then enlarged during treatment	1
Bled during treatment, then continued to enlarge	1
Bled during treatment, after enlarging	1
Bled during treatment, then early excision	2
Bled following treatment, then early excision	1
Never bled, early excision	1
Never bled, but enlarged or unchanged during or after treatment	7
Never bled, became smaller or disappeared during or after treatment	10
Total	28

Source: Brust JCM, Dickinson PCT, Hughes JEO, Holtzman RHH. The diagnosis and treatment of cerebral mycotic aneurysm. Ann Neurol 1990; 27:238.

Table 3–14. Causes of Death in Tetanus Patients at Harlem Hospital Center

Heroin Users	
Inadequately controlled tetanospasms	5
Infection	3
Pulmonary embolism	1
Cardiac arrest	
Secondary to respiratory insufficiency	3
Without apparent cause	9
Nonheroin Users	
Perforated viscus	1
Stroke	1

Source: Brust JCM, Richter RW. Tetanus in the inner city. N Y State J Med 1974; 74:1735.

aggravates anerobic conditions, further encourages bacillus growth.[341–343] At Harlem Hospital Center, of 34 patients with tetanus seen during a period of 8 years, 30 were heroin users. The case fatality rate was 70% for the drug users and 50% for the nondrug users. Among the drug users, curarization was frequently necessary to control tetanospasms, and even well-controlled patients often had unexplained cardiac arrest (Table 3–14).[341] Fatal tetanus occurred in a parenteral heroin user whose tetanus antibody titers (prior to administration of tetanus immune globulin) were 16 times the level considered protective.[344]

Botulism

During the 1990s wound botulism with dysphagia, dysphonia, diplopia, mydriasis, and descending paralysis was increasingly encountered in parenteral drug users in the United States and Europe.[345–352] Of 102 cases of wound botulism in California between 1951 and 1998, 101 were in parenteral drug abusers.[352a] California wound botulism is associated with subcutaneous or intramuscular injection of "black tar" heroin, a gummy form of the drug produced in Mexico and contaminated with ground paper fiber soaked in black shoe polish and possibly with soil.[353] A parenteral heroin user with wound botulism was treated with intravenous immunoglobulin for "Miller Fisher variant of the Guillain-Barré syndrome" until day 14 of his illness, when drainage of abscesses on his buttocks revealed *Clostridium botulinum*.[353a] A California heroin injector had recurrent wound botulism a year after

his initial bout.[353b] Botulism occurred in a pregnant heroin user, necessitating cesarian delivery at 34 weeks gestation.[354] In Washington State within a 5-day period botulism developed in four non-intravenous injectors of black tar heroin.[354a]

Immunosuppression and Infection

Heroin users are immunocompromised even in the absence of HIV infection.[355,356] Endogenous opioids regulate the activation of natural killer (NK) cells and the proliferation of T lymphocytes, and morphine suppresses interferon levels in mice.[357,358] Tuberculosis and fungal infections are therefore frequent in HIV-negative heroin users; reports include devastating cerebral mucormycosis, intravertebral candidiasis, cryptococcal meningitis, nocardial brain abscess, and brainstem chromoblastomycosis.[359–364]

Local or disseminated candidiasis in Europe is associated with the practice of dissolving Iranian "brown heroin" in lemon juice, an excellent culture medium for various *Candida* species.[365–368] Disseminated candidiasis occurred in a Swiss man who injected buprenorphine tablets dissolved in bottled lemon juice, culture of which grew *Candida albicans*.[369] *Candida* endophthalmitis has been reported from both Germany and Spain.[370,371] British and Dutch heroin samples were found contaminated with aflatoxin, which could further contribute to immunosuppression.[372]

HIV Infection and AIDS

As of 2000 in the United States nonhomosexual parenteral drug abusers constituted 25% of the 765,559 adults and adolescents with AIDS reported to the Centers for Disease Control (CDC) (and half of reported women with AIDS). Male homosexual drug abusers constituted another 6%. During the 1990s the rate of growth of the AIDS epidemic decreased among male homosexuals but increased among parenteral drug abusers.[373,374] In 1982, 29% of patients in a New York methadone maintenance treatment program had antibodies to HIV; 2 years later the figure was 87%,[375] and 75% of hospitalized parenteral drug abusers had inverted helper-suppressor T lymphocyte ratios.[376] A survey of 242 North Italian heroin users in 1989 revealed HIV seropositivity in 76%.[377] The prevalence of HIV infection is especially high in communities where needles are shared; in "shooting galleries" drug users rent unsterile equipment previously used by others.[378,379] Such practices contribute to the higher incidence of AIDS among male compared with female drug abusers.

Needle sharers have increasingly taken to cleaning their equipment with bleach, and needle exchange programs in Europe and the United States have led to reduced sharing.[380–382] A 1999 survey of 110 needle exchange programs in the United States revealed that during the previous year nearly 20 million syringes had been exchanged; additionally the distribution centers provided bleach and condoms, referred addicts to treatment, tested for HIV and hepatitis B and C, and screened for tuberculosis and sexually transmitted disease. Political ideology remains an obstacle to expansion of such programs.

For a variety of reasons—saturation of high-risk behavior groups, loss of HIV-seropositive drug users from the pool of active drug abusers, entry of HIV-seronegative new drug abusers into the pool, and conscious reduction of risky behavior—by 1987 HIV seroprevalence among parenteral drug abusers in New York City appeared to have stabilized at approximately 60%.[382a] Similar stabilization was evident in other cities in the United States and Europe, even as other communities during the 1990s experienced the AIDS epidemic for the first time. The worldwide linkage of AIDS and drug abuse was reflected in outbreaks of HIV infection in India and China along overland heroin trafficking routes originating in Burma and Laos.[383]

Because AIDS is a sexually transmitted disease and affects heterosexual partners of carriers and because one-third of women entering treatment for opioid abuse engage in prostitution, the disease claims victims lacking the usual risk factors.[384] In the United States, AIDS develops in 13% to 30% of children born to HIV-seropositive mothers, the great majority of whom are either parenteral drug abusers or sexual partners of parenteral drug abusers.[373]

Parenteral drug abusers have the same neurological complications of HIV infection that afflict other risk groups, including CNS opportunistic infections, neoplasms, stroke, peripheral neuropathy, vacuolar myelopathy, and primary HIV encephalopathy (Table 3–15). Of special concern is tuberculosis, the prevalence of which had declined steadily in the United States until it rose sharply in the late 1980s.[385] Clinically apparent tuberculosis develops

Table 3–15. Major Neurological Complications of HIV Infection

HIV meningitis
Peripheral neuropathy
    Early, Guillain-Barré-like
    Late, sensory, painful
Herpes zoster
Opportunistic CNS infection
Toxoplasmosis
Cryptococcal meningitis or granuloma
Progressive multifocal leukoencephalopathy
Cytomegalovirus
Candida, Mucor, Nocardia, and other fungi
Herpes simplex
Tuberculosis (meningitis, Pott's disease, brain abscess, or intraparenchymal tuberculoma)
Syphilis
CNS lymphoma
Stroke (nonbacterial thrombotic endocarditis, cerebral vasculitis, intracranial hemorrhage)
Vacuolar myelopathy
    HIV encephalopathy (AIDS–dementia complex)

in 10% of HIV-infected patients, and parenteral drug abusers are especially at risk; extrapulmonary tuberculosis—including meningitis, Pott's disease, and CNS tuberculoma or abscess—is encountered far more frequently than in HIV-negative patients with tuberculosis.[386–389] Purified protein derivative (PPD) tuberculin tests are frequently negative in HIV-seropositive parenteral drug abusers, who should be considered positive with 2 mm induration (rather than the usual 5 mm); they should also undergo anergy testing.[390] As if immunosuppression were not enough, in the early 1990s AIDS patients were increasingly infected with tubercle bacilli resistant to conventional antimicrobials.[391] During 1990, tuberculosis was diagnosed in 263 patients at Harlem Hospital Center; 81% were HIV seropositive.

Also of concern is syphilis.[392–401] Genital ulcers and promiscuous behavior are added risk factors for HIV infection in drug abusers. Syphilitic meningitis, meningovascular syphilis, and general paresis cause symptoms similar to those of other AIDS-related infections (including HIV encephalopathy); the diagnosis is therefore easy to miss.[392] Moreover, syphilis in HIV-seropositive subjects is reportedly characterized by negative serology (including negative CSF VDRL in the presence of neurosyphilis),[393] an aggressive course,[394] and treatment failures necessitating maintenance therapy.[395] In a study from Miami, 12 of 829 AIDS patients (1.5%) had neurosyphilis; at least four were parenteral drug abusers, and four had been treated for early syphilis.[396] Of 42 patients from Houston with combined HIV infection and neurosyphilis, five had abnormal CSF but were asymptomatic, nine had meningitic symptoms, five of these nine plus 15 others had cranial neuropathies, and 11 had strokes.[397] A recommended alternative to maintenance penicillin in uncomplicated early syphilis is three doses of 2.4×10^6 units of benzathine penicillin; for neurosyphilis, 12 to 24×10^6 units of penicillin daily for 10 days is required.[398]

More than 90% of patients with AIDS have neuropathological abnormalities at autopsy, and up to 92% have neurological symptoms and signs.[402–409] The latter high figure is from a prospective study of symptomatic HIV-seropositive patients at Harlem Hospital Center.[409] A retrospective survey of AIDS cases reported to the CDC suggested that parenteral drug abusers are more likely than other risk groups to have cryptococcal meningitis and CNS toxoplasmosis.[410] The Harlem Hospital Center study found no difference between parenteral drug abusers and nondrug-abusing homosexuals in the prevalence of these infections or of such neurological symptoms as dementia, hemiparesis, seizures, ataxia, or peripheral neuropathy.[409] In Baltimore, controlled neuropsychological studies of asymptomatic HIV-seropositive parenteral drug abusers found that they—similar to nondrug-abusing asymptomatic HIV-seropositive homosexuals—had no evidence of significant cognitive impairment.[411] The occurrence and progression of cognitive decline secondary to HIV infection is similar among HIV-infected parenteral drug users and other risk groups.[412]

A Canadian study found that "use of various recreational drugs" did not increase the risk of AIDS developing in men seropositive for HIV,[413] and a Baltimore study found that over an 18-month period CD4 cell counts fell no faster among HIV-seropositive parenteral drug abusers than among other HIV-seropositive groups.[414] A New York City study found no difference in the rate of acceleration to AIDS between HIV-seropositive parenteral drug abusers and nondrug abusers; among drug abusers, however, there was higher pre-AIDS morbidity and mortality, especially from bacterial infection.[415]

Co-infection with HIV and cytomegalovirus, each presumably from needle sharing, occurred in two intravenous drug abusers. The mononucleosis-like illness that followed perhaps resulted from enhancement of each virus's replication by the other.[416]

HTLV-I and HTLV-II

Parenteral drug abusers are also subject to infection with either human T cell lymphotropic virus (HTLV)-I or HTLV-II retroviruses.[417–420] In a CDC survey of 3217 parenteral drug abusers in 29 American treatment centers, HTLV seroprevalence rates ranged from 0.4% to 18%, with the highest in Los Angeles, New Orleans, and Seattle; 84% of the positive samples were HTLV-II.[420] Similar prevalence and HTLV-II preponderance were reported in northern Italian parenteral drug abusers.[421] Myelopathy evidently due to HTLV-I has been reported in parenteral drug abusers from Louisiana, Florida, and Washington, DC.[422–426] Myelopathy associated with HTLV-II infection was reported in a parenteral drug abuser from Baltimore.[427] From a different vantage, of 25 patients with HTLV-I-associated myelopathy reported to the CDC from 1988 to 1990, three were parenteral drug abusers.[428]

Stroke

Case Reports

Heroin users are prone to stroke unrelated to liver or kidney disease, endocarditis, or AIDS. A report from Harlem Hospital Center involved six patients aged 25 to 38 years.[429] Four, all normotensive, had cerebral infarcts in association with loss of consciousness after intravenous heroin. In one of these, cerebral angiography was normal. In another, there was stenosis of the internal carotid artery at the siphon and of the early anterior cerebral artery, plus occlusion of the middle cerebral artery; the changes suggested primary vessel disease rather than emboli. Two other active heroin users had occlusive strokes that did not follow overdose or even a recent injection. In one, who was normotensive, cerebral angiography was consistent with widespread small vessel arteritis. Suggesting hypersensitivity, one of the patients had blood eosinophilia, hypergammaglobulinemia, and a positive direct Coombs test, and another had an elevated erythrocyte sedimentation rate and positive latex fixation.

Other reports of occlusive stroke in heroin users include a 19-year-old boy who had taken heroin intravenously for a year, plus intermittent lysergic acid diethylamide (LSD), and developed sudden global aphasia; cerebral angiography suggested diffuse angiitis.[430] A 21-year-old woman developed hemiparesis 2 weeks after starting daily heroin and 6 hours after an intravenous injection; accompanying symptoms suggested anaphylaxis, with eosinophilia and angiographic changes consistent with cerebral arteritis.[431] Cerebral infarction followed the first heroin injection in several months in a 20-year-old man whose cerebral angiogram showed arterial "beading."[432] A 34-year-old man developed hemiparesis while sniffing heroin; cerebral angiography was normal.[433] Another young man had infarction in the territory of the left anterior choroidal artery after sniffing heroin.[434] Two Danish patients, aged 30 and 35 years, awakened from presumed overdose with aphasia and right hemiparesis; cerebral angiography was normal in each.[435] Acute severe cerebellar ataxia followed intra-arterial injection of heroin.[436] Intracerebral hemorrhage occurred in a young German within minutes of intravenous heroin.[437] A middle-aged woman who had taken daily heroin intranasally for many years had rupture of a cerebellar vascular malformation.[438] Other heroin-associated infarcts resulted in aphasia and cortical blindness.[439,440] A young heroin user with border-zone infarcts had occlusive disease of the basal cerebral arteries and moyamoya-like collaterals; the primary event was considered vasculitis.[446a]

A man using intravenous heroin after 2 years of abstinence developed nalorphine-responsive coma and apnea and then, over several hours, progressive quadriparesis, anarthria, dysphagia, and sensory loss, suggesting a ventral pontine lesion; it was unclear if the cause was vascular.[441]

Stroke Mechanisms

Heroin could cause stroke by several mechanisms (Table 3–16).[142,442] Hypoventilation causes hypotension and decreased cerebral perfusion, and bilateral globus pallidus infarction is common at heroin-user autopsies.[443,444] Hemiplegia has appeared on awakening from naloxone-responsive coma, and overdose has produced dementia, spastic quadriparesis,

Table 3–16. Possible Causes of Stroke in Heroin Abusers

Hypertension (nephropathy)
Clotting derangement (liver disease, thrombocytopenia)
Endocarditis (embolic infarction, ruptured mycotic aneurysm)
Overdose, hypoperfusion
Particle embolism
Allergic vasculitis
Toxic vasculitis

deafness, seizures, dystonia, and ballism.[445,446] Magnetic resonance imaging has shown border-zone infarction in the cerebrum and the spinal cord.[446a] In some cases, an awkward posture of the neck during overdose coma might have kinked the carotid artery and further decreased cerebral perfusion.[435] Delayed post-anoxic encephalopathy also occurs.[447]

Refractile particles are observed in the skin of heroin users, and jugular vein injectors sometimes accidentally hit the carotid artery, yet embolization of foreign material to the brain has rarely been documented in heroin users.[448,449] It more often affects parenteral abusers of other drugs.[141,450] In the 1970s, pentazocine (Talwin) and tripelennamine (Pyribenzamine)—"T's and blues"—were widely abused in Chicago and other midwestern cities.[451,452] Crushed oral tablets were suspended in water, passed through cotton or a cigarette filter, and injected intravenously. Cerebral hemorrhages and infarcts resulted.[453] At autopsy, there was often pulmonary arteriolar occlusion by microcrystalline cellulose or particulate magnesium silicate (talc).[454,455] Such microemboli are especially likely to reach the brain when multiple lung emboli have caused pulmonary hypertension and opened functional pulmonary arteriovenous shunts.[142] Lesions consistent with cerebral vasculitis are seen angiographically in T's and blues stroke patients.

Talc microemboli were present at autopsy in the liver, spleen, and brain of a parenteral paregoric abuser.[456] A young man who frequently injected pulverized unfiltered meperidine tablets intravenously had occasional seizures after injection and then impaired memory and visual blurring; there were fundal hemorrhages and arteriolar occlusions, and symptoms improved with abstinence.[457] Posterior cerebral artery occlusion follwed intravenous injection of a hydromorphone suppository, probably by paradoxical embolism of the product's cocoa butter content.

Consistent with allergic vasculitis are frequent immunological abnormalities in heroin users—for example, altered complement, hypergammaglobulinemia (including elevated immunoglobulin M [IgM] independent of IgG and IgA), circulating immune complexes, antibodies to smooth muscle and lymphocyte membranes, and false-positive serology for syphilis.[458] Opium, morphine, codeine, and meperidine have caused urticaria, angioneurotic edema, and anaphylaxis.[459] Morphine binding by gamma-globulin has been observed in addicts and experimental animals.[460,461]

During heroin withdrawal, platelet alpha$_2$-adrenoceptors and epinephrine-induced platelet aggregation are increased.[462] Clotting is deliberately impaired in parenteral addicts who add heparin or other anticoagulants to their drug mixture.[463]

Heroin Myelopathy

Possibly vascular in origin is heroin myelopathy. Acute paraparesis, sensory loss, and urinary retention usually occur shortly after injection and often follow a period of abstinence.[464–475] Symptoms are sometimes present on awakening from coma. Preserved proprioception in some suggests infarction in the territory of the anterior spinal artery, and in a patient with bilateral pallidal infarction there was also magnetic resonance imaging (MRI) evidence of spinal cord border zone infarction.[444] A man who awoke several hours after snorting heroin with flaccid paralysis of the legs and urinary retention had MRI evidence of mid-thoracic acute transverse myelitis.[476] In one autopsy, there was necrosis "confined almost entirely" to the upper thoracic cord gray matter, and in another there was also involvement of the anterior aspect of the posterior columns and a pyramidal tract in the lower thoracic cord.[471] Possible causes of these lesions, as with heroin cerebral strokes, include "borderzone" cord infarction during a period of coma and hypotension, embolism of foreign material, and direct toxicity or hypersensitivity. Consistent with the latter was a man who, remaining awake, had episodic numbness and weakness of both legs for a few minutes after each injection.[472] An adolescent 11 days after injection developed a rash on his chest and feet and then, following a second injection 6 days later, paraplegia.[474] Cord biopsy in another patient showed vasculitis affecting mainly small arteries

and arterioles, with "double refractile fragments" in inflamed tissues.[468] A patient at Harlem Hospital Center developed paraparesis and urinary retention after a friend injected heroin into a vessel over his midthoracic spine; myelography was normal, and it was presumed that the common intercostal origins of the posterior cutaneous and spinal arteries or veins had allowed access of the injected material. In another case, an anterior spinal artery syndrome with quadriplegia followed supraclavicular heroin injection.[477]

Peripheral Nerve Lesions

A number of other neurological complications affect heroin users (Table 3–17). Risk factors for developing polyneuropathy include AIDS, antiretroviral therapy, concomitant ethanol abuse, and malnutrition.[477a] Guillain-Barré neuropathy is described.[478–480] Peripheral nerves are also damaged by direct injection, by local infection, or by pressure palsies during coma.[481] Bilateral ulnar palsy developed secondary to osteomyelitis affecting the ulnar diaphysis.[482] Two cases of iliopsoas infarction were diagnosed by CT and biopsy; in one, there was also femoral neuropathy.[483] Painful brachial and lumbosacral plexopathies resemble neuralgic amyotrophy, suggesting an immunological origin.[484–491] Brachial plexopathies have also resulted from septic aneurysm of the subclavian or axillary arteries;[492] angiography should be considered in patients with appropriate symptoms. Persistent vocal cord paralysis has followed repeated jugular vein injections,[493,494] and a

Table 3–17. Noninfectious Neurological Complications of Heroin Abuse

Stroke
Myelopathy
Seizures
Peripheral nerve injury
Peripheral neuropathy
Brachial and lumbar plexopathy
Cranial neuropathy
Rhabdomyolysis
Fibrotic myositis
Quinine amblyopia
Lead poisoning
Chloroquine encephalopathy
Spongiform encephalopathy
MPTP parkinsonism

young Thai, taking his first heroin dose in several months, awoke with bilateral, severe, permanent sensorineural deafness; the site of pathology was not determined.[495]

Myopathy

Rhabdomyolysis and myoglobinuria with renal failure can follow prolonged coma and is likely the result of direct muscle compression. It also follows injection without loss of consciousness, suggesting hypersensitivity;[485,487,496–510] in one instance, recurrent myoglobinuria followed a repeat injection.[504] In two cases rhabdomyolysis accompanied brachial or lumbosacral plexopathy.[489,510] Rhabdomyolysis has also followed heroin sniffing.[511] In some cases, myocardial involvement with acute ventricular failure has accompanied rhabdomyolysis.[512] A young man with rhabdomyolysis following heroin overdose had the highest serum myoglobin level ever recorded in a survivor (>400,000 μg/L); his course was complicated by hyperkalemic cardiac arrest and hypercalcemia with diffuse tissue deposition of calcium.[513] Heroin-induced rhabdomyolysis can affect only the legs, mimicking transverse myelitis.[514] Compartment syndromes following heroin injection can require fasciotomy to prevent loss of a limb.[515,516]

A Harlem Hospital Center patient who chronically injected heroin into his deltoids developed fibrotic myositis and abduction contracture of the shoulders.[517] It was unclear if the myopathy was due to nonspecific repeated needle trauma or local toxicity of heroin or an adulterant, but studies of animals receiving systemic morphine suggest chemical toxicity to muscles.[518]

Quinine Amblyopia

Optic atrophy occurred in a Harlem Hospital Center patient whose heroin mixture provided huge doses of quinine: about 5 g daily. A dealer as well as an addict, he was able to serve as his own control by preparing his heroin without quinine. Vision then improved.[519] A man who took 6 g quinine sulfate for relief of muscle cramps accompanying heroin detoxification developed similar visual loss.[520] A report from Sri Lanka indicated that dyschromatopsia affected 83% of heroin addicts.

Quinine was not mentioned, and 40% of patients inhaled the drug.[521]

Lead Poisoning

Abdominal pain and ascending tetraplegia occurred in several Italians who used a batch of unrefined brown heroin contaminated with lead salts.[522] Lead-contaminated heroin caused bilateral brachial plexopathy in another Italian[523] and colic and encephalopathy in a Spaniard.[524]

Chloroquine Poisoning

Adulteration of heroin with chloroquine caused headache, confusion, and visual disturbance in a British user.[525]

Spongiform Encephalopathy

Spongiform encephalopathy affected 47 Dutch heroin smokers practicing the technique of "chasing the dragon."[526] Symptoms began with apathy, bradyphrenia, and cerebellar dysarthria and ataxia; some patients then developed spastic hemiparesis or quadriparesis, tremor, chorea, myoclonus, pseudobulbar palsy, fever, blindness, and, in 11 instances, death. CT showed cerebral and cerebellar white matter lucency, and at autopsy there was edema and spongiform white matter degeneration, including the spinal cord. All heroin samples had come from Amsterdam and contained variable amounts of procaine, phenacetin, caffeine, antipyrine, strychnine, quinine, lidocaine, and diethylcarbonate. The disease could not be reproduced in rats or rabbits, and the responsible toxin was not identified. Five similar cases subsequently appeared in Turin, where it was shown that brainstem auditory evoked potentials were frequently prolonged in asymptomatic "dragon chasers."[527,528] Two German "Chinese blowers" developed severe persistent cerebellar signs, and MRI revealed white matter abnormalities.[529] A Swiss man who had dragon-chased for 15 years developed progressive spastic paraparesis, sensory loss, and urinary incontinence, and imaging revealed lesions predominantly in the lateral and dorsal columns of the spinal cord.[529a] Subsequent reports appeared from Taiwan, the

United States, Canada, Britain, and Ireland, during which time dragon chasing became the most widely used method of heroin use worldwide.[530–536]

Two New York City dragon chasers developed ataxia, dysmetria, and dysarthria, and one progressed to akinetic mutism, decorticate posturing, and subsequent spastic quadriparesis.[536] MRI showed typical leukoencephalopathy in the cerebral hemispheres and cerebellum as well as the posterior limb of the internal capsule and areas of the brainstem. Magnetic resonance spectroscopy showed elevated brain lactate. Clinical improvement followed treatment with antioxidants including coenzyme Q, suggesting mitochondrial dysfunction. The contribution of the metal on which the heroin is heated to the pathologically observed myelin splitting is obscure; aluminum foil, not tin foil, is used. Moreover, leukoencephalopathy was reported after intravenous injection of heroin[537,538] and in a 2-year-old whose route of exposure was presumably oral.[539]

MPTP and Parkinsonism

In 1979, severe parkinsonism was reported in a young Maryland graduate student who manufactured and self-injected a meperidine analog, 1-methyl-4-propionoxy-piperidine (MPPP).[540] He later died of a drug overdose, and at autopsy destruction of the substantia nigra zona compacta was evident; other areas usually involved in Parkinson's disease, such as the locus ceruleus and the dorsal motor nucleus of the vagus, were spared. Parkinsonism then began appearing in the San Francisco Bay area among users of MPPP sold as "synthetic heroin," and the responsible toxin was identified as a by-product of MPPP synthesis, 1-methyl-4-phenyl-1,2,3,6-tetrahydropyridine (MPTP).[541–544] Used commercially as a chemical intermediate, MPTP has also caused parkinsonism in laboratory workers accidentally contaminated by inhalation or skin contact.[545] Bradykinesia and rigidity are severe, with muteness and inability to swallow; one patient could move nothing but his eyes.[541,546] Dementia and autonomic impairment do not occur, however. Appearing within a few days of using the drug, symptoms sometimes progress for a few days after it is stopped.[541] Improvement is then rare, but levodopa/carbidopa and bromocriptine provide

relief, often dramatically, and in some instances are probably life-saving.[545,547] Typical side effects of therapy include dyskinesia, on-off phenomenon, and psychiatric symptoms, and attempts after more than a year to wean patients off levodopa/carbidopa have been unsuccessful.[548]

The CSF of affected patients contains elevated protein levels and, as in Parkinson's disease, decreased homovanillic acid levels, but unlike Parkinson's disease, CSF 3-methoxy-4-hydroxyphenyl glycol (MHPG) is normal, implying sparing of norepinephrine systems.[547] In monkeys given MPTP, toxicity is restricted to dopaminergic neurons of the nigrostriatal system.[548–550]

Heroin users exposed to single doses of MPTP have not developed parkinsonian symptoms, but it is feared that the disease might emerge with advancing age and "normal" decreases in dopaminergic activity.[549] Symptoms have been reported in previously asymptomatic patients,[545,548] and positron-emission tomography (PET) (using 18F-dopa) of asymptomatic drug users exposed to MPTP showed decreased numbers of dopamine-containing neurons.[551]

Parkinsonism caused by MPTP has implications beyond drug abuse. Although species vary greatly in the neurological signs produced by MPTP, with primates most prominently affected, striatal dopamine depletion occurs in every animal studied, including rat, mouse, guinea pig, and frog.[548] MPTP is metabolized to 1-methyl-4-phenylpyridinium (MMP+).[552] This reaction and the ability of MPTP to deplete dopamine, destroy neurons, and produce parkinsonism is blocked by the type B monoamine oxidase (MAO) inhibitors pargyline and deprenyl.[553] MPP+ but not MPTP is selectively taken up by dopaminergic neurons; probably MPTP enters glia (the receptor for it being MAO itself) and is biotransformed there to MPP+, which then enters nigral dopaminergic neurons by way of the dopamine uptake system. MPP+ inhibits ATP production and stimulates formation of superoxide radicals, which react with nitric oxide to form peroxynitrite, which in turn, by oxidation and nitration, damages proteins—including tyrosine hydroxylase (the rate-limiting enzyme in dopamine synthesis) and alpha-synuclein (a major constituent of Lewy bodies in Parkinson's disease). MPP+ also activates apoptotic genetic programs.[554] Thus, a serendipitous appearance of a West Coast "designer drug" led to new insights into the possible patho-physiology of Parkinson's disease.

Seizures

A case–control study at Harlem Hospital Center found that heroin use, both past and current, was a risk factor for new-onset seizures independent of overdose, head injury, infection, stroke, alcohol, or other illicit drugs.[555] In animals, opioids can be convulsant, anticonvulsant, or both and can modify post-ictal phenomena; these effects are variably blocked or not blocked by opioid antagonists. Effects depend on the opioid used, dose, route of administration, seizure type, and opioid receptor subtype.[556–564]

Tourette Syndrome

A few months after beginning to smoke heroin, a woman with Tourette syndrome developed malignant coprolalia, which was refractory to treatment and did not improve after she became abstinent.[568a]

Effects on Cognition

As with other drugs of abuse, the effects of chronic opioid use on cognition is difficult to quantitate, for premorbid baselines are seldom available, and confounders abound, including comorbid psychiatric illness, polysubstance use (including ethanol), street drug adulterants, and previous overdose. Neuropsychological testing suggests different patterns of cognitive dysfunction in chronic heroin users compared with psychostimulant users.[565] Levels of *N*-acetylaspartate (a marker of neuronal viability) were reduced in the frontal cortex of 12 heroin addicts, most of whom, however, used other drugs, including ethanol.[566] In adult rats chronic administration of morphine or heroin inhibits neurogenesis in the hippocampus.[567] Neurofilament proteins were reduced in number and abnormally phosphorylated in the prefrontal cortex of human addicts following heroin or methadone overdose.[568] The clinical significance of these observations is uncertain. Consistent with the apparently normal cognition and productivity of addicts who received maintenance morphine in the past and today receive maintenance methadone, there is to date little evidence that chronic administration of opioids per se causes lasting cognitive or psychiatric dysfunction.

Other Related Agents

During the 1990s American physicians were increasingly willing to treat unrelieved pain, especially from cancer, with opioid analgesics, and the prescribing of morphine, methadone, fentanyl, hydromorphone, and oxycodone increased substantially. During the same period, however, even as heroin use rose steadily, abuse of these agents as reflected in the Drug Abuse Warning Network (DAWN) did not increase.[569] Abuse of opioids other than heroin was not insignificant, however, and as we shall see with oxycodone, the extent of abuse was not reflected in DAWN data.

Strategies for treating chronic pain with opioids, including "opioid rotation," are reviewed elsewhere.[569a]

Pentazocine

MPPP-MPTP and T's and blues demonstrate that when other opioids are more available than heroin, they are abused (see above). The mixed agonist-antagonist pentazocine does not suppress morphine abstinence symptoms and in fact may precipitate them even though it does not antagonize morphine's respiratory depression; it is not liked by heroin addicts.[570] Nonetheless, oral and parenteral abuse do occur independently of T's and blues, and both psychic and physical dependence develops in patients originally taking it for analgesia.[571,572] At low doses, pentazocine causes euphoria, lightheadedness, sedation, impotence, and anhidrosis; higher doses cause headache, nausea, vomiting, blurred vision, diplopia, increased heart rate and blood pressure, urinary retention, respiratory depression, and dysphoric psychotomimetic symptoms including delusions and hallucinations. Seizures occur. In contrast to morphine and heroin, there appears to be a maximally tolerated dose. Withdrawal symptoms are milder than with heroin but include prominent drug-seeking behavior. Treatment of pentazocine withdrawal is with gradually decreasing doses of pentazocine itself.

Pentazocine abusers who inject the drug subcutaneously or intramuscularly develop severe focal skin and muscle fibrosis. Pentazocine injected intramuscularly into all four limbs and the trunk—in one case even the back—has produced symptoms suggesting the stiff man syndrome with hard, tender muscles and disabling contractures. Focal precipitation of acidic pentazocine is probably responsible.[573–575]

T's and blues seem to be a descendent of "blue velvet" (tripelennamine and paregoric) abuse in the 1950s; the combination is believed to avoid both the sedation of the opioid and the occasional stimulation of the antihistamine (although sedation with this agent is actually more common).[452,455,576] In studies with volunteers, tripelennamine in the usual street ratio of 1:2 did increase the euphoric effects of pentazocine.[577] Pentazocine and tripelennamine each cause seizures and psychosis, and in mice the two agents combined are considerably more lethal than either.[451,578]

Respiratory insufficiency is common.[579] Staphylococcal infections occur less often in T's and blues users than in heroin users, but *Pseudomonas* infections are more common, perhaps because tripelennamine is inhibitory to the former but not the latter.[580] In 1983, the manufacturer added naloxone to pentazocine tablets. T's and blues abuse then declined but did not disappear—perhaps because naloxone does not block pentazocine's sigma receptor actions and has no effect on tripelennamine.[581,582]

Butorphanol

Like pentazocine, butorphanol is an agonist at κ-receptors and a mixed agonist/antagonist at μ-receptors. During the 1980s roughly 60 adverse reactions from intramuscular butorphanol (Stadol) were reported annually to the U.S. Food and Drug Administration (FDA), mostly psychological disturbances (including confusion, paranoia, and hallucinations). Less than six reports of dependence or addiction occurred yearly, although the medical literature did document recreational abuse and dependence.[583–585] Reminiscent of T's and blues, parenteral abuse of butorphanol mixed with diphenhydramine was described in Mississippi adolescents.[586] In 1991 a nasal spray of Stadol was

approved by the FDA as a non-scheduled drug and promoted for migraine. Five times more potent than the parenteral preparation, the new preparation led to an upsurge in reported adverse reactions from 60 to 400 per year, with reports of dependence/addiction occurring roughly twice weekly.[587] In 1996, under pressure from the media and the American Academy of Neurology, the FDA agreed to schedule the drug.[588]

Meperidine

Meperidine (Demerol) was originally introduced (like heroin) as a "nonaddicting" analgesic, and its ready availability soon produced a plethora of addicted physicians and nurses.[589] Its action is similar to morphine's despite chemical dissimilarity (Figure 3–3), but it has a shorter duration of action (2 to 4 hours) and is less likely to produce miosis. A toxic metabolite, normeperidine, causes tremor, agitation, confusion, delirium, hallucinations, myoclonus, and seizures.[590–592] (Normeperidine's biological half-life is greatly prolonged in patients with renal failure, sickle cell disease, and cancer; repetitive doses of meperidine should be avoided in such settings.[172]) The combination of meperidine with MAO inhibitors exacerbates symptoms and can be fatal.[593] An elderly man who took 4000 mg meperidine over 9 days for postoperative pain developed severe parkinsonism that responded to levodopa/carbidopa; symptoms did not recur when treatment was stopped.[594] As with pentazocine, widespread fibrotic myositis complicates parenteral meperidine abuse.[595] Symptoms of meperidine abstinence usually appear within 3 hours after the last dose, peak at 8 to 12 hours, and decline over 4 to 5 days. There may be intense craving, nervousness, and muscle twitching but often little nausea, vomiting, diarrhea, or mydriasis.[1]

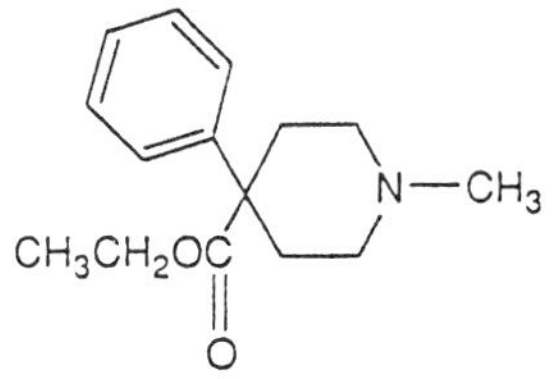

Figure 3–3. Meperidine.

Propoxyphene

The low abuse potential of propoxyphene (Darvon), an analgesic about as strong as aspirin, is countered by its ready availability, and in 1980 the FDA, concerned about illicit use, recommended that prescriptions for it not be refillable.[596–599] Abuse may be oral or intravenous.[600] Propoxyphene is often implicated in drug-related deaths, especially in association with ethanol or tranquilizers, but its prevalence as a street drug is less certain.[601–603] Among adolescents arrested for ethanol-related offenses, propoxyphene is often abused but usually along with other drugs.[604] Similarly, propoxyphene or its metabolites were frequently identified at medical examiner autopsies, but when deaths were attributed to drug toxicity, multiple substances (e.g., benzodiazepines, barbiturates, amitriptyline, or ethanol) were present in 89%; although 30% had a history of ethanol or drug abuse, only 1.8% abused propoxyphene alone.[605,606] Propoxyphene abuse seems to occur most often among patients who take it initially for pain and then gradually increase the dose.[599] Intolerable subjective discomfort and craving may be resistant to even very gradual drug withdrawal.[607] Overdose causes delusions, hallucinations, and seizures, and death is often preceded by naloxone-resistant cardiodepression or pulmonary edema.[1,171,602,608–610] High doses cause peripheral deafness.[611]

Hydromorphone

Hydromorphone (Dilaudid) abuse, often parenteral, also spread during the late 1970s.[612] In Washington, DC, during 1987, there was a sharp increase in deaths related to hydromorphone, pills of which were crushed and sold as heroin.[613] High doses of hydromorphone can cause vivid visual hallucinations in the absence of delirium or other symptoms of overdose.[614] In 2000 a New York City physician and two pharmacists were arrested for diverting huge quantities of Dilaudid (wholesale price US$3 to US$5 per tablet) to Virginia (street price US$25 to US$60 per tablet).[615]

Codeine

During the 1980s, New York City, New Jersey, Pennsylvania, and Los Angeles witnessed a rising popularity of glutethimide combined with codeine ("hits," "sets," "loads") or with acetaminophen plus codeine ("4's and doors").[616–618] The euphoric effect of these combinations resembles heroin's but is longer lasting. In 1980–1981 in northeast New Jersey, 236 deaths were attributed to "hits," compared with 126 for heroin and 46 for methadone.[619] In 1985–1987, nine such deaths occurred in Erie, Pennsylvania.[620] The abuse potential of codeine alone is quite low; it partially suppresses morphine withdrawal, and large doses (1200–1800 mg daily) produce a mild abstinence syndrome.[621] Upper extremity gangrene followed intra-arterial self-injection of crushed codeine tablets.[622] Reports from Australia describe abuse of codeine linctus, a mixture of codeine phosphate and squill oxymel, a cardiac glycoside; complications include diffuse myopathy with myasthenic features and cardiac atrioventricular dissociation.[623–625]

Oxycodone

Oxycodone is the principal ingredient of a number of combination analgesics such as Percocet and Tylox, which are popular oral or nasal recreational drugs in areas of rural America. In 1996, Oxy-Contin was promoted as a time-release analgesic with low abuse potential. Whereas Tylox contains 5 mg of oxycodone, Oxy-Contin pills contain 20, 40, and 80 mg. It was quickly discovered that crushing the tablets destroyed the time-release matrix and that the resulting powder could be snorted or, mixed with water, injected. Following its introduction, prescriptions for Oxy-Contin doubled every year; in 2000 six-and-a-half million were written. Widespread abuse, which began in Appalachi "hillbilly heroin" quickly spread across the United States, with over 200,000 addicted users, many of whom moved on to heroin. In 2002 the FDA identified 464 Oxy-Contin overdose deaths during the previous 2 years, and in Florida a physician who had prescribed Oxy-Contin to hundreds of patients, four of whom died from overdose, was convicted of manslaughter.[626–628] In 2004 a Federal District Court concluded that Purdue Pharma, the maker of Oxy-Contin, had deliberately misled federal officials to win patents protecting the drug.[628a]

Not surprisingly, other long-acting opioid analgesics—notably sustained relief morphine sulfate and methadone—when prescribed for conditions such as chronic daily headache, also carry risk for dosage escalation and psychic and physical dependence.[629]

Hydrocodone

Hydrocodone, comparable to codeine in analgesic potency, has a greater addiction liability. Two migraineurs who became addicted to a hydrocodone/acetaminophen mixture (Vicodin) developed peripheral deafness.[630] DAWN reports of hydrocodone-related emergency room encounters increased 31% from 1999 to 2000.[630a]

Methadone

Illegal diversion of methadone dispensed in methadone maintenance treatment programs has been a longstanding concern (see later). Until recently, however, the abuse potential of methadone was considered low; available as 5 or 10 mg pills for analgesia or in a liquid form for treating addiction, methadone has a delayed effect that precludes a potent "high." However, pills can be ground up and either inhaled or, dissolved in water, injected, and "take home" methadone from treatment programs can be sold for street use. During the late 1990s, as opioid treatment of chronic pain became more acceptable (and as oxycodone warn-ings made physicians wary of prescribing it), methadone as an analgesic became increasingly popular. At the same time, the rising epidemic of heroin addiction led to more methadone maintenance treatment programs. As with oxycodone, widespread methadone abuse made its first appearance in rural areas of the United States such as Appalachia and Maine. In North Carolina deaths caused by methadone rose from 7 in 1997 to 58 in 2001. In Florida methadone-related deaths increased from 209 in 2000 to 357 in 2001 to 254 in the first 6 months of 2002. The DAWN reported 10,725 emergency room visits related to methadone abuse in 2001, nearly double the number in 1999.[630a,630b] A particular hazard of oral methadone is that by the time its delayed action peaks, users may have left the scene of administration (e.g., a party), with no

one to witness their collapse. A complication of injecting crushed pills is pulmonary granulomatous disease.[630c]

Antidiarrheal opioids

A woman became addicted to a kaolin and morphine antidiarrheal mixture and developed fatal hypokalemic myocardial necrosis.[631] High doses of the antidiarrheal opioid diphenoxylate produce euphoria and physical dependence, but low aqueous solubility prevents parenteral abuse. Even less likely to be abused is the antidiarrheal opioid loperamide, which is neither euphorigenic nor water-soluble.[1]

Fentanyl

In 1979, deaths began occurring among Southern California drug users who had thought they were taking high-grade Southeast Asian "China White" heroin but who in fact had been sold alpha-methyl-fentanyl, an analog of fentanyl (Figure 3–4).[632] Used as an anesthetic in major surgery, fentanyl is sometimes abused by health care professionals.[320,321,633–635] Commercially available derivatives include sufentanil, alfentanil, and Innovar (fentanyl plus droperidol, a neuroleptic). Abuse of alpha-methyl-fentanyl spread up the California coast and eastward to Arizona; at the time of its appearance, it was entirely legal, being unclassified as a scheduled drug. It and similar fentanyl analogs are easy and inexpensive to manufacture; chemicals and equipment worth US$200 can produce US$2 million worth of street drug.[636] More than 1400 potential analogs of fentanyl exist, and at least 10, some of which are thousands of times more potent than heroin, have appeared in the street, accounting for numerous overdose

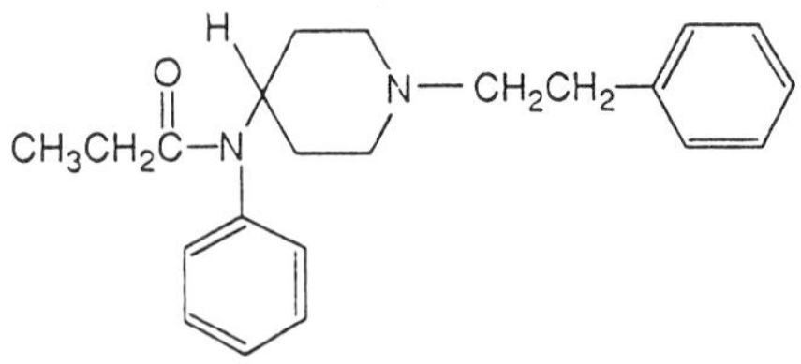

Figure 3–4. Fentanyl.

deaths.[637] They are usually taken intravenously but are sometimes snorted. Users describe effects different from heroin's: a "fainter rush," longer nod, and more gradual "comedown."[636] By the mid-1980s, fentanyl analog "designer drugs" were taken by an estimated 20% of California's 100,000 "heroin" users, especially in suburban areas. Their use then declined sharply in the U.S. West coast, only to emerge in the East.[638–641] During 1988, 16 deaths from methyl-fentanyl were reported from Pittsburgh alone, and during a single weekend in 1991, more than 100 cases of overdose from methyl-fentanyl (nicknamed "Tango and Cash") were treated in New York City, New Jersey, and Connecticut; at least 12 ended fatally.[642]

Myoclonus has been described in patients withdrawing from transdermal fentanyl.[614a]

Lofetamine

In the 1950s, lofetamine, a drug that seems to combine opioid and amphetamine-like effects, was widely abused in Japan. In 1989, lofetamine abuse was reported in Italy.[643] Lofetamine may be a partial agonist; it relieves opioid withdrawal, its effects are reversed by naloxone, and pentazocine can be substituted for it.

Opium

Opium, smoked or ingested, has become increasingly popular in the United States and Europe with the arrival of large numbers of émigrés from Asia. It can be prepared from home-grown poppies, and its source can sometimes be identified by its opioid content and its impurities. Complications include increased risk for esophageal cancer and toxicity from deliberately added arsenic.[644,645]

Poppy seeds can also be made into tea with significant morphine content.[646] A baker whose daily morphine dose by this route was 280 mg had a new-onset grand mal seizure. The possible contribution of other alkaloids in the mixture—e.g., noscapine, papaverine—is uncertain.[647]

Satisfying a penchant for Victorian chic, laudanum became a popular drug among artists in the Seattle area during the 1990s.[648]

Dextromethorphan

The cough-suppressant dextromethorphan is popular among middle-class American teenagers, who can purchase it through the internet. Although not an analgesic, and lacking significant dependence liability, it can cause euphoria and hallucinations.[649]

Tramadol

Psychic and physical dependence on the atypical μ-agonist tramadol are described in case reports from France, Germany, and China.[650,651] Fatal status epilepticus occurred in an alcoholic man taking tramadol plus venlafaxine, trazodone, and quetiapine.[652]

Long-Term Treatment

Drug-Free Therapy, Psychotherapy, and Other Approaches

The central controversy of whether opioid abuse is a social, a psychological, or a metabolic problem has produced different approaches to treatment.[653] Chronic drug-seeking behavior could be the result of protracted abstinence, consistent with the view that such subjects have a permanent opioid deficiency disease analogous to insulin-dependent diabetes mellitus,[192,654] or it could be related more to environmental psychological conditioning, as exemplified by detoxified patients who relapse into drug craving on returning to their old neighborhoods.[655] A powerful reinforcer might be not only the euphoria or relief of abstinence symptoms following drug intake, but also, as noted in Chapter 1, the risky goal-directedness that fills an abuser's days. Many so-called addicts take far too little heroin to cause severe physical dependence and obtain opioid-like euphoria self-injecting saline ("needle freaks").[656] Similarly open to more than one explanation are the tendency of some opioid addicts to "mature out" in middle age,[657] the infrequency with which American soldiers physically dependent on heroin in Vietnam used the drug on returning to the United States,[658] and the rarity with which hospitalized cancer patients physically dependent on opioids experience drug craving after discharge.[40,659] (In a study of 38 out-patients with chronic noncancer pain who received opioid analgesics orally for several years, only two—both previous drug abusers—developed craving and dose escalation.[660])

Psychological and social factors are considered paramount by advocates of drug-free therapy. Data supporting such an approach, however, are either discouraging or difficult to obtain. Relapse occurs in the vast majority of opioid addicts after either voluntary hospitalization or imprisonment (euphemistically called "civil commitment programs").[661–663]

Whatever the role of psychological factors, most workers agree that psychotherapy, including "cognitive behavior therapy" and "motivational enhancement therapy," and strategies such as contingency contracts and vouchers, have only an ancillary role in the treatment of opioid abuse.[654,664–667] As with drug abusers generally, no "addictive personality" defines opioid users, although a wide variety of psychiatric disturbances are overrepresented among them, especially major depression and antisocial personality.[668–671] Whether a psychiatric illness precedes or follows opioid abuse can be difficult to determine; as would be expected, psychiatric disturbance predicts poor response to therapy of any kind.

As noted above and in Chapter 2, family, twin, and adoption studies have established drug dependence in general and opioid dependence in particular as genetically influenced. As with other complex disorders, the genes involved are likely numerous, and they have yet to be identified. Recognizing the respective roles of genes and environment in opioid dependence has not so far led to innovations in treatment.[87,672–677]

Drug-free communities such as Synannon, Day-top, Odyssey House, and Phoenix House reach only a small percentage of abusers and are costly. Data relating to them, although sparse, reveal extremely high relapse rates after patients leave a program.[99,678,679]

Studies of acupuncture in opioid addiction have been either negative or badly designed.[680]

Although chronic opioid use leads to social withdrawal and decreased physical activity, mental performance remains unimpaired. Legalized morphine or heroin, practiced in the United States before restrictive legislation and more recently in Britain, demonstrated that stable daily doses of heroin or morphine are compatible with social productivity.[104,681–684] For reasons discussed later, however, today most British opioid users registered in governmental programs take methadone.[685–687]

Opioid Antagonist Therapy

Proponents of opioid antagonist treatment view opioid abuse as a chronic relapsing, frequently temporary self-limited condition. Naloxone, a pure antagonist, has weak oral efficacy and a short duration of action. Naltrexone, another pure antagonist, is orally effective and at a dose of 150 mg daily blocks heroin effects for 72 hours.[688,689] In 1984 the FDA approved naltrexone for maintenance treatment of opioid dependence. Taken three times weekly, naltrexone precipitates withdrawal in patients who have not been abstinent for at least 7 days. Side effects include nausea, epigastric pain, headache, nervousness, fatigue, and insomnia. Hepatotoxicity can follow large doses. Up-regulation of opioid receptors during chronic naltrexone therapy increases the risk of overdose even several days after stopping therapy.[690]

Despite its FDA approval naltrexone has limited usefulness in opioid dependence. Randomized trials reveal retention rates as low as 2% and no better efficacy than placebo.[689,691] Contributing to patient noncompliance could be dysphoria secondary to blockade of endorphins.[692] Naltrexone might be an appropriate treatment for selected highly motivated patients, including health care professionals. The efficacy of naltrexone reportedly increased when it was combined with fluoxetine and regular counseling.[692a]

Methadone Maintenance Therapy

Methadone maintenance therapy is based on the premise that opioid abuse is a chronic metabolic disorder and that methadone not only substitutes for a patient's endogenous deficiency but also "blocks" the effects of other exogenously administered opioids.[693] Cross-tolerant to heroin and morphine, methadone is taken orally in gradually increasing doses, usually up to 80–120 mg daily. Although tolerance develops to methadone sedation, euphoria, and analgesia, it does not develop to "blockade." Moreover, methadone is taken up and then slowly released by the liver. Therefore, in contrast to heroin, single daily doses produce high steady-state tissue levels without "cycling between abstinence and narcosis."[693] If someone receiving methadone takes heroin, it may produce paresthesias (caused by histamine release) but not euphoria—at least with heroin doses affordable by most addicts. Methadone itself produces little psychic effect of its own and only minor and acceptable side effects such as constipation, nausea, diaphoresis, weight gain, decreased libido, and menstrual irregularities secondary to hyperprolactinemia.[689] Sleep architecture disturbance and sleep apnea are described.[694] Plasma levels of methadone are increased by concomitant administration of cimetidine, erythromycin, ketoconazole, and fluvoxamine. They are decreased by concomitant administration of ethanol, barbiturates, phenytoin, carbamazepine, isoniazid, rifampin, retinovir, nevirapine, and possibly efavirenz. Unexplained deaths occurred in several Australians who had recently begun methadone maintenance therapy; all had chronic hepatitis, which possibly caused fatally high methadone tissue levels.[695] A racemic compound, methadone's D-isomer, is an antagonist at glutamate NMDA receptors, an action that might give it additional analgesic potency compared with morphine.[696] In contrast to heroin, methadone does not impair NK lymphocyte activity.[697] Impaired cognitive function in patients receiving methadone maintenance treatment correlates with a history of ethanol dependence, repeated exposure to heroin overdose, and co-morbid psychiatric disorders rather than with methadone per se.[698]

The abstinence rate of Dole and Nyswander's original methadone maintenance pilot study was 98% at 1 year and 60% at 3 years, with striking decreases in arrests and increases in employment or return to school.[699] Other programs with less strict entry requirements have had lower retention rates, but they are still severalfold higher (and at considerably less expense) than documented retention rates (and social rehabilitation) of any abstinence program.[700–702] A study of 633 patients in six methadone programs in New York, Philadelphia, and Baltimore found that parenteral drug use decreased to 29% at 4 years for those who continued treatment, compared with 82% for those who discontinued treatment.[689] In another report of 727 patients, weekly heroin use dropped from 89% before treatment to 28% at 1 year.[703] A randomized

controlled study found that patients receiving methadone maintenance treatment had better treatment retention and lower heroin use rates compared with those who underwent detoxification plus intensive psychosocial therapy.[704] Methadone maintenance is associated with reduced illegal activity and reduced risk behavior for HIV infection.[703–706]

More than 900 methadone maintenance programs exist in the United States, and more than 150,000 Americans currently receive methadone maintenance therapy, yet it remains a controversial approach.[707–710] Criticisms of methadone maintenance therapy include the objection to keeping someone physically dependent; the observation that some subjects receiving methadone continue to take heroin and may take other illicit drugs (especially cocaine, marijuana, and benzodiazepines) or become ethanol dependent;[711–713] the occurrence among patients of psychic changes, including apathy, daytime "nodding," hypochondriasis, and drug craving as well as impaired male sexual performance; accidental ingestion by children; the fact that methadone does not address socioeconomic or psychological factors; and diversion of methadone into illicit use.[711–717]

These criticisms draw the following rejoinders. First, methadone maintenance is a specific treatment for opioid abuse. Nonopioid abuse, other medical illness, unemployment, or antisocial behavior are separate problems requiring additional supportive services, which governmental regulations hinder. (As Jaffe put it, "The best that we can do is get someone to become what they might have been if they had never become a heroin addict."[708]) Addressing the need for comprehensive medical care, an American study—following existing practices in Britain—demonstrated the feasibility of treating selected methadone-maintenance patients in a physician's office, with monthly visits and take-home medication.[718,719] As for other illicit drug use, in reports from New York City and Baltimore cocaine use decreased among heroin addicts when they began methadone maintenance.[720,721] New or continued cocaine use is not unusual, however, especially among depressed patients,[722] and in animal studies methadone increased cocaine conditioned place preference, indicating enhancement of cocaine reinforcement.[723] Illicit benzodiazepine use—especially diazepam, lorazepam, and alprazolam—is also common among patients receiving methadone, and ethanol abuse is not unusual.[724–726] (Alcoholism in former heroin addicts carries a sad irony; from a medical standpoint, ethanol is a far more harmful drug than heroin.)

Second, heroin abuse among these patients is often, although not always, due to inadequate methadone dosage (i.e., less than 50 mg daily), insufficient to produce the blood concentration of 200 µg/mL necessary for effective blockade.[667,726–728] Low dosage—based, it would appear, on moral posturing rather than medical data[729,730,730a]—leads to dropout and recidivism. In a randomized, double-masked trial lasting 40 weeks, patients receiving 80–100 mg methadone daily had significantly lower rates of opioid-positive urine samples (53%) than those receiving 40–50 mg daily (62%).[731] Some patients have inadequate blood concentrations even at conventional higher dosage. In a study of 500 patients receiving maintenance methadone, 18 continued to use heroin despite doses of 80–100 mg daily; very low serum methadone levels were found, indicating aberrant metabolism and the need for either higher dosage or alternate treatment.[732] Patients with Axis I psychiatric comorbidity often require especially high doses, sometimes over 150 mg per day.[733]

Not only do patients require adequate doses of methadone, but also the great majority must continue maintenance therapy indefinitely. As Dole stressed, the treatment is "corrective but not curative," and recidivism among addicts who try to stop or taper methadone is 70% to 80%.[693,707] Newman suggests that judging methadone maintenance treatment by the number of addicts who relapse when dosage is lowered or terminated is analogous to judging birth control pills by counting the number of pregnancies after treatment is stopped.[734] The goal of methadone maintenance treatment is "rehabilitation, not abstinence."[707] (In 1984, because of budgetary restrictions, California instituted a 2-year limit on methadone maintenance for those unable to pay US$200 a month. The result was a predictable fiasco of heroin relapse, with projected savings offset by the cost of incarceration, legal supervision, and medical treatment.[735])

As to diversion for street use, such methadone is most often taken orally by patients themselves to prevent withdrawal or to detoxify.[736] Street sales do occur, however, perhaps increasingly since the late 1990s, when policies requiring daily visits were relaxed. "Take home" methadone is associated with better program compliance and vocational rehabilitation.[630a] For example, a study comparing not only dosages but also clinic attendance requirements found that patients receiving 80 mg daily had better outcomes than those receiving 50 mg daily and that at either dosage patients attending a clinic twice weekly had better outcomes than those attending five times per week.[737] Noting that methadone is "not often diverted for recreational or casual use but rather by individuals with opioid dependence who lack access to methadone maintenance treatment programs," a National Consensus Panel sponsored by the National Institutes of Health in 1998 called for reduction of unnecessary regulation of methadone maintenance programs in order to increase access to treatment for all who need it.[736] Following this recommendation, the Substance Abuse and Mental Health Services Administration in 2001 lengthened from 6 to 31 the number of daily doses selected patients could take home. The degree to which this contributed to the jump in illicit methadone use nationwide is unclear. However, the great majority of recent recruits to recreational methadone appear to be using pills, not the liquid preparation used for methadone maintenance treatment.[630]

Methadone maintenance therapy during pregnancy raises questions as to its possible adverse effects on offspring.[738] Withdrawal symptoms are possibly more severe when the mother takes methadone than when she takes heroin.[244,739] Such symptoms can persist for several months, and affected infants have impaired fetal respiratory movements, are small, and may be prone to sudden infant death and later impaired perceptual-motor performance.[244,740,741] In one study, infants of mothers who conceived while taking heroin and were then treated with methadone had smaller birth weight, length, and head circumference than non-drug controls; at 9 months of age, weight and length had caught up to control levels, but at 2 years, head circumference remained smaller than that of controls even though psychomotor development appeared normal.[742] In another study, infants of mothers maintained on methadone had lower weight and smaller head circumference at birth but by 6 months of age were no different developmentally from drug-free controls.[743] Another study found no difference in withdrawal symptoms between heroin-exposed and methadone-exposed infants and no neonatal complications other than withdrawal in methadone-exposed infants.[744] Factors other than in utero opioid exposure could of course be responsible for neonatal or development abnormalities.[256,260,745,746] Birth weight was significantly lower, however, in methadone-treated monkeys compared with controls.[747]

These concerns—and the inconsistency of the data—must be weighed against the hazard of opioid detoxification during pregnancy. With close supervision, however, such can be accomplished without detrimental effects on the fetus.[748]

Methadone maintenance treatment of breast-feeding mothers carries little risk to their infants, at least up to 80 mg daily, although some recommend monitoring of infant blood methadone levels.[749]

The AIDS epidemic brought a new urgency to the controversy over methadone maintenance therapy.[750] In New York City in 1990, fewer than 10% of heroin addicts enrolled in methadone maintenance programs before 1980 were HIV-seropositive compared with 60% enrolled after 1987.[710] Similar figures have been reported from other American cities and from Europe.[751–754] Not only does methadone maintenance reduce parenteral drug abuse, but also the setting provides opportunities for counseling and other AIDS risk reduction.[755]

A young man developed choreic movements of the arms, torso, and muscles of speech after 2 years of maintenance methadone; chorea disappeared when treatment was discontinued.[756] Transient choreoathetosis occurred during rapid methadone dose adjustment in a heroin- and cocaine-abuser.[757] A 71-year-old man developed bilateral ballism during methadone withdrawal.[758]

Of 390 patients receiving methadone maintenance therapy, 37% reported chronic moderate-to-severe pain syndromes. Pain management becomes especially challenging in patients already receiving opioids.[758a]

LAAM

L-α-acetylmethadol (LAAM), a long-acting derivative of methadone, was approved by the FDA for maintenance treatment in 1993. Available in oral and parenteral preparations, it can be taken every 2 to 3 days. A meta-analysis of 14 randomized controlled trials comparing LAAM with methadone maintenance found a trend toward greater decrease in illicit drug use with LAAM.[759] As with methadone, clinical efficacy depends on adequate dosage.[760] A disadvantage of LAAM compared with methadone is the longer period needed to achieve the targeted maintenance dose (9 vs. 5 days), leading to greater dropout rates early in treatment.[761] In one study increasing the dose too rapidly resulted in respiratory depression.[762] High doses of LAAM have been associated with electrocardiographic changes of torsades de pointes.[763] LAAM appears not to suppress plasma testosterone levels.[764] For most patients, LAAM's advantages outweigh its disadvantages, and its underuse in most American treatment programs is principally the result of regulatory red tape.[689]

Buprenorphine

Buprenorphine is a partial agonist at μ-opioid receptors and a weak antagonist at κ-receptors, and it has a slow rate of dissociation from opioid receptors. The result is a long duration of action, milder withdrawal symptoms, less respiratory depression or likelihood of overdose, and less potential for abuse.[689] In France, where it has been used to treat opioid addiction since 1996, buprenorphine is available as a sublingual tablet and a sublingual tablet containing naloxone. (The naloxone would not be absorbed sublingually, but if the combined tablet were injected, the naloxone would precipitate withdrawal.[765]) As with LAAM, maintenance buprenorphine can be administered three times per week.[766,767] Trials comparing buprenorphine with placebo demonstrate efficacy; trials comparing buprenorphine with methadone or LAAM are less consistent, describing either equal, greater, or lesser efficacy. As with methadone, adequate dosage is essential.[766,768–771,771a] Side effects include sedation, anxiety, nausea, constipation, and headache. Respiratory depression occurs with overdose, and, because buprenorphine is a partial μ-agonist, naloxone may not reverse it. Reports of hepatotoxicity may or may not signify cause and effect.[771a]

It is controversial whether buprenorphine is more effective than other agents in treating combined heroin and cocaine ("speedball") abuse.[768,772,773] In monkeys buprenorphine suppressed self-administration of both cocaine and the opioid alfentanil, but much higher doses were required to suppress cocaine reinforcement.[774] Others observed buprenorphine suppression of cocaine self-administration in monkeys,[775] but a possible interpretation is that the rate of self-administration decreases because buprenorphine and cocaine are *additively* rewarding.[776]

The dependence liability of buprenorphine is considered low and its abstinence symptoms mild, but abuse and severe withdrawal have been widely reported.[777–789] In rats, buprenorphine lowered the threshold for brain self-stimulation reward.[790] In baboons, buprenorphine is mildly reinforcing, maintaining moderate levels of self-injection in some animals and none in others.[791] In monkeys, buprenorphine is reinforcing but, similar to methadone, less so than heroin.[792]

A man who took a single dose of buprenorphine for pain developed auditory hallucinations and attempted suicide.[793]

Despite the presence of nearly 900 methadone maintenance centers in the United States, only 14% of opioid-dependent patients receive such treatment. Treatment availability is limited by geographical constraints and political ideology.[794] As a particularly egregious example, New York's Mayor Rudolf Giulianni in 1998 attempted to close down all methadone maintenance treatment centers in the 11 public hospitals under his jurisdiction. A timely and well-publicized report by a National Institutes of Health Consensus Panel attesting to the benefits of such therapy resulted in the mayor ultimately changing his mind.[736,795,796] Studies demonstrate that maintenance programs operating through primary care physicians' offices lead to increased enrollment and retention.[689,766,794,797] In October 2000 Congress passed the Drug Addiction Treatment Act, which allows office-based physicians to prescribe schedule III, IV, and V medications approved for detoxification and treatment of opioid dependence. On the basis of randomized placebo-controlled trials demonstrating efficacy, in 2002 the FDA approved buprenorphine (Subutex) and buprenorphine/naloxone (Suboxone) as Schedule III drugs.[797a–d] Each is available as 2 mg or 8 mg sublingual tablets.

Heroin Maintenance Therapy

Around the same time that federal law enforcers (with the approval of the American Medical Association) shut down morphine maintenance programs in the United States, the Rolleston Commission in the United Kingdom authorized physicians to prescribe maintenance opioids, including heroin, for dependent patients.[798] Heroin must be taken two or three times daily, and oral efficacy requires very high doses.[207] It tends to produce lethargy, irritability, and hypochondriasis, and users vary widely in what they consider optimal dosage, leading to frequent illegal supplementation.[683] With the upsurge in heroin abuse by Americans and Europeans during the 1960s, much legally prescribed heroin found its way into the black market, and as a consequence in the UK restrictions were placed on who could dispense it and where. By the mid-1990s less than 1% of the 16,500 British patients being treated pharmacologically for opioid dependence received heroin.[799] Most were prescribed methadone.[800]

Nonetheless, the failure of many hard-core addicts to benefit from methadone maintenance or other treatment approaches has rekindled interest in the use of pharmaceutical heroin. During the 1990s in Switzerland 1035 patients with treatment-refractory heroin dependence received injectable heroin up to three times daily, often combined with take-home oral methadone. Patients were stabilized on 500–600 mg heroin daily without evidence of further tolerance. At 6 months, retention in the program was 89%; at 18 months it was 69%. Other drug use was affected little if at all. The death rate was 1% per year, but no deaths were from heroin overdose. Unexpectedly, at 12 months 60% of patients discharged from the program went on to other treatments, including methadone maintenance (37%) and drug-free programs (22%).[801] An extension of the study in which 1969 patients received heroin found similarly favorable outcomes, with 75% retention at 18 months.[802]

This study had no control subjects, for all the patients were previous treatment failures. In Geneva during the same period, however, patients who had failed at least two prior attempts at drug treatment were randomly assigned to receive either intravenous heroin three times daily ($n = 27$) or other drug treatment (usually methadone) ($n = 24$). After 6 months one subject receiving heroin still used street heroin compared with 10 of the control subjects.[803]

These studies have generated considerable controversy. A World Health Organization (WHO) evaluation declared that the data do not allow one to ascribe the observed benefits to heroin prescribing per se rather than to "the overall treatment programme."[804] Others noted such design weaknesses as uncorroborated self-reports.[805] Advocates of the Swiss approach stress the need for alternative therapies in patients for whom methadone has not worked.[806]

In 2003 two open-label randomized controlled trials in the Netherlands compared inhalable heroin or injectable heroin plus methadone with methadone alone. After 12 months of treatment both forms of combined therapy were significantly more effective than methadone alone, and discontinuation of the co-prescribed heroin resulted in rapid deterioration in 82% of those who had responded to it.[806a] As of 2003, further studies of prescription heroin were either planned or under way in Germany, Spain, and Australia.[807]

Potential Therapies

Suggested but as yet untested potential pharmacotherapies for opioid dependence include γ-hydroxybutyric acid,[808] opioid κ-antagonists,[809] baclofen,[810] γ-vinyl–γ-aminobutyric acid,[811] and ibogaine.[812]

References

1. Reisine T, Pasternak G. Opioid analgesics and antagonists. In: Hardman JG, Limbird LE, eds. Goodman and Gilman's The Pharmacological Basis of Therapeutics, 9th edn. New York: McGraw-Hill, 1996:521.
2. Martin WR. Pharmacology of opioids. Pharmacol Rev 1984; 35:283.
3. Pert CB, Snyder SH. Opiate receptor demonstration in nervous tissue. Science 1973; 179:1011.
4. Simon EJ, Hiller JM, Edelman I. Stereospecific binding of the potent narcotic analgesic ^{3}H-etorphine to rat brain homogenate. Proc Natl Acad Sci USA 1973; 70:1947.
5. Terenius L. Stereospecific interaction between narcotic analgesics and a synaptic plasma membrane fraction of rat cerebral cortex. Acta Pharmacol Toxicol 1973; 32:317.
6. Hughes J, Smith TW, Kosterlitz HW, et al. Identification of two related pentapeptides from the brain with potent opiate agonist activity. Nature 1975; 258:577.
7. Wise RA. Opiate reward: sites and substrates. Neurosci Biobehav Rev 1989; 13:129.
8. Zukin RS, Zukin SR. The case for multiple opiate receptors. Trends Neurosci 1984; 7:160.
9. Kosterlitz AW, Corbett AD, Paterson SJ. Opioid receptors and ligands. NIDA Res Monogr 1990; 95:159.
10. Shippenberg TS, Elmer GI. The neurobiology of opiate reinforcement. Crit Rev Neurobiol 1998; 12:267.
11. Smith AP, Lee NM. Pharmacology of dynorphin. Annu Rev Pharmacol Toxicol 1988; 28:123.
11a. Rowbotham DJ. Endogenous opioids, placebo response, and pain. Lancet 2001; 357:1901.
12. Weitz CJ, Lowney LI, Faull KF, et al. 6-Acetyl morphine: a natural product present in mammalian brain. Proc Natl Acad Sci USA 1988; 85:5335.
13. Cox BM, Goldstein A, Li CH. Opioid activity of a peptide, beta-lipotropin (61-91) derived from beta-lipotropin. Proc Natl Acad Sci USA 1976; 73:1821.
14. Henderson G, McKnight AT. The orphan opioid receptor and its endogenous ligand-nociceptin/orphanin FQ. Trends Pharmacosci 1997; 18:293.
15. Darland T, Heinricher MM, Grandy DK. Orphanin FQ/nociceptin: a role in pain and analgesia, but so much more. Trends Neurosci 1998; 21:215.
16. Walker JR, Ahmed SH, Gracy KN, Koob GF. Microinjections of an opiate receptor antagonist into the bed nucleus of the stria terminalis suppress heroin self-administration in dependent rats. Brain Res 2000; 854:85.
17. Ciccocioppo R, Angeletti S, Panocka I, Massi M. Nociceptin/orphanin FQ and drugs of abuse. Peptides 2000; 21:1071.
18. Lazarus LH, Bryant SD, Salvadori S, et al. Opioid infidelity; novel opioid peptides with dual high affinity for δ- and μ-receptors. Trends Neurosci 1996; 19:31.
19. Zaki PA, Bilsky EJ, Venderah TW, et al. Opioid receptor types and subtypes; the δ receptor as a model. Annu Rev Pharmacol Toxicol 1996; 36:379.
20. Raffa RB. The actions of FMRF-NH2 and FMRF-NH2 related peptides on mammals. NIDA Res Monogr 1991;105:243.
21. Malin DH, Lake JR, Fowler DE, et al. FMRF-NH2-like mammalian peptide precipitates opiate withdrawal syndrome in the rat. Peptides 1990; 11:277.
22. Mansour A, Khachaturian H, Lewis ME, et al. Anatomy of CNS opioid receptors. Trends Neurosci 1988; 11:308.
23. Fujimoto JM, Arts KS. Intracerebroventricular (ICV) clonidine produces an antianalgesic effect through spinal dynorphin A (1–17) mediation. NIDA Res Monogr 1990; 95:306.
24. Faden AL. Opioid and nonopioid mechanisms may contribute to dynorphin's pathophysiological actions in spinal cord injury. Ann Neurol 1990; 27:67.
25. Porreca F, Mosberg HI, Omnaas JR, et al. Supraspinal and spinal potency of selective opioid agonists in the

mouse writhing test. J Pharmacol Exp Ther 1987; 240:890.

26. Sora I, Takahashi N, Funada M, et al. Opiate receptor knockout mice define μ receptor roles in endogenous nociceptive responses and morphine-induced analgesia. Proc Natl Acad Sci USA 1997; 94:1544.

27. Adler MW, Geller EB. The opioid system and temperature regulation. Annu Rev Pharmacol Toxicol 1988; 28:429.

28. Ling GSF, MacLeod JM, Lee S, et al. Separation of morphine analgesia from physical dependence. Science 1984; 226:462.

29. Law P-Y, Wong YH, Loh HH. Molecular mechanisms and regulation of opioid receptor signaling. Annu Rev Pharmacol Toxicol 2000; 40:389.

30. Schuller AG, King MA, Zhang J, et al. Retention of heroin and morphine-6-beta-glucaronide analgesia in a new line of mice lacking exon 1 of MOR-1. Nat Neurosci 1999; 2:151.

31. Elmer GI, Evans JL, Goldberg SR, et al. Transgenic superoxide dismutase mice: increased opioid mesolimbic mu-opioid receptors results in greater opioid-induced stimulation and opioid-reinforced behavior. Behav Pharmacol 1996; 7:628.

32. Matthes HW, Maldonado R, Simonin F, et al. Loss of morphine-induced analgesia, reward effect, and withdrawal symptoms in mice lacking the mu-opioid receptor gene. Nature 1996; 383:819.

33. Snyder SH. Drugs and neurotransmitter receptors in the brain. Science 1984; 224:22.

34. Traynor J. Subtypes of the κ-opioid receptor: fact or fiction? Trends Pharmacol Sci 1989; 10:52.

35. Simmons ML, Chavkin C. Endogenous opioid regulation of hippocampal function. Int Rev Neurobiol 1996; 39:145.

35a. Morris BJ, Johnston HM. A role for hippocampal opioids in long-term functional plasticity. Trends Neurosci 1995; 18:350.

36. Pan ZZ. μ-opposing actions of the κ-opioid receptor. Trends Neurosci 1998; 19:94.

37. Basbaum Al, Fields HL. Endogenous pain control systems: brainstem spinal pathways and endorphin circuitry. Annu Rev Neurosci 1984; 7:309.

38. Vaccarino AL, Olson GA, Olson RD, Kastin AJ. Endogenous opiates: 1998. Peptides 1999; 20:1527.

39. Zubieta J-K, Smith YR, Bueller JA, et al. Regional mu opioid receptor regulation of sensory and effective dimensions of pain. Science 2001; 293:311.

40. Melzack R. The tragedy of needless pain. Sci Am 1990; 262:27.

41. Alderson HL, Parkinson JA, Robbins TW, Everitt BJ. The effects of excitotoxic lesions of the nucleus accumbens core or shell regions on intravenous heroin self-administration in rats. Psychopharmacology 2001; 153:455.

42. Napier TC, Mitrovic I. Opioid modulation of ventral pallidal inputs. Ann N Y Acad Sci 1999; 877:176.

43. Olmstead MC, Munn EM, Franklin KB, Wise RA. Effects of pedunculopontine nucleus lesions on responding for intravenous heroin under different schedules of reinforcement. J Neurosci 1998; 18:5035.

44. Devine DP, Leone P, Pocock D, Wise RA. Differential involvement of ventral tegmental μ-, δ-, and κ-opioid receptors in modulation of basal mesolimbic dopamine release: in vivo microdialysis studies. J Pharmacol Exp Ther 1993; 266:1236.

45. Tanda G, Di Chiara G. A dopamine-mu$_1$ opioid link in the rat ventral tegmentum shared by palatable food (/Fonzies) and non-psychostimulant drugs of abuse. Eur J Neurosci 1998; 10:1179.

46. Tanda G, Pontieri FFE, Chiara G. Cannabinoid and heroin activation of mesolimbic dopamine transmission by a common mu$_1$ opioid receptor mechanism. Science 1997; 276:2048.

47. Gonzales RA, Weiss F. Suppression of ethanol-reinforced behavior by naltrexone is associated with attenuation of ethanol-induced dopamine release in the nucleus accumbens. J Neurosci 1998; 18:10663-10671.

48. Franklin KBJ. Analgesia and abuse potential: an accidental association or a common substrate. Pharmacol Biochem Behav 1998; 59:993.

49. Martin TJ, Kim SA, Cannon DG, et al. Antagonism of delta (2)-opioid receptors by naltrindole-5′-isothiocyanate attenuates heroin self-administration but not antinociception in rats. J Pharmacol Exp Ther 2000; 294:975.

50. Bozarth MA, Wise RA. Anatomically distinct opiate receptor fields mediate reward and physical dependence. Science 1984; 224:514.

51. Hand TL, Stinus L, LeMoal M. Differential mechanisms in the acquisition and expression of heroin-induced place preference. Psychopharmacology 1989; 98:61.

52. Dai S, Corrigall WA, Coen K-M, Kalant H. Heroin self-administration by rats: influence of dose and physical dependence. Pharmacol Biochem Behav 1989; 32:1009.

53. Wise RA. Addictive drugs and brain stimulation reward. Annu Rev Neurosci 1995; 19:319.

54. Maldonado R. Participation of noradrenergic pathways in the expression of opiate withdrawal: biochemical and physical evidence. Neurosci Biochem Rev 1997; 21:91.

55. Koob GF, Stinus L, LeMoal M, Bloom FE. Opponent process theory of motivation: neurobiological evidence from studies of opiate dependence. Neurosci Biobehav Rev 1989; 13:135.

56. Christie MJ, Chester GB. Physical dependence on physiologically released endogenous opiates. Life Sci 1982; 30:1173.

57. Myer EC, Morris DL, Brase DA, et al. Naltrexone therapy of apnea in children with elevated cerebrospinal fluid beta-endorphin. Ann Neurol 1990; 27:75.

58. Sweep CG, Weigant VM, DeVry J, Van Ree JM. Beta-endorphin in brain limbic structures as a neurochemical

correlate of psychic dependence on drugs. Life Sci 1989; 44:1133.

59. O'Brien CP, Terenius LY, Nyberg F, et al. Endogenous opioids in cerebrospinal fluid opioid-dependent humans. Biol Psychiatry 1988; 24:649.

60. Clement-Jones V, McLaughlin L, Lowry PJ, et al. Acupuncture in heroin addicts: changes in met-enkephalin and endorphin in blood and cerebrospinal fluid. Lancet 1979; II:380.

61. Facchinetti F, Volpe A, Nappi G, et al. Impairment of adrenergic-induced proopiomelanocortin-related peptide release in heroin addicts. Acta Endocrinol 1985; 108:1.

62. O'Brien CP, Terenius L, Wahlstrom A, et al. Endorphin levels in opioid-dependent human subjects: longitudinal study. Ann N Y Acad Sci 1982; 398:377.

63. Sharpe LG, Pickworth WB. Morphine abstinence syndrome: cholinergic mechanisms in the ventral peri-aqueductal gray of the dog. NIDA Res Monogr 1984; 49:143.

64. Collier HOJ, Tucker JF. Novel form of drug-dependence-on adenosine in guinea pig ileum. Nature 1983; 302:618.

65. Trujillo KA, Akil H. Inhibition of morphine tolerance and dependence by the NMDA receptor antagonist MK-801. Science 1991; 251:85.

66. Wiertelak EP, Maier SF, Watkins LR. Cholecystokinin antianalgesia: safety cues abolish morphine analgesia. Science 1992; 256:830.

67. Aghajanian GK. Tolerance of locus coeruleus neurones to morphine and suppression of withdrawal response by clonidine. Nature 1978; 276:186.

68. Gold MS, Redmond DE, Kleber HD. Clonidine blocks acute opiate-withdrawal symptoms. Lancet 1978; II:599.

69. Shearman G, Hynes M, Fielding S, Lal H. Clonidine self-administration in the rat: a comparison with fentanyl self-administration. Pharmacologist 1977; 19:171.

70. Woolverton WL, Wessinger WD, Balster RL. Reinforcing properties of clonidine in rhesus monkeys. Psychopharmacology 1982; 77:17.

71. Christie MJ, Williams JT, Osborne PB, Bellchambecs CE. Where is the locus of opioid withdrawal? Trends Pharmacosci 1997; 18:134.

72. Aston-Jones G, Delfs JM, Druhan J, Zhu Y. The bed nucleus of the stria terminalis. A target site for nora-drenergic actions in opiate withdrawal. Ann N Y Acad Sci 199; 877:486.

73. Wang Y, Joharchi N, Fletcher PJ, et al. Further studies to examine the nature of dexfenfluramine-induced suppression of heroin self-administration. Psychopharmacology 1995; 120:134.

74. Tao R, Auerbach S. Anesthetics block morphine-induced increases in serotonin release in rat CNS. Synapse 1994; 18:307.

75. DeVries TJ, Shippenberg TS. Neural systems underlying opiate addiction. J Neurosci 2002; 22:3321.

76. Connor M, Christie MJ. Opioid receptor signaling mechanisms. Clin Exp Pharmacol Physiol 1999; 26:493.

77. Sharma SK, Bhatia M, Ralhan R. Mechanism of development of tolerance and dependence in neuroblastoma × glioma hybrid cells and mice. NIDA Res Monogr 1988; 87:157.

78. Self DW, Terwilliger RZ, Nestler EJ, Stein L. Inactivation of G_i and G_o proteins in nucleus accumbens reduces both cocaine and heroin reinforcement. J Neurosci 1994; 14:6239.

79. Sim-Selley LJ, Selley DE, Vogt LJ, et al. Chronic heroin self-administration desensitizes μ-opioid receptor-activated G-proteins in specific regions of rat brain. J Neurosci 2000; 20:4555.

80. Zhang J, Ferguson SSG, Barak LS, et al. Role for G protein-coupled receptor kinase in agonist-specific regulation of μ-opioid receptor responsiveness. Proc Natl Acad Sci USA 1998; 12:7157.

81. Bohn LM, Lefkowitz RJ, Gainetdinov RR, et al. Enhanced morphine analgesia in mice lacking β-arrestin 2. Science 1999; 286:2495.

82. Maldonado R, Blendy JA, Tzavara E, et al. Reduction of morphine abstinence in mice with a mutation in the gene encoding CREB. Science 1996; 273:657.

83. Bohn LM, Gainetdinov RR, Lin F-T, et al. μ-opioid receptor desensitization by β-arrestin-2 determines morphine tolerance but not dependence. Nature 2000; 408:720.

84. Bhargava HN. Diversity of agents that modify opioid tolerance, physical dependence, abstinence syndrome, and self-administrative behavior. Pharmacol Rev 1994; 46:293.

85. Salmon AM, Damaj MI, Marubio LM, et al. Altered neuroadaptations in opiate dependence and neurogenic inflammatory nociception in alpha CGRP-deficient mice. Nat Neurosci 2001; 4:357.

86. Murtra P, Sheasby AM, Hunt SP, DeFelipe C. Rewarding effects of opiates are absent in mice lacking the receptor for substance P. Nature 2000; 405:180.

87. Tsuang MT, Lyons MJ, Faraone SV. Using twin data to define drug abuse phenotypes. Am J Med Genet 2000; 96:474.

88. Mas M, Sabater E, Olaso MJ, et al. Genetic variability in morphine sensitivity and tolerance between different strains of rats. Brain Res 2000; 866:109.

89. LaForge KS, Yuferov V, Kreek MJ. Opioid receptor and peptide gene polymorphisms: potential implications for addictions. Eur J Pharmacol 2000; 410:249.

90. Lichtermann D, Franke P, Maier W, et al. Pharmacogenetics and addiction to opiates. Eur J Pharmacol 2000; 410:269.

91. Lawford BR, Young RM, Noble EP, et al. The D(2) dopamine receptor A(1) allele and opioid dependence: association with heroin use and response to methadone treatment. Am J Med Genet 2000; 96:592.

92. Horowitz R, Kotler M, Shufman E, et al. Confirmation of an excess of the high enzyme activity COMT val

allele in heroin addicts in a family-based haplotype relative risk study. Am J Med Genet 2000; 96:599.

93. Tyndale RF, Droll KP, Sellers EM. Genetically deficient CYP2D6 metabolism provides protection against oral opiate dependence. Pharmacogenetics 1997; 7:375.

94. Emboden W. Narcotic Plants. New York: Macmillan, 1979:26.

95. Kerimi N. Opium use in Turkmenistan: a historical perspective. Addiction 2000; 95:1319.

96. Paulshock BZ. William Heberden and opium—some relief to all. N Engl J Med 1983; 308:53.

97. Haller JS. Heroin addiction, insights from Alexis de Tocqueville. N Y State J Med 1986; 86:121.

98. Miller RJ, Tran PB. More mysteries of opium reveal'd: 300 years of opiates. Trends Pharmacol Sci 2000; 21:299.

99. Brecher EM. Licit and Illicit Drugs. Boston: Little, Brown, 1972.

100. Musto D. Opium, cocaine, and marijuana in American history. Sci Am 1991; 265:40.

101. Higby GJ. Heroin and medical reasoning: the power of analogy. N Y State J Med 1986; 86:137.

102. Sneader W. The discovery of heroin. Lancet 1998; 352:1697.

103. Penfield W. Halsted of Johns Hopkins. The man and his problem as described in the secret records of William Osler. JAMA 1969; 210:2214.

104. Blaine JD, Bozetti LP, Ohlson KE. The narcotic analgesics: the opiates. In: Drug Use in America: Problem in Perspective. The Technical Papers of the Second Report of the National Commission on Marijuana and Drug Abuse. Washington, DC: US Government Printing Office, 1973:60.

105. Hughes PH, Barker NW, Crawford GA, Jaffe JH. The natural history of a heroin epidemic. Am J Public Health 1972; 62:995.

106. Stimmel B. The socioeconomics of heroin dependency. N Engl J Med 1972; 287:1275.

107. Kandel DB. Epidemiological trends and implications for understanding the nature of addiction. In: O'Brien CP, Jaffe JH, eds. Addictive States. Res Publ Assoc Res Nerv Ment Dis 1992; 70:23.

108. Halloway M. Treatment for addiction. Sci Am 1991; 265:94.

109. Maitland L, Nossiter BD. U.S. tries new tack in drug fight as global supply and use mount. NY Times, January 30, 1983.

110. Treaster JB. A more potent heroin makes a comeback in a new, needleless form. NY Times, April 28, 1991.

111. Alvarez L. The middle class rediscovers heroin. NY Times, August 14, 1995.

112. Schemo DJ. Heroin is proving a growth industry for Colombia. NY Times, March 30, 1997.

113. Brzezinski M. Re-engineering the drug business. NY Times Magazine, June 23, 2002.

114. Forero J, Weiner T. Latin American poppy fields undermine U.S. drug battle. NY Times, June 8, 2003.

115. Hamid A. The heroin epidemic in New York City: current status and prognosis. J Psychoactive Drugs 1997; 29:375.

116. DesJarlais DC, Perlis T, Friedman SR, et al. Behavioral risk reduction in a declining HIV epidemic: injection drug users in New York City, 1990-1997. Am J Public Health 2000; 90:1112.

117. Hickman M, Seaman S deAngelis D. Estimating the relative incidence of heroin use: application of a method for adjusting observed reports of first visits to specialized drug treatment agencies. Am J Epidemiol 1002; 153:632.

118. Kline A, Mammo A, Culleton R, et al. Trends in injection drug use among persons entering addiction treatment—New Jersey, 1992–1999. MMWR 2001; 50:378.

119. Schwartz RH. Adolescent heroin use: a review. Pediatrics 1998; 102:1461.

120. Wren CS. Face of heroin: it's younger and suburban. NY Times, April 25, 2000.

121. Heroin overdose deaths—Multnomah County, Oregon, 1993–1999. MMWR 2000; 49:633.

122. Unintentional opiate overdose deaths—King County, Washington, 1990–1999. MMWR 2000; 49:636.

123. Mark TL, Woody GE, Juday T, Kleber HD. The economic costs of heroin addiction in the United States. Drug Alcohol Dep 2001; 61:19.

124. Dean M. Britain on the brink of a new heroin epidemic. Lancet 1999; 353:1947.

125. Golden T. A war on terror meets a war on drugs. NY Times, Nov 25, 2001.

126. Golden T. U.S. fears a glut of heroin from a volatile Afghanistan. NY Times, April 1, 2002.

126a. Kristof ND. A scary Afghan road. NY Times, November 13, 2003.

127. Skolnick JH. The limits of narcotics law enforcement. J Psychoact Drugs 1984; 16:119.

128. Nicholi AM. The non-therapeutic use of psychoactive drugs. A modern epidemic. N Engl J Med 1983; 308:925.

129. Robertson JR. Drug users in contact with general practice. BMJ 1984; 290:34.

130. Blachy PH. Naloxone for diagnosis in methadone programs. JAMA 1973; 244:334.

131. Harding G. Patterns of heroin use: what do we know? Br J Addict 1988; 83:1247.

132. Hser YI, Hoffman V, Grella CE, et al. A 33-year follow-up of narcotics addicts. Arch Gen Psychiatry 2001; 58:503.

133. Musto DF. The American Disease: Origins of Narcotic Control. New Haven, CT: Yale University Press, 1973.

134. Nurco DN, Ball JC, Shaffer JW, Hanton TE. The criminality of narcotic addicts. J Nerv Ment Dis 1985; 173:94.

135. Shaffer JW, Nurco DN, Ball JC, et al. The relationship of preaddiction characteristics to the types and

amounts of crime committed by narcotic addicts. Int J Addict 1987; 22:153.

136. Martin WR, Fraser HF. A comparative study of physiological and subjective effects of heroin and morphine administered intravenously in postaddicts. J Pharmacol Exp Ther 1961; 133:388.

137. Levine MN, Sackett DL, Bush H. Heroin vs morphine for cancer pain? Arch Intern Med 1986; 146:353.

138. Hubner CB, Kornetsky C. Heroin, 6-acetylmorphine and morphine effects on threshold for rewarding and aversive brain stimulation. J Pharmacol Exp Ther 1992; 260:562.

139. Rady JJ, Roerig SC, Fujimoto JM. Heroin acts on different opioid receptors than morphine in Swiss Webster and ICR mice to produce antinociception. J Pharmacol Exp Ther 1991; 256:448.

139a. Vanderenne M, Vendenbussche H, Verstraete A. Detection time of drugs of abuse in urine. Acta Clin Belg 200; 55:323.

140. Sjøgren P, Thuneborg LP, Christup L, et al. Is development of hyperalgesia, allodynia and myoclonus related to morphine metabolism during long-term administration? Six case histories. Acta Anaesthesiol Scand 1998; 42:1070.

141. Sapira JD. The narcotic addict as a medical patient. Am J Med 1968; 45:555.

142. Caplan LR, Hier DB, Banks G. Stroke and drug abuse. Stroke 1982; 13:869.

143. Eskes D, Brown JK. Heroin–caffeine–strychnine mixtures—where and why? Bull Narc 1975; 27:67.

144. French JF, Stafford J. AIDS and intranasal heroin. Lancet 1989; I:1082.

145. Casriel C, Rockwell R, Stepherson B. Heroin sniffers: between two worlds. J Psychoactive Drugs 1988; 20:437.

146. Gossop M, Griffiths P, Strang J. Chasing the dragon: characteristics of heroin chasers. Br J Addict 1988; 83:1159.

147. Madden S. Chasing the dragon and syringe-exchange programs. Br J Addict 1989; 84:697.

148. Strang J, Gossop M, Griffiths P, Farrel M. The technology of dragon chasing. Br J Addict 1989; 84:699.

149. London M, O'Reagan T, Aust P, Stackford A. Poppy tea drinking in East Anglia. Br J Addict 1990; 85:1345.

150. Kalant H. Opium revisited: a brief review of its nature, composition, non-medical use and relative risks. Addiction 1997; 92:267.

151. Perlman DC, Perkins MP, Paone D, et al. "Shotgunning" as an illicit drug smoking. J Subst Abuse Treat 1997; 14:3.

152. Foley KM. Opioids. In: Brust JCM, ed. Neurologic Complications of Drug and Alcohol Abuse. Neurol Clin 1993; 11:503–522.

153. Fraser HF, Isbell H. Comparative effects of 290 mg morphine sulfate in non-addicts and former morphine addicts. J Pharmacol Exp Ther 1952; 105:498.

154. Creighton FJ, Ghodse AH. Naloxone applied to conjunctiva as a test for physical opiate dependence. Lancet 1989; I:748.

155. Kay DC, Eisenstein RB, Jasinski DR. Morphine effects on human REM state, waking time, and NREM sleep. Psychopharmacologia 1969; 14:404.

156. Frenk H, Liban A, Balamuth R, Urca G. Opiate and non-opiate aspects of morphine induced seizures. Brain Res 1982; 253:253.

157. Volavka J, Zaks A, Roubicek J, Fink M. Electroencepha-lographic effects of diacetylmorphine (heroine) and naloxone in man. Neuropharmacology 1970; 9:587.

158. Larpin R, Vincent A, Perret C. Morbidité et mortalité hospitalières de l'intoxication aigué par les opices. Presse Med 1990; 19:1403.

159. McCann SM, Lumpkin MD, Mizunuma H, et al. Peptidergic and dopaminergic control of prolactin release. Trends Neurosci 1984; 7:127.

160. Tagliero F, Capra F, Dorizzi R, et al. High serum calcitonin levels in heroin addicts. J Endocrinol Invest 1984; 7:331.

161. Vescovi PP, Girasole G, Caccavari R, et al. Metyrapone effects on beta-endorphin, ACTH, and cortisol levels after chronic opiate receptor stimulation in man. Neuropeptides 1990; 15:129.

162. Genazzami AR, Petraglia F. Opioid control of luteinizing hormone secretion in humans. J Steroid Biochem 1989; 33:751.

163. Buffum JC. Pharmacosexuality update: heroin and sexual function. J Psychoact Drugs 1983; 15:317.

164. Mendelson JH, Mello NK. Hormones and psychosexual development in young men following chronic heroin use. Neurobehav Toxicol Teratol 1982; 4:441.

165. Ceriello A, Dello Russo P, Curcio F, et al. Depressed antithrombin III biological activity in opiate addicts. J Clin Pathol 1984; 37:1040.

166. Giugliano D. Morphine, opioid peptides, and pancreatic islet function. Diabetes Care 1984; 7:92.

167. Passariello N, Gugliano I, Ceriello A, et al. Increased platelet aggregation in opiate addicts. Blood 1982; 60:276.

168. Higgins ST, Stitzer ML, McCaul ME, et al. Pupillary response to methadone challenge in heroin users. Clin Pharmacol Ther 1985; 37:460.

169. O'Brien CP. Drug addiction and drug abuse. In: Hardman JG, Limbird LE, eds. Goodman and Gilman's The Pharmacological Basis of Therapeutics, 9th edition. New York: McGraw-Hill, 1996:557.

170. Haertzen CA, Hooks NT. Changes in personality and subjective experience associated with the chronic administration and withdrawal of opiates. J Nerv Ment Dis 1969; 148:606.

171. Khantzian EJ, McKenna GJ. Acute toxic and withdrawal reactions associated with drug use and abuse. Ann Intern Med 1979; 90:361.

172. Nelson LS. Opioids. In: Goldfrank LR, Flomenbaum NE, Levin NA, et al, eds. Toxicologic Emergencies, 6th edition. Stamford, CT: Appleton & Lange, 1998:975.

173. Sporer KA. Acute heroin overdose. Ann Intern Med 1999; 130:584.

174. Winek CL, Wahba WW, Rozin L. Heroin fatality due to penile injection. Am J Forensic Med Pathol 1999; 20:90.

175. Darke S, Ross J. Fatal heroin overdoses resulting from non-injecting routes of administration. Addiction 2000; 95:569.

176. Wyler D, Zollinger V. The "golden sniff": suicide by sniffing heroin. Archiv Kriminol 1997; 200:154.

177. Gaeta TJ, Capodano RJ, Spevack CO. Potential danger of nalmefene use in the emergency department. Ann Emerg Med 1997; 29:193.

178. Edston E, van Hage-Hamsten M. Anaphylactoid shock—a common cause of death in heroin addicts? Allergy 1997; 52:950.

179. Nolan AG. Recreational drug misuse: issues for the cardiologist. Heart 2000; 83:627.

180. Choudry N, Doe J. Inadvertent abuse of amphetamines in street heroin. Lancet 1986; II:817.

181. Kramer TH, Fine J, Bahari B, Ottomanelli G. Chasing the dragon: the smoking of heroin and cocaine. J Subst Abuse Treatment 1990; 7:65.

182. Duvauchelle CL, Sapoznik T, Koornetsky C. The synergistic effects of combining cocaine and heroin ("speedball") using a progressive-ratio schedule of drug reinforcement. Pharmacol Biochem Behav 1998; 61:297.

183. Hemby SE, Co C, Dworkin SI, Smith JE. Synergistic elevations in nucleus accumbens extracellular dopamine concentrations during self-administration of cocaine/heroin combinations (Speedball) in rats. J Pharmacol Exp Ther 1999; 288:274.

184. Kreek MJ. Opioid interaction with alcohol. Adv Alcohol Subst Abuse 1984; 3:35.

185. Rooney S, Kelly G, Bamford L, et al. Co-abuse of opiates and benzodiazepines. Irish J Med Sci 1999; 168:36.

186. Ross J, Darke S, Hall W. Transitions between routes of benzodiazepine administration among heroin users in Sydney, Australia. Addiction 1997; 92:697.

187. Darke S, Ross J. The use of antidepressants among injecting drug users in Sydney, Australia. Addiction 2000; 95:407.

188. Sorensen SC, Mattison K. Naloxone as an antagonist in severe alcohol intoxication. Lancet 1978; II:688.

189. Perrone J, Shaw L, DeRoos F. Laboratory confirmation of scopolamine co-intoxication in patients using tainted heroin. J Toxicol Clin Toxicol 1999; 37:491.

190. Hamilton RJ, Perrone J, Hoffman R, et al. A descriptive study of an epidemic of poisoning caused by heroin adulterated with scopolamine. J Toxicol Clin Toxicol 2000; 38:597.

191. Himmelsbach CK. The morphine abstinence syndrome, its nature and treatment. Ann Intern Med 1941; 15:829.

192. Jasinski DR. Opiate withdrawal syndrome: acute and protracted aspects. Ann N Y Acad Sci 1981; 362:183.

193. Nash P, Colasanti B, Khazan N. Long-term effects of morphine on the electroencephalogram and behavior of the rat. Psychopharmacologia 1973; 29:271.

194. Goldberg SR, Schuster CR. Nalorphine: increased sensitivity of monkeys formerly dependent on morphine. Science 1969; 166:1548.

195. Carlson KR, Cooper DO. Morphine dependence and protracted abstinence. Regional alternations in CNS radioligand binding. Pharmacol Biochem Behav 1985; 23:1059.

196. Liebmann PM, Lehofer M, Moser M, et al. Persistent analgesia in former opiate addicts is resistant to blockade of endogenous opioids. Biol Psychiatry 1997; 42:962.

197. Kosten TR, O'Connor PG. Management of drug and alcohol withdrawal. N Engl J Med 2003; 348:1786.

198. Liu SJ, Wang RI. Case report of barbiturate-induced enhancement of methadone metabolism and withdrawal syndrome. Am J Psychiatry 1984; 141:1287.

199. Tong TG, Pond SM, Kreek MJ, et al. Phenytoin-induced methadone withdrawal. Ann Intern Med 1981; 94:349.

200. Saxon AJ, Whittaker S, Hawkes CS. Valproic acid, unlike other anticonvulsants, has no effect on methadone metabolism: two cases. J Clin Psychiatry 1989; 50:228.

201. Kennedy JA, Harman N, Sbriglio R, et al. Metyrapone-induced withdrawal symptoms. Br J Addict 1990; 85:1133.

202. Cochin J, Kornetsky C. Development and loss of tolerance to morphine in rat after single and multiple injections. J Pharmacol Exp Ther 1964; 145:1.

203. Wright C, Bigelow GE, Stitzer ML. Acute physical dependence in man: repeated naloxone-precipitated withdrawal after a single dose of methadone. NIDA Res Monogr 1990; 95:395.

204. Bickel WK, Stitzer ML, Liebson IA, Bigelow GE. Acute physical dependence in man: effects of naloxone after brief morphine exposure. J Pharmacol Exp Ther 1988; 244:126.

205. Heishman SJ, Stitzer ML, Bigelow GE, Liebson IA. Acute opioid physical dependence: naloxone dose effects after brief morphine exposure. J Pharmacol Exp Ther 1989; 248:127.

206. FDA Regulations Governing Methadone. In: Federal Register, vol XXXVII, section 130. 44, 1972.

207. Ghodse AH, Creighton FJ, Bhat AV. Comparison of oral preparations of heroin and methadone to stabilize opiate misusers as inpatients. BMJ 1990; 300:719.

208. Cami J, DeTorres S, San L, et al. Efficacy of clonidine and of methadone in the rapid detoxification of patients dependent on heroin. Clin Pharmacol Ther 1985; 38:336.

209. Jasinski DR, Johnson RE, Kocher TR. Clonidine in morphine withdrawal. Arch Gen Psychiatry 1985; 42:1063.

210. Lin SK, Strang J, Su LW, et al. Double-blind randomized controlled trial of lofexidine versus clonidine in the treatment of heroin withdrawal. Drug Alcohol Dep 1997; 48:127.

211. Lauzon P. Two cases of clonidine abuse/dependence in methadone-maintained patients. J Subst Abuse Treat 1992; 9:125.

212. Schubert H, Fleischhacker WW, Meise V, Theohar C. Preliminary results of guanfacine treatment of acute opiate withdrawal. Am J Psychiatry 1984; 141:1271.

213. Soler-Insa PA, Bedate-Villar J, Theohar C, Yotis A. Treatment of heroin withdrawal with guanfacine: an open clinical investigation. Can J Psychiatry 1987; 32:679.

214. San L, Cami J, Peri JM, et al. Efficacy of clonidine, guanfacine, and methadone in the rapid detoxification of heroin addicts: a controlled clinical trial. Br J Addict 1990; 85:141.

215. O'Connor PG, Waugh ME, Carroll KM, et al. Primary care-based ambulatory opioid detoxification: the results of a clinical trial. J Gen Intern Med 1995; 10:255.

216. Vining E, Kosten TR, Kleber HD. Clinical utility of rapid clonidine naltrexone detoxification for opioid abusers. Br J Addict 1988; 83:567.

217. Buntwal N, Bearn J, Gossop M, Strang J. Naltrexone and lofexidine treatment for in-patient opiate detoxification. Drug Alcohol Dep 2000; 59:183.

218. O'Connor PG, Carroll KM, Shi JM, et al. Three methods of opioid detoxification in a primary care setting. A randomized trial. Ann Intern Med 1997; 127:526.

219. Kosten TR, Kleber HD. Buprenorphine detoxification from opioid dependence. A pilot study. Life Sci 1988; 42:635.

220. Bell JR, Young MR, Masterman SC, et al. A pilot study of naltrexone-accelerated detoxification in opioid dependence. Med J Aust 1999; 171:26.

221. Lawental E. Ultra-rapid opiate detoxification as compared to 30-day inpatient detoxification program—a retrospective follow-up study. J Subst Abuse 2000; 11:173.

222. O'Connor PG, Kosten TR. Rapid and ultrarapid opioid detoxification techniques. JAMA 1998; 279:229.

223. Cuccia AT, Monnat M, Spagnoli J, et al. Ultra-rapid opiate detoxification using deep sedation with oral midazolam: short- and long-term results. Drug Alcohol Dep 1998; 52:243.

224. Zielbauer P. State knew of risky heroin treatment before patient deaths. NY Times, October 31, 1999.

225. Alper KR, Lotsof HS, Frenken GM, et al. Treatment of opioid withdrawal with ibogaine. Am J Addict 1999; 8:234.

226. Bisaga A, Gianelli P, Popik P. Opiate withdrawal with dextromethorphan. Am J Psychiatry 1997; 154:584.

227. Foley KM, Houde RW. Methadone in cancer pain management: individualize dose and titrate to effect. J Clin Oncol 1998; 16:3213.

228. Newmeyer JA, Johnson G, Klot S. Acupuncture as a detoxification modality. J Psychoact Drugs 1984; 16:241.

229. Auriacombe M, Tignol J, LeMoal M, Stinus L. Transcutaneous electrical stimulation with Limoge current potentiates morphine analgesia and attenuates opiate abstinence syndrome. Biol Psychiatry 1990; 28:650.

230. Chiriboga CA, Ferriero DM. Neurologic complications of maternal drug abuse. In: Berg BO, ed. Principles of Child Neurology. New York: McGraw-Hill, 1996:1363.

231. Kandall SR. Treatment strategies for drug-exposed neonates. Clin Perinatol 1999; 26:231.

232. Kahn EJ, Newman LL, Polk G. The course of the heroin withdrawal syndrome in newborn infants treated with phenobarbital or chlorpromazine. J Pediatr 1969; 75:495.

233. Klenka HM. Babies born in a district general hospital to mothers taking heroin. BMJ 1986; 293:745.

234. Zelson C, Lee SJ, Casalino M. Neonatal narcotic addiction: comparative effects of maternal intake of heroin and methadone. N Engl J Med 1973; 289:1216.

235. Fulroth R, Phillips B, Durand DJ. Perinatal outcome of infants exposed to cocaine and/or heroin in utero. Am J Dis Child 1989; 143:905.

236. Rementeria JL, Nunag NN. Narcotic withdrawal in pregnancy: stillbirth incidence with a case report. Am J Obstet Gynecol 1973; 116:1152.

237. Thomas CS, Osborn M. Inhaling heroin during pregnancy. BMJ 1988; 296:1672.

238. Rosen TS, Johnson HL. Children of methadone maintained mothers: follow-up to 18 months of age. J Pediatr 1982; 101:192.

239. Kandall SR, Doberczak TM, Jantunen M, Stein J. The methadone-maintained pregnancy. Clin Perinatol 1999; 26:173.

240. Pacifico P, Nardelli E, Pantarotto MF. Neonatal heroin withdrawal syndrome: evaluation of different pharmacological treatments. Pharmacol Res 1989; 21:63.

241. Kandall SR, Doberczak TM, Mauer KR, et al. The comparative effects of opiates vs central nervous system depressant treatment on neonatal drug withdrawal. Am J Dis Child 1983; 137:378.

241a. Osborn DA, Jeffrey HE, Cole MJ. Sedatives for opiate withdrawal in newborn infants. Cochrane Database of Systematic Reviews 2002; (3) CD002053.

242. Finnegan LP. The effects of narcotics and alcohol on pregnancy and the newborn. Ann N Y Acad Sci 1981; 362:136.

243. Chasnoff IJ, Burns WJ. The Moro reaction: a scoring system for narcotic withdrawal. Dev Med Child Neurol 1984; 26:484.

244. Peterson DR. SIDS in infants of drug-dependent mothers. J Pediatr 1980; 96:734.

245. Wilson GS, Desmond MM, Verniaud WM. Early development of infants of heroin-addicted mothers. Am J Dis Child 1973; 126:457.

246. Kletter R, Jeremy RJ, Rumsey C, et al. Developmental decline in infants born to HIV-infected intravenous drug-using mothers. NIDA Res Monogr 1990; 95:409.

247. Kirby MC. Effects of morphine on spontaneous activity of 18-day rat fetus. Dev Neurosci 1979; 2:238.

248. Taeusch HW, Carson SH, Wang NS, Avery ME. Heroin induction of lung maturation and growth retardation in fetus rabbits. J Pediatr 1972; 82:869.

249. Malanga CJ, Kosofsky BE. Mechanisms of action of drugs of abuse on the developing fetal brain. Clin Perinatol 1999; 26:17.

250. Nassogne MC, Gressens P, Evrard P, Courtoy PJ. In contrast to cocaine, prenatal exposure to methadone does not produce detectable alterations in the developing mouse brain. Brain Res Dev Brain Res 1998; 110:61.

251. Steingart RA, Abu-Roumi M, Newman ME, et al. Neurobehavioral damage to cholinergic systems caused by prenatal exposure to heroin or phenobarbital: cellular mechanisms and the reversal of deficits by neural grafts. Brain Res Dev Brain Res 2000; 122:125.

252. Piatti E, Rizzi R, Chiesara E. Genotoxicity of heroin and cannabinoids in humans. Pharmacol Res 1989; 21:59.

253. Fischman HK, Roizin L, Moralishvili E, et al. Clastogenic effects of heroin in pregnant monkeys and their offspring. Mut Res 1983; 118:77.

254. Shafer DA, Falek A, Donahoe RM, Madden JJ. Biogenetic effects of opiates. Int J Addict 1990–91; 25:1.

255. Maynard EC. Material abuse of cocaine and heroin. Am J Dis Child 1990; 144:520.

256. Kaltenbach K, Finnegan LP. Developmental outcome of children born to methadone maintained women: a review of longitudinal studies. Neurobehav Toxicol Teratol 1984; 6:271.

257. Marcus J, Hans SL, Jeremy RJ. A longitudinal study of offspring born to methadone-maintained women. III. Effects of multiple risk factors on development at 4, 8, and 12 months. Am J Drug Alcohol Abuse 1984; 10:195.

258. Oats JN, Beischer NA, Breheny JE, Pepperell RJ. The outcome of pregnancies complicated by narcotic drug addiction. Aust N Z J Obstet Gynaecol 1984; 24:14.

259. Strauss ME, Reynolds KS. Psychological characteristics and development of narcotic-addicted infants. Drug Alcohol Depend 1983; 12:381.

260. Lifeschitz MH, Wilson GS, Smith EO, Desmond MM. Factors affecting head growth and intellectual function in children of drug addicts. Pediatrics 1985; 75:269.

261. Eyler FD, Behnke M. Early development of infants exposed to drugs prenatally. Clin Perinatol 1999; 26: 107.

261a. Lester BM, Lagasse L, Seifer R, et al: The Maternal Lifestyle Study (MLS): effects of prenatal cocaine or opiate exposure on auditory brain response at one month. J Pediatr 2003; 142:279.

262. Barr HL, Antes D, Oldenberg DJ, Rosen A. Mortality of treated alcoholics and drug addicts: the benefits of abstinence. J Stud Alcohol 1984; 45:440.

263. Cherubin CE. The medical sequelae of narcotic addiction. Ann Intern Med 1967; 67:23.

264. Ghodse AH, Sheehan M, Taylor C, Edwards G. Deaths of drug addicts in the United Kingdom, 1967–1981. BMJ 1985; 290:425.

265. Haastrop S, Jepson PW. Seven year follow-up of 300 young drug abusers. Acta Psychiatr Scand 1984; 70:503.

266. Steentoft A, Worm K, Christensen H. Morphine concentrations in autopsy material from fatal cases after intake of morphine and/or heroin. J Forensic Sci Soc 1988; 28:87.

267. Ruttenber AJ, Luke JL. Heroin-related deaths: new epidemiologic insight. Science 1984; 226:14.

268. Centers for Disease Control. Heroin-related deaths—District of Colombia, 1980–1982. MMWR 1983; 32:321.

269. Darke S, Hall W. Weatherburn D, Lind B. Fluctuations in heroin purity and the incidence of fatal heroin overdose. Drug Alcohol Depend 1999; 54:155.

270. Ruttenber AJ, Kalter HD, Santinga P. The role of ethanol abuse in the etiology of heroin-related death. J Forens Sci 1990; 35:891.

271. Introna F, Smialek JE. The "mini-packer syndrome." Fatal injection of drug containers in Baltimore, Maryland. Am J Forens Med Pathol 1989; 10:21.

272. Stewart A, Heaton ND, Hognin B. Body packing—a case report and review of the literature. Postgrad Med J 1990; 66:659.

272a. Traub SJ, Hoffman RS, Nelson LS: Body packing–the internal concealment of illicit drugs. N Engl J Med 2003; 349:2519.

273. Wetli CV, Rao A, Rao VJ. Fatal heroin body packing. Am J Forensic Med Pathol 1997; 18:312.

274. Joynt BP, Mikhael NZ. Sudden death of a heroin body packer. J Anal Toxicol 1985; 9:238.

275. Simpson LR. Sudden death while attempting to conceal drugs; laryngeal obstruction by a package of heroin. J Forens Sci 1976; 21:378.

276. Baker A. Boy sickened by heroin he swallowed. NY Times, April 12, 2002.

277. Wren CS. A pipeline of the poor feeds the flow of heroin. NY Times, February 21, 1999.

277a. Wetli CV, Rao A, Rao VJ. Fatal heroin body packing. Am J Forensic Med Pathol 1997; 18:312.

278. Sperry K. An epidemic of intravenous narcoticism deaths associated with the resurgence of black tar heroin. J Forens Sci 1988; 33:1156.

279. Monforte JR. Some observations concerning blood morphine concentrations in narcotic addicts. J Forens Sci 1977; 22:718.

280. Osler W. Oedema of left lung—morphia poisoning. Montreal Gen Hosp Rep 1880; 1:291.

281. Levine LH, Hiroch CS, White LW. Quinine cardiotoxicity: a mechanism for sudden death in narcotic addicts. J Forensic Sci 1973; 18:167.

282. Labi M. Paroxysmal atrial fibrillation in heroin intoxication. Ann Intern Med 1969; 71:951.

283. Lipaki J, Stimmel B, Donoso E. The effect of heroin and multiple drug abuse on the electrocardiogram. Am Heart J 1973; 86:663.

284. Hughes S, Calverley PM. Heroin inhalation and asthma. BMJ 1988; 297:1511.

285. Kurtin P, Wagner J. Deep vein thrombosis in intravenous drug abusers presenting as a systemic illness. Am J Med Sci 1984; 287:44.

286. Magnan A, Ottomani A, Garbe L, et al. Détresse éspiratoire chez une heroinomane seropositive pour le virus de l'immunodeficience humaine. Ann Fr Anesth Reanim 1991; 10:74.

287. deAraujo MS, Gerard F, Chossegros P, et al. Vascular hepatotoxicity related to heroin addiction. Virchows Arch [A] 1990; 417:497.

288. Sandgren JE, McPhee MS, Greenberger NJ. Narcotic bowel syndrome treatment with clonidine. Ann Intern Med 1984; 101:331.

289. Pastan RS, Silverman SL, Goldenberg DL. A musculoskeletal syndrome in intravenous heroin users. Association with brown heroin. Ann Intern Med 1977; 87:22.

290. Dettmeyer R, Stojanovski G, Madea B. Pathogenesis of heroin-associated glomerulonephritis. Correlation between the inflammatory activity and renal deposits of immunoglobulin and complement? Forensic Sci Int 2000; 113:227.

291. Cunningham EE, Brentjens JR, Zielezny MA, et al. Heroin nephropathy: a clinicopathologic and epidemiologic study. Am J Med 1980; 47:58.

292. Dubrow A, Mittman N, Ghali V, Flamenbaun W. The changing spectrum of heroin-associated nephropathy. Am J Kidney Dis 1985; 5:36.

293. Overland ES, Nolan AJ, Hopewell PC. Alteration of pulmonary function in intravenous drug abusers: prevalence, severity, and characterization of gas exchange abnormalities. Am J Med 1980; 68:231.

294. Giugliano D, Quatraro A, Ceriello A, D'Onofrio F. Endogenous opiates, heroin addiction, and non-insulin dependent diabetes. Lancet 1985; II:769.

295. Savona S, Nardi MA, Lennette ET, Karpatkin S. Thrombocytopenia purpura in narcotic addicts. Ann Intern Med 1985; 102:737.

296. Brown LS, Kreek MJ, Trepo C, et al. Human immunodeficiency virus and viral hepatitis seroepidemiology in New York City intravenous drug abusers (IVDAs). NIDA Res Monogr 1990; 95:443.

297. van den Hoek JA, van Haastrecht HJ, Goudsmit J, et al. Prevalence, incidence, and risk factors of hepatitis C virus infection among drug users in Amsterdam. J Infect Dis 1990; 162:823.

298. Gimeno V, Escudero A, Gonzales R, et al. Hepatitis agunda en heroinomanos: estudio etiologico y evolutivo de 110 casos. Rev Clin Esp 1989; 184:360.

299. Shade CP, Komorwska D. Continuing outbreak of hepatitis A, linked with intravenous drug abuse in Multnomah County. Public Health Rep 1988; 105:452.

300. Purchase D, Mottram K, Miron C, et al. Hepatitis B vaccination for injection drug users–Pierce County, Washington, 2000. MMWR 2001; 50:388.

301. Davis GL, Rodrique JR. Treatment of chronic hepatitis C in active drug users. N Engl J Med 2001; 345:215.

302. Thomas DL, Vlahov D, Solomon L, et al. Correlates of hepatitis C virus infections among injection drug users. Medicine 1995; 74:212.

303. Lorvick J, Kral AH, Seal K, et al. Prevalence and duration of hepatitis C among injection drug users in San Francisco, Calif. Am J Public Health 2001; 91:46.

304. Appel PW, Joseph H, Richman BL. Causes and rates of death among methadone maintenance patients before and after the onset of the HIV/AIDS epidemic. Mt Sinai J Med 2000; 67:444.

304a. Stephenson J. Former heroin addicts face barriers to treatment for HCV. JAMA 2001; 285:1003.

304b. Edlin BR, Seal KH, Lorvick J, et al. Is it justifiable to withhold treatment for hepatitis C from illicit drug users? N Engl J Med 2001; 345:211.

305. Ciccarone D, Bamberger JD, Kral AH, et al. Soft tissue infections among injection drug users-San Francisco, California, 1996–2000. MMWR 2001; 50:381.

306. Gattell JM, Miro JM, Para C, Garcia-San Miguel J. Infective endocarditis in drug addicts. Lancet 1984; I:228.

307. Hubbell G, Cheitlin MD, Rapaport E. Presentation, management, and follow-up of infective endocarditis in drug addicts. Am Heart J 1981; 138:85.

308. Novick DM, Ness GL. Abuse of antibiotics by abusers of parenteral heroin or cocaine. South Med J 1984; 77:302.

309. Tuazo n CU, Sheagren JN. Staphylococcal endocarditis in parenteral drug abusers: source of the organism. Ann Intern Med 1975; 82:788.

310. Reyes MP, Palutke WA, Wylin RF, et al. *Pseudomonas endocarditis* in the Detroit Medical Center, 1969–1972. Medicine 1973; 52:173.

311. Harris PD, Yeoh CB, Breault J, et al. Fungal endocarditis secondary to drug addiction. Recent concepts in diagnosis and therapy. J Thorac Cardiovasc Surg 1972; 6:980.

312. Pollack S, Magtader A, Lange M. *Neisseria subflava* endocarditis. Case report and review of the literature. Am J Med 1984; 76:752.

313. Vartian CV, Shlaes DM, Padhye AA, Ajello L. *Wangiella dermatitides* endocarditis in an intravenous drug user. Am J Med 1985; 78:703.

314. Ubeda Ruiz P, Gutierrez Martin I, Ramirez Galleymore D, et al. Endocarditis due to *Gemella*

morbillorum in a parenteral drug-abuse addict. Rev Clin Espanola 2000; 200:176.

315. Bick RL, Anhalt JE. Malaria transmission among narcotic addicts: a report of 10 cases and review of the literature. Calif Med 1971; 115:56.

316. Gonzalez-Garcia JJ, Arnalich F, Pena JM, et al. An outbreak of *Plasmodium vivax* malaria among heroin users in Spain. Trans R Soc Trop Med Hyg 1986; 80:549.

317. Lopez-Cortes L, Lozamo deLeon F, Gomez-Mateos JM, et al. Tick-borne relapsing fever in intravenous drug abusers. J Infect Dis 1989; 159:804.

318. Christie B. Gangrene bug killed 35 heroin users. West J Med 2000; 173:82.

319. Ringertz SH, Hoiby EA, Jenenius M, et al. Injectional anthrax in a heroin skin-popper. Lancet 2000; 356:1574.

320. Maki DG, Klein BS, McCormick RD, et al. Nosocomial *Pseudomonas pickettii* bacteremias traced to narcotic tampering: a case for selective drug screening of health care personnel. JAMA 1991; 265:981.

321. Ostrowsky BE, Whitener C, Bredenberg HK. *Serratia marcescens* bacteremia traced to an infused narcotic. N Engl J Med 2002; 346:1529.

322. Koppel BS, Tuchman AJ, Mangiardi JR, et al. Epidural spinal infection in intravenous drug abusers. Arch Neurol 1988; 45:1331.

323. Jabbari B, Pierce JF. Spinal cord compression due to *Pseudomonas* in a heroin addict. Neurology 1977; 27:1034.

324. Kaplan SS. *Pseudomonas* disc space infection in an occasional heroin user. Ariz Med 1974; 31:916.

325. Messer HD, Litvinoff J. Pyogenic cervical osteomyelitis. Arch Neurol 1976; 33:571.

326. Endress C, Guyot DR, Fata J, Salciccioli G. Cervical osteomyelitis due to IV heroin use: radiologic findings in 14 patients. AJR Am J Roentgenol 1990; 155:133.

327. Lewis R, Gorback S, Alter P. Spinal *Pseudomonas* chondroosteomyelitis in heroin users. N Engl J Med 1972; 286:1330.

328. Wiesseman GJ, Wood VE, Kroll LL. *Pseudomonas* vertebral osteomyelitis in heroin addicts: report of five cases. J Bone Joint Surg Am 1973; 55:1416.

329. Smith MA, Trowers NRH, Klein RS. Cervical osteomyelitis caused by *Pseudomonas cepecia* in an intravenous drug abuser. J Clin Microbiol 1985; 21:445.

330. Sverzut JM, Laval C, Smadja P, et al. Spinal cord abscess in a heroin addict. Case report. Neuroradiology 1998; 40:455.

331. Derkinderen P, Bruneel F, Bouchaud O, Regnier B. Spondylodiscitis and epidural abscess due to *Candida albicans*. Eur Spine J 2000; 9:72.

332. Amine AB. Neurosurgical complications of heroin addiction: brain abscess and mycotic aneurysm. Surg Neurol 1977; 7:385.

333. Gilroy J, Andaya L, Thomas VJ. Intracranial mycotic aneurysms and subacute endocarditis in heroin addiction. Neurology 1973; 23:1193.

334. Greenman RL, Arcey SM, Gutterman DA, Zweig RM. Twice-daily intramuscular ceforanide therapy of *Staphylococcus aureus* endocarditis in parenteral drug abusers. Antimicrob Agents Chemother 1984; 25:16.

335. Jaffe RB. Cardiac and vascular involvement in drug abuse. Semin Roentgenol 1983; 18:207.

336. Brust JCM, Dickinson PCT, Hughes JEO, Holtzman RHH. The diagnosis and treatment of cerebral mycotic aneurysm. Ann Neurol 1990; 27:238.

337. Ho K, Rassekh Z. Mycotic aneurysm of the right subclavian artery. A complication of heroin addiction. Chest 1978; 74:116.

338. Ledgerwood AM, Lucas CE. Mycotic aneurysm of the carotid artery. Arch Surg 1974; 109:496.

339. Navarro C, Dickinson PCT, Kondlapoedi P, Hagstrom JW. Mycotic aneurysm of the pulmonary arteries in intravenous drug addicts. Report of three cases and review of the literature. Am J Med 1984; 76:1124.

340. Talan DA, Maran GJ. Tetanus among injecting drug users—California, 1997. Ann Emerg Med 1998; 32:385.

341. Brust JCM, Richter RW. Tetanus in the inner city. N Y State J Med 1974; 74:1735.

342. Heurich AE, Brust JCM, Richter RW. Management of urban tetanus. Med Clin North Am 1973; 57:1373.

343. Redmond J, Stritch M, Blaney P. Severe tetanus in a narcotic addict. Ir Med J 1984; 77:325.

344. Abrahamian FM, Pollack CV, LoVecchio F, et al. Fatal tetanus in a drug abuser with "protective" antitetanus antibodies. J Emerg Med 2000; 18:189.

345. Jensen T, Jacobsen D, von der Lippe E, et al. Clinical wound botulism in injecting drug addicts. Tidsskr Norske Laegeforen 1998; 118:4363.

346. Hiersemenzel LP, Jermann M, Waespe W. Descending paralysis caused by wound botulism. A case report. Nervenarzt 2000; 71:130.

347. Martin C, Schaller MD, Lepori M, Liaudet L. Cranial nerve palsies and descending paralysis in a drug abuser resulting from wound botulism. Intensive Care Med 1999; 25:765.

348. Mulleague L, Bonner SM, Samuel A, et al. Wound botulism in drug addicts in the United Kingdom. Anaesthesia 2001; 56:120.

349. Werner SB, Passaro D, McGee J, et al. Wound botulism in California, 1951–1998: recent epidemic in heroin injectors. Clin Infect Dis 2000; 31:1018.

350. Jensenius M, Lovstad RZ, Dhaenens G, Rorvik IM. A heroin user with a wobbly head. Lancet 2000; 356:1160.

351. MacDonald KL, Rutherford GW, Friedman SM, et al. Botulism and botulism-like illness in chronic drug abusers. Ann Intern Med 1985; 102:616.

352. Elston HR, Wang M, Loo LK. Arm abscesses caused by *Clostridium botulinum*. J Clin Microbiol 1991; 29:2678.

352a. Werner SB, Passaro D, McGee J, et al. Wound botulism in California, 1951–1998: recent epidemic in heroin injectors. Clin Infect Dis 2000; 31:1018.

353. Kao AW, Bonovich D, Solbrig M, et al. Wound botulism among "skin-popping" injection drug-users: a case series 1991–2002. Neurology 2003; 60 (Suppl 1): A104.

353a. Passaro DJ, Werner SB, McGee J, et al. Wound botulism associated with black tar heroin among injecting drug users. JAMA 1998; 279:859.

353b. Merrison AFA, Chidley KE, Dunnett J, et al. Wound botulism associated with subcutaneous drug use. BMJ 2002; 325:1020.

354. Robin L, Herman D, Redett R. Botulism in a pregnant woman. N Engl J Med 1996; 335:823.

354a. Wound botulism among black tar heroin users? Washington, 2003. MMWR 2003; 52:885.

355. Weber RJ, Band LC, de Costa B, et al. Neural control of immune function: opioids, opioid receptors and immunosuppression. NIDA Res Monogr 1991; 105:96.

356. Govitrapong P, Suttitum T, Kotchabhakdi N, Uneklabh T. Alterations of immune function in heroin addicts and heroin withdrawal subjects. J Pharmacol Exp Ther 1998; 286:883.

357. Chang K-J. Opioid peptides have actions on the immune system. Trends Neurosci 1984; 7:234.

358. Novick DM, Ochshorn M, Ghali V, et al. Natural killer cell activity and lymphocyte subsets in parenteral heroin abusers and long-term methadone maintenance patients. J Pharmacol Exp Ther 1989; 250:606.

359. Chmel H, Grieco MH. Cerebral mucormycosis and renal aspergillosis in heroin addicts without endocarditis. Am J Med Sci 1973; 266:225.

360. Hershewe GL, Davis LE, Bicknell JM. Primary cerebellar brain abscess from nocardiosis in a heroin addict. Neurology 1988; 38:1655.

361. Kasantikul V, Shuangshoti S, Taecholarn C. Primary phycomycosis of the brain in heroin addicts. Surg Neurol 1987; 28:468.

362. Morrow R, Wong B, Finkelstein WE, et al. Aspergillosis of the cerebral ventricles in a heroin abuser. Case report and review of the literature. Arch Intern Med 1983; 143:161.

363. Pierce PF, Soloman SL, Kaufman L, et al. *Zygomycetes* brain abscesses in narcotic addicts with serological diagnosis. JAMA 1982; 248:2881.

364. Kasantikul V, Shuangshoti S, Sampatanukul P. Primary chromoblastomycosis of the medulla oblongata: complication of heroin addiction. Surg Neurol 1988; 29:319.

365. Etienne M, Nemery A, Darcis JM, et al. Disseminated candidiasis in heroin addicts. Report of two cases and review of the literature. Acta Clin Belg 1986; 41:18.

366. Hay RJ. Systemic candidiasis in heroin addicts. BMJ 1986; 292:1096.

367. Rowe IF, Wright ED, Higgens CS, Burnie JP. Intravertebral infection due to *Candida albicans* in an intravenous heroin abuser. Ann Rheum Dis 1988; 47:522.

368. Leclech C, Cimon B, Chennebault JM, Verret JL. Pustular candidiasis in heroin addicts. Ann Dermatol Venereol 1997; 124:157.

369. Scheidegger C, Frei R. Disseminated candidiasis in a drug addict not using heroin. J Infect Dis 1989; 159:1007.

370. Klein A, Haller-Schober EM, Faulborn J. *Candida* endophthalmitis in drug abuse: case report. Ophthalmologe 2000; 97:619.

371. Martinez-Vazquez C, Fernandez-Ulloa J, Bardon J, et al. *Candida albicans* endophthalmitis in brown heroin: response to early vitrectomy preceded and followed by antifungal therapy. Clin Infect Dis 1998; 27:1134.

372. Hendrickse RG, Maxwell SM, Young R. Aflatoxins and heroin. BMJ 1989; 299:492.

373. Anderson RM, May RM. Understanding the AIDS epidemic. Sci Am 1992; 267:58.

374. Centers for Disease Control. HIV/AIDS Surveillance. Year End Edition. Atlanta, GA: DHHS, 1992.

375. Spira TJ, DesJarlais DC, Marmor M, et al. Prevalence of antibody to lymphadenopathy-associated virus among drug-detoxification patients in New York. N Engl J Med 1984; 311:467.

376. Layon J, Idris A, Warzyunski M, et al. Altered T-lymphocyte subsets in hospitalized intravenous drug abusers. Arch Intern Med 1984; 144:1376.

377. Mandelli C, Cesana M, Ferroni P, et al. HBV, HDV, and HIV infections in 242 drug addicts: two-year follow-up. Eur J Epidemiol 1988; 4:318.

378. Schoenbaum EE, Hartel D, Selwyn PA, et al. Risk factors for human immunodeficiency virus infection in intravenous drug users. N Engl J Med 1989; 321:874.

379. Schrager L, Friedland G, Feiner C, Kahl P. Demographic characteristics, drug use, and sexual behavior of IV drug users with AIDS in Bronx, New York. Public Health Rep 1991; 106:78.

380. Saxon A, Calsyn DA, Whittaker S, Freeman G. Needle obtainment and cleaning habits of addicts. NIDA Res Monogr 1990; 95:418.

381. Ingold FR, Ingold S. The effects of the liberalization of syringe sales on the behavior of intravenous drug users in France. Bull Narc 1989; 41:67.

382. Singh MP, McKnight CA, Paone D, et al. Update: syringe exchange programs—United States, 1998. MMWR 1999; 50:384.

382a. DesJarlais DC, Friedman SR, Novick DM, et al. HIV-1 infection among intravenous drug users in Manhattan, New York City, from 1977 through 1987. JAMA 1989; 261:1008.

383. Beyrer C, Razak MH, Lisam K, et al. Overland heroin trafficking routes and HIV-I spread in south and southeast Asia. AIDS 2000; 14:75.

384. Brookmeyer R. Reconstruction and future trends of the AIDS epidemic in the United States. Science 1991; 253:37.

385. Friedman LN, Williams MT, Singh TP, et al. Tuberculosis, AIDS, and death among substance abusers on welfare in New York City. N Engl J Med 1996; 334:828.

386. Bishburg E, Sunderam G, Reichman LB, Kapila R. Central nervous system tuberculosis with the acquired immunodeficiency syndrome and its related complex. Ann Intern Med 1986; 105:210.

387. Mallolas J, Gatell JM, Rovira M, et al. Vertebral arch tuberculosis in two human immunodeficiency virus-seropositive heroin addicts. Arch Intern Med 1988; 148:125.

388. Barnes PF, Bloch AB, Davidson PT, Snider DE. Tuberculosis in patients with human immunodeficiency virus infection. N Engl J Med 1991; 324:1644.

389. Havlir DV, Barnes PF. Tuberculosis in patients with human immunodeficiency virus infection. N Engl J Med 1999; 340:367.

390. Graham NMH, Nelson KE, Solomon L, et al. Prevalence of tuberculin positivity and skin test anergy in HIV-l-seropositive and seronegative intravenous drug users. JAMA 1992; 267:369.

391. Frieden TR, Sterling T, Pablos-Mendez A, et al. The emergence of drug-resistant tuberculosis in New York City. N Engl J Med 1993; 328:521.

392. Lukehart SA, Hook EW, Baker-Zander SA, et al. Invasion of the central nervous system by T. pallidum: implications for diagnosis and treatment. Ann Intern Med 1988; 109:855.

393. Feraru ER, Aronow HA, Lipton RB. Neurosyphilis in AIDS patients: initial CSF VDRL may be negative. Neurology 1990; 49:541.

394. Johns DR, Tierney M, Felsenstein D. Alteration in the natural history of neurosyphilis by concurrent infection with the human immunodeficiency virus. N Engl J Med 1987; 316:1569.

395. Berry CD, Hooten TM, Collier AC, Lukehart SA. Neurologic relapse after benzathine penicillin therapy for secondary syphilis in a patient with HIV infection. N Engl J Med 1987; 316:1587.

396. Katz DA, Berger JR. Neurosyphilis in acquired immunodeficiency syndrome. Arch Neurol 1989; 46:895.

397. Musher DM, Hammill RJ, Baughn RE. The effect of human immunodeficiency virus infection on the course of syphilis and the response to treatment. Ann Intern Med 1990; 113:872.

398. Musher DM. Syphilis, neurosyphilis, penicillin, and AIDS. J Infect Dis 1991; 163:1201.

399. Berger JR. Neurosyphilis in human immunodeficiency virus type 1-seropositive individuals. Arch Neurol 1991; 48:700.

400. Katz DA, Berger JR, Duncan RC. Neurosyphilis. A comparative study of the effects of infection with human immunodeficiency virus. Arch Neurol 1993; 50:243.

401. Lopez-Zetina J, Ford W, Weber M, et al. Predictors of syphilis seroreactivity and prevalence of HIV among street recruited injection drug users in Los Angeles County, 1994–6. Sex Transm Infect 2000; 76:462.

402. Anders KH, Guerra WF, Tomiyasu U, et al. The neuropathology of AIDS. UCLA experience and review. Am J Pathol 1986; 124:537.

403. Anders K, Verity MA, Concilla PA, Vinters HV. Acquired immune deficiency syndrome (AIDS): neuropathologic studies. J Neuropathol Exp Neurol 1984; 43:315.

404. Berger JR, Moskowitz L, Fischl M, Kelly RE. Neurologic disease as the presenting manifestation of acquired immunodeficiency syndrome. South Med J 1987; 80:683.

405. Britton CB. HIV infection. In: Brust JCM, ed. Neurologic Complications of Drug and Alcohol Abuse. Neurol Clin 1993; 11:605–624.

406. Porter SB, Sande MA. Toxoplasmosis of the central nervous system in the acquired immunodeficiency syndrome. N Engl J Med 1992; 327:1643.

407. Koppel BS, Wormser GP, Tuchman AJ, et al. Central nervous system involvement in patients with acquired immune deficiency syndrome. Acta Neurol Scand 1983; 71:337.

408. McArthur JC. Neurologic manifestations of AIDS. Medicine 1987; 66:407.

409. Malouf R, Dobkin J, Jacquette G, Brust JCM. Neurologic complications of HIV infection in parenteral drug abusers. Arch Neurol 1990; 47:1002.

410. Levy RM, Janssen RS, Bush TJ, Rosenbaum ML. Neuroepidemiology of acquired immunodeficiency syndrome. AIDS 1988; 1:31.

411. Concha M, Selnes OA, Munoz A, et al. Factors associated with neuropsychological performance in a cohort of intravenous drug users (IVDUs) infected with HIV-1. Neurology 1992; 42 (Suppl 3):192.

412. Selnes OA, Galai N, McArthur JC, et al. HIV infection and cognition in intravenous drug users: long-term follow-up. Neurology 1997; 48:223.

413. Coates RA, Farewell VT, Raboud J, et al. Co-factors of progression to acquired immunodeficiency syndrome in a cohort of male sexual contacts of men with human immunodeficiency virus disease. Am J Epidemiol 1990; 132:717.

414. Margolick JB, Munoz A, Vlahov D, et al. Changes in T-lymphocyte subsets in intravenous drug users with HIV-1 infection. JAMA 1992; 267:1631.

415. Selwyn PA, Alcabes P, Hartel D, et al. Clinical manifestations and predictors of disease progression in drug users with human immunodeficiency virus infection. N Engl J Med 1992; 327:1697.

416. Bonetti A, Weber R, Vogt MW, et al. Co-infection with human immunodeficiency virus type 1 (HIV-1) and cytomegalovirus in two intravenous drug users. Ann Intern Med 1989; 111:293.

417. Lee H, Swanson P, Shorty VS, et al. High rate of HTLV-II infection in seropositive IV drug abusers in New Orleans. Science 1989; 244:471.

418. Robert-Guroff M, Weiss SH, Giron JA. Prevalence of antibodies to HTLV-I, II, and III in intravenous drug abusers from an AIDS epidemic region. JAMA 1986; 255:3133.

419. Gradilone A, Zani M, Barillari G, et al. HTLV-I and HIV infection in drug addicts in Italy. Lancet 1986; II:753.

420. Khabbaz RF, Onorato IM, Cannon RO, et al. Seroprevalence of HTLV-I and HTLV-II among intravenous drug users and persons in clinics for sexually transmitted diseases. N Engl J Med 1992; 326:375.

421. Zanetti AR, Galli C. Seroprevalence of HTLV-I and HTLV-II. N Engl J Med 1992; 326:1783.

422. Parry GJ, Erlemeier S, Malamut R, Garcia C. HTLV-I-associated myelopathy (HAM) in native Louisiana drug abusers. Neurology 1990; 40 (Suppl): 239.

423. Honig LS, Lipka JJ, Young KK, et al. HTLV-I-associated myelopathy in a Californian: diagnosis by reactivity to a viral recombinant antigen. Neurology 1991; 41:448.

424. McKendall RR, Oas J, Lairmore MD. HTLV-I-associated myelopathy endemic in Texas-born residents and isolation of virus from CSF cells. Neurology 1991; 41:831.

425. Berger JR, Svenningsson A, Raffanti S, Resnick L. Tropical spastic paraparesis-like illness occurring in a patient dually infected with HIV-I and HTLV-II. Neurology 1991; 41:85.

426. Berger JR, Svenningsson A, McCarthy M, et al. The role of HTLV in HIV-I neurologic disease. Neurology 1991; 41:197.

427. Jacobson S, Lehky T, Nishimura M, et al. Isolation of HTLV-II from a patient with chronic progressive neurological disease clinically indistinguishable from HTLV-I-associated myelopathy/tropical spastic paraparesis. Ann Neurol 1993; 33:392.

428. Janssen RS, Kaplan JE, Khabbaz RF, et al. HTLV-I-associated myelopathy/tropical spastic paraparesis in the United States. Neurology 1991; 41:1355.

429. Brust JCM, Richter RW. Stroke associated with addiction to heroin. J Neurol Neurosurg Psychiatry 1976; 39:194.

430. Lignelli GJ, Buchheit WA. Angiitis in drug abusers. N Engl J Med 1971; 284:112.

431. Woods BT, Strewler GJ. Hemiparesis occurring six hours after intravenous heroin injection. Neurology 1972; 22:863.

432. King J, Richards M, Tress B. Cerebral arteritis associated with heroin abuse. Med J Aust 1978; 2:444.

433. Herskowitz A, Gross E. Cerebral infarction associated with heroin sniffing. South Med J 1973; 66:778.

434. Bartolomei F, Nicoli F, Swaider L, et al. Accident vasculaire cérébral ischémique après prise nasale d'heroine. Une nouvelle observation. Presse Med 1992; 21:983.

435. Jensen R, Olsen TS, Winther BB. Severe non-occlusive ischemic stroke in young heroin addicts. Acta Neurol Scand 1990; 81:354.

436. Celius EG. Neurologic complications in heroin abuse: illustrated by two unusual cases. Tidsskrift Norske Laegeforen 1997; 117:356.

437. Knoblauch AL, Buchholz M, Koller MG, Kistler H. Hemiplegie nach Injektion von Heroin. Schweiz Med Wochenschr 1983; 113:402.

438. Sloan MA, Kittner SJ, Rigamonti D, Price TR. Occurrence of stroke associated with use/abuse of drugs. Neurology 1991; 41:1358.

439. Kortikale Blindheit nach Heroin intoxication. Nukleomedizin 2000; 2:N16-N19.

440. Munoz Casares FC, Serrano Castro P, Linan Lopez M, et al. Sudden aphasia in a young woman. Rev Clin Esp 1999; 199:325.

440a. Niehaus L, Meyer BU: Bilateral borderzone brain infarctions in association with heroin abuse, J Neurol Sci 1998; 160:180.

441. Hall JH, Karp HR. Acute progressive ventral pontine disease in heroin abuse. Neurology 1973; 23:6.

442. Brust JCM. Stroke and substance abuse. In: Barnett HJM, Mohr JP, Stein BM, Yatsu FM, eds. Stroke: Pathophysiology, Diagnosis, and Management, 3rd edn. New York: Churchill-Livingstone, 1998:979.

443. Niehaus L, Roricht S, Meyer BU, et al. Nuclear magnetic resonance tomography detection of heroin-associated CNS lesions. Akt Radiol 1997; 7:309.

444. Anderson SN, Skullerud K. Hypoxic/ischemic brain damage, especially pallidal lesions, in heroin addicts. Forensic Sci Int 1999; 102:51.

445. Vila N, Chamorro A. Balistic movements due to ischemic infarcts after intravenous heroin overdose: report of two cases. Clin Neurol Neurosurg 1997; 99:259.

446. Schoser BG, Groden C. Subacute onset of oculogyric crises and generalized dystonia following intranasal administration of heroin. Addiction 1999; 94:431.

446a. Niehaus L, Roricht S, Meyer BU, et al. Nuclear magnetic resonance tomography detection of heroin-associated CNS lesions. Aktuel Radiol 1997; 7:309.

447. Protass LM. Delayed post-anoxic encephalopathy after heroin use. Ann Intern Med 1971; 74:738.

448. Hirsch CS. Dermatopathology of narcotic addiction. Hum Pathol 1972; 3:37.

449. Ostor A. The medical complications of narcotic addiction. Med J Aust 1977; 1:497.

450. Atlee W. Talc and cornstarch emboli in eyes of drug abusers. JAMA 1972; 219:49.

451. Lahmeyer HW, Steingold RG. Pentazocine and tripelennamine: a drug abuse epidemic? Int J Addict 1980; 15:1219.

452. Wadley C, Stillie GD. Pentazocine (Talwin) and tripelennamine (Pyribenzamine): a new drug combination or just a revival? Int J Addict 1980; 15:1285.

453. Caplan LR, Thomas C, Banks G. Central nervous system complications of addiction to "T's and Blues." Neurology 1982; 32:623.

454. Houck RJ, Bailey G, Daroca P, et al. Pentazocine abuse. Chest 1980; 77:227.

455. Szwed JJ. Pulmonary angiothrombosis caused by "blue velvet" addiction. Ann Intern Med 1970; 73:771.

456. Butz WC. Disseminated magnesium and silicate associated with paregoric addiction. J Forens Sci 1970; 15:581.

457. Lee J, Sapira JD. Retinal and cerebral microembolization of talc in a drug abuser. Am J Med Sci 1973; 265:75.

457a. Biter S, Gomez CR: Stroke following injection of a melted suppository. Stroke 1993; 24:741.

458. Ortona L, Laghi V, Cauda R. Immune function in heroin addicts. N Engl J Med 1979; 300:45.

459. Shaikh WA. Allergy to heroin. Allergy 1990; 45:555.

460. Ryan JJ, Parker CW, Williams RL. Gamma-globulin binding of morphine in heroin addicts. J Lab Clin Med 1972; 80:155.

461. Baranek JT. Morphine binding by serum globulins from morphine-treated rabbits. Fed Proc 1974; 33:474.

462. Garcia-Sevilla JA, Ugedo L, Ulibarri I, Guitierrez M. Platelet alpha-2 adrenoceptors in heroin addicts during withdrawal and after treatment with clonidine. Eur J Pharmacol 1985; 114:365.

463. Maqbool Z, Billett HH. Unwitting heparin abuse in a drug addict. Ann Intern Med 1982; 96:790.

464. Ell JJ, Unley D, Silver JR. Acute myelopathy in association with heroin addiction. J Neurol Neurosurg Psychiatry 1981; 44:448.

465. Goodhart LC, Loizou LA, Anderson M. Heroin myelopathy. J Neurol Neurosurg Psychiatry 1982; 45:562.

466. Grassa C, Montanari E, Scaglioni A, et al. Acute heroin myelopathy—case report. Ital J Neurol Sci 1984; 5:63.

467. Guidotti M, Passerini D, Brambilla M, Landi G. Heroin myelopathy. A case report. Ital J Neurol Sci 1985; 6:99.

468. Judice DJ, LeBlanc HJ, McGarry PA. Spinal cord vasculitis presenting as spinal cord tumor in a heroin addict. J Neurosurg 1978; 48:131.

469. Krause GS. Brown-Sequard syndrome following heroin injection. Ann Emerg Med 1983; 12:581.

470. Lee MC, Randa DC, Gold LH. Transverse myelopathy following the use of heroin. Minn Med 1976; 59:82.

471. Pearson J, Richter RW, Baden MM, et al. Transverse myelopathy as an illustration of the neurologic and neuropathologic features of heroin addiction. Hum Pathol 1972; 3:109.

472. Richter RW, Rosenberg RN. Transverse myelitis associated with heroin addiction. JAMA 1968; 206:1255.

473. Rodriguez E, Smokvina M, Sokolow J, Grynbaum BB. Encephalopathy and paraplegia occurring with the use of heroin. N Y State J Med 1971; 71:2879.

474. Schein PS, Yessayun L, Mayman CI. Acute transverse myelitis associated with intravenous opium. Neurology 1971; 21:101.

475. Thompson WR, Waldman MB. Cervical myelopathy following heroin administration. J Med Soc N J 1970; 67:223.

476. McCreary M, Emerman C, Hanna J, Simon J. Acute myelopathy following intranasal insufflation of heroin: a case report. Neurology 2000; 55:31.

477. Fleishon H, Mandel S, Arenas A. Anterior spinal artery syndrome after cervical injection of heroin. Arch Neurol 1982; 39:739.

477a. Berger AR, Schaumburg HH, Gourevitch MN, et al: Prevalence of peripheral neuropathy in injection drug users. Neurology 1999; 53:592.

478. Smith WR, Wilson AF. Guillain-Barré syndrome in a heroin addict. JAMA 1975; 231:1367.

479. Ammueilaph R, Boongird P, Leechawengwongs M, Vejjajiva A. Heroin neuropathy. Lancet 1973; I:1517.

480. Loizou LA, Boddie HG. Polyradiculoneuropathy associated with heroin abuse. J Neurol Neurosurg Psychiatry 1978; 41:855.

481. Ritland D, Butterfield W. Extremity complications of drug abuse. Am J Surg 1973; 126:639.

482. Colavita N, Orazi C, LaVecchia G, et al. An unusual kind of muscular and skeletal involvement in a heroin addict. Arch Orthop Trauma Surg 1984; 103:140.

483. Kaku DA, So YT. Acute femoral neuropathy and iliopsoas infarction in intravenous drug abusers. Neurology 1990; 40:1317.

484. Challenor YB, Richter RW, Bruun B, Pearson J. Non-traumatic plexitis and heroin addiction. JAMA 1973; 225:958.

485. Herdmann J, Benecke R, Meyer BU, Freund HJ. Erfolgreiche Kortikeidbehandlung einer lumbosakralen Plexusneuropathie bei Heroinabusus. Klinik, Electrophysiologie, Therapie und Verlauf. Nervenarzt 1988; 59:683.

486. Stamboulis E, Psimaris A, Malliara-Loulakaki S. Brachial and lumbar plexitis as a reaction to heroin. Drug Alcohol Depend 1988; 22:205.

487. Hecker E, Friedli WG. Plexusiasionen, Rhabdomyolysis, und Heroin. Schweiz Med Wochenschr 1988;118: 1982.

488. Delcker A, Dux R, Diener HC. Akute Plexuslasionen bei Heroinabhangigkeit. Nervenarzt 1992; 63:240.

489. Diaz Guzman J, Valverde CP, Grande RG, et al. Rhabdomyolysis and lumbosacral plexopathy in intravenous drug addict. Report of a case. Ann Med Interne (Paris) 1996; 13:84.

490. Riggs JE, Schochet SS, Hogg JP. Focal rhabdomyolysis and brachial plexopathy: an association with heroin and chronic ethanol use. Military Med 1999;164:228.

491. Wemeau J, Montagne B, Hazzen Decarpentry C. Parsonage-Turner amyotrophic neuralgia in 2 heroin addicts. Presse Med 1997; 26:165.

492. Miller CM, Sangiulo P, Schanzer H, et al. Infected false aneurysms of the subclavian artery: a complication in drug addicts. J Vasc Surg 1984; 1:684.

493. Raz S, Ramanathan V. Injection injuries of the recurrent laryngeal nerve. Laryngoscope 1984; 94:197.

494. Hillstrom RP, Cohn AM, McCarroll KA. Vocal cord paralysis resulting from neck injections in the

intravenous drug use population. Laryngoscope 1990; 100:503.

495. Polpathapee S, Tuchinda P, Chiwapong S. Sensorineural hearing loss in a heroin addict. J Med Assoc Thai 1984; 67:57.

496. Aeschlimann A, Mall T, Sandoz P, Probst A. Course and complications of rhabdomyolysis following heroin poisoning. Schweiz Med Wochenschr 1984; 114:1236.

497. Nolte KB, McDonough ET. Rhabdomyolysis and heroin abuse. Am J Forensic Med Pathol 1991; 12:273.

498. deGans J, Stan J, Van Winjungaarden GK. Rhabdomyolysis and neurological lesions after intravenous heroin abuse. J Neurol Neurosurg Psychiatry 1985; 48:1057.

499. Fames M, Radu EW, Harder F. Rabdomyolyse und Kompartment-syndrome bei Heroinabusus. Helv Chir Acta 1984; 50:745.

500. Gibb WR, Shaw IC. Myoglobinuria due to heroin abuse. J R Soc Med 1985; 78:862.

501. Kathrein H, Kirchmair W, Koning P, Diettrich P. Rhabdomyolyse mit akuten Nierenversagen nach Heroinintoxikation. Dtsch Med Wochenschr 1983; 108:464.

502. Owen CA, Mubarak SJ, Hargens AR, et al. Intramuscular pressures with limb compression. N Engl J Med 1979; 300:1169.

503. Penn AS, Rowland LP, Fraser DW. Drugs, coma, and myoglobinuria. Arch Neurol 1972; 26:336.

504. Richter RW, Challenor YB, Pearson J, et al. Acute myoglobinuria associated with heroin addiction. JAMA 1971; 216:1172.

505. Schreiber SN, Liebowitz MR, Bernstein LH. Limb compression and renal impairment (crush syndrome) following narcotic and sedative overdose. J Bone Joint Surg Am 1972; 54:1683.

506. Schwartzfarb L, Singh G, Marcus D. Heroin-associated rhabdomyolysis with cardiac involvement. Arch Intern Med 1977; 137:1255.

507. Chan YF, Wong PK, Chow TC. Acute myoglobinuria as a fatal complication of heroin addiction. Am J Forensic Med Pathol 1990; 11:160.

508. Claros-Gonzolez I, Banos-Gallardo M, Forascepi-Roza R, Arguelles-Torana M. Rabdomiolisis atraumatica y fracaso renal agudo secundario a sobredosis de heroina. Rev Clin Esp 1988; 182:338.

509. Richards JR. Rhabdomyolysis and drugs of abuse. J Emerg Med 2000; 19:51.

510. Rice EK, Isbel NM, Becker GJ, et al. Heroin overdose and myoglobinuric acute renal failure. Clin Nephrol 2000; 54:449.

511. Aunane D, Teboul JF, Richard C, Auzepy P. Severe rhabdomyolysis related to heroin sniffing. Intens Care Med 1990; 16:410.

512. Scherrer P, Delaloye-Bishchof A, Turini G, Perret C. Participation myocardique à la rhabdomyolyse non traumatique après surdosage aux opiaces. Schweiz Med Wochenschr 1985; 115:1116.

513. Kumar R, West DM, Jingree M, Laurence AS. Unusual consequences of heroin overdose: rhabdomyolysis, acute renal failure, paraplegia and hypercalcaemia. Br J Anaesth 1999; 83:496.

514. Yang CC, Yang GY, Ger J, et al. Severe rhabdomyolysis mimicking transverse myelitis in a heroin addict. J Toxicol Clin Toxicol 1995; 33:59.

515. Klockgether T, Weller M, Haarmeier T, et al. Gluteal compartment syndrome due to rhabdomyolysis after heroin abuse. Neurology 1997; 48:275.

516. Funk L, Grover D, deSilva H. Compartment syndrome of the hand following intraarterial injection of heroin. J Hand Surg [Br] 1999; 24:366.

517. Louis EO, Bodner R, Challenor Y, Brust JCM. Focal myopathy induced by chronic intramuscular heroin injection. Muscle Nerve 1994; 17:550.

518. Pena J, Aranda C, Luque E, Vaamonde R. Heroin-induced myopathy in rat skeletal muscle. Acta Neuropathol 1990; 80:72.

519. Brust JCM, Richter RW. Quinine amblyopia related to heroin addiction. Ann Intern Med 1971; 74:84.

520. Feeney GFX, Lee GA, O'Connor PA. Quinine-induced blindness during attempted heroin withdrawal. Med J Aust 1999; 170:449.

521. Dias PLR. Dyschromatopsia in heroin addicts. Br J Addict 1990; 85:241.

522. Dalessandro-Gandolfo L, Macci A, Biolcati G, et al. Inconsueta modalita d'intossicazione da piombo. Presentazione di un caso. Recenti Prog Med 1989; 80:140.

523. Antonini G, Palmieri G, Spagnoli G, Millefiorini M. Lead brachial neuropathy in heroin addiction. A case report. Clin Neurol Neurosurg 1989; 91:167.

524. Parras F, Patier JL, Ezpeteta C. Lead-contaminated heroin as a source of inorganic-lead intoxication. N Engl J Med 1987; 316:755.

525. O'Gorman P, Patel S, Notcutt S, Wicking J. Adulteration of "street" heroin with chloroquine. Lancet 1987; I:746.

526. Wolters ECH, Van Winjungaarden GK, Stam FC, et al. Leukoencephalopathy after inhaling "heroin pyrolysate." Lancet 1982; II:1233.

527. Schiffer D, Brignolio F, Giordena MT, et al. Spongiform encephalopathy in addicts inhaling pre-heated heroin. Clin Neuropathol 1985; 4:174.

528. Bianco C, Cocito D, Benna P, et al. Brain-stem auditory evoked potential alterations in heroin addicts. J Neurol 1985; 232:262.

529. Hungerbuhler H, Waespe W. Leukoencephalopathie nach Inhalation von Heroin-Pyrolysat. Schweiz Med Wochenschr 1990; 120:1801.

529a. Nyffeler T, Stabba A, Sturzenegger M: Progressive myelopathy with selective involvement of the lateral and posterior columns after inhalation of heroin vapor. J Neurol 2003; 250:496.

530. Strang J, Griffiths P, Gossop M. Heroin smoking by "chasing the dragon": origins and history. Addiction 1997; 92:673.

531. Chang YJ, Tsai CH, Chen CJ. Leukoencephalopathy after inhalation of heroin vapor. J Formosa Med Assoc 1997; 96:758.

532. Stohler R, Dursteler-MacFarland KM, Gramespacker C, et al. A comparison of heroin chasers with heroin injectors in Switzerland. Eur Addict Res 2000; 6:154.

533. Smyth BP, O'Brien M, Barry J. Trends in opiate misuse in Dublin: the emergence of chasing the dragon. Addiction 2000; 95:1217.

534. Chen CY, Lee KW, Lee CC, et al. Heroin-induced spongiform leukoencephalopathy: value of diffusion MR imaging. J Comp Assist Tomogr 2000; 24:73.

535. Hill MD, Cooper PW, Perry JR. Chasing the dragon—neurological toxicity associated with inhalation of heroin vapour: case report. Can Med Assoc J 2000; 162:236.

536. Kriegstein AR, Shungu DC, Millar WS, et al. Leukoencephalopathy and raised brain lactate from heroin vapor inhalation ("chasing the dragon"). Neurology 1999; 53:1765.

537. Rizzuto N, Marbin M, Ferrari S, et al. Delayed spongiform leukoencephalopathy after heroin abuse. Acta Neuropathol 1997; 94: 87.

538. Maschke M, Fehlings T, Kastrup O, et al. Toxic leukoencephalopathy after intravenous consumption of heroin and cocaine with unexpected clinical recovery. J Neurol 1999; 246:850.

539. Roulet Perez E, Maeder P, Rivier L, et al. Toxic leukencephalopathy after heroin ingestion in a $2\frac{1}{2}$-year-old child. Lancet 1992; 340:729.

540. Davis GC, Williams AC, Markey SP, et al. Chronic parkinsonism secondary to intravenous injection of meperidine analogues. Psychiatry Res 1979; 1:249.

541. Langston JW, Ballard P, Tetrud JW, Irwin I. Chronic parkinsonism in humans due to a product of meperidine-analog synthesis. Science 1983; 219: 9789.

542. Leads from the MMWR. Street drug contaminant causing parkinsonism. JAMA 1984; 252:331.

543. Stern Y. MPTP-induced parkinsonism. Prog Neurobiol 1990; 34:107.

544. Wright JM, Wall RA, Perry TL, Paty DW. Chronic parkinsonism secondary to intranasal administration of a product of meperidine-analogue synthesis. N Engl J Med 1984; 310:325.

545. Langston JW, Ballard PA. Parkinson's disease in a chemist working with 1-methyl-4-phenyl-1,2,5,6-tetrahydropyridine. N Engl J Med 1983; 309:310.

546. Ballard PA, Tetrud JW, Langston JW. Permanent human parkinsonism due to 1-methyl-4-phenyl-1,2,3, 6-tedrahydropyridine (MPTP): seven cases. Neurology 1985; 35:949.

547. Langston JW, Ballard P. Parkinsonism induced by 1-methyl-4-phenyl-1,2,3,6-tetrahydropyridine (MPTP): implications for treatment and the pathogenesis of Parkinson's disease. Can J Neurol Sci 1984; 11:160.

548. Langston JW. MPTP and Parkinson's disease. Trends Neurosci 1985; 8:79.

549. Burns RS, LeWitt PA, Ebert MH, et al. The clinical syndrome of striatal dopamine deficiency. Parkinsonism induced by 1-methyl-4-phenyl-1,2,3,6-tetrahydropyridine (MPTP). N Engl J Med 1985; 312:1418.

550. Langston JW, Forno LS, Rebert CS, Irwin I. Selective nigral toxicity after systemic administration of 1-methyl-4-phenyl-1,2,5,6-tetrahydropyridine (MPTP) in the squirrel monkey. Brain Res 1984; 292: 390.

551. Calne DB, Langston JW, Stoessl AJ, et al. Positron emission tomography after MPTP. Observations relating to the cause of Parkinson's disease. Nature 1986; 317:246.

552. Markey SP, Johannessen JN, Chiveh CC, et al. Intraneuronal generation of a pyridinium metabolite may cause drug-induced parkinsonism. Nature 1984; 311:464.

553. Heikkila RE, Manzino L, Cabbat FS, Duvoisin RC. Protection against the dopaminergic neurotoxicity of 1-methyl-4-phenyl-1,2,5,6-tetrahydropyridine by monoamine oxidase inhibitors. Nature 1984; 311:467.

554. Przedborski S, Vila M. MPTP: a review of its mechanisms of neurotoxicity. Clin Neurosci Res 2001; 1:407.

555. Ng SKC, Brust JCM, Hauser WA, Susser M. Illicit drug use and the risk of new onset seizures: contrasting effects of heroin, marijuana, and cocaine. Am J Epidemiol 1990; 40:1017.

556. Bohaus DW, Rigsbee LC, McNamara JO. Intranigral dynorphin 1–13 suppressed kindled seizures by a naloxone-sensitive mechanism. Brain Res 1987; 405:358.

557. Dua AK, Pinsky C, LaBella FS. Mu- and delta-opioid receptor mediated epileptoid responses in morphine-dependent and nondependent rats. Electroencephalogr Clin Neurophysiol 1985; 61:569.

558. Frey HH. Interactions between morphine-like analgesics and anticonvulsant drugs. Pharmacol Toxicol 1987; 60:210.

559. Garant DS, Gale K. Infusion of opiates into substantia nigra protects against maximal electroshock seizures in rats. J Pharmacol Exp Ther 1985; 234:45.

560. Ikonomidou-Turski C, Cavalheiro EA, Turski WA, et al. Convulsant action of morphine, [D-Ala2,-D-Leu5] enkephalin and naloxone in the rat amygdala: electroencephalographic, morphological, and behavioral sequelae. Neuroscience 1987; 20:671.

561. Tortella FC. Endogenous opioid peptides and epilepsy: quieting the seizing brain? Trends Pharmacol Sci 1988; 9:366.

562. Tortella FC, Robles L, Holaday JW. U50,488, a highly selective kappa opioid: anticonvulsant profile in rats. J Pharmacol Exp Ther 1986; 237:49.

563. Tortella FC, Robles L, Mosberg HI. Evidence for mu opioid receptor mediation of enkephalin-induced electroencephalographic seizures. J Pharmacol Exp Ther 1987; 240:571.

564. Walker GE, Yaksh TL. Studies on the effects of intrathecally injected DADL and morphine on nociceptive

thresholds and electroencephalographic activity: a thalamic delta receptor syndrome. Brain Res 1986; 383:1.

565. Ornstein TJ, Iddon JL, Baldacchino AM, et al. Profiles of cognitive dysfunction in chronic amphetamine and heroin abusers. Neuropsychopharmacology 2000; 23:113.

566. Haselhorst R, Dürsteler-MacFarland KM, Scheffler K, et al. Frontocortical *N*-acetylaspartate reduction associated with long-term IV heroin use. Neurology 2002; 58:305.

567. Eisch AJ, Barrot M, Schad CA, et al. Opiates inhibit neurogenesis in the adult rat hippocampus. Proc Natl Acad Sci USA 2000; 97:7579.

568. Ferrer-Alcon M, Garcia-Sevilla JA, Jaquet PE, et al. Regulation of nonphosphorylated and phosphorylated forms of neurofilament proteins in the prefrontal cortex of human opioid addicts. J Neurosci Res 2000; 61:338.

568a. Berthier ML, Campos VM, Kulisevsky J, Valero JA: Heroin and malignant coprolalia in Tourette's syndrome. J Neuropsychiatr Clin Neurosci 2003; 15:116.

569. Joranson DE, Ryan KM, Gilson AM, Dahl JI. Trends in medical use and abuse of opioid analgesics. JAMA 2000; 283:1710.

569a. Ballantyne JC, Mao J. Opioid therapy for chronic pain. N Engl J Med 2003; 349:1943.

570. Schuster CR, Smith BB, Jaffe JH. Drug abuse in heroin users: an experimental study of self-administration of methadone, codeine, and pentazocine. Arch Gen Psychiatry 1971; 24:359.

571. Lewis JR. Misprescribing analgesics. JAMA 1974; 228:1155.

572. Sandoval RG, Wang RIH. Tolerance and dependence on pentazocine. N Engl J Med 1969; 280:1391.

573. Choucair AK, Ziter FA. Pentazocine abuse masquerading as familial myopathy. Neurology 1984; 34:524.

574. Schlicher JE, Zuchlke RL, Lynch PJ. Local changes at the site of pentazocine injection. Arch Dermatol 1971; 104:90.

575. Steiner JC, Winkelman AC, deJesus PV. Pentazocine-induced myopathy. Arch Neurol 1973; 28:408.

576. Shannon HF, Su TP. Effects of the combination of tripelennamine and pentazocine at the behavioral and molecular levels. Pharmacol Biochem Behav 1982; 17:789.

577. Jasinski DR, Boren JJ, Henningfield JE, et al. Progress report from the NIDA Addiction Research Center, Baltimore, MD. In: Harris LS, ed. Problems of Drug Dependence 1983. Washington, DC: NIDA Research Monograph 49, DHHS, 1984:69.

578. Waller DP, Katz NL, Morris RW. Potentiation of lethality in mice by combinations of pentazocine and tripelennamine. Clin Toxicol 1980; 16:17.

579. Itkonen J, Schnoll S, Daghestani A, Glassroth J. Accelerated development of pulmonary complications due to illicit intravenous use of pentazocine and triplennamine. Am J Med 1984; 76:617.

580. Botsford KB, Weinstein RA, Nathan CR, Kabins SA. Selective survival in pentazocine and triplennamine of *Pseudomonas aeruginosa* serotype Oii from drug addicts. J Infect Dis 1985; 151:209.

581. Baum C, Hsu JP, Nelson RC. The impact of the addition of naloxone on the use and abuse of pentazocine. Public Health Rep 1987; 102:426.

582. Reed DA, Schnoll SH. Abuse of pentazocine-naloxone combination. JAMA 1986; 256:2562.

583. Evans WS, Bowen JN, Giordano FK, Clark BA. A case of Stadol dependence. JAMA 1985; 253:2191.

584. Brown GR. Stadol dependence: another case. JAMA 1985; 254:910.

585. Austin RP. Diversion of butorphanol. Am J Hosp Pharm 1983; 40:1306.

586. Smith SG, Davis WM. Nonmedical use of butorphanol and diphenhydramine. JAMA 1984; 252:1010.

587. Fisher MA, Glass S. Butorphanol (Stadol): a study in problems of current drug information and control. Neurology 1997; 48:1156.

588. AAN. Public relations efforts result in restrictions on migraine drug. AAN News 1997; 10:1.

589. Rasor RW, Orecraft HJ. Addiction to meperidine (Demerol) hydrochloride. JAMA 1955; 157:654.

590. Hershey LA. Meperidine and central neurotoxicity. Ann Intern Med 1983; 98:548.

591. Hochman MS. Meperidine-associated myoclonus and seizures in long-term hemodialysis patients. Ann Neurol 1983; 14:593.

592. Kaiko RF, Foley KM, Grabinski PY, et al. Central nervous system excitatory effects of meperidine in cancer patients. Ann Neurol 1983; 13:180.

593. Meyer D, Halfin V. Toxicity secondary to meperidine in patients on monoamine oxidase inhibitors: a case report and critical review. J Clin Psychopharmacol 1981; 1:319.

594. Lieberman AN, Goldstein M. Reversible parkinsonism related to meperidine. N Engl J Med 1985; 312:509.

595. Aberfeld DC, Bienenstock H, Shapiro MS, et al. Diffuse myopathy related to meperidine addiction in a mother and daughter. Arch Neurol 1968; 19:384.

596. Collins GB, Kiefer KS. Propoxyphene dependence. Postgrad Med J 1981; 70:57.

597. Lader M. Abuse of weak opioid analgesics. Hum Toxicol 1984; 3 (Suppl):2295.

598. Anon. Physicians asked to write "no refill" on propoxyphene Rxes. FDA Drug Bull 1980; 10:11.

599. Wall R, Linford SMJ, Akhter M. Addiction to Distalgesic (dextropropoxyphene). BMJ 1980; I:1213.

600. Chambers CD, Taylor WJR. Patterns of propoxyphene abuse. Int J Clin Pharmacol 1971; 4:240.

601. Chard P. Darvon dependence: three case studies. Chem Depend 1980; 4:65.

602. Finkle BS. Self-poisoning with dextropropoxyphene and dextropropoxyphene compounds: the USA experience. Hum Toxicol 1984; 3 (Suppl):115S.

603. Hooper HE, Santo Y. Use of propoxyphene (Darvon) by adolescents admitted to drug programs. Contemp Drug Prob 1980; 9:357.

604. Schuckit MA, Morrisey ER. Propoxyphene and phencyclidine (PCP) use in adolescents. J Clin Psychiatry 1978; 39:7.

605. Finkle BS, Caplan YH, Garriott JC, et al. Propoxyphene in postmortem toxicology, 1976–1978. J Forens Sci 1981; 26:739.

606. Litman RE, Diller J, Nelson F. Deaths related to propoxyphene or codeine or both. J Forens Sci 1983; 28:128.

607. D'Adadie NB, Lenton JD. Propoxyphene dependence: problems in management. South Med J 1984; 77:229.

608. Young RJ. Dextropropoxyphene overdosage. Pharmacological considerations and clinical management. Drugs 1983; 26:70.

609. Amsterdam EA, Rendig SV, Henderson L, Mason DT. Depression of myocardial contractile function by propoxyphene and norpropoxyphene. J Cardiovasc Pharmacol 1981; 3:129.

610. Henry JA, Cassidy SL. Membrane stabilizing activity: a major cause of fatal poisoning. Lancet 1986; I:1414.

611. Harrell M, Shea JJ, Emmett JR. Total deafness with chronic propoxyphene abuse. Laryngoscope 1978; 88:1518.

612. McBride DC, McCoy CB, Rivers JE, Lincoln LA. Dilaudid use: trends and characteristics of users. Chem Depend 1980; 4:85.

613. Leads from the MMWR. Dilaudid-related deaths—District of Colombia, 1987. JAMA 1988; 260:903.

614. Bivera E, Schoeller T, Montejo G. Organic hallucinosis in patients receiving high doses of opiates for cancer pain. Pain 1992; 48:397.

614a. Han PK, Arnold R, Bond G, et al: Myoclonus secondary to withdrawal from transdermal fentanyl: case report and literature review. J Pain Sympt Management 2002; 23:66.

615. Sullivan J. Doctor and 2 pharmacists charged in suspected prescription drug scheme. NY Times, February 17, 2000.

616. Feuer E, French J. Descriptive epidemiology of mortality in New Jersey due to combinations of codeine and glutethimide. Am J Epidemiol 1984; 119:202.

617. Shamoian CA. Codeine and glutethimide: euphoretic, addicting combination. NY State J Med 1975; 75:97.

618. Sramek JJ, Khajawall A. "Loads." N Engl J Med 1981; 305:231.

619. Feuer E, French J. Death related to narcotics overdose in New Jersey. J Med Soc N J 1984; 81:291.

620. Bender FH, Cooper JV, Dreyfus R. Fatalities associated with an acute overdose of glutethimide (Doriden) and codeine. Vet Hum Toxicol 1988; 30:322.

621. Murray RM. Minor analgesic abuse: the slow recognition of a public health problem. Br J Addict 1980; 75:9.

622. Goldberg I, Bahar A, Yosipovitch Z. Gangrene of the upper extremity following intra-arterial injection of drugs. A case report and review of the literature. Clin Orthop 1984; 188:223.

623. Curry KH, Stanhope JM. Codeine linctus and myopathy. Med J Aust 1984; 140:247.

624. Kilpatrick C, Braund W, Burns R. Myopathy with myasthenic features possibly induced by codeine linctus. Med J Aust 1982; 2:410.

625. Seow SS. Abuse of APF Linctus codeine and cardiac glycoside toxicity. Med J Aust 1984; 140:54.

626. Tough P. The alchemy of OxyContin. NY Times Magazine, July 29, 2001.

627. Meier B. Doctor guilty in 4 deaths tied to a drug. NY Times, February 20, 2002.

628. Meier B. OxyContin deaths may top early count. NY Times, April 15, 2002.

628a. Harris G: Judge says maker of OxyContin misled officials to win patents. NY Times January 6, 2004.

629. Chabal C, Miklavz E, Jacobson L, et al. Prescription opiate abuse in chronic pain patients: clinical criteria, incidence, and predictors. Clin J Pain 1997; 13:150.

630. Oh AK, Ishiyama A, Baloh RW. Deafness associated with abuse of hydrocadone/acetaminophen. Neurology 2000; 54:2345.

630a. Belluck J, Methadone, once the way out, suddenly grows as a killer drug. NY Times, February 9, 2003.

630b. Fiellin DA, O'Connor PG. Office-based treatment of opioid-dependent patients. N Engl J Med 2002; 347:817.

630c. Sieniewitz DJ, Nidecker AC. Conglomerate pulmonary disease: a form of talcosis in intravenous methadone abusers. AJR Am J Roentgenol 1980; 135:697.

631. Barragry JM, Morris DV. Fatal dependence on kaolin and morphine mixture. Postgrad Med J 1980; 56:180.

632. Ayres WA, Starsiak MJ, Sokolay P. The bogus drug: 3-ethyl and alpha-methyl fentanyl sold as "China White." J Psychoact Drugs 1981; 13:91.

633. Silsby HD, Kruzich DJ, Hawkins MR. Fentanyl citrate abuse among health care professionals. Milit Med 1984; 149:227.

634. Berens AI, Voets AJ, Dennedts P: Illicit fentanyl in Europe. Lancet 1996; 347:1334-1335.

635. Hays L, Stillner V, Littrell R. Fentanyl dependence associated with oral ingestion. Anesthesiology 1992; 77:819.

636. LaBarbera M, Wolfe T. Characteristics, attitudes, and implications of fentanyl use based on reports from self-identified fentanyl users. J Psychoact Drugs 1983; 15:293.

637. Carroll FL, Boldt KG, Huang PT, et al. Synthesis of fentanyl analogs. NIDA Res Monogr 1990; 95:497.

638. Henderson GL. Designer drugs: past history and future prospects. J Forens Sci 1988; 33:569.

639. Martin M, Hecker J, Clark R, et al. China White epidemic: an eastern United States emergency department experience. Ann Emerg Med 1991; 20:158.

640. Hibbs J, Perper J, Winek CL. An outbreak of designer drug-related deaths in Pennsylvania. JAMA 1991; 265:1011.

641. Smialek JE, Levien B, Chin L, et al. A fentanyl epidemic in Maryland, 1992. J Forensic Sci 1994; 39:159.

642. Nieves E. Toxic heroin has killed 12, officials say. NY Times, February 4, 1991.

643. Mannelli P, Janiri L, DeMarinis M, Tempesta E. Lofetamine: new abuse of an old drug: clinical evaluation of opioid activity. Drug Alcohol Depend 1989; 24:95.

644. Soyibo K, Lee MG. Use of illicit drugs among high-school students in Jamaica. Bull WHO 1999; 77:258.

645. Kalant H. Opium revisited: a brief review of its nature, composition, non-medical use and relative risks. Addiction 1997; 92:267.

646. London M, O'Reagan T, Aust P, Stockford A. Poppy tea drinking in East Anglia. Br J Addict 1990; 85:1345.

647. King MA, McDonough MA, Drummer OH, Berkovic SF. Poppy tea and the baker's first seizure. Lancet 1997; 350:716.

648. Hamilton K, Rossi M, Gegax TT. Back to Xanadu, via Seattle. Newsweek, August 29, 1994.

649. Jacobs A. Ailing New Jersey prep schoolers bought drug through Internet. NY Times, May 26, 2000.

650. Aknine X, Varescon-Pousson I, Boissonnas A. Dépendence au tramadol (Topalgic). A propos d'un cas chez un ancien héroinomone. Ann Med Interne 2000; 151 (Suppl B):B3.

651. Liu ZM, Zhou WH, Lian Z, et al. Drug dependence and abuse potential of tramadol. Acta Pharmacol Sinica 1999; 20:52.

652. Ripple MG, Pestnaer JP, Levine BS, et al. Lethal combination of tramadol and multiple drugs affecting serotonin. Am J Forensic Med Pathol 2000; 21:370.

653. Meyer RE. What treatments for the heroin addict? JAMA 1986; 256:511.

654. Dole VP. Addictive behavior. Sci Am 1980; 243:18.

655. Wikler A. Dynamics of drug dependence. Implications of a conditioning theory for research and treatment. Arch Gen Psychiatry 1973; 28:611.

656. Levine DG. Needle freaks. Compulsive self-injection by drug abusers. Am J Psychiatry 1974; 131:297.

657. Musto DF, Ramos MR. Notes on American medical history. A follow-up study of the New Haven morphine maintenance clinic of 1920. N Engl J Med 1981; 304:1071.

658. O'Brien CP, Nace EP, Mintz J, et al. Follow-up of Vietnam veterans. 1. Relapse to drug use after Vietnam service. Drug Alcohol Depend 1980; 5:333.

659. Foley KM. The treatment of cancer pain. N Engl J Med 1985; 313:84.

660. Portenoy RK, Foley KM. Chronic use of opioid analgesics in non-malignant pain: report of 38 cases. Pain 1986; 25:171.

661. Baganz PC, Maddux JF. Employment status of narcotic addicts one year after hospital discharge. Public Health Rep 1965; 80:615.

662. Vaillant G. A 20-year follow-up of New York narcotic addicts. Arch Gen Psychiatry 1973; 29:237.

663. Kramer JC, Bass RA. Institutionalization patterns among civilly committed addicts. JAMA 1969; 208:2297.

664. Kosten TR, Rounsaville BJ, Kleber HD. A 2.5 year follow-up of depression, life crises, and treatment effects on abstinence among opioid addicts. Arch Gen Psychiatry 1986; 43:733.

665. Rounsaville BJ, Kleber HD. Psychotherapy/counseling for opiate addicts: strategies for use in different treatment settings. Int J Addict 1985; 20:869.

666. Woody GE, McLellan AT, Luborsky L, et al. Severity of psychiatric symptoms as a predictor of benefits from psychotherapy: the Veterans Administration-Penn Study. Am J Psychiatry 1984; 141:1172.

667. Preston KL, Umbricht A, Epstein DH. Methadone dose increase and abstinence reinforcement for treatment of continued heroin use during methadone maintenance. Arch Gen Psychiatry 2000; 57:395.

668. Anglin MD, Weisman CP, Fisher DG. The MMPI profiles of narcotics addicts. I. A review of the literature. Int J Addict 1989; 24:867.

669. Rounsaville BJ, Kosten TR, Weissman MM, et al. Psychiatric disorders in relatives of probands with opiate addiction. Arch Gen Psychiatry 1991; 48:33.

670. Khantzian EJ, Treece C. DSM-III psychiatric diagnosis of narcotic addicts: recent findings. Arch Gen Psychiatry 1985; 42:1067.

671. Rounsaville BJ, Weissman MM, Kleber HD, Wilber CH. Heterogeneity of psychiatric diagnosis in treated opiate addicts. Arch Gen Psychiatry 1982; 39:161.

672. Tsuang MT, Lyons MJ, Meyer JM, et al. Co-occurrence of abuse of different drugs in men: the role of drug-specific and shared vulnerability. Arch Gen Psychiatry 1998; 55:967.

673. Tsuang MT, Lyons MJ, Mayer JM, et al. Genetic influences on DSM-III R drug abuse and dependence: a study of 3372 twin pairs. Am J Med Genet Neuropsychol Genet 1996; 67:473.

674. Goldman D, Bergen A. General and specific inheritance of substance abuse and alcoholism. Arch Gen Psychiatry 1998; 55:964.

675. Kendler KS, Karkowski L, Prescott CA. Hallucinogen, opiate, sedative and stimulant use and abuse in a population-based sample of female twins. Acta Psychiatr Scand 1999; 99:368.

676. Merikangas KR, Stolar M, Stevens DE, et al. Familial transmission of substance use disorders. Arch Gen Psychiatry 1998; 55:973.

677. Kendler KS, Karkowski LM, Neale MC, Prescott LA. Illicit psychoactive substance use, heavy use, abuse, and dependence in a U.S. population-based sample of male twins. Arch Gen Psychiatry 2000; 57:261.

678. Bale RN, Zarcone VP, Van Stone WW, et al. Three therapeutic communities. A prospective controlled study of narcotic addiction treatment: process and

two-year follow-up results. Arch Gen Psychiatry 1984;41:185.

679. DeLeon G, Schwartz S. Therapeutic communities: what are the retention rates? Am J Drug Alcohol Abuse 1984; 10:267.

680. Ter-Riet G, Kleijnen J, Knipschild P. A meta-analysis of studies into the effect of acupuncture on addiction. Br J Gen Pract 1990; 40:379.

681. Koran LM. Heroin maintenance for heroin addicts: issues and evidence. N Engl J Med 1973; 288:654.

682. Pillard RC. Shall we allow heroin maintenance? N Engl J Med 1973; 288:682.

683. Hawks D. The proposal to make heroin available legally to intravenous drug abusers. Med J Aust 1988; 149:455.

684. Parry A. Taking heroin maintenance seriously: the politics of tolerance. Lancet 1992; 339:350.

685. Burr A. A British view of prescribing pharmaceutical heroin to opiate addicts: a critique of the "heroin solution" with special reference to the Piccadilly and Kensington Market drug scenes in London. Int J Addict 1986; 21:83.

686. Connell PH, Mitcheson M. Necessary safeguards when prescribing opioid drugs to addicts: experience of drug dependence clinics in London. BMJ 1984; 288:767.

687. Bayer R. Heroin maintenance: an historical perspective on the exhaustion of liberal narcotics reform. J Psychedelic Drugs 1976; 8:157.

688. Gonzalez JP, Brogden RN. Naltrexone: a review of its pharmacodynamic and pharmacokinetic properties and therapeutic efficacy in the management of opioid dependence. Drugs 1988; 35:192.

689. O'Connor PG, Fiellin DA. Pharmacologic treatment of heroin-dependent patients. Ann Intern Med 2000; 133:40.

690. Spanagel R. Is there a pharmacological basis for therapy with rapid opioid detoxification? Lancet 1999; 354:2017.

691. San L, Pomarol G, Peri JM, et al. Follow-up after a six-month maintenance period on naltrexone versus placebo in heroin addicts. Br J Addict 1991; 86:983.

692. Crowley TJ, Wagner JE, Zebe G, et al. Naltrexone-induced dysphoria in former opioid addicts. Am J Psychiatry 1985; 142:1081.

692a. Lanabaso MA, Iraurgi I, Jimenez-Lerma JM, et al. A randomized trial of adding fluoxetine to a naltrexone treatment programme for heroin addicts. Addiction 1998; 93:739.

693. Dole VP. Implications of methadone maintenance for theories of narcotic addiction. JAMA 1988; 260:3025.

694. Teichtahl H, Prodomidis A, Miller B, et al. Sleep-disordered breathing in stable methadone programme patients: a pilot study. Addiction 2001; 96:395.

695. Drummer OH, Syrjanen M, Opeskin K, Cordner S. Deaths of heroin addicts starting on a methadone maintenance program. Lancet 1990; I:108.

696. Davis AM, Inturrisi CE. D-methadone blocks morphine tolerance and N-methyl-D-aspartate-induced hyperalgesia. J Pharmacol Exp Ther 199; 289:1048.

697. Novick DM, Ochshorn M, Ghali V, et al. Natural killer cell activity and lymphocyte subsets in parenteral heroin abusers and long-term methadone maintenance patients. J Pharmacol Exp Ther 1989; 250:606.

698. Specka M, Finkbeiner T, Lodemann E, et al. Cognitive-motor performance of methadone-maintained patients. Eur Addic Res 2000; 6:8.

699. Dole VP, Nyswander ME. Methadone maintenance treatment: a ten-year perspective. JAMA 1976; 235:2117.

700. Gerstein DR, Lewin LS. Treating drug problems. N Engl J Med 1990; 323:844.

701. Schwartz RP, Brooner RK, Montoya ID, et al. A 12-year follow-up of a methadone medical maintenance program. Am J Addict 1999; 8:293.

702. Ward J, Mattick JJP, Hall W, Darke S. The effectiveness and safety of methadone maintenance. Addiction 1996; 91:1727.

703. Hubbard RL, Craddock SG, Flynn PM, et al. Overview of 1-year follow-up outcomes in the Drug Abuse Treatment Outcome Study (DATOS). Psychology of Addictive Behaviors 1997; 11:261.

704. Sees KL, Delucchi KL, Masson C, et al. Methadone maintenance vs 180-day psychosocially enriched detoxification for treatment of opioid dependence. A randomized controlled trial. JAMA 2000; 283:1303.

705. Metzger DS, Navaline H, Woody CE. Drug abuse treatment as AIDS prevention. Public Health Rep 1998; 113 (Suppl 1):97.

706. Zaric CS, Barnett PG, Brandeau ML. HIV transmission and the cost-effectiveness of methadone maintenance. Am J Public Health 2000; 90:1100.

707. Zweben JE. Methadone maintenance in the treatment of opioid dependence. A current perspective. West J Med 1990; 152:588.

708. Kirn TF. Methadone maintenance treatment remains controversial after 23 years of experience. JAMA 1988; 260:2970.

709. Liappas JA, Jenner FA, Viente B. Literature on methadone maintenance clinics. Int J Addict 1988; 23:927.

710. Newman RE. Advocacy for methadone treatment. Ann Intern Med 1990; 113:819.

711. Kolar AF, Brown BS, Weddington WW, Ball JC. A treatment crisis: cocaine use by clients in methadone maintenance programs. J Subst Abuse Treat 1990; 7:101.

712. Saxon AJ, Calsyn DA, Blaes PA, et al. Marijuana use by methadone maintenance patients. NIDA Res Monogr 1991; 105:306.

713. Lehman WE, Barrett ME, Simpson DD. Alcohol use by heroin addicts 12 years after drug abuse treatment. J Stud Alcohol 1990; 51:233.

714. Bell J, Zador D. A risk-benefit analysis of methadone maintenance treatment. Drug Safety 2000; 22:179.

715. Green H, James RA, Gilbert JD, et al. Methadone maintenance programs—a two-edged sword? Am J Forensic Med Pathol 2000; 21:359.

716. Heinemann A, Iversen-Bergmann S, Stein S, et al. Methadone-related fatalities in Hamburg 1990–1999: implications for quality standards in maintenance treatment? Forensic Sci Int 2000; 113:449.

717. Caplehorn JR, Drummer OH. Mortality associated with New South Wales methadone programs in 1994: lives lost and saved. Med J Aust 1999; 170:104.

718. Novick DM, Pascarelli EF, Joseph H, et al. Methadone maintenance patients in general medical practice. A preliminary report. JAMA 1988; 259:3299.

719. Wesson DR. Revival of medical maintenance in the treatment of heroin dependence. JAMA 1988; 259:3314.

720. Hanbury R, Sturiano V, Cohen M, et al. Cocaine use in persons on methadone maintenance. Adv Alcohol Subst Abuse 1986; 6:97.

721. Nurco DN, Kinlock TW, Hanlon TE, Ball JC. Non-narcotic drug use over an addiction career—a study of heroin addicts in Baltimore and New York City. Compr Psychiatry 1988; 29:450.

722. Batki SL, Sorensen JL, Gibson DR, Maude-Griffin P. HIV-infected IV drug users in methadone treatment: outcome and psychological correlates—a preliminary report. NIDA Res Monogr 1990; 95:405.

723. Bilsky EJ, Montegut MJ, Delong CL, et al. Opioidergic modulation of cocaine conditioned place preference. Life Sci 1992; 50:85.

724. Iguchi MY, Griffiths RR, Bickel WK, et al. Relative abuse liability of benzodiazepines in methadone maintained population in three cities. NIDA Res Monogr 1990; 95:364.

725. Anglin MD, Almog IJ, Fisher DG, Peters KR. Alcohol use by heroin addicts: evidence for an inverse relationship. A study of methadone maintenance and drug-free treatment samples. Am J Drug Alcohol Abuse 1989; 15:191.

726. Bell J, Bowron P, Lewis J, Batey R. Serum levels of methadone in maintenance clients who persist in illicit drug use. Br J Addict 1990; 85:1599.

727. Caplehorn JR, Bell J. Methadone dosage and retention of patients in maintenance treatment. Med J Aust 1991; 154:195.

728. Wolff K, Hay AW, Vail A, et al. Non-prescribed drug use during methadone treatment by clinic—and community-based patients. Addiction 1996; 91:1699.

729. D'Aunno T, Vaughn TE. Variations in methadone treatment practices. Results from a national study. JAMA 1992; 267:253.

730. Cooper JR. Ineffective use of psychoactive drugs. Methadone treatment is no exception. JAMA 1992; 267:281.

730a. D'Aunno T, Pollack HA. Changes in methadone treatment practices. Results from a national panel study, 1988–2000. JAMA 2002; 288:850.

731. Strain EC, Bigelow GE, Liebson IA, et al. Moderate- vs. high-dose methadone in the treatment of opioid dependence. A randomized trial. JAMA 1999; 281:1000.

732. Tennant FS. Inadequate plasma concentrations in some high dose methadone patients. Am J Psychiatry 1987; 144:1349.

733. Maremmanil I, Zolesi O, Aglietti M, et al. Methadone dose and retention during treatment of heroin addicts with Axis I psychiatric comorbidity. J Addict Dis 2000; 19:29.

734. Newman RG. Methadone treatment: defining and evaluating success. N Engl J Med 1987; 317:447.

735. Murphy S, Rosenbaum M. Money for methadone. II. Unintended consequences of limited-duration methadone maintenance. J Psychoact Drugs 1988; 20:397.

736. National Consensus Development Panel on Effective Medical Treatment of Opiate Addiction. Effective medical treatment of opiate addiction. JAMA 1998; 280:1936.

737. Rhoades HM, Creson D, Elk R, et al. Retention, HIV risk, and illicit drug use during treatment: methadone dose and visit frequency. Am J Public Health 1998; 88:34.

738. Kandall SR, Doberczak TM, Jantunen M, Stein J. The methadone-maintained pregnancy. Clin Perinatol 1999; 26:171.

739. Mass U, Kattner E, Weighart-Jesse B, et al. Infrequent neonatal opiate withdrawal following maternal methadone detoxification during pregnancy. J Perinat Med 1990; 18:111.

740. Richardson BS, O'Grady JP, Olsen GD. Fetal breathing movements and the response to carbon dioxide in patients on methadone maintenance. Am J Obstet Gynecol 1984; 150:400.

741. Davis DD, Templer DI. Neurobehavioral functioning in children exposed to narcotics in utero. Addict Behav 1988; 13:275.

742. Chasnoff IJ, Burns KA, Burns WJ, Schnoll SH. Prenatal drug exposure: effects on neonatal and infant growth and development. Neurobehav Toxicol Teratol 1986; 8:357.

743. Kaltenbach K, Finnegan LP. Perinatal and development outcome of infants exposed to methadone in utero. NIDA Res Monogr 1987; 76: 276.

744. Stimmel B, Goldberg J, Reisman A, et al. Fetal outcome in narcotic-dependent women: the importance of the type of maternal narcotic used. Am J Drug Alcohol Abuse 1982–1983; 9:383.

745. Edelin KC, Gurganious L, Golar K, et al. Methadone maintenance in pregnancy: consequences to care and outcome. Obstet Gynecol 1988; 71:399.

746. Brown HL, Britton KA, Mahaffey D, et al. Methadone maintenance in pregnancy: a reappraisal. Am J Obstet Gynecol 1998; 179:459.

747. Hein PR, Schatorje J, Frencken HJ. The effect of chronic methadone treatment on intra-uterine growth

of the cynomolgus monkey (*Macaca fascicularis*). Eur J Obstet Gynecol Reprod Biol 1988; 27:81.

748. Mass U, Kattner E, Weingert-Jesse B, et al. Infrequent neonate opiate withdrawal following maternal detoxification during pregnancy. J Perinatol Med 1990; 18:111.

749. Ito S. Drug therapy for breast-feeding women. N Engl J Med 2000; 343:118.

750. Cooper JR. Methadone treatment and the acquired immunodeficiency syndrome. JAMA 1989; 262:1664.

751. Dole VP. Methadone treatment and the acquired immunodeficiency syndrome epidemic. JAMA 1989; 262:1681.

752. Novick DM, Joseph H, Croxson TS, et al. Absence of antibody to human immunodeficiency virus in long-term, socially rehabilitated methadone maintenance patients. Arch Intern Med 1990; 150:97.

753. Bourne PG. AIDS and drug use. An international perspective. J Psychoact Drugs 1988; 20:153.

754. Serraino D, Franceschi S. Methadone maintenance programs and AIDS. Lancet 1989; II:1522.

755. Magura S, Grossman JI, Lipton S, et al. Correlates of participation in AIDS education and HIV antibody testing by methadone patients. Public Health Rep 1989; 104:231.

756. Wasserman S, Yahr MD. Choreic movements induced by the use of methadone. Arch Neurol 1980; 37:727.

757. Bonnet U, Banger M, Wolstein J, Gastpar M. Choreoathetoid movements associated with rapid adjustment to methadone. Pharmacopsychiatry 1998; 31:143.

758. Palmer W-R, Haferkame G. Involuntary movements associated with methadone. Arch Neurol 1981; 38:737.

758a. Rosenblum A, Joseph H, Fong C, et al. Prevalence and characteristics of chronic pain among chemically dependent patients in methadone and residential treatment facilities. JAMA 2003; 289:2370.

759. Glantz M, Klawansky S, McAullife W, Chalmers T. Methadone vs. L-alpha-acetylmethadol (LAAM) in the treatment of opiate addiction. A meta-analysis of the randomized, controlled trials. Am J Addict 1997; 6:339.

760. Eissenberg T, Bigelow GE, Strain ED, et al. Dose-related efficacy of levomethadyl acetate for treatment of opioid dependence. A randomized clinical trial. JAMA 1997; 277:1945.

761. Johnson RE, Chutuape MA, Strain EC, et al. A comparison of levomethadyl acetate, buprenorphine, and methadone for opioid dependence. N Engl J Med 2000; 343:1290.

762. Eissenberg T, Stitzer ML, Bigelow GE, et al. Relative potency of levo-alpha-acetylmethadol and methadone in humans under acute dosing conditions. J Pharmacol Exp Ther 1999; 289:936.

763. Deamer RL, Wilson DR, Clark DS, et al. Torsades de pointes associated with high dose levomethadyl acetate (ORLAAM). J Addict Dis 2001; 20.

764. Mendelson JH, Ellingboe J, Judson B, Goldstein A. Plasma testosterone and luteinizing hormone levels during levo-alpha-acetylmethadol maintenance and withdrawal. Clin Pharmacol Ther 1984; 36:239.

765. Mendelson J, Jones RT, Welm S, et al. Buprenorphine and naloxone combination. Psychopharmacology 1999; 141:37.

766. O'Connor PG, Oliveto AH, Shi JM, et al. A randomized trial of buprenorphine maintenance for heroin dependence in a primary care clinic for substance users vs. a methadone clinic. Am J Med 1998; 105:100.

767. Schottenfeld RS, Pakes JR, Oliveto AH, Shi JM, et al. Buprenorphine vs. methadone maintenance treatment for concurrent opioid dependence and cocaine abuse. Arch Gen Psychiatry 1997; 54:713.

768. Schottenfeld RS, Pakes J, O'Connor P, et al. Thrice-weekly versus daily buprenorphine maintenance. Biol Psychiatry 2000; 47:1072.

769. Petitjean S, Stohler R, Deglon JJ, et al. Double-blind randomized trial of buprenorphine and methadone in opiate dependence. Drug Alcohol Dep 2001; 62:97.

770. Ling W, Charuvastra C, Collins JF, et al. Buprenorphine maintenance treatment of opiate dependence: a multicenter, randomized clinical trial. Addiction 1998; 93:475.

771. Fischer G, Gombas W, Eder H, et al. Buprenorphine versus methadone maintenance for the treatment of opioid dependence. Addiction 1999; 94:1337.

771a. Buprenorphine for opioid dependence. Med Lett Oct 30, 2002.

772. Kosten TR, Kleber HD, Morgan CH. Treatment of cocaine abuse using buprenorphine. Biol Psychiatry 1989; 26:637.

773. Mendelson JH, Mello NK, Teoh SK, et al. Buprenorphine treatment for concurrent heroin and cocaine dependence: Phase I study. In: Harris L, ed. Problems of Drug Dependence 1990. DHHS, Rockville, MD: NIDA Research Monograph 105, 1991:196.

774. Winger G, Skjoldager P, Woods JH. Effects of buprenorphine and other opioid agonists and antagonists on alfentanil- and cocaine-reinforced responding in rhesus monkeys. J Pharmacol Exp Ther 1992; 261:311.

775. Mello NK, Mendelson JH, Bree MP, Lukas SE. Buprenorphine suppresses cocaine self-administration by rhesus monkeys. Science 1989; 245:859.

776. Brown EE, Finlay JM, Wong JTF, et al. Behavioral and neurochemical interactions between cocaine and buprenorphine: implications for the pharmacotherapy of cocaine abuse. J Pharmacol Exp Ther 1991; 256:119.

777. O'Connor JJ, Moloney E, Travers R, Campbell A. Buprenorphine abuse among opiate addicts. Br J Addict 1988; 83:1085.

778. Quigley AJ, Bredemeyer DE, Seow SS. A case of buprenorphine abuse. Med J Aust 1984; 140:425.

779. Rainey HB. Abuse of buprenorphine. N Z Med J 1986; 99:72.

780. Richert S, Strauss A, von Arnim T, et al. Drug dependence of buprenorphine. MMWR 1983; 125:1195.

781. Robertson JR, Bucknall ABV. Burprenorphine: dangerous drug or over-looked therapy? BMJ 1986; 292:1465.

782. San Molina L, Porta-Serra M. Addiction to buprenorphine. Rev Clin Esp 1987; 181:288.

783. Strang J. Abuse of buprenorphine. Lancet 1985; II:725.

784. Wodak AD. Buprenorphine: new wonder drug or new hazard? Med J Aust 1984; 140:389.

785. Lewis JW. Buprenorphine. Drug Alcohol Depend 1985; 14:362.

786. Chowdhury AN, Chowdhury S. Buprenorphine abuse: report from India. Br J Addict 1990; 85:1349.

787. San L, Tremoleda J, Olle JM, et al. Prevalencia del consumo de buprenorphina en heroinomanos en tratamiento. Med Clin 1989; 93:645.

788. San L, Cami J, Fernandez T, et al. Assessment and management of opioid withdrawal symptoms in buprenorphine-dependent subjects. Br J Addict 1992; 87:55.

789. Lavelle TL, Hammersley R, Forsyth A, Bain D. The use of buprenorphine and temazepam by drug injectors. J Addict Dis 1991; 10:5.

790. Hubner CB, Kornetsky C. The reinforcing properties of the mixed agonist-antagonist buprenorphine as assessed by brain-stimulation reward. Pharmacol Biochem Behav 1988; 30:195.

791. Lukas SE, Brady JV, Griffiths RR. Comparison of opioid self-injection and disruption of schedule-controlled performance in the baboon. J Pharmacol Exp Ther 1986; 238:924.

792. Mello NK, Lukas SE, Bree MP, Mendelson JH. Progressive ratio performance maintained by buprenorphine, heroin and methadone in macaque monkeys. Drug Alcohol Depend 1988; 21:81.

793. Paraskevaides EC. Near fatal auditory hallucinations after buprenorphine. BMJ 1988; 296:214.

794. Rounsaville BJ, Kosten TR. Treatment for opioid dependence. Quality and access. JAMA 2000;283:1337.

795. MacFarquhar N. Report backs methadone for addicts. NY Times, Dec 9, 1998.

796. Brust JCM. Substance abuse, neurobiology, and ideology. Arch Neurol 1999; 56:1528.

797. Weinrich M, Stuart M. Provision of methadone treatment in primary care medical practices. Review of the Scottish experience and implications for U.S. policy. JAMA 2000; 283:1343.

797a. Markel H. For addicts, relief may be an office visit away. NY Times, October 27, 2002.

797b. Krook AL, Brørs O, Dahlberg J, et al. A placebo-controlled study of high dose buprenorphine in opiate dependents waiting for medication-assisted rehabilitation in Oslo, Norway. Addiction 2002; 97:533.

797c. Kakko J, Svanborg KD, Kreek MJ, et al. One-year retention and social functioning after buprenorphine-assisted relapse prevention treatment for heroin dependence in Sweden: a randomised, placebo-controlled trial. Lancet 2003; 361:662.

797d. Fudala PJ, Bridge TP, Herbert S, et al. Office-based treatment of opiate addiction for heroin dependence with a sublingual tablet formulation of buprenorphine and naloxone. N Engl J Med 2003; 349:949.

798. Drucker E. Drug prohibition and public health: 25 years of evidence. Public Health Rep 1999; 114:14.

799. Strong J, Sheridan J. Heroin prescribing in the British system of the mid-1990s. Data from the 1995 survey of community pharmacies in England and Wales. Drug Alcohol Rev 1997; 16:7.

800. Bammer G, Dobler-Mikola A, Fleming PM, et al. The heroin prescribing debate: integrating science and politics. Science 1999; 284:1277.

801. Uchlenhagen A, Gurzwiller F, Dobler-Mikola A, eds. Programme for a medical prescription of narcotics: final report of the research representatives. Summary of the synthesis report. Zurich: University of Zurich, 1997.

802. Rehm J, Gschwend P, Steffen T, et al. Feasibility, safety, and efficacy of injectable heroin prescription for refractory opioid addicts: a follow-up study. Lancet 2001; 358:1417.

803. Perneger TV, Giner F, del Rio M, Mino A. Randomized trial of heroin maintenance programme for addicts who fail in conventional drug treatments. BMJ 1998; 317:13.

804. Report of the External Panel on the Evaluation of the Swiss Scientific Studies of Medically Prescribed Narcotics to Drug Addicts. Geneva: World Health Organization, 1999.

805. Satel SL, Aeschbach E. The Swiss heroin trials. Scientifically sound? J Subst Abuse Treat 1999; 17:331.

806. Nadelmann E. Commonsense drug policy. Foreign Affairs 1998; 77:111.

806a. van don Brink W, Hendrinks VM, Blanken P, et al. Medical prescription of heroin to treatment resistant heroin addicts: two randomised controlled trials. BMJ 2003; 327:310.

807. Drucker E, Vlahav D. Controlled clinical evaluation of diacetyl morphine for treatment of intractable opiate dependence. Lancet 1999; 353:1543.

808. Gallimberti L, Spella MR, Soncini CA, Gessa GL. Gamma-hydroxybutyric acid in the treatment of alcohol and heroin dependence. Alcohol 2000; 20:257.

809. Rothman RB, Gorelick DA, Heishman SJ, et al. An open-label study of a functional opioid kappa antagonist in the treatment of opioid dependence. J Subst Abuse Treat 2000; 18:27.

810. Zi ZX, Stein EA. Baclofen inhibits heroin self-administration behavior and mesolimbic dopamine release. J Pharmacol Exp Ther 1999; 290:1369.

811. Gerasimov MR, Dewey SL. Gamma-vinyl gamma-aminobutyric acid attenuates the synergistic elevations of nucleus accumbens dopamine produced by a cocaine/ heroin (speedball) challenge. Eur J Pharmacol 1999; 380:1.

812. Popik P, Layer RT, Skolnick P. 100 years of ibogaine: Neurochemical and pharmacological actions of a putative anti-addictive drug. Pharmacol Rev 1995; 47:235.

Chapter 4
Amphetamine and Other Psychostimulants

I love coffee! I love tea!
I love the Java jive, and it loves me!
—The Ink Spots

Who put the Benzedrine in Mrs. Murphy's Ovaltine?
—Harry "The Hipster" Gibson

Speed kills.
—DEA slogan

This chapter discusses drugs that are taken for psychostimulation, especially amphetamine and related indirect bioamine agonists[1,2] but also other substances with different pharmacological properties. (Cocaine, because in the 1980s it became a major American preoccupation, is considered separately in Chapter 5.) Amphetamine-like drugs are used for narcolepsy and attention deficit disorder. It was long believed that their anorectic effects wear off in a matter of weeks, yet a 1992 study found that weight loss was sustained as long as the drugs were taken.[3] They are rarely of value in depressive disorders. Although their manufacture decreased following regulatory legislation in the 1960s and 1970s,[4] amphetamine-like psychostimulants are still produced in huge quantities, both legally and illegally (Table 4–1, Figure 4–1).

Pharmacology and Animal Studies

Acute Effects and Self-administration

Amphetamine is both a central stimulant and a peripheral sympathomimetic. In animals, it raises systolic and diastolic blood pressure. Low doses

Table 4–1. Amphetamine and Related Agents

Amphetamine (Benzedrine)
Dextroamphetamine (Dexedrine)
Amphetamine and dextroamphetamine (Biphetamine)
Methamphetamine (Methedrine; Desoxyn; Fetamin)
Ephedrine
Pseudoephedrine
Methylphenidate (Ritalin)
Pemoline (Cylert)
Phenmetrazine (Preludin; Prelu-2)
Diethylpropion (Tenuate; Tepanil)
Benzphetamine (Didrex)
Fenfluramine (Pondimin) (withdrawn)
Dexfenfluramine (Redux) (withdrawn)
Phendimetrazine (Plegine; Bontril)
Phentermine (Ionamin; Wilpo; Adipex-P; Fastin)
Mazindol (Sanorex; Mazanor)
Phenylpropanolamine (Propadrine; Propagest; and in decongestants and diet pills) (withdrawn)
Propylhexedrine (Benzedrex nasal inhaler)
Naphzoline (Privine nasal solution; Naphcon ophthalmic solution)
Tetrahydrozoline (Tyzine nasal solution; Visine ophthalmic solution)
Oxymetazoline (Afrin nasal solution; Ococlear ophthalmic solution)
Xylometazoline (Otrivin nasal solution)
Phenoxazoline (nasal solutions)

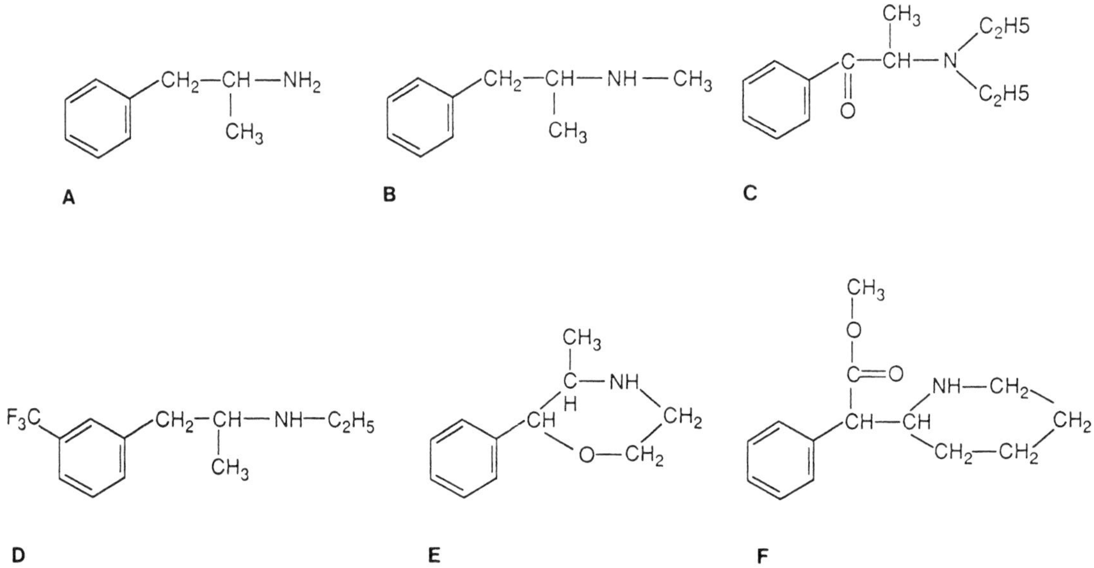

Figure 4–1. Amphetamine (A), Methamphetamine (B), Diethylpropion (C), Fenfluramine (D), Phenmetrazine (E), and Methylphenidate (F).

reflexly slow the heart rate; higher doses cause tachycardia or cardiac arrhythmia. Stimulation of the medullary respiratory center increases the rate and depth of respiration, and excitatory actions on the brainstem, diencephalon, and cerebrum produce increased locomotor activity, sleeplessness, and increased body temperature.[2,5] Higher or repeated doses cause stereotypic motor behavior (exploration, nose poking, head bobbing) and then tremor, dyskinesias, or catalepsy. Seizures are less frequent than with cocaine; in fact, amphetamine raises the threshold for electroshock seizures. Also in contrast to cocaine, amphetamine increases the cerebral metabolic rate for oxygen ($CMRO_2$).[6] As a central nervous system (CNS) stimulant, the D-isomer of amphetamine (dextroamphetamine) is 4 times more potent than the L-isomer. Methamphetamine is more potent than either.

Amphetamine produces appetite suppression and weight loss by inhibiting the lateral hypothalamic feeding center. By unclear mechanisms it potentiates the analgesic effects of opioids, and it is itself analgesic.[7,8]

Similar to cocaine, amphetamine enhances an animal's rate of self-stimulation through electrodes implanted in the medial forebrain bundle, and rats or monkeys self-inject the drug either systemically or directly into the nucleus accumbens (NA).[9]

Preferring amphetamine to food or water, animals eventually develop fatal seizures and hyperthermia.[10] (Perhaps relevant to human psychostimulant abuse, animals with pre-existing pronounced locomotor responses to novel stimuli are more likely to self-administer amphetamine compulsively.[11]) Animals also self-administer methamphetamine, methylphenidate, phentermine, diethylpropion, phenmetrazine, phendimetrazine, benzphetamine, methylenedioxyamphetamine (MDA), methylenedioxymethamphetamine (MDMA), and, to a lesser degree, ephedrine, clotermine, and chlorphentermine. They do not self-administer fenfluramine, methoxyamphetamine, 2,5-dimethoxy-4-methyl-amphetamine (DOM), or dimethoxyethylamphetamine (DOET).[12]

Pharmacological Mechanisms

The psychostimulants enhance the synaptic activity of biogenic amines: norepinephrine, dopamine, and serotonin.[13] Peripheral cardiovascular effects depend on norepinephrine, which probably also contributes to alerting, anorexia, and locomotor stimulation. Stereotypy and dyskinesias are related to neostriatal dopamine. Reinforcement (self-administration) depends on dopaminergic neurons in the mesencephalic ventral tegmental area (VTA) projecting to the NA and medial prefrontal cortex[14] (see Chapter 2). Dopamine-depleting lesions of either the VTA or the NA disrupt self-administration of amphetamine by animals. Lesions of the norepinephrine system (locus ceruleus) do not. Dopamine antagonists increase response rates for intravenous self-administration of amphetamine (presumably a compensatory response). Norepinephrine antagonists have no effect.[9,15]

The role of serotonin in the effects of psychostimulants differs among agents. It is reasonable to speculate that serotonin contributes to amphetamine-induced psychosis and hallucinations. Self-administration of amphetamine by rats is reduced by pretreatment with L-tryptophan (a serotonin precursor) or fluoxetine (a serotonin reuptake blocker) and enhanced by dihydroxytryptamine (which selectively destroys serotonergic neurons).[16] Serotonin probably contributes little to the subjective effects of amphetamine in humans. With MDA and MDMA its contribution is greater, and with those agents not self-administered by animals (e.g., DOM) it plays a dominant role. (In humans, such drugs produce lysergic acid diethylamide (LSD)-like effects; see Chapter 8.)

The psychostimulants have been subdivided into two pharmacologically distinct groups, based on whether the increased locomotor activity and stereotypies produced in animals are blocked by reserpine.[17] The *nonamphetamine class* of stimulants (methylphenidate, pipradrol, nomifensine, mazindol, cocaine) are inhibited by pretreatment with reserpine, which depletes nerve endings of catecholamines in the granular (storage) pool. The *amphetamine class* of stimulants (amphetamine, methamphetamine, phenmetrazine, pemoline) are not inhibited by reserpine. By contrast, alpha-methyltyrosine (AMT), which blocks catecholamine synthesis, inhibits the amphetamine class of stimulants but not the nonamphetamine class. Similarly, amphetamine-induced release of dopamine into cat lateral ventricle is enhanced by reserpine and inhibited by AMT; methylphenidate release of dopamine is inhibited by reserpine but not by AMT. Amphetamine's mechanism of action thus depends on the cytoplasmic, newly synthesized, rapidly metabolized pool of dopamine. Methylphenidate's mechanism of action depends on the granular storage pool.[18,19] Both mechanisms require the presynaptic dopamine uptake transporter, which carries dopamine in either direction across presynaptic nerve endings.[20,21] Once it has entered nerve terminals, amphetamine inhibits storage of dopamine by the granular pool and degradation of dopamine by monoamine oxidase, thereby increasing levels of dopamine in the cytoplasmic pool. Binding to the transporter, dopamine is then carried out into the synaptic cleft.[22,23] By contrast, methylphenidate (and cocaine) block reuptake of dopamine from the synaptic cleft back into the nerve ending.[24] This blockade then makes the granular storage pool of dopamine available for release, accounting for the ability of reserpine and the inability of AMT to block methylphenidate's action.[17]

Tolerance and Sensitization

With both classes of psychostimulants, there is tolerance to the anorectic, cardiovascular, hyperthermic, and lethal effects but sensitization (reverse tolerance) to dyskinesias, psychotomimetic effects, and seizures. As noted in Chapter 2, sensitization is the "progressive enhancement of a behavioral, physiological, or neurochemical response to repeated administration of a fixed dose of drug."[25] With psychostimulants once-daily dosage for a week or two in rodents results in increased locomotor and stereotypic responses to subsequent single doses of the drug, and this behavioral enhancement persists for over a year.[26] Pretreatment with amphetamine also facilitates the later acquisition of drug self-administration and so in humans might play a critical role in the development of persistent drug craving. The physiological basis of sensitization to amphetamines (and to other drugs) is uncertain. In rats intra-VTA injections of amphetamine every other day for four doses potentiates the locomotor responses to systemically administered amphetamine 2 weeks later, and this behavioral sensitization is then apparent with morphine as well.[27] Selective dopamine D_1 antagonists prevent this behavioral sensitization; dopamine D_2 antagonists do not.[28] Repeated injections of amphetamine into the NA do not result in sensitization, but repeated injections into the VTA produce sensitization to later administration of amphetamine into the NA. The VTA thus appears to be involved in the induction of behavioral sensitization and the NA in its expression.[29]

N-methyl-D-aspartate (NMDA) receptor antagonists inhibit the induction but not the expression of amphetamine behavioral sensitization. Blockade of AMPA glutamate receptors abolishes the expression of amphetamine sensitization.[25] The prefrontal cortex (PFC) provides a major excitatory glutamatergic projection to the VTA, and lesions of the PFC block sensitization to amphetamine.[30] Excitatory synapses on VTA neurons exhibit both long-term potentiation (LTP) and long-term depression (LTD); amphetamine blocks LTD, and the resulting increased excitatory drive to dopaminergic neurons—i.e., unopposed LTP—might contribute to sensitization.[31] A further possibility is that increased glutamate activity recruits neurotrophic and neuroprotective substances which produce long-lasting neuronal adaptations that underlie sensitization.[32]

Although dopamine D_1 receptor antagonists prevent sensitization to amphetamine, D_1 receptor knockout mice paradoxically exhibit sensitization to the drug.[33] Thus, although dopamine clearly plays a critical role in the induction and expression of amphetamine sensitization, the precise mechanism remains elusive.[34] One hypothesis focuses on the dopamine D_3 receptor, which has far greater affinity for dopamine than do D_1 and D_2 receptors and which, in contrast to D_1 and D_2 receptors, inhibits locomotion. The hypothesis proposes that amphetamine sensitization is the consequence of selective down-regulation of D_3 receptors, leaving locomotor and other effects of D_1 and D_2 receptors unopposed.[26]

Neurotoxicity

In monkeys, chronic amphetamine or methamphetamine administration damages brain dopaminergic nerve terminals, with lasting depletion of brain dopamine.[35,36] In rats, methamphetamine similarly affects both dopaminergic and serotonergic nerves, and silver staining shows destruction of dopamine terminals.[37] Methylphenidate displays no such toxicity to either neurotransmitter system. It would appear that the cytoplasmic, newly synthesized transmitter pool is required for amphetamine and methamphetamine neurotoxicity, which is blocked

by inhibition of dopamine synthesis.[13] The mechanism of damage is unknown.[38] Excitatory neurotransmitters could play a role.[25] In mice, the NMDA receptor blockers MK-801 and phencyclidine protect against methamphetamine neurotoxicity,[39] and methamphetamine-induced dopaminergic neurotoxicity does not occur in either knockout mice lacking neuronal nitric oxide synthase or transgenic mice overproducing superoxide dismutase.[40–42] Knockout mice lacking the p53 gene are protected against delayed methamphetamine toxicity—evidence that apoptosis is a pathological feature.[43] Methamphetamine-induced reactive oxygen and nitrogen species might, in different dosing schedules, result in variable necrotic and apoptotic cascades.[36] The presence of dopamine itself contributes to oxidative stress by producing toxic metabolites, including hydroxyl and superoxide radicals, hydrogen peroxide, and dopamine quinones; shifting dopamine from vesicles to cytoplasm, amphetamine accelerates the formation of these free radicals.[44] Depletion of dopamine protects against methamphetamine toxicity, and administration of L-DOPA reinstates it.[45] When mitochondrial function is pharmacologically compromised, dopaminergic neurons exposed to methamphetamine demonstrate a marked increase in cell death.[44]

Historical Background and Epidemiology

In the 1920s, the search for an oral antiasthmatic led to the discovery of ephedrine in the ma huang plant (*Ephedra vulgaris*), which had been used for that purpose in China for centuries. In 1932, the synthetic ephedrine analog, amphetamine, was introduced and sold in over-the-counter form in Benzedrine inhalers; 250 mg of the drug was contained in a cotton plug. The ability of amphetamine to ward off sleep and elevate mood was quickly recognized, and users learned either to extract drug from the plug or to ingest it whole.[45,46] By the late 1930s, warnings appeared in medical journals of amphetamine's abuse liability.[47] During the Second World War, amphetamine was provided to soldiers of both sides and in Japan to the civilian population as well. (The most famous wartime amphetamine addict was Adolf Hitler, who, after his assassination attempt, took daily cocaine as well.[48]) Following the war, Japanese pharmaceutical companies continued to promote the drug, leading to an epidemic of amphetamine abuse in which 5% of all Japanese aged 16 to 25 years became physically dependent.[45] The epidemic subsided following passage of stringent control laws.

During the 1950s, drug companies tried to develop amphetamine analogs with selective effects, either stimulation without appetite suppression (e.g., methylphenidate) or appetite suppression without stimulation (e.g., phenmetrazine, diethylpropion, or phendimetrazine). Among the latter group, selective action proved less than claimed. In Sweden during the 1950s, amphetamine was regulated but phenmetrazine was not, and an epidemic of phenmetrazine abuse led to removal of the drug from the market.[49] (Another amphetamine analog, fenfluramine, does suppress appetite without CNS stimulation and perhaps for that reason has never been very popular among the obese.)

Attempts to temper amphetamine stimulation by combining it with a sedative were also fruitless. During the 1950s in Britain, a mixture of amphetamine and amobarbital (Drinamyl, "purple hearts") was widely abused.

'In the United States, amphetamine was available in over-the-counter form until 1954, and with or without a prescription, its popularity continued among students and truck drivers who wanted to stay alert, athletes who sought increased endurance, and dieters who actually used it for mood elevation, often in conjunction with sedatives or ethanol.[50–53] Acute intoxication was an ongoing accompaniment.[54–56] Oral amphetamines were also common illicit street drugs ("uppers," "ups," "bennies," "black beauties," "dexies," "pep pills," "jelly beans").

Amphetamine began to be used intravenously by American servicemen in Korea and Japan during the early 1950s. Presaging the current "speedball," it was often combined with heroin. The practice was then taken up in the San Francisco Bay area, where, in addition, intravenous amphetamine was prescribed illegally by physicians to "treat" heroin addicts. By the 1960s, intravenous abuse of amphetamine and methamphetamine ("speed," "crank," "crystal meth," "tina") was a well-publicized problem in the United States, resulting in removal of Desoxyn ampules from the market and restriction of Methedrine ampules to hospitals.[57] In 1965, the Federal Drug Abuse Control Amendments further restricted manufacture and distribution of

amphetamines, and supply shifted to illicit manufacture ("speed labs"). Although seemingly overshadowed by the cocaine epidemic of the 1980s, abuse of amphetamine and methamphetamine has remained a major drug problem in the United States and other countries. In 1982, an estimated 13 million Americans had used amphetamine or methamphetamine without medical supervision, including over one-third of high school seniors.[58] In a 1988 survey of 1152 parenteral drug abusers in a Stockholm prison, 958 had used amphetamine, compared with only 194 who had used heroin.[59] In 1987, 2900 urine toxicology profiles were performed at the University of California Medical Center in San Diego, and 290 (10%) were positive for amphetamine or methamphetamine, a prevalence comparable to cocaine's.[60] Twelve percent of positive urine tests were from neonates. By 1989, in Hawaii smokable methamphetamine ("ice") had replaced smokable cocaine ("crack") as the drug of choice.[61]

During the 1990s, as cocaine use waned, the popularity of methamphetamine surged, especially in rural Midwest and Southwest America and in cities on the West Coast.[61a, 62] Particularly attracted to the drug are habitués of gay clubs and members of motorcycle gangs. By the end of the 1990s the drug was considered the fastest-growing illegal drug in the United States, Canada, and parts of Europe. Methamphetamine is injected, snorted, smoked, and drunk in beverages, and preferred routes of administration vary with locale. Injection is common in Denver, Seattle, and San Francisco. Inhalation and smoking are preferred in the East and Midwest United States. In San Francisco young urban professionals put methamphetamine into coffee ("bikers' coffee"). In Houston, methamphetamine is mixed with finely ground glass, causing the inhaled mixture to scratch the nasal mucosa, and facilitating absorption. A powdered form of methamphetamine is a staple of the dance scene, where it is rubbed onto the gums, added to alcoholic drinks, or "bombed" (wrapped in cigarette paper and swallowed). The drug is often taken with heroin ("speedball") or sedatives.[63–65]

Whereas most methamphetamine marketed in Europe is in pills made in Southeast Asia, most American methamphetamine is sold as a powder made in clandestine laboratories, many of which are in California and operated by Mexicans who formerly trafficked in Colombia-grown cocaine. Other laboratories are found across the United States, especially in the Midwest. In 1998 the U.S. Drug Enforcement Agency identified 454 such laboratories in Missouri, Kansas, and Nebraska.[66] Methamphetamine costs US$1300 to US$1800 a pound to produce. Its wholesale price ranges from US$4500 to US$8000 a pound in California and US$15,000 to US$20,000 a pound on the East Coast.

Ephedrine is used in the manufacture of methamphetamine, and in 1995 the U.S. Food and Drug Administration directed that over-the-counter bronchodilators no longer contain ephedrine.[63] Deliberately added constituents of illicit methamphetamine include iodine crystals, ephedrine, pseudoephedrine, caffeine, phenylpropanolamine, dextromethorphan, pool acid, and red phosphorus contained in road flares.[63,64] Unintended byproducts include hydrochloric acid and phosphine.[66]

Acute Effects

Initial Symptoms and Signs

In human novices, 10–30 mg oral dextroamphetamine produces alertness, euphoria, increased motor activity, improved coordination, and greater physical endurance, but the feeling of well-being can lead to overconfidence and impaired judgment.[67] Some subjects are initially drowsy, becoming hyperalert only after 1 or 2 hours.[68] Some experience agitation, dysphoria, confusion, headache, palpitations, and fatigue. Systolic blood pressure is raised, often with reflex bradycardia, and there is mild pupillary dilatation.[69] Sleep is reduced as well as the percentage of time spent in the rapid eye movement (REM) phase, and there is a shift toward higher frequencies in the resting electroencephalogram.[2]

Intravenous amphetamine produces a brief "flash" or "rush," a sharp awakening that may be compared to an electric shock or orgasm but is qualitatively different from an opioid "rush." Because the transit time from lung to brain is shorter than from antecubital vein to brain, the rush is even more rapid and powerful following inhalation of "ice." With either route of administration, there is a lingering euphoria. Amphetamine's biological half-life is about 8 hours, and methamphetamine's is about 12 hours; powerful psychic effects can therefore last several hours (compared with 30 to

90 minutes for cocaine).[70] With repeated use, moreover, drug accumulation occurs. Amphetamine delays genital orgasm and heightens it when it occurs.[71]

Tolerance and Sensitization

Tolerance to these effects develops rapidly. Although 100 mg amphetamine can be fatal to a novice, addicts have taken thousands of milligrams daily. Intravenous users of amphetamines ("speed freaks") often take the drug in a familiar pattern.[72] After a period of oral use, injections begin. There then develops a "run": several days of intravenous injections every 2 or 3 hours in increasing dosage up to 100–300 mg per injection, during which time the subject is continuously awake. Toxic symptoms appear: tremor, bruxism, dystonia, choreoathetosis, picking and excoriations, sweating, thirst, difficulty with micturition, and sometimes cardiac arrhythmia. Anorexia leads to marked weight loss when "runs" occur successively. Suspiciousness and rapid mood changes occur as well as preoccupation with one's thoughts and a sense of profundity. Stereotyped repetitive behavior might consist of taking apart and trying to put together mechanical objects or stringing beads for hours. Paranoia eventually develops in nearly all chronic abusers, and frank psychosis is common. Hallucinations are auditory, visual, olfactory, or haptic (the feeling of bugs or vermin crawling over and under the skin). The emergence of dyskinesias and psychosis during chronic amphetamine use is a good example of drug sensitization (reverse tolerance), all the more striking when it occurs while tolerance is developing to "rush," euphoria, anorexia, hyperthermia, cardiovascular effects, and lethality.[73] A contributor to tolerance may be anorexia, which causes ketosis and increases amphetamine excretion. More important, however, is cellular responsiveness (pharmacodynamic tolerance), not tissue levels of drug (pharmacokinetic tolerance). Dyskinesias usually resolve within a few days of stopping amphetamine but can last weeks, months, or even years.[74,75,75a]

Relationship to Schizophrenia

In subjects tolerant to cardiovascular effects, amphetamine may be overlooked as the cause of schizophrenic symptoms,[2] although the extent to which psychotic symptoms actually resemble schizophrenia is disputed.[76,77] Amphetamine produces positive schizophrenic symptoms (e.g., paranoia, hallucinations) but in contrast to phencyclidine does not produce negative symptoms (e.g., emotional withdrawal, motor retardation) or a formal thought disorder.[78] Paranoia sometimes leads to violence, including suicide and homicide. Subjects carry weapons and attack strangers who fit into their persecutory delusions.[76] Psychosis may emerge gradually over months or occur during a single "run." Amphetamine exacerbates psychotic symptoms in most schizophrenics, and premorbid psychopathology is common in chronic abusers, but psychosis also occurs in apparently normal subjects, and it is unusual for psychotic symptoms to persist after the drug is stopped.[73,77] Moreover, some schizophrenic patients receiving amphetamines have had symptomatic improvement.[77–79] In one report, schizophrenic patients already receiving haloperidol became more active and had improved performance on the Wisconsin Card Sorting Test after receiving amphetamine; the authors proposed that the combined treatment selectively enhanced cortical dopaminergic activity.[80]

Overdose

Acute overdose of amphetamine or methamphetamine causes excitement, confusion, headache, chest pain, hypertension, tachycardia, flushing, profuse sweating, and mydriasis, progressing to delirium, hallucinations, hyperpnea, cardiac arrhythmia, hyperpyrexia (sometimes over 109°F [42.7°C]), seizures, shock, coma, and death.[81–87] (In rats the brain warms before the body, indicating that hyperthermia is neurally triggered rather than movement driven.)[87a] Acute pulmonary edema may be the principal manifestation,[88] and autopsy often indicates a non-cardiac origin.[89] Small children display head banging, mutilation of digits by biting, and violent purposeless movements.[82] Myoglobinuria occurs, and shock has resulted from loss of intravascular volume into necrotic muscle. Some subjects have acute pyrogenic reactions following previously tolerated doses.[90] Disseminated intravascular coagulation may be secondary to hyperthermia, and death may be from heat stroke itself. At autopsy, diffuse cerebral edema and petechiae are found.[56,81]

Dogs and rabbits given lethal doses of ampheta had severe hyperpyrexia and, at autopsy, subendocardial and epicardial hemorrhage, myocardial fiber necrosis, and neuronal degeneration in the cerebral cortex and cerebellum.[91,92] Curare prevented the fever and the fatal course, suggesting that muscle hyperactivity was critical.[93] Fever may have contributed to similar pathological findings in the brains of cats receiving chronic methamphetamine, although in that study neuronal catecholamine depletion was considered the primary cause.[94]

Seizures are less frequent among amphetamine users than cocaine users. In a report from San Francisco General Hospital of 49 recreational drug-induced seizures, 11 occurred in users of amphetamine, either alone (8) or with cocaine, phencyclidine, or heroin. Seizures occurred in both first-time and chronic users, were independent of route of administration (intravenous, intranasal, or oral), and were not always associated with other signs of overdose.[95]

The usual fatal dose of amphetamine for a nontolerant adult is 20–25 mg/kg and for children 5 mg/kg, but idiosyncratic reactions sometimes follow low doses. Qualitative urine testing for amphetamines is of no value in the acute setting, and serum drug screens are unreliable, so diagnosis is based on history and examination.[96]

Treatment of overdose usually begins with reducing excitement and protecting against injury.[96] Because psychostimulant poisoning is infrequently lethal, physical restraints and sedation should be used only as necessary.[86,97] One should try to maintain verbal contact with the patient in a quiet, lighted room. The combination of hyperthermia and agitation can be rapidly fatal, however, requiring rapid external cooling and sedation.[96] Barbiturates can aggravate delirium, potentiate postexcitatory depression, and, if amphetamine has been taken with a sedative, precipitate stupor or coma. Neuroleptics also have drawbacks, especially if the diagnosis is uncertain or amphetamine has been taken with another drug. They can precipitate seizures in cocaine intoxication, aggravate delirium in anticholinergic intoxication, contribute to myoglobinuria in phencyclidine intoxication, and produce hypotension in any setting. Chlorpromazine effectively reversed delirium and self-injury in a series of small children poisoned by amphetamine, methamphetamine, or phenmetrazine.[82] Others recommend haloperidol on the grounds that chlorpromazine prolongs the half-life of amphetamine.[98] The current sedative of choice in most emergency rooms, however, is an intravenous benzodiazepine, rapidly titrated until the patient is calm. Very large doses may be necessary, for example more than 100 mg of diazepam.[96]

Cardiorespiratory support is provided as needed. Seizures are treated conventionally with a benzodiazepine and phenytoin. For severe hypertension, beta-blockers carry the risk of unopposed alpha-adrenergic activity and aggravation of blood pressure. The combined alpha- and beta-blocking drug labatalol has greater beta- than alpha-blocking properties. Preferable are alpha-blockers (e.g., phenoxybenzamine or phentolamine) or direct vasodilators (e.g., nitroprusside).[99] Forced diuresis and acidification of urine enhance drug excretion, but acidification is given only in the absence of metabolic acidosis and myoglobinuria.[100] For severe refractory cases, peritoneal dialysis or hemodialysis can be instituted.[82]

Concomitant use of methamphetamine and ethanol aggravates both cardiac and psychotomimetic effects.[101]

Dependence and Withdrawal

Amphetamines produce psychic and probably physical dependence, and there are often only a few months between first exposure and chronic use.[71] Withdrawal from prolonged use is followed by depression, fatigue, and increased appetite and sleep, including time spent in the REM phase.[101] Following a "run," the subject, because of tenseness, paranoia, or exhaustion, stops taking the drug and falls asleep for usually 12 to 18 hours ("crashing"). Sometimes sedatives are taken to induce sleep, but usually drowsiness occurs within a few hours of the last "fix" and cannot be resisted without taking more stimulant. Longer "runs" are followed by more prolonged sleep, sometimes lasting several days. Psychotic symptoms are usually absent on awakening, but there is hunger (often ravenous), lethargy, and depression. Injections are then resumed, and a new "run" begins.

Withdrawal symptoms are not life-threatening, but depression, sometimes suicidal, can last for weeks, requiring hospitalization and treatment with tricyclic antidepressants. Drug craving and dysphoria can wax and wane for months.[36] In contrast to opioid addicts, amphetamine abusers tend to "burn out" after a few years.[71]

Medical and Neurological Complications

Systemic Toxicity

Parenteral psychostimulant use leads to many of the same medical sequelae that beset parenteral abusers of other drugs. Infections often involve unusual organisms and affect the nervous system.[102,103] There is also, of course, a risk for human immunodeficiency virus (HIV) infection from either parenteral use or from risky sexual behavior during intoxication.[62]

A 19-year-old boy developed pneumomediastinum while snorting amphetamine.[104]

Hepatocellular toxicity has been associated with both acute and chronic amphetamine use. Proposed mechanisms include a direct toxic effect, hepatotoxic contaminants, hypotension, hepatic vasoconstriction, vasculitis, and viral hepatitis.[105]

Myocardial infarction is less often associated with amphetamine than with cocaine. It has occurred in young, otherwise healthy men taking amphetamine alone or with heroin[106,107] and has followed snorting of methamphetamine.[108,109] Acute cardiomyopathy with normal coronary angiography has followed intravenous amphetamine use,[110] and congestive cardiomyopathy has followed chronic oral amphetamine use.[111] An autopsy study suggested that chronic methamphetamine use increases the risk of coronary artery atherosclerosis.[89]

Stroke

A frequent complication of amphetamine abuse is stroke, both occlusive and hemorrhagic. More than 50 patients, ages 16 to 60 years, have been reported with intracranial hemorrhage after amphetamine use.[89,109,112–150] Routes of administration have been oral, intravenous, or nasal. Most patients were chronic users, but in five, stroke followed first exposure. Dosage was usually unknown but in one case was less than 80 mg. Some also took methylphenidate, phenmetrazine, LSD, DOM, cocaine, heroin, or barbiturates. Symptoms usually began with severe headache within minutes of drug use. Blood pressure was elevated in more than half, with diastolic pressure as high as 120 mmHg. Computed tomography (CT) has shown intracerebral hemorrhage (often lobar), intraventricular hemorrhage, subarachnoid hemorrhage, or no abnormality. Cerebral angiography in 12 patients showed irregular narrowing ("beading") of distal cerebral vessels, consistent with vasculitis, which was found at autopsy in several patients.[149] In several others a cerebral vascular malformation or saccular aneurysm was identified at angiography, CT, or autopsy.[89,150]

High fever and disturbed clotting were not noted in any of these patients. Some of the hemorrhages appeared to be secondary to acute hypertension, some to vasculitis, and some to a combination of the two, but in others neither feature was apparent. Moreover, acute hypertension could have been either causal or a transient result of the stroke, and fleeting blood pressure elevations could have been missed.

Amphetamine-induced cerebral vasculitis has caused occlusive as well as hemorrhagic stroke and appears to be of more than one type. Necrotizing angiitis occurred in 14 Los Angeles abusers of multiple drugs, including amphetamine, methamphetamine, barbiturates, chlordiazepoxide, diazepam, marijuana, hydroxyzine, LSD, heroin, meperidine, mescaline, oxycodone, oxymorphone, DOM, and strychnine.[151] All but two patients used methamphetamine, and one used it exclusively. Five patients were asymptomatic, and in others there were a variety of systemic symptoms and signs, including skin rash, anemia, hypertension, arthralgia, pneumonitis, renal failure, and peripheral neuropathy. One, with "progressive encephalopathy," at autopsy had vasculitis affecting pontine arterioles. Another, with "mental obtundation," had brain vasculitis with cerebral and brainstem infarcts and cerebellar hemorrhage. Vessel changes affected only muscular arteries and arterioles and were considered typical for polyarteritis nodosa, although unassociated with Australia antigen.[152,153]

Such brain lesions have been observed pathologically in other amphetamine or methamphetamine abusers.[126,149,154,155] Sometimes, however, cerebral arteritis has been presumed on the basis of cerebral angiography, and the relation to amphetamine has not always been obvious.[118–120,124,125,131] Widespread angiographic beading of cerebral arteries, with multiple occlusion of arterioles, was reported in 19 young drug abusers (mostly intravenous methamphetamine) admitted for coma or stroke.[156] Ischemic stroke has followed intranasal inhalation of methamphetamine, with intervals from last use to stroke ranging from 12 hours to 2 weeks. Angiographically occluded or "beaded" vessels have included the extracranial and supraclinoid internal carotid, distal middle cerebral, lenticulostriate, and thalamoperforating arteries.[157,158]

Monkeys given intravenous methamphetamine underwent serial angiograms.[159] Some showed beaded small cerebral vessels at 10 minutes with a return to normal at 24 hours. In others, both small and large vessels were affected, and the changes persisted or progressed over a 2-week period. Clinically there was hypertension and behavioral change. At autopsy, some animals had subarachnoid hemorrhage with brain petechiae, infarcts, microaneurysms, and perivascular white cell cuffing. More severe vasculitic changes occurred in a later study of monkeys receiving intravenous methamphetamine three times weekly for up to a year.[160] In rats given intravenous methamphetamine, electron microscopy revealed endothelial cell changes in vessels too small (under 100 μm) to be seen angiographically. Angiographic and histological changes have also occurred in monkeys and rats receiving intravenous methylphenidate.[160]

These lesions differ from those of polyarteritis nodosa, in which elastic arteries, capillaries, and veins are spared. It is unclear whether they are the result of hypersensitivity or direct toxicity or whether subarachnoid hemorrhage itself contributes.

A young man developed a Brown–Séquard syndrome after unsuccessfully attempting to inject methamphetamine into his jugular vein. The mechanism was probably direct injection into an artery supplying the cervical spinal cord, with the drug acting as either a sclerosant or a vasoconstrictor.[160a]

Systemic Vasculopathy

In an adolescent amphetamine abuser with mononeuritis multiplex, sural nerve biopsy showed apparent hypersensitivity angiitis of medium and small arteries, arterioles, venules, and veins; there were no CNS symptoms.[161] Amphetamine-induced angiitis has also caused renal failure.[162] Other vasculopathies include aortic dissection and ischemic colitis.[96,150]

Movement Disorders

Tourette syndrome has been exacerbated and precipitated by amphetamine, methylphenidate, and pemoline, sometimes clearing with discontinuation of the drug but sometimes persisting.[163–165] Also occasionally persistent are the bruxism and choreiform movements that develop with chronic amphetamine use.[74] An amphetamine addict with intractable bruxism was successfully treated with botulinum toxin.[75a]

Lead Poisoning

Two methamphetamine users from Oregon developed lead poisoning. One had hallucinations, constipation, hepatic tenderness, and jaundice initially misdiagnosed as infectious hepatitis; the other had weakness, malaise, headache, abdominal pain, myalgia, chills, sweating, and weight loss. Lead acetate had been used in the illicit manufacture of the drug.[166]

Chronic Neurotoxicity

Similar to chronically exposed animals, human methamphetamine users have brain alterations that suggest long-lasting neurotoxicity.[36] Autopsy studies demonstrate reduction in striatal levels of dopamine and dopamine transporter (DAT).[167] Positron emission tomography studies also show reduced striatal DAT binding.[168] In one study the reduction was present after 3 years of abstinence.[169] Chronic users also have reduced glucose metabolism in the thalamus and striatum but increased glucose metabolism in the cerebral cortex.[170] Studies with magnetic resonance spectroscopy (MRS) demonstrate metabolic abnormalities in the presence of normal structural magnetic resonance imaging.[171] Whether such alterations cause clinically significant cognitive or behavioral abnormalities is uncertain. Reports are largely anecdotal, and formal studies have been methodologically flawed.[172]

Also unknown is whether methamphetamine-induced striatal abnormalities increase the risk of Parkinson's disease with advancing age.[36,173,173a]

Obstetric and Pediatric Aspects

At the Presbyterian Hospital in New York, amphetamine metabolites were detected in 13% of more than 500 women admitted for delivery (compared with 10% for cocaine). The screens did not distinguish between metabolites of amphetamine and other drugs such as cold remedies. Medical histories predicted none of the amphetamine-positive samples.[174]

Newborns of methamphetamine-using mothers have abnormal sleep patterns, poor feeding, tremor, and hypertonia as well as higher than expected rates of prematurity, intrauterine growth retardation, and smaller head circumference.[175,176] An anecdotal report described dysgenesis of the corpus callosum following in utero exposure to amphetamine and septo-optic dysplasia following in utero exposure to the amphetamine-like agent phenylpropanolamine.[177] In another study, echoencephalographic abnormalities were found in nine of 24 neonates exposed to methamphetamine, including white matter cavities (1), white matter densities (3), intraventricular hemorrhage (4), subarachnoid hemorrhage (4), subependymal hemorrhage (3), and ventricular enlargement (2).[178] Other anecdotally reported anomalies and adverse outcomes include cleft lip, cardiac defects, low birth weight, reduced head circumference, biliary atresia, prematurity, stillbirth, hyperbilirubinemia, and undescended testes.[179] Amphetamine precipitated eclampsia in a 19-year old.[180] Permanent visual and cognitive impairment and altered behavior were observed in a 14-year follow-up study of Swedish children exposed in utero to amphetamine.[181] Methamphetamine-exposed newborns demonstrate impaired visual recognition memory compared with controls.[182] Young children with a history of such exposure had metabolic abnormalities in the striatum as demonstrated by MRS without any visible abnormalities on magnetic resonance imaging.[183] Confounders in these reports include inadequate prenatal care, use of other substances, and social environment. For example, in the Swedish study 80% of the mothers used ethanol, tobacco, or both.

Clefting, cardiac anomalies, and growth retardation have been reproduced in animal studies (rats, mice, rabbits, chicks), some but not all of which used pair-fed controls (especially relevant in studying an anorexigenic drug). Also observed are abnormalities of notochord and neural tube, exencephaly, and malformed limbs and eyes.[179] In rats long-term reductions in dopamine and serotonin transporters possibly accounted for impaired motor performance and learning.[184,185] Central monoaminergic pathways develop early in ontogeny and plausibly modulate the development of other neural elements.[45] In gerbils receiving single doses of amphetamine as juveniles (corresponding to late gestation in humans), reduced hippocampal granule cell numbers, altered prefrontal cortex circuitry, and cognitive deficits were observed during adulthood.[186] In sheep methamphetamine causes vasoconstriction in uterine and placental vessels and fetal hypertension.[187] These animal studies lend support to the validity of reports in humans.

Other Related Agents

Phenylpropanolamine

Phenylpropanolamine (PPA), a drug similar to but less potent than amphetamine, was marketed, sometimes combined with ephedrine or caffeine, in over-the-counter diet pills (e.g., Dex-a-diet, Dexatrim, Anorexin, Maxi-slim) and decongestants (Table 4–2).[188] During the 1980s and 1990s an estimated 5 billion doses of PPA were used annually

Table 4–2. "Cold" or Allergy Medications that Contained Phenylpropanolamine

Alka-Seltzer Plus Cold Medicine
Allerest
Bayer Children's Cold Tablets
Children's CoTylenol
Comtrex
Contac
Coricidin-D
Coryban-D
Deconex
Dehist
Dimetapp
Duadacin
Four-Way Cold Tablets
Histabid Duracap
Naldecon Pediatric Syrup
Noraminic
Oraminic
Ornade
Sinarest
Sine-off Sinus Medicine
Sinubid
Spect-T Decongestant Lozenges
St. Joseph's Cold Tablets for Children
Sucrets Cold Decongestant
Triaminic

in the United States. Animal studies suggest that the addiction liability of PPA is low—it is not self-administered by pigeons or monkeys[189]—and studies with human volunteers reveal little stimulant or euphoric properties at therapeutic doses.[190] (In one such study, very high doses of PPA produced "arousal" and "vigor" but in contrast to amphetamine did not cause euphoria.[191]) Nonetheless, PPA, alone or combined with ephedrine or caffeine, was a well-known illicit street drug, often misrepresented as amphetamine ("look-alike pills," "pseudospeed," "pea shooters"). PPA was also sold by mail order as a "legal stimulant."[192,192a]

A narrow margin of safety exists between recommended and toxic doses of PPA, and in a study of normal volunteers there was considerable variability between subjects in PPA pressor effects.[193] Complications of PPA include acute hypertension and severe headache;[194–198] intractable nausea and vomiting;[199] cardiac arrhythmia;[200–201] hallucinations, paranoia, and homicidal behavior;[202–204] and seizures.[195,204-206] Hemorrhagic stroke, intracerebral and subarachnoid, has followed recommended as well as excessive dosage.[199,207–223,223a] Of those with intracerebral hemorrhage, several have had multiple simultaneous lesions, suggesting diffuse vessel abnormalities, and vasculitis has been both implied angiographically and demonstrated pathologically. A young woman, 3 weeks postpartum, had an intracerebral hemorrhage following a single dose of Dexatrim, Extra Strength; leptomeningeal and brain biopsy demonstrated necrotizing vasculitis of small arteries and veins with infiltration of polymorphonuclear leukocytes.[213] PPA with caffeine, from a commercial diet preparation, caused subarachnoid hemorrhage in rats receiving it parenterally in several times the recommended dose.[188]

Ischemic stroke and transient ischemic attack are also reported.[224] Headache persisting for more than a week after a single dose of a non-prescription allergy medication containing PPA was associated with diffuse vasospasm at cerebral angiography.[225]

An epidemiological study in 1984 found no association between stroke and PPA but had design limitations.[220] In 2000 a case–control study involving 43 U.S. hospitals found that appetite suppressants containing PPA increase the risk of subarachnoid hemorrhage in women (odds ratio 16.58). No men in that study used PPA-containing diet pills, but a trend toward increased risk of hemorrhagic stroke was observed in men and women using PPA-containing cough and cold remedies. The greater risk associated with diet pills was attributed to higher daily doses.[226] Strokes did occur, however, after first use of PPA and in recommended doses. Based on this study it was estimated that between 200 and 400 PPA-related strokes occur annually in the United States.[227] That year the Food and Drug Administration (FDA) ordered products containing PPA to be withdrawn from the market.[228,229]

In contrast to its ban on PPA-containing diet remedies, the FDA's ban on cough or cold remedies containing PPA was based on a trend that fell short of conventional statistical significance. A report from Mexico described 16 consecutive patients with hemorrhagic (15) or ischemic (1) stroke temporally associated (30 minutes to 24 hours) with use of over-the-counter cough and cold drugs containing PPA. Some strokes occurred after a single dose and in recommended dosage. Cerebral angiography was either normal or showed vasospasm or beading.[230] Although anecdotal, this report does lend support for the FDA's decision.[231]

Developed as a potential anorectic, 4-methylaminorex is an easily manufactured cyclic derivative of PPA. As a street drug nicknamed "U4Euh," it became popular in Florida during the 1980s. A fatality followed co-ingestion of 4-methylaminorex and diazepam.[231a] In 1994, 4-methylaminorex was declared a Schedule I drug.[231b]

Ephedrine and Pseudoephedrine

Ephedrine and pseudoephedrine are also present in over-the-counter decongestants and bronchodilators. Ephedrine's margin of safety is similar to phenylpropanolamine's; pseudoephedrine's is greater, but both agents have caused anxiety, headache, tachyarrhythmia, and hypertensive crisis.[192,211,219,232,233] The abuse potential of these drugs is low, but dependence occurs.[222,234] Ephedrine is also taken by athletes to enhance performance.[53] Psychosis is described in abusers of ephedrine or pseudoephedrine either alone or in combination with other agents (e.g., Actifed, containing pseudoephedrine and triprolidine.)[235–237] In Britain, over-the-counter Do-Do tablets containing ephedrine, caffeine, and theophylline, are a popular form of stimulant abuse.[237] Both ischemic and hemorrhagic

strokes are described in ephedrine users.[238] A young man who had previously used "speed" and LSD had a subarachnoid hemorrhage within an hour of ingesting pills that turned out to be ephedrine; cerebral angiography, initially normal, a week later showed beading and branch occlusions, and biopsy of normal-appearing skin revealed deposits of immunoglobulin M (IgM) and the C3 component of complement in dermal vessels, suggesting circulating immune complexes.[239] Intracranial hemorrhage has also followed pseudoephedrine use.[230,240]

Dietary supplements containing ephedra alkaloids ("ma huang") are popular in the U.S. for energy enhancement and weight reduction. After passage in 1994 of the Federal Dietary Supplement Health and Education Act, which reduced the FDA's control over "food additives," there was a nationwide surge in sales of these products, marketed as legal stimulants with names such as "Cloud 9," "Herbal Ecstasy," "Ultimate Euphoria," and "Up Your Gas". An estimated 12 million people used these supplements in 1999.[241] In the U.K. Herbal Ecstasy is a popular drug at "raves" (a dance event where loud fast music is played non-stop for hours at a time); it contains herbs from around the world, including Tibetan Ma Huang, Chinese Black Ginseng Root, German Wild Ginko Biloba, African Raw Cola Nut, Wild Brazilian Guarana, Indonesian Green Tea Extract, Russian Golu-Kola, Australian Fo-Ti Tieng, and Rou Gui Cinnemonum Cassia. Such products often contain caffeine. Psychosis, cardiotoxicity (including sudden death), and ischemic and hemorrhagic stroke are reported in users of dietary ephedra.[242–248,248a] A review of 140 adverse events associated with ephedra use and reported to the FDA revealed stroke in 10 and seizures in 7.[241] A case–control study did not find an association between use of ephedra-containing products and risk of hemorrhagic stroke, but a trend was observed for doses of more than 32 mg per day.[248b]

In 1996 such products were banned in New York and other U.S. states. Although "food additives" can be marketed without safety or efficacy studies, the FDA can ban them on the grounds of unreasonable risk of harm at recommended doses; political pressure tends to prevent such action, however. (For example, Metabolife, the nation's leading seller of ephedra products, spent millions of dollars between 1998 and 2003 lobbying against state and federal regulations and contributing to political parties.[248c]) In 2003 the FDA finally banned products containing ephedra.

Diet Pills

A number of other amphetamine-like drugs are promoted mainly as diet pills, and they vary in their abuse potential (which in turn correlates loosely with their Drug Enforcement Administration [DEA] scheduling). Phenmetrazine, which is self-administered by animals and causes psychostimulation and euphoria in humans, is widely abused, including parenterally.[65,190,249,250] So is phentermine, inadvertent arterial injection of which has caused subclavian and carotid mycotic aneurysms.[251] Phentermine was also implicated in occlusive stroke in two young women, one of whom also took phendimetrazine and oral contraceptives and whose angiogram showed changes consistent with vertebrobasilar angiitis.[252] Less often abused is diethylpropion and then usually orally.[253,254] Mania and paranoid psychosis with auditory and visual hallucinations have affected diethylpropion users.[255,256] Intracerebral hemorrhage occurred following ingestion of diethylpropion by a 60-year-old normotensive man.[133] The anorectic benzphetamine is self-administered by animals and produces amphetamine-like effects in humans, but abuse seems to be rare.[190] The anorectic mazindol (which does not structurally resemble amphetamine) is self-administered by monkeys,[250] yet in humans it not only fails to produce euphoria but also in one study was dysphoric.[190,191] (The rarity of mazindol abuse shows that animal studies do not always predict human dependence liability.) Also more often dysphoric than euphoric is fenfluramine, which is not self-administered by animals;[2] nonetheless, abuse of fenfluramine—taken in large oral doses for its psychic effects—was reported among young South Africans.[257] An 11-year-old girl taking phentermine and propylhexedrine suffered fatal heat stroke while hiking.[258] Intracerebral hemorrhage occurred in a middle-aged woman taking fenfluramine and phentermine.[259] A cohort study of subjects taking appetite suppressants found that phentermine, fenfluramine, and dexfenfluramine increased the risk of stroke (odds ratio 2.4), but confidence intervals were wide.[260] Two young women taking fenfluramine developed multifocal small cerebral infarcts, neurosensory hearing loss, and retinal arteriolar occlusions.[261]

In 1997, because of reports of valvular heart disease and pulmonary hypertension in people using dexfenfluramine or fenfluramine, these drugs were withdrawn from the U.S. market.[262]

In animals fenfluramine and dexfenfluramine in doses of the same order as recommended in humans cause long-lasting damage to brain serotonin neurons.[263,264]

Methylphenidate, Pemoline

Classified as a Schedule II drug, methylphenidate, like cocaine, blocks the dopamine transporter, and is self-administered by animals.[265,266] The drug is prescribed for 7% of American school-aged children for attention deficit hyperactivity disorder (ADHD), and oral recreational use is frequent among adolescents and college students.[267,268] As a street drug ("Vitamin R," "Skippy," "poor man's cocaine," the "smart drug") crushed tablets are snorted or injected intravenously.[269–271] As with other psychostimulants it is often combined with heroin.[65]

Methylphenidate is often prescribed by unwary physicians in drug-seeking scams. Of 22 methylphenidate abusers in Baltimore, nine had children who were taking methylphenidate for "hyperactivity."[272] A Wisconsin survey of children who had been prescribed methylphenidate found that 20% had been approached to sell or trade their medication.[273] In Seattle, methylphenidate abuse was especially common among patients receiving methadone maintenance therapy.[274] Water-insoluble constituents of the tablets lead to a high incidence of pulmonary complications, including chest pain, wheezing, hemoptysis, abnormal pulmonary function tests, and eventually fibrosis or even fatal pulmonary hypertension.[272,275] Deep neck abscesses in methylphenidate abusers are also attributed to foreign body reaction to tablet fillers followed by superinfection.[276] Other users have developed a syndrome of fever, myalgia, arthralgia, and eosinophilia.[277] Methylphenidate neuropsychiatric toxicity is similar to that of other psychostimulants. Acutely syncope is common, and dyskinesias and psychosis develop during the course of a binge.[278–280] Seizures, appearing as a late complication, suggest the "kindling" pattern seen with cocaine.

Cerebrovascular complications are also reported. Right hemiplegia in a young woman followed attempted injection into the left jugular vein of crushed methylphenidate tablets; 2 weeks later, left hemiplegia followed a similar right injection.[281] Talc microemboli have been seen in the fundi of intravenous methylphenidate abusers, sometimes with retinal and vitreous hemorrhages and neovascularization; in one such patient, who had not had a clinical stroke, talc and cornstarch emboli were also present in brain and lung.[282,283] Infarction of the medulla followed intravenous methylphenidate in a young woman; at autopsy, there were talc deposits in small vessels around the infarct.[284] A 12-year-old boy taking methylphenidate orally in prescribed dosage for ADHD developed hemiparesis and aphasia; angiography revealed occlusion of the anterior cerebral artery and a branch of the middle cerebral artery, plus vessel irregularities suggestive of arteritis.[285]

Children with ADHD are at increased risk for later drug abuse, but the effect of therapy is disputed. Some workers believe treatment with methylphenidate reduces the risk; others believe it increases the risk.[286]

Pemoline, used to treat attention deficit disorder, is considered to have much less addiction liability than methylphenidate, but it has been abused. Choreoathetosis severe enough to cause myoglobinuria followed ingestion of more than 1000 mg pemoline within 24 hours in a middle-aged man without other signs of toxicity.[287]

Bronchodilators and Nasal Sprays

Propylhexedrine and 1-desoxyephedrine replaced amphetamine in Benzedrex inhalers, and complications of oral or parenteral abuse include psychosis, myocardial infarction, cardiomyopathy, pulmonary hypertension, and sudden death.[46,288–291] An adolescent who had previously used cocaine and amphetamine developed headache, nausea, numbness of hands and feet, precordial chest pain, and palpitations after intravenously injecting epinephrine from a bronchodilator inhaler.[292] Cerebral infarction and retinal artery branch occlusion were reported in chronic intranasal abusers of sprays and drops containing phenoxazoline or oxymetazoline.[293,294]

Khat, Methcathinone

Khat (*Catha edulis*) is a shrub indigenous to East Africa and the Arabian peninsula; its leaves contain cathinone, a compound similar to amphetamine.[295] Animals self-administer cathinone at rates higher than amphetamine but lower than cocaine.[296] Cathinone's duration of action is shorter than amphetamine's, and tolerance develops more rapidly to its anorectic effects. Today several million people in East Africa (especially Ethiopia and Kenya) and the southwest Arabian peninsula (especially Yemen) chew khat leaves for their stimulating properties.[297] Users include participants in social "khat sessions," where the goal is euphoria and loquacity, and farmers and manual laborers, who use the drug to reduce hunger and fatigue. Khat's toxic psychic effects are limited by its bulkiness and by the slow absorption and rapid metabolism of the psychoactive cathinone, but aggressive behavior, hallucinatory psychosis, and fatal hyperthermia have occurred.[298,299] Similarly, although withdrawal symptoms are usually mild, severe depression, suicide, and homicide have followed abstinence. Bilateral optic atrophy with central scotomas was reported in several khat users, in one of whom electroretinography suggested retinal toxicity in addition to optic neuropathy.[300,301] A single case report from the UK described rapidly progressive leukoencephalopathy in a daily khat chew; magnetic resonance imaging and brain biopsy revealed abnormalities similar to those seen with leukoencephalopathy resulting from inhalation of heroin pyrolysate (see Chapter 3), but use of other drugs was denied.[302]

Although prohibited in a number of African and Arabian countries, khat use increased in that part of the world during the 1980s. Moreover, although the leaves lose their effect within a few days of harvesting, air travel and creative gardening have allowed khat chewing to spread beyond its originally indigenous areas.[303,304] Psychosis has been reported in users in Italy, Britain, and the United States.[305–308]

Methcathinone, the methyl-derivative of cathinone, is a designer drug synthesized from ephedrine. Also known as ephedrane, its potency is similar to that of methamphetamine. Methcathinone has been widely abused in the former Soviet Union since the 1970s. Street-named "cat" or "Jeff," methcathinone has become popular in the United States, especially in the Midwest.[309–311]

MDA, MDMA, MDEA

In the 1960s 3,4-methylenedioxyamphetamine (MDA) became a popular street drug, and it was soon evident that it was a different kind of agent than either amphetamine or the so-called hallucinogenic amphetamines such as mescaline or dimethoxymethylamphetamine (DOM).[312,313] At low doses, MDA produces decreased anxiety and a sense of self-awareness, with a desire to talk with other people (the "love drug").[314] As the dose is increased, the drug becomes hallucinogenic and then psychostimularory.[315] MDA abuse continues in the United States, but in the 1980s its popularity was exceeded by a similar drug, 3,4-methylene-dioxymethamphetamine (MDMA, Figure 4–2). Developed in 1914 as an appetite suppressant, MDMA for many years was legally available and occasionally used in psychiatric treatment for its ability to create a pleasant state of introspection and facilitate communication.[316] By the 1980s it was widely abused, especially on college campuses, and in 1985 the DEA made it a Schedule I controlled substance.[317]

Animals trained to discriminate MDA generalize to MDMA and vice versa but not to amphetamine or typical hallucinogens.[312] Animals self-administer MDA and MDMA but not hallucinogens.[318,319] MDMA-induced locomotor stimulation in animals is blocked by the serotonin antagonist methysergide, suggesting reduced serotonergic modulation of dopaminergic neurons. This and other evidence suggests that MDA and MDMA act predominantly as serotonin agonists with only weak dopaminergic activity.[9,320–322]

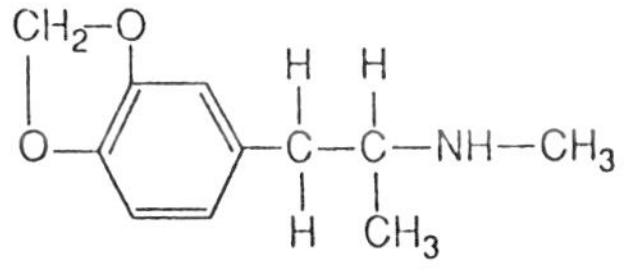

Figure 4–2. 3,4-Methylendioxymethamphetamine (MDMA).

MDMA is known as "Ecstasy" (and also as "Adam," "XTC," "M&M," "the Yuppie Drug," "Essence," "Clarity," "Venus," "Zen," and "Doctor"); a similar drug, 3,4-methylenedioxyethy-amphetamine (MDEA), is known as "Eve."[323–325] MDA, MDMA, and MDEA, like methcathinone, are "designer amphetamines," congeners of phenylethylamine, of which over 200 psychoactive variants exist.[96,326] MDMA and MDEA pharmacologically possess properties of both psychostimulants and hallucinogens, and are referred to as "entactogens" (Latin: "to be moved"; Greek: "within").[326a] (Those used recreationally for their hallucinogenic rather than their psychostimulatory or euphoriant effects are discussed in Chapter 8.) They are usually taken in group sessions; during the 1990s their popularity in the United States, Europe, and Australia at "raves," house parties, and dance clubs became epidemic, especially among college students.[96,327] By the end of the 1990s, as the price of a tablet fell from US$25 to US$8, their use in the United States spread beyond the college and club scene. Most Ecstasy is produced in the Netherlands or Belgium and smuggled into the United States by Israeli or Russian gangs. (Couriers are often dancers at topless nightclubs.) In 1997 the U.S. Customs Service seized 400,000 ecstasy pills; in 2000 it seized 9.3 million. A national survey in 2000 found that 8% of American 12th graders had used Ecstasy during the previous year, up from 3.5% in 1998.[328]

MDMA comes as a powder which can be pressed into pills of usually 100 mg. The usual dose is 100 to several hundred milligrams, taken over 30 to 120 minutes. The drug is ingested orally, placed under the tongue, added to juice or a soft drink, or snorted intranasally. It is rarely taken parenterally, and compulsive use is infrequent. What is sold as MDMA often contains (or is replaced by) MDA, MDEA, ephedrine, amphetamine, ketamine, LSD, caffeine, or lactose. "Candy flipping" refers to the intentional combination of Ecstasy with LSD. "Staking" refers to taking several tablets at once or mixing the drug with alcohol, marijuana, dextromethorphan, or other psychoactive agents.[326,329] In Australia MDMA is often taken with the potent designer hallucinogen, para-methoxyamphetamine (PMA).[330] Onset of action is within 30 minutes; elimination half-life is 7 hours, but the elimination half-life of an active metabolite is 16 to 38 hours.

A designer drug analog of MDMA, 4-bromo-3, 4-dimethoxyphenylethylamine ("nexus," "2CB") was declared a Schedule I drug by the DEA in 1994.[330a]

Desired effects of MDMA include "enhanced communication, empathy, or understanding;" euphoria or ecstasy; and "transcendental or religious experiences."[323,331,331a] Perceptual changes include vivid color enhancement, illusions, and, at higher doses, hallucinations (visual, tactile, auditory, olfactory, or gustatory); visual hallucinations are either formed or unformed, and polyopia is reported. Formed hallucinations are experienced more often with MDA than with MDMA or MDEA, which tend to cause visual distortions.[332] Undesirable side effects include anxiety, tremor, muscle tightness, jaw clenching, diaphoresis, profuse salivation, blurred vision, ataxia, tachycardia, hypertension, and nausea. Mydriasis and horizontal or vertical nystagmus are seen.[333] Effects usually disappear within 24 hours, but users have reported jaw tightness, blurred vision, fatigue, nausea, anxiety, depression, or insomnia lasting days or even weeks, and "flashbacks" occur.[334,334a] Tolerance may develop more rapidly to MDMA's desirable effects than to its undesirable effects.[335]

As with amphetamine, overdose with MDA, MDMA, or MDEA causes hypertensive crisis, tachyarrhythmia, panic, paranoia, psychosis, and delirium.[332] Symptoms suggest the serotonin syndrome.[335a] Hyperthermia, especially in someone participating in a non-stop "rave," can be severe, resulting in rhabdomyolysis, disseminated intravascular coagulation, seizures, coma, and death.[334–340] Suicidal ingestion of 50 tablets produced a temperature of 106°F (41.1°C) and seizures; the patient survived.[341] Seizures can also occur as the only CNS complication of MDMA ingestion.[341a] A 16-year-old girl who ingested 30 tablets of MDMA had myoclonus of her legs while remaining awake.[341b] Liver failure can follow hyperthermia but has also occurred, sometimes fatally, in its absence.[342] Pancreatic necrosis and aplastic anemia are also described.[332] Hypoglycemia, hypernatremia, and hyponatremia are common. Hyponatremia may be the consequence of either inappropriate secretion of antidiuretic hormone or excessive water drinking; it has resulted in fatal cerebral edema.[343,343a] A report from the United Kingdom described 81 MDMA-related deaths during a 3-year period; causes included malignant hyperthermia, disseminated intravascular coagulation, rhabdomyolysis, cardiac arrhythmia, hepatic necrosis, stroke, traffic fatalities, and suicide.[343b]

MDMA and amphetamine overdose are treated similarly. Alkalinization of the urine for myoglobinuria will prolong the elimination half-life of MDMA, but acidification will precipitate myoglobin in the renal tubules.[339] On theoretical grounds the nonselective serotonin antagonists methysergide and cyproheptadine have been recommended for temperature control. So has the muscle relaxant dantrolene. Agitation or seizures are managed with parenteral benzodiazepines; haloperidol, which interferes with heat dissipation and lowers seizure threshold, should be avoided. Severe hypertension can be treated with sodium nitroprusside.[326]

Ischemic stroke, hemorrhagic stroke, and cerebral venous sinus thrombosis have followed MDMA use.[344–346,346a–346f] Basilar artery occlusion occurred in a 25-year-old woman who used both MDMA and cocaine.[346g] Rupture of a middle cerebral artery saccular aneurysm occured in an 18-year-old MDMA user.[346c]

Transient parkinsonism was reported in a healthy 29-year-old following MDMA use; he was also using "thermadrine" (ephedrine, caffeine, and aspirin).[347] Parkinsonism unresponsive to levodopa developed in a 19-year-old man who had used MDMA twice monthly for 6 months and whose father and uncle had Parkinson's disease.[347a] Parkinsonism was also described in a 38-year-old man who reported Ecstasy use and whose symptoms responded to levodopa and subthalamic nucleus stimulation.[347b] In these cases MDMA use was not verified toxicologically. A report that usual recreational doses of MDMA caused parkinsonism in primates was retracted when methodological errors were discovered.[347c,347d] In primates made parkinsonian with 1-methyl-4-phenyl-1,2,3,6-tetrahydropyridine (MPTP), MDMA relieved L-DOPA-induced dyekinesias.[347e]

In contrast to amphetamine, which damages dopaminergic nerve terminals, and methamphetamine, which damages both dopaminergic and serotonergic nerve terminals, MDMA and MDA (and, less potently, MDEA) selectively destroy serotonin axons and axon terminals in rat and primate brain.[348,349] In monkeys, this effect requires only two to three times the usual human dose. As with amphetamine, the mechanism of neurotoxicity is unclear, but it is prevented if serotonin uptake blockers such as fluoxetine are administered within

12 hours of MDMA administration.[350] It is also prevented by combined pretreatment with parachlorophenylalanine and reserpine, which deplete both releasable and storage serotonin.[351] The damage, moreover, is partially reversible—a year later serotonin uptake sites return to control levels, yet the content of serotonin in these areas remains lower than normal.[352] In rats and monkeys whose brains were examined 12 to 18 months after exposure to MDMA there was substantial serotonergic axonal sprouting, but, especially in monkeys, the reinnervation pattern was very abnormal, with denervation of distant targets and hyperinnervation of proximal targets.[353] In some regions of cerebral cortex in monkeys, density of serotonin axons remained reduced after 7 years.[354]

These abnormalities follow administration of doses much larger than encountered with recreational use. A study of humans using single photon emission computed tomography and a serotonin transporter-binding ligand found that compared with moderate MDMA users (average lifetime dose 27 tablets), heavy users (average lifetime dose 530 tablets) had decreased transporter density.[355] Positron emission tomography (PET) studies showed similar reductions, which also correlated with extent of previous use.[356] Autopsy of a heavy chronic MDMA user revealed reduced striatal levels of serotonin with preserved levels of dopamine.[357] Compared with controls, heavy MDMA users receiving transcranial magnetic stimulation to the occipital cortex had significantly lower thresholds for experiencing visual phosphenes; frequency of use correlated with the presence of visual hallucinations. The authors speculated that MDMA-induced acute release and reuptake inhibition of serotonin inhibited GABAergic neurons containing $5\text{-HT}_{2A/2C}$ receptors, causing cortical hyperexcitability, and that with chronic exposure to the drug axonal serotonergic degeneration would result in cortical underactivity.[357a]

Compared with non-MDMA users, heavy MDMA users abstinent for at least 2 weeks had impaired immediate verbal memory and delayed visual memory, and the degree of impairment correlated with cerebrospinal fluid levels of the serotonin metabolite 5-hydroxyindoleacetic acid.[358] In that study neither semantic nor procedural memory nor other cognitive domains were tested, leaving uncertain how specific the cognitive impairment was to working and episodic memory.[357,358a]

In another study MDMA users were tested cognitively a year apart, on each occasion abstinent for at least 2 weeks; continued use of MDMA was associated with progressive decline in immediate and delayed recall.[359] Others have described similar memory impairment in MDMA users.[360–362b] In one report even moderate use (average dose 350–490 mg/month) was associated with impaired cognitive performance.[363] Retraction of the study associating MDMA with parkinsonism led some investigators to challenge as well studies associating MDMA with lasting alterations in brain serotonin and with cognitive impairment.[363a,363b,363c]

Piperazine Drugs

A number of compounds that contain a piperazine moiety in their molecule bind to serotonin receptors, and reports from Europe describe their legal promotion on the Internet as recreational drugs. 1-Benzyl-piperazine (BZP), 1-[3-chlorophenyl]-piperazine (mCPP), and 1-[4-methoxyphenyl]-piperazine (mMeOPP) are examples. These designer drugs are claimed to mimic the effects of MDMA. It remains to be seen if that is the case and if their popularity will spread across the Atlantic.[364]

Modafinil

The mechanism of action of Modafinil, a Schedule IV drug used to treat narcolepsy, is uncertain. It is mildly reinforcing in monkeys, but in this regard is 200 times less potent than amphetamine and 15 times less potent than ephedrine. Its physicochemical properties prevent intravenous use or inhalation. Human recreational use has not been described.[365]

Monoamine Oxidase Inhibitors

Similar to psychostimulant drugs, monoamine oxidase inhibitors increase the availability of biogenic amines at synapses, and so it is not surprising that some users experience amphetamine-like effects: euphoria and a sense of increased energy. Tranylcypromine (Parnate) abuse, with craving and dose escalation, was reported in three patients who received the drug for treatment of depression associated with amphetamine abuse.[366] Taking tranylcypromine, they developed progressive irritability, violent outbursts, and paranoia. Interestingly, none had complications when ingesting tyramine-containing cheese or wine. Other reports describe psychological dependence on tranylcypromine or phenylzine, with withdrawal depression, irritability, and "shivering."[367–370] One woman who abused tranylcypromine developed status epilepticus on abrupt discontinuation.[371] Other monoamine oxidase inhibitor users have reportedly had delirium, hallucinations, and paranoid psychosis following withdrawal.[372] It can be difficult distinguishing the symptoms of antidepressant withdrawal from the symptoms that led to taking antidepressants in the first place.

Amitriptyline, Nomifensine

Oral abuse of the tricyclic antidepressant amitriptyline (Elavil) is well recognized, although whether it is taken for its effects on biogenic amines or for its anticholinergic properties is uncertain.[373] Amitriptyline has sedative effects, and its abuse is largely limited to abusers of other drugs. In a survey of 346 patients enrolled in a New York City methadone maintenance treatment program, 86 (25%) admitted to taking amitriptyline for its euphoric properties.[374] Overdose resembles atropine poisoning (see Chapter 11), and abrupt cessation has precipitated panic, headache, myalgia, nausea, vomiting, diarrhea, sweating, tremor, and palpitations—symptoms considered to be withdrawal phenomena and not simply reappearance of predrug anxiety or depression.[372–376]

The antidepressant nomifensine blocks synaptic reuptake of norepinephrine but has only slight dopamine-releasing effects. In normal humans, it "enhances drive" without producing euphoria.[377] Abuse of nomifensine, with dosage escalation, was reported in a woman who had previously abused sedatives.[378]

Yohimbine

Yohimbine, derived from the bark of *Corynanthe yohimbi* in West and Central Africa, has been touted (probably incorrectly) as an aphrodisiac for more than a century. In the United States, it can be purchased without prescription from mail-order companies. An alpha$_2$-adrenergic receptor antagonist, yohimbine produces nervousness, palpitations, hot and cold flashes, tremor, piloerection, and systolic hypertension. It precipitates panic attacks in patients suffering from panic disorders and in fact is considered the best current pharmacological model of anxiety.[379,380] At high doses, it also causes a dissociative mental state and hallucinations. As a street drug, it is known as "yo-yo."[381]

Ginseng

For thousands of years, ginseng root preparations have been used as all-purpose tonics in Asia. The plant—genus *Panax*, that is, panacea—also grows in the United States, and between 5 and 6 million Americans use ginseng. Preparations include roots, capsules, tablets, teas, extracts, cigarettes, chewing gum, and candy; routes of administration include oral, intranasal, smoking, and intravenous.[382] The desired effects are stimulation and euphoria, but the pharmacological mechanisms are uncertain; ginseng contains a variety of glycosides and steroidal saponins. Chronic users experience nervousness, insomnia, diarrhea, tachycardia, and hypertension, and abrupt withdrawal has precipitated weakness, tremor, and hypotension.[382–384]

Animal studies suggest that ginseng inhibits behavioral sensitization to morphine, cocaine, and methamphetamine and blocks conditioned place preference to psychostimulants, raising the possibility of therapeutic potential.[385]

Betel

In East Africa, India, Southeast Asia, Indonesia, and the Philippines, 200 million people chew betel made from the nut of the palm, *Areca catechu;* the preparation also contains quicklime and leaves from nutmeg or other local psychoactive plants. Active ingredients from the palm nut include arecholine and arecaidine. The effect is psychostimulation, often with ataxia and tremor, followed the next day by fatigue, apathy, and headache. Addiction occurs, with ability to work dependent

Table 4–3. Herbal Preparations Sold as Stimulants in the United States

Herb	Source	Active Ingredients	Use
Cinnamon	*Cinnamon camphora*	Unknown. Contains tannins and oils	Bark smoked, often with marijuana
Hydrangea	*Hydrangea paniculata*	Hydrangin glycoside, saponin, cyanogenic glycoside	Smoke (marijuana substitute)
Damiana	*Turnera diffusa aphrodisiaca*	Unknown. Contains volatile oils, resins tannins, and "damianin"	Liquid, pill, smoke (marijuana substitute)
Passion flower	*Passiflora caerulea*	Harmine alkaloids, cyanogenic glycosides	Capsules, tea, smoke (marijuana substitute)
Prickly poppy	*Argemona mexicana*	Isoquinolone alkaloids, prolopine, berberine	Smoke seeds

Source: Hung OL, Lewin NA, Howland MA. Herbal preparations. In: Goldfrank LR, Flomenbaum NE, Levin NA, et al., eds. Goldfrank's Toxicologic Emergencies, 6th edition. Stamford, CT: Appleton & Lange, 1998:1221.

on the drug. High doses cause toxic psychosis and auditory hallucinations. Betel stains the teeth red and increases the risk of oral cancer.[386,386a]

Kratour

An unusual substance abuse has been studied in Malaysia and Thailand. Leaves of the kratour tree (*Mitragyna speciosa*) are chewed as an opium substitute, with a mild opioid-like withdrawal syndrome, yet acute effects are both stimulating and calming, comparable to chewing coca leaves and smoking opium simultaneously. The active agent is an indole, mitragynine.[387,388]

Other Herbal Products

A large number of herbal preparations are sold in the United States as capsules, teas, and cigarettes, many for their euphoriant and stimulating effects. Some contain such well-defined ingredients as ephedrine, nutmeg, or yohimbine; others produce their effects by unclear mechanisms (Table 4–3).[383,389]

Caffeine

The most widely used psychoactive drug in the world is caffeine (Figure 4–3). Tea, prepared from leaves of the bush *Thea sinensis*, originated in China probably thousands of years ago and today is consumed by more than half the world's population. Coffee, made from the fruit of *Coffea arabica*, first appeared in Ethiopia more than 1000 years ago and today is the major source of caffeine in the United States; coffee is drunk in 98% of American households, and 30% of adult Americans drink three to five cups a day. Other sources of caffeine include cola-flavored drinks (containing extracts of the nut of *Cola acuminata*), cocoa and chocolate (from seeds of *Theobroma cacao* and containing theobromine plus small amounts of caffeine), and both prescription and over-the-counter medications (Table 4–4).[390,391]

Similar to theophylline and theobromine, caffeine is a methylxanthine. Its actions include inhibition of cyclic nucleotide phosphodiesterases and adenosine; the latter action probably accounts for most of its pharmacological effects.[392] Adenosine receptors, which are of two major types, are ubiquitous throughout the body and are believed to regulate oxygen availability and utilization. Among many actions, adenosine dilates cerebral blood vessels and decreases neuronal firing rates in the CNS. Adenylyl cyclase is inhibited by A-1 receptors and stimulated by A-2 receptors. At concentrations

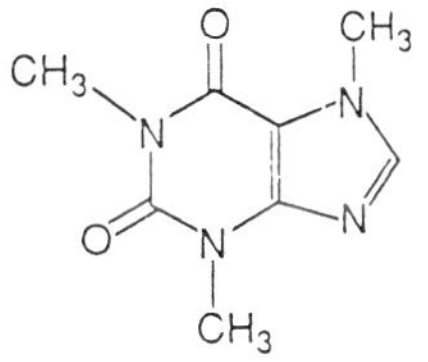

Figure 4–3. Caffeine.

Table 4–4. Caffeine Concentrations in Beverages and Pharmaceuticals

Product	Caffeine Concentration
Beverage and Food (mg/100 mL)	
Coffee	
Brewed	40–120 (usual cup: about 85 mg)
Decaffeinated	1–3
Tea	13–60 (usual cup: about 50 mg)
Cola drinks	10–15
Cocoa	4–10
Milk chocolate	20
Prescription Medication (mg/tablet)	
Cafergot	100
Darvon compound	32
Synalgos	30
Fiorinal	40
Migral	50
Migraine	100
Over-the-Counter Preparation (mg/tablet)	
Anacin	32
Midol	32
Excedrin	65
Cope, Easy Mens	32
Many cold preparations	40
Dristan	16.2
Prolamine	140
Spantrol	150
Vanquish	33
No-Doz	100

Source: Modified from Lewin NA. Caffeine. In: Goldfrank LR, Flomenbaum NE, Lewin NA, et al., eds. Goldfrank's Toxicologic Emergencies, 6th edition. Stamford, CT: Appleton & Lange, 1998:651, with permission of the publisher.

within the therapeutic range, caffeine antagonizes both actions. Whether it does so by binding to adenosine receptors is disputed.[390,393]

In animals, caffeine stimulates locomotor activity.[394] In knockout mice lacking adenosine A_{2A} receptors it no longer does so.[395] In drug discrimination studies, low doses generalize not only to other methylxanthines, but also to amphetamine, methylphenidate, and cocaine; high doses generalize only to other methylxanthines.[396] Self-administration studies have been inconsistent.

Both primates and rats show wide individual differences, and many animals develop preference for caffeine only after forced exposure, suggesting that physical dependence potentiates reinforcement. Caffeine maintains self-administration much less reliably than amphetamine or cocaine.[397] Animal studies using radioactive glucose showed that caffeine caused increased metabolic activity in the striatum but not the nucleus accumbens (NA). Human studies using PET similarly found no change in NA activity. The authors concluded that the alerting action of caffeine does not involve the reward system.[398] Others, however, found that enhanced dopaminergic neurotransmission does contribute to the behavioral effects of caffeine.[399]

Tolerance develops to caffeine-stimulated locomotor activity, without cross-tolerance to non-methylxanthine psychostimulants. By contrast, tolerance to caffeine's rate-decreasing effects on food-reinforced operant responding generalizes both to methylxanthine and to nonmethylxanthine psychostimulants.[394]

In humans, caffeine reduces drowsiness and fatigue and improves the flow of thought. Heart rate and blood pressure increase moderately, gastric acid and pepsin secretion is stimulated, and there is diuresis. The oils of coffee cause diarrhea; the tannins of tea cause constipation. Higher doses of caffeine cause nervousness, anxiety, tremor, insomnia, tachycardia, and ventricular premature contractions. Caffeine seems to be an example of a drug that produces craving independent of euphoria or otherwise pleasant effects; in some individuals, consumption continues in the face of increasing dysphoria.[397]

Toxic doses of caffeine cause agitation, dry mouth, dysesthesias, myalgia, "restless legs," tinnitus, ocular dyskinesias, scotomas, nausea, vomiting, and cardiac arrhythmia.[390,400–403] Panic attacks have been induced and schizophrenic symptoms exacerbated. Very high doses of caffeine cause delirium, seizures, and coma. Fatalities are rare but have been reported in both children and adults.[404–411] The lethal dose in adults has usually been 5–10 g, but serious toxicity can follow ingestion of only 1 g. Treatment includes induced vomiting if the patient is seen early; activated charcoal; catharsis; and respiratory, cardiac, and blood pressure support. Resin hemoperfusion has been used, and antacids and ranitidine are given for gastritis. Benzodiazepines can be used for sedation and, with phenytoin or phenobarbital, for seizures.

Peak serum levels of caffeine occur after 30 to 60 minutes, and its half-life is 3 to 7 hours.[390] Metabolites include theophylline and theobromine. Both tolerance and physical dependence develop to caffeine. Withdrawal symptoms include headache, yawning, drowsiness, irritability, difficulty concentrating, depression, diarrhea, and nausea.[390,412] In a double-blind, placebo-controlled study, such symptoms occurred even after low to moderate caffeine intake—mean 235 mg daily, equivalent to 2.5 cups of coffee.[413] Headache can be severe, and symptoms are sometimes called 'flu-like.' Neonatal caffeine withdrawal causes irritability, jitteriness, and vomiting.[414]

Abuse of caffeine-containing "legal stimulants," with dosage escalation to more than 1 g daily, has been reported in abusers of other drugs and in alcoholics.[411,415] A middle-aged woman began using No Doz and Vivarin during periods of cocaine unavailability.[415] Death resulted from coffee enemas in a health food faddist.[409]

Although an association of caffeine and cardiovascular disease has been claimed,[416] the weight of evidence is against caffeine carrying risk for myocardial infarction, peripheral vascular disease, hypertension, or stroke.[390,417,418] A study of ambulatory volunteers, however, found small increases in blood pressure (average 6 mmHg systolic, 5 mmHg diastolic) that correlated with systemic caffeine concentrations; increases of 2–4 mmHg persisted for several hours after consumption. An epidemiological review concluded that these modest effects could translate across populations into significant risk factors for heart disease and stroke.[418a] Coffee raises serum levels of both high-density and low-density lipoprotein cholesterol; the effect seems to be independent of caffeine.[419] In a population-based cohort study caffeine reduced the risk of type 2 diabetes mellitus.[419a] In rodents, caffeine reduces ischemic damage, perhaps by up-regulating adenosine receptors.[420–422] In a study with rats ethanol plus caffeine ("caffeinol") reduced cerebral infarct volume; ethanol alone aggravated ischemic damage, and caffeine alone had no effect.[422a]

An alleged association of caffeine with pancreatic or renal cancer was refuted by subsequent studies.[423] Huge doses of caffeine are teratogenic in mammals, but the amounts consumed in beverages or medications do not appear to increase the risk for fetal malformations or low birth weight.[404] Caffeine increases the risk of osteoporosis in the elderly.[424]

A case–control study found coffee-drinking to reduce the risk of developing Parkinson's disease.[425] A prospective cohort study found a similar inverse association between Parkinson's disease and caffeine consumption, whether coffee or tea.[426] Premorbid personality traits were offered as a possible mechanism, but it was noted that adenosine A_{2A} receptors modulate the nigrostriatal dopamine system and that adenosine antagonists might be useful in the treatment of Parkinson's disease.[427] In the prospective Nurses' Health Study caffeine reduced the risk of Parkinson's disease among women who did not use postmenopausal hormones but increased the risk of those who used them.[427a]

Seventy-five percent of American pregnant women drink caffeinated beverages, yet for the past two decades the FDA has advised pregnant women "to avoid caffeine-containing foods and drugs."[428,429] Case–control studies have shown caffeine to increase the risk of spontaneous abortion. In one study the risk occurred in the first trimester and affected only nonsmokers.[430] (Smoking accelerates the elimination of caffeine.) In another study, the risk occurred in the second trimester and affected only those who drank more than six cups of coffee per day.[431] A meta-analysis concluded that women consuming more than 150 mg caffeine daily are at increased risk for both spontaneous abortion (odds ratio 1.4) and a low birth weight baby (odds ratio 1.5).[432] Animals exposed to moderate-to-high doses of caffeine in utero or during early postnatal life manifest decreased brain weight and impaired learning and memory.[433]

References

1. Foltin RW, Fischman MW. Assessment of abuse liability of stimulant drugs in humans: a methodological survey. Drug Alcohol Dep 1991; 28:3.
2. Hoffman BB. Catecholamines, sympathomimetic drugs, and adrenergic receptor antagonists. In: Hardman JG, Limbird LE, eds. Goodman and Gilman's The Pharmacological Basis of Therapeutics, 10th edition. New York: McGraw-Hill, 2001:215.
3. Weintraub M. Long-term weight control study: conclusions. Clin Pharmacol Ther 1992; 51:642.

4. Treffert DA, Johanson D. Restricting amphetamines. JAMA 1981; 245:1336.

5. Hill H, Horita A. Inhibition of amphetamine hyperthermia by blockade of dopamine receptors in rabbits. J Pharm Pharmacol 1971; 23:715.

6. Berntman L, Carlsson C, Hagerdal M, Siesjo BK. Excessive increase in oxygen uptake and blood flow in the brain during amphetamine intoxication. Acta Physiol Scand 1976; 97:264.

7. Franklin KB. Analgesia and abuse potential: an accidental association or a common substrate? Pharmacol Biochem Behav 1998; 59:993.

8. Dalal S, Melzack R. Potentiation of opioid drugs by psychostimulant drugs: a review. J Pain Sympt Management 1998; 16:245.

9. Gold LH, Geyer MA, Koob GF. Neurochemical mechanisms involved in behavioral effects of amphetamines and related designer drugs. NIDA Res Monogr 1989; 94:146.

10. Pickens R, Harris WC. Self-administration of *d*-amphetamine by rats. Psychopharmacologia 1968; 12:158.

11. Piazza PV, Deminiere J-M, LeMoal M, Simon H. Factors that predict individual vulnerability to amphetamine self-administration. Science 1989; 245:1511.

12. Sannerud CA, Brady JV, Griffiths RR. Self-injection in baboons of amphetamines and related designer drugs. NIDA Res Monogr 1989; 94:30.

13. Seiden LS, Kleven MS. Methamphetamine and related drugs: toxicity and resulting behavioral changes in response to pharmacological probes. NIDA Res Monogr 1989; 94:146.

14. Moghaddam B, Bunney BS. Differential effect of cocaine on extracellular dopamine levels in rat medial prefrontal cortex and nucleus accumbens: comparison to amphetamine. Synapse 1989; 4:156.

15. Lyness WH, Friedle NM, Moore KE. Increased self-administration of d-amphetamine after destruction of 5-hydroxydopamine neurons. Pharmacol Biochem Behav 1980; 12:937.

16. Leccese AP, Lyness WH. The effects of putative 5-hydroxytryptamine receptor active agents on d-amphetamine median forebrain bundle lesions. 'Brain Res 1984; 303:153.

17. McMillen BA. CNS stimulants: two distinct mechanisms of action for amphetamine-like drugs. Trends Pharmacol Sci 1983; 4:429.

18. Schmitz Y, Lee CJ, Schmauss C, et al. Amphetamine distorts stimulation-dependent dopamine outflow: effects on D2 autoreceptors, transporters, and synaptic vesicle stores. J Neurosci 2001; 21:5916.

19. Anderson BB, Chen G, Gutman DA, et al. Dopamine levels of two classes of vesicles are differentially depleted by amphetamine. Brain Res 1998; 788:294.

20. Jones SR, Gainetdinov RR, Wightman RM, Caron MG. Mechanisms of amphetamine action revealed in mice lacking the dopamine transporter. J Neurosci 1998; 18:1979.

21. Gatley SJ, Volkow ND, Gifford AN, et al. Dopamine-transporter occupancy after intravenous doses of cocaine and methylphenidate in mice and humans. Psychopharmacology 1999; 146:93.

22. Sulzer D, Chen T-K, Lau YY, et al. Amphetamine redistributes dopamine from synaptic vesicles to the cytosol and promotes reverse transport. J Neurosci 1995; 15:4102.

23. Floor E, Meng L. Amphetamine releases dopamine from synaptic vesicles by dual mechanisms. Neurosci Lett 1996; 215:53.

24. Madras BK, Fahey MA, Bergman J, et al. Effects of cocaine and related drugs in non-human primates. 1.[3-H]Cocaine binding sites in caudate-putamen. J Pharmacol Exp Ther 1989; 251:131.

25. Rockhold RW. Glutamatergic involvement in psychomotor stimulant action. Prog Drug Res 1998; 50:155.

26. Ricktand NM, Woods SC, Berger SP, Strakowski SM. D3 dopamine receptor, behavioral sensitization, and psychosis. Neurosci Biobehav Rev 2001; 25:427.

27. Bjijou Y, Stinus L, Le Moal M, Cador M. Evidence for selective involvement of dopamine D1 receptors of the ventral tegmental area in the behavioral sensitization induced by intra-ventral tegmental area injections of D-amphetamine. J Pharmacol Exp Ther 1996; 277:1177.

28. Vezina P. D1 dopamine receptor activation is necessary for the induction of sensitization by amphetamine in the ventral tegmental area. J Neurosci 1996; 16:241.

29. Cador M, Bjijou Y, Stinus L. Evidence of a complete independence of the neurobiological substrates for the induction and expression of behavioral sensitization to amphetamine. Neuroscience 1995; 65:385.

30. Wolf ME, Xue CJ. Amphetamine-induced glutamate efflux in the rat ventral tegmental area is prevented by MK-801, SCH 23390, and ibotenic acid lesions of the prefrontal cortex. J Neurochem 1999; 73:1529.

31. Jones S, Kornblum JL, Kauer JA. Amphetamine blocks long-term synaptic depression in the ventral tegmental area. J Neurosci 2000; 20:5575.

32. Flores C, Stewart J. Basic fibroblast growth factor as a mediator of the effects of glutamate in the development of long-lasting sensitization to stimulant drugs: studies in the rat. Psychopharmacology 2000; 151:152.

33. Xu M, Guo Y, Vorhees CV, Zhang J. Behavioral responses to cocaine and amphetamine administration in mice lacking the dopamine D1 receptor. Brain Res 2000; 852:198.

34. Vanderschuren LJ, Kalivas PW. Alterations in dopaminergic and glutamatergic transmission in the induction and expression of behavioral sensitization: a critical review of preclinical studies. Psychopharmacology 2000; 151:99.

35. Villemagne V, Yuan J, Wong DF, et al. Brain dopamine neurotoxicity in baboons treated with doses of methamphetamine comparable to those recreationally used by humans: evidence from [11C]WIN-35, 428

positron emission tomography studies and direct in vitro determinations. J Neurosci 1998; 18:419.

36. Davidson C, Gow AJ, Lee TH, Ellinwood EH. Methamphetamine neurotoxicity: necrotic and apoptotic mechanisms and relevance to human abuse and treatment. Brain Res Rev 2001; 36:1.

37. Ricaurte GA, Seiden LS, Schuster CR. Further evidence that amphetamines produce long-lasting dopamine neurochemical deficits by destroying dopamine nerve fibers. Brain Res 1984; 303:359.

38. Gawin FH, Ellinwood EH. Cocaine and other stimulants. Actions, abuse, treatment. N Engl J Med 1988; 318:1173.

39. Sonsalla PK, Nicklas WJ, Heikkila RE. Role for excitatory amino acids in methamphetamine-induced nigrostriatal toxicity. Science 1989; 243:398.

40. Iman SZ, el-Yazal J, Newport GD, et al. Methamphetamine-induced dopaminergic neurotoxicity: role of peroxynitrite and neuroprotective role of antioxidants and peroxynitrite decomposition catalysts. Ann N Y Acad Sci 2001; 939:366.

41. Itzhak Y, Gandia C, Huang PL, Ali SF. Resistance of neuronal nitric oxide synthase-deficient mice to methamphetamine-induced dopaminergic neurotoxicity. J Pharmacol Exp Ther 1998; 284:1040.

42. Cadet JL, Sheng S, Ali R, et al. Attenuation of methamphetamine-induced neurotoxicity in copper/zinc superoxide dismutase transgenic mice. J Neurochem 1994; 62:380.

43. Hirata H, Cadet JL. p53 knockout mice are protected against the long-term effects of methamphetamine on dopaminergic terminals and cell bodies. J Neurochem 1997; 69:780.

44. Lotharius J, O'Malley KL. Role of mitochondrial dysfunction and dopamine-dependent oxidative stress in amphetamine-induced toxicity. Ann Neurol 2001; 49:79.

45. Frost DO, Cadet J-L. Effects of methamphetamine-induced neurotoxicity on the development of neural circuitry: a hypothesis. Brain Res Rev 2000; 34:103.

46. Anderson RJ, Reed WG, Hillis LD, et al. History, epidemiology, and medical complications of nasal inhaler abuse. J Toxicol Clin Toxicol 1982; 19:95.

47. Munroe RR, Drell HJ. Use of stimulants obtained from inhalers. JAMA 1937; 135:909.

48. Post JM. Drunk with power. Alcohol and drug abuse among the leadership elite. Washington Post National Weekly Edition, February 5, 1990:39.

49. Cohen S. Stimulant abuse in Sweden. In: Drug Dependence, no. 2, National Clearinghouse for Mental Health Information. Bethesda, MD: National Institute of Mental Health, 1969:30.

50. Brecher EM. Licit and Illicit Drugs. Boston: Little, Brown, 1972:267.

51. Kalant OJ. The Amphetamines: Toxicity and Addiction, 2nd edition. Springfield, IL: Charles C Thomas, 1973.

52. Scarpino V, Arrigo A, Benzi G, et al. Evaluation and prevalence of "doping" among Italian athletes. Lancet 1990; 336:1048.

53. Catlin DH, Hatton CK. Use and abuse of anabolic and other drugs for athletic enhancement. Adv Intern Med 1991; 36:399.

54. Smith LC. Collapse with death following the use of amphetamine sulfate. JAMA 1939; 113:1022.

55. Norman J, Shea JT. Acute hallucinosis as a complication of addiction to amphetamine sulfate. N Engl J Med 1945; 233:270.

56. Harvey JK, Todd CW, Howard JH. Fatality associated with Benzedrine ingestion. A case report. Delaware State M J 1949; 21:111.

57. Grinspoon L, Hedblom P. The Speed Culture: Amphetamine Use and Abuse in America. Cambridge, MA: Harvard University Press, 1975.

58. Nicholi AM. The nontherapeutic use of psychoactive drugs. N Engl J Med 1984; 16:241.

59. Kall KI, Olin RG. HIV status and changes in risk behavior among intravenous drug users in Stockholm 1987-1988. AIDS 1990; 4:153.

60. Bailey DN. Amphetamine detection during toxicology screening of a university medical center patient population. Clin Toxicol 1987; 25:399.

61. Jackson JG. Hazards of smokable methamphetamine. N Engl J Med 1989; 321:907.

61a. Butterfield F: Across rural America, drug casts a grim shadow. NY Times January 4, 2004.

62. Jacobs A: The beast in the bathhouse. Crystal meth use by gay men threatens to re-ignite an epidemic. NY Times January 12, 2004.

63. National Institute on Drug Abuse. Epidemiologic trends in drug abuse. Community Epidemiologic Work Group, 1998. Vol I: Highlights and Executive Summary. Bethesda, MD: NIH, 1998.

64. National Institute on Drug Abuse. Epidemiologic trends in drug abuse. Community Epidemiologic Work Group, 1998. Vol II: Proceedings. Bethesda, MD: NIH, 1998.

65. Luna GC. Use and abuse of amphetamine-type stimulants in the United States of America. Pan Am J Public Health 2001; 9:114.

66. Nieves E. Drug labs in valley hideouts feed nation's habit. NY Times, May 13, 2001.

67. Weiss B, Laties VG. Enhancement of human performance by caffeine and the amphetamines. Pharmacol Rev 1962; 14:1.

68. Tecce JJ, Cole JO. Amphetamine effects in man: paradoxical drowsiness and lowered electrical brain activity (CNV). Science 1974; 185:451.

69. Martin WR, Sloan JW, Sapira JD, Jasinski DR. Physiologic, subjective, and behavioral effects of amphetamine, methamphetamine, ephedrine, phenmetrazine, and methylphendiate in man. Clin Pharmacol Ther 1971; 12:245.

70. Cook CE, Jeffcoat AR, Perez-Reyes M, et al. Plasma levels of methamphetamine after smoking methamphetamine hydrochloride. NIDA Res Monogr 1991; 105:578.

71. Kramer JC, Fischman VS, Littlefield DC. Amphetamine abuse: patterns and effects of high doses taken intravenously. JAMA 1967; 201:305.

72. Cox C, Smart RG. The nature and extent of speed use in North America. Can Med Assoc J 1970; 102:724.

73. Yui K, Goto K, Ikemoto S, et al. Neurobiological basis of relapse prediction in stimulant-induced psychosis and schizophrenia: the role of sensitization. Mol Psychiatr 1999; 4:512

74. Lundh H, Tunving K. An extrapyramidal choreiform syndrome caused by amphetamine addiction. J Neurol Neurosurg Psychiatry 1981; 44:728.

75. Rhee KJ, Albertson TE, Douglas JC. Choreoathetoid disorder associated with amphetamine-like drugs. Am J Emerg Med 1988; 6:131.

75a. See SJ, Tan EK: Severe amphetamine-induced bruxism: treatment with botulinum toxin. Acta Neurol Scand 2003; 107:161.

76. Bell DS. Comparison of amphetamine psychosis and schizophrenia. Br J Psychiatry 1965; 111:701.

77. Angrist B, van Kammen DP. CNS stimulants as tools in the study of schizophrenia. Trends Neurosci 1984;7:388.

78. Javitt DC, Zukin SR. Recent advances in the phency-clidine model of schizophrenia. Am J Psychiatry 1991; 148:1301.

79. van Kammen D, Bunney WE, Docherty JP, et al. D-amphetamine-induced heterogeneous changes in psychotic behavior in schizophrenia. Am J Psychiatry 1982; 139:991.

80. Goldberg TE, Bigelow LB, Weinberger DR, et al. Cognitive and behavioral effects of the coadministration of dextroamphetamine and haloperidol in schizophrenia. Am J Psychiatry 1991; 178:78.

81. Zalis EG, Parmley LF. Fatal amphetamine poisoning. Arch Intern Med 1963; 112:822.

82. Espelin DE, Done AK. Amphetamine poisoning. N Engl J Med 1968; 278:1361.

83. Edison GR. Amphetamines. A dangerous illusion. Ann Intern Med 1971; 74:605.

84. Cohen S. Amphetamine abuse. JAMA 1975; 231:414.

85. Kojima T, Une I, Yashiki M, et al. A fatal methamphet-amine poisoning associated with hyperpyrexia. Forensic Sci Int 1984; 24:87.

86. Derlet RW, Rice P, Horowitz BZ, Lord RV. Amphetamine toxicity: experience with 127 cases. J Emerg Med 1989; 7:157.

87. Chan P, Chen JH, Lee MH, et al. Fatal and nonfatal methamphetamine intoxication in the intensive care unit. J Toxicol Clin Toxicol 1994; 32:147.

87a. Brown PL, Wise RA, Kiyatkin EA. Brain hyperthermia is induced by methamphetamine and exacerbated by social interaction. J Neurosci 2003; 23:3924.

88. Nestor TA, Tamamoto WI, Kam TH. Acute pulmonary oedema caused by crystalline methamphetamine. Lancet 1989; II:1277.

89. Karch SB, Stephens BG, Ho C-H. Methamphetamine-related deaths in San Francisco: demographic,

90. Kendrick WC, Hull AR, Knochel JP. Rhabdomyolysis and shock after intravenous amphetamine administration. Ann Intern Med 1977; 86:381.

91. Kasirsky G, Zaidi IH, Tansy MF. LD50 and pathologic effects of acute and chronic administration of methamphetamine HCl in rabbits. Res Commun Chem Pathol Pharmacol 1972; 3:215.

92. Zalis EG, Lundberg GD, Knutson RA. The pathophysiology of acute amphetamine poisoning with pathologic correlation. J Pharmacol Exp Ther 1967; 158:115.

93. Zalis EG, Kaplan G, Lundberg GD, Knutson RA. Acute lethality of the amphetamines in dogs and its antagonism with curare. Proc Soc Exp Biol Med 1965; 18:557.

94. Duarte Escalante O, Ellinwood EH. Central nervous system cytopathological changes in cats with chronic methedrine intoxication. Brain Res 1970; 21:151.

95. Alldredge BK, Lowenstein DH, Simon RP. Seizures associated with recreational drug abuse. Neurology 1989; 39:1037.

96. Chiang WK. Amphetamines. In: Goldfrank LR, Flomenbaum NE, Lewin NA, et al., eds. Goldfrank's Toxicologic Emergencies, 6th edition. Stamford, CT: Appleton & Lange, 1998:1091.

97. Albertson TE, Derlet RW, Van Hoozen BE. Methamphetamine and the expanding complications of amphetamines. West J Med 1999; 170:21.

98. Lemberger L, Witt EP, David J, Kopin IJ. The effects of haloperidol and chlorpromazine on amphetamine metabolism and amphetamine stereotype behavior in rat. J Pharmacol Exp Ther 1970; 174:428.

99. Ghuran A, Nolan J. Recreational drug misuse: issues for the cardiologist. Heart 2000; 83:627.

100. Khantzian EJ, McKenna GJ. Acute toxic and withdrawal reactions associated with drug use and abuse. Ann Intern Med 1979; 90:361.

101. Mendelson J, Jones RT, Upton R, Jacob P III. Methamphetamine and ethanol interactions in humans. Clin Pharm Ther 1995; 57:559.

102. Kantor HL, Emsellem HA, Hogg JE, Simon GL. Candida albicans meningitis in a parenteral drug abuser. South Med J 1984; 77:404.

103. Brooks GF, O'Donoghue JM, Rissing JP, et al. Eikenella corrodens, a recently recognized pathogen: infections in medical-surgical patients and in association with methylphenidate abuse. Medicine 1974; 53:325.

104. Seaman ME. Barotrauma related to inhalational drug abuse. J Emerg Med 1990; 8:141.

105. Jones AK, Jarvic DR, McDermid G, Proudfoot AT. Hepatocellular damage following amphetamine intoxication. J Toxicol Clin Toxicol 1994; 32:435.

106. Carson P, Oldroyd K, Phadke K. Myocardial infarction due to amphetamine. BMJ 1987; 294:1525.

107. Packe GE, Garton MJ, Jennings K. Acute myocardial infarction caused by intravenous amphetamine abuse. Br Heart J 1990; 64:23.

pathologic, and toxicologic profiles. J Forensic Sci 1999; 44:359.

108. Furst SR, Fallon SP, Reznik GN, Shah PK. Myocardial infarction after inhalation of methamphetamine. N Engl J Med 1990; 323:1147.

109. Waksman J, Taylor RN, Bodor GS, et al. Acute myocardial infarction associated with amphetamine use. Mayo Clin Proc 2001; 76:323.

110. Call TD, Hartneck J, Dickinson WA, et al. Acute cardiomyopathy secondary to intravenous amphetamine abuse. Ann Intern Med 1982; 97:559.

111. Smith HJ, Roche AHG, Jagusch MF, Hersdon PB. Cardiomyopathy associated with amphetamine administration. Am Heart J 1976; 91:792.

112. Poteliakhoff A, Roughton BC. Two cases of amphetamine poisoning. BMJ 1956; I:26.

113. Lloyd JTA, Walker DRH. Death after combined dexamphetamine and phenylzine. BMJ 1965; II:168.

114. Coroner's report. Amphetamine overdose kills boy. Pharmaceut J 1967; 198:172.

115. Kane FJ, Keeler MH, Reifler CB. Neurological crisis following methamphetamine. JAMA 1969; 210:556.

116. Goodman SJ, Becker DP. Intracranial hemorrhage associated with amphetamine abuse. JAMA 1970; 212:480.

117. Weiss SR, Raskind R, Morganstern NL, et al. Intracerebral and subarachnoid hemorrhage following use of methamphetamine ("speed"). Int Surg 1970; 53:123.

118. Margolis MT, Newton TH. Methamphetamine ("speed") arteritis. Neuroradiology 1971; 2:179.

119. Tibbetts JC, Hinck VC. Conservative management of a hematoma in the fourth ventricle. Surg Neurol 1973; 1:253.

120. Chynn KY. Acute subarachnoid hemorrhage. JAMA 1973; 233:55.

121. Hall CD, Blanton DE, Scatliff JH, Morris CE. Speed kills: fatality from the self administration of methamphetamine intravenously. South Med J 1973; 66:650.

122. Yatsu FM, Wesson DR, Smith DE. Amphetamine abuse. In: Richter RW, ed. Medical Aspects of Drug Abuse. Hagerstown, MD: Harper & Row, 1975:50.

123. Olsen ER. Intracranial hemorrhage and amphetamine usage. Angiology 1977; 28:464.

124. Yarnell PR. "Speed" headache and hematoma. Headache 1977; 17:69.

125. Edwards K. Hemorrhagic complications of cerebral arteritis. Arch Neurol 1977; 34:549.

126. Kessler JT, Jortner BS, Adapon BD. Cerebral vasculitis in a drug abuser. J Clin Psychiatry 1978; 39:559.

127. LoVerme S. Complications of amphetamine abuse. In: Culebras A, ed. Clini-Pearls, vol 2, no. 8. Syracuse, NY: Creative Medical Publications, 1979:5.

128. Delaney P, Estes M. Intracranial hemorrhage with amphetamine abuse. Neurology 1980; 30:1125.

129. Gericke OL. Suicide by ingestion of amphetamine sulfate. JAMA 1980; 128:1125.

130. D'Souza T, Shraberg D. Intracranial hemorrhage associated with amphetamine use. Neurology 1981; 31:922.

131. Cahill DW, Knipp H, Mosser J. Intracranial hemorrhage with amphetamine abuse. Neurology 1981; 31:1058.

132. Shukla D. Intracranial hemorrhage associated with amphetamine use. Neurology 1982; 32:917.

133. Harrington H, Heller HA, Dawson D, et al. Intracerebral hemorrhage and oral amphetamine. Arch Neurol 1983; 40:503.

134. Yu YJ, Cooper DR, Wallenstein DE, Block B. Cerebral angiitis and intracerebral hemorrhage associated with methamphetamine abuse. J Neurosurg 1983; 58:109.

135. Lukes SA. Intracerebral hemorrhage from an arteriovenous malformation after amphetamine injection. Arch Neurol 1983; 40:60.

136. Matick H, Anderson D, Brumlik J. Cerebral vasculitis associated with oral amphetamine overdose. Arch Neurol 1983; 40:253.

137. Salanova V, Taubner R. Intracerebral hemorrhage and vasculitis secondary to amphetamine use. Postgrad Med J 1984; 60:429.

138. Imanse J, Vanneste J. Intraventricular hemorrhage following amphetamine abuse. Neurology 1990; 40:1318.

139. Delaney P. Intracranial hemorrhage associated with amphetamine use. Neurology 1981; 31:923.

140. Dinnen A. Cerebral hemorrhage due to stimulants. Med J Aust 1971; 2:101.

141. Lessing MP, Hyman NM. Intracranial haemorrhage caused by amphetamine abuse. J R Soc Med 1989; 82:766.

142. El-Omar MM, Ray K, Geary R. Intracerebral haemorrhage in a young adult: consider amphetamine abuse. Br J Clin Pract 1996; 50:115.

143. Conci F, D'Angelo V, Tampieri D, et al. Intracerebral hemorrhage and angiographic beading following amphetamine abuse. Ital J Neurol Sci 1988; 9:77.

144. Selmi F, Davies KG, Sharma RR, et al. Intracerebral hemorrhage due to amphetamine abuse: report of two cases with underlying arteriovenous malformations. Br J Neurosurg 1995; 9:9.

145. Goplen AK, Berg-Johnson J, Dullerud R. Fatal cerebral hemorrhage in young amphetamine addicts. Tidsskr Nor Laegeforen 1995; 115:832.

146. Chaudhuri C, Salahudeen AK. Massive intracerebral hemorrhage in an amphetamine addict. Am J Med Sci 1999; 317:350.

147. Buxton N, McConachie NA. Amphetamine abuse and intracranial hemorrhage. J R Soc Med 2000; 93:472.

148. McEvoy AW, Kitchen ND, Thomas DGT. Intracerebral hemorrhage in young adults: the emerging importance of drug misuse. BMJ 2000; 320:132.

149. Shibata S, Mori K, Sekine I, Suyama H. Subarachnoid and intracerebral hemorrhage associated with necrotizing angiitis due to methamphetamine abuse—an autopsy case. Neurol Med Chir Tokyo 1991; 31:45.

150. Davis GG, Swalwell CI. Acute aortic dissections and ruptured berry aneurysms associated with methamphetamine abuse. J Forensic Sci 1994; 39:1481.

151. Citron BP, Halpern M, McCarron M, et al. Necrotizing angiitis associated with drug abuse. N Engl J Med 1970; 283:1003.

152. Citron BP, Peters RL. Angiitis in drug abusers. N Engl J Med 1971; 284:112.

153. Gocke DJ, Christian CL. Angiitis in drug abusers. N Engl J Med 1971; 284:112.

154. Bostwick DG. Amphetamine induced cerebral vasculitis. Hum Pathol 1981; 12:1031.

155. Gautier J-C. L'angiopathie cérébrale moniliforme des toxicomanes. Signification physiopathologique. Rôle possible du spasm. Bull Nat Acad Med 1988; 172:87.

156. Rumbaugh CL, Bergeron RT, Fang HCH, McCormick R. Cerebral angiographic changes in the drug abuse patient. Radiology 1971; 101:335.

157. Rothrock JF, Rubenstein R, Lyden PD. Ischemic stroke associated with methamphetamine inhalation. Neurology 1988; 38:589.

158. Sachdeva K, Woodward KG. Caudal thalamic infarction following intranasal methamphetamine use. Neurology 1989; 39:305.

159. Rumbaugh CL, Bergeron T, Scanlon RL, et al. Cerebral vascular changes secondary to amphetamine abuse in the experimental animal. Radiology 1971; 101:345.

160. Rumbaugh CL, Fang HCH, Higgins RE, et al. Cerebral microvascular injury in experimental drug abuse. Invest Radiol 1976; 11:282.

160a. Hwang W, Ralph J, Marco E, et al. Incomplete Brown-Séquard syndrome after methamphetamine injection into the neck. Neurology 2003; 60:2015.

161. Stafford CR, Bogdanoff BM, Green L, Spector HB. Mononeuropathy multiplex as a complication of amphetamine angiitis. Neurology 1975; 25:570.

162. Rifkin SI. Amphetamine-induced angiitis leading to renal failure. South Med J 1977; 70:108.

163. Golden GS. Gilles de la Tourette's syndrome following amphetamine administration. Dev Med Child Neurol 1976; 16:76.

164. Pollack MA, Cohen NL, Friedhoff AJ. Gilles de la Tourette's syndrome: familial occurrence and precipitation by methylphenidate therapy. Arch Neurol 1977; 34:630.

165. Bonthala CM, West A. Pemoline induced chorea and Gilles de la Tourette's syndrome. Br J Psychiatry 1983; 143:300.

166. Allcott JV, Barnhart RA, Mooney LA. Acute lead poisoning in two users of illicit methamphetamine. JAMA 1987; 258:510.

167. Wilson JM, Kalasinsky KS, Levey AI, et al. Striatal dopamine nerve terminal markers in human, chronic methamphetamine users. Nat Med 1996; 2:699.

168. Volkow ND, Chang L, Wang GJ, et al. Association of dopamine transporter reduction with psychomotor impairment in methamphetamine abusers. Am J Psychol 2001; 158:377.

169. McCann UD, Wong DF, Yokoi F, et al. Reduced striatal dopamine transporter density in abstinent methamphetamine and methcathinone users: evidence from positron emission tomography studies with [11C] WIN-35, 428. J Neurosci 1998; 18:841.

170. Volkow ND, Chang L, Wang GJ, et al. Higher cortical and lower subcortical metabolism in detoxified methamphetamine abusers. Am J Psychol 2001; 158:383.

171. Ernst T, Chang L, Leonido-Yee M, et al. Evidence for long-term neurotoxicity associated with methamphetamine abuse: a 1H-MRS study. Neurology 2000; 54:134.

172. Weinrieb RM, O'Brien CP. Persistent cognitive deficits attributed to substance abuse. In: Brust JCM, ed. Neurologic Complications of Drug and Alcohol Abuse. Neurol Clin 1993; 11:663.

173. Guilarte TR. Is methamphetamine abuse a risk factor in parkinsonism? Neurotoxicology 2001; 22:725.

173a. Moszczynska A, Fitzmaurice P, Ang L, et al. Why is Parkinsonism not a feature of human methamphetamine users? Brain 2004; 127:363.

174. Matera C, Warren WB, Moomjy M, et al. Prevalence of use of cocaine and other substances in an obstetrics population. Am J Obstet Gynecol 1990; 163:797.

175. Oro AS, Dixon SD. Perinatal cocaine and methamphetamine exposure: maternal and neonatal correlates. J Pediatr 1987; 11:571.

176. Eriksson M, Larsson G, Zetterstrom R. Amphetamine addiction and pregnancy. Acta Obstet Gynecol Scand 1981; 60:253.

177. Dominguez R, Vila-Coro AA, Slopis JM, Bohan TP. Brain and ocular abnormalities in infants with in utero exposure to cocaine and other street drugs. Am J Dis Child 1991; 145:688.

178. Dixon SD, Bejar R. Echoencephalographic findings in neonates associated with maternal cocaine and methamphetamine use: incidence and clinical correlates. J Pediatr 1989; 115:770.

179. Plessinger MA. Prenatal exposure to amphetamines. Obst Gynecol Clin North Am 1998; 25:119.

180. Elliott RH, Rees GB. Amphetamine ingestion presenting as eclampsia. Can J Anaesth 1990; 37:130.

181. Cernerud L, Eriksson M, Jonsson B, et al. Amphetamine addiction during pregnancy: 14 year follow-up of growth and school performance. Acta Paediatr 1996; 85:204.

182. Hansen RL, Struthers JM, Gospe SMJ. Visual evoked potentials and visual processing in stimulant drug-exposed infants. Dev Med Child Neurol 1993; 35:798.

183. Smith LM, Chang ML, Yonekura ML, et al. Brain proton magnetic resonance spectroscopy in children exposed to methamphetamine in utero. Neurology 2001; 57:255.

184. Acuff-Smith K. Schilling MA, Fisher JE, et al. Stage-specific effects of perinatal d-methamphetamine exposure on behavioral and eye development in rats. Neurotoxicol Teratol 1996; 18:199.

185. Seiden LS, Sabol KE, Ricaurte GA: Amphetamine: effects on catecholamine systems and behavior. Annu Rev Pharmacol Toxicol 1993; 32:639.

186. Dawirs RR, Teuchert-Noodt G. A novel pharmacologic concept in an animal model of psychosis. Acta Psychiatr Scand, Suppl 2001; 408:10.

187. Burchfield DJ, Lucas VW, Abrams RM, et al. Disposition and pharmacodynamics of methamphetamine in pregnant sheep. JAMA 1991; 265:196.

188. Mueller SM, Muller J, Asdell SM: Cerebral hemorrhage associated with propanolamine in combination with caffeine. Stroke 1984; 15:119–123.

189. Woolverton WL, Johanson CE, de la Garza R, et al. Behavioral and neurochemical evaluation of phenylpropanolamine. J Pharmacol Exp Ther 1986; 237:926.

190. Chait LD, Uhlenhuth EH, Johanson CE. Reinforcing and subjective effects of several anorectics in normal human volunteers. J Pharmacol Exp Ther 1987; 242:777.

191. Chait LD, Uhlenhuth EH, Johanson CE. The discriminative stimulus and subjective effects of phenylpropanolamine, mazindol, and *d*-amphetamine in humans. Pharmacol Biochem Behav 1986; 24:1665.

192. Pentel P. Toxicity of over-the-counter stimulants. JAMA 1984; 252:1898.

192a. Tinsley JA, Watkins DD. Over-the-counter stimulants: abuse and addiction. Mayo Clin Proc 1998; 73:977.

193. O'Connell MB, Pentel PR, Zimmerman CL. Individual variability in the blood pressure response to intravenous phenylpropanolamine: a pharmacokinetic and pharmacodynamic investigation. Clin Pharmacol Ther 1989; 45:252.

194. Bernstein E, Diskant B. Phenylpropanolamine, a potentially hazardous drug. Ann Emerg Med 1982; 11:315.

195. Bale JF, Fountain MT, Shaddy R. Phenylpropanolamine associated CNS complications in children and adolescents. Am J Dis Child 1984; 138:683.

196. Waggoner WC. Phenylpropanolamine overdosage. Lancet 1983; II:1503.

197. Mueller SM. Neurologic complications of phenylpropanolamine use. Neurology 1983; 33:650.

198. Hyams JS, Leichtner AM, Breiner RG, et al. Pseudopheochromocytoma and cardiac arrest associated with phenylpropanolamine. JAMA 1985; 253:1609.

199. LeCoz P, Woimant F, Rougemont D, et al. Angiopathies cérébrales bénignes et phenylpropanolamine. Rev Neurol 1988; 144:295.

200. Peterson RB, Vasquez LA. Phenylpropanolamine-induced arrhythmias. JAMA 1973; 233:324.

201. Woo OF, Benowitz NL, Baily FW, et al. Atrioventricular conduction block caused by phenylpropanolamine. JAMA 1985; 253:2646.

202. Norvenius G, Widerlov E, Lonnerholm G. Phenylpropanolamine and mental disturbances. Lancet 1979; II:1367.

203. Schaffer CB, Pauli MW. Psychotic reaction caused by proprietary oral diet agents. Am J Psychiatry 1980; 137:1256.

204. Cornelius JR, Soloff PH, Reynolds CF. Paranoia, homicidal behavior and seizures associated with phenylpropanolamine. Am J Psychiatry 1984; 141:120.

205. Mueller SM, Solow EB. Seizures associated with a new combination "pick-me-up" pill. Ann Neurol 1982; 11:322.

206. Howrie DL, Wokfson JM. Phenylpropanolamine-induced seizure. J Pediatr 1983; 102:143.

207. King J. Hypertension and cerebral hemorrhage from Trimolets ingestion. Med J Aust 1979; 2:258.

208. Lovejoy FH. Stroke and phenylpropanolamine. Pediatr Alert 1981; 12:45.

209. Mueller SM, Muller J, Asdell SM. Cerebral hemorrhage associated with phenylpropanolamine in combination with caffeine. Stroke 1984; 15:119.

210. Mesnard B, Ginn DR. Excessive phenylpropanolamine ingestion followed by subarachnoid hemorrhage. South Med J 1984; 77:939.

211. Stoessl AJ, Young GB, Feasby TE. Intracerebral hemorrhage and angiographic beading following ingestion of catecholaminergics. Stroke 1985; 16:734.

212. Kikta DG, Devereaux MW, Chandar K. Intracranial hemorrhages due to phenylpropanolamine. Stroke 1985; 16:510.

213. Fallis RJ, Fisher M. Cerebral vasculitis and hemorrhage associated with phenylpropanolamine. Neurology 1985; 35:405.

214. Kizer KW. Intracranial hemorrhage associated with overdose of decongestant containing phenylpropanolamine. Am J Emerg Med 1986; 2:180.

215. Kase CS, Foster TE, Reed JE, et al. Intracerebral hemorrhage and phenylpropanolamine use. Neurology 1987; 37:399.

216. Maertens P, Lum G, Williams JP, et al. Intracerebral hemorrhage and cerebral angiopathic changes in a suicidal phenylpropanolamine poisoning. South Med J 1987; 80:584.

217. Glick R, Hoying J, Cerullo L, Perlman S. Phenylpropanolamine: an over-the-counter drug causing central nervous system vasculitis and intracerebral hemorrhage. Neurosurgery 1987; 20:969.

218. Forman HP, Levin S, Stewart B, et al. Cerebral vasculitis and hemorrhage in an adolescent taking diet pills containing phenylpropanolamine: case report and review of literature. Pediatrics 1989; 83:737.

219. Sloan MA, Kittner SJ, Rigamonti D, Price TR. Occurrence of stroke associated with use/abuse of drugs. Neurology 1991; 41:1358.

220. Jick H, Aselton P, Hunter JR. Phenylpropanolamine and cerebral hemorrhage. Lancet 1984; 1071:345.

221. McDowell JR, LeBlanc HJ. Phenylpropanolamine and cerebral hemorrhage. West J Med 1985; 35:404.

222. Maher LM. Postpartum intracranial hemorrhage and phenylpropanolamine use. Neurology 1987; 37:1686.

223. Lake CR, Gallant S, Masson E, Miller P. Adverse drug effects attributed to phenylpropanolamine: a review of 142 case reports. Am J Med 1990; 89:195.

223a. Chung Y-T, Hung D-Z, Hsu C-P, et al. Intracerebral hemorrhage in a young woman with arteriovenous malformation after taking diet control pills containing phenylpropanolamine. A case report. Chung Hua I Hsuch Tas Chih (Taipei) 1998; 61:432.

224. Johnson DA, Etter HS, Reeves DM. Stroke and phenylpropanolamine use. Lancet 1983; 56: 970.

225. Traynelis VC, Brick JF. Phenylpropanolamine and vasospasm. Neurology 1986; 36:593.

226. Kerman WN, Viscoli CM, Brass LM, et al. Phenylpropanolamine and the risk of hemorrhagic stroke. N Engl J Med 2000; 343:1826.

227. Fleming GA. The FDA, regulation, and the risk of stroke. N Engl J Med 2000; 343:188.

228. Stolberg SG. FDA ban sought on chemical used for cold remedies. NY Times, October 20, 2000.

229. Mersfelder TL. Phenylpropanolamine and stroke: the study, the FDA ruling, the implications. Cleveland Clin J Med 2001; 68:213.

230. Cantu C, Arauz A, Murillo-Bonilla LM, et al. Stroke associated with sympathomimetics contained in over-the-counter cough and cold drugs. Stroke 2003; 34:1667.

231. Brust JCM. Over-the-counter cold remedies and stroke. Stroke 2003; 34:1673.

231a. Davis FT, Brewster ME. A fatality involving U4Euh, a cyclic derivative of phenylpropanolamine. J Forensic Sci 1988; 33:549.

231b. Karch S. Aminorex banned. Forensic Drug Abuse Advisor (FDAA) 1994; 6:38.

232. Garcia-Albea E. Subarachnoid hemorrhage and nasal vasoconstrictor abuse. J Neurol Neurosurg Psychiatry 1983; 46:875.

233. Mariani PJ. Pseudoephedrine-induced hypertensive emergency: treatment with labetalol. Am J Emerg Med 1986; 4:141.

234. Pugh CR, Howie SM. Dependence on pseudo-ephedrine. Br J Psychiatry 1986; 149:789.

235. Lambert MT. Paranoid psychosis after abuse of proprietary cold remedies. Br J Psychiatry 1987; 151:548.

236. Whitehorse M, Duncan JM. Ephedrine psychosis rediscovered. Br J Psychiatry 1987; 150:258.

237. Loosmore S, Armstrong D. Do-Do abuse. Br J Psychiatry 1990; 157:278.

238. Bruno A, Nolte KB, Chapin J. Stroke associated with ephedrine use. Neurology 1993; 43:1313.

239. Wooten MR, Khangure MS, Murphy MJ. Intracerebral hemorrhage and vasculitis related to ephedrine abuse. Ann Neurol 1983; 13:337.

240. Loizou LA, Hamilton JG, Tsementzis SA. Intracranial hemorrhage in association with pseudoephedrine overdose. J Neurol Neurosurg Psychiatry 1982; 45:471.

241. Haller CA, Benowitz NL. Adverse cardiovascular and central nervous system events associated with dietary supplements containing ephedra alkaloids. N Engl J Med 2000; 343:1833.

242. Anon. Adverse events associated with ephedrine-containing products-Texas, December 1993-September 1995. JAMA 1996; 276:1711.

243. Theoharides TC. Sudden death of a healthy college student related to ephedrine toxicity from a ma huang-containing drink. J Clin Psychopharmacol 1997; 17:437.

244. Josefson D. Herbal stimulant causes U.S. deaths. BMJ 1996; 312:1378.

245. Zahn KA, Li RL, Purssell RA. Cardiovascular toxicity after ingestion of "herbal ecstasy." J Emerg Med 1999; 17:289.

246. Zacks SM, Klein L, Tan CD, et al. Hypersensitivity myocarditis associated with ephedra use. J Toxicol Clin Toxicol 1999; 37:485.

247. Vahedi K, Domigo V, Amerenco R, Bousser MG. Ischaemic stroke in a sportsman who consumed MaHuang extract and creatine monohydrate for body building. J Neurol Neurosurg Psychiatry 2000; 68:112.

248. Shekelle PG, Hardy ML, Morton SC, et al. Efficacy and safety of ephedra and ephedrine for weight loss and athletic performance. A meta-analysis. JAMA 2003; 289:1537.

248a. Capwell RR. Ephedrine-induced mania from an herbal diet supplement. Am J Psychiatry 1995; 152:647.

248b. Morganstern MD, Viscoli CM, Kernan WN, et al. Use of Ephedra-containing products and risk for hemorrhagic stroke. Neurology 2003; 60:132.

248c. Wolfe SM. Ephedra-scientific evidence versus money/politics. Science 2003; 300:437.

248d. The ephadra ban is not enough. NY Times, January 5, 2004.

249. Mellar J, Hollister LE. Phenmetrazine: an obsolete problem drug. Clin Pharmacol Ther 1982; 32:671.

250. Corwin RL, Woolverton WL, Schuster CR, Johanson CE. Anorectics: effects on food intake and self-administration in rhesus monkeys. Alcohol Drug Res 1987; 7:351.

251. Hamer R, Phelp D. Inadvertent intra-arterial injection of phentermine. A complication of drug abuse. Ann Emerg Med 1981; 10:148.

252. Kokkinos J, Levine SR. Possible association of ischemic stroke with phentermine. Stroke 1993; 24:310.

253. Caplan J. Habituation to diethylpropion (Tenuate). Can Med Assoc J 1963; 88:943.

254. Cohen S. Diethylpropion (Tenuate): an infrequently abused anorectic. Psychosomatics 1977; 18:28.

255. Carney MWP. Diethylpropion and psychosis. Clin Neuropharmacol 1988; 11:183.

256. Rosse RB, Johri SK, Deutsch SI. Pupillary changes associated with the development of stimulant-induced mania: a case report. Clin Neuropharmacol 1997; 20:270.

257. Levin A. The non-medical use of fenfluramine by drug-dependent young South Africans. Postgrad Med J 1975; 51:186.

258. Kew MC, Hopp M, Rothberg A. Fatal heat stroke in a child taking appetite-suppressant drugs. S Afr Med J 1982; 62:905.

259. Wen PY, Feske S, Teoh SK. Cerebral hemorrhage in a patient taking fenfluramine and phentermine for obesity. Neurology 1987; 49:63.

260. Derby LE, Myers MW, Jick H. Use of dexfenfluramine, fenfluramine and phentermine and the risk of stroke. Br J Clin Pharmacol 1999; 47:565.

261. Schwitter J, Agosti R, Ott P, et al. Small infarctions of cochlear, retinal, and encephalic tissue in young women. Stroke 1992; 23:903.

262. Jick H, Vasilakis C, Weinrauch LA, et al. A population-based study of appetite-suppressant drugs and the risk of cardiac valve regurgitation. N Engl J Med 1998; 339:719.

263. Bennett-Clarke CA, Leslie MJ, Lance RD, Rhoades RW. Fenfluramine depletes serotonin from the developing cortex and alters thalamocortical organization. Brain Res 1995; 702:255.

264. McCann UD, Seiden LS, Rubin LJ, Ricuarte GA. Brain serotonin neurotoxicity and primary pulmonary hypertension from fenfluramine and dexfenfluramine. A systematic review of the evidence. JAMA 1997; 278:666.

265. Volkow ND, Fowler JS, Gatley JS, et al. Comparable changes in synaptic dopamine induced by methylphenidate and cocaine in the baboon brain. Synapse 1999; 31:59.

266. Kollins SH, MacDonald EK, Rush CR. Assessing the abuse potential of methylphenidate in nonhuman and human subjects. A review. Pharm Biochem Behav 2001; 68:611.

267. Weiner AL. Emerging drugs of abuse in Connecticut. Conn Med 2000; 64:19.

268. Klein-Schwartz W. Abuse and toxicity of methylphenidate. Curr Opin Pediatr 2002; 14:219.

269. Garland EJ. Intranasal abuse of prescribed methylphenidate. J Am Acad Child Adolesc Psychiatry 1998; 37:573.

270. Massello W, Carpenter DA. A fatality due to intranasal abuse of methylphenidate (Ritalin). J Forensic Sci 1999; 44:220.

271. Llana ME, Crismon ML. Methylphenidate: increased abuse or appropriate use? J Am Pharm Assoc 1999; 39:526.

272. Parran TV, Jasinski DR. Intravenous methylphenidate abuse. Arch Intern Med 1991; 151:781.

273. Musser CJ, Ahmann FW, Mundt P, et al. Stimulant use and the potential for abuse in Wisconsin as reported by school administrators and longitudinally followed children. J Dev Behav Pediatr 1998; 19:187.

274. Raskind M, Bradford T. Methylphenidate (Ritalin) abuse and methadone maintenance. Dis Nerv Syst 1975; 36:9.

275. Lewman LV. Fatal pulmonary hypertension from intravenous injection of methylphenidate (Ritalin) tablets. Hum Pathol 1972; 3:67.

276. Zemplenyi J, Colman MF. Deep neck abscesses secondary to methylphenidate (Ritalin) abuse. Head Neck Surg 1984; 6:858.

277. Wolf J, Fein A, Fehrenbacher L. Eosinophilic syndrome with methylphenidate abuse. Ann Intern Med 1978; 89:224.

278. Spensley J, Rockwell DA. Psychosis during methylphenidate abuse. N Engl J Med 1972; 286:880.

279. Hahn HH, Schweid AI, Beaty HN. Complications of injecting dissolved methylphenidate tablets. Arch Intern Med 1969; 123:656.

280. Extein I. Methylphenidate-induced choreoathetosis. Am J Psychiatry 1978; 135:252.

281. Chillar RK, Jackson AL. Reversible hemiplegia after presumed intracarotid injection of Ritalin. N Engl J Med 1981; 304:1305.

282. Atlee W. Talc and cornstarch emboli in eyes of drug abusers. JAMA 1972; 219:49.

283. Tse DT, Ober RR. Talc retinopathy. Am J Ophthalmol 1980; 90:624.

284. Mizutami T, Lewis R, Gonatas N. Medial medullary syndrome in a drug abuser. Arch Neurol 1980; 37:425.

285. Trugman JM. Cerebral arteritis and oral methylphenidate. Lancet 1988; I:584.

286. Holden C. Putting kids on drugs to fight drugs. Science 1999; 285:1007.

287. Briscoe JG, Curry SC, Gerkin RD, Ruiz RR. Pemoline-induced choreoathetosis and rhabdomyolysis. Med Toxicol 1988; 3:72.

288. McIntyre D. Psychosis due to nasal decongestant abuse. Br J Psychiatry 1976; 112:93.

289. White L, DiMiao VJM. Intravenous propylhexedrine and sudden death. N Engl J Med 1977; 297:1071.

290. Anderson R, Garza H, Garriott JC, DiMaio V. Intravenous propylhexedrine (Benzedrex) abuse and sudden death. Am J Med 1979; 67:15.

291. Croft CH, Firth BG, Hillis LP. Propylhexedrine-induced left ventricular dysfunction. Ann Intern Med 1982; 97:560.

292. Hall AH, Kulig KW, Rumack BH. Intravenous epinephrine abuse. Am J Emerg Med 1987; 5:64.

293. Margaral LE, Sandborn GE, Donoso LA, Gander JR. Branch retinal artery occlusion after excessive use of nasal spray. Ann Ophthalmol 1985; 17:500.

294. Montalban J, Ibanez L, Rodriguez C, et al. Cerebral infarction after excessive use of nasal decongestants. J Neurol Neurosurg Psychiatry 1989; 52:541.

295. Brenneisen R, Fisch HU, Koelbing U, et al. Amphetamine-like effects in humans of the khat alkaloid cathinone. Br J Clin Pharmacol 1990; 30:825.

296. Yanagita T. Intravenous self-administration of cathinone and of 2-amino-(2,5-dimethyl-4-methyl)-phenylpropane in rhesus monkeys. Drug Alcohol Depend 1986; 17:135.

297. Kalix P. Khat, an amphetamine-like stimulant. J Psychoactive Drug 1994; 26:69.

298. Pantelis C, Hindler C, Taylor J. Use and abuse of khat: distribution, pharmacology, side effects and description

of psychosis attributed to khat chewing. Psychol Med 1989; 19:657.

299. Yousef G, Huq Z, Lambert T. Khat chewing as a cause of psychosis. Br J Hosp Med 1995; 54:322.

300. Baird DA. A case of optic neuritis in a khat addict. East Afr Med J 1952; 29:325.

301. Roper JP. The presumed neurotoxic effects of Catha edulis–an exotic plant now available in the United Kingdom. Br J Ophthalmol 1986; 70:779.

302. Morrish PK, Nicolaou N, Brakkenberg P, Smith PEM. Leukoencephalopathy associated with khat misuse. J Neurol Neurosurg Psychiatry 1999; 67:556.

303. Browne DL. Qat use in New York City. NIDA Res Monogr 1991; 105:464.

304. Griffiths P, Gossop M, Wickenden S, et al. A transcultural pattern of drug use: qat (khat) in the UK. Br J Psychiatry 1997; 170:281.

305. Giannini AJ, Castelanni S. A manic-like psychosis due to khat (Catha edulis). J Toxicol Clin Toxicol 1982; 19:455.

306. Gough SP, Cookson IB. Khat-induced schizophreniform psychosis in UK. Lancet 1984; I:455.

307. Mayberry J, Morgan G, Perkin E. Khat-induced schizophreniform psychosis in UK. Lancet 1984; I:455.

308. Nencini P, Grassi M, Botan A, et al. Khat chewing spread to the Somali community in Rome. Drug Alcohol Depend 1989; 23:255.

309. Emerson TS, Cisek JE. Methcathinone ("cat"): a Russian designer amphetamine infiltrates the rural midwest. Ann Emerg Med 1993; 22:1897.

310. Glennon RA, Yousif M, Naiman N, et al. Methcathinone: a new and potent amphetamine-like agent. Pharmacol Biochem Behav 1987; 26:547.

311. Young R, Glennon RA. Cocaine-stimulus generalization to two new designer drugs: methcathinone and 4-methyl-aminorex. Pharmacol Biochem Behav 1993; 45:229.

312. Nichols DE, Oberlender R. Structure-activity relationships of MDMA-like substances. NIDA Res Monogr 1989; 94:1.

313. Jackson B, Reed A. Another abusable amphetamine. JAMA 1970; 211:830.

314. Weil A. The love drug. J Psychoact Drugs 1976; 8:335.

315. Climko RP, Roehrich H, Sweeney DR, Al-Rari J. Ecstasy: a review of MDMA and MDA. Int J Psychiatr Med 1986; 16:359.

316. Grinspoon L, Bakalar JB. Can drugs be used to enhance the psychotherapeutic process? Am J Psychother 1986; 15:393.

317. Peroutka SJ. Incidence of recreational use of 3,4-methylenedimethoxymethamphetamine (MDMA, "Ecstasy") on an undergraduate campus. N Engl J Med 1987; 317:1542.

318. Beardsley PM, Balster RL, Harris LS. Self-administration of methylenedioxymethamphetamine (MDMA) by Rhesus monkeys. Drug Alcohol Depend 1986; 18:149.

319. Lamb RJ, Griffiths RR. Self-injection of d,1-3,4-methylenedioxymethamphetamine (MDMA) in the baboon. Psychopharmacology 1987; 91:268.

320. Gold LH, Koob GF, Geyer MA. Stimulant and hallucinogenic behavioral profiles of 3,4-methylenedioxymethamphetamine (MDMA) and N-ethyl-3,4-methylenedioxyamphetamine (MDEA) in rats. J Pharmacol Exp Ther 1988; 247:547.

321. Stone D, Stahl D, Hanson G, Gibb J. The effects of 3,4-methylenedioxymethamphetamine and 3,4- methylenedioxyamphetamine (MDA) on monoaminergic systems in the rat brain. Eur J Pharmacol 1986; 128:41.

322. Oberlender R, Nichols DE. (+)-N-Methyl-1-(1,3-benzodioxol-5-yl)-2-butanamine as a discriminative stimulus in studies of 3,4-methylenedioxymethamphetamine-like behavioral activity. J Pharmacol Exp Ther 1990; 255:1098.

323. Siegel RK. MDMA. Nonmedical use and intoxication. J Psychoact Drugs 1986; 18:349.

324. Bost RO. 3,4-Methylenedioxymethamphetamine (MDMA) and other amphetamine derivatives. J Forensic Sci 1988; 33:576.

325. Boja JW, Schechter MD. Behavioral effects of N-ethyl-3,4-methylenedioxyamphetamine (MDEA; "Eve"). Pharmacol Biochem Behav 1987; 28:153.

326. Doyen S. The many faces of ecstasy. Curr Opin Pediatr 2001; 13:170.

326a. Kovar K-A. Chemistry and pharmacology of hallucinogens, entactogens, and stimulants. Pharmacopsychiatry 1999: 31 (Suppl):69.

327. Christophersen AS. Amphetamine designer drugs-an overview and epidemiology. Toxicol Lett 2000; 112–13:127.

328. Butterfield F. Violence rises as club drug spreads out into the streets. NY Times, June 24, 2001.

329. Rome E. It's a rave new world: rave culture and illicit drug use in the young. Cleveland Clin J Med 2001; 68:541.

330. White JM, Bochner F, Irvine RJ. The agony of "Ecstasy." Med J Aust 1997; 166:117.

330a. Karch S. Nexus banned by DEA. Forensic Drug Abuse Advisor (FDAA) 1994; 6:12.

331. Peroutka SJ, Newman H, Harris H. Subjective effects of 3,4-methylenedioxymethamphetamine in recreational users. Neuropsychopharmacology 1988; 1:273.

331a. Harris DS, Baggott M, Mendelson JH, et al. Subjective and hormonal effects of 3,4-methylenedioxymethamphetamine (MDMA) in humans. Psychopharmacology 2002; 162:396.

332. Hegadoren KM, Baker GB, Baurin M. 3,4-Methylenedioxy analogues of amphetamine: defining the risks to humans. Neurosci Biobehav Rev 1999; 23:539.

333. Brown C, Osterloh J. Multiple severe complications from recreational ingestion of MDMA ("Ecstasy"). JAMA 1987; 258:780.

334. Hayner GN, McKinney H. MDMA. The dark side of ecstasy. J Psychoact Drugs 1986; 18:341.

334a. Kalant H. The pharmacology and toxicology of "ecstasy" (MDMA) and related drugs. Can Med Assoc J 2001; 165:917.

335. Dowling GP, McDonough ET, Bost RO. "Eve" and "Ecstasy"–Garden of Eden or serpent? A report of five deaths associated with the use of MDEA and MDMA. JAMA 1987; 257:1615.

335a. Gillman PK. Ecstasy, serotonin syndrome and the treatment of hyperpyrexia. Med J Aust 1997; 167:109.

336. Suarez RV, Riemorsma R. "Ecstasy" and sudden cardiac death. Am J Forensic Med Pathol 1988; 9:339.

337. Whitaker-Azmitia PM, Aronson TA. "Ecstasy" (MDMA)-induced panic. Am J Psychiatry 1989; 146:119.

338. Ramsey JD, Butcher MA, Murphy MF, et al. A new method to monitor drugs at dance venues. BMJ 2001; 323:603.

339. Shannon M. Methylenedioxymethamphetamine (MDMA, "ecstasy"). Pediatr Emerg Care 2000;16:377.

340. Ramcharan S, Munhorst PL, Otten JM, et al. Survival after massive ecstasy overdose. J Toxicol Clin Toxicol 1998; 36:727.

341. Regenthal R, Kruger M, Rudolf K, et al. Survival after massive "ecstasy" (MDMA) ingestion. Intensive Care Med 1999; 25:640.

341a. Zagnami PG, Albano C. Psychostimulants and epilepsy. Epilepsia 2002; 43 (Suppl 2):2.

341b. Hinkelbein J, Gabel A, Volz M, Ellinger K: Suicide attempt with high dose ecstasy. Anaeshetist 2003; 52:51.

342. Case Records of the Massachusetts General Hospital. N Engl J Med 2001; 344:591.

343. Henry JA, Fallon JK, Kieman AT, et al. Low dose MDMA ("ecstasy") induces vasopressin secretion. Lancet 1998; 351:1784.

343a. O'Connor A, Cluroe A, Couch R, et al. Death from hyponatremia-induced cerebral oedema associated with MDMA ("ecstasy") use. N Z Med J 1999; 112:255.

343b. Schifano F, Oyefeso A, Webb L, et al. Review of deaths related to taking ecstasy, England and Wales, 1997-2000. BMJ 2003; 326:80.

344. Reneman L, Habraken JB, Majoie CB, et al. MDMA ("Ecstasy") and its association with cerebrovascular accidents: preliminary findings. Am J Neuroradiol 2000; 21:1001.

345. McCann U, Slate SO, Ricaurte GA. Adverse reaction with 3,4-methylenedioxymethamphetamine (MDMA, ecstasy). Drug Saf 1996; 15:107.

346. Hanyu S, Ikeguchi K, Imai H, et al. Cerebral infarction associated with 3,4-methylenedioxymethamphetamine ("Ecstasy") abuse. Eur Neurol 1995; 35:173.

346a. Manchada S, Connolly MJ. Cerebral infarction in association with Ecstasy abuse. Postgrad Med J 1993; 69:874.

346b. McEvoy AW, Kitchen ND, Thomas DG. Intracerebral hemorrhage and drug abuse in young adults. Br J Neurosurg 2000; 14:449.

346c. Auer J, Berent R, Weber T, et al. Subarachnoid hemorrhage with "Ecstasy" abuse in a young adult. Neurol Sci 2002; 23:199.

346d. Harries DP, DeSilva R. "Ecstasy" and intracerebral hemorrhage. Scott Med J 1992; 37:150.

346e. Gledhill JA, Moore DF, Bell D, et al. Subarachnoid hemorrhage associated with MDMA abuse. J Neurol Neurosurg Psychiatry 1993; 56:1036.

346f. Hughes JC, McCabe M, Evans RJ. Intracranial hemorrhage associated with ecstasy." Arch Emerg Med 1993; 10:372.

346g. Vallée J-N, Crozier S, Guillevin R, et al. Acute basilar artery occlusion treated by thromboaspiration in a cocaine and ecstasy abuser. Neurology 2003; 61:839.

347. Mintzer S, Hickenbottom S, Gilman S. Parkinsonism after taking ecstasy. N Engl J Med 1999; 340:1443.

347a. Kuniyoshi SM, Jankovic J. MDMA and parkinsonism. N Engl J Med 2003; 349:96.

347b. O'Suilleabhain P, Giller C. Rapidly progressive parkinsonism in a self-reported abuser of Ecstasy and other drugs. Mov Disord 2003; 18:1378.

347c. Ricaurte GA, Yuan J, Hatzidimitrious G, et al. Severe dopaminergic neurotoxicity in primates after a common recreational dose regimen of MDMA ("ecstasy"). Science 2002; 297:2260.

347d. Holden C. Paper on toxic party drug is pulled over vial mix-up. Science 2003; 301:1454.

347e. Iravani MM, Jackson MJ, Juoppamaki M, et al: 3,4-methylenedioxymethamphetamine (ecstasy) inhibits dyskinesia expression and normalizes motor activity in 1-methyl-4-phenyl-1,2,3,6-tetrahydropyridine-treated primates. J Neurosci 2003; 23:9107.

348. Battaglia G, Yeh SY, O'Hearn E, et al. 3,4-methylenedioxymethamphetamine and 3,4-methylenedioxyamphetamine destroy serotonin terminals in rat brain: quantification of neurodegeneration by measurement of [3H]paroxetine-labelled serotonin uptake sites. J Pharmacol Exp Ther 1987; 242:911.

349. Ricaurte GA, Forno LS, Wilson MA, et al. 3,4-methylenedioxymethamphetamine selectively damages central serotonergic neurons in nonhuman primates. JAMA 1988; 260:51.

350. Schmidt CJ. Neurotoxicity of the psychedelic amphetamine, methylenedioxymethamphetamine. J Pharmacol Exp Ther 1986; 240:1.

351. Molliver ME, Mamounas LA, Wilson MA. Effects of neurotoxic amphetamines on serotonergic neurons: immunocytochemical studies. NIDA Res Monogr 1989; 94:270.

352. DeSouza EB, Battaglia G. Effects of MDMA and MDA on brain serotonin neurons: evidence from neurochemical and autoradiographic studies. NIDA Res Monogr 1989; 94:196.

353. Fischer C, Hatzidimitriou G, Wlos J, et al. Reorganization of ascending 5-HT axon projections in animals previously exposed to the recreational drug (I)

3,4-methylenedioxymethamphetamine (MDMA, "Ecstasy"). J Neurosci 1995; 15:5476-5485.

354. Hazidimitriou G, McCann UD, Ricuarte GA. Altered serotonin innervation patterns in the forebrain of monkeys treated with (I) 3,4-methylendioxymethamphetamine seven years previously: factors influencing abnormal recovery. J Neurol 1999; 19:5096.

355. Reneman L, Booij J, deBruin K, et al. Effects of dose, sex, and long-term abstention from use on toxic effects of MDMA (ecstasy) on brain serotonin neurons. Lancet 2001; 358:1864.

356. McCann UD, Szabo Z, Scheffel U, et al. Positron emission tomographic evidence of toxic effect of MDMA ("Ecstasy") on brain serotonin neurons in human beings. Lancet 1998; 352:1433.

357. Kish SJ, Furukawa Y, Ang L, et al. Striatal serotonin is depleted in brain of a human MDMA (Ecstasy) user. Neurology 2000; 55:294.

357a. Oliveri M, Calvo G. Increased visual cortical excitability in ecstasy users: a transcranial magnetic stimulation study. J Neurol Neurosurg Psychiatry 2003; 74:1136.

358. Bolla KI, McCann UD, Ricuarte GA. Memory impairment in abstinent MDMD ("Ecstasy") users. Neurology 1998; 51:1532.

358a. D'Esposito M. Serotonin neurotoxicity. Implications for cognitive neuroscience and neurology. Neurology 1998; 51:1529.

359. Zakzanis KK, Young DA. Memory impairment in abstinent MDMA ("Ecstasy") users: a longitudinal investigation. Neurology 2001; 56:966.

360. Morgan MJ. Memory deficits associated with recreational use of "ecstasy" (MDMA). Psychopharmacology 1999; 141:30.

361. Parrott AC, Lees A, Garnham NJ, et al. Cognitive performance in recreational users of MDMA ("ecstasy"): evidence for memory deficits. J Psychopharmacol 1998; 12:79.

362. Morland J. Toxicity of drug abuse-amphetamine designer drugs (ecstasy): mental effects and consequences of single dose use. Toxicol Lett 2000; 112-113:147.

362a. Fox HC, McLean A, Tumer JJD, et al: Neuropsychological evidence of a relatively selective profile of temporal dysfunction in drug free MDMD ("Ecstasy") polydrug users. Psychopharmacology 2002; 162:203.

362b. Parrott A: Cognitive deficits and cognitive normality in recreational cannabis and Ecstasy/MDMA users. Hum Psychopharmacol 2003; 18:89.

363. Gouzoulis-Mayfrank E, et al. Impaired cognitive performance in drug-free users of recreational ecstasy (MDMA). J Neurol Neurosurg Psychiatry 2000; 68:719.

363a. McNeil DG. Research on Ecstasy is clouded by errors. NY Times, December 2, 2003.

363b. Verbaten MN. Specific memory deficits in Ecstasy users? The results of a meta-analysis. Hum Psychopharmacol 2003; 18:281.

363c. Kish SJ. What is the evidence that Ecstasy (MDMA) can cause Parkinson's disease? Mov Disord 2003; 18:1219.

364. DeBoer D, Bosman IJ, Hidvégi E, et al. Piperazine-like compounds: a new group of designer drugs-of-abuse on the European market. Forensic Sci Int 2001; 121:47.

365. Jasinski DR, Kovacevic-Ristanovic R. Evaluation of the abuse liability of modafinil and other drugs for excessive daytime sleepiness associated with narcolepsy. Clin Neuropharmacol 2000; 23:149.

366. Shopsin B, Kline NS. Monoamine oxidase inhibitors: potential for drug abuse. Biol Psychiatr 1976; 11:451.

367. Ben-Arie O, George GCW. A case of tranylcypromine (Parnate) addiction. Br J Psychiatry 1979; 135:273.

368. Griffin N, Draper RJ, Webb MGT. Addiction to tranylcypromine. BMJ 1981; 283:346.

369. Pitt B. Withdrawal symptoms after stopping phenelzine? BMJ 1974; 2:332.

370. LeGassicke J, Ashcrof GW, Eccelston D, et al. The clinical state, sleep, and amine metabolism of a tranylcypromine (Parnate) addict. Br J Psychiatry 1965; 111:357.

371. Vartzopoulos D, Krull F. Dependence on monoamine oxidase inhibitors in high dose. Br J Psychiatry 1991; 158:856.

372. Dilsaver SC. Heterocyclic antidepressant, monoamine oxidase inhibitor and neuroleptic withdrawal phenomena. Prog Neuropsychopharmacol Biol Psychiatry 1990; 14:137.

373. Cohen MJ, Hanbury R, Stimmel B. Abuse of amitriptyline. JAMA 1978; 240:1372.

374. Cantor R. Methadone maintenance and amitriptyline. JAMA 1979; 241:2378.

375. Bialos D, Giller E, Jatlow P, et al. Recurrence of depression after long-term amitriptyline treatment. Am J Psychiatry 1982; 139:325.

376. Charney DS, Heninger GR, Sternberg DE, Landis H. Abrupt discontinuation of tricyclic antidepressant drugs-evidence for noradrenergic hyperactivity. Br J Psychiatry 1982; 141:377.

377. Siegfried K, Taeuber K. Pharmacodynamics of nomifensine: a review of studies in healthy subjects. J Clin Psychiatry 1984; 45:33.

378. Boning J, Fuchs G. Nomifensine and psychological dependence-a case report. Pharmacopsychiatry 1986; 19:386.

379. Charney DS, Heninger GR, Breier A. Noradrenergic function on panic anxiety. Effects of yohimbine in healthy subjects and patients with agoraphobia and panic disorder. Arch Gen Psychiatry 1984; 41:751.

380. Lader M, Bruce M. States of anxiety and their induction by drugs. Br J Clin Pharmacol 1986; 22:251.

381. Linden CH, Vellman WP, Rumrack B. Yohimbine: a new street drug. Ann Emerg Med 1985; 14:1002.

382. Siegel RK. Ginseng abuse syndrome. Problems with the panacea. JAMA 1979; 241:1614.

383. Hung OL, Lewin NA, Howland MA. Herbal preparations. In: Goldfrank LR, Flomenbaum NE, Lewin NA, et al., eds. Toxicologic Emergencies, 6th edition. Stamford, CT: Appleton & Lange, 1998:1221.

384. Plotnikoff GA, George J. Herbalism in Minnesota. Minn Med 1999; 82:13.

385. Takahashi M, Tokuyama S. Pharmacological and physiological effects of ginseng on actions induced by opioids and psychostimulants. Meth Find Exp Clin Pharmacol 1998; 20:77.

386. Cawte J. Psychoactive substances of the South Seas: betel, kava and pituri. Aust N Z J Psychiatry 1985; 19:83.

386a. Croucher R, Islam S. Socio-economic aspects of areca nut use. Addict Biol 2002; 7:139.

387. Suwanlert S. A study of Kratom eaters in Thailand. Bull Narc 1975; 27:21.

388. Jansen KLR, Prast CJ. Psychoactive properties of mitragynine (Kratom). J Psychoact Drugs 1988; 20:455.

389. Siegel RK. Herbal intoxication. Psychoactive effects from herbal cigarettes, tea, and capsules. JAMA 1976; 236:473.

390. Undem BJ, Lichtenstein LM. Drugs used in the treatment of asthma. In: Hardman JG, Limbird LE, eds. Goodman and Gilman's The Pharmacological Basis of Therapeutics, 10th edition. New York: McGraw-Hill, 2001:733.

391. Graham DM. Caffeine–its identity, dietary sources, intake and biological effects. Nutr Rev 1978; 36:97.

392. Williams M, Jarvis MF. Adenosine antagonists as potential therapeutic agents. Pharmacol Biochem Behav 1988; 29:433.

393. Katz JL, Prada JA, Goldberg SR. Effects of adenosine analogs alone and in combination with caffeine in the squirrel monkey. Pharmacol Biochem Behav 1988; 29:429.

394. Holtzman SG, Finn IB. Tolerance to behavioral effects of caffeine in rats. Pharmacol Biochem Behav 1988; 29:411.

395. Khakh BS, Kennedy C. Adenosine and ATP: progress in their receptors' structures and functions. Trends Pharmacol Sci 1998; 19:39.

396. Mumford GK, Holtzman SG. Quantitative differences in the discriminative stimulus effects of low and high doses of caffeine in the rat. J Pharmacol Exp Ther 1991; 258:857.

397. Griffiths RR, Woodson PP. Reinforcing properties of caffeine: studies in humans and laboratory animals. Pharmacol Biochem Behav 1988; 29:419.

398. Service RF: Coffee cravers are not addicts. Science 1999; 284:244.

399. Holtzman SG. Discriminative effects of CGS 15943, a competitive adenosine receptor antagonist, have a dopamine component in monkeys. Eur J Pharmacol 1999; 376:7.

400. Myers MG. Effects of caffeine on blood pressure. Arch Intern Med 1988; 148:115.

401. Myers MG. Caffeine and cardiac arrhythmias. Chest 1988; 94:4.

402. Lutz EG. Restless legs, anxiety, and caffeinism. J Clin Psychiatry 1978; 39:693.

403. Charney DS, Heninger GR, Jatlow PI. Increased anxiogenic effects of caffeine in panic disorders. Arch Gen Psychiatry 1985; 42:233.

404. Curatolo PW, Robertson D. The health consequences of caffeine. Ann Intern Med 1983; 98:641.

405. DiMaio VJM, Garriott JC. Lethal caffeine poisoning in a child. Forensic Sci Int 1974; 3:275.

406. Turner JE, Cravey RH. A fatal ingestion of caffeine. Clin Toxicol 1977; 10:341.

407. Sullivan JL. Caffeine poisoning in an infant. J Pediatr 1977; 90:1022.

408. Banner W, Czajka PA. Acute caffeine overdose in a neonate. Am J Dis Child 1980; 134:495.

409. Eisele JW, Reay DT. Deaths related to coffee enemas. JAMA 1980; 244:1608.

410. Zimmerman PM, Pulliam J, Schwengels J, MacDonald SE. Caffeine intoxication. A near fatality. Ann Emerg Med 1985; 14:1227.

411. Garriott JC, Simmons LM, Poklis A, Mackell MA. Five cases of fatal overdose from caffeine-containing "look-alike" drugs. J Anal Toxicol 1985; 9:141.

412. Hughes JR, Higgins ST, Bickel WK, et al. Caffeine self-administration, withdrawal, and adverse effects among coffee drinkers. Arch Gen Psychiatry 1991; 48:611.

413. Silverman K, Evans SM, Strain EC, Griffiths RR. Withdrawal syndrome after the double-blind cessation of caffeine consumption. N Engl J Med 1992; 327:1110.

414. McGowan JD, Altman RE, Kanto WP. Neonatal withdrawal symptoms after chronic maternal ingestion of caffeine. South Med J 1988; 81:1092.

415. Russ NW, Sturgis ET, Malcolm RJ, Williams L. Abuse of caffeine in substance abusers. J Clin Psychiatry 1988; 49:457.

416. LaCroix AZ, Mead LA, Liang K-Y, et al. Coffee consumption and the incidence of coronary heart disease. N Engl J Med 1986; 315:977.

417. Dawber TR, Kannel WB, Gordon T. Coffee and cardiovascular disease. Observations from the Framingham Study. N Engl J Med 1974; 291:871.

418. Grobbee DE, Rimm EB, Giovannucci E, et al. Coffee, caffeine, and cardiovascular disease in men. N Engl J Med 1990; 323:1026.

418a. James JE. Is habitual caffeine use a preventable cardiovascular risk factor? Lancet 1997; 349:279.

419. Fried RE, Levine DM, Kwiterovich PO, et al. The effect of filtered-coffee consumption on plasma lipid levels. Results of a randomized clinical trial. JAMA 1992; 267:811.

419a. van Dam RM, Feskens EJM. Coffee consumption and risk of type 2 diabetes mellitus. Lancet 2002; 360:1477.

420. Rudolphi KA, Keil M, Fastbom J, Fredholm BB. Ischaemic damage in gerbil hippocampus is reduced

following upregulation of adenosine (A1) receptors by caffeine treatment. Neurosci Lett 1989; 103:275.

421. Li H, Bruederlin B, Buchan AM. Chronic caffeine protects hippocampal CA1 cells from severe forebrain ischemia. Stroke 1991; 22:132.

422. Sutherland GR, Peeling J, Lesiuk HJ, et al. The effects of caffeine on ischemic neuronal injury as determined by magnetic resonance imaging and histopathology. Neuroscience 1991; 42:171.

422a. Aronowski J, Strong R, Shirzadi A, et al. Ethanol plus caffeine (caffeinol) for treatment of ischemic stroke. Preclinical experience. Stroke 2003; 34:1246.

423. Michaud DS, Giovannucci E, Willett WC, et al. Coffee and alcohol consumption and the risk of pancreatic cancer in two prospective United States cohorts. Cancer Epidemic Biomark Prevent 2001; 10:429.

424. Kiel DP, Felson DT, Hannan MT. Caffeine and the risk of hip fracture: the Framingham Study. Am J Epidemiol 1990; 132:675.

425. Benedetti MD, Bower JH, Maraganore DM, et al. Smoking, alcohol, and coffee consumption preceding Parkinson's disease. A case-control study. Neurology 2000; 55:1350.

426. Ross GW, Abbott RD, Petrovitch H, et al. Association of coffee and caffeine intake with the risk of Parkinson's disease. JAMA 2000; 283:2674.

427. Richardson PJ, Kase H, Jenner PG. Adenosine A2A receptor antagonists as new agents for the treatment of Parkinson's disease. Trends Pharmacol Sci 1997; 18:338.

427a. Ascherio A, Chen H, Schwarzschild MA, et al. Caffeine, postmenopausal estrogen, and risk of Parkinson's disease. Neurology 2003; 60:790.

428. Nehlig A. Are we dependent upon coffee and caffeine? A review on human and animal data. Neurosci Biobehav Rev 1999; 23:563.

429. Eskenazi B. Caffeine-filtering the facts. N Engl J Med 1999; 341:1688.

430. Cnattingíus S, Signorello LB, Annerén G, et al. Caffeine intake and the risk of first-trimester spontaneous abortion. N Engl J Med 2000; 343:1839.

431. Klebanoff MA, Levine RJ, DerSimonian R, et al. Maternal serum paraxanthine, a caffeine metabolite, and the risk of spontaneous abortion. N Engl J Med 1999; 341:1639.

432. Fernandez O, Sabhorwal M, Smiley T, et al. Moderate to heavy coffee consumption during pregnancy and relationship to spontaneous abortion and abnormal fetal growth: a meta-analysis. Reprod Toxicol 1998; 12:435.

433. Nehelig A, Debry G. Potential teratogenic and neurodevelopmental consequences of coffee and caffeine exposure: a review on human and animal data. Neurotoxicol Teratol 1994; 16:531.

Chapter 5
Cocaine

If you are forward you will see who is the stronger, a gentle little girl who doesn't eat enough or a big wild man who has cocaine in his body.
—Sigmund Freud to his fiancée Martha Bernays

I would rather live ten years with coca than one million centuries without coca.
—Italian neurologist Paolo Mantegazza, 1859

If coke is a lady, crack is a bitch.
—Anonymous West Coast user

Cocaine, the only naturally occurring local anesthetic, is also a central nervous system (CNS) stimulant (Figure 5–1). Pharmacologically it is similar to amphetamine and related psychostimulants (see Chapter 4). In the 1980s, cocaine became the most feared illicit drug in the United States. It thereby merits its own chapter.

Pharmacology and Animal Studies

Acute Effects and Self-Administration

In animals, cocaine produces an alerting response with increased exploration, locomotion, grooming, and rearing.[1,2] Repeated administration leads to stereotypic movements, and seizures occur at previously subthreshold doses (kindling).[3,4] Cocaine's local anesthetic properties may contribute to seizures; similar kindling occurs with other local anesthetics that do not produce locomotor or stereotypic effects.[5,6] Kindled seizures and progressive stereotypy (and in humans, progressive psychosis)

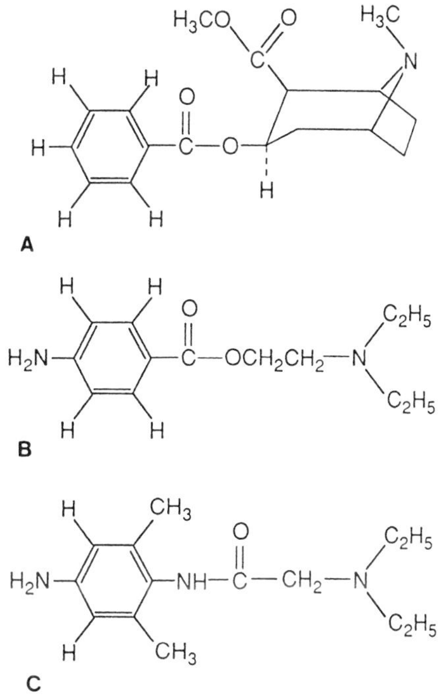

Figure 5–1. Cocaine (A), Procaine (B), and Lidocaine (C).

are examples of reverse tolerance. Cocaine's acute rewarding effects and cardiovascular actions, by contrast, are more likely to demonstrate tolerance.[7]

Cocaine is highly reinforcing in every species tested, using conditioned place preference, self-stimulation, and self-administration designs.[2] As with amphetamine, animals self-inject cocaine even when they receive electric shocks, and in preference to food and water until they die.[2,8,9] In one experiment, rats self-administering heroin established a stable pattern of use with gradually increasing intake and preserved grooming, body weight, and general health; by contrast, rats self-administering cocaine did so erratically and excessively and tended to cease grooming, to lose weight, and to deteriorate in general health. After 30 days, mortality was 36% for the heroin animals and 90% for the cocaine animals.[10] Others have shown—with obvious relevance to human patterns of use—that when access in animals is limited to a few hours daily, stable regular patterns of self-injection ensue, but when access is unlimited, such stability disappears and the drug is taken erratically, excessively, and fatally.[11]

Self-administration studies of this type carry the confounding factor of direct cocaine effects, which produce increased responding independent of re-inforcement. The dose–response curve of cocaine self-administration, moreover, is often an inverted U: at high doses, direct cocaine effects *reduce* response rates.[2] The problem of separating cocaine's direct stimulant effects from reinforcement per se can be circumvented by measuring the break point in progressive ratio schedules rather than the rate of responding.[12] In one such study, monkeys responded up to 12,800 times for each 0.48 mg/kg dose of cocaine.[13]

Effects on Neurotransmitter and Signal Transduction Systems

Dopamine and Cocaine

1. Cocaine's principal synaptic action is to block reuptake of dopamine, norepinephrine, and serotonin, acting through cocaine-binding sites on bioamine uptake transporters.[14,15] (Complementary DNAs for the cocaine-sensitive dopamine and norepinephrine transporters have been cloned and, interestingly, have homology to the γ-aminobutyric acid [GABA] transporter.[16–18]) In addition, cocaine—like methylphenidate but unlike amphetamine—releases dopamine from granular storage vesicles.[19] Cocaine affects three major dopaminergic systems: the mesolimbic pathway (ventral tegmental area [VTA] to nucleus accumbens [NA] and other limbic areas), the mesocortical pathway (VTA to medial prefrontal cortex [mPFC] and orbitofrontal cortex), and the nigrostriatal pathway. Studies in animals and humans implicate the mesolimbic pathway in drug reward (euphoria in humans, increased locomotor activity in animals), drug-related memories, and conditioned responses. The mesocortical pathway is implicated in compulsive drug taking and loss of inhibitory control. The nigrostriatal pathway is implicated in habit formation and stereotypy.[20–24]

2. In discriminative stimulus (DS) studies, animals that have learned to discriminate cocaine from saline to obtain a reward generalize to other stimulants that share its dopaminergic effects (amphetamine, methamphetamine, diethylpropion, phenmetrazine, phentermine, cathinone, and methylphenidate) but not to stimulants that do not (fenfluramine, strychnine).[25,26] Substitution occurs with selective agonists for dopamine D_1, D_2, and D_3 receptors, and these effects are blocked by selective D_1, D_2, and D_3 antagonists.[20] Alpha-adrenergic and beta-adrenergic receptor blockers and acetylcholine and serotonin receptor blockers do not affect cocaine DS.[26] Consistent with cocaine's greater pharmacological resemblance to methylphenidate than to amphetamine (see Chapter 4), reserpine, which depletes dopamine from granular storage vesicles, blocks cocaine DS but not amphetamine DS,[2] and conversely alpha-methyltyrosine (AMT), which depletes newly formed dopamine, blocks amphetamine DS but not cocaine DS.[23] Some DS studies suggest that dopamine alone cannot account for all of cocaine's effects. In one study, procaine but not lidocaine partially substituted for cocaine,[27] whereas in another study, lidocaine partially substituted.[28]

3. Rats self-inject the dopamine D_2 receptor agonists apomorphine and piribedil,[29] and monkeys self-administer these agents but not the noradrenergic uptake blocker nisoxetine.[30,31] The potencies of cocaine and related drugs in

self-administration studies correlate with their potencies in inhibiting the binding of [^{3}H]mazindol to dopamine transport sites in rat striatum[32] and with extracellular release of dopamine in the NA.[33] Dopamine receptor blockers (chlorpromazine, perphenazine, sulpiride, alphaflupenthixol) alter cocaine self-administration by animals;[2] alpha-adrenergic and beta-adrenergic blockers do not.[31] In rhesus monkeys antagonists for either dopamine D_1 or dopamine D_2 receptors reduce the reinforcing efficacy of smoked cocaine base.[34] In squirrel monkeys abstinent after a period of chronic intravenous cocaine self-administration, relapse following a priming dose of cocaine was facilitated by a dopamine D_2 agonist and inhibited by a D_2 antagonist.[35] (Interestingly, by contrast, a D_1 agonist and a D_1 antagonist each inhibited relapse.)

4. Dopamine D_3 receptors co-localize with D_1 receptors in the NA, and in mice a selective D_3 partial agonist reduced cocaine-associated cue-conditioned behavior without altering the unconditioned effects of cocaine itself and without producing any primary rewarding effect of its own.[36] As a partial agonist the drug has high affinity for the receptor but low intrinsic activity, and in the presence of cocaine it acts as a receptor antagonist.[37]

5. Studies involving intracranial self-administration demonstrate maximal cocaine effects after injection into the mPFC. Local injection of the dopamine antagonist sulpiride blocks such effects; blockers of alpha-noradrenergic and beta-noradrenergic and cholinergic receptors do not.[38,39] Although earlier studies reported negative results, cocaine is also self-administered into the NA.[40] It has been suggested that the prefrontal cortex initiates cocaine effects, whereas the NA maintains them.[2] Systemic administration causes increased levels of extracellular dopamine in the NA but decreased levels in the mPFC.[41] Dopamine in the mPFC has an inhibitory effect on NA dopamine levels and on locomotor activity.[42]

6. In rats, 6-hydroxydopamine lesions in the NA (which selectively destroy dopaminergic nerve terminals) decrease self-administration of cocaine but not of food or water and do not affect the descending limb of the dose–response curve (which reflects direct rate-decreasing effects of

cocaine).[43] Lesions in the ventral pallidum (to which the NA projects) and the VTA also disrupt cocaine self-administration.[44,45] In rats 6-hydroxydopamine lesions of the mPFC *enhanced* cocaine-induced locomotor activity. A possible explanation is that dopamine in the mPFC normally inhibits glutamatergic excitatory output to the NA; loss of this inhibition would increase dopaminergic neurotransmission in the NA.[46] Such a mechanism would not explain why cocaine is self-administered into the mPFC.

7. Cocaine's rewarding properties involve both D_1 and D_2 dopamine receptors, but the relative importance of each is uncertain (see Chapter 2). Although D_1 and D_2 receptor agonists are each self-administered by animals and reliably substitute for cocaine on DS tests, they have opposite effects on cocaine "priming," the relapse into cocaine-seeking behavior triggered by environmental stimuli associated with the drug or by low doses of the drug itself. In rodents, dopamine D_2 agonists induced their own priming and enhanced priming induced by cocaine; D_1 agonists did not induce priming, and they prevented cocaine-seeking behavior induced by cocaine.[47] In rats self-administering cocaine intravenously, D_2-receptor agonists, when substituted for cocaine, maintained responding, but D_1-receptor agonists did not.[48] In both mice and monkeys D_1 receptor agonists and antagonists produced unexpectedly different results in different experimental settings; D_1 dopaminergic actions were evident in the effects of cocaine on locomotor activity, less evident in discriminative stimulus effects, and least evident in effects on operant responses.[49] On the other hand, cocaine sensitization develops in animals after several days of abstinence but not at shorter intervals, and sensitization in this model correlates temporally with persistent increases in D_1 but not D_2 receptors in the NA.[50]

8. During cocaine administration neuroadaptations are evident within dopamine-receptive neurons in the NA and the striatum, and during withdrawal from cocaine neuroadaptations are found in dopaminergic neurons of the VTA. The striatum is organized into two compartments. The striosomal compartment receives input from limbic cortex and projects to the substantia

nigra; the matrix compartment receives input from sensory, motor, and association cortex and projects to the pallidum.[51] When cocaine is administered in a schedule that results in expression of Fos-related antigens (FRAs) in striatal neurons receiving dopaminergic input, sensitization (as evidenced by increased locomotor activity) is accompanied by a shift of FRAs from a largely matrix pattern to a largely striosomal pattern.[52] In rats during continuous systemic administration of cocaine (which causes tolerance to cocaine-induced hyperactivity) there is dopamine autoreceptor supersensitivity on dopaminergic neurons of the VTA and consequent inhibition of neuronal firing.[53] During withdrawal from cocaine there is a transient increase followed by a long-lasting decrease in dopamine transporters and dopamine efflux in the shell of the NA (but not in nigrostriatal dopaminergic nerve terminals).[52,54,55] In humans adaptations in dopaminergic neurons are reflected in imaging studies that show decreased cocaine uptake and decreased dopaminergic responsiveness in the brains of detoxified cocaine users.[56,57]

9. Like methylphenidate (but unlike amphetamine), cocaine does not cause morphological damage to dopamine nerve terminals.[19] However, cocaine does deplete dopamine in rat frontal cortex and hypothalamus and reduces tyrosine hydroxylase in rat striatum.[58,59] Some investigators attribute these reductions to supersensitivity of dopamine D_2 inhibitory autoreceptors.[60] Dopamine receptors are supersensitive in animals chronically receiving cocaine, and if inhibitory dopamine autoreceptors are more supersensitive than postsynaptic dopamine receptors, the net effect would be decreased dopaminergic neurotransmission at the mPFC and the NA.

Glutamate and Cocaine

1. Glutamate receptor stimulation increases the firing rate of dopaminergic neurons in the VTA. In mice cocaine-induced locomotor activity was blocked by the *N*-methyl-D-aspartate (NMDA) glutamate receptor antagonist dizocilpine.[61] In another study a glutamate receptor antagonist blocked the initiation but not the expression of sensitization to cocaine.[62] In other studies glutamate receptor antagonists prevented both the initiation and the expression of sensitization to cocaine.[63,64] In mice both cocaine and stress sensitized the response of VTA dopaminergic neurons to glutamate for up to a week.[65] Consistent with such observations, the enhancement of cocaine-induced locomotor response in animals with selective dopaminergic lesions in the mPFC is attributed to disinhibition of glutamatergic neurons in the mPFC, which receive direct inhibitory dopaminergic projections from the VTA. These glutamatergic neurons project to numerous structures, including the NA, where they facilitate dopaminergic neurotransmission from neurons in the VTA.[46]

2. A single dose of cocaine enhances glutamatergic transmission in the VTA for several days. The mechanism is not simply increased glutamate release into synapses; postsynaptic effects are similar to those associated with long-term potentiation (LTP) in the hippocampus (see Chapter 2). That is to say, cocaine, by uncertain mechanisms, indirectly activates glutamate AMPA receptors on dopaminergic neurons in the VTA, setting in motion a train of events that ultimately produces LTP-like increased synaptic efficacy.[66,67]

3. As with other reinforcing drugs, chronic exposure to cocaine induces the persistent expression of the transcription factor ΔfosB in the NA, and this expression correlates with a markedly increased locomotor response when animals receive cocaine.[68] Among its actions, ΔfosB genetically alters the makeup of glutamate AMPA receptors, thereby reducing the sensitivity of projecting GABAergic spiny neurons in the NA to glutamate. Inhibition of these NA GABAergic neurons is considered a key step in drug reward, and so ΔfosB expression, by influencing glutamate neurotransmission in this manner, increases an animal's responsiveness to reward and locomotor-activating effects of cocaine.[68–70]

4. In rats, extinction training (a form of inhibitory learning that progressively reduces cocaine-seeking behavior in the absence of cocaine reward) induces increases in the GluR1 and GluR2/3 subunits of AMPA receptors in the NA. Viral-mediated overexpression of GluR1 and GluR2 in NA neurons facilitates extinction of cocaine-seeking responses.[71]

5. Acute and chronic cocaine administration produces alterations in subtype composition of AMPA, NMDA, and metabotropic glutamate receptors in other areas as well, including the VTA and the mPFC.[72,73]

6. Relapse into cocaine self-administration in animals and cocaine craving in humans can be triggered by emotional stress, social setting, visual cues, or a small amount of the drug itself. Although electrical stimulation of reward circuits in the median forebrain bundle (MFB) is rewarding, it does not trigger relapse in animals previously exposed to cocaine. By contrast, electrical stimulation of the hippocampus elicited cocaine-seeking behavior in such animals, a response dependent on glutamatergic projections from the hippocampus to the VTA. Stimulation of either area leads to increased firing of dopaminergic cells in the VTA and increased release of dopamine in the NA, but the dopamine release after hippocampal stimulation is considerably more sustained (30 minutes) than after MFB stimulation (less than 5 seconds). Although hippocampal electrical self-stimulation is much less reinforcing than MFB self-stimulation, hippocampal stimulation seems to trigger memories integral to craving, conveying the information via its glutamatergic output to the VTA.[74,75]

7. In animals the glutamate NMDA receptor antagonists dizocilpine and phencyclidine prevent the development of both cocaine-induced seizures and cocaine-induced stereotypy.[76]

Opioids and Cocaine

1. In animals naloxone, which blocks μ- and δ-opioid receptors, reduces the rewarding effects of cocaine on electrical self-stimulation as well as the rewarding effects of cocaine self-administration.[77]

2. In mice cocaine greatly enhances morphine analgesia,[78] and in rats cocaine blocks the development of tolerance to morphine analgesia.[79]

3. Unlike μ- and δ-opioid receptor agonists, κ-receptor agonists—including the endogenous opioid peptide dynorphin—are not reinforcing. In fact, κ-receptor agonism appears to counter cocaine sensitization.[80] During chronic cocaine administration κ-receptors within the NA are increased, and prodynorphin gene expression and dynorphin immunoreactivity are elevated. Intravenously administered κ-receptor agonists inhibit glutamate neurotransmission in the VTA, thereby reducing firing of dopaminergic cells in the VTA and dopamine release in the NA. The result is blockade of behavioral sensitization. Kappa-receptor agonists do not block the locomotor activating effects of an acute cocaine challenge. Kappa-receptor agonists delivered directly into the NA similarly block sensitization, but when delivered into the mPFC they exacerbate sensitization and increase NA dopamine levels. A proposed explanation is that, as with 6-hydroxydopamine lesions of the mPFC, κ-receptor agonists reduce dopaminergic firing in the mPFC, with disinhibition of mPFC glutamatergic output to the NA.[81]

4. In rats withdrawal from chronically administered cocaine produced a biphasic pattern of μ-opioid expression, with up-regulation followed by down-regulation.[82]

Serotonin and Cocaine

1. Cocaine has a higher affinity for the serotonin transporter than for the dopamine transporter, but purely serotonergic agonists are not self-administered by animals or abused by humans. The role of serotonin in cocaine reward is uncertain. Part of the problem is the diversity of serotonin receptors (at least 14).[83] In animals with dihydroxytryptamine lesions of the serotonin system, cocaine reinforcement is increased (as evidenced by an increased break point for cocaine self-administration).[84] Moreover, knockout mice lacking the $5HT_{1B}$ receptor respond to cocaine in a manner resembling wild-type mice already sensitized to the drug, and they have increased levels of ΔfosB transcription factors in the NA.[85,86] On the other hand, a $5HT_{1B}$ agonist partially substituted for cocaine in drug discrimination studies and potentiated the rewarding effects of cocaine administered intravenously.[85,87] A proposed mechanism for this effect is that $5HT_{1B}$ receptors inhibit GABAergic terminals on dopaminergic neurons of the VTA; $5HT_{1B}$ agonists would therefore indirectly increase firing of these VTA dopaminergic neurons.[88]

A proposed mechanism for the paradoxical findings in $5HT_{1B}$ receptor knockout mice—enhanced cocaine reinforcement—is that effects of the knockout lead to compensatory mechanisms during development.[85] Unexpectedly, although $5HT_{1B}$ knockout mice self-administer cocaine, they fail to display conditioned place preference for stimuli associated with cocaine.[89]

2. In rats, a selective $5HT_{1A}$ receptor agonist enhanced the development of sensitization to cocaine. A proposed mechanism is that stimulation of $5HT_{1A}$ autoreceptors on brainstem dorsal raphe serotonergic neurons inhibited them; these neurons are believed to send inhibitory projections to the VTA, and so their inhibition would result in disinhibition of VTA dopaminergic neurons.[90]

3. In animals cocaine reinforcement is enhanced by a $5HT_2$ receptor agonist and reduced by a $5HT_2$ receptor antagonist.[91] A $5HT_{2A}$ receptor agonist enhanced NA dopamine release in rats receiving cocaine.[92]

4. In rats cocaine sensitization is blocked by ondansetron, a $5HT_3$ receptor antagonist.[93]

5. In rats injection of a $5HT_4$ antagonist into the NA shell attenuated cocaine-induced locomotor activity.[94]

GABA and Cocaine

1. Cocaine sensitization is associated with decreased number and function of $GABA_A$ receptors in the striatum,[95] yet in other studies, unexpectedly, there was decreased GABA release in the striatum.[96] (Decreased neurotransmitter release should cause up-regulation, not down-regulation, of receptors.) In the septal nucleus chronic cocaine administration caused reduced $GABA_B$ receptor function and increased GABA release.[97] These somewhat paradoxical findings might be related to different intraterminal neurotransmitter pools in GABAergic neurons or to GABA autoreceptors.[96]

2. In knockout mice lacking the $GABA_A$ receptor beta 3 subunit, locomotor stimulation following acute cocaine was greater in –/– mice than +/+ mice, whereas behavioral responses to chronically administered cocaine were greater in +/+ than –/– mice.[98]

3. In rats the $GABA_B$ receptor agonist baclofen reduced cocaine self-administration.[99,100]

Cocaine and Acetylcholine (ACh)

1. The NA contains cholinergic interneurons, and cocaine self-administration increased acetylcholine (ACh) levels in the NA.[101]

2. In rats, injections of scopolamine into the mPFC produced increased locomotor activity; when the animals received systemic cocaine, however, intra-mPFC scopolamine reduced locomotor activity. The manner in which muscarinic cholinergic neurotransmission regulates cocaine responses is uncertain.[102]

3. Knockout mice lacking the M_5 muscarinic cholinergic receptor lose conditioned place preference for cocaine and are disinclined to self-administer it.[103,103a]

Cocaine and Norepinephrine

Cocaine blocks norepinephrine uptake, accounting for much of its effects on peripheral and cerebral circulation, but as with serotonin agonists, purely adrenergic agonists are not self-administered by animals or abused by humans. Knockout mice lacking norepinephrine transporters, however, display enhanced locomotion to cocaine administration, accompanied by dopamine D_2/D_3 supersensitivity.[104]

Cocaine and Cannabinoids

In rats a CB_1 receptor agonist provoked relapse to cocaine-seeking after prolonged withdrawal periods, and a CB_1 receptor antagonist prevented relapse triggered by re-exposure to cocaine-associated cues or to cocaine itself (but not relapse triggered by stress).[105]

Cocaine and DARPP-32

1. When phosphorylated at threonine-34 by protein kinase A (PKA), dopamine- and cyclic AMP-regulated phosphoprotein-32 (DARPP-32) inhibits protein phosphatase-1 (PP-1), causing numerous target proteins of PP-1 (including ion channels and transcription factors) to remain phosphorylated. Stimulation of dopamine D_1 receptors activates PKA, leading to phosphorylation and activation of DARPP-32. Removal of DARPP-32's phosphate groups at threonine-34 by other phosphatases blocks DARPP-32

inhibition of PP-1 and counteracts the effects of PKA. Mice lacking the DARPP-32 gene exhibit enhanced behavioral responses to chronic cocaine administration, suggesting that the dopamine D_1–PKA–DARPP-32 pathway serves as a negative homeostatic feedback to cocaine's behavioral effects.[106,107]

2. Cyclin-dependent kinase 5 (Cdk5), restricted to brain, is involved in neurodevelopment. A target of the transcription factor ΔfosB, Cdk5 as a consequence is elevated in the striatum of rats receiving chronic cocaine. Cdk5 phosphorylates DARPP-32 at threonine-75, preventing its phosphorylation at threonine-34 and blocking the action of PKA. The result is similar to DARPP-32 knockout, i.e., potentiation of chronic cocaine behavioral effects. Such observations provide further evidence that PKA–DARPP-32 is a negative feedback to chronic cocaine effects and suggest that ΔfosB stimulation of Cdk5 production might play a role in cocaine sensitization.[108]

Cocaine and CART

A peptide called cocaine- and amphetamine-regulated transcript (CART) is increased in the striatum, the amygdala, the NA, and other brain areas following cocaine administration. The role of CART peptide in psychostimulant drug action is uncertain, but it appears to be a neuromodulator co-localized with GABA in axon terminals.[109,110]

Cocaine and Glia-derived Neurotrophic Factor

Infusion of glia-derived neurotrophic factor (GDNF) into the VTA in mice blocks the rewarding effects of cocaine, and intra-VTA infusion of an anti-GDNF antibody enhances cocaine responses. Chronic cocaine administration decreases levels of a protein kinase that mediates GDNF signaling, suggesting that cocaine-induced reduction of GDNF signaling in the VTA contributes to sensitization.[111]

Cocaine and Glucocorticoids

In rhesus monkeys self-administration of cocaine produces dose-dependent increases in cortisol and ACTH.[112] In rats, cocaine withdrawal produces increased release of corticotropin releasing factor (CRF).[113] In rats, stress (intermittent footshock) reinstates cocaine-seeking behavior after prolonged drug-free periods.[114] Intracerebroventricular administration of a CRF receptor antagonist blocks this reinstatement.[115] In yoked rats—such that one rat actively self-administered cocaine (contingent administration) while the other received it passively (non-contingent administration)—plasma corticosterone levels were higher in the rat receiving contingent cocaine.[116]

Cocaine and Structural Proteins

Like other drugs, cocaine induces the expression of immediate early genes (IEGs) such as c-*fos* and *junB*, which code for transcription factors. One IEG induced by cocaine codes for Arc, a cytoskeletal protein present in the nucleus and dendrites of striatal neurons. Interestingly, cocaine and amphetamine produce different striosome/matrix patterns of Arc expression, perhaps reflecting differences in their behavioral effects.[117]

Cocaine and Nitric Oxide

Infusion of a nitric oxide synthase inhibitor into the VTA blocks the development of behavioral sensitization to cocaine.[118]

Pharmacokinetics

Following any route of administration, the plasma half-life of cocaine is about 40 to 60 minutes; it is detectable in urine for up to 36 hours.[119] Cocaine is metabolized by liver and plasma cholinesterases mainly to benzoylecgonine and ecgonine methyl ester, with smaller amounts of ecgonine, norcocaine, and other hydroxylated products.[120] Benzoylecgonine is itself a potent CNS stimulant and persists in the brain long after cocaine has disappeared. It is usually detectable in plasma for 2 to 3 days but in heavy users has been identified after 3 weeks.[121] Fetuses, infants, elderly men, pregnant women, and patients with liver disease have low plasma cholinesterase levels and are sensitive to low doses of cocaine, as are those with congenital cholinesterase deficiency.[122]

Benzoylecgonine and other metabolites can be detected in hair and fingernails after blood and urine tests have become negative.[123-125] Use of this technique confirms that self-reporting greatly underestimates cocaine use.[126]

Historical Background and Epidemiology

Cocaine is obtained from the South American shrub, *Erythroxylon coca*, leaves of which have been chewed by South American Indians for many centuries.[2] (In an imaginative study, hair was analyzed from eight Chilean mummies dating between 2000 and 1500 BC; all were positive for benzoylecgonine.[127]) The Incas considered the coca plant a gift of the Sun God, and its use was restricted to priests and the ruling class. Following the conquest of the Incas by the Spanish in the 16th century, coca use was at first banned as idolatrous but later encouraged when it was recognized that Inca slaves worked harder when it was available. Then, as today, the leaves were chewed with lime or ash to increase the release of cocaine.

Perhaps because the plant decayed on passage from South America and was difficult to grow in the European climate, coca did not become popular in Europe until after the isolation of cocaine by Niemann in 1855. Vin Mariani, a coca wine developed by Angelo Mariani, became enormously popular in Europe and the United States; enthusiasts included President William McKinley, Thomas Edison, and the Czar of Russia, and Mariani received a medal of appreciation from the Pope. In 1886, John Pemberton of Georgia introduced Coca Cola, originally an elixir containing both cocaine and caffeine and promoted as a headache remedy and stimulant.[128] Alcohol was removed in 1888 and cocaine in 1906 (the year the Pure Food and Drug Act was passed).

In 1884, Sigmund Freud published "Ueber Coca," in which he referred to cocaine as "a far more potent and far less harmful stimulant than alcohol."[129] In this and later papers, Freud recommended cocaine as a stimulant and aphrodisiac and for treatment of digestive disorders, cachexia, asthma, and addiction to ethanol and morphine. It was Freud's colleague Karl Koller, however, who successfully developed cocaine as a local anesthetic, which quickly became recognized as its only legitimate medical use.[130] (It was as an anesthetic that cocaine came to the attention of the ophthalmologist A. Conan Doyle; Sherlock Holmes was a celebrated recreational user.) In the meantime, Freud had treated his friend Ernst Fleishl's morphine addiction with cocaine, only to convert Fleishl into a cocaine addict.[131] (In a reversed approach, the surgeon William Halsted treated his own cocaine addiction with morphine and became a morphine addict.[132]) As early as 1886, the Viennese chemist Erlenmeyer had labeled cocaine "the third scourge of humanity," along with ethanol and morphine.[130]

An international coca market flourished during the first three decades of the 20th century; the major exporters were Peru, Bolivia, Java, and Formosa, and the major consumers North America and Europe. In 1911–12 the Hague Opium Convention initiated international regulation of the production and distribution of opium, morphine, heroin, and cocaine. In 1914 the United States fulfilled its obligation by passing the Harrison Narcotic Act, which banned the use of cocaine in proprietary medicines and strictly regulated its importation, manufacture, and medical use.[133]

From the 1920s to the 1960s, recreational use of cocaine in the United States was largely restricted to jazz musicians, actors, and the "cultural avant garde." Its cost limited spread and made it a status drug for the affluent. In the early 1970s, there began a steady rise in the prevalence of cocaine use that continued over the next two decades. The number of Americans who had tried cocaine at least once rose from 5.4 million in 1974 to 21.6 million in 1982, including up to 20% of high school seniors and 28% of those aged 18 to 25 years.[134] It was estimated that if the cocaine industry were included in American corporate listings, it would, with at least US$27 billion annual gross income, rank seventh, between Gulf Oil and the Ford Motor Company.[135]

The appearance in 1985 of commercially manufactured alkaloidal cocaine ("crack") led to acceleration of the epidemic and with it lawlessness and violence in American cities reminiscent of Prohibition in the 1920s. By 1988, in the United States there were 5000 new cocaine users daily, 6 million people were regular users, and nearly 1 million were "compulsive users."[136]

Estimates of cocaine-related fatality have been based on figures from the Center for Disease Control's National Center for Health Statistics (NCHS), which monitors death certificates, and the Drug Abuse Warning Network (DAWN), which surveys hospital emergency rooms and medical examiners' and coroners' offices. During the 6-year period 1983 to 1988, NCHS reported that cocaine-related deaths increased fivefold, from 218 to 1179, and DAWN reported a sixfold increase from 314 to 1952. Seventy-nine percent of NCHS deaths and 69% of DAWN deaths were attributed to poisoning; the rest were ascribed to injury or disease.[137] A review of forensic cases from Arizona, Utah, Virginia, New York City, Michigan, and San Diego implied even higher mortality rates than these federal estimates would indicate;[138-144] for example, of 151 cocaine intoxication deaths reported by the New York City Medical Examiner during 1986, only seven were identified by NCHS.[141]

As with other drugs (including ethanol and tobacco), cost and availability determine prevalence of use. A study of veterans with schizophrenia found that cocaine use (and psychiatric symptoms) increased at the start of each month.[145] A subsequent study observed that the number of deaths in the United States increased in the first week of each month and that deaths related to substance abuse in general contributed to the increase.[146] The authors of these reports speculated that diversion of disability and other support payments into drug procurement accounted for the pattern.

In 1986, one-third of male homicides in Manhattan were drug related.[147] In New York City in 1987, more than 40% of all felony indictments were for drug law violations, and a 1988 study by the National Institute of Justice in 10 large American cities revealed that one-half to three-quarters of all arrestees were taking illicit drugs (excluding marijuana).[148,149] During 1989 in Atlanta, Georgia, 40% of 224 homicide victims tested had cocaine metabolites in their blood.[150] In Memphis, 46 of 84 cocaine-related deaths were homicides, and cocaine metabolites were present in 17% of all homicide victims.[151]

Violence is related to drug abuse in three different ways.[152] *Pharmacological violence* refers to violent behavior induced by the drugs themselves. *Economic compulsive violence* refers to violent crime committed to obtain drugs. *Systemic violence* refers to violence intrinsic to the lifestyles and business methods of drug traffickers. Although most ethanol-related violence is pharmacological in origin, cocaine-related violence is overwhelmingly of the systemic type.[153] An example, familiar to municipal hospitals, is adolescent cocaine runners

with leg or spinal gunshot wounds incurred during territorial wars. Sometimes the spinal cord is deliberately cut ("pithing").

From 1984 to 1987, a quarter of New York City drivers aged 16 to 45 years who died in automobile accidents had cocaine or a metabolite in blood or urine.[154]

Increased cocaine consumption in the United States occurred despite enormous expenditures that were mainly targeted at crop eradication in South America, interdiction at United States borders, and local law enforcement. During 1990, federal expenditures for the "War on Drugs" amounted to nearly US$10 billion, of which nearly US$4 billion were for criminal justice activities and more than US$2 billion were for drug interdiction programs.[155] (A high point of the latter effort was the military kidnapping and extradition on drug trafficking charges of the Chief of State of Panama—an event apparently without historical precedent.)

Approximately 2.5 million square miles of South American land are potentially cultivatable for coca. During the peak of the crack epidemic, however, less than 800 square miles were being used for that purpose.[149] By the 1990s, as military pressure was increasing against distribution centers in Medellin, Colombia, and cultivation areas in Peru and Bolivia, distribution shifted to the Colombian city of Cali, and both cultivation and distribution spread to other South American countries, including Venezuela, Brazil, Ecuador, Uruguay, and Suriname.[156] *Erythroxylon coca* also grows abundantly in Mexico, the West Indies, and Indonesia.[157] As for interdiction, cocaine is easy to smuggle (in contrast to bulky marijuana), and huge profits provide big incentives. In 1991, 1 kg of cocaine purchased for US$1200 in Colombia sold wholesale in the United States for approximately US$20,000; after conversion to "crack," its retail value (at about US$5.00 per vial) was roughly three times that amount.[158]

In the United States casual use of cocaine, estimated by the National Household Survey, and high school use, estimated by the High School Senior Survey, peaked during the mid-1980s[159,160] The major factor for the subsequent decline appeared to be reduced demand—the result of education and changing attitudes, including the predictable decline of a fad—rather than reduced supply.[161] Indeed, although federal appropriations for drug control were targeted at interdiction, cocaine continued to be plentiful and cheap throughout the "War on Drugs," and compulsive use, especially within inner cities—the poor, the homeless, high school dropouts, and arrestees—declined far less.[160,162,163] During 1998 nearly 2 million Americans were regular cocaine users, roughly the same as in 1991.[159,160,164] In fact, between 1994 and 1998 the number of new cocaine users per year increased from 514,000 to 934,000 (82%).[165]

The degree to which the "War on Drugs" contributed to the reduction of violent crime in the United States is therefore controversial. Increases in homicide did occur in city after city as crack made its appearance in the 1980s, leading to draconian laws (e.g., mandatory life imprisonment for repeated possession of crack—but not for possession of cocaine hydrochloride) and an expansion of the prison population from less than 400,000 in 1970 to 2.1 million in 2000.[166] During the 1990s the United States built more prisons than schools, and the United States currently has the second highest incarceration rate in the world. By 2002 it was estimated that 28% of black and 16% of Hispanic men will enter a state or federal prison during their lifetime. For whites the figure is 4%.[166] Other factors undoubtedly contributed to the decline in violent crime, however, including a healthy economy and a drop in unemployment rates, stricter gun laws, and the more delayed effect of legalized abortion. In fact, it has been suggested that police action against crack markets actually increased homicide rates by replacing older, established dealers with inner city, violence-prone teenagers.[167]

During the early 1990s 80% of cocaine smuggled into the United States was controlled by the Cali drug cartel, which, because of stepped-up interdiction efforts in Florida, passed most of it through Mexico. By 1995, Mexican entrepreneurs had taken control of a significant portion of this trafficking. With annual profits of US$30 billion, Mexican traffickers, engaging in bribery and assassination, quickly achieved considerable influence in both the private business sector and the federal government of Mexico.[168,169] At the same time, Dominican drug gangs became increasingly visible. During 1998 Dominican drug traffickers transported nearly one-third of the approximately 300 metric tons of cocaine that entered the United States.[170] In Europe, the collapse of the Soviet Union and its empire was followed by an increased flow of South American cocaine through Russia, Poland, Hungary, Romania, and Bulgaria.[171]

Meanwhile, with the breakup of the Medellin and Cali cartels in the mid-1990s, the cocaine industry in Colombia entered a new phase. The dozens of smaller trafficking groups that sprang up became controlled by a left-wing insurgency organization, the Revolutionary Armed Forces of Colombia (FARC) and paid taxes on drug income to the guerrillas in return for protection. Operating freely in nearly 40% of Colombian territory, the rebels thus took control of production and distribution of 500 tons of cocaine yearly—90% of the world's supply.[172] (Right-wing paramilitary death squads opposing the FARC are also heavily financed by cocaine.) The response of the United States government was US$1.3 billion in military aid to bolster the Colombian army and to defoliate the cocaine fields ("Plan Colombia"). The most tangible effect of this policy was to drive up the price of coca, with increased production in Peru, Bolivia, and Ecuador and little change in production within Colombia itself.[173] In Bolivia, for example, although U.S.-led coca eradication and crop substitution programs had been accompanied by substantial reductions in coca cultivation, by 2003 crop substitution was clearly an economic failure, coca production was sharply rising, and grass-roots opposition to U.S. political influence was becoming galvanized.[174,174a]

Preparation and Methods of Use

Cocaine is effective orally, and its absorption by South American natives who chew coca leaves is probably from swallowed saliva as well as across oral mucous membranes. Harvested leaves are soaked in alkali; kerosene and sulfuric acid (and sometimes potassium permanganate) are then added, producing semisolid "coca-paste," which contains alkaloidal ("free-base") cocaine, plus impurities. Coca-paste ("bazooka") is widely smoked in South America, and, less commonly, in Panama, the Caribbean, the Netherlands, and the United States.[175] Further refining produces cocaine hydrochloride, which is then adulterated with inactive substances such as mannitol, boric acid, lactose, dextrose, sucrose, inositol, talc, flour, or corn starch, and active substances such as procaine, lidocaine, benzocaine, ephedrine, amphetamine, phenylpropanolamine, caffeine, or strychnine.[176] Street preparations ("snow," "flake," "coke," "girl," "lady," "dama blanca," "blow," "jam," "happy trails," "rock," "nose candy," "leaf," "gold," "dust") sell by the gram, with purity ranging from 7% to 100%.[177]

When cocaine is inhaled nasally (snorting), users usually lay out a "line" of powder (20–50 mg) and sniff it through a straw. It can also be taken parenterally, usually intravenously; more than 80% of New York City heroin users concomitantly inject cocaine ("speedball").[177] Because cocaine hydrochloride is destroyed at very high temperatures, smoking requires conversion back to "free-base," which before the emergence of "crack" was made from cocaine hydrochloride using commercially available extraction kits. To make "free-base," cocaine hydrochloride is dissolved in water and converted to the alkaloidal form by adding a strong base such as ammonium hydroxide. The alkaloid is extracted with an organic solvent such as petroleum ether, and the free-base is then crystallized. In the process, most adulterants are left behind.[178] The preparation of crack is even simpler: Adding baking soda or sodium bicarbonate to cocaine hydrochloride in heated water precipitates alkaloidal cocaine, which is then dried by evaporation into a cake-like solid. In this process, adulterants are more likely to be co-precipitated. (The basis of the term *crack* is disputed. One version is that the small "rocks" sold are "cracked" off larger pieces. Another is that when smoked in a pipe, it makes a crackling sound.) Usually 50–120 mg of free-base or "crack" is inhaled per "hit," sometimes repeated every few minutes in binges (resembling amphetamine "runs") lasting 30 minutes to 96 hours. Sometimes single binges last days, separated by a few days of abstinence. During binges, all thoughts are focused on the drug; food, sleep, family, and even survival become secondary.[179] Tolerance leads to higher doses, and 3000 mg have been taken in a single "hit."

Intranasal snorting of 96 mg cocaine hydrochloride produced peak plasma levels of 150–200 ng/mL. Intravenous injection of 32 mg cocaine produced peak levels of 300 ng/mL. Chronic smoking of alkaloidal cocaine produced plasma levels of 800–900 ng/mL 3 hours after smoking.[180]

"Doing a shotgun" refers to the practice of exhaling smoked drug into the mouth of another user.[181]

Cocaine has also been taken rectally, sublingually, vaginally, and intraurethrally, and sudden death has followed such routes of administration.[182–184]

Psychosis, seizures and death have even followed topical application of TAC (tetracaine, adrenaline, cocaine) or AC (adrenaline, cocaine) solution to wounds or mucous membranes.[185,186] The slow rise in tissue levels achieved by oral cocaine probably explains its unpopularity, even though levels are eventually as high as by other routes.[187]

A special form of administration is "body packing," in which smuggled cocaine is swallowed or inserted rectally in packets wrapped with latex, and "body stuffing," in which packaged cocaine is more hurriedly swallowed to avoid detection. Rupture of packets in the gastrointestinal tract of smugglers ("mules") causes severe toxicity, sometimes fatal, and bowel obstruction can require surgery.[188]

Acute Effects

Intended Intoxication

Injected or smoked cocaine produces, similar to amphetamine, a brief "rush," peaking at one-half to 2 minutes and followed by euphoria, excitement, garrulousness, and a sense of increased mental and physical powers.[178,189] Experienced users are often unable to tell the drugs apart except that cocaine's effects are shorter lived, lasting usually 20 to 40 minutes.[190] (The rapid transit time from lung to brain—5 to 10 seconds—means cocaine smoking can produce an even more intense "rush" than intravenous use.[191]) Snorted cocaine produces qualitatively similar stimulation for up to 90 minutes without the initial "rush," peaking at about 30 minutes and lasting about 1 hour.[189] (Snorted cocaine limits its own absorption by causing vasoconstriction of the nasal mucosa.) As with amphetamine, a cocaine user's sense of increased mental power is not borne out with objective testing.[190]

Low doses of cocaine slow the heart rate (because of vagal stimulation); higher doses cause symptoms and signs of sympathetic overactivity: tachycardia, tachypnea, and hypertension. (In dogs, the hypertensive response to cocaine is reduced by pretreatment with the ganglionic blocker hexamethonium, suggesting that cocaine increases sympathetic activity through CNS actions.[192]) In rats, cocaine's pressor effects depend on alpha$_1$-adrenergic vasoconstriction and are two-phased, with a centrally mediated initial peak response and a peripherally-mediated sustained but more modest response.[193,194] Skin pallor is secondary to vaso-constriction. Other symptoms of mild to moderate overdose are most often cardiopulmonary, psychiatric, or neurological and can occur alone or together (Table 5–1). Of 233 visits to Grady Memorial Hospital in Atlanta for "cocaine-related medical problems," the most common symptoms were chest pain (40%) (most often considered nonischemic), shortness of breath (22%), palpitations (21%), anxiety (22%), dizziness (13%), and headache (12%). Only 10% of patients required admission.[195] Cocaine-associated chest pain accompanied by "J-point/ST-segment elevation" most often signifies "benign early repolarization," a common finding in young people.[196]

"Punding" refers to stereotypic motor behavior characterized by repetitive examination and handling of external objects or parts of the body.[197] With chronic cocaine use symptoms can progress to multifocal tics, dystonia, chorea ("crack dancing"), and opsoclonus-myoclonus.[198-200] Obsessive-compulsive disorder can also develop.[201]

Acute Overdose

More severe symptoms can be life-threatening, and some, including psychiatric and neurological, show sensitization (reverse tolerance) with repeated cocaine use.[202-206] Patients may be agitated, combative, paranoid, depressed, lethargic, or comatose. There may be hyperreflexia, tremor, stereotypic movements, dystonia, chorea, myoclonus, or seizures. Metabolic acidosis can be marked, and cardiac arrhythmia or pulmonary edema can precede cardiac arrest. In the Atlanta series, the heart rate ranged from 34 to 168/minute, the systolic blood pressure from 70 to 240 mmHg, and the respiratory rate from 6 to 50/minute.[195] Fever can be high enough to suggest heat stroke, and rhabdomyolysis causes renal failure.[207-215b] Disseminated intravascular coagulation occurs.[216]

Headache

Migraine-like headaches, sometimes accompanied by hemiparesis or vertigo, are especially common during cocaine binges, whether snorting, smoking, or parenterally injecting.[217,218] They are often promptly relieved by additional cocaine, perhaps attributable to blockade of serotonin reuptake.[219] Dependency developed in a patient who began using cocaine as a treatment for migraine.[220]

Table 5–1. Acute Toxic Effects of Cocaine

Cardiopulmonary
Chest pain
Shortness of breath
Palpitations
Diaphoresis
Pulmonary edema
Cardiac arrhythmia
Myocardial infarction
Cardiac arrest

Psychiatric
Anxiety
Insomnia
Paranoia
Agitation, violence
Depression, suicide
Hallucinations
Psychosis

Neurological
Dizziness, syncope
Vertigo
Paresthesias
Headache
Tremor
Stereotypy
Bruxism
Chorea
Dystonia
Myoclonus
Seizures
Lethargy
Coma
Ischemic or hemorrhagic stroke

Other
Throat tightness
Blurred vision (mydriasis)
Nasal congestion
Nausea, vomiting
Abdominal pain
Weakness
Fever
Chills
Myalgia
Back pain
Rhabdomyolysis

Source: Modified from Brody SL, Slovis CM, Wrenn KD. Cocaine-related medical problems: consecutive series of 233 patients. Am J Med 1990; 88:325, with permission of the publisher.

Behavioral Change and Psychosis

In volunteers, 4-hour infusions of cocaine induced suspiciousness,[221] and chronic users are increasingly likely to develop pathological behavior.[222] At first there is irritability, hyperactivity, impaired interpersonal relations, and disturbed eating and sleeping. Symptoms then progress to anxiety, stereotypic compulsive behavior, confusion, paranoia, and frank psychosis. Hallucinations are visual ("snow lights"), auditory, gustatory, olfactory, or tactile ("cocaine bugs," the sensation of insects crawling beneath the skin).[1,2,60] Psychosis occurs regardless of predrug personality. (On the other hand, comorbid substance abuse is very common among schizophrenics, who, when cocaine-intoxicated, are especially likely to have hallucinations.[223]) During an epidemic of free-base use in the Bahamas, paranoia and bizarre violent behavior in some patients lasted several weeks.[224] Similar protracted psychopathology accompanied an epidemic of coca paste smoking in Peru.[225] A patient receiving repeated topical anesthesia containing 3 mL of 10% cocaine developed psychosis that lasted 60 hours.[226]

Seizures

Seizures occur immediately or within a few hours of cocaine administration with or without other signs of toxicity.[227-237] Single major motor seizures are most common, but focal seizures occur, and status epilepticus is sometimes refractory to anticonvulsant therapy. Among 32 cases of cocaine-related seizures seen at San Francisco General Hospital, routes of administration included intranasal, intravenous, smoking, and oral, and seizures occurred from 10 minutes to "under 24 hours" after use.[233] Nine patients used additional drugs, including marijuana, amphetamine, phencyclidine, methylphenidate, and LSD. Of 474 patients seen at Hennepin County Medical Center in Minneapolis for acute cocaine intoxication, 44(9.3%) had seizures within 90 minutes of cocaine use.[234] In 32, seizures were new onset, and of these the great majority were induced by either intravenous or "crack" cocaine. In 12, seizures occurred in patients who had previous seizures unrelated to cocaine, and among these patients intranasal use

was more common than intravenous or "crack" cocaine. In both groups, 40% of seizures followed first-time cocaine use.

In a subsequent report from Minneapolis, seizures occurred in 98 (10%) of 945 patients admitted for cocaine intoxication, with striking sex differences: 18.4% of women but only 6.2% of men had seizures. Patients with single generalized seizures (the most common type) all had normal cranial CT scans and electroencephalography. Patients with new-onset focal seizures had evidence of cerebral infarction or hemorrhage. Four patients with status epilepticus had ingested massive (2–8 g) doses of cocaine, were resistant to treatment, and had considerable morbidity and mortality.[238]

The prevalence of seizures among cocaine-intoxicated patients is higher in the Minneapolis series than in others. At Bronx Municipal Hospital in New York, only four of 283 (1.4%) hospitalized cocaine users had seizures,[230] and at San Francisco General Hospital, seizures occurred in 29 of 1275 (2.3%) cocaine users.[228] Telephone surveys of users detect much higher seizure prevalences.[239] A large survey of adolescent drug abusers in Virginia found that seizures occurred in none of the intranasal cocaine users, in 1% of "experimental" crack smokers, and in 9% of heavy crack smokers.[240] In a case–control series of new-onset seizures from Harlem Hospital Center, cocaine use was not identified as a risk factor; the reasons for this surprising finding are probably that only incident (new-onset) seizures were included and the study was conducted before the advent of "crack."[241] In fact, the Harlem Hospital study would have excluded most of the patients reported from Minneapolis.

A young woman who smoked "crack" over 3 days developed bizarre behavior that turned out to be complex partial status epilepticus, a diagnosis easy to overlook in patients with other reasons for behavioral abnormality.[242]

Relevant to the observation that seizures sometimes occur several hours or more after use of cocaine are studies in rats that demonstrate epileptogenicity of the cocaine metabolite benzoylecgonine. In contrast to cocaine-induced seizures, those associated with benzoylecgonine had longer latencies and less often resulted in death.[243]

In mice, diazepam and phenobarbital failed to protect against cocaine-induced seizures, whereas glutamate NMDA antagonists were highly protective.[244] Animal studies also support a role for serotonergic neurotransmission in cocaine-induced seizures, which in mice are aggravated by selective serotonin reuptake inhibitors (SSRIs).[245]

Consistent with animal studies that demonstrate a kindling pattern of cocaine-induced seizures,[245a] a young woman would experience grand mal seizures immediately after smoking "crack," but after 2 years she began having seizures no longer temporally associated with acute cocaine use, and her electroencephalogram demonstrated spikes. Phenytoin (which is largely ineffective in electrically kindled animals) did not control her seizures, whereas carbamazepine (which is much more effective in kindled animals) did.[246]

Abnormal Movements

Acute dystonia and chorea following cocaine use usually last minutes to a few days and in some instances have emerged during early abstinence.[247-252] During withdrawal from "crack" smoking a young woman experienced "serpentine" movements of her trunk which she controlled by increasing her use of cocaine; the movements persisted after 20 months of abstinence and were accompanied by "severe obsessional thoughts and compulsive behaviors."[253]

Cocaine reportedly exacerbated symptoms in a patient with idiopathic dystonia and in another with neuroleptic-induced tardive dystonia.[254] Haloperidol has precipitated acute dystonia in heavy cocaine users,[255] and patients with Tourette syndrome, well controlled with haloperidol, have developed severe tics and vocalizations after using cocaine intranasally.[256-258] Tics have also followed cocaine use in previously asymptomatic patients.[257] Diffuse myoclonus and opsoclonus followed cocaine snorting in a young woman, clearing over 4 weeks.[200]

Rhabdomyolysis

Rhabdomyolysis can occur without other symptoms or signs of toxicity and has been attributed to both muscle ischemia[207] and direct toxicity to skeletal muscle.[259] In one case it recurred with repeated cocaine use.[215] Elevated serum creatine kinase and even myoglobinuria can occur in the absence of any muscle symptoms.[260-263] Combined muscle and skin infarction was also reported.[264]

Fatalities

The lethal dose of cocaine in human novices is about 500–800 mg but is quite variable and can follow any route of administration.[190,265,266] As much as 14 g alkaloidal cocaine has been smoked daily without serious complications, yet death has followed intravenous injection of only 20 mg. In rats, the lethal dose ranges from 35 to 100 mg/kg and in dogs from 16.5 to 24.4 mg/kg. Postmortem blood levels in human overdose have usually ranged from 1 to 25 µg/ml.[267] A young man who died after swallowing a bag of cocaine to avoid arrest had a blood level of 212 mg/L.[268] Sudden death may be from ventricular fibrillation or, rarely, anaphylactic response to impurities.[202,205] Patients with blood levels much lower than those associated with true overdose have suddenly died following delirium and extreme hyperthermia resembling the neuroleptic malignant syndrome.[269-272] Unlike neuroleptic malignant syndrome, however, most patients with cocaine-induced hyperthermia have flaccid limbs or dystonic posturing rather than rigidity.[273,274] A patient with a rectal temperature of 114°F (45.5°C) survived.[275] A crack-using schizophrenic taking risperidone had a temperature of 109.4°F (43°C), acute disseminated intravascular coagulation, and rhabdomyolysis and recovered with a permanent pancerebellar syndrome.[276] In some fatalities, autopsy reveals pulmonary edema and ascites, perhaps neurogenic in origin.[277]

Most cocaine overdose victims are chronic users, and autopsies reveal increased cocaine recognition sites on dopamine transporters (DAT)[278] and up-regulation dopamine D_3 receptors in the NA and of κ-opioid receptors in the amygdala and other limbic areas.[279,280] Cardiac enlargement is also often present, especially in cases of sudden death.[266]

Some investigators divide acute cocaine fatalities into two distinct syndromes, namely, fatal overdose and fatal excited delirium.[280a] The excited delirium syndrome is more likely to be accompanied by hyperthermia and rhabdomyolysis, is less likely to be associated with seizures, occurs especially in "chronic and intense" parenteral users of crack smokers, and might be a consequence of altered dopamine processing. Victims of fatal excited delirium have reduced numbers of dopamine D_2 receptors in temperature regulatory centers of the hypothalamus.[280b] Moreover, whereas cocaine users without excited delirium have increased cocaine recognition sites on striatal dopamine transporters, victims of excited delirium do not.[280c] DAT mRNA levels are significantly decreased in midbrains of cocaine users who die following a period of agitated delirium; levels are normal in cocaine users who die simply of "overdose."[281] These observations are consistent with reduced ability to clear synaptic dopamine.[282] It thus appears that chronic cocaine use leads to adaptive changes in the brain and the heart that lower the threshold for psychosis, delirium, arrhythmia, and lethality.[282]

In many fatal cases unexpectedly high levels of the metabolite norcocaine are present.[283]

Other drugs could play a role in cocaine-related fatalities, and psychosis predisposes to violence, accidental death, and suicide.[284-288] Of 925 persons dying in New York City with cocaine in their bodies, death was attributed to cocaine overdose in 4% and to combined cocaine and heroin overdose in 12%; 38% were attributed to homicide, 7% to suicide, and 8% to accidents.[140] It is estimated that 60% to 80% of cocaine users consume ethanol at the same time.[289] Users have taken cocaine with organophosphates—creating their own pseudo-cholinesterase deficiency to prolong the drug's half-life.[156] Cocaine toxicity is also enhanced by concomitant use of monoamine oxidase inhibitors, cyclic antidepressants, phenylpropanolamine, alpha-methyldopa, and reserpine.[156] Adulteration of intranasally-administered cocaine with atropine resulted in agitation, mydriasis, dry flushed skin, and absence of bowel sounds.[290] Adulteration with a warfarin-containing rodenticide, brodifacoum, caused epistaxis and retroperitoneal hemorrhage.[291] Adulteration with arsenic caused vomiting, diarrhea, anemia, and a sensorimotor polyneuropathy.[292] Hypoglycemia presenting as acute psychosis was misdiagnosed as cocaine intoxication.[293]

Treatment of Overdose

Treatment of cocaine overdose depends on symptoms and signs and may require sedation, bicarbonate for acidosis, artificial ventilation, oxygen, blood pressure support, antihypertensives, cardiac monitoring, or antiarrhythmia drugs.[227,294] Hyperthermia can be treated with an ice water bath and a fan, plus sedation.[189]

The choice of specific medications is controversial, for animal studies are conflicting and human studies anecdotal. In rats, dogs, swine, and primates, diazepam and other sedatives prevent seizures and death.[295-298] On theoretical grounds phenytoin, which like cocaine blocks sodium channels, is often avoided in cocaine-intoxicated patients, and in fact animal studies show that sodium channel antagonists including lamotrigine, topiramate, and zonisamide are ineffective against cocaine-induced seizures. (By contrast, GABA-enhancing drugs including felbamate, gabapentin, and vigabatrim are protective.)[299]

Neuroleptics, which would theoretically have antidopaminergic, antiadrenergic, sedative, and antihyperthermic effects, are not very effective in cocaine poisoning. In cocaine-intoxicated primates, chlorpromazine unexpectedly did raise rather than lower the seizure threshold.[298] In dogs, all animals developed seizures, yet chlorpromazine prevented mortality.[300] In rats, haloperidol, a dopamine D_2 antagonist, had no effect on cocaine lethality, and the D_1 antagonist SCH23390 was effective only if given before the cocaine.[301] In swine, haloperidol did not prevent cocaine-induced seizures.[297] In resting human volunteers, domperidone, a D_2 antagonist, did not prevent cocaine-induced hypertension, tachycardia, or elevated catecholamine levels, and with exercise domperidone actually aggravated these responses, a finding of obvious relevance to agitated patients.[302]

In mice, propranolol reduced pulmonary edema and ascites and improved survival.[277] Reports on the use of propranolol in humans are conflicting, however; in some cases, nonselective beta blockade seems to leave alpha stimulation unopposed, causing a further increase in blood pressure.[303] Beta blockade also potentiates cocaine-induced coronary vasoconstriction.[304] Although promoted as a combined beta- and alpha-adrenergic blocker, labetolol has more beta- than alpha-antagonism,[305] and case reports claiming efficacy of labetolol are countered by animal studies showing no benefit.[297,306] Although the use of beta-blockers—especially beta-1 cardioselective agents such as atenolol, metoprolol, and esmolol—still has its advocates,[307] vasodilators such as nitroprusside or alpha-adrenergic blockers such as phentolamine are currently recommended for cocaine-induced hypertensive crisis.[189]

Animal studies with calcium channel blockers are also conflicting. In one report, nitrendipine suppressed cardiac arrhythmias and seizures and increased survival in cocaine-intoxicated rats.[308] In another study, pretreatment of rats with diltiazem, nifedipine, or verapamil potentiated seizures and death.[309] (In that study, both calcium channel blockers and cocaine were given intraperitoneally, raising the possibility that local vasodilatation increased cocaine absorption.)

In mice acute cocaine lethality was reduced by the opioid partial agonist buprenorphine but not by the pure antagonists naloxone or naltrexone, suggesting that buprenorphine might be useful in cases of combined heroin–cocaine ("speedball") toxicity.[310] Other reportedly beneficial agents are pancuronium (which prevented fatalities in dogs without affecting cardiovascular signs)[295,300] and tricyclic antidepressants (which, despite aggravation of some effects, decreased cocaine's cardiac actions in rats).[311] Although the drug of choice for ventricular arrhythmias, lidocaine exacerbated seizures and death in cocaine-intoxicated rats.[312]

Table 5-2 summarizes currently recommended therapy for acute cocaine intoxication. Patients should receive oxygen, sedation with a benzodiazepine, and sodium bicarbonate for acidosis. Hypertension is treated with nitroprusside or phentolamine (or if the patient is pregnant hydralazine). Myocardial ischemia is treated with nitrates and calcium channel blockers. Atrial tachyarrhythmias unresponsive to sedation or cooling are treated with calcium channel blockers. Ventricular dysrhythmias (other than torsade de pointes) are treated with lidocaine, pacing, and sodium bicarbonate.[305]

A young woman repeatedly developed catatonia during "crack" binges; symptoms were unaffected by haloperidol but cleared promptly following parenteral lorazepam.[313]

Recovery from cocaine overdose is usually within a few hours unless there is hypoxic-ischemic brain damage.[202]

In rats butyrylcholinesterase protected against cocaine cardiovascular toxicity by hastening clearance of cocaine and shifting cocaine metabolism from pharmacologically active metabolites (benzoylecgonine, norcocaine) to inactive metabolites (ecgonine, ecgonine methyl ester).[314] Cocaine-induced seizures are also attenuated by 5-HT_2 antagonists,[315] by glutamate NMDA receptor antagonists,[316] and by sigma receptor ligands.[317] Such approaches await trials in humans.

When other drugs are taken with cocaine, they confuse the clinical picture and complicate treatment.[318] Ethanol reportedly enhances cocaine toxicity, perhaps because in the presence of ethanol cocaine is metabolized to cocaethylene, which binds to the dopamine transporter and blocks dopamine reuptake as avidly as cocaine itself.[289,319] (Although some animal and human studies suggested that cocaine combined with ethanol is more reinforcing than cocaine alone,[320,321] others found cocaethylene itself to be less potent than cocaine.[322]) Cocaine is often injected with heroin, and heroin–cocaine mixtures are smoked. Volunteers receiving intravenous cocaine and morphine combinations had cardiovascular effects similar to those caused by cocaine alone and subjective effects reflecting the particular "highs" of each drug.[323] Methadone maintenance patients frequently use cocaine,[324] which both acutely and chronically reduces the severity of naloxone-precipitated opioid withdrawal.[325] Parenteral cocaine users and crack smokers often take sedatives to induce sleep. Crack cocaine is also often smoked with marijuana ("grimmie"),

Table 5–2. Treatment of Cocaine Overdose

Sedation with intravenous benzodiazepine; avoid restraints if possible

High-flow oxygen

Sodium bicarbonate for acidosis

Anticonvulsants (diazepam, lorazepam, phenobarbital); general anesthetics for refractory seizures

Antihypertensives (nitroprusside or phentolamine; if pregnant, hydralazine)

For pulmonary edema: furosemide, morphine sulfate

Artificial ventilation

Blood pressure support

Cardiac monitoring

For atrial arrhythmia: cooling if febrile, calcium channel blockers

For ventricular arrhythmia: sodium bicarbonate, lidocaine

For torsades de pointes: magnesium, overdrive pacing, avoid bicarbonate

Urinary acidification (unless already acidosis or rhabdomyolysis)

For hyperthermia: ice water bath, fan, sedation

For rhabdomyolysis: vigorous hydration, sodium bicarbonate

tobacco ("caviar" or "cavies"), or phencyclidine ("whack" or "spacebase").[178]

Dependence and Withdrawal

The "high" of snorted or intravenous cocaine usually lasts less than an hour and is followed by fatigue and depression. Effects of intramuscular or subcutaneous injection are longer lasting, whereas those of smoking are more intense but shorter.[326] In volunteers, 4-hour cocaine infusions maintained the drug euphoric "high" but not the initial "rush"; haloperidol pretreatment did not affect the cocaine "rush" but partially attenuated the euphoric "high."[327]

As with amphetamine, there seems to be tolerance for subjective and cardiovascular effects, including lethality, and reverse tolerance for psychosis, stereotypic movements, and seizures.[190,328] In one study, a single intranasal 96-mg dose produced acute tolerance to heart rate and subjective effects.[329] Another study found tolerance to heart rate but not to pressor effects.[330] Another found tolerance to neither.[331] Panic attacks following cocaine snorting have emerged after years of daily use, sometimes persisting after the drug was stopped.[332]

Signs of physical dependence are difficult to demonstrate, and abrupt discontinuation of cocaine is not dangerous. Chronic use causes abstinence symptoms, however, and these have been divided into three phases.[178] In phase one—the "crash"—there is an abrupt decline in mood and energy, with depression, anxiety, agitation, and drug craving. Suspiciousness and paranoia are common, and the severity of depression correlates with the intensity of the high produced by cocaine.[333] Studies using single photon emission computed tomography (SPECT) revealed altered CNS serotonin transporter binding in such subjects.[334] Over the next few hours, cocaine craving decreases, replaced by exhaustion and the desire for sleep. Users often take sedatives, ethanol, marijuana, or opioids at this point, and when sleep is achieved, there is rapid eye movement rebound and frequent awakening, with continued depressed mood and hunger. Hypersomnolence lasting several days can be severe ("cocaine washout syndrome").[335] Phase two then emerges, a protracted period of dysphoria, lack of motivation, and a return of cocaine craving, which may be intensified by environmental (conditioned) cues. If abstinence is maintained, dysphoria lasts up to 12 weeks. During phase three, dysphoria clears, but intermittent conditioned cocaine craving can continue for months or years.[178]

Depression in cocaine users thus has several causes. It may be a pre-existing condition being "treated" with cocaine, a psychological reaction to inability to overcome addiction, or a physiological feature of cocaine withdrawal. Decreased dopamine release in chronic cocaine users might result in decreased activation of reward circuits by normal physiological reinforcers and might perpetuate cocaine use as a means of compensating for the deficit.[336] Depression in cocaine users can be severe, and suicide by cocaine overdose is probably underreported.[288]

In subjects studied with positron emission tomography (PET), cue-induced cocaine craving was associated with metabolic activation of the amygdala and the anterior cingulate.[337] Cocaine users are often tobacco smokers, and nicotine aggravates cue-induced cocaine craving, whereas the nicotine antagonist mecamylamine attenuates it.[338]

Patterns of cocaine use include experimental (short-term), recreational (in social settings), circumstantial (to stimulate work or relieve depression), intensified (3 to 20 times daily), and compulsive ("dominates the individual's life and precludes other social functioning").[339] Recreational intranasal users are usually able to titrate and control their doses without escalation, and although insomnia, lassitude, irritability, anxiety, rhinitis, and weight loss are common, toxic psychosis is not. Intravenous users and smokers are likely to escalate use—sometimes at a cost of thousands of dollars per week—and to develop psychopathology and impaired social functioning. Variably present are chronic headache, exhaustion, tremor, grimacing, paranoia, hallucinations (visual, auditory, olfactory, and tactile), panic attacks, and sometimes violent or suicidal behavior.[340] Psychosocial disruption is not dependent on route of administration, however. Before the appearance of "crack," it was estimated that the average duration from first cocaine use to functional deterioration was 4 years in adults and 18 months in adolescents.[341] A survey of adolescent users found that more than half progressed to at least weekly use.[342]

Cocaine Substitutes

Local anesthetics have reinforcing effects in animals,[343] and in human volunteers, intravenous procaine produced a "high" and was misidentified as cocaine.[344] Intranasal lidocaine also reportedly caused a cocaine-like "high" in humans, but in that study a placebo effect could not be excluded.[345] Although such drugs do not appear to be deliberately abused by humans, they are commonly used to adulterate or even substitute for cocaine in street preparations and could contribute to complications such as psychosis or seizures.[176,346] They (and other adulterants) may be present in "crack."[347] Thallium poisoning occurred in three subjects after snorting what they believed was cocaine.[348]

Other "cocaine substitutes," legally sold in paraphernalia stores as incenses but usually taken intranasally, include such products as "Cocaine Snuff" (caffeine and citric acid), "Coca Leaf Incense" (procaine, tetracaine, and caffeine), "Coke-snuff" (ground tobacco, menthol), "Ma-Huang Incense" (ephedrine), and "Yocaine Snuff" (yohimbine hydrochloride, coryanthine).[349] Conversely, "Health Inca Tea" and "Mate De Coca," commercially available in health food stores, do contain cocaine (despite disclaimers by the sellers) and have been abused.[350,351]

Other Medical and Neurological Complications

Because of vasoconstriction, chronic intranasal cocaine causes rhinitis, anosmia, epistaxis, and rarely perforated nasal septum, cerebrospinal fluid rhinorrhea, iritis, midline nasopharyngeal ulceration, central facial destructive granuloma, naso-oral fistula, osteolytic sinusitis with bilateral optic neuropathy, and even brain abscess.[202,352-358] Deliberate intranasal impaction of "crack" cocaine caused necrotizing infection of the nose, upper lip, cheeks, forehead, and temples.[359] Wound botulism, with dysphagia, dysarthria, diplopia, and descending paralysis, affects parenteral cocaine users,[360,361] and botulism has accompanied maxillary sinusitis in intranasal users.[362,363] A contributing factor might be local vasoconstriction and reduced tissue oxygen tension.

"Crack" smokers develop hoarseness, tracheobronchitis with dark sputum, dyspnea, and impaired pulmonary function. Oropharyngeal and tracheal thermal injuries include accidental inhalation of metal filtration devices in crack cocaine pipes.[364] Pulmonary complications include pneumomediastinum, pneumopericardium, bronchiolitis obliterans, organizing pneumonia, and alveolar hemorrhage.[365,366] Reports of cocaine-associated lung disease include Churg–Strauss vasculitis and a syndrome mimicking sarcoidosis.[367,368] A telltale sign of crack smoking is madarosis—loss of eyebrow and eyelash hair.[369]

Dopamine is present in high concentrations in the retina, and compared with controls abstinent cocaine users have impaired blue-yellow color vision and reduced blue cone electroretinogram responses.[370,371] Also reported are acute angle glaucoma precipitated by intranasal application of cocaine[372] and "crack eye syndrome"—corneal epithelial defect and infiltration following crack use and eye rubbing.[373]

Acutely cocaine stimulates release of adrenocorticotrophic hormone (ACTH), luteinizing hormone (LH), and follicle stimulating hormone (FSH) and suppresses release of prolactin. Enhancement of sexual drive was depicted in the sexually explicit pottery and sculpture of the Peruvian Moche culture 1000 years before the Incas.[374] Both men and women frequently combine cocaine with ethanol for sexual enhancement.[375] Chronic use, however, causes hyperprolactinemia and decreased libido, amenorrhea in women, and impotence and gynecomastia in men, sometimes persisting for months after abstinence.[376,377] In eight cocaine-using men, blood levels of prolactin were elevated, whereas levels of LH, testosterone, and cortisol were normal.[378] It is possible that hyperprolactinemia contributes not only to sexual dysfunction, but also to impaired immune function.[379]

Degree and duration of the "high" elicited by cocaine is reportedly greater in women than in men, and female rats are more sensitive than males to cocaine's locomotor stimulatory effects. Ovariectomized rats had reduced cocaine-induced hyperactivity, which was restored by administration of estrogen but not progesterone. The mechanism of interaction is unclear.[380]

Cocaine caused refractory priapism in three men seen in a single emergency deportment over a period of several months.[381]

Cocaine unmasked and then exacerbated myasthenia gravis in a young snorting woman.[382] The cause may have been cocaine's local anesthetic actions on motor nerves coupled with decreased end plate reserve. Cocaine has also caused hypokalemic periodic paralysis in subjects not otherwise affected; a possible explanation is intracellular shift of potassium secondary to the adrenergic effects of cocaine.[382a]

Cocaine hepatotoxicity is probably secondary to the metabolite norcocaine, which binds to hepatic proteins; it is produced in greater amounts in subjects with pseudocholinesterase deficiency. Ethanol potentiates cocaine-induced liver disease.[2,383,384]

Cocaine impairs renal function in a number of ways, including acute rhabdomyolysis, malignant hypertension, and acute and chronic ischemia. The drug is implicated in cases of interstitial nephritis and anti-glomerular basement membrane nephritis, and it enhances renal mRNA expression of tissue inhibitors of metalloproteinase-2, resulting in increased matrix accumulation as seen in diabetes mellitus. Cocaine also increases oxidative stress in the kidney.[385]

Several case reports describe scleroderma in cocaine users, some of whom developed scleroderma renal crisis.[386]

Cocaine precipitated acute symptoms in a patient with variegate porphyria.[387]

Cocaine affects the immune system in complex ways. It increases interferon-gamma secretion and decreases interleukin-10 secretion, thus enhancing Th1-type immune responses while inhibiting Th2-type responses.[388] Intravenous cocaine users are at greater risk for endocarditis than are parenteral abusers of other drugs.[389] Parenteral cocaine users are also at particular risk for acquired immunodeficiency syndrome (AIDS) and perhaps other retroviral infections, for the drug is often taken in "shooting galleries" with shared needles and paraphernalia.[390,391] In addition, "crack" smoking is a risk factor for AIDS and other sexually transmitted diseases, including syphilis, gonorrhea, chlamydia, herpes simplex, and hepatitis B.[392-395] "Crack dens" are centers of promiscuity; sexual services are exchanged for drugs, and genital ulcers facilitate transmission of human immunodeficiency virus (HIV).[390,396,397] (Enormous increases in the prevalence of syphilis and other sexually transmitted diseases paralleled the crack epidemic of the 1980s.) Furthermore, cocaine increases susceptibility to HIV infection by down-regulating HIV-suppressing chemokines and upregulating HIV entry co-receptors,[398] and it opens the blood–brain barrier to HIV invasion by damaging brain microvascular endothelial cells and by inducing proinflammatory cytokines and chemokines.[399]

Cardiovascular Effects

Heart

Although acute chest pain after cocaine use is usually noncardiac in origin,[400,401] it signifies myocardial infarction in some patients, including those who are young and lack other evidence of coronary artery disease.[164,402-405] By 1991, 114 cases of cocaine-induced myocardial infarction had been reported, and of the 92 who received angiography or autopsy, 35 (age range 21 to 60 years, average 32) had normal coronary arteries. Most were also moderate to heavy cigarette smokers.[405a] In several cases, symptoms of cardiac ischemia recurred when cocaine use was resumed.[406] Cardiac catheterization studies demonstrate that cocaine causes coronary artery constriction in humans,[407,408] and in dogs cocaine increases myocardial oxygen demand while simultaneously preventing compensatory coronary artery vasodilatation.[192] Cocaine also promotes coronary thrombosis in the absence of coronary artery constriction.[409] Episodic electrocardiographic evidence of myocardial ischemia persisted for several weeks after cessation of heavy chronic cocaine use in 8 of 21 subjects.[410] A middle-aged man had a myocardial infarction 3 days after he stopped using cocaine.[411]

Cocaine users also develop myocardial contraction band necrosis, myocarditis, and dilated cardiomyopathy.[412-416] Acutely cocaine depresses myocardial function independently of ischemia.[417] In dogs cocaine decreased coronary artery diameter and left ventricular ejection fraction; when ethanol was given, myocardial function decreased further without additional coronary vasoconstriction.[418] Fatal arrhythmia, including asystole, ventricular tachycardia, and ventricular fibrillation, results from combinations of increased sympathetic tone, local anesthetic effects, myocardial ischemia, and myocarditis.[2,189,227,412,419-421] Syncope, which is common following acute cocaine use, is probably cardiogenic in many instances.[189,422] In dogs, cocaine's acute negative cardiac inotropic effects were prevented by pretreatment with nifedipine but not when nifedipine was given after cocaine administration.[423]

Systemic Circulation

Acute aortic dissection and rupture have occurred,[424-428] as has aortic thrombosis.[429] Bowel ischemia and gangrene can follow either oral or intravenous cocaine,[430,431] and perforated gastric ulcer has followed crack smoking.[432] Renal, splenic, and bowel infarction, limb gangrene, and rupture of a splenic aneurysm are also reported.[433-437a] Peripheral limb ischemia resembling Buerger disease has been described,[438] and in one report pathophysiology was confounded by the deliberate addition of arsenic to the cocaine.[292] Pulmonary artery hypertrophy affects chronic users,[439] and alveolar hemorrhage after freebase smoking could be secondary to pulmonary vasoconstriction and tissue hypoxia.[440]

Stroke

Reported Cases. Parenteral cocaine users are at risk for stroke related to infection: endocarditis, AIDS, and hepatitis. They also have strokes caused by the drug itself, whether taken intranasally, intravenously, or intramuscularly or smoked as "crack."[441] The first report of a cocaine-related stroke was in 1977 from Harlem Hospital Center: A middle-aged, mildly hypertensive man drank a bottle of wine and injected cocaine intramuscularly and an hour later abruptly developed aphasia and right hemiparesis; cerebrospinal fluid was normal, and cerebral angiography was refused.[442] The same year fatal rupture of a cerebral saccular aneurysm occurred in a young cocaine snorter.[443] Further cocaine strokes were not reported until the mid-1980s, but by mid-2002, more than 600 cases had been described, about half occlusive and half hemorrhagic (Tables 5–3, 5–4).[414,441-510,510a-510i]

Ischemic strokes include transient ischemic attacks and infarction of cerebrum, thalamus, brainstem, spinal cord, retina, orbit and peripheral oculomotor nerve.[460,461,479,493,497,511-516e] Infarction has occurred in pregnant women and both antenatally and perinatally in newborns whose mothers used cocaine shortly before delivery.[441,447,490]

Table 5–3. Cocaine-related Stroke: Reports

	Type (no. of cases)	Special Features	Route
1977			
Brust, Richter[442]	CI		IM
Lundberg[443]	SAH (1)	Aneurysm	IN
1982			
Caplan et al.[444]	ICH (1)	Negative angiogram	IN
1984			
Schwartz, Cohen[445]	CI (1)	Angiogram: narrow MCA, ACA; occluded PCA	IN
	SAH (1)	Aneurysm	IN
	ICH (1)	Negative angiogram	IN
Lichtenfeld et al.[446]	SAH (1)	Aneurysm	IN
	ICH (1)	AVM	IN
1986			
Chasnoff et al.[447]	CI (1)	Newborn, maternal use	IN
Golbe, Merlin[448]	CI (1)	Angiogram: narrow ICA, distal branch occlusion	Crack
Rogers et al.[450]	SAH (1)	Aneurysm	Not stated
1987			
Altes-Capella et al.[451]	SAH (1)	Aneurysm	IV
Levine et al.[452]	Infarct (3)	Cerebral 1, VB 2	Crack 3
Wojak, Flamm[453]	ICH (4)	Glioma 1, hemorrhagic infarct 1	IN 2, 2 not stated
	SAH (2)	Aneurysm 2	Free-base 1, IN
Kaye, Feinstat[454]	SAH? (1)	Vasospasm?	IN
Cregler, Mark[455]	SAH (1)	Angiogram not done	IN

Continued

Table 5–3. *Continued*

	Type (no. of cases)	Special Features	Route
Mittelman, Wetli[456]	ICH (4)	AVM 2	Not stated
	SAH (1)	Aneurysm	Not stated
Lowenstein et al.[457]	TIA (8)		Free-base 3, IV 3, IN 2
	Infarct (1)		IN
	ICH (2)	AVM 2	IN 1, IV 1
	SAH (1)	Aneurysm	IV
Lehman[458]	ICH (1)	Angiogram not done	IN
1988			
Mangiardi et al.[459]	ICH (4)	AVM 2	IV 2, crack 2
	SAH (5)	Aneurysm 1, angiogram not done 3	IV 3, crack 2
Devenyi[460]	Infarct (1)	Central retinal artery occlusion	IV
Mody et al.[461]	TIA (2)	Cerebral 1, VB 1	Crack 2
	Infarct (3)	Cerebral 2, VB 1	IN 1, crack 1
	Infarct (1)	Anterior spinal artery	Crack
	ICH (3)	AVM (1)	Crack 3
Weingarten[462]	Infarct? (1)	MRI white matter lesions	IN
Toler[463]	Infarct (1)	3 months after last use: lupus anticoagulant present	IV
Devore, Tucker[464]	Infarct (1)	Pontine	Not stated
Henderson, Torbey[465]	SAH (1)	Aneurysm, during pregnancy	Crack
Tenorio et al.[466]	Infarct (1)	Intrauterine exposure	Not stated
1989			
Nails et al.[469]	ICH (4)	AVM? 1, radiographic vasculitis? 3	Not stated
Peterson, Moore[470]	SAH or ICH (13)	Aneurysm 3, AVM 2	Crack 13
Moore, Peterson[471]	TIA or CI (21)		Not stated
Mast et al.[482]	Periventricular Leukomalacia (5)	Newborn, maternal use	Not stated
	Infarct (8)		
	Intraventricular Hemorrhage (7)		Not stated
	ICH (6)		Not stated
Tardiff et al.[472]	SAH or ICH (9)	Aneurysm 6	Not stated
Klonoff et al.[473]	SAH or ICH (7)	Aneurysm 3	Crack 1, IN 3, IV 2, ? 1
Rowley et al.[474]	Infarct (2)		IN 2
	ICH (1)	Angiogram not done	IN 2
De Broucker et al.[475]	ICH (1)		IN
Jacobs et al.[476]	Infarct (8)		Crack 4, IN 1
	ICH (4)	AVM 1	Crack 2, IV 2
	SAH (4)	Aneurysm 2	Crack 3, IV 1
Mercado et al.[477]	ICH (1)	Post-partum, negative angiogram	Not stated
Nolte, Gelman[478]	ICH (1)	Autopsy: no vasculitis	IV
Engstrand et al.[479]	Infarct (8)	Cerebral 5, VB 2, spinal cord 1	Crack 4, IN 1, IV 1, ? 2
Spires et al.[480]	ICH (1)	Newborn, maternal use	Not stated
Meza et al.[481]	Infarct (1)		IN
Dixon, Bejar[483]	Infarct and/or hemorrhage (13)	Combinations of CI, SAH ICH, IVH	Not stated
1990			
Seaman[484]	Infarct (1)		Not stated
Levine et al.[441]	Infarct (18)	VB 4; autopsy 1: no vasculitis	Crack
	ICH (5)	AVM 1	Crack
	SAH (5)	Aneurysm 1	Crack

Continued

Table 5–3. *Continued*

	Type (no. of cases)	Special Features	Route
Deringer et al.[486]	Infarct (1)	Last used 6 months previously	Not stated
Green et al.[487]	ICH (1)		Negative
Krendel et al.[488]	Infarct (2)	Biopsy: vasculitis	Crack 2
		Autopsy: vasculitis	
Hall[505]	Infarct (1)		Not stated
Petty et al.[414]	Infarct (1)	Cardiomyopathy, embolic	Crack
Kaku, Lowenstein[489]	Infarct (7)		Not stated
	ICH (10)	AVM 1	Not stated
	SAH (6)	Aneurysm 5	Not stated
Hoyme et al.[490]	SAH (1)	Neonatal	Not stated
	Infarct (1)	Antenatal	
Simpson et al.[485]	SAH (17)	Aneurysm 16, AVM 1	IV
Kramer et al.[491]	Infarct (1)	Perinatal, bilateral MCA	Crack
Guidotti, Zanesi[504]	Infarct (2)		IN 1, crack 1
Sawaya, Kaminski[516]	Infarct (1)	Spinal cord	Not stated
1991			
Harruff et al.[492]	ICH (2)		Not stated
Peterson et al.[493]	Infarct (19)		IN 1, freebase 2, crack 16
	ICH (7)	Pontine 1, spinal cord 1	Freebase 1, crack 6
	SAH (8)	Aneurysm 5	IN 1, crack 7
Ramadan et al.[494]	ICH (1)	Pontine	Crack
Sloan et al.[495]	Infarct (3)		IN 3
	SAH (2)	Aneurysm 2	IV 1, IN 1
Sauer[496]	Infarct (1)	Cardiomyopathy, embolic	IV
Daras et al.[497]	Infarct (18)	Anterior spinal artery 2	IN 4, IV 3, crack 9
		Coexistent meningovascular syphilis 1	
Hamer et al.[498]	Infarct (1)		Not stated
	SAH (1)		Not stated
Heier et al.[499]	Infarct (17)	Antenatal	Not stated
Fredericks et al.[500]	Infarct (1)	Multifocal; biopsy: vasculitis	IN and IV
Dominguez et al.[501]	Infarct (5)	Antenatal	IV 2, crack 2, Not stated 1
Chadan et al.[506]	SAH (1)	Aneurysm	IV
1992			
Sloan[502]	Infarct (1)	Concurrent myocardial and	IN
		cerebral infarcts	
Konzen et al.[503]	Infarct (3)	Autopsy 1: marked vasospasm,	Crack 3
		no vasculitis	
Nwosu et al.[510a]	Infarct (1)	Mitral valve prolapse	IN
Brown et al.[513]	Infarct (26)	AVM 3, neoplasm 2, aneurysm 12	Not stated
	ICH (18)		
	SAH (12)		
Koppel et al.[510c]	Infarct (1)	Strokes occurred during	Not stated
	ICH (1)	pregnancy	
	SAH (1)		
1993			
Libman et al.[510b]	TIA (1)	Transient monocular blindness	Not stated
1994			
Casas Parera et al.[510d]	Infarct (2)	AVM	Not stated
	ICH (2)		
Baquero, Alfaro[510h]	ICH (1)	Thalamic	Not stated

Continued

Table 5–3. *Continued*

	Type (no. of cases)	Special Features	Route
Daras et al.[510e]	Infarct (25)	AVM 3	Smoke 26
	ICH (16)	Aneurysm 4	Snort 10
	SAH (9)		IV 12
	IVH (5)		
Mena et al.[515]	Infarct (3)		Not stated
	ICH (2)		
1995			
Merkel et al.[519a]	ICH (2)	Vasculitis	IN
Reeves et al.[510f]	Infarct (1)		Not stated
Kibayashi et al.[530]	ICH (26)		
	SAH (26)	Aneurysm 26	Not stated
1996			
Nolte et al.[510]	ICH (7)		IV or not stated
	SAH (3)	Aneurysm 3	
Davis Swalwell[529]	SAH (3)	Aneurysm 3	Not stated
Samkoff et al.[528]	Spontaneous spinal epidural hematoma		Smoke or IN
Martinez et al.[510g]	Infarct (2)		IN
1997			
Migata et al.[512]	Oculomotor nerve infarct		Smoke
Keller, Chappell[527]	Spontaneous subdural hematoma		Not stated
Edigo-Herrero, Gonzalez[525]	ICH	Pontine	Not stated
DiLazzaro et al.[511]	Spinal TIA or infarct		Not stated
Effiong et al.[523]	TIA	Vasoconstriction aggravated by hyperkalemia	Smoke
Fessler et al.[508]	Infarct (7)		Not stated
	ICH (6)	Aneurysm 14	
	SAH (16)		
1998			
Khellaf, Fénelon[524]	Cerebellar hemorrhage	Cocaine injected with heparinoid	IV
Giess et al.[516b]	Infarcts, TIAs (1)		Not stated
1999			
LaMonica et al.[521]	Infarct (1)		Smoke
Domingo et al.[516c]	Infarct (1)		Not stated
Munoz Casares et al.[516d]	TIA (1)		Not stated
Cuervo Pinna et al.[559]	Infarct (1)	Lupus anticoagulant	Not stated
2000			
Storen et al.[507]	Infarct (1)	Moyamoya in both cases	Smoke
	SAH (1)		
Witlin et al.[510i]	ICH (1)	Post-partum	Not stated
Strupp et al.[522]	Mesencephalic infarct	Concomitant amphetamine	IN
Tolat et al.[509]	Infarct (2)		Smoke
	SAH (1)		
Nanda et al.[533]	SAH (14)	Aneurysm 14	
2001			
Conway, Tamargo[532]	SAH (27)	Aneurysm 27	Not stated
2002			
Van Stavern Gorman[516a]	Infarct	Intraocular and orbital structures	IN

CI, cerebral infarct; SAH, subarachnoid hemorrhage; ICH, intracerebral hemorrhage; IVH, intraventricular hemorrhage; TIA, transient ischemic attack; MCA, middle cerebral artery; ACA, anterior cerebral artery; PCA, posterior cerebral artery; AVM, arteriovenous malformation; VB, vertebrobasilar; IM, intramuscular; IN, intranasal; IV, intravenous.

Table 5–4. Cocaine-related Stroke: Types and Numbers of Reported Cases

Occlusive	261
TIA	15
Infarct	230
TIA or infarct	21
Occlusive and/or hemorrhagic	13
Hemorrhagic	202
ICH	150
SAH	173
ICH or SAH	29
Intraventricular hemorrhage	12
Aneurysm	157
AVM	23
Total stroke	629

TIA, Transient ischemic attack; ICH, intracerebral hemorrhage; SAH, subarachnoid hemorrhage; AVM, arteriovenous malformation.

In an ultrasound study of 26 newborns exposed to cocaine, five had "periventricular leukomalacia"; eight, cerebral infarction; seven, intraventricular hemorrhage; and six, intracerebral hemorrhage.[482]

In some cases, cerebral infarction has been attributed to vasculitis on the basis of angiographic findings;[454] such changes, however, probably represented vasospasm following undiagnosed subarachnoid hemorrhage[516a] or direct vasoconstriction caused by the drug.[473,517] Autopsies usually show histologically normal cerebral vessels,[441,468] although in six cases mild cerebral vasculitis was observed at biopsy or autopsy.[488,500,518,519,519a] In two of these cases cerebral angiography showed beading or narrowing of cerebral vessels; in the other four, angiography was negative. ESR was elevated (32–108 mm/h) in three[500,519a] and normal in one. All six cases had small vessel angiitis, with lymphocyte preponderance in four[488,500,519] and polymorphonuclear predominance in two.[519a] Giant cells were not seen, and only one case had vessel wall necrosis.[519a] Four patients received glucocorticoids.[488,500,519a] In contrast to these cases a man with multiple cerebral infarcts clinically and by magnetic resonance imaging (MRI) had "multifocal areas of segmental stenosis and dilation" by angiography, yet brain biopsy revealed no evidence of vasculitis.[520]

A cocaine user with rhabdomyolysis and renal failure simultaneously developed "leukocytoclastic vasculitis" of the skin.[519b]

A young man who used alkaloidal cocaine "regularly" for 10 years insidiously developed personality change, reduced attention, and impaired memory; computed tomography (CT) revealed patchy areas consistent with infarction, and cerebral angiography showed markedly narrowed internal carotid and middle cerebral arteries, with prominent lenticulostriate networks and pial collaterals ("moyamoya-like"). The degree of collateralization, as well as the history, suggested a slowly progressive rather than an acute event.[507]

A 35-year-old woman with 12 years of "crack" use developed progressive mental alteration over several weeks; compulsive behavior, choreiform movements, irritability, and inappropriate laughter culminated, after a 3-day binge, in garbled words, abnormal repetitive movements, and then muteness. CT showed diffuse cerebral atrophy, but SPECT showed focal reductions in perfusion involving both frontal lobes and the left temporal lobe. Symptoms did not improve over the next 6 months.[521]

Five minutes after intranasally inhaling a mixture of cocaine and amphetamine, a 16-year-old boy developed unsteadiness and diplopia, and MRI revealed infarction in the mesencephalon.[522]

A patient receiving long-term hemodialysis developed hemiplegia, rhabdomyolysis, and severe hyperkalemia while using "crack." No lesion was seen at CT, and the hemiplegia resolved following correction of the hyperkalemia. The authors suggested that the hemiplegia was ischemic in origin but worsened by the hyperkalemia.[523]

Two reported strokes were likely embolic secondary to cocaine-related cardiomyopathy.[414,496] In another report a 20-year-old with no other risk factors had superior cerebellar artery occlusion 6 months after last use, raising the possibility of delayed effects.[486] In a 27-year-old cocaine sniffer with "heaviness and paresthesias" in the legs and occasional "forgetfulness," MRI revealed multiple periventricular white matter lesions.[462]

Intracerebral or subarachnoid hemorrhage has occurred during or within hours of cocaine use or with a less clear temporal relationship. Often there has been other substance use, especially ethanol. A young woman with a cerebellar hemorrhage had mixed her cocaine with enoxaparin (a low-molecular-weight heparin) to facilitate intravenous administration.[524] Intraparenchymal hemorrhages have been cerebral, brainstem, and cerebellar.[508-510,513,515,524-526] Also described are spontaneous acute subdural hematoma, spontaneous spinal epidural hematoma, superior sagittal sinus thrombosis with hemorrhagic venous infarction, dural arteriovenous fistula, and mycotic aneurysm rupture.[513,527,528] More than half the patients with hemorrhagic stroke who underwent cerebral angiography had saccular aneurysms or vascular malformations. Other hemorrhages include bleeding into embolic infarction or glioma.[453] Cerebral hemorrhages have occurred in newborns and in pregnant and postpartum women.[441,465,477,480,482,490]

During 1 year, 10 of 17 cases of fatal nontraumatic intracranial hemorrhage investigated by the Connecticut Chief Medical Examiner were associated with cocaine abuse. Seven were intraparenchymal and three subarachnoid secondary to ruptured saccular aneurysm. In none did vessels show vasculitis.[510] In a 7-year survey in Alabama, three cases of fatal ruptured cerebral aneurysm were identified. Thirty-nine had toxicological analysis; cocaine was found in three (and methamphetamine in six). In none was there vasculitis.[529] In a 3-year autopsy survey by the New York City Medical Examiner's Office, there were 26 cases of "cocaine-induced" intracerebral hemorrhage and 26 cases of "cocaine-induced" cerebral aneurysm rupture. Patients with intracerebral hemorrhage were significantly more likely to be hypertensive. In none was there evidence of vasculitis.[530] Fourteen other cases of cocaine-associated intracranial hemorrhage were specifically examined for vasculitis, which was absent in all.[531] Autopsy on a patient with multiple cerebral hemorrhages after smoking "crack" also revealed histologically normal cerebral vessels.[487]

In a retrospective survey of 150 consecutive patients admitted for subarachnoid hemorrhage, 17 had used intravenous cocaine within 72 hours. Mortality and morbidity were worse among the cocaine users, perhaps as a consequence of drug-aggravated vasospasm.[485]

In another study, however, 27 of 440 patients with "aneurysmal subarachnoid hemorrhage" (6.1%) had used cocaine within 72 hours, and while vasospasm was significantly more likely among the cocaine users (63% vs 30%), there was no difference in clinical outcome.[532]

In two studies comparing ruptured aneurysms associated or not associated with cocaine, the cocaine-associated aneurysms were significantly smaller and the patients were younger.[508,533]

A case–control study from Atlanta failed to find any association between "crack use at any time or acute crack use" and "stroke or cerebral infarction."[534] Cases were "patients aged 20 to 39 years with a diagnosis of stroke" and controls were inpatients with "noncocaine-related diagnoses." Sixty-six of 144 cases (32%) and 99 of 147 controls (43%) had used crack at any time (odds ratio 0.7); 12 of 56 cases (21%) and 11 of 67 controls (16%) had used crack within the last 4 hours (odds ratio 1.9). This potentially influential study has been appropriately criticized on several grounds.[535] First, information about any use of crack was missing in 54.2% of cases and 32.7% of controls; information about acute crack use was missing in 61.1% of cases and 54.4% of controls. Second, nearly half of the controls with information available had used crack, and many were acute users, raising the possibility that crack users are more likely than non-users to be admitted to the hospital for a variety of reasons. Third, the study found no association of stroke with several established risk factors, including tobacco and diabetes mellitus.

Another case–control study, from California, compared 347 cases (incident strokes in women aged 15 to 44 years) and 1021 controls (randomly chosen members of the same health plan—i.e., outpatients). Use of cocaine, amphetamine, or both was a strong risk factor for stroke (after adjusting for confounders, odds ratio 13.9 for cocaine and 3.8 for amphetamine).[536]

Stroke Pathophysiology. The mechanisms of cocaine-related stroke are diverse. Striking, considering that cocaine and amphetamine have similar actions and effects, are the high frequency of underlying aneurysm or vascular malformation in hemorrhagic strokes of cocaine users compared with amphetamine users and, conversely, the frequency of vasculitis in amphetamine users compared with cocaine users.[537] Cocaine hydrochloride is more often associated with hemorrhagic than occlusive stroke, whereas hemorrhagic and occlusive strokes occur with roughly equal frequency in "crack" users, but the rising prevalence of stroke since the appearance of "crack" is probably attributable to wider use and higher dosage rather than to a peculiarity of "crack" itself.[538] Cocaine-induced myocardial infarction, cardiac arrhythmia, and cardiomyopathy carry a risk for embolic stroke. More significant, however, is cocaine's effects on the systemic and cerebral circulation. By blocking reuptake of norepinephrine from sympathetic nerve endings (and probably also by affecting calcium flux), cocaine is a vasoconstrictor.[539,540,540a] Although chronic cocaine use does not seem to cause chronic hypertension,[541] acute hypertension can lead to intracranial hemorrhage, especially in subjects with underlying aneurysms or vascular malformations. Animal and in vitro studies suggest that cocaine-induced peripheral vasoconstriction is mediated at least in part by inhibition of local vasodilatory nitric oxide.[541a]

Compared with controls, newborns exposed to cocaine in utero had increased mean arterial blood pressure and cerebral blood flow velocity during the first day of life, with levels becoming normal on the second day; such changes would increase the risk of perinatal cerebral hemorrhage.[542]

Cerebral vasoconstriction probably causes occlusive stroke, and cocaine metabolites, which in some chronic users are detectable in urine for weeks, also cause cerebral vasospasm.[326,543] In healthy young cocaine users, intravenous infusion of cocaine (0.2 or 0.4 mg/kg) caused dose-related cerebral vasoconstriction (as detected by magnetic resonance angiography), and the likelihood of vasoconstriction was greatest in those with the heaviest lifetime cocaine use, suggesting a cumulative residual effect.[517] Vasoconstriction was greater in men than in women, in whom it occured only during their luteal menstrual cycle phase.[543a] Doppler sonography studies in cocaine users reveal increased cerebrovascular resistance which persists for at least a month during abstinence.[544] Cocaine stimulates central sympathetic outflow,[545] but in a study using isolated rat carotid arteries, cocaine also caused vasoconstriction, indicating a peripheral effect, and the vasoconstriction was blocked by prazosin, phentolamine, and 6-hydroxydopamine.[546] In other animal studies cocaine-induced vasoconstriction in tissues lacking sympathetic innervation was not blocked by prazosin or phentolamine but was prevented by pretreatment with a calcium channel blocker, suggesting a direct action of cocaine on calcium flux.[539] Serotonin reuptake blockade may also contribute to cocaine's vasoconstrictor effects.[547] Street cocaine is sometimes adulterated with amphetamine,[2] and in rabbits neither drug

alone caused significant basilar artery spasm, whereas the two drugs in combination did.[548]

A 34-year-old woman had thrombosis of the internal carotid artery; at emergency thrombectomy the arterial wall was grossly normal. A 32-year-old woman had multiple hemorrhagic infarcts; at autopsy, there was no vasculitis, but large cerebral arteries were markedly narrowed with infolded and frayed internal elastic lamina. In these two cases, thrombosis and infarction could have been the result of severe vasospasm, with hemorrhage occurring during reperfusion.[503] During an attack of transient monocular blindness in a heavy cocaine user, funduscopic examination revealed "diffuse severe narrowing of the retinal arterioles" in the affected eye.[510b] In volunteers using cocaine intranasally, transcranial Doppler ultrasound revealed increased cerebral blood velocities, consistent with increased distal arteriolar resistance.[549]

In addition to direct vasoconstriction and the secondary effects of hypertension and cardiac disease, cocaine affects the cerebral circulation in diverse ways. Although intraluminal cocaine constricted cat and rat pial vessels in vitro, topical cocaine dilated pial vessels in adult cats and in fetal and neonatal sheep, and this effect was prevented by the beta-blocker propranolol.[540,543,550,551] The cocaine metabolite ecgonine methyl ester is a cerebral vasodilator whereas the metabolite benzoylecgonine is a cerebral vasoconstrictor, and species vary in their production of different cocaine metabolites.[551] In pigs, intravenously administered cocaine caused carotid artery constriction, but in vitro there was no response, suggesting that in this species the vasoconstriction effect was indirect, through "release of humoral and/or neural vasoactive substances."[552]

Cocaine increases endothelial release of endothelin, probably by acting on sigma receptors,[553] and in rabbits cocaine-induced cerebral vasospasm was prevented by administration of an endothelin receptor antagonist.[553a] In vascular smooth muscle cells cocaine causes a rise in intracellular free calcium and a loss of intracellular magnesium.[554]

In vitro, cocaine enhances the response of platelets to arachidonic acid, promoting aggregation.[555] In healthy volunteers intranasal cocaine activated platelets and increased the formation of circulating platelet aggregates.[555a] However, cocaine also inhibited fibrinogen binding to activated platelets and caused dissociation of preformed platelet aggregates,[556] and severe destructive thrombocytopenia responsive to corticosteroids or splenectomy was reported in six HIV-negative cocaine users (none of whom had a stroke).[557] In rabbits, repeated cocaine injections caused arteriosclerotic aortopathy.[558] In a cocaine user with symptoms of coronary artery disease, protein C and antithrombin III were depleted and returned to normal, with clearing of symptoms, when drug use was discontinued.[415] Antiphospholipid antibodies have been found in occasional cocaine users.[495,559] In human long-term cocaine users intranasal or intravenous cocaine administration acutely caused erythrocytosis and increased levels of von Willebrand factor without affecting white blood cell or platelet counts.[560]

Cognitive Effects

As with amphetamine and other stimulants, it is unclear whether chronic cocaine use causes lasting mental abnormalities. Protracted depression in abstinent users has been attributed, without much evidence, to permanent depletion of limbic dopamine. An autopsy study found that levels of a neuronal protein, VMAT2, were reduced in dopaminergic cells of the ventral striatum in cocaine users compared with controls, and that the reduction was greatest in those with depression.[561,561a] This finding does not answer whether cocaine caused depression in these patients or whether they were drawn to cocaine use because they were depressed. Psychological impairment and poor work performance were described in South American coca leaf chewers, but these studies, like those involving other recreational drugs, did not account for pre-cocaine cognitive capacity, acute drug effects, or other confounders.[562,563]

Human studies using controls suggest that chronic cocaine use produces impairment in short-term auditory recall, concentration, and reaction time.[564-567] Other studies found abstinent cocaine users deficient, compared with controls, in tests of executive functioning, visuoperception, psychomotor speed, and manual dexterity.[568,569] A study comparing cocaine abusers during a 45-day abstinence period with controls found lasting impairment on tests of nonverbal declarative memory; on tests of procedural memory (motor

learning), however, the cocaine users performed better than the controls, even when adjustment was made for tobacco use.[570,571] This unexpected performance improvement was tentatively attributed to dopamine receptor hypersensitivity during the abstinence period.

Psychometric testing of cocaine-dependent and nonsubstance-abusing schizophrenics found similar patterns of impaired learning and recall performance, but the comorbid patients were more markedly impaired.[572] Persistent schizophrenic symptoms reportedly emerged in a group of long-term (6 or more years) psychostimulant abusers.[573]

A study of chronic cocaine users during 4 weeks of abstinence found worse neuropsychological performance among those who also consumed large amounts of ethanol. This apparent additive effect was thought to be related to cocaethylene.[574]

Chronic cocaine users have diffuse electroencephalographic theta activity, which increases with continuous use.[575] In a CT study, habitual cocaine users (at least twice weekly for 2 years or more) had significant degrees of cerebral atrophy (enlargement of the lateral ventricles and widening of the sylvian fissures) compared with first-time users and nonusers; subjects were between 20 and 40 years of age, and those with alcoholism, polydrug abuse, and HIV seropositivity were excluded.[576] In a later report, however, the same investigators found neurocognitive impairment in chronic cocaine users, but they did not find cerebral atrophy when adjustments were made for tobacco, ethanol, other drugs, nutrition, head injury, and HIV.[577]

Another study, using MRI, found accelerated loss of temporal lobe volume with age in chronic cocaine and amphetamine users.[578] The same investigators reported abnormal cerebral white matter signals in asymptomatic chronic cocaine users; the lesions were considered consistent with "subclinical vascular events" that could contribute to cognitive dysfunction as the subjects aged.[579,580]

Following 3 to 4 months of abstinence from chronic cocaine use, PET demonstrated decreased metabolic activity in the frontal lobes.[581] Similar findings were reported using SPECT, and some of these subjects had normal CT and MRI scans and no other evidence of neurological disease.[582] Of 18 subjects with abnormal brain perfusion patterns on SPECT, 13 had mild and five had moderate deficits on psychometric testing, especially spatial learning, organization, perseveration, set maintenance, verbal learning, and concept attainment.[583] In a PET study, glucose metabolism was reduced over the entire cerebral cortex, thalamus, and midbrain following the acute administration of cocaine.[584]

Twenty-six of 57 neurologically normal chronic cocaine users had abnormal visual evoked responses.[585] Cocaine-dependent subjects had delayed event-related potentials in response to a novel auditory stimulus.[586]

Compared with controls, chronic cocaine users had reduced N-acetyl aspartate (NAA) peaks (a neuronal/ axonal marker, measured by magnetic resonance spectroscopy) in the thalamus but not the basal ganglia.[587] (The authors noted that thalamus and basal ganglia activation correlates with cocaine "rush" but not with cocaine craving.[588]) Magnetic resonance spectroscopy also identified abnormal levels of creatine and myoinositol but normal levels of NAA in the white matter of "heavy" cocaine users, suggesting damage to non-neuronal brain tissue.[589,590] Diffusion tensor imaging identified "white matter microstructural abnormalities" in inferior frontal brain regions, but not in the temporal lobes, of heavy cocaine users.[590a]

The evidence thus supports the view that cocaine does cause lasting cognitive impairment and that the damage might be secondary to cerebral ischemia. It has been suggested that antiplatelet drugs or neuroprotective agents might benefit cocaine users with cerebral perfusion defects.[590b]

Obstetric and Pediatric Aspects

In the United States, cocaine use during pregnancy is common and underreported, and "crack babies" have received considerable media attention. At Parkland Hospital in Dallas, 10% of pregnant women reported cocaine use,[591] and at Boston City Hospital's prenatal unit, 17% of urine samples were positive for cocaine or its metabolites.[592] At several public and private prenatal facilities in Pinellas County, Florida, urine samples reflected cocaine use in 1.9% of white women and 7.5% of black women.[593] Cocaine-exposed newborns have filled pediatric hospital units ("crack boarders"); in 1990, it was estimated that more than 100,000 such infants had been born in the United States and that by the year 2000 the number of American children

exposed prenatally to cocaine would be as high as 4 million, in some school districts constituting more than half of all classrooms. As these children began to enter nursery and primary schools, the media publicized their functional disabilities and their custodial and educational costs. For example, in Los Angeles in 1990, it reportedly cost US$3500 a year to educate each normal child in a regular classroom while the cost of each drug-exposed child was US$15,000.[594] Such alarms resulted in a voluminous literature on cocaine's perinatal and neonatal effects.[595,596,596a]

Reports describe increased spontaneous abortion,[597,598] abruptio placentae,[598-600] premature delivery, retarded fetal growth, low birth weight, and decreased head circumference.[598,600-604,604a] Reported congenital malformations include genitourinary[600,605-607] and cardiovascular anomalies (pulmonary artery atresia or stenosis and atrial or ventricular septal defects),[490,597,608] skull defects,[597,609] spinal anomalies,[482] intestinal atresia or necrotizing enterocolitis,[610] congenital limb reduction defects,[490,611] iris vessel tortuosity,[612] and developmental retinopathy.[613]

Neonatal tremor, irritability, brisk tendon reflexes, and hypertonia are frequently observed in cocaine-exposed infants, clearing in a few days.[602] Also described in neonates are "depression of interactive behavior and poor organizational response to environmental stimuli."[600] In a study using the Bayley Mental and Motor Scales of Infant Development cocaine-exposed infants often scored below average compared with 390 controls.[614] After excluding users of other illicit drugs and controlling for the effects of ethanol and tobacco, another study found that cocaine use in the third trimester adversely affected neonatal body length, head circumference, attention, and responsiveness.[615,616] Others, controlling for birth weight, gestational age, maternal age, and ethanol, cannabis, and tobacco use, found, at 3 weeks of age, "poorer state regulation and greater excitability" in infants with prenatal cocaine exposure; the effects were dose-related.[617] Others reported similar findings as well as synergistic effects of cocaine with ethanol and cannabis.[618]

A neonatal "withdrawal syndrome" purportedly resembles heroin's but lacks gastrointestinal symptoms; cardiac arrhythmia and seizures are described.[482] Sixteen infants exposed to cocaine in utero had seizures at birth, and eight of them continued to have seizures after the first month of life.[619] Even in the absence of seizures, electroencephalograms have shown spikes and sharp waves lasting several months.[620] In contrast to the opioid neonatal withdrawal syndrome, these symptoms and signs, if they are attributable to cocaine per se, are likely the result of direct toxicity, not abstinence. Moreover, although neonatal opioid withdrawal is a frequently lethal emergency, signs of neonatal cocaine toxicity seldom require vigorous treatment.

Babies exposed to cocaine during the first trimester had less well developed spectral correlations between homologous brain regions at birth and lower spectral electroencephalographic power at 1 year of age, implying "fewer interhemispheric connections" at birth and "fewer neuronal aggregates" at 1 year.[621]

Cocaine-exposed neonates had increased plasma norepinephrine concentrations, which correlated with neurobehavioral disturbance at 1 to 3 days but not at 2 weeks.[622] Possible mechanisms for the elevation include uterine vasoconstriction and catecholamine release in response to hypoxemia and central dopamine depletion with loss of dopaminergic inhibitory modulation of sympathetic tone.

In a prospective study of 30 cocaine-exposed newborns at Harlem Hospital, intrauterine growth retardation, small head circumference, and diffuse or axial hypertonus severe enough to label "hypertonic tetraparesis" were significantly more common among patients than among controls.[623] In a later study by the same investigators, 136 cocaine-unexposed infants were compared with 104 infants in whom cocaine exposure was not only verified but quantitated as mild or severe by maternal hair analysis. In this study, which excluded mothers with alcoholism, parenteral drug use, and AIDS and controlled for tobacco use (identified by self-report), impaired fetal head growth, and abnormalities of muscle tone, movement, and posture were associated with cocaine exposure in a dose-dependent fashion.[624] At 24 months of age, however, hypertonus was no longer detectable in children with prenatal cocaine exposure. It is uncertain whether these neonatal signs predict later developmental difficulties.[625,626]

A study from San Francisco, in which prenatal tobacco use was identified by urine assays of the nicotine metabolite cotinine rather than by self-report, found that tobacco exposure was a better predictor of abnormal muscle tone in neonates than was cocaine.[627] In that study, however, cocaine exposure was based on meconium levels of benzoylecgonine rather than hair analysis; thus, while tobacco use may have been underestimated in the Harlem Hospital study, cocaine use may have been underestimated in the San Francisco study.

Again using maternal hair analysis and adjusting for ethanol, tobacco, marijuana, and opioids, the Harlem Hospital investigators found that head circumference decreased with increasing cocaine dose during pregnancy.[628] Moreover, head circumference was disproportionately smaller than predicted by birth weight, suggesting that cocaine acts directly to inhibit fetal brain growth rather than indirectly by causing vasoconstriction of placental vessels.

As noted, strokes occur both perinatally and neonatally in cocaine-exposed infants. In an ultrasound study of neonates exposed in utero to cocaine or methamphetamine there was evidence of ischemic or hemorrhagic stroke in over one-third.[483] In another report of 49 exposed infants, CT or MRI in more than half suggested periventricular leukomalacia, cerebral infarction, intraventricular hemorrhage, or intraparenchymal hemorrhage.[482] Not all infants so diagnosed have displayed neonatal behavioral abnormalities.[483] Brainstem auditory evoked response testing revealed prolonged latencies indicative of brainstem or cerebral damage in 18 cocaine-exposed infants.[629] An ultrasound study in which meconium levels of benzoylecgonine were used to quantitate cocaine exposure found that heavy but not light exposure was associated with subependymal hemorrhage.[630]

In a radiological review (sonography, CT, or MRI) of 43 consecutive newborns of cocaine-using mothers, cerebral infarction occurred in 17% and congenital anomalies in 12%, compared with 2% and 0 in controls. Malformations included encephalocele, holoprosencephaly, intraspinal lipoma, and hypoplastic cerebellum. The authors speculated that strokes were caused by placental and cerebral vasospasm in the third trimester and that malformations were the result of vasospasm in the first trimester.[499] Others, however, expressed doubt that first-trimester malformations are ischemic in origin.[631]

Sudden infant death syndrome (SIDS) was reported in 15% of 66 infants exposed to cocaine in utero,[632] and abnormal cardiorespiratory patterns were described in exposed neonates whether or not they subsequently developed apnea.[599] Subsequent studies, however, found only a small increase in SIDS among infants prenatally exposed to cocaine,[633] and a study of premature infants found that in utero cocaine exposure actually *decreased* the risk of respiratory distress syndrome.[634] A meta-analysis of 10 published studies on SIDS concluded that intrauterine exposure to drugs in general was a risk factor but that an increased risk could not be attributed to cocaine alone.[635]

Cocaine-using mothers are likely to avoid prenatal care, to be malnourished, to abuse other substances including tobacco and ethanol, and to underreport cocaine use.[636,637] (In a case–control study of spontaneous abortion, maternal hair analysis was more than four times as likely to be positive as self-reports of cocaine use, and only when the hair analysis figures were used did cocaine emerge as a significant risk factor.[638]) Cocaine users have a high prevalence of sexually transmitted disease, including HIV and syphilis, which they transmit to offspring.[639,639a] They are socio-economically impoverished. Such factors confound attempts to determine the true risk of in utero cocaine exposure.[633] Although most workers concur that cocaine causes spontaneous abortion, abruptio placentae, intrauterine growth retardation, and decreased head circumference, some have found no increase in prematurity,[598,603] congenital anomalies,[592,603,640] or abnormal neonatal behavior.[641] Some, observing intrauterine growth restriction, describe "catch-up growth" by 12 to 18 months.[642] One study, using maternal hair analysis, found heavy but not light use of cocaine was associated with intrauterine growth retardation, and exposure late in pregnancy was necessary for the association.[643] In one report, "social users" who stopped taking cocaine when they realized they were pregnant did not have an increased incidence of "adverse pregnancy outcome."[644] One study found decreased intrauterine growth associated with prenatal cocaine exposure in women with and without prenatal care, and the adequacy of prenatal care did not influence the difference between cocaine-exposed and unexposed infants.[645] Another study found cranial ultrasound abnormalities in nearly two-thirds of inner city neonates whether they had been exposed to cocaine or not, with no significant difference between the two groups,

suggesting that abnormalities reported by others are not cocaine-specific.[646] One group of investigators even charged that studies failing to find a causal relationship between maternal cocaine use and fetal health problems are frequently rejected by journal reviewers on ideological grounds.[647]

In 1991, 20 scientific reports of cocaine use during pregnancy were subjected to meta-analysis.[648] Fifteen were prospective cohort studies, four were retrospective cohort studies, and one was a case–control study; case reports were excluded, as were studies that did not separate cocaine users from other drug users and studies without control groups. Although the odds ratios for such outcomes as spontaneous abortion, abruptio placentae, prematurity, low birth weight, and malformations were elevated in cocaine users compared with drug-free controls, statistically significant risk was identified only for genitourinary malformations and intrauterine death. Comparing polydrug users who used cocaine with polydrug users who did not use cocaine, only the odds ratio for genitourinary malformations was significant. The authors stressed the difficulty in defining the role of cocaine alone in adverse pregnancy outcomes.

An extensive review of studies published between 1989 and 1999 acknowledged the difficulty in isolating cocaine effects.[649] For example, of 16 studies that evaluated cocaine-exposed neonates using the Brazelton Neonatal Behavioral Assessment Scale, half had no controls for other drug use. Some (but not all) studies that attempted such controls did find adverse effects, variably involving "habituation, orientation, motor maturity, number of abnormal reflexes, range of state, depressed and excitable scores, ... alert responsiveness, ... autonomic regulation, ... [and] state regulation." Some studies found increased effects related to amount and duration of exposure, and some found interactions of cocaine with ethanol or tobacco. Among studies of infants aged 3 to 24 months using Bayley Scales of Infant Development (which assess cognition and behavior), half found no differences between prenatally exposed infants and controls.

Another review stressed the failure of many studies to measure "specific domains of function" that might be affected by prenatal cocaine exposure, for example, motor performance, reactivity, attention, regulation, arousal modulation, or executive function.[650] These reviewers acknowledged that cocaine-exposed children often have compromised neuropsychological performance but considered them to be "part of a much larger group of high-risk children who would benefit from broad-based interventional services." When proper adjustments are made, they concluded, impoverished bac grounds are more important than cocaine exposure per se.

In a more recent review of 74 reports published during 1984 through 2000, 38 were excluded on methodological grounds (failure to mask investigators to children's cocaine status, lack of a control group, absence of prospective recruitment, or inclusion of children exposed in utero to opioids, amphetamines, or phencyclidine or whose mothers were infected with HIV).[651] Systematic analysis of the remaining 36 studies failed to identify a "consistent negative association between prenatal cocaine exposure and physical growth, developmental tests scores, or receptive or expressive language" after controlling for tobacco, ethanol, marijuana, or the quality of the child's environment. Possible effects of cocaine on motor skills during the first year of life could not be separated from equally likely effects of tobacco. Cocaine effects on "attentiveness and emotional expressivity" and on neurophysiological measurements (electroencephalogram, rapid eye movement, or brainstem auditory evoked responses) were inconsistently reported and "of uncertain clinical importance."

In criticizing prior studies, the authors of this review singled out a meta-analysis of six reports associating in utero cocaine exposure with impaired expressive and receptive language function, an association which, it was claimed, could cost up to US$352 million annually in special education services.[652] Appearing in a leading journal, this paper received considerable media attention, yet five of the six studies reviewed were retrospective, two did not use masked examiners, two included children exposed to opioids and amphetamines, and none controlled for tobacco exposure.

A prospective study of 658 infants exposed prenatally to cocaine found that at 1 month of age, compared with controls, they had "lower arousal, poor quality of movement and self-regulation, higher excitability, more hypertonia, and more nonoptimal reflexes." Cocaine exposure was based on meconium assay, and "adjustment for co-variates"—including maternal ethanol, tobacco, and marijuana

use during pregnancy—was based on "the hospital interview."[653]

A study of 4-year-olds exposed prenatally to cocaine found no difference, compared with controls, in intelligence testing.[654] A similar study found difficulty sustaining attention in prenatally exposed young children but no significant effects on growth, intelligence, achievement, or classroom behavior.[655] Among schoolchildren aged 6 to 9 years there was no difference in IQ scores between those with and without prenatal cocaine exposure.[656] Comparable studies on older children have not been done, and it is possible that cognitive or behavioral abnormalities will become evident during adolescence. It is clear, however, that if prenatal exposure to cocaine has detrimental effects on the brain, they are not only less than previously claimed but also small compared with the effects of tobacco and ethanol.[166] Nonetheless, over 200 American women have been criminally prosecuted for using cocaine while pregnant, and governmental programs have been instituted that offer crack-using women cash incentives to become sterilized. The University of South Carolina even adopted a policy of screening selected pregnant patients for cocaine and reporting positive results to the police.[657] No one in America (so far) has been prosecuted for using tobacco or ethanol during pregnancy.

Animal studies support the contention that cocaine damages fetuses. In utero cocaine exposure to mice or rats causes soft tissue and skeletal anomalies, reduced fetal weight, fetal edema, abruptio placentae, and intracranial hemorrhage.[658-662] Impaired learning has followed doses too small to produce grossly evident abnormalities.[660] Other reported abnormalities include deficient conditioning to noxious stimuli,[663] enhanced cocaine (and ethanol) self-administration during adulthood,[664,665] decreased exploratory behavior and grooming,[666] delayed eye maturation,[666] congenital hearing loss,[666] attentional disorder,[667] enhanced susceptibility to cocaine-induced seizures later in life,[668] and perinatal mortality.[669] Reported morphological abnormalities include hippocampal dysplasia[670] and neurodegeneration in the habenula.[671] In animals, cocaine decreases uterine and placental blood flow,[672-674] and serum cholinesterase levels are decreased during pregnancy.[675]

Animal studies also suggest that males exposed to cocaine before mating have an increased incidence of offspring with developmental abnormalities.[676]

Cocaine binds to spermatozoa, which could act as a vector to transport cocaine into an ovum.[677]

Several broad questions arise regarding cocaine's fetal effects in animals:

1. Are the effects secondary to uterine, placental, or fetal cerebrovascular vasoconstriction and CNS hypoxia, to direct neurotoxicity, or to both?[551,678,679] Does maternal malnutrition (aggravated by cocaine's anorexiogenic effects) contribute? Are indirect effects mediated through cocaine-induced cardiotoxicity? (Cocaine causes apoptosis in fetal cardiac cells.[680])

2. Does damage occur early in gestation, late in gestation, or both? Early damage would affect cytogenesis and cell migration; later damage would affect brain growth and differentiation. Evidence supports damage at both stages.[681,682]

3. Does the damage involve dopamine, serotonin, or other neurotransmitters (which early in development act as trophic factors)? Early in gestation, before CNS monoamine neurons are formed, systemic catecholamines can cross an immature fetal blood–brain barrier to influence neurodevelopment in a global fashion. Later, with formation of specific monoamine systems, the influence of dopamine and serotonin on brain development becomes more local. Cocaine (which, in the developing brain, binds more strongly to the serotonin transporter than the dopamine transporter[683]) could have disruptive effects at either stage.[684]

4. Do cocaine metabolites contribute to damage? In cultures of fetal rat mesencephalic neurons the cocaine metabolite norcocaine—but not cocaine itself—was cytotoxic to dopaminergic neurons, and fetal brains of rats prenatally exposed to cocaine had norcocaine concentrations capable of causing such cytotoxicity.[685]

5. Does activation by cocaine of immediate early genes in the developing brain alter gene expression and neuronal phenotype?[686] Cocaine inhibited DNA synthesis in fetal rat brain and the incorporation of thymidine in cultured glial cells.[687] By such a mechanism, effects on neurotransmitters could be indirect; for example, it has been suggested that cocaine-induced reduction of dopamine in developing brain is secondary to cocaine-induced reduction of glial cell line-derived neurotrophic factor (GDNF).[688] In monkeys, fetal midbrain levels of tyrosine hydroxylase (the rate-limiting enzyme in dopamine synthesis) are reduced and rostral forebrain levels of dopamine D_1 and D_2 receptors, preprodynorphin, and preproenkephalin are elevated.[689] Similarly in monkeys, fetal cocaine exposure increases levels of dopamine transporter mRNA in midbrain but not in striatum or rostral forebrain.[690]

6. Does fetal cocaine exposure produce neurochemical changes not evident at birth but appearing with maturity? In rats exposed prenatally to cocaine, basal levels of serotonin in multiple brain regions and of dopamine in striatum were reduced in adult animals but not immature animals.[691]

Maternal cocaine use is associated with congenital syphilis among newborns, and postnatal cocaine exposure carries its own hazards, especially upper and lower respiratory symptoms.[692] Infants have had tremor or seizures during nursing by cocaine-using mothers.[693,694] A 9-month-old developed status epilepticus after accidental ingestion of cocaine powder, and seizures occurred in an infant and a 2-year-old who passively inhaled "crack" smoke.[695] In a report from Boston City Hospital, cocaine metabolites were present in six of 250 (2.4%) urine assays of small children seen in the emergency room for problems unrelated to cocaine. Possible exposure routes included breast-feeding, intentional administration, accidental ingestion of the drug or of cocaine-contaminated dust, and passive inhalation of "crack" smoke.[696] Dramatically illustrating the spectrum of pediatric cocaine catastrophes, one report described six fatal cases: intrauterine death of a 35-week fetus, anoxic encephalopathy at birth with 3 months' vegetative survival, traumatic asphyxia in a 4-month-old, infectious cardiomyopathy at age 21 months following maternal cocaine abuse at birth, malnutrition and dehydration in a 7-week-old, and poisoning of a 6-week-old by his teenage brother.[697]

Long-term Treatment

The Limits of Analogy

The long-term treatment of cocaine addiction is unsatisfactory (Table 5–5). Three types of pharmacotherapy are used to treat substance abuse, namely agonists (methadone for heroin, nicotine patch for tobacco); antagonists (naltrexone for

Table 5–5. Long-term Treatment

Dopamine agonism
Tricyclic antidepressants
Bromocriptine
Amantadine
Methylphenidate
Mazindol
Bupropion
Indatraline
Monoamine oxidase inhibitors
L-dopa
Cocaine analogs
Cocaethylene
Dopamine antagonism and partial agonism
Phenothiazines
Haloperidol
Flupenthixol
Raclopride
Serotonin agonism
Selective serotonin reuptake inhibitors (SSRIs)
Fenfluramine
Serotonin antagonism
Para-chlorophenylalanine
Ritanserin
Opioid agonism and antagonism
Methadone
Buprenorphine
Kappa receptor agonists
Naltrexone
Anticonvulsant and GABAergic agents
Carbamazepine
Gamma-vinyl-GABA
Baclofen
Gabapentin
Benzodiazepines
Glutamate inhibition
Lamotrigine
Memantine
Dextromethorphan
Acamprosate
Other
Methyllycacotinine
Disulfiram
Cannabinoids
Ibogaine
Sigma receptor ligands
Calcium channel blockers
Immunotherapy
For pre-existing psychiatric disorder
Desipramine
Lithium
Methylphenidate
Acupuncture
Psychotherapy
Contingency contracts
Self-help groups

heroin), and metabolic modulators (disulfiram for ethanol).[698] For cocaine, identification of an effective agent in any of these three categories has proved elusive.

Environmental Confounders

Animal studies reveal a myriad of environmental variables that affect cocaine self-administration, the efficacy of different pharmacological agents, or both.[699,700]

1. Unit dose of cocaine self administration. As noted above, with increasing dose cocaine self-administration demonstrates an "inverted U-shaped" dose–response curve. The descending limb could represent a satiation effect, motor or aversive effects, or both. The efficacy of dopamine agonists and dopamine antagonists in reducing self-administration becomes less as unit dose increases.

2. Schedule of cocaine self-administration. The efficacy of dopamine antagonists, the selective serotonin reuptake inhibitor fluoxetine, and the opioid partial agonist buprenorphine vary markedly with dosage schedule. Not only are there differences that depend on whether animals are responding under fixed ratio schedules, fixed interval schedules, or progressive ratio schedules (see Chapter 2), but within each type of schedule, varying the response rate or interval that produces reward can determine whether an agent reduces self-administration.

3. Schedule of nondrug stimuli. Punishment (e.g., electric shock) accompanying cocaine self-administration facilitates pharmacological efficacy; so do alternative reinforcers (e.g., food). (Extrapolating such observations to humans, availability of alternative reinforcers could be made contingent on participating in a treatment program.)

4. Conditioned stimuli. Presentation of drug-paired stimuli during various schedules of cocaine delivery increases self-administration (see Chapter 2).

5. Food deprivation. Rates of cocaine self-administration are much higher in food-deprived rats than in satiated rats.

6. Environmental stressors. Physical stress (footshock), emotional stress (observing another rat receiving footshock), and social stress (an

aggressive same-sex intruder) enhance cocaine self-administration.

7. Rearing environment. Evidence is conflicting as to whether animals reared in isolation are more or less likely than those reared in groups to respond differently to psychostimulants, to self-administer cocaine, or to be affected by pharmacological therapy.

Pharmacotherapies

The sheer number of pharmacotherapies that have been studied or recommended for cocaine addiction reflects their collective ineffectiveness.

Direct or Indirect Dopamine Agonists

Desirable features of agonist substitution therapy are moderate agonism and slow onset of action. Numerous agents with different modes of action have been tried.

a. Bromocriptine, a direct agonist, suppressed cocaine self-administration in animals only at doses that caused stereotypic movements, and in human studies, some of which were placebo-controlled, a reduction in cocaine craving was offset by side effects.[702,703] In subsequent double-blind placebo-controlled trials, moreover, bromocriptine did not reduce cocaine subjective effects, craving, or use.[704-706]

b. Amantadine, an indirect dopamine agonist, appeared promising in early studies[707] but in properly controlled trials of sufficient duration was no better than placebo in reducing cocaine craving or use.[708,709]

c. Pergolide, a direct agonist, reduced insomnia and craving during cocaine withdrawal without causing side effects as often as bromocriptine.[710] Subsequent double-blind, placebo-controlled trials, however, failed to demonstrate efficacy.[711,712] In one study it was discovered that pergolide was being diverted for use as a street drug.[713]

d. Methylphenidate, an indirect agonist, actually increased cocaine craving in one study.[714] In a double-blind trial it was no better than placebo in affecting either retention or benzoylecgonine-positive urine screens.[715] (See below for methylphenidate's use in cocaine-using patients with attention deficit hyperactivity disorder.)

e. Desipramine is a tricyclic antidepressant that acts primarily as an inhibitor of norepinephrine reuptake. Early open-label trials with desipramine (and with other antidepressants, including imipramine, maprotiline, and trazodone) reported attenuated cocaine euphoria and reduced craving.[698,716,717] However, several double-blind, placebo-controlled trials of desipramine found no benefit.[698,718,719] Desipramine's usefulness in treating withdrawal depression is limited by a 1- to 2-week delay in onset of action. Moreover, some patients experience the "early tricyclic jitteriness syndrome," with symptoms resembling mild cocaine intoxication and paradoxically triggering craving.[720] Desipramine can potentiate cocaine's pressor effects.[721]

f. Mazindol, a dopamine reuptake blocker that appears free of abuse potential, was promising in a preliminary study lasting 4 weeks.[722] Subsequent trials failed to confirm benefit.[723,724] Similarly ineffective was the reuptake blocker bupropion.[725] In monkeys the long-acting nonselective monoamine reuptake inhibitor indatraline reduced cocaine self-administration, but it also reduced food intake and produced behavioral stereotypies.[726]

g. Monoamine oxidase inhibitors are indirectly dopaminergic. An early trial with phenylzine was promising.[727] A later trial with selegiline found no benefit.[728]

h. A single trial of L-DOPA/carbidopa similarly found no benefit.[729]

i. Cocaine itself is orally psychoactive, and its slow onset of action minimizes abuse liability by this route, as exemplified by coca leaf chewers and coca tea drinkers in South America. In a study lasting 2 weeks, oral cocaine (up to 100 mg four times daily) attenuated the acute psychological effects of an intravenous cocaine (25 or 50 mg) challenge. In nonhuman primates several cocaine analogs reduced cocaine self-administration.[730]

j. In rats, cocaine and cocaethylene produced equivalent degrees of behavioral activation and increased brain extracellular dopamine levels; rapid tolerance developed to cocaethylene effects, with diminished subsequent response to a cocaine challenge. Such tolerance did not occur in the cocaine-receiving rats, suggesting potential for cocaethylene as an agonist therapy.[731]

Two Cochrane reviews concluded that evidence does not support the use of either dopamine agonists or antidepressants to treat cocaine dependence.[731a,731b] A possible reason for the lack of benefit might be that such agents in sensitized patients either directly trigger craving or enhance responses to external cocaine cues.[22]

Dopamine Antagonists and Partial Agonists

a. In animals chlorpromazine decreased cocaine self-administration only at doses that reduced food responding as well.[701] In humans phenothiazines and haloperidol did not completely block cocaine euphoria and aggravated anhedonic withdrawal symptoms.[732]
b. Flupenthixol, a xanthine antidepressant, at low doses selectively blocks dopamine D_2 autoreceptors (thereby acting as an indirect dopamine agonist at the level of the nucleus accumbens). A preliminary study with cocaine outpatients was promising,[733] but subsequent studies did not bear out the promise.[698]
c. As noted above, drugs acting as selective dopamine D_3-receptor partial agonists reduce cocaine self-administration in animals.[36,37] D_3-receptor antagonists, including raclopride and nafodotride, attenuate cocaine craving in humans. A D_3-receptor antagonist is currently undergoing clinical trial.[103a,734]

Serotonin Agonists

a. Fluoxetine, a selective serotonin reuptake inhibitor (SSRI), attenuated the subjective effects of cocaine in human volunteers.[735] Early open-label studies were also promising.[698] Subsequent double-blind placebo-controlled trials, however, were largely negative.[736,737] One study did suggest efficacy of fluoxetine in cocaine abusers receiving methadone maintenance therapy.[738] In an open-label study of cocaine abusers with comorbid depression who had failed treatment with desipramine the SSRI venlafaxine appeared to be of benefit.[739] In a study of cocaine abusers and comorbid depression and alcoholism fluoxetine was no better than placebo.[740]
b. In an open-label trial the serotonin agonist fenfluramine combined with the dopamine agonist phentermine attenuated cocaine withdrawal symptoms but was no more effective than placebo in promoting abstinence.[741] (This drug combination was subsequently withdrawn from the market because of its association with valvular heart disease. See Chapter 4.)

Serotonin Antagonists

a. In rats, para-chlorophenylalanine, a tryptophan hydroxylase inhibitor, decreased cocaine-seeking behavior. Human studies have not been conducted.
b. In a placebo-controlled, double-blind trial, ritanserin, a $5HT_2$ receptor antagonist, reduced cocaine craving but not cocaine use.[741a]

Opioid Agonists

a. In effective methadone maintenance programs (i.e., dosages of 60–120 mg daily: see Chapter 3) more patients stop regular cocaine use (69%) than start it (10%).[742]
b. Buprenorphine, a partial μ-receptor agonist and κ-receptor antagonist, acts as a μ-antagonist in the presence of high levels of μ-receptor ligands. In monkeys, buprenorphine reduced cocaine self-administration,[743] and early clinical trials suggested that it might be superior to methadone for patients dependent on both heroin and cocaine.[744] Subsequent clinical trials, however, showed buprenorphine was no better than methadone in preventing cocaine abuse (and inferior to methadone in treating heroin dependence).[745]
c. Kappa-receptor agonists such as dynorphin A are non-reinforcing and in animals decrease cocaine self-administration and block the development of sensitization.[746] The mechanism is probably a lowering of dopaminergic tone, either directly or indirectly (see Chapter 2). A number of κ-receptor agonists have been studied in animals, but human trials have not been conducted.[747] The observation that dopamine D_1 receptor stimulation is linked with dynorphin production suggests that selective D_1 receptor agonists, by indirectly facilitating κ receptors, might be useful in treating cocaine dependence.[748]

d. In patients with comorbid ethanol and cocaine dependence the μ-receptor antagonist naltrexone was no more effective than placebo.[749]

e. In monkeys self-administering "speedball" combinations of heroin and cocaine, the dopamine antagonist flupenthixol combined with the opioid antagonist quadazocine reduced self-administration, whereas neither agent was effective alone.[750]

Anticonvulsant and GABAergic Agents

a. On the basis of its anti-kindling properties, carbamazepine was selected as a potential treatment for cocaine dependence. Early studies, including a 12-week double-blind, placebo-controlled trial, were promising,[751] but a recent review of five randomized controlled trials concluded that carbamazepine is no better than placebo.[752]

b. Gamma-vinyl-GABA (GVG, Vigabatrin) inhibits GABA transaminase, thereby increasing GABAergic inhibition of dopaminergic neurotransmission in animals receiving cocaine and heroin.[753] In rats, GVG blocks cocaine-induced locomotor activity, position place preference, and cocaine self-administration.[754] Clinical trials are under way.[755]

c. As noted above, the GABA$_B$ receptor agonist baclofen reduces cocaine self-administration.[99,100] Baclofen attenuate cocaine craving in humans.[103a] Clinical trials are anticipated.

d. Gabapentin increases GABA turnover. A depressed cocaine-dependent woman discovered that her husband's gabapentin was an effective cocaine substitute, reducing her craving and anxiety. Clinical trials with gabapentin have been proposed.[756]

e. Benzodiazepines such as diazepam enhance GABA neurotransmission by binding nonspecifically to omega 1- and omega 2-receptors. The nonbenzodiazepine zolpidem binds only to omega 1-receptors (see Chapter 6). In rats diazepam prevented cocaine-induced place preference. Zolpidem did not.[757] There are no clinical studies, however, that support the use of benzodiazepines in cocaine dependence.

Drugs Affecting Glutamate Neurotransmission

Mice lacking a particular glutamate receptor, mGluR5, never become dependent on cocaine no matter how much they are given.[758] In rats, stimulation of the glutamatergic pathway from the hippocampal subiculum to the midbrain ventral tegmental area causes previously cocaine-addicted animals to resume self-administration.[759] In humans, however, lamotrigine, a glutamate release inhibitor, altered neither the subjective ratings nor the physiological responses to cocaine,[760] and memantine, a glutamate NMDA antagonist, increased cocaine's positive subjective ratings.[761] The NMDA antagonists phencyclidine and dizocilpine have unacceptable side effects that preclude clinical use. A less potent NMDA receptor blocker, dextromethorphan (present in over-the-counter cough remedies) attenuates cocaine-seeking in rats and might prove useful in humans. Acamprosate, which blocks glutamate release, reduces craving in alcoholics and might be effective in treating other dependencies.[762]

Agents Affecting Nicotinic Acetylcholine Receptors

In rats, intravenous infusion of cotinine, the major metabolite of nicotine, inhibited both nicotine- and cocaine-induced release of dopamine in the nucleus accumbens.[763] Methyllycaconitine, a selective antagonist of alpha 7 nicotinic ACh receptors, attenuated the reinforcing effects of both nicotine and cocaine.[764]

Disulfiram

Disulfiram inhibits dopamine beta-hydroxylase as well as acetaldehyde dehydrogenase (see Chapter 12). Giving disulfiram to human volunteers receiving cocaine increased their plasma cocaine concentrations, heart rates, blood pressures, and anxiety, suggesting that the presence of such negative effects coupled with inability to temper them with ethanol might be therapeutically useful.[765] In a double-blind placebo-controlled trial, however, disulfiram did not alter behavioral responses to cocaine.[766] In a study of methadone-maintained heroin addicts, disulfiram was associated with decreased use of cocaine, whether or not ethanol was also abused.[767] Similar findings occurred in a study of buprenorphine-maintained patients receiving disulfiram.[768]

Cannabinoids

As noted above, animals abstinent from cocaine will resume cocaine self-administration upon exposure to stress, presentation of cocaine-associated cues, or administration of low doses of cocaine. A cannabinoid receptor agonist (HU-210) also precipitates relapse, and a cannabinoid receptor antagonist (SR141716A) prevents relapse precipitated by cocaine or cocaine-associated cues (but not stress).[769] The antagonist has no effect on cocaine self-administration, i.e., it attenuates craving during abstinence but does not mediate the primary effects of the drug. The mechanism of cocaine–cannabinoid interaction is uncertain. Dopamine elicits anandamide (an endogenous cannabinoid ligand) in the striatum, and anandamide indirectly facilitates dopamine release by inhibiting inhibitory GABAergic interneurons.[770] Whether such observations will prove therapeutically useful remains to be seen.

Ibogaine

An indole alkaloid found in the West African shrub, *Tabernanthe iboga*, ibogaine produces complex psychic effects, including hallucinations (see Chapter 8). Multiple sites of action are described, including dopamine transporters, muscarinic cholinergic receptors, glutamate NMDA receptors, opioid κ receptors, serotonin receptors, ζ receptors, voltage-dependent sodium and calcium channels, and neurotensin and substance P systems.[771-774] In rats ibogaine enhances sensitivity to the psychomotor stimulant effects of cocaine, but only in animals receiving cocaine chronically and only with low cocaine dosage.[775] It inhibits cocaine self-administration in rodents.[776] Ibogaine engendered considerable media attention as a possible treatment for multiple drug dependencies, including cocaine. Anecdotal reports in humans described interruption of drug-seeking behavior for several months after a single dose.[777] A Schedule I drug, ibogaine causes whole-body tremors and at high doses cerebellar damage.[778] These problems have spawned a search for more effective and safer structural derivatives.

Sigma-Receptor Ligands

The physiological role of ζ receptors remains uncertain, but ζ-receptor ligands attenuate the locomotor stimulatory effects of cocaine.[779]

Calcium Channel Blockers

In rats isradipine (an L-type calcium channel blocker) decreased cocaine-induced place preference.[780] In humans a related drug amlodipine reduced craving, but side effects (flushing, headache, fatigue) were common.[781]

Immunotherapy

Cocaine is hydrolyzed by liver carboxylesterases and plasma butyrylcholinesterase (BChE) (also known as pseudocholinesterase) to benzoylecgonine and ecgonine methyl ester. (A lesser metabolic pathway in the liver generates norcocaine.) In rodents, pretreatment with BChE attenuates the acute physiological and behavioral effects of cocaine. The effect lasts for only a few days, however.[782] Another approach is immunotherapy; both active and passive immunization with cocaine vaccines have been studied in animals.[783,784] A problem with this approach is that cocaine can bind 250 times its weight in antibody, and so large doses would likely overwhelm circulating antibody levels. A novel strategy is to use catalytic antibodies that cleave cocaine into inactive fragments and are then free to repeat the process many times per second.[785,786] Passive immunization with such an agent could last weeks.

Acupuncture

Among cocaine-dependent, methadone-maintained patients, those receiving acupuncture were more likely than no-needle controls to produce cocaine-negative urine; moreover, those whose needles were inserted in a part of the ear considered specific for the treatment of drug abuse were less likely to use cocaine than those whose needles were inserted in "non-specific" auricular areas.[787] Another study, less surprisingly, found no difference between "specific" and "non-specific" ear points.[788] (It goes without saying that the concept of "ear point specificity" in the treatment of substance abuse subverts much of what we know about mammalian anatomy and physiology.)

Comorbidity

Some cocaine users appear to be self-medicating pre-existing psychiatric illness. Studies estimate that depressive disorders are present in 30% of users, bipolar disorders in 20%, and attention deficit disorder in 5%; it is obviously difficult in some instances to tell cause from effect.[789] Both favorable and unfavorable results have been reported on the use of desipramine in those with pre-existing depression; lithium in those with bipolar disorder; methylphenidate, pemoline, or bromocriptine in those with attention deficit disorder; and neuroleptics in those with schizophrenia.[790-796] Cocaine use fluctuated with depressed mood in two patients with seasonal affective disorder.[797]

Anorexia nervosa and bulimia also occur with unexpected frequency among cocaine users.[798] So do alcoholism, anxiety disorders, antisocial personality, pathological gambling, and sensation seeking.[789,799-802] In one report, alcoholism was currently present in 29% of cocaine users seeking treatment, with a lifetime prevalence of 62%, "nearly twice the rate of alcoholism seen in opioid addicts."[789] In contrast to opioid addicts, cocaine users tended to become alcoholic after abusing cocaine, perhaps as a means of reducing cocaine-induced anxiety and insomnia.

Psychotherapy

As with other substance abuse, psychotherapy may have adjunctive benefit but is of little value used alone.[803] The role of pavlovian conditioning in craving is the basis for extinction therapy: presenting cocaine-associated stimuli until they lose their ability to provoke conditioned responses.[804] Other approaches include cognitive therapy, "supportive-expressive psychodynamic therapy," "group drug counseling," and residential programs. Whatever approach or medication is used, outpatients require regular physician visits, urine testing, counseling, and education (which should include other family members). Medication can be given for 4 to 6 months, with retreatment for relapse. Given the frustrations of medical therapy, it is not surprising that self-help and peer groups (Cocaine Anonymous) have proliferated.[805-807]

References

1. Bozarth MA. New perspectives on cocaine addiction: recent findings from animal research. Can J Physiol Pharmacol 1989; 67:1158.

2. Johanson C-E, Fischman MW. The pharmacology of cocaine related to its abuse. Pharmacol Rev 1989; 41:3.

3. Post RM, Rose H. Increasing effects of repetitive cocaine administration in the rat. Nature 1976; 260:731.

4. Karler R, Petty C. Calder L, Turkanis SA. Proconvulsant and anticonvulsant effects in mice of acute and chronic treatment with cocaine. Neuropharmacology 1989; 28:709.

5. Post RM, Weiss SRB. Psychomotor stimulant vs. local anesthetic effects of cocaine: role of behavioral sensitization and kindling. NIDA Res Monogr 1988; 88:217.

6. Reith MEA, Meisler BE, Lajtha A. Locomotor effects of cocaine, cocaine congeners and local anesthetics in mice. Pharmacol Biochem Behav 1985; 23:831.

7. Ambre JJ, Belknap SSM, Nelson J, et al. Acute tolerance to cocaine in humans. Clin Pharmacol Ther 1988; 44:1.

8. Aigner TC, Balster RL. Choice behavior in rhesus monkeys: cocaine versus food. Science 1978; 201:534.

9. Johanson CE. Assessment of the dependence potential of cocaine in animals. NIDA Res Monogr 50, 1984; 50:54.

10. Bozarth MA, Wise RA. Toxicity associated with long-term intravenous heroin and cocaine self-administration in the rat. JAMA 1985; 254:81.

11. Johanson C-E, Balster RL, Bonese K. Self-administration of psychomotor stimulant drugs: the effects of unlimited access. Pharmacol Biochem Behav 1976; 4:45.

12. Winger GD, Woods JH. Comparison of fixed-ratio and progressive ratio schedules of maintenance of stimulant drug-reinforced responding. Drug Alcohol Depend 1985; 15:123.

13. Yanagita T. An experimental framework for evaluation of dependence liability in various types of drugs in monkeys. Bull Narc 1973; 25:57.

14. Lakoski JM, Cunningham KA. Cocaine interaction with central monoaminergic systems: electrophysiological approaches. Trends Pharmacol Sci 1988; 9:177.

15. Ritz MC, Lamb RJ, Goldberg SR, Kuhar MJ. Cocaine receptors on dopamine transporters are related to self-administration of cocaine. Science 1987; 237:1219.

16. Shimada S, Kitayama S, Lin C-L, et al. Cloning and expression of a cocaine-sensitive dopamine transporter complementary DNA. Science 1991; 254:576.

17. Kilty JE, Lorang D, Amara SG. Cloning and expression of a cocaine-sensitive rat dopamine transporter. Science 1991; 254:578.

18. Pacholczyk T, Blakely RD, Amara SG. Expression cloning of a cocaine- and antidepressant-sensitive human noradrenaline transporter. Nature 1991; 350:350.

19. Seiden LS, Kleven MS. Lack of toxic effects of cocaine on dopamine or serotonin neurons in the rat brain. NIDA Res Monogr 1988; 88:276.

20. Callahan PM, delaGarza R, Cunningham KA. Mediation of the discriminative stimulus properties of cocaine by mesocorticolimbic dopamine systems. Pharmacol Biochem Behav 1999; 57:601.

21. Wise R, Bozarth MA. A psychomotor theory of addiction. Psychol Rev 1987; 94:469.

22. Childress AR, Mozley PD, McElgin W, et al. Limbic activation during cue-induced cocaine craving. Am J Psychiatry 1999; 156:11.

23. Volkow ND, Fowler JS. Addiction, a disease of compulsion and drive: involvement of the orbitofrontal cortex. Cereb Cortex 2000; 10:318.

24. Volkow ND, Fowler JS, Wang G-J. Role of dopamine in drug reinforcement and addiction in humans: results from imaging studies. Behav Pharmacol 2002; 13:355.

25. Wood DM, Emmett-Oglesby MW. Substitution and cross-tolerance profiles of anorectic drugs in rats trained to detect the discriminative stimulus properties of cocaine. Psychopharmacology 1988; 95:364.

26. McKenna ML, Ho BT. The role of dopamine in the discriminative stimulus properties of cocaine. Neuropharmacology 1980; 19:297.

27. de la Garza R, Johanson C-E. Discriminative stimulus properties of cocaine in pigeons. Psychopharmacology 1985; 85:23.

28. Huang J, Wilson MC. Comparative stimulus properties of cocaine and other local anesthetics in rats. Res Commun Subst Abuse 1982; 3:120.

29. Yokel RA, Wise RA. Amphetamine-type reinforcement by dopaminergic agonists in the rat. Psychopharmacology 1978; 58:289.

30. Woolverton WL, Goldberg LI, Ginos JZ. Intravenous self-administration of dopamine receptor agonists by rhesus monkeys. J Pharmacol Exp Ther 1984; 230:678.

31. Woolverton WL. Evaluation of the role of norepinephrine in the reinforcing effects of psychomotor stimulants in rhesus monkeys. Pharmacol Biochem Behav 1987; 26:835.

32. Ritz MC, Lamb RJ, Goldberg SR, Kuhar MJ. Cocaine receptors on dopamine transporters are related to self-administration of cocaine. Science 1987; 237:1219.

33. Pettit HD, Justice JB. Effect of dose on cocaine self-administration behavior and dopamine levels in the nucleus accumbens. Brain Res 1991; 539:94.

34. Campbell UC, Rodefer JS, Carroll ME. Effects of dopamine antagonists (D_1 and D_2) on the demand for smoked cocaine base in rhesus monkeys. Psychopharmacology 1999; 144:381.

35. Khroyan TV, Barrett-Larimore RL, Rowlett JK, Spealman RD. Dopamine D_1- and D_2-like receptor mechanisms in relapse to cocaine-seeking behavior: effects of selective antagonists and agonists. J Pharmacol Exp Ther 2000; 294:680.

36. Pilla M, Perahon S, Sautel F, et al. Selective inhibition of cocaine-seeking behavior by a partial dopamine D_3 receptor agonist. Nature 1999; 400:371.

37. Koob GF, Caine SB. Cocaine addiction therapy—are we partially there? Nat Med 1999; 5:993.

38. Goeders NE, Smith JE. Reinforcing properties of cocaine in the medial prefrontal cortex: primary action on presynaptic dopaminergic terminals. Pharmacol Biochem Behav 1986; 25:191.

39. Goeders NE, Dworkin SI, Smith JE. Neuropharmacological assessment of cocaine self-administration into the medial prefrontal cortex. Pharmacol Biochem Behav 1986; 24:1429.

40. McBride WJ, Murphy JM, Ikemoto S. Localization of brain reinforcement mechanism: intracranial self-administration and intracranial place-conditioning studies. Behav Brain Res 1999; 101:129.

41. Prasad BM, Hochstatter T, Sorg BA. Expression of cocaine sensitization: regulation by the medial prefrontal cortex. Neuroscience 1999; 88:765.

42. Hedou G, Feldon J, Heidbreder CA. Effects of cocaine on dopamine in subregions of the rat prefrontal cortex and their efferents to subterritories of the nucleus accumbens. Eur J Pharmacol 1999; 372:143.

43. Dworkin SI, Smith JE. Neurobehavioral pharmacology of cocaine. NIDA Res Monogr 1988; 88:185.

44. Roberts DCS, Koob GF. Disruption of cocaine self-administration following 6-hydroxydopamine lesions of the ventral tegmental area in rats. Pharmacol Biochem Behav 1982; 17:901.

45. Hubner CB, Koob GF. Ventral pallidal lesions produce decreases in cocaine and heroin self-administration in the rat. Soc Neurosci Abstr 1987; 13:1717.

46. Beyer CE, Steketee JD. Dopamine depletion in the medial prefrontal cortex induces sensitized-like behavioral and neurochemical responses to cocaine. Brain Res 1999; 833:133.

47. Self DW, Barnhart WJ, Lehman DA, Nestler EJ. Opposite modulation of cocaine-seeking behavior by D_1- and D_2-like dopamine receptor agonists. Science 1996; 271:1586.

48. Caine SB, Negus SS, Mello NK, Bergman J. Effects of dopamine D_1-like and D_2-like agonists in rats that self-administer cocaine. J Pharmacol Exp Ther 1999; 291:353.

49. Katz JL, Kopajtic TA, Myers KA, et al. Behavioral effects of cocaine: interactions with D_1 dopaminergic antagonists and agonists in mice and squirrel monkeys. J Pharmacol Exp Ther 1999; 291:265.

50. Neisewander JL, Lucki JL, McGonigle P. Time-dependent changes in sensitivity to apomorphine and monoamine receptors following withdrawal from continuous cocaine administration in rats. Synapse 1994; 16:1.

51. Gerfen CR. The neostriatal mosaic: multiple levels of compartmental organization in the basal ganglia. Annu Rev Neurosci 1992; 15:285.

52. Pilotte NS. Neurochemistry of cocaine withdrawal. Curr Opin Neurol 1997; 10:534.

53. King GR, Xiong Z, Douglas S, et al. The effects of continuous cocaine dose on the induction of behavioral tolerance and dopamine autoreceptor function. Eur J Pharmacol 1999; 376:207.

54. Kuhar MJ, Pilotte NS. Neurochemical changes in cocaine withdrawal. Trends Pharmacol Sci 1996; 17:260.

55. Moratalla R, Elibol B, Vallejo M, Graybiel AM. Network-level changes in expression of inducible fos-jun proteins in the striatum during chronic cocaine treatment and withdrawal. Neuron 1996; 17:147.

56. Volkow ND, Wang GJ, Fowler JS, et al. Decreased striatal dopaminergic responsiveness in detoxified cocaine-dependent subjects. Nature 1997; 386:830.

57. Volkow ND, Wang GJ, Fischman MW, et al. Relationship between subjective effects of cocaine and dopamine transporter occupancy. Nature 1997; 386:827.

58. Trulson MB, Babb S, Joe JC, et al. Chronic cocaine administration depletes tyrosine hydroxylase immunore-activity in the rat brain nigrostriatal system: quantitative light microscopic studies. Exp Neurol 1986; 94:744.

59. Wyatt RJ, Karuum F, Suddath R, et al. Persistently decreased brain dopamine levels and cocaine. JAMA 1988; 259:2996.

60. Gawin F, Ellinwood E. Cocaine and other stimulants. N Engl J Med 1988; 318:1173.

61. Uzbay IT, Wallis CJ, Lal H, Forster MJ. Effects of NMDA receptor blockers on cocaine-stimulated locomotor activity in mice. Behav Brain Res 2000; 108:57-61.

62. Druhan JP, Wilent WB. Effects of the competitive N-methyl-D-aspartate receptor antagonist, CPP, on the development and expression of conditioned hyperac-tivity and sensitization induced by cocaine. Behav Brain Res 1999; 102:195.

63. Karler R, Calder LD, Chaudhry IA, Turkanis SA. Blockade of "reverse tolerance" to cocaine and amphetamine by MK-801. Life Sci 1989; 45:599.

64. Kalivas PW, Alesdatter JE. Involvement of N-methyl-D-aspartate receptor stimulation in the ventral tegmen-tal area and amygdala in behavioral sensitization to cocaine. J Pharmacol Exp Ther 1993; 267:486.

65. Saal D, Dong Y, Bonci A, et al. Drugs of abuse and stress trigger a common synaptic adaptation in dopamine neurons. Neuron 2003; 37:577.

66. Unglass MA, Whistler JL, Malenka RC, et al. Single cocaine exposure in vivo induces long-term potentia-tion in dopamine neurons. Nature 2001; 411:583.

67. Nestler EJ. Total recall–the memory of addiction. Science 2001; 292:2266.

68. Kelz MB, Chen J, Carlezon WA, et al. Expression of the transcription factor ΔfosB in the brain controls sensitivity to cocaine. Nature 1999; 401:272.

69. White FJ, Hu XT, Zhang XF. Neuroadaptations in nucleus accumbens neurons resulting from repeated cocaine administration. Adv Pharmacol 1998; 42:1006.

70. Peoples LL, Uzwiak AJ, Guyette FX, West MO. Tonic inhibition of single nucleus accumbens neurons in the rat: a predominant but not exclusive firing pattern induced by cocaine self-administration sessions. Neuroscience 1998; 86:13.

71. Sutton MA, Schmidt EF, Choi K-H, et al. Extinction-induced upregulation in AMPA receptors reduces cocaine-seeking behavior. Nature 2003; 421:70.

72. Ghasemzadeh MB, Nelson LC, Lu X-Y, Kalivas PW. Neuroadaptations in ionotropic and metabotropic glu-tamate receptor mRNA produced by cocaine treatment. J Neurochem 1999; 72:157.

73. Churchill L, Swanson CJ, Urbina M, Kalivas PW. Repeated cocaine alters glutamate receptor subunit levels in the nucleus accumbens and ventral tegmental area of rats that develop behavioral sensitization. J Neurochem 1999; 72:2397.

74. Holden C. Zapping memory center triggers drug craving. Science 2001; 292:1039.

75. Vorel SR, Liu X, Hayes RJ, et al. Relapse to cocaine-seeking after hippocampal theta burst stimulation. Science 2001; 292:1175.

76. Witkin JM, Tortella FC. Modulators of N-methyl-D-aspartate protect against diazepam- or phenobarbi-tal-resistant cocaine convulsions. Life Sci 1991; 48:PL51.

77. Hurd YL. Cocaine effects on dopamine and opioid peptide neural systems: implications for human cocaine abuse. NIDA Res Monogr 1996; 163:94.

78. Yoburn BC, Luffy K, Sierra V. In vitro d-amphetamine and cocaine increase opioid binding in mouse brain homogenate. NIDA Res Monogr 1991; 105:522.

79. Misra AL, Pontani RB, Vadlamani NL. Blockade of tolerance to morphine analgesia by cocaine. Pain 1989; 38:77.

80. Shippenberg TS, Rea W. Sensitization and behavioral effects of cocaine: modulation by dynorphin and kappa-opioid receptor agonists. Pharmacol Biochem Behav 1997; 57:449.

81. Chefer V, Thompson AC, Shippenberg TS. Modula-tion of cocaine-induced sensitization by kappa-opioid receptor agonists. Ann N Y Acad Sci 2001; 937:803.

82. Sharpe LG, Pilotte NS, Shippenberg TS, et al. Autoradiographic evidence that prolonged withdrawal from intermittent cocaine reduces mu-opioid receptor expression in limbic regions of the rat brain. Synapse 2000; 37:292.

83. White FJ. Cocaine and the serotonin saga. Nature 1998; 393:118.

84. Loh EA, Roberts DC. Break-points on a progressive ratio schedule reinforced by intravenous cocaine increase following depletion of forebrain serotonin. Psychopharmacology 1990; 101:262.

85. Rocha BA, Scearce-Levie K, Lucas JJ, et al. Increased vulnerability to cocaine in mice lacking the serotonin-1B receptor. Nature 1998; 393:175.

86. Shippenberg TS, Hen R, He M. Region-specific enhancement of basal extracellular and cocaine-evoked dopamine levels following constitutive deletion of the serotonin-1B receptor. J Neurochem 2000; 75:258.

87. Callahan PM, Cunningham KA. Modulation of the dis-criminative stimulus properties of cocaine by 5-HT1B and 5-HT2C receptors. J Pharmacol Exp Ther 1995; 274:1414.

88. Cameron DL, Williams JT. Cocaine inhibits GABA release in the VTA through endogenous 5-HT. J Neurosci 1994; 14:3763.

89. Belzung C, Scearce-Levie K, Barreau S, Hen R. Absence of cocaine-induced place conditioning in serotonin 1B receptor knockout mice. Pharmacol Biochem Behav 2000; 66:221.

90. De la Garza R, Cunningham KA. The effects of the 5-hydroxytryptamine$_{1A}$ agonist 8-hydroxy-2-(di-n-propylamino)tetralin on spontaneous activity, cocaine-induced hyperactivity, and behavioral sensitization: a microanalysis of locomotor activity. J Pharmacol Exp Ther 2000; 292:610.

91. Walsh SL, Cunningham KA. Serotonergic mechanisms involved in the discriminative stimulus, reinforcing, and subjective effects of cocaine. Psychopharmacology 1997; 130:41.

92. Yan Q, Reith ME, Yan S. Enhanced accumbal dopamine release following 5-HT (2A) receptor stimulation in rats pretreated with intermittent cocaine. Brain Res 2000; 863:254.

93. King GR, Xiong Z, Douglass S, Ellinwood EH. Long-term blockade of the expression of cocaine sensitization by ondansetron, a 5HT (3) receptor antagonist. Eur J Pharmacol 2000; 394:97.

94. McMahon LR, Cunningham KA. Antagonism of 5-hydroxytryptamine (4) receptors attenuates hyperactivity induced by cocaine: putative role for 5-hydroxytryptamine (4) receptors in the nucleus accumbens shell. J Pharmacol Exp Ther 1999; 291:300.

95. Peris J. Repeated cocaine injections decrease the function of striatal gamma-aminobutyric acid$_A$ receptors. J Pharmacol Exp Ther 1996; 276:1002.

96. Jung BJ, Dawson R, Sealey SA, Peris J. Endogenous GABA release is reduced in the striatum of cocaine-sensitized rats. Synapse 1999; 34:103.

97. Shoji S, Simms D, McDaniel WC, Gallagher JP. Chronic cocaine enhances gamma-aminobutyric acid and glutamate release by altering presynaptic and not postsynaptic gamma-aminobutyric acid$_B$ receptors within the rat dorsolateral septal nucleus. J Pharmacol Exp Ther 1997; 280:129.

98. Resnick A, Homanics GE, Jung BE, Peris J. Increased acute cocaine sensitivity and decreased cocaine sensitization in GABA(A) receptor beta3 subunit knockout mice. J Neurochem 1999; 73:1539.

99. Campbell UC, Lac ST, Carroll ME. Effects of baclofen on maintenance and reinstatement of intravenous cocaine self-administration in rats. Psychopharmacology 1999; 143:209.

100. Brebner K, Phelan R, Roberts DC. Effect of baclofen on cocaine self-administration in rats reinforced under fixed-ratio 1 and progressive-ratio schedules. Psychopharmacology 2000; 148:314.

101. Mark GP, Kinney AE, Grubb MC, Keys AS. Involvement of acetylcholine in the nucleus accumbens in cocaine reinforcement. Ann N Y Acad Sci 1999; 877:792.

102. Ikemoto S, Goeders NE. Intra-medial prefrontal cortex injections of scopolamine increase instrumental responses for cocaine: an intravenous self-administration study in rats. Brain Res Bull 2000; 51:151.

103. Zhang W, Yamada M, Gomeza J, et al. Multiple muscarinic acetylcholine receptor subtypes modulate striatal dopamine release, as studied with M1-M5 muscarinic receptor knock-out mice. J Neurosci 2002; 22:6347.

103a. Moyer P. Addiction: new clues from neuroscience. Neurology Today, April 2003:29.

104. Xu F, Gainetdinov RR, Wetsel WC, et al. Mice lacking the norepinephrine transporter are supersensitive to psychostimulants. Nat Neurosci 2000; 3:465.

105. DeVries TJ, Shaham Y, Homberg JR, et al. A cannabinoid mechanism in relapse to cocaine seeking. Nat Med 2001; 7:1151.

106. Hiroi N, Fienberg AA, Haile CN, et al. Neuronal and behavioral abnormalities in striatal function in DARPP-32-mutant mice. Eur J Neurosci 1999; 11:1114.

107. Gupta A, Tsai L-H. A kinase to dampen the effects of cocaine? Science 2001; 292:236.

108. Bibb JA, Chen J, Taylor JR, et al. Effects of chronic exposure to cocaine are regulated by the neuronal protein Cdk5. Nature 2001; 410:376.

109. Koylu EO, Couceyro PR, Lambert PD, Kuhar MJ. Cocaine- and amphetamine-regulated transcript peptide immunohistochemical localization in the rat brain. J Comp Neurol 1998; 391:115.

110. Adams RD, Gong W, Vechia SD, et al CART: from gene to function. Brain Res 1999; 848:137.

111. Messer CJ, Eisch AJ, Carlezon WA. Role for GDNF in biochemical and behavioral adaptations to drugs of abuse. Neuron 2000; 26:247.

112. Broadbear JH, Winger G, Cicero TJ, Woods JH. Effects of self-administered cocaine on plasma adrenocorticotropic hormone and cortisol in male rhesus monkeys. J Pharmacol Exp Ther 1999; 289:1641.

113. Richter RM, Weiss F. In vivo CRF release in rat amygdala is increased during cocaine withdrawal in self-administering rats. Synapse 1999; 32:254.

114. Shaham Y, Erb S, Stewart J. Stress-induced relapse to heroin and cocaine seeking in rats: a review. Brain Res Rev 2000; 33:13.

115. Erb S, Stewart J. A role for the bed nucleus of the stria terminalis, but not the amygdala, in the effects of corticotropin-releasing factor on stress-induced reinstatement of cocaine seeking. J Neurosci 1999; 19:RC35.

116. Galici R, Pechnick RN, Poland RE, France CP. Comparison of noncontingent versus contingent cocaine administration on plasma corticosterone levels in rats. Eur J Pharmacol 2000; 387:59.

117. Tan A, Moratalla R, Lyford GA, et al. The activity-regulated cytoskeletal-associated protein arc is expressed in different striosome-matrix patterns following exposure to amphetamine and cocaine. J Neurochem 2000; 74:2074.

118. Byrnes JJ, Pantke MM, Onton JA, Hammer JP. Inhibition of nitric oxide synthase in the ventral tegmental area attenuates cocaine sensitization in rats. Prog Neuropsychopharmacol Biol Psychiatry 2000; 24:261.

119. Javaid JI, Musa MN, Fischman MW, et al. Kinetics of cocaine in humans after intravenous and intranasal administration. Biopharm Drug Dispos 1983; 4:9.

120. Busto U, Bendayan R, Sallers EM. Clinical pharmacokinetics of non-opiate abused drugs. Clin Pharmacokin 1989; 16:1.

121. Weiss RD, Gawin FH. Protracted elimination of cocaine metabolites in long-term, high-dose cocaine abusers. Am J Med 1988; 85:879.

122. Devenyi P. Cocaine complications and cholinesterase. Ann Intern Med 1989; 110:167.

123. Graham K, Koren G, Klein J, et al. Determination of gestational cocaine exposure by hair analysis. JAMA 1989; 262:3328.

124. Weinhaus SB, Tzanani N, Dogan S, et al. Fast analysis of drugs in a single hair. J Am Soc Mass Spectrom 1998; 9:1311.

125. Garside D, Ropero-Miller JD, Goldberger BA, et al. Identification of cocaine analytes in fingernail and toenail specimens. J Forensic Sci 1998; 43:974.

126. Fendrich M, Johnson TP, Sudman S, et al. Validity of drug use reporting in a high-risk community sample: a comparison of cocaine and heroin survey reports with hair tests. Am J Epidemiol 1999; 149:955.

127. Cartmell LW, Aufderhide A, Weems C. Cocaine metabolites in pre-Colombian mummy hair. J Okla State Med Assoc 1991; 84:11.

128. Schoenberg BS. Coke's the one: the centennial of the "ideal brain tonic" that became a symbol of America. South Med J 1988; 81:70.

129. Freud S. Über Coca. Zentralbl Ther 1884; 2:289.

130. Goldberg MF. Cocaine: the first local anesthetic and the "third scourge of humanity." Arch Ophthalmol 1984; 102:1143.

131. Gay P. Freud. A Life for Our Time. New York: WH Norton Co, 1988.

132. Penfield W. Halsted of Johns Hopkins. The man and his problem as described in the secret records of William Osler. JAMA 1969; 210:2215.

133. Musto DF. International traffic in coca through the early 20th century. Drug Alcohol Dep 1998; 49:145.

134. O'Malley PM, Bachman JG, Johnson LD. Period, age, and cohort effects on substance use among American youth, 1976–1982. Am J Public Health 1984; 74:682.

135. Van Dyck C, Byck R. Cocaine. Sci Am 1982; 246:128.

136. Barnes DM. Drugs: running the numbers. Science 1988; 240:1729.

137. Pollock DA, Holmgreen P, Lui K-J, Kirk ML. Discrepancies in the reported frequency of cocaine-related deaths, United States, 1983 through 1988. JAMA 1991; 266:2233.

138. Rogers JN, Henry TE, Jones AM, et al. Cocaine-related deaths in Pima County, Arizona, 1982-1984. J Forensic Sci 1986; 31:1404.

139. Sander R, Ryser MA, Lamoreaux TC, Raleigh K. An epidemic of cocaine-associated deaths in Utah. J Forensic Sci 1985; 30:478.

140. Cornwell PD, Valentour JC. Cocaine deaths in Virginia. Med Leg Bull 1986; 35:1.

141. Tardiff K, Gross E, Wu J, et al. Analysis of cocaine positive fatalities. J Forensic Sci 1989; 34:53.

142. Bailey DN, Shaw RF. Cocaine- and methamphetamine-related deaths in San Diego County (1984): homicides and accidental overdoses. J Forensic Sci 1989; 34:407.

143. Hood I, Ryan D, Monforte J, Valentour J. Cocaine in Wayne County medical examiner's cases. J Forensic Sci 1990; 35:591.

144. McKelway R, Vieweg V, Westerman P. Sudden death from acute cocaine intoxication in Virginia in 1988. Am J Psychiatry 1990; 147:1667.

145. Shaner A, Eckman TA, Roberts LJ, et al. Disability income, cocaine use, and repeated hospitalization among schizophrenic cocaine abusers: a government-sponsored revolving door. N Engl J Med 1995; 333:777.

146. Phillips DP, Christenfield N, Ryan NM. An increase in the number of deaths in the United States in the first week of the month. An association with substance abuse and other causes of death. N Engl J Med 1999; 341:93.

147. Tardiff K, Gross EM, Messner SF. A study of homicides in Manhattan. Am J Public Health 1986; 76:139.

148. Marshall E. Testing urine for drugs. Science 1988; 214:150.

149. Nadelmann EA. Drug prohibition in the United States: costs, consequences, and alternatives. Science 1989; 245:939.

150. Hanzlick R, Gowitt GT. Cocaine metabolite detection in homicide victims. JAMA 1991; 265:760.

151. Haruff RC, Francisco JT, Elkins SK, et al. Cocaine and homicide in Memphis and Shelby County: an epidemic of violence. J Forensic Sci 1988; 33:1231.

152. Goldstein PJ. The drugs–violence nexus: a tripartite conceptual framework. J Drug Issues 1985; 15:493.

153. De La Rosa M, Lambert EY, Gropper B, eds. Drugs and Violence: Causes, Correlates, and Consequences. NIDA Res Monogr 1990:103.

154. Marzuk PM, Tardiff K, Leon AC, et al. Prevalence of recent cocaine use among motor vehicle fatalities in New York City. JAMA 1990; 263:250.

155. Shenon P. The score on drugs: it depends on how you see the figures. NY Times, April 22, 1990.

156. Lane C, Waller D, Larmer B, Katel P. The newest war. Newsweek, January 6, 1992.

157. Hollander JE, Hoffman RS. Cocaine. In: Goldfrank LR, Flomenbaum NE, Lewin NA, et al. Goldfrank's Toxicologic Emergencies, 6th Edition. Stamford, CT, Appleton & Lange, 1998: 1071.

158. Stone M. Coke Inc. New York Magazine, July 16, 1990.

159. Kleber HD. Tracking the cocaine epidemic. JAMA 1991; 266:2272.

160. Massing M. Whatever happened to the "War on Drugs"? New York Review of Books, June 11, 1992.

161. Treaster JB. Drop in youths' cocaine use may reflect a societal shift. NY Times, January 25, 1991.

162. Jarvik ME. The drug dilemma: manipulating the demand. Science 1990; 250:387.

163. Gelb LH. Yet another summit. NY Times, November 3, 1991.

164. Califano JA: Substance abuse and addiction—the need to know. Am J Public Health 1998; 88:9.

165. Lange RA, Hillis LD. Cardiovascular complications of cocaine use. N Engl J Med 2001; 345:351-358.

166. Doyle R: Why do prisons grow? Sci Am 2001; December:28.

167. Helmuth L. Has America's tide of violence receded for good? Science 2000; 289:582.

168. Golden T. Mexican connection grows as cocaine supplier to U.S. NY Times, July 30, 1995.

169. Dillon S. Bribes and publicity mark fall of Mexican drug lord. NY Times, May 12, 1995.

170. Krauff C, Rahter L. Dominican drug traffickers tighten grip on the northeast. NY Times, October 11, 1998.

171. Bonner R. Poland becomes a major conduit for drug traffic. NY Times, December 30, 1993.

172. Rohter L. A web of drugs and strife in Colombia. NY Times, April 21, 2000.

173. Forero J. Farmers in Peru are turning again to coca crop. NY Times, February 14, 2002.

174. Lifsher M. In U.S. drug war, ally Bolivia loses ground to farmers. Wall St. Journal, May 13, 2003.

174a. Zurita-Vargas L. Coca culture. NY Times, October 15, 2003.

175. ElSohly MA, Brenneisen R, Jones AB. Coca paste: chemical analysis and smoking experiments. J Forensic Sci 1991; 36:93.

176. Shannon M. Clinical toxicity of cocaine adulterants. Ann Emerg Med 1988; 17:1243.

177. DesJarlais DC, Friedman SR. Intravenous cocaine, crack, and HIV infection. JAMA 1988; 259:1945.

178. Wesson DR, Washburn P. Current patterns of drug abuse that involve smoking. NIDA Res Monogr 1990; 99:5.

179. Gawin FG: Cocaine addiction: psychology and neurophysiology. Science 1991; 251:1580.

180. Perez-Reyes M, DiGuiseppi S, Ondrusek G, et al. Freebase cocaine smoking. Clin Pharmacol Ther 1982; 32:459.

181. Perlman DC, Henman AR, Kochems L, et al. Doing a shotgun: a drug use practice and its relationship to sexual behaviors. Soc Sci Med 1999; 48:1441.

182. Mahler JC, Perry S, Sutton B. Intraurethral cocaine administration. JAMA 1988; 259:3126.

183. Ettinger TB, Stine RJ. Sudden death temporally related to vaginal cocaine abuse. Am J Emerg Med 1989; 7:129.

184. Doss PL, Gowitt GT. Investigation of a death caused by rectal insertion of cocaine. Am J Forensic Med Pathol 1988; 9:336.

185. Tripp M, Dowd DD, Eitel DR. TAC toxicity in the emergency department. Ann Emerg Med 1991; 20:106.

186. Barnett P. Cocaine toxicity following dermal application of adrenaline–cocaine preparation. Pediatr Emerg Care 1998; 14:280.

187. Wilkinson P, Van Dyke C, Jatlow P, et al. Intranasal and oral cocaine kinetics. Clin Pharmacol Ther 1980; 27:386.

188. Caruana DS, Weinbach B, Goerg D, Gardner LB. Cocaine packet ingestion. Diagnosis, management, and natural history. Ann Intern Med 1984; 100:73.

189. Goldfrank LR, Hoffman RS. The cardiovascular effects of cocaine. Ann Emerg Med 1991; 20:165.

190. Fischman MW, Schuster CR. Acute tolerance to cocaine in humans. NIDA Res Monogr 1981; 34:241.

191. Jones RT. The pharmacology of cocaine smoking in humans. NIDA Res Monogr 1990; 99:30.

192. Wilkerson RD. Cardiovascular effects of cocaine in conscious dogs: importance of fully functional autonomic and central nervous systems. J Pharmacol Exp Ther 1988; 246:466.

193. Knuepfer MM, Branch CA. Cardiovascular responses to cocaine are initially mediated by the central nervous system in rats. J Pharmacol Exp Ther 1992; 263:734.

194. Branch CA, Knuepfer MM. Adrenergic mechanisms underlying cardiac and vascular responses to cocaine in conscious rats. J Pharmacol Exp Ther 1992; 263:742.

195. Brody SL, Slovis CM, Wrenn KD. Cocaine-related medical problems: consecutive series of 233 patients. Am J Med 1990; 88:325.

196. Hollander JE, Lozano M, Fairweather P, et al. "Abnormal" electrocardiograms in patients with cocaine-associated chest pain are due to "normal" variants. J Emerg Med 1994; 12:199.

197. Rylander G. Psychosis and the punding and choreiform syndromes in addictions to central stimulant drugs. Psychiatry Neurol Neurochir 1972; 75:203.

198. Daras M, Koppel BS, Atos-Radzion E. Cocaine-induced choreoathetoid movements ("crack dancing"). Neurology 1994; 44:751.

199. Bartzokis G, Beckson M, Wirshing DA, et al. Choreoathetoid movements in cocaine dependence. Biol Psychiatry 1999; 45:1630.

200. Scharf D. Opsoclonus–myoclonus following the intranasal use of cocaine. J Neurol Neurosurg Psychiatry 1989; 52:1447.

201. Crum RM, Anthony JC. Cocaine use and other suspected risk factors for obsessive-compulsive disorder: a prospective study with data from the Epidemiologic Catchment Area surveys, Drug Alcohol Depend 1993; 31:281.

202. Gay GR. Clinical management of acute and chronic cocaine poisoning. Ann Emerg Med 1982; 11:562.

203. Merab J. Acute dystonic reaction to cocaine. Am J Med 1988; 84:564.

204. Brower KJ, Blow FC, Beresford TP. Forms of cocaine and psychiatric symptoms. Lancet 1988; I:50.

205. Derlet RW, Albertson TE. Emergency department presentation of cocaine intoxication. Ann Emerg Med 1989; 18:542.

206. Garland JS, Smith DS, Rice TB, Siker D. Accidental cocaine intoxication in a nine-month-old infant. Presentation and treatment. Pediatr Emerg Care 1989; 5:245.

207. Roth D, Alarcon FJ, Fernandez JA, et al. Acute rhabdomyolysis associated with cocaine intoxication. N Engl J Med 1988; 319:673.

208. Herzlich BC, Arsura EL, Pagala M, Grob D. Rhabdomyolysis related to cocaine abuse. Ann Intern Med 1988; 109:335.

209. Menashe PI, Gottlieb JE. Hyperthermia, rhabdomyolysis, and myoglobinuric renal failure after recreational use of cocaine. South Med J 1988; 81:379.

210. Anand V, Siami G, Stone WJ. Cocaine-associated rhabdomyolysis and acute renal failure. South Med J 1989; 82:67.

211. Pogue VA, Nurse HM. Cocaine-associated acute myoglobinuric renal failure. Am J Med 1989; 86:183.

212. Rubin RB, Neugarten J. Cocaine-induced rhabdomyolysis masquerading as myocardial ischemia. Am J Med 1989; 86:551.

213. Singhal P, Horowitz B, Quinnones MC, et al. Acute renal failure following cocaine abuse. Nephron 1989; 52:76.

214. Howard RL, Kaehny WD. Cocaine and rhabdomyolysis. Ann Intern Med 1989; 110:90.

215. Horst E, Bennett RL, Barrett O. Recurrent rhabdomyolysis in association with cocaine use. South Med J 1991; 84:269.

215a. Counselman FL, McLaughlin EW, Kardon EM, Bhambhani-Bharnani AS. Creatine phosphokinase elevation in patients presenting to the emergency department with cocaine-related complaints. Am J Emerg Med 1997; 15:221.

215b. Horowitz BZ, Panacek EA, Jouriles NJ. Severe rhabdomyolysis with renal failure after intranasal cocaine use. J Emerg Med 1997; 15:833.

216. Campbell BG. Cocaine abuse and hyperthermia, seizures, and fatal complications. Med J Aust 1988; 149:387.

217. Lipton RB, Choy-Kwong M, Solomon S. Headaches in hospitalized cocaine users. Headache 1989; 29:225.

218. Satel SL, Gawin FH. Migraine-like headache and cocaine use. JAMA 1989; 261:2995.

219. Cunningham KA, Lakoski JM. Electrophysiological effects of cocaine and procaine on dorsal raphe serotonin neurons. Eur J Pharmacol 1988; 148:457.

220. Brower KJ. Self-medication of migraine headaches with freebase cocaine. J Subst Abuse Treat 1988; 5:23.

221. Sherer MA, Kumor KM, Cone EJ, Jaffe JH. Suspiciousness induced by four-hour infusions of cocaine. Arch Gen Psychiatry 1988; 45:673.

222. Satel SL, Southwick SM, Gawin FH. Clinical features of cocaine-induced paranoia. Am J Psychiatry 1991; 148:495.

223. Serper MR, Chou J C-Y, Allen MH, et al. Symptomatic overlap of cocaine intoxication and acute schizophrenia at emergency presentation. Schiz Bull 1999; 25:387.

224. Manschreck TC, Allen DF, Neville M. Freebase psychosis: cases from a Bahamian epidemic of cocaine abuse. Comp Psychiatry 1987; 28:555.

225. Jeri FR, Sanchez CC, del Pozo T, et al. Further experience with the syndromes produced by coca paste smoking. Bull Narc 1978; 30:1.

226. Lesko LM, Fischman MW, Javaid JR, Davis JM. Iatrogenic cocaine psychosis. N Engl J Med 1982; 307:1153.

227. Jonnson S, O'Meara M, Young JB. Acute cocaine poisoning. Importance of treating seizures and acidosis. Am J Med 1983; 75:1061.

228. Lowenstein DH, Massa SM, Rowbotham MC, et al. Acute neurologic and psychiatric complications associated with cocaine abuse. Am J Med 1987; 83:841.

229. Myers JA, Earnest MP. Generalized seizures and cocaine abuse. Neurology 1984; 34:675.

230. Choy-Kwong M, Lipton RB. Seizures in hospitalized cocaine users. Neurology 1989; 39:425.

231. Schwartz RH, Estroff T, Hoffman NG. Seizures and syncope in adolescent cocaine abusers. Am J Med 1988; 85:462.

232. Harden CL, Montjo RE, Tuchman AJ, Daras M. Seizures provoked by cocaine use. Ann Neurol 1990; 28:263.

233. Alldredge BK, Lowenstein DH, Simon RP. Seizures associated with recreational drug abuse. Neurology 1989; 39:1037.

234. Pascual-Leone A, Dhuna A, Altafullah I, Anderson DC. Cocaine-induced seizures. Neurology 1990; 40:404.

235. Kramer LD, Locke GE, Ogunyemi A, Nelson L. Cocaine-related seizures in adults. Am J Drug Alcohol Abuse 1990; 16:307.

236. Holland RW, Marx JA, Earnest MP, Ranniger S. Grand mal seizures temporally related to cocaine use: clinical and diagnostic features. Ann Emerg Med 1992; 21:772.

237. Winberg S, Blaho K, Logan B, Geraci S. Multiple cocaine-induced seizures and corresponding cocaine and metabolite concentrations. Am J Emerg Med 1998; 16:529.

238. Dhuna A, Pascual-Leone A, Langendorf F, Anderson DC. Epileptogenic properties of cocaine in humans. Neurotoxicology 1991; 16:621.

239. Washton AM, Tatarsky A. Adverse effects of cocaine abuse. In: Harris L, ed. Problems of Drug Dependence 1983. Washington, DC: NIDA Res Monogr 1984; 49:247.

240. Schwartz RH, Luxenberg MG, Hoffman NG. Crack use by American middle-class adolescent polydrug abusers. J Pediatr 1991; 118:150.

241. Ng SKC, Brust JCM, Hauser WA, Susser M. Illicit drug use and the risk of new-onset seizures. Am J Epidemiol 1990; 132:47.

242. Ogunyemi AO, Locke GE, Kramer LD, Nelson L. Complex partial status epilepticus provoked by "crack" cocaine. Ann Neurol 1989; 26:785.

243. Konkol RJ, Erickson BA, Doerr JK, et al. Seizures induced by the cocaine metabolite benzoylecgonine in rats. Epilepsia 1992; 33:420.

244. Witkin JM, Gasior M, Heifets B, Tortella FC. Anticonvulsant efficacy of N-methyl-D-aspartate antagonists against convulsions induced by cocaine. J Pharmacol Exp Ther 1999; 289:703.

245. O'Dell LE, George FR, Ritz MC. Antidepressant drugs appear to enhance cocaine-induced toxicity. Exp Clin Psychopharmacol 2000; 8:133.

245a. Miller KA, Witkin JM, Ungared JT, Gasior M. Pharmacological and behavioral characterization of cocaine kindled seizures in mice. Psychopharmacology 2000; 148:78.

246. Dhuna A, Pascual-Leone A, Langendorf F. Chronic, habitual cocaine abuse and kindling-induced epilepsy: a case report. Epilepsia 1991; 32:890.

247. Rebischung D, Daras M, Tuchman AJ. Dystonic movements associated with cocaine use. Ann Neurol 1990; 28:267.

248. Kumor K. Cocaine withdrawal dystonia. Neurology 1990; 40:863.

249. Farrell PE, Diehl AK. Acute dystonic reaction to crack cocaine. Ann Emerg Med 1991; 20:322.

250. Choy-Kwong M, Lipton RB. Dystonia related to cocaine withdrawal: a case report and pathogenic hypothesis. Neurology 1989; 39:996.

251. Catalano G, Catalano MC, Rodriguez R. Dystonia associated with crack cocaine use. South Med J 1997; 90:1050.

252. Fines RE, Brady WJ, DeBehnke DJ. Cocaine-associated dystonic reaction. Am J Emerg Med 1997; 15:513.

253. Weiner WJ, Rabinstein A, Lewin B, et al. Cocaine-induced persistent dyskinesias. Neurology 2001; 56:964.

254. Cardoso F, Jankovic J. Movement disorders. In: Brust JCM, ed. Neurologic Complications of Drug and Alcohol Abuse. Neurol Clin 1993; 11:625.

255. Kumor K, Sherer M, Jaffe J. Haloperidol-induced dystonia in cocaine addicts. Lancet 1986; II2:1341.

256. Mesulam M-M. Cocaine and Tourette's syndrome. N Engl J Med 1986; 315:398.

257. Pascual-Leone A, Dhuna A. Cocaine-associated multifocal tics. Neurology 1990; 40:999.

258. Factor SA, Sanchez-Ramos JR, Wiener WJ. Cocaine and Tourette's syndrome. Ann Neurol 1988; 23:423.

259. Richards JR. Rhabdomyolysis and drugs of abuse. J Emerg Med 2000; 19:51.

260. Welch RD, Todd K, Krause GS. Incidence of cocaine-associated rhabdomyolysis. Ann Emerg Med 1991; 20:154.

261. Parks JM, Reed G, Knochel JP. Case report: cocaine-associated rhabdomyolysis. Am J Med 1989; 297:334.

262. Steingrub JS, Sweet S, Teres D. Crack-induced rhabdomyolysis. Crit Care Med 1989; 17:1073.

263. Guerin JM, Lustman C, Barbotin-Larrieu F. Cocaine-associated acute myoglobinuric renal failure. Am J Med 1989; 87:248.

264. Zamora-Quezada JC, Dinerman H, Stadecker MJ, Kelly J. Muscle and skin infarction after free-basing cocaine (crack). Ann Intern Med 1988; 108:564.

265. Wetli CV, Wright RK. Deaths caused by recreational cocaine use. JAMA 1979; 241:2519.

266. Karch S, Stephens B, Ho CH. Relating cocaine blood concentrations to toxicity—an autopsy study of 99 cases. J Forensic Sci 1998; 43:41.

267. Smart RG, Anglin L. Do we know the lethal dose of cocaine? J Forensic Sci 1987; 32:303.

268. Amon CA, Tate LG, Wright RK, Matusiak W. Sudden death due to ingestion of cocaine. J Anal Toxicol 1986; 10:217.

269. Loghmanee F, Tobak M. Fatal malignant hyperthermia associated with recreational cocaine and ethanol abuse. Am J Forensic Pathol 1986; 7:246.

270. Wetli CV, Fishbain DA. Cocaine induced psychosis and sudden death in recreational cocaine users. J Forensic Sci 1985; 30:873.

271. Ruttenber AJ, Lawler-Heavner J, Yin M, et al. Fatal excited delirium following cocaine use: epidemiologic findings provide new evidence for mechanisms of cocaine toxicity. J Forensic Sci 1997; 42:25.

272. Calloway CW, Clarke RF. Hyperthermia in psychostimulant overdose. Ann Emerg Med 1994; 24:68.

273. Kosten TR, Kleber HD. Sudden death in cocaine abusers: relation to neuroleptic malignant syndrome. Lancet 1987; I:1198.

274. Daras M, Kakkouras L, Tuchman AJ, Koppel BS. Rhabdomyolysis and hyperthermia after cocaine abuse: a variant of the neuroleptic malignant syndrome? Acta Neurol Scand 1995; 92:161.

275. Roberts JR, Quattrocchi E, Howland MA. Severe hyperthermia secondary to intravenous drug abuse. Am J Emerg Med 1984; 2:373.

276. Tanvetyanon T, Dissin J, Selcer VM. Hyperthermia and pancerebellar syndrome after cocaine abuse. Arch Intern Med 2001; 161:608.

277. Robin ED, Wong RJ, Ptashne KA. Increased lung water and ascites after massive cocaine overdosage in mice and improved survival related to beta-adrenergic blockage. Ann Intern Med 1989; 110:202.

278. Staley JK, Hearn WL, Ruttenber AJ, et al. High affinity cocaine recognition sites on the dopamine transporter

are elevated in fatal cocaine overdose victims. J Pharmacol Exp Ther 1994; 271:1678.

279. Staley JK, Rothman RB, Rice KC, et al. Kappa-2 opioid receptors in limbic areas of the human brain are upregulated by cocaine in fatal overdose victims. J Neurosci 1997; 17:8225.

280. Mash DC, Staley JK. D_3 dopamine and kappa opioid receptor alterations in human brain of cocaine-overdose victims. Ann N Y Acad Sci 1999; 877:507.

280a. Ruttenber AJ, McAnally HB, Wetli CV. Cocaine-associated rhabdomyolysis and excited delirium: different stages of the same syndrome. Am J Forensic Med Pathol 1999; 20:120.

280b. Wetli CV, Mash D, Karch SB. Cocaine-associated agitated delirium and the neuroleptic malignant syndrome. Am J Emerg Med 1996; 14:425.

280c. Staley J, Hearn W, Ruttenber A, et al. High affinity cocaine recognition sites on the dopamine transporter are elevated in fatal cocaine overdose victims. J Pharmacol Exp Ther 1994; 271:1678.

281. Chen L, Segal DM, Moraes CT, Mash DC. Dopamine transporter mRNA in autopsy studies of chronic cocaine users. Brain Res Mol Brain Res 1999; 73:181.

282. Karch SB. Interpretation of blood cocaine and metabolite concentrations. Am J Emerg Med 2000; 18:635.

283. Blaho K, Logan B, Winbery S, et al. Blood cocaine and metabolite concentrations, clinical findings, and outcome of patients presenting to an ED. Am J Emerg Med 2000; 18:593.

284. Clarke MJ. Suicide and cocaine. JAMA 1988;260:2506.

285. Honer WG, Gewirtz G, Turey M. Psychosis and violence in cocaine smokers. Lancet 1987; II:451.

286. Mittleman RE, Wetli CV. Death caused by recreational cocaine use: an update. JAMA 1984; 252:1889.

287. Press S. Crack and fatal child abuse. JAMA 1988; 260:3132.

288. Sperry K. Suicide with, and because of, cocaine. JAMA 1988; 259:2995.

289. Randell T. Cocaine and alcohol mix in body to form even longer lasting, more lethal drug. JAMA 1992; 267:1043.

290. Weiner AL, Bayer MJ, McKay CA, et al. Anticholinergic poisoning with adulterated intranasal cocaine. Am J Emerg Med 1998; 16:517.

291. Waien SA, Hayes D, Leonardo JM. Severe coagulopathy as a consequence of smoking crack laced with rodenticide. N Engl J Med 2001; 345:700.

292. Lombard J, Levin IH, Weiner WJ. Arsenic intoxication in a cocaine abuser. N Engl J Med 1989; 320:869.

293. Brady WJ, Duncan CW. Hypoglycemia masquerading as acute psychosis and cocaine intoxication. Am J Emerg Med 1999; 17:318.

294. Brust JCM. Acute neurologic complications of drug and alcohol abuse. Neurol Clin North Am 1998; 16:503.

295. Catravas JD, Waters IW. Acute cocaine intoxication in the conscious dog: studies on the mechanism of lethality. J Pharmacol Exp Ther 1981; 217:350.

296. Derlet RW, Albertson TE. Diazepam in the prevention of seizures and death in cocaine-intoxicated rats. Ann Emerg Med 1989; 18:542.

297. Spivey WH, Schoffstall JM, Kirkpatrick, et al. Comparison of labatelol, diazepam, and haloperidol for the treatment of cocaine toxicity in the swine model. Ann Emerg Med 1990; 19:467.

298. Guinn MM, Bedford JA, Wilson JC. Antagonism of intravenous cocaine lethality in nonhuman primates. Clin Toxicol 1980; 16:499.

299. Gasior M, Ungard JT, Witkin JM. Pre-clinical evaluation of newly approved and potential antiepileptic drugs against cocaine-induced seizures. J Pharmacol Exp Ther 1999; 290:1148.

300. Catravas JD, Waters IW, Walz MA, et al. Acute cocaine intoxication in the conscious dog: pathophysiologic profile of acute lethality. Arch Int Pharmacodyn Ther 1978; 235:328.

301. Witkin JM, Goldberg SR, Katz JL. Lethal effects of cocaine are reduced by the dopamine-1 receptor antagonist SCH 23390 but not by haloperidol. Life Sci 1989; 44:1285.

302. Mercuro G, Gessa G, Rivano CA, et al. Evidence for a dopaminergic control of sympathoadrenal catecholamine release. Am J Cardiol 1988; 62:827.

303. Romoska E, Sacchetti AD. Propranolol-induced hypertension in the treatment of cocaine intoxication. Ann Emerg Med 1985; 14:1112.

304. Lang RA, Cigarroa RG, Flores ED, et al. Potentiation of cocaine-induced coronary vasoconstriction by beta-adrenergic blockade. Ann Intern Med 1990; 112:897.

305. Hollander JE, Hoffman RS. Cocaine. In: Goldfrank LR, Flomenbaum NE, Lewin NA, et al., eds. Goldfrank's Toxicologic Emergencies, 6th edition, Stamford, CT: Appleton & Lange, 1998:1071.

306. Gay GR, Loper KA. The use of labatalol in the management of cocaine crisis. Ann Emerg Med 1988; 17:282.

307. Leikin JB. Cocaine and β-adrenergic blockers: a remarriage after a decade-long divorce? Crit Care Med 1999; 27:688.

308. Nahas G, Trouve R, Demus JF, von Sitbon M. A calcium-channel blocker as antidote to the cardiac effects of cocaine intoxication. N Engl J Med 1985; 313:520.

309. Derlet RW, Albertson TE. Potentiation of cocaine toxicity with calcium channel blockers. Am J Emerg Med 1989; 7:464.

310. Shukla VK, Goldfrank LR, Turndorf H, Bansinath M. Antagonism of acute cocaine toxicity by buprenorphine. Life Sci 1991; 49:1887.

311. Antelman SM, Kocan D, Rowland N, et al. Amitriptyline provides long-lasting immunization against sudden cardiac death from cocaine. Eur J Pharmacol 1981; 69:119.

312. Derlet RW, Albertson T. Lidocaine potentiation of cocaine toxicity. Ann Emerg Med 1991; 20:135.

313. Gingrich JA, Rudnick-Levin F, Almeida C, et al. Cocaine and catatonia. Am J Psychiatry 1998; 155:1629.

314. Mattes CE, Lynch TJ, Singh A, et al. Therapeutic use of butyrylcholinesterase for cocaine intoxication. Toxicol Appl Pharmacol 1997; 145:372.

315. O'Dell LE, Kreifeldt MJ, George FR, Ritz MC. The role of serotonin (2) receptors in mediating cocaine-induced convulsions. Pharmacol Biochem Behav 2000; 65:677.

316. Brackett RL, Pouw B, Blyden JF, et al. Prevention of cocaine-induced convulsions and lethality in mice: effectiveness of targeting different sites on the NMDA receptor complex. Neuropharmacology 2000; 39:407.

317. McCracken KA, Bowen WD, deCosta BR, Matsumoto RR. Two novel sigma receptor ligands, BD1047 and LR172, attenuate cocaine-induced toxicity and loco-motor activity. Eur J Pharmacol 1999; 370:225.

318. Miller NS, Gold MS, Belkin BM. The diagnosis of alcohol and cannabis dependence in cocaine dependence. Adv Alcohol Subst Abuse 1990; 8:33.

319. Hearn WL, Flynn DD, Hime GW, et al. Cocaethylene: a unique cocaine metabolite displays high affinity for the dopamine transporter. J Neurochem 1991; 56:698.

320. Raven MA, Necessary BD, Danluck DA, Ettenberg A. Comparison of the reinforcing and anxiogenic effects of intravenous cocaine and cocaethylene. Exp Clin Psychopharmacol 2000; 8:117.

321. McCance-Katz EF, Kosten TR, Jatlow P. Concurrent use of cocaine and alcohol is more potent and poten-tially more toxic than use of either alone–a multiple dose study. Biol Psychiatry 1998; 44:250.

322. Hart CL, Jatlow P, Severino KA, McLance-Katz EF. Comparison of intravenous cocaethylene and cocaine in humans. Psychopharmacology 2000; 149:153.

323. Foltin RW, Fischman MW. The cardiovascular and subjective effects of intravenous cocaine and morphine combinations in humans. J Pharmacol Exp Ther 1992; 261:623.

324. Cushman P. Cocaine use in a population of drug abusers on methadone. Hosp Community Psychiatry 1988; 39:1205.

325. Kosten TA. Cocaine attenuates opiate withdrawal in human and rat. In: Harris L, ed. Problems of Drug Dependence 1989. Washington, DC: NIDA Res Monogr 1990; 95:361.

326. Siegel RK. Cocaine free base use. J Psychoact Drugs 1982; 14:311.

327. Sherer MA. Intravenous cocaine: psychiatric effects, biological mechanisms. Biol Psychiatry 1988; 24:865.

328. Zahniser NR, Peris J, Dwoskin LP, et al. Sensitization to cocaine in the nigrostriatal dopamine system. In: Clouet D, Asghar K, Brown R, eds. Mechanisms of Cocaine Abuse and Toxicity. NIDA Res Monogr 1988; 88:55.

329. Fischman MW, Schuster CR, Javaid J, et al. Acute tolerance development to the cardiovascular and subjective effects of cocaine. J Pharmacol Exp Ther 1985; 235:677.

330. Foltin RW, Fischman MW, Pedroso JJ, Pearlson GD. Repeated intranasal cocaine administration. Lack of tolerance to pressor effects. Drug Alcohol Depend 1988; 22:169.

331. Kumor K, Sherer M, Thompson L, et al. Lack of cardiovascular tolerance during intravenous cocaine infusions in human volunteers. Life Sci 1988; 42:2063.

332. Louie AK, Lannon RA, Kettler TA. Treatment of cocaine-induced panic disorder. Am J Psychiatry 1989; 146:40.

333. Uslaner J, Kalechstein A, Richter T, et al. Association of depressive symptoms during abstinence with the subjective high produced by cocaine. Am J Psychiatry 1999; 156:1444.

334. Jacobsen LK, Staley JK, Malison RT, et al. Elevated central serotonin transporter availability in acutely abstinent cocaine-dependent patients. Am J Psychiatry 2000; 157:1134.

335. Roberts JR, Greenberg MI. Cocaine washout syn-drome. Ann Intern Med 2000; 132:679.

336. Volkow ND, Fowler JS, Wang GJ. Imaging studies on the role of dopamine in cocaine reinforcement and addiction in humans. J Psychopharmacol 1999; 13:337.

337. Childress AR, Mozley PD, McElgin W, et al. Limbic activation during cue-induced cocaine craving. Am J Psychiatry 1999; 156:11.

338. Reid MS, Mickalian JD, Delucchi KL, Berger SP. A nicotine antagonist, mecamylamine, reduces cue-induced cocaine craving in cocaine-dependent subjects. Neuropsychopharmacology 1999; 20:297.

339. Siegel RK. Changing patterns of cocaine use: longitu-dinal observations, consequences, and treatments. NIDA Res Monogr 1984; 50:92.

340. Schwartz RH, Luxenberg MG, Hoffman NG. "Crack" use by American middle-class adolescent polydrug abusers. J Pediatr 1991; 118:150.

341. Washton AM, Gold MS, Pottash AC, Semitz L. Adolescent cocaine abusers. Lancet 1984; II:746.

342. Smith DE, Schwartz RH, Martin DM. Heavy cocaine use by adolescents. Pediatrics 1989; 83:539.

343. Johanson CE. The reinforcing properties of procaine, chloroprocaine, and proparacaine in rhesus monkeys. Psychopharmacology 1980; 67:189.

344. Fischman MW, Schuster CR, Rajfer S. A comparison of the subjective and cardiovascular effects of cocaine and procaine in humans. Pharmacol Biochem Behav 1983; 18:711.

345. Van Dyck C, Jatlow P, Ungerer J, et al. Cocaine and lidocaine have similar psychological effects after intranasal application. Life Sci 1979; 24:271.

346. Klatt EC, Montgomery S, Namiki T, Noguchi TT. Misrepresentation of stimulant street drugs: a decade of experience in an analysis program. J Toxicol Clin Toxicol 1986; 24:441.

347. Shannon M, Lacouture PG, Roa J, Woolf A. Cocaine exposure among children seen at a pediatric hospital. Pediatrics 1989; 83:337.

348. Insley BM, Grufferman S, Ayliffe HE. Thallium poisoning in cocaine abusers. Am J Emerg Med 1986; 4:545.

349. Siegel RK. Herbal intoxication. Psychoactive effects from herbal cigarettes, tea, and capsules. JAMA 1976; 236:473.

350. Siegel RK, Elsohly MA, Plowman T, et al. Cocaine in herbal tea. JAMA 1986; 255:40.

351. Engelke BF, Gentner WA. Determination of cocaine in "Mate de Coca" herbal tea. J Pharmaceut Sci 1991; 80:96.

352. Sawicka EH, Trosser A. Cerebrospinal fluid rhinorrhea after cocaine sniffing. BMJ 1983; 284:1476.

353. Wang ES. Cocaine-induced iritis. Ann Emerg Med 1991; 20:192.

354. Becker GD, Hill S. Midline granuloma due to illicit cocaine use. Arch Otolaryngol Head Neck Surg 1988; 114:90.

355. Newman NM, DiLoreto DA, Ho JT, et al. Bilateral optic neuropathy and osteolytic sinusitis. Complications of cocaine abuse. JAMA 1989; 259:72.

356. Rao AN. Brain abscess; a complication of cocaine inhalation. N Y State J Med 1988; 88:548.

357. Sittel C, Eckel HE. Nasal cocaine abuse presenting as a central facial destructive granuloma. Eur Arch Otorhinolaryngology 1998; 255:446.

358. Lancaster J, Belloso A, Wilson CA, McCormick M. Rare case of nasal-oral fistula with extensive osteocartilaginous necrosis secondary to cocaine abuse: review of otorhinolaryngological presentations in cocaine addicts. J Laryngol Otol 2000; 114:630.

359. Tierney BP, Stadelmann WK. Necrotizing infection of the face secondary to intranasal impaction of "crack" cocaine. Ann Plastic Surg 1999; 43:640.

360. MacDonald KL, Cohen ML, Blake PA. The changing epidemiology of adult botulism in the United States. Am J Epidemiol 1986; 124:794.

361. Rapoport S, Watkins PB. Descending paralysis resulting from occult wound botulism. Ann Neurol 1984; 16:359.

362. Kudrow DB, Henry DA, Haake DA, et al. Botulism associated with *Clostridium botulinum* sinusitis after intranasal cocaine use. Ann Intern Med 1988; 109:984.

363. MacDonald KL, Rutherford GW, Friedman SM, et al. Botulism and botulism-like illness in chronic drug abusers. Ann Intern Med 1985; 102:616.

364. Ludwig WG, Hoffner RJ. Upper airway burn from crack cocaine pipe screen ingestion. Am J Emerg Med 1999; 17:108.

365. Ettinger NA, Albin RJ. A review of the respiratory effects of smoking cocaine. Am J Med 1989; 87:664.

366. Haim DY, Lippmann ML, Goldberg SK, Walkenstein MD. The pulmonary complication of crack cocaine: a comprehensive review. Chest 1995; 107:233.

367. Orriols R, Munoz X, Ferrer J, et al. Cocaine-induced Churg–Strauss vasculitis. Eur Respir J 1996; 9:175.

368. Dispinigaitis PV, Jones JG, Frymus MM, Folkert WW. "Crack" cocaine-induced syndrome mimicking sarcoidosis. Am J Med Sci 1999; 317:416.

369. Tames SM, Goldenring JM. Madarosis from cocaine use. N Engl J Med 1986; 314:1324.

370. Desai P, Roy M, Roy A, et al. Impaired color vision in cocaine-withdrawn patients. Arch Gen Psychiatry 1997; 54:696.

371. Roy M, Roy A, Williams J, et al. Reduced blue cone electroretinogram in cocaine-withdrawn patients. Arch Gen Psychiatry 1997; 54:153.

372. Hari CK, Roblin DG, Clayton MI, Nair RG. Acute angle glaucoma precipitated by intranasal application of cocaine. J Laryngol Otol 1999; 113:250.

373. Colatrella N, Daniel TE. Crack eye syndrome. J Am Optometr Assoc 1999; 70:193.

374. Siegel RK. Cocaine and sexual dysfunction: the curse of Mama Coca. J Psychoact Drugs 1982; 14:71.

375. Smith DE, Wesson DR, Apter-Marsh M. Cocaine- and alcohol-induced sexual dysfunction in patients with addictive disease. J Psychoact Drugs 1984; 16:359.

376. Mello JH, Mendelson JH. Cocaine's effects on neuroendocrine systems. Clinical and preclinical studies. Pharmacol Biochem Behav 1997; 57:571.

377. Concores JA, Dackis CA, Gold MS. Sexual dysfunction secondary to cocaine abuse in two patients. J Clin Psychiatry 1986; 47:384.

378. Mendelson JH, Teoh SK, Lange U, et al. Anterior pituitary, adrenal, and gonadal hormones during cocaine withdrawal. Am J Psychiatry 1988; 145:1094.

379. Mendelson JH, Mello NK, Teoh SK, et al. Cocaine effects on pulsatile secretion of anterior pituitary, gonadal, and adrenal hormones. J Clin Endocrinol Metab 1989; 69:1256.

380. Sell SL, Scalzitti JM, Thomas ML, Cunningham KA. Influence of ovarian hormones and estrous cycle on the behavioral response to cocaine in female rats. J Pharmacol Exp Ther 2000; 293:879.

381. Altman AL, Seftel AD, Brown SL, Hampel N. Cocaine associated priapism. J Urol 1999; 161:1817.

382. Berciano J, Oterino A, Rebollo M, Pascual J. Myasthenia gravis unmasked by cocaine abuse. N Engl J Med 1991; 325:892.

382a. Lajara-Nanson WA: Cocaine induced hypokalemic periodic paralysis. J Neurol Neurosurg Psychiatry 2002; 73:92.

383. Ponsada X, Bart R, Jover R, et al. Increased toxicity of cocaine on human hepatocytes induced by ethanol: role of GSH. Biochem Pharmacol 1999; 58:1579.

384. Oztecan S, Dogru-Abbasoglu S, Mutlu-Turkoglu U, et al. The role of stimulated lipid peroxidation and impaired calcium sequestration in the enhancement of cocaine-induced hepatotoxicity by ethanol. Drug Alcohol Dep 2000; 58:77.

385. Nzerve CM, Hewan-Lowe K, Riley LJ. Cocaine and the kidney: a synthesis of pathophysiologic and clinical perspectives. Am J Kidney Dis 2000; 35:783.

386. Attoussi S, Faulkner ML, Oso A, Umoru B. Cocaine-induced scleroderma and scleroderma renal crisis. South Med J 1998; 91:961.

387. Dick AD, Prentice MG. Cocaine and acute porphyria. Lancet 1987; II:1150.

388. Gan X, Zhang L, Newton T, et al. Cocaine infusion increases interferon-gamma and decreases interleukin-10 in cocaine-dependent subjects. Clin Immunol Immunopathol 1998; 89:181.

389. Chambers HF, Morris DL, Tauber MG, Modin G. Cocaine use and the risk for endocarditis in intravenous drug users. Ann Intern Med 1987; 106:833.

390. Chaisson RE, Bacchetti P, Osmond D, et al. Cocaine use and HIV infection in intravenous drug users in San Francisco. JAMA 1989; 261:561.

391. Schoenbaum EE, Hartel D, Selwyn PA, et al. Risk factors for human immunodeficiency virus infection in intravenous drug users. N Engl J Med 1989; 321:874.

392. Lerner WD. Cocaine abuse and acquired immunodeficiency syndrome: a tale of two epidemics. Am J Med 1989; 87:661.

393. Fullilove RE, Fullilove MT, Bowser BP, Gross SA. Risk of sexually transmitted disease among black adolescent crack users in Oakland and San Francisco, Calif. JAMA 1990; 263:851.

394. Comer GM, Mittal MK, Donelson SS, Lee TP. Cluster of fulminant hepatitis B in crack users. Am J Gastroenterol 1991; 86:331.

395. Alternative case-finding methods in a crack-related syphilis epidemic—Philadelphia. MMWR 1991; 40:77.

396. Weiss RD. Links between cocaine and retroviral infection. JAMA 1989; 261:607.

397. DesJarlais DC, Abdul-Quader A, Minkoff H, et al. Crack use and multiple AIDS risk behaviors. J AIDS 1991; 4:446.

398. Nair MP, Chadha KC, Hewitt RG, et al. Cocaine differentially modulates chemokine production by mononuclear cells from normal donors and human immunodeficiency virus type 1-infected patients. Clin Diagn Lab Immunol 2000; 7:96.

399. Zhang L, Looney D, Taub D, et al. Cocaine opens the blood–brain barrier to HIV-1 invasion. J Neurovirol 1998; 4:619.

400. Gitter MJ, Goldsmith SR, Dunbar DN, Sharkey SW. Cocaine and chest pain: clinical features and outcome of patients hospitalized to rule out myocardial infarction. Ann Intern Med 1991; 115:277.

401. Weber JE, Shofer FS, Larkin GL, et al. Validation of a brief observation period for patients with cocaine-associated chest pain. N Engl J Med 2003; 348:510.

402. Amin M, Gabelman G, Kaspel J, Buttrick P. Acute myocardial infarction and chest pain syndromes after cocaine use. Am J Cardiol 1990; 66:1434.

403. Isner JM, Chokshi SK. Cardiovascular complications of cocaine. Curr Prob Cardiol 1991; 16:89.

404. Hollander JE, Hoffman RS, Gennis P, et al. Prospective multicenter evaluation of cocaine-associated chest pain. Acad Emerg Med 1994; 1:330.

405. Mittleman MA, Mintzer D, MacLure M, et al. Triggering of myocardial infarction by cocaine. Circulation 1999; 99:2737.

405a. Minor RL, Scott BD, Brown DD, Winniford MD. Cocaine-induced myocardial infarction in patients with normal coronary arteries. Ann Intern Med 1991; 115:797.

406. Zimmerman FH, Gustafson GM, Kemp HG. Recurrent myocardial infarction associated with cocaine abuse in a young man with normal coronary arteries: evidence for coronary artery spasm culminating in thrombosis. J Am Coll Cardiol 1987; 9:964.

407. Lange RA, Cigarroa RG, Yancy CW, et al. Cocaine-induced coronary-artery vasoconstriction. N Engl J Med 1989; 321:1558.

408. Moliterno DJ, Willard JE, Lange RA, et al. Coronary vasoconstriction induced by cocaine, cigarette smoking, or both. N Engl J Med 1994; 330:454.

409. Gardezi N. Cardiovascular effects of cocaine. JAMA 1987; 257:979.

410. Nadamanee K, Gorelick DA, Josephson MA, et al. Myocardial ischemia during cocaine withdrawal. Ann Intern Med 1989; 111:876.

411. Del Aguila C, Rosman H. Myocardial infarction during cocaine withdrawal. Ann Intern Med 1990; 112:712.

412. Isner JJM, Estes NAM, Thompson PD, et al. Acute cardiac events temporally related to cocaine abuse. N Engl J Med 1986; 315:1438.

413. Karch SB, Billingham ME. The pathology and etiology of cocaine-induced heart disease. Arch Pathol Lab Med 1988; 112:225.

414. Petty GW, Brust JCM, Tatemichi TK, Barr ML. Embolic stroke after smoking "crack" cocaine. Stroke 1990; 21:1632.

415. Chokshi SK, Moore R, Pandian NG, Isner JM. Reversible cardiomyopathy associated with cocaine intoxication. Ann Intern Med 1989; 111:1039.

416. Peng SK, French WJ, Pelikan PC. Direct cocaine cardiotoxicity demonstrated by endomyocardial biopsy. Arch Pathol Lab Med 1989; 113:842.

417. Pitts WR, Vongpatanasin W, Cigarroa JE, et al. Effects of the intracoronary infusion of cocaine on left ventricular systolic and diastolic function in humans. Circulation 1998; 97:1270.

418. Uszenski RT, Gillis RA, Schaer GL, et al. Additive myocardial depressant effects of cocaine and ethanol. Am Heart J 1992; 124:1276.

419. Kabas JS, Blanchard SM, Matsuyama Y, et al. Cocaine-mediated impairment of cardiac conduction in the dog: a potential mechanism for sudden death after cocaine. J Pharmacol Exp Ther 1990; 252:185.

420. Jain RK, Jain MK, Bachenheimer LC, et al. Factors determining whether cocaine will potentiate the cardiac effects of neurally released norepinephrine. J Pharmacol Exp Ther 1990; 252:147.

421. Kerns W, Garvey L, Owens J. Cocaine-induced wide complex dysrhythmia. J Emerg Med 1997; 15:321.

422. Castro VJ, Nacht R. Cocaine-induced bradyarrhythmia: an unsuspected cause of syncope. Chest 2000; 117:275.

423. Hale SL, Alker KJ, Rezkalla SH, et al. Nifedipine protects the heart from the acute deleterious effects of cocaine if administered before but not after cocaine. Circulation 1991; 83:1437.

424. Edwards J, Rubin RN. Aortic dissection and cocaine abuse. Ann Intern Med 1987; 107:779.

425. Barth CW, Bray M, Roberts WC. Rupture of the ascending aorta during cocaine intoxication. Am J Cardiol 1986; 57:496.

426. Madu EC, Shala B, Beugh D. Crack-cocaine-associated aortic dissection in early pregnancy. A case report. Angiology 1999; 50:163.

427. Fikar CR, Koch S. Etiologic factors of acute aortic dissection in children and young adults. Clin Pediatr 2000; 39:71.

428. Nallimothu BK, Saint S, Kolias TJ, Eagle KA. Of nicks and time. N Engl J Med 2001; 345:359.

429. Webber J, Kline RA, Lucas CE. Aortic thrombosis associated with cocaine use: report of two cases. Ann Vasc Surg 1999; 13:302.

430. Freudenberger RS, Cappell MS, Huff DA. Intestinal infarction after intravenous cocaine administration. Ann Intern Med 1990; 113:715.

431. Papi C, Candia S, Masci P, et al. Acute ischemic colitis following intravenous cocaine use. Ital J Gastroenterol Hepatol 1999; 31:305.

432. Abramson DL, Gertler JP, Lewis T, Kral JG. Crack-related perforated gastropyloric ulcer. J Clin Gastroenterol 1991; 13:17.

433. Sharff JA. Renal infarction associated with intravenous cocaine use. Ann Emerg Med 1984; 13:1145.

434. Novielli KD, Chambers CV. Splenic infarction after cocaine use. Ann Intern Med 1991; 114:251.

435. Berger JL, Nimier M, Desmonts JM. Continuous axillary plexus block in treatment of accidental intra-arterial injection of cocaine. N Engl J Med 1988; 318:930.

436. Mines D. Splenic artery aneurysm rupture. Am J Emerg Med 1991; 9:74.

437. Mirzayan R, Hanks SE, Weaver FA. Cocaine-induced thrombosis of common iliac and popliteal arteries. Ann Vasc Surg 1998; 12:476.

437a. Hoang MP, Lee EL, Anand A. Histologic spectrum of arterial and arteriolar lesions in acute and chronic cocaine-induced mesenteric ischemia: report of three cases and literature review. Am J Surg Pathol 1998; 22:1404.

438. Marder VJ, Mellinghoff IK. Cocaine and Buerger disease: is there a pathogenetic association? Arch Intern Med 2000; 160:2057.

439. Murray R, Simialek J, Golle M, et al. Pulmonary artery medial hypertrophy without foreign particle microembolization in cocaine users. Chest 1988; 94S:48.

440. Godwin JE, Hasle RA, Miller KS, et al. Cocaine, pulmonary hemorrhage, and hemoptysis. Ann Intern Med 1989; 110:843.

441. Levine SR, Brust JCM, Futrell N, et al. Cerebrovascular complications of the use of the "crack" form of alkaloidal cocaine. N Engl J Med 1990; 323:699.

442. Brust JCM, Richter RW. Stroke associated with cocaine abuse? N Y State J Med 1977; 77:1473.

443. Lundberg GD, Garriott JC, Reynolds PC, et al. Cocaine-related death. J Forensic Sci 1977; 22:402.

444. Caplan LR, Hier DB, DeCruz I. Cerebral embolism in the Michael Reese Stroke Registry. Stroke 1983; 14:530.

445. Schwartz ICA, Cohen JA. Subarachnoid hemorrhage precipitated by cocaine snorting. Arch Neurol 1984; 41:705.

446. Lichtenfield PJ, Rubin DB, Feldman RS. Subarachnoid hemorrhage precipitated by cocaine snorting. Arch Neurol 1984; 41:223.

447. Chasnoff IJ, Bussey ME, Savich R, Stack CM. Perinatal cerebral infarction and maternal cocaine use. J Pediatr 1986; 108:456.

448. Golbe LI, Merkin MD. Cerebral infarction in a user of free-base cocaine ("crack"). Neurology 1986; 36:1602.

449. Cregler LL, Mark H. Medical complications of cocaine abuse. N Engl J Med 1986; 315:1495.

450. Rogers JN, Henry TE, Jones AM, et al. Cocaine-related deaths in Pima County, Arizona, 1982–1984. J Forensic Sci 1986; 31:1404.

451. Altes-Capella J, Cabezudo-Artero JM, Forteza-Rei J. Complications of cocaine abuse. Ann Intern Med 1987; 107:940.

452. Levine SR, Washington JM, Jefferson MF, et al. "Crack" cocaine-associated stroke. Neurology 1987; 37:1849.

453. Wojak JC, Flamm ES. Intracranial hemorrhage and cocaine use. Stroke 1987; 18:712.

454. Kaye BR, Fainstat M. Cerebral vasculitis associated with cocaine abuse. JAMA 1987; 258:2104.

455. Cregler LI, Mark H. Relation of stroke to cocaine abuse. N Y State J Med 1987; 87:128.

456. Mittleman RE, Wetli CV. Cocaine and sudden "natural" death. J Forensic Sci 1987; 32:11.

457. Lowenstein DH, Massa SM, Rowbotham MC, et al. Acute neurologic and psychiatric complications associated with cocaine abuse. Am J Med 1987; 83:841.

458. Lehman LB. Intracerebral hemorrhage after intranasal cocaine use. Hosp Phys 1987; 7:69.

459. Mangiardi JR, Daras M, Geller ME, et al. Cocaine-related intracranial hemorrhage: report of nine cases and review. Acta Neurol Scand 1988; 77:177.

460. Devenyi P, Schneiderman JF, Devenyi RG, Lawby L. Cocaine-induced central retinal artery occlusion. Can Med Assoc J 1988; 138:129.

461. Mody CK, Miller BL, McIntyre HB, et al. Neurologic complications of cocaine abuse. Neurology 1988; 38:1189.

462. Weingarten KO. Cerebral vasculitis associated with cocaine abuse or subarachnoid hemorrhage? JAMA 1988; 259:1658.

463. Toler KA, Anderson B. Stroke in an intravenous drug user secondary to the lupus anticoagulant. Stroke 1988; 19:274.

464. Devore RA, Tucker HM. Dysphagia and dysarthria as a result of cocaine abuse. Otolaryngol Head Neck Surg 1988; 98:174.

465. Henderson CE, Torbey M. Rupture of intracranial aneurysm associated with cocaine use during pregnancy. Am J Perinatol 1988; 5:142.

466. Tenorio GM, Nazvi M, Bickers GH, Hubbird RH. Intrauterine stroke and maternal polydrug abuse. Clin Pediatr 1988; 27:565.

467. Rowbotham MC. Neurologic aspects of cocaine abuse. West J Med 1988; 149:442.

468. Levine SR, Welch KM. Cocaine and stroke. Stroke 1988; 19:779.

469. Nalls G, Disher A, Darabagi J, et al. Subcortical cerebral hemorrhages associated with cocaine abuse. CT and MR findings. J Comput Assist Tomogr 1989; 13:1.

470. Peterson PL, Moore PM. Hemorrhagic cerebrovascular complications of crack cocaine abuse. Neurology 1989; 39 (Suppl 1):302.

471. Moore PM, Peterson PL. Nonhemorrhagic cerebrovascular complications of cocaine abuse. Neurology 1989; 39 (Suppl 1):302.

472. Tardiff K, Gross E, Wu J, et al. Analysis of cocaine-positive fatalities. J Forensic Sci 1989; 34:53.

473. Klonoff DC, Andrews BT, Obana WG. Stroke associated with cocaine use. Arch Neurol 1989; 46:989.

474. Rowley HA, Lowenstein DH, Rowbotham MC, Simon RP. Thalamomesencephalic strokes after cocaine abuse. Neurology 1989; 39:428.

475. DeBroucker, Verstichel P, Cambier J, DeTruchis P. Accidents neurologiqes après prise de cocaine. Presse Med 1989; 18:541.

476. Jacobs IG, Roszler MH, Kelly JK, et al. Cocaine abuse: neurovascular complications. Radiology 1989; 170:223.

477. Mercado A, Johnson G, Calver D, Sokol RJ. Cocaine, pregnancy, and postpartum intracerebral hemorrhage. Obstet Gynecol 1989; 73:467.

478. Nolte KB, Gelman BB. Intracerebral hemorrhage associated with cocaine abuse. Arch Pathol Lab Med 1989; 113:812.

479. Engstrand BC, Daras M, Tuchman AJ, et al. Cocaine-related ischemic stroke. Neurology 1989; 39 (Suppl 1):186.

480. Spires MC, Gordon EF, Choudhuri M, et al. Intracranial hemorrhage in a neonate following prenatal cocaine exposure. Pediatr Neurol 1989; 5:324.

481. Meza I, Estrad CA, Montalvo JA, et al. Cerebral infarction associated with cocaine use. Henry Ford Hosp Med J 1989; 37:50.

482. Mast J, Carpanzamo CR, Hier L. Maternal cocaine use: neurologic effects on offspring. Neurology 1989; 30 (Suppl 1):187.

483. Dixon SD, Bejar R. Echoencephalographic findings in neonates associated with maternal cocaine and methamphetamine use: incidence and clinical correlates. J Pediatr 1989; 115:770.

484. Seaman ME. Acute cocaine abuse associated with cerebral infarction. Ann Emerg Med 1990; 19:34.

485. Simpson RK, Fischer DK, Narayan RK, et al. Intravenous cocaine abuse and subarachnoid hemorrhage: effect on outcome. Br J Neurosurg 1990; 4:27.

486. Deringer PM, Hamilton LL, Whelan MA. A stroke associated with cocaine use. Arch Neurol 1990; 47:502.

487. Green R, Kelly KM, Gabrielson T, et al. Multiple intracerebral hemorrhages after smoking "crack" cocaine. Stroke 1990; 21:957.

488. Krendel DA, Ditter SM, Frankel MR, Ross WK. Biopsy-proven cerebral vasculitis associated with cocaine abuse. Neurology 1990; 40:1092.

489. Kaku DA, Lowenstein DH. Emergence of recreational drug abuse as a major risk factor for stroke in young adults. Ann Intern Med 1990; 113:821.

490. Hoyme HE, Jones KL, Dixon SD, et al. Prenatal cocaine exposure and fetal vascular disruption. Pediatrics 1990; 85:743.

491. Kramer LD, Locke GE, Ogunyemi A, Nelson L. Neonatal cocaine-related seizures. J Child Neurol 1990; 5:60.

492. Harruff RC, Phillips AM, Fernandez GS. Cocaine-related deaths in Memphis and Shelby County. Ten-year history, 1980–1989. J Tenn Med Assoc 1991; 84:66.

493. Peterson PL, Roszler M, Jacobs I, Wilner HI. Neurovascular complications of cocaine abuse. J Neuropsychiatr 1991; 3:143.

494. Ramadan N, Levine SR, Welch KMA. Pontine hemorrhage following "crack" cocaine use. Neurology 1991; 41:946.

495. Sloan MA, Kittner SJ, Rigamonti D, Price TR. Occurrence of stroke associated with use/abuse of drugs. Neurology 1991; 41:1358.

496. Sauer CM. Recurrent embolic stroke and cocaine-related cardiomyopathy. Stroke 1991; 22:1203.

497. Daras M, Tuchman AJ, Marks S. Central nervous system infarction related to cocaine abuse. Stroke 1991; 22:1320.

498. Hamer JJ, Kamphuis DJ, Rico RE. Cerebral hemorrhages and infarcts following use of cocaine. Ned Tijdschr Geneeskd 1991; 135:333.

499. Heier LA, Carpanzano CR, Mast J, et al. Maternal cocaine abuse: the spectrum of radiologic abnormalities in the neonatal CNS. AJR Am J Roentgenol 1991; 157:1105.

500. Fredericks RK, Lefkowitz DS, Challa VER, Troost BT. Cerebral vasculitis associated with cocaine abuse. Stroke 1991; 22:1437.

501. Dominguez R, Vila-Coro AA, Slopis JM, Bohan TP. Brain and ocular abnormalities in infants with in utero exposure to cocaine and other street drugs. Am J Dis Child 1991; 145:688.

502. Sloan MA, Mattioni TA. Concurrent myocardial and cerebral infarctions after intranasal cocaine use. Stroke 1992; 23:427.

503. Konzen JP, Levine SR, Charbel FT, Garcia JH. The mechanisms of alkaloidal cocaine-related stroke. Neurology 1992; 42 (Suppl 3):249.

504. Guidotti M, Zanasi S. Cocaine use and cerebrovascular disease: Two cases of ischemic stroke in young adults. Ital J Neurol Sci 1990; 11:153.

505. Hall JAS: Cocaine-induced stroke: first Jamaican case. J Neurol Sci 1990; 98:347.

506. Chadan N, Thierry A, Sautreaux JL, et al. Rupture aneurysmale et toxicomanie à la cocaine. Neurochirurgie 1990; 37:403.

507. Storen EC, Wijdicks EFM, Crum BA, Schultz G. Moyamoya-like vasculopathy from cocaine dependency. AJNR Am J Neuroradiol 2000; 21:1008.

508. Fessler RD, Esshaki CM, Stankewitz RC, et al. The neurovascular complications of cocaine. Surg Neurol 1997; 47:339.

509. Tolat D, O'Dell WO, Golamco-Estrella SP, Avella H. Cocaine-associated stroke: three cases and rehabilitation considerations. Brain Inj 2000; 14:383.

510. Nolte KB, Brass LM, Fletterick CF. Intracranial hemorrhage associated with cocaine abuse. A prospective autopsy study. Neurology 1996; 46:1291.

510a. Nwosu CM, Nwabueze AC, Ikeh VO. Stroke at the prime of life: a study of Nigerian Africans between the ages of 16 and 45 years. E Afr Med J 1992; 69:384.

510b. Libman RB, Masters SR, de Paola A, Mohr JP. Transient monocular blindness associated with cocaine abuse. Neurology 1993; 43:228.

510c. Koppel B, Daras M, Kaminsky S, et al. Cerebrovascular complications of pregnancy. Ann Neurol 1992; 32:239.

510d. Casas Parera I, Gatto E, Fernandez Pardal MM, et al. Complicaciones neurologicas por abuso de cocaine. Medicina 1994; 54:35.

510e. Daras M, Tuchman AJ, Koppel BS, et al. Neurovascular complications of cocaine. Acta Neurol Scand 1994; 90:124-129.

510f. Reeves RR, McWilliams ME, Fitz-Gerald MJ. Cocaine-induced ischemic cerebral infarction mistaken for a psychiatric syndrome. South Med J 1995; 88:352.

510g. Martinez N, Diez-Tejedor E, Frank A. Vasospasm/thrombus in cerebral ischemia related to cocaine abuse. Stroke 1996; 27:147.

510h. Baquero M, Alfaro A. Progressive bleeding in spontaneous thalamic hemorrhage. Neurologia 1994; 9:364.

510i. Witlin AG, Mattar F, Sibai BM. Postpartum stroke: a twenty-year experience. Am J Obstet Gynecol 200; 183:83.

511. DiLazzaro V, Restuccia D, Oliviero A, et al. Ischaemic myelopathy associated with cocaine: clinical, neurophysiological, and neuroradiological features. J Neurol Neurosurg Psychiatry 1997; 63:531.

512. Migita DS, Devereaux MW, Tomsak RL. Cocaine and pupillary-sparing oculomotor paresis. Neurology 1997; 49:1466.

513. Brown E, Prajer J, Lee HY, Ramsey RG. CNS complications of cocaine abuse: prevalence, pathophysiology, and neuroradiology. AJR Am J Roentgenol 1992; 159:137.

514. DeVore RA, Tucker HM. Dysphagia and dysarthria as a result of cocaine abuse. Otolaryngol Head Neck Surg 1998; 98:174.

515. Mena I, Giombetti RJ, Miller BL, et al. Cerebral blood flow changes with acute cocaine intoxication: clinical correlations with SPECT, CT, and MRI. NIDA Res Monogr 1994; 138:161.

516. Sawaya GR, Kaminski MJ. Spinal cord infarction after cocaine use. South Med J 1990; 83:601.

516a. Levine SR, Welch KMA, Brust JCM. Cerebral vasculitis associated with cocaine abuse or subarachnoid hemorrhage. JAMA 1988; 259:1648.

516b. Giess R, Rieckmann P, Mullges W. Juvenile cerebral ischaemia caused by designer drugs. Dtsch Med Wochenschr 1998; 123:1308.

516c. Domingo J, Menendez JL, Cerrada E, del Ser T. Cerebral infarction caused after cocaine consumption. Neurologia 1999; 14:45.

516d. Munoz Casares FC, Serrano Castro P, Linan Lopez M, et al. Sudden aphasia in a young woman. Rev Clin Esp 1999; 199:325.

516e. Van Stavern GP, Gorman M: Orbital infarction after cocaine use. Neurology 2002; 59:642.

517. Kaufman MJ, Levin JM, Ross MH, et al. Cocaine-induced cerebral vasoconstriction detected in humans with magnetic resonance angiography. JAMA 1998; 279:376.

518. Case records of the Massachusetts General Hospital: N Engl J Med 1993; 329:117.

519. Morrow PL, McQuillan JB. Cerebral vasculitis associated with cocaine abuse. J Forensic Sci 1993; 38:732.

519a. Merkel PA, Koroshetz WJ, Irizarry MC, et al. Cocaine-associated cerebral vasculitis. Semin Arthritis Rheum 1995; 25:172.

519b. Enriquez R, Palacios FO, Gonzolez CM, et al. Skin vasculitis, hypokalemia and acute renal failure in rhabdomyolysis associated with cocaine. Nephron 1991; 59:336.

520. Martin K, Rogers T, Kavanaugh A. Central nervous system angiopathy associated with cocaine abuse. J Rheumatol 1995; 22:780.

521. LaMonica G, Donatelli A, Katz JL. A case of mutism subsequent to cocaine abuse. J Subst Abuse Treat 1999; 17:109.

522. Strupp M, Hamann GF, Brandt T. Combined amphetamine and cocaine abuse caused mesencephalic ischemia in a 16-year-old boy—due to vasospasm? Eur Neurol 2000; 43:181.

523. Effiong C, Ahuja TS, Wagner JD, et al. Reversible hemiplegia as a consequence of severe hyperkalemia and cocaine abuse in a hemodialysis patient. Am J Med Sci 1997; 314:408.

524. Khellaf M, Fénelon G. Intracranial hemorrhage associated with cocaine abuse. Neurology 1998; 50:1519.

525. Egido-Herrero JA, Gonzalez JL. Pontine hemorrhage after abuse of cocaine (Hemorragia pontina tras abuso de cocaine). Rev Neurol 1997; 25:137.

526. Oyesiku NM, Colohan AR, Barrow DL, Reisner A. Cocaine-induced aneurysmal rupture: an emergent factor in the natural history of intracranial aneurysms? Neurosurgery 1993; 32:518.

527. Keller TM, Chappell ET. Spontaneous acute subdural hematoma precipitated by cocaine abuse: case report. Surg Neurol 1997; 47:12.

528. Samkoff LM, Daras M, Kleiman A, Koppel BS. Spontaneous spinal epidural hematoma: another neurologic complication of cocaine? Arch Neurol 1996; 53:819.

529. Davis GG, Swalwell CI. The incidence of acute cocaine or methamphetamine intoxication in deaths due to ruptured cerebral (berry) aneurysms. J Forensic Sci 1996; 41:626.

530. Kibayashi K, Mastri AR, Hirsch CS. Cocaine induced intracerebral hemorrhage: analysis of predisposing factors and mechanisms causing hemorrhagic strokes. Hum Pathol 1995; 26:659.

531. Aggarwal SK, Williams V, Levine SR, et al. Cocaine-associated intracranial hemorrhage: absence of vasculitis in 14 cases. Neurology 1996; 46:1741.

532. Conway JE, Tamargo RJ. Cocaine use is an independent risk factor for cerebral vasospasm after aneurysmal subarachnoid hemorrhage. Stroke 2001; 32:2338.

533. Nanda A, Vannemreddy PS, Polin RS, Willis BK. Intracranial aneurysms and cocaine abuse: analysis of prognostic indicators. Neurosurgery 2000; 46:1063.

534. Qureshi AI, Akbar MS, Czander E, et al. Crack cocaine use and stroke in young patients. Neurology 1997; 48:341.

535. Riggs JE, Gutmann L. Crack cocaine use and stroke in young patients. Neurology 1997; 49:1473.

536. Petitti DB, Sidney S, Quesenberry C, Bernstein A. Stroke and cocaine or amphetamine use. Epidemiology 1998; 9:596.

537. Brust JCM. Vasculitis owing to substance abuse. Neurol Clin 1997; 15:945.

538. Levine SR, Brust JCM, Futrell N, et al. A comparative study of the cerebrovascular complications of cocaine: alkaloidal versus hydrochloride—a review. Neurology 1991; 41:1173.

539. Isner JM, Chokshi SK. Cocaine and vasospasm. N Engl J Med 1989; 321:1604.

540. Huang QF, Gebrewold A, Altura BT, Altura BM. Cocaine-induced cerebral vascular damage can be ameliorated by Mg^{2+} in rat brain. Neurosci Lett 1990; 109:113.

540a. Johnson BA, Devous MD, Ruiz P, et al. Treatment advances for cocaine-induced ischemic stroke: focus on dihydropyridine-class calcium channel antagonists. Am J Psychiatry 2001; 158:1191.

541. Brecklin CS, Gopaniuk-Folga A, Kravetz T, et al. Prevalence of hypertension in chronic cocaine users. Am J Hypertens 1998; 11:1279.

541a. Mo W, Singh AK, Arruda JA, et al. Role of nitric oxide in cocaine-induced acute hypertension. Am J Hypertens 1998; 11:708.

542. van de Bor M, Walther FJ, Sims ME. Increased cerebral blood flow velocity in infants of mothers who abuse cocaine. Pediatrics 1990; 85:733.

543. Powers RH, Madden JA. Vasoconstrictive effects of cocaine, metabolites and structural analogs on cat cerebral arteries. FASEB J 1990; 4:A1095.

543a. Kaufman MJ, Levin JM, Mass LC, et al: Cocaine-induced cerebral vasoconstriction differs as a function of sex and menstrual cycle phase. Biol Psychiatry 2001; 49:774.

544. Herning RI, King DE, Better WE, Cadet JL. Neurovascular deficits in cocaine users. Neuropsychopharmacology 1999; 21:110.

545. Vongpatanasin W, Monsour Y, Chavoshan B, et al. Cocaine stimulates the human cardiovascular system via a central mechanism of action. Circulation 1999; 100:497.

546. Mo W, Arruda JA, Dunea G, Singh AK. Cocaine-induced hypertension: role of the peripheral sympathetic system. Pharmacol Res 1999; 40:139.

547. Zhang X, Schrott LM, Spaber SB. Evidence for a serotonin-mediated effect of cocaine causing vasoconstriction and herniated umbilici in chicken embryos. Pharmacol Biochem Behav 1998; 59:585.

548. Wang AM, Suojanen JN, Colucci VM, et al. Cocaine- and methamphetamine-induced acute cerebral vasospasm: an angiographic study in rabbits. AJNR Am J Neuroradiol 1990; 11:1141.

549. Fayad PB, Price LH, McDougle CJ, et al. Acute hemodynamic effects of intranasal cocaine on the cerebral and cardiovascular systems. Stroke 1992; 23:26.

550. Dohi S, Jones D, Hudak ML, Traystman RJ. Effects of cocaine on pial arterioles in cats. Stroke 1990; 21:1710.

551. O'Brien TP, Pane MA, Traystman RJ, Gleason CA. Propranolol blocks cocaine-induced cerebral vasodilation in newborn sheep. Crit Care Med 1999; 27:784.

552. Nunez BD, Miao L, Ross JN, et al. Effects of cocaine on carotid vascular reactivity in swine after balloon vascular injury. Stroke 1994; 25:631.

553. Wilbert-Lampen U, Seliger C, Zilker T, Arendt RM. Cocaine increases the endothelial release of immuno-reactive endothelin and its concentration in human plasma and urine: reversal by coincubation with sigma-receptor antagonists. Circulation 1998; 98:385.

553a. Fandino J, Sherman JD, Zuccarello M, et al. Cocaine-induced endothelin-1-dependent spasm in rabbit basilar artery in vivo. J Cardiovasc Pharmacol 2003; 41:158.

554. Zhang A, Cheng TP, Altura BT, Altura BM. Acute cocaine results in rapid rises in free calcium concentration in canine cerebral vascular smooth muscle cells: possible relation to etiology of stroke. Neurosci Lett 1996; 215:57.

555. Togna G, Tempesta E, Togna AR, et al. Platelet responsiveness and biosynthesis of thromboxane and prostacyclin in response to in vitro cocaine treatment. Haemostasis 1985; 15:100.

555a. Heesch CM, Wilhelm CR, Ristich J, et al. Cocaine activates platelets and increases the formation of circulating platelet containing aggregates. Heart (Br Cardiac Soc) 2000; 83:688.

556. Jennings LK, White MM, Sauer CM, et al. Cocaine-induced platelet defects. Stroke 1993; 24:1352.

557. Leissinger CA. Severe thrombocytopenia associated with cocaine use. Ann Intern Med 1990; 112:708.

558. Langner RO, Bement CL, Perry LE. Arteriosclerotic toxicity of cocaine. NIDA Res Monogr 1987; 88:325.

559. Cuervo Pinna MA, Calvo Romero JM, Ramos Salada JL. The association between cocaine consumption and lupus anticoagulant as the probable cause of ischemic stroke. Rev Clin Esp 1999; 199:329.

560. Siegel AJ, Sholar MB, Mendelson JH, et al. Cocaine-induced erythrocytosis and increase in von Willebrand factor: evidence for drug-related blood doping and prothrombotic effects. Arch Intern Med 1999; 159:1925.

561. Little K, Krolewski DM, Zhang L, et al. Loss of striatal vesicular monoamine transporter protein (VMAT2) in human cocaine users. Am J Psychiatry 2003; 160:47.

561a. Little KY, Krolewski DM, Zhang L, et al. Loss of striatal vesicular monoamine transporter protein (VMAT2) in human cocaine users. Am J Psychiatry 2003; 160:47.

562. Buck AA, Sasaki TT, Hewitt JJ, Macrae AA. Coca chewing and health. An epidemiologic study among residents of a Peruvian village. Am J Epidemiol 1968; 88:159.

563. Negrete JC, Murphy HBM. Psychological deficit in chewers of coca leaf. Bull Narc 1967; 19:11.

564. Weinrieb RM, O'Brien CP. Persistent cognitive deficits attributed to substance abuse. In: Brust JCM, ed. Neurological Complications of Drug and Alcohol Abuse. Neurol Clin 1993; 11:663.

565. Ardila A, Roselli M, Strumwasser S. Neuropsychological deficits in chronic cocaine abusers. Int J Neurosci 1991; 57:73.

566. O'Malley S, Adamse M, Heaton RK, Gawin FH. Neuropsychological impairment in chronic cocaine abusers. Am J Drug Alcohol Abuse 1992; 18:131.

567. Smelson DA, Roy A, Santana S, Engelhart C. Neuropsychological deficits in withdrawn cocaine-dependent males. Am J Drug Alcohol Abuse 1999; 25:377.

568. Bolla KI, Rothman R, Cadet JL. Dose-related neurobehavioral effects of chronic cocaine use. J Neuropsychiatr Clin Neurosci 1999; 11:361.

569. Hoff AL, Riordan H, Morris L, et al. Effects of crack cocaine on neurocognitive function. Psychiatry Res 1996; 60:167.

570. Van Gorp WG, Wilkins JN, Hinkin CH, et al. Declarative and procedural memory functioning in abstinent cocaine abusers. Arch Gen Psychiatry 1999; 56:85.

571. Van Gorp WG, Hull J, Wilkins JN, et al. Nicotine dependence and withdrawal in cocaine-dependent patients. Arch Gen Psychiatry 2000; 57:512.

572. Serper MR, Bergman A, Copersino ML, et al. Learning and memory impairment in cocaine-dependent and comorbid schizophrenic patients. Psychiatry Res 2000; 93:21.

573. McLellan AT, Woody GE, O'Brien CP. Development of psychiatric disorders in drug abusers. N Engl J Med 1979; 301:1310-1313.

574. Bolla KI, Funderburk FR, Cadet JL. Differential effects of cocaine and cocaine plus alcohol on neurocognitive performance. Neurology 2000; 54:2285.

575. Pascual-Leone A, Dhuna A. EEG in cocaine addicts. Ann Neurol 1990; 28:250.

576. Pascual-Leone A, Dhuna A, Anderson DC. Cerebral atrophy in habitual cocaine abusers: a planimetric CT study. Neurology 1991; 41:34.

577. Langendorf FG, Tupper DE, Rottenberg DA, et al. Does chronic cocaine exposure cause brain atrophy? A quantitative MRI study. Neurology 2000 (Suppl 3); 54:A442.

578. Bartzokis G, Beckson M, Lu PH, et al. Age-related brain volume reductions in amphetamine and cocaine addicts and normal controls: implications for addiction research. Psychiatry Res 2000; 98:93.

579. Bartzokis G, Goldstein IB, Hance DB, et al. The incidence of T2-weighted MR imaging signal abnormalities in the brain of cocaine-dependent patients is age-related and region-specific. AJNR Am J Neuroradiol 1999; 20:1628.

580. Bartzokis G, Beckson M, Hance DB, et al. Magnetic resonance imaging evidence of "silent" cerebrovascular toxicity in cocaine dependence. Biol Psychiatry 1999; 45:1203.

581. Volkow ND, Hitzemann R, Wang G-J, et al. Long-term frontal metabolic changes in cocaine abusers. Synapse 1992; 11:184.

582. Tumeh SS, Nagel JS, English RJ, et al. Cerebral abnormalities in cocaine abusers: demonstration by

SPECT perfusion brain scintigraphy. Radiology 1990; 176:821.

583. Holman BL, Carvalho PA, Mendelson J, et al. Brain perfusion is abnormal in cocaine-dependent polydrug users: a study using technetium-99m-HMPAO and ASPECT. J Nucl Med 1991; 32:1206.

584. London ED, Cascella NG, Wong DF, et al. Cocaine-induced reduction of glucose utilization in human brain. Arch Gen Psychiatry 1990; 47:567.

585. Levisohn PM, Kramer RE, Rosenberg NL. Neurophysiology of chronic cocaine and toluene abuse. Neurology 1992; 42 (Suppl 3):434.

586. Biggins CA, MacKay S, Clark W, Fein G. Event-related potential evidence for frontal cortex effects of chronic cocaine dependence. Biol Psychiatry 1997; 42:472.

587. Li S-J, Wang Y, Pankiewicz J, Stein EA. Neurochemical adaptation to cocaine abuse: reduction of N-acetyl aspartate in thalamus of human cocaine abusers. Biol Psychiatry 1999; 45:1481.

588. Breiter HC, Gollub RL, Weisskoff RM, et al. Acute effects of cocaine on human brain activity and emotion. Neuron 1997; 19:591.

589. Chang L, Mehringer CM, Ernst T, et al. Neurochemical alterations in asymptomatic abstinent cocaine users: a proton magnetic resonance spectroscopy study. Biol Psychiatry 1997; 42:1105.

590. Chang L, Ernst T, Strickland T, Mahringer CM. Gender effects on persistent cerebral metabolic changes in the frontal lobes of abstinent cocaine users. Am J Psychiatry 1999; 156:716.

590a. Lim KO, Chois SJ, Pomara N, et al: Reduced frontal white matter integrity in cocaine dependence: a controlled diffusion tensor imaging study. Biol Psychiatry 2002; 51:890.

590b. Kosten TR. Pharmacotherapy of cerebral ischemia in cocaine dependence. Drug Alcohol Dep 1998; 49:133.

591. Little BB, Snell LM, Klein VR, Gilstrap LC. Cocaine abuse during pregnancy: maternal and fetal implications. Obstet Gynecol 1989; 73:157.

592. Frank DA, Zuckerman BS, Amaro H, et al. Cocaine use during pregnancy: prevalence and correlates. Pediatrics 1988; 82:888.

593. Chasnoff IJ, Landress HJ, Barrett ME. The prevalence of illicit-drug or alcohol use during pregnancy and discrepancies in mandatory reporting in Pinellas County, Florida. N Engl J Med 1990; 322:1202.

594. Chira S. Crack babies turn 5 and schools brace. NY Times, May 25, 1990.

595. Heagarty M. Crack cocaine: a new danger for children. Am J Dis Child 1990; 144:756.

596. Chiriboga CA. Fetal effects. In: Brust JCM, ed. Neurologic Complications of Drug and Alcohol Abuse. Neurol Clin 1993; 11:707.

596a. Chiriboga CA. Fetal alcohol and drug effects. Neurologist 2003; 9:257.

597. Bingol H, Fuchs M, Diaz V, et al. Teratogenicity of cocaine in humans. J Pediatr 1987; 110:93.

598. Hadeed AJ, Siegel SR. Maternal cocaine use during pregnancy: effect on the newborn infant. Pediatrics 1989; 84:205.

599. Chasnoff IJ, Burns WJ, Schnoll SH, Burns KA. Cocaine use in pregnancy. N Engl J Med 1985; 313:666.

600. Chasnoff IJ, Griffiths DR, MacGregor S, et al. Temporal patterns of cocaine use in pregnancy. Perinatal outcome. JAMA 1989; 261:1741.

601. Chouteau M, Brickner P, Namerow PB, Leppert P. The effect of cocaine abuse on birth weight and gestational age. Obstet Gynecol 1988; 72:351.

602. Cherukuri R, Minkoff H, Feldman J, et al. A cohort study of alkaloidal cocaine ("crack") in pregnancy. Obstet Gynecol 1988; 72:147.

603. Zuckerman B, Frank DA, Hingson R, et al. Effects of marijuana and cocaine use on fetal growth. N Engl J Med 1989; 320:762.

604. Fulroth R, Phillips B, Durand BJ. Perinatal outcome of infants exposed to cocaine and/or heroin in utero. Am J Dis Child 1989; 143:905.

604a. Bandstra ES, Morrow CE, Anthony JC, et al. Intrauterine growth of full-term infants: impact of prenatal cocaine exposure. Pediatrics 2001; 108:1309.

605. Ryan L, Ehrlich S, Finnegan L. Cocaine abuse in pregnancy: effects on the fetus and newborn. Neurotoxicol Teratol 1987; 9:295.

606. Chasnoff IJ, Chisum GM, Kaplan WE. Maternal cocaine use and genitourinary tract malformations. Teratology 1988; 37:201.

607. Urogenital anomalies in the offspring of women using cocaine during early pregnancy—Atlanta, 1968–1980. MMWR 1989; 38:536.

608. Lipschultz SE, Frassica JJ, Orav EJ. Cardiovascular abnormalities in infants prenatally exposed to cocaine. J Pediatr 1991; 118:44.

609. Esmer MC, Rodriquez-Soto G, Carrasco-Daza D, et al. Cloverleaf skull and multiple congenital anomalies in a girl exposed to cocaine in utero: case report and review of the literature. Childs Nerv Syst 2000; 16:176.

610. Downing GJ, Horner SR, Kilbride HW. Characteristics of perinatal cocaine-exposed infants with necrotizing enterocolitis. Am J Dis Child 1991; 145:26.

611. Bays J. Fetal vascular disruption with prenatal exposure to cocaine or methamphetamine. Pediatrics 1991; 87:416.

612. Spierer A, Isenberg SJ, Inkelis SH. Characteristics of the iris in 100 neonates. J Pediatr Ophthalmol Strabismus 1989; 26:28.

613. Teske MP, Trese MT. Retinopathy of prematurity-like fundus and persistent hyperplastic primary vitreous associated with maternal cocaine use. Am J Ophthalmol 1987; 103:719.

614. Singer L, Arendt R, Yamashita, et al. Development of infants exposed in utero to cocaine. Pediatr Res 1992; 31:260A.

615. Eyler FD, Behnke M, Conlon M, et al. Birth outcomes from a prospective, matched study of prenatal crack/cocaine use. I. Interactive and dose effects on health and growth. Pediatrics 1998; 101:229.

616. Eyler FD, Behnke M, Conlon M, et al. Birth outcomes from a prospective, matched study of prenatal crack/cocaine use. II. Interactive and dose effects on neurobehavioral assessment. Pediatrics 1998; 101:237.

617. Tronick EZ, Frank DA, Cabral H, et al. Late dose-response effects of prenatal cocaine exposure on newborn neurobehavioral performance. Pediatrics 1996; 98:76.

618. Napiorkowski B, Lester BM, Freier MC, et al. Effects of in utero substance exposure on infant neurobehavior. Pediatrics 1996; 98:71.

619. Kramer LD, Locke GE, Ogunyemi A, Nelson L. Neonatal cocaine-related seizures. J Child Neurol 1990; 5:60.

620. Doberczak TM, Shanzer S, Senie RT, Kandall SR. Neonatal neurologic and electroencephalographic effects of intrauterine cocaine exposure. J Pediatr 1988; 113:354.

621. Scher MS, Richardson GA, Day NL. Effects of prenatal cocaine/crack and other drug exposure on electroencephalographic sleep studies at birth and one year. Pediatrics 2000; 105:39.

622. Mirochnick M, Meyer J, Frank D, et al. Elevated plasma norepinephrine after in utero exposure to cocaine and marijuana. Pediatrics 1997; 99:555.

623. Chiriboga CA, Bateman D, Brust JCM, Hauser WA. Neurological outcome of neonates exposed in-utero to cocaine. Pediatr Neurol 1993; 9:115.

624. Chiriboga CA, Brust JCM, Bateman D, Hauser WA. Dose-response effect of fetal cocaine exposure on newborn neurologic function. Pediatrics 1999; 103:79.

625. Chiriboga CA, Bateman D, Brust JCM, Hauser WA. Neurological findings in cocaine-exposed infants. Pediatr Neurol 1993; 9:115.

626. Chiriboga CA, Vibbert M, Malour R, et al. Neurological correlates of fetal cocaine exposure: transient hypertonia of infancy and early childhood. Pediatrics 1995; 96:1070.

627. Dempsey DA, Hajnal BL, Partridge JC, et al. Tone abnormalities are associated with maternal cigarette smoking during pregnancy in utero cocaine-exposed infants. Pediatrics 2000; 106:79.

628. Bateman DA, Chiriboga CA. Dose-response effect of cocaine in newborn head circumference. Pediatrics 2000; 106:e33.

629. Shih L, Cone-Wesson B, Reddix B. Effects of maternal cocaine abuse on neonatal auditory system. Int J Pediatr Otorhinolaryngol 1988; 15:245.

630. Frank DA, McCarten KM, Robson CD, et al. Level of in utero cocaine exposure and neonatal ultrasound findings. Pediatrics 1999; 104:1101.

631. Volpe BJ. Effect of cocaine use on the fetus. N Engl J Med 1992; 327:399.

632. Chasnoff IJ, Hunt CE, Kletter R, Kaplan D. Prenatal cocaine exposure is associated with respiratory pattern abnormalities. Am J Dis Child 1989; 143:583.

633. Mayes LC, Granger RH, Bornstein RH, Zuckerman B. The problem of prenatal cocaine exposure. JAMA 1992; 267:406.

634. Zuckerman B, Maynard EC, Cabral H. A preliminary report of prenatal cocaine exposure and respiratory distress syndrome in premature infants. Am J Dis Child 1991; 145:696.

635. Fares I, McCulloch KM, Raju TN. Intrauterine cocaine exposure and the risk for sudden infant death syndrome: a meta-analysis. J Perinatol 1997; 17:179.

636. Miller JM, Boudreaux MC, Regan FA. A case–control study of cocaine use during pregnancy. Am J Obstet Gynecol 1995; 172:180.

637. Plessinger MA, Wopods JR. Cocaine in pregnancy. Recent data on maternal and fetal risks. Obstet Gynecol Clin North Am 1998; 25:99.

638. Ness RB, Grisso JA, Hirschinger N, et al. Cocaine and tobacco use and the risk of spontaneous abortion. N Engl J Med 1999; 340:333.

639. Congenital syphilis—New York City, 1986–1988. MMWR 1989; 38:825.

640. Madden JD, Payne TF, Miller S. Maternal cocaine abuse and effect on the newborn. Pediatrics 1986; 77:209.

641. Neuspiel DR, Hamel SC, Hochberg E, et al. Maternal cocaine use and infant behavior. Neurotoxicol Teratol 1991; 13:229.

642. Bauer CR. Perinatal effects of prenatal drug exposure: neonatal aspects. Clin Perinatol 1999; 26:87.

643. Kuhn L, Kline J, Ng S, et al. Cocaine use during pregnancy and intrauterine growth retardation: new insights based on maternal hair tests. Am J Epidemiol 2000; 152:112.

644. Graham K, Dimitrakoudis D, Pellegrini E, Koren G. Pregnancy outcome following first trimester exposure to cocaine in social users in Toronto, Canada. Vet Hum Toxicol 1989; 31:143.

645. Richardson GA, Hamel SC, Goldschmidt L, Day NL. Growth of infants prenatally exposed to cocaine/crack: comparison of a prenatal care and no prenatal care sample. Pediatrics 1999; 104:e293.

646. Frank DA, McCarten K, Cahral H, et al. Cranial ultra-sounds in term newborns: failure to replicate excess abnormalities in cocaine exposed. Pediatr Res 1992; 31:247A.

647. Koren G, Shear H, Graham K, Einarson T. Bias against the null hypothesis: the reproductive hazards of cocaine. Lancet 1989; II:440.

648. Lutiger B, Graham K, Einarson TR, Koren G. Relationship between gestational cocaine use and pregnancy outcome: a meta-analysis. Teratology 1991; 44:405.

649. Eyler FD, Behnke M. Early development of infants exposed to drugs prenatally. Clin Perinatol 1999; 26:107.

650. Tronick EZ, Beeghly M. Prenatal cocaine exposure, child development, and the compromising effects of cumulative risk. Clin Perinatol 1999; 26:151.

651. Frank DA, Augustyn M, Knight WG, et al. Growth, development, and behavior in early childhood following prenatal cocaine exposure. A systematic review. JAMA 2001; 285:1613.

652. Lester BM, LaGasse LL, Seifer R. Cocaine exposure and children: the meaning of subtle effects. Science 1998; 282:633.

653. Lester BM, Tronick EZ, LaGasse L, et al. The Maternal Lifestyle Study: effects of substance exposure during pregnancy on neurodevelopmental outcome in 1-month-old infants. Pediatrics 2002; 110:1182.

654. Hurt H, Malmed E, Betancourt L, et al. Children with in utero cocaine exposure do not differ from control subjects on intelligence testing. Arch Pediatr Adolesc Med 1997; 151:1237.

655. Richardson GA, Coroy ML, Day NL. Prenatal cocaine exposure: effects on the development of school-age children. Neurotoxicol Teratol 1996; 18:627.

656. Wasserman GA, Kline JK, Bateman DA, et al. Prenatal cocaine exposure and school-age intelligence. Drug Alcohol Dep 1998; 50:203.

657. Annas GJ. Testing poor pregnant women for cocaine—physicians as police investigators. N Engl J Med 2001; 344:1729.

658. Mahalik MP, Gautieri RF, Mann DE. Teratogenic potential of cocaine hydrochloride in CF-1 mice. J Pharmacol Sci 1980; 69:703.

659. Fantel AG, Macphail T. The teratogenicity of cocaine. Teratology 1982; 26:17.

660. Spear LP, Kirstein C, Bell J, et al. Effects of prenatal cocaine on behavior during the early postnatal period in rats. Teratology 1987; 35:BTS12.

661. Church MW, Dintcheff BA, Gessner PK. Dose-dependent consequences of cocaine on pregnancy outcome in the Long-Evans rat. Neurotoxicol Teratol 1988; 10:51.

662. el-Bizri H, Guest I, Varma DR. Effects of cocaine on rat embryo development in vivo and in cultures. Pediatr Res 1991; 29:187.

663. Wilkins AS, Genova LM, Posten W, et al. Transplacental cocaine exposure. 1. A rodent model. Neurotoxicol Teratol 1998; 20:215.

664. Hecht GS, Spear NE, Spear LP. Alterations in the reinforcing efficacy of cocaine in adult rats following prenatal exposure to cocaine. Behav Neurosci 1998; 112:410.

665. Kelley BM, Groseclose CH, Middaugh LD. Prenatal cocaine exposure increases the reinforcing strength of oral ethanol in C57 mice. Neurotoxicol Teratol 1997; 19:391.

666. Church MW, Crossland WJ, Holmes PA, et al. Effects of prenatal cocaine on hearing, vision, growth, and behavior. Ann N Y Acad Sci 1998; 846:12.

667. Mactutus CF. Prenatal intravenous cocaine adversely effects attentional processing in preweanling rats. Neurotoxicol Neuroteratol 1999; 21:539.

668. Snyder-Keller A, Sam C, Keller RW. Enhanced susceptibility to cocaine and pentylenetetrazol-induced seizures in prenatally cocaine-treated rats. Neurotoxicol Teratol 2000; 22:231.

669. Iso A, Nakahara K, Barr GA, et al. Long-term intravenous perinatal cocaine exposure on the mortality of rat offspring. Neurotoxicol Teratol 2000; 22:165.

670. Baraban SC, Wenzel HJ, Castro PA, Schwartzkroin PA. Hippocampal dysplasia in rats exposed to cocaine in utero. Brain Res Dev Brain Res 1999; 117:213.

671. Murphy CA, Ghazi I, Kokabi A, Ellison G. Prenatal cocaine produces signs of neurodegeneration in the lateral habenula. Brain Res 1999; 851:175.

672. Woods J, Plessinger M, Clark KE. Effects of cocaine on uterine blood flow and fetal oxygenation. JAMA 1987; 257:957.

673. Moore T, Sorg J, Miller L, et al. Hemodynamic effects of intravenous cocaine on the pregnant ewe and fetus. Am J Obstet Gynecol 1986; 155:883.

674. Morgan MA, Silavin SL, Randolf M, et al. Effect of intravenous cocaine on uterine blood flow in the gravid baboon. Am J Obstet Gynecol 1991; 164:1021.

675. Stewart DJ, Inaba T, Lucassen M, et al. Cocaine metabolism: cocaine and novocaine hydrolysis by liver and serum esterases. Clin Pharmacol Ther 1979; 25:464.

676. Abel EL, Moore C, Waselewsky D, et al. Effects of cocaine hydrochloride on reproductive function and sexual behavior of male rats and on the behavior of their offspring. J Androl 1989; 10:17.

677. Yazigi RA, Odem RR, Polakoski KL. Demonstration of specific binding of cocaine to human spermatozoa. JAMA 1991; 266:1956.

678. Patel TG, Laungani RC, Grose EA, Dow-Edwards DL. Cocaine decreases uteroplacental blood flow in the rat. Neurotoxicol Teratol 1999; 21:559.

679. Glezer II, Toporovsky IM, Lima V, Yablonsky-Alter E. Cocaine adversely affects development of cortical embryonic neurons in vitro: immunocytochemical study of calcium-binding proteins. Brain Res 1999; 815:389.

680. Xiao Y, He J, Gilbert RD, Zhang L. Cocaine induces apoptosis in fetal myocardial cells through a mitochondrial-dependent pathway. J Pharmacol Exp Ther 2000; 292:8-14.

681. Lidow MS. Nonhuman primate model of the effect of prenatal cocaine exposure on cerebral cortical development. Ann N Y Acad Sci 1998; 846:182.

682. Jones LB, Stanwood GD, Reinoso BS, et al. In utero cocaine-induced dysfunction of dopamine D_1 receptor signaling and abnormal differentiation of cerebral cortical neurons. J Neurosci 2000; 20:4606.

683. Whitaker-Azmitia PM. Role of the neurotrophic properties of serotonin in the delay of brain maturation induced by cocaine. Ann N Y Acad Sci 1998; 846:158.

684. Bloom FE. Keynote address. Ann N Y Acad Sci 1998; 846:xix.

685. Sanchez-Ramos J, Song S, Weiner W, Busto R. Potential cytotoxicity of norcocaine for developing dopaminergic neurons. Neurology 1992; 42 (Suppl 3):406.

686. Nassogne M-C, Evrard P, Courtoy PJ. Selective direct toxicity of cocaine on fetal mouse neurons. Teratogenic implications of neurite and apoptotic neuronal loss. Ann N Y Acad Sci 1998; 846:51.

687. Li J-H, Lin L-F. Genetic toxicology and abused drugs: a brief review. Mutagenesis 1998; 13:557.

688. Lipton JW, Ling Z, Vu TQ, et al. Prenatal cocaine exposure reduces glial cell line-derived neurotrophic factor (GDNF) in the striatum and the carotid body of the rat: implications for DA neurodevelopment. Dev Brain Res 1999; 118:231.

689. Ronnekleiv OK, Fang Y, Choi WS, Chai L. Changes in the midbrain–rostral forebrain dopamine circuitry in the cocaine-exposed primate fetal brain. Ann N Y Acad Sci 1998; 846:165.

690. Fang Y, Ronnekleiv OK. Cocaine upregulates the dopamine transporter in fetal rhesus monkey brain. J Neurosci 1999; 19:8966.

691. Cabrera-Vera TM, Garcia F, Pinto W, Battaglia G. Neurochemical changes in brain serotonin neurons in immature and adult offspring prenatally exposed to cocaine. Brain Res 2000; 870:1.

692. Chasnoff IJ, Lewis DE, Squires L. Cocaine intoxication in a breast-fed infant. Pediatrics 1987; 80:836.

693. Chaney NE, Franke J, Wadlington WB. Cocaine convulsions in a breast-feeding baby. J Pediatr 1988; 112:134.

694. Rivkin M, Gilmore HE. Generalized seizures in an infant due to environmentally acquired cocaine. Pediatrics 1989; 84:1100.

695. Bateman DA, Heagarty MC. Passive freebase cocaine ("crack") inhalation by infants and toddlers. Am J Dis Child 1989; 143:25.

696. Kharasch SJ, Glotzer D, Vinci R, et al. Unsuspected cocaine exposure in young children. Am J Dis Child 1991; 145:204.

697. Sturner WQ, Sweeney KG, Callery RT, Haley NR. Cocaine babies: the scourge of the '90s. J Forensic Sci 1991; 36:34.

698. Stitzer ML, Walsh SL. Psychostimulant abuse: the case for combined behavioral and pharmacological treatments. Pharmacol Biochem Behav 1997; 57:457.

699. LeSage MG, Stafford D, Glowa JR. Preclinical research on cocaine self-administration: environmental determinants and their interaction with pharmacological treatment. Neurosci Biobehav Rev 1999; 23:717.

700. Mello NK, Negus SS. Preclinical evaluation of pharmacotherapies for treatment of cocaine and opioid abuse using drug self-administration procedures. Neuropsychopharmacology 1996; 14:375.

701. Winger G. Pharmacological modifications of cocaine and opioid self-administration. In: Clouet D, Asghar K, Brown R, eds. Mechanisms of Cocaine Abuse and Toxicity. NIDA Res Monogr 1988; 88:125.

702. Kosten TR, Schumann B, Wright D. Bromocriptine treatment of cocaine abuse in patients maintained on methadone. Am J Psychiatry 1988; 145:381.

703. Extein IL, Gross DA, Gold MS. Bromocriptine treatment of cocaine withdrawal symptoms. Am J Psychiatry 1989; 146:403.

704. Kranzler HR, Bauer LO. Effects of bromocriptine on subjective and autonomic responses to cocaine-associated stimuli. NIDA Res Monogr 1991; 105:505.

705. Preston KL, Sullivan JT, Strain EC, Bigelow GE. Effects of cocaine alone and in combination with bromocriptine in human cocaine abusers. NIDA Res Monogr 1991; 105:507.

706. Handelsman L, Rosenblum A, Palij M, et al. Bromocriptine for cocaine dependence. A controlled clinical trial. Am J Addict 1997; 6:54.

707. Giannini AJ, Folts DJ, Feather JN, Sullivan BS. Bromocriptine and amantadine in cocaine detoxification. Psychiatr Res 1989; 29:11.

708. Handelsman L, Limpitlaw L, Williams D, et al. Amantadine does not reduce cocaine use or craving in cocaine-dependent methadone-maintenance patients. Drug Alcohol Depend 1995; 39:173.

709. Kampman K, Volpicelli JR, Alterman AL, et al. Amantadine in the early treatment of cocaine dependence: a double-blind, placebo-controlled trial. Drug Alcohol Dep 1996; 41:25.

710. Malcolm R, Hutto BR, Phillips JD, Ballenger JC. Pergolide mesylate treatment of cocaine withdrawal. J Clin Psychiatry 1991; 52:39.

711. Levin FR, McDowell D, Evans SM, et al. Pergolide mesylate for cocaine abuse: a controlled preliminary trial. Am J Addict 1999; 8:120.

712. Malcolm R, Herron J, Sutherland SE, Brady KT. Adverse outcomes in a controlled trial of pergolide for cocaine dependence. J Addict Dis 2001; 20:81.

713. Malcolm R, Moore JW, Kajdasz DK, et al. Pergolide mesylate. Adverse events occurring in the treatment of cocaine dependence. Am J Addict 1997; 6:117.

714. Kleber H. Psychopharmacological trials in cocaine abuse treatment. Am J Drug Alcohol Abuse 1986; 12:235.

715. Grabowski J, Roache JD, Schmitz JM, et al. Replacement medication for cocaine dependence: methylphenidate. J Clin Psychopharmacol 1997; 17:485.

716. Gawin FH, Kleber HD, Byck R, et al. Desipramine facilitation of initial cocaine abstinence. Arch Gen Psychiatry 1989; 46:117.

717. Brotman AW, Witkie SM, Gelenberg AJ, et al. An open trial of maprotiline for the treatment of cocaine abuse: a pilot study. J Clin Psychopharmacol 1988; 8:125.

718. Hall SM, Tunis S, Triffleman E, et al. Continuity of care and desipramine in primary cocaine abusers. J Nerv Ment Dis 1994; 182:570.

719. Carroll KM, Rounsaville BJ, Gordon LT, et al. Psychotherapy and pharmacotherapy for ambulatory cocaine abusers. Arch Gen Psychiatry 1994; 51:177.

720. Weiss RD. Relapse to cocaine abuse after initiating desipramine treatment. JAMA 1988; 260:2545.

721. Kosten T, Gawin FH, Silverman DG, et al. Intravenous cocaine challenges during desipramine maintenance. Neuropsychopharmacology 1992; 7:169.

722. Berger P, Gawin F, Kosten TR. Treatment of cocaine abuse with mazindol. Lancet 1989; I:283.

723. Margolin A, Avants SK, Kosten TR. Mazindol for relapse prevention to cocaine abuse in methadone maintenance patients. Am J Drug Alcohol Abuse 1995; 21:469.

724. Stine SM, Krystal JH, Kosten TR, Charney DS. Mazindol treatment for cocaine dependence. Drug Alcohol Depend 1995; 39:245.

725. Gorelick DA. The rate hypothesis and agonist substitution approaches to cocaine abuse treatment. Adv Pharmacol 1998; 42:995.

726. Negus SS, Brandt MR, Mello NK. Effects of long-acting monoamine inhibitor indatraline on cocaine self-administration in rhesus monkeys. J Pharmacol Exp Ther 1999; 291:60.

727. Golwyn DH. Cocaine abuse treated with phenylzine. Int J Addict 1988; 23:897.

728. Haberny KA, Walsh SL, Ginn DH, et al. Absence of acute interactions with the MAO-B inhibitor selegiline. Drug Alcohol Dep 1995; 39:55.

729. Rosen H, Flemenbaum A, Slater VL. Clinical trial of carbidopa–L-DOPA combination for cocaine abuse. Am J Psychiatry 1986: 143:149.

730. Howell LL, Eilcox KM. The dopamine transporter and cocaine medication development: drug self-administration in non-human primates. J Pharmacol Exp Ther 2001; 298:1.

731. Bradberry CW, Lee T, Jatlow P. Rapid induction of behavioral and neurochemical tolerance to cocaethylene, a model compound for agonist therapy of cocaine dependence. Psychopharmacology 1999; 146:87.

731a. Soares BG, Lima MS, Reisser AA, et al. Dopamine agonists for cocaine dependence. Cochrane Database of Systematic Reviews (4): CD00352, 2001.

731b. Lima MS, Reisser AA, Soares BG, et al. Antidepressants for cocaine dependence. Cochrane Database of Systematic Reviews (4): CD002950, 2001.

732. Wise RA. Neural mechanisms and reinforcing action of cocaine. NIDA Res Monogr 1984; 50:15.

733. Gawin FH, Allen D, Humblestone B. Outpatient treatment of "crack" cocaine smoking with flupenthixol decanoate. A preliminary report. Arch Gen Psychiatry 1989; 46:322.

734. LeFoll B, Schwartz JC, Sokoloff P. Dopamine D3 receptor agents as potential new medications for drug addiction. Eur Psychiatry 2000; 15:140.

735. Walsh SL, Preston KL, Sullivan JT, et al. Fluoxetine alters the effects of intravenous cocaine in humans. J Clin Psychopharmacol 1994; 14:396.

736. Covi L, Hess JM, Kreitr NA, Haertzen CA. Effects of combined fluoxetine and counseling in the outpatient treatment of cocaine abusers. Am J Drug Alcohol Abuse 1995; 21:327.

737. Grabowski J, Rhoades H, Elk R, et al. Fluoxetine is ineffective for treatment of cocaine dependence or concurrent opiate and cocaine dependence: two placebo-controlled, double-blind trials. J Clin Psychopharmacol 1995; 15:163.

738. Batki SL, Manfredi L, Jacob P, et al. Double-blind fluoxetine treatment of cocaine dependence in methadone maintenance (MMT) patients. Interim analysis. NIDA Res Monogr 1993; 132:102.

739. McDowell DM, Levin FR, Seracini AM, Nunes EV. Venlafaxine treatment of cocaine abusers with depressive symptoms. Am J Drug Alcohol Abuse 2000; 26:25.

740. Cornelius JR, Salloum IM, Thase ME, et al. Fluoxetine versus placebo in depressed alcoholic cocaine abusers. Psychopharmacol Bull 1998; 34:117.

741. Kampman KM, Rukstalis M, Pettinati H, et al. The combination of phentermine and fenfluramine reduced cocaine withdrawal symptoms in an open trial. J Subst Abuse Treat 2000; 19:77.

741a. Johnson BA, Chen YR, Swann AC, et al. Ritanserin in the treatment of cocaine dependence. Biol Psychiatry 1997; 42:932.

742. Borg L, Brow DM, Ho A, Kreek MJ. Cocaine abuse sharply reduced in an effective methadone maintenance program. J Addict Dis 1999; 18:63.

743. Mello NK, Mendelson JH, Bree MP, et al. Bupremorphine suppresses cocaine self-administration by rhesus monkeys. Science 1989; 245:859.

744. Mello NK, Mendelson JH, Lukas SE, et al. Bupremorphine treatment of opiate and cocaine abuse: clinical and preclinical studies. Harv Rev Psychiatry 1993; 1:168.

745. Schottenfeld RS, Pakes JR, Oliveto A, et al. Bupremorphine vs methadone maintenance treatment for concurrent opioid dependence and cocaine abuse. Arch Gen Psychiatry 1997; 54:713.

746. Schenk S, Partridge B, Shippenberg TS. U69593, a kappa-opioid agonist, decreases cocaine self-administration and decreases cocaine-produced drug seeking. Psychopharmacology 1999; 144:339.

747. Neumeyer JL, Mello NK, Negus SS, Bidlack JM. Kappa opioid agonists as targets for pharmacotherapies in cocaine abuse. Pharmaceut Acta Helv 2000; 74:337.

748. Kreek MJ. Opiate and cocaine addictions: challenge for pharmacotherapies. Pharmacol Biochem Behav 1997; 57:551.

749. Hersh D, Van Kirk JR, Kranzler HR. Naltrexone treatment of comorbid alcohol and cocaine disorders. Psychopharmacology 1998; 139:44.

750. Mello NK, Negus SS. Effects of flupenthixol and quadazocine on self-administration of speedball combinations of cocaine and heroin by rhesus monkeys. Neuropsychopharmacology 1999; 21:575.

751. Halikas JA, Crosby RD, Pearson VL, Graves NM. A randomized double-blind study of carbamazepine in the treatment of cocaine abuse. Clin Pharmacol Ther 1997; 62:89.

752. Lima AR, Lima MS, Soares BG, et al. Carbamazepine for dependence. Cochrane Database of Systematic Reviews 2000; 2:CD002023.

753. Gerasimov MR, Dewey SL. Gamma-vinyl-gamma-aminobutyric acid attenuates the synergistic elevations of nucleus accumbens produced by a cocaine/heroin (speedball) challenge. Eur J Pharmacol 1999; 380:1-.

754. Kushner SA, Dewey SL, Kornetsky C. The irreversible gamma-aminobutyric acid (GABA) transaminase inhibitor gamma-vinyl-GABA blocks cocaine self-administration in rats. J Pharmacol Exp Ther 1999; 290:797.

755. Dewey SL, Morgan AE, Ashby CR, et al. A novel strategy for the treatment of cocaine addiction. Synapse 1998; 30:119.

756. Markowitz JS, Finkenbine R, Myrick H. Gabapentin abuse in a cocaine user: implications for treatment? J Clin Psychopharmacol 1997; 17:423.

757. Mericinne E, Kankaapaa A, Lillsunde P, Seppala T. The effects of diazepam and zolpidem on cocaine- and amphetamine-induced place preference. Pharmacol Biochem Behav 1999; 62:159.

758. Powledge TM. Beating abuse. Glutamate may hold a key to drug addiction. Sci Am 2002; 286:20.

759. Dave A. New addiction research unlikely to be applied. Nat Med 2001; 7:757.

760. Winther LC, Saleem R, McCance-Katz EF, et al. Effects of lamotrigine on behavioral and cardiovascular responses to cocaine in human subjects. Am J Drug Alcohol Abuse 2000; 26:47.

761. Collins ED, Ward AS, McDowell DM, et al. The effects of memantine on the subjective, reinforcing and cardiovascular effects of cocaine in humans. Behav Pharmacol 1998; 9:587.

762. McGeehan AJ, Olive MF. The anti-relapse compound acamprosate inhibits the development of a conditioned place preference to ethanol and cocaine but not morphine. Br J Pharmacol 2003; 138:9.

763. Sziraki I, Sershen H, Benuck M, et al. The effect of cotinine on nicotine- and cocaine-induced dopamine release in the nucleus accumbens. Neurochem Res 1999; 24:1471.

764. Panagis G, Kastellakis A, Spyraki C, Nomikes G. Effects of methyllycacotinine (MLA), an alpha 7 nicotine receptor antagonist, on nicotine- and cocaine-induced potentiation of brain stimulation reward. Psychopharmacology 2000; 149:388.

765. McCance-Katz EF, Kosten TR, Jatlow P. Chronic disulfiram treatment effects on intranasal cocaine administration: initial results. Biol Psychiatry 1998; 43:540.

766. McCance-Katz EF, Kosten TR, Jatlow P. Disulfiram effects on acute cocaine administration. Drug Alcohol Dep 1998; 52:27.

767. Petrakis IL, Carroll KM, Nich C, et al. Disulfiram treatment for cocaine dependence in methadone-maintained opioid addicts. Addiction 2000; 95:219.

768. George TP, Chawarski MC, Pakes J, et al. Disulfiram versus placebo for cocaine dependence in buprenorphine-maintained subjects: a preliminary trial. Biol Psychiatry 2000; 47:1080.

769. DeVries TJ, Shaham Y, Homberg JR, et al. A cannabinoid mechanism in relapse to cocaine addiction. Nat Med 2001; 7:1151.

770. Piomelli D. Cannabinoid activity curtails cocaine craving. Nat Med 2001; 7:1099.

771. Popik P, Layer RT, Skolnick P. 100 years of ibogaine: neurochemical and pharmacological actions of a putative anti-addictive drug. Pharmacol Rev 1995; 47:235.

772. Sershen H, Hashim A, Lajtha A. Ibogaine for cocaine abuse: pharmacological interactions at dopamine and serotonin receptors. Brain Res Bull 1997; 42:161.

773. Alburges ME, Hanson GR. Ibogaine pretreatment dramatically enhances the dynorphin response to cocaine. Brain Res 1999; 847:139.

774. Alburges ME, Ramos BP, Bush L, Hanson GR. Responses of the extrapyramidal and limbic substance P systems to ibogaine on cocaine treatments. Eur J Pharmacol 2000; 390:119.

775. Szumlinski KK, Maisonneuve IM, Glick SD. Pretreatment with the putative anti-addictive drug, ibogaine, increases the potency of cocaine to elicit locomotor responding: a study with acute and chronic cocaine-treated rats. Psychopharmacology 1999; 145:227.

776. Glick SD, Kuehne ME, Raucci J, et al. Effects of iboga alkaloids on morphine and cocaine self-administration in rats: relationship to tremorigenic effects and to effects on dopamine release in nucleus accumbens and striatum. Brain Res 1994; 657:14.

777. Alburges ME, Hanson GR. Differential responses by neurotensin systems in extrapyramidal and limbic structures to ibogaine and cocaine. Brain Res 1999; 818:96.

778. Glick SD, Maisonneuve IM. Development of novel medications for drug addiction. The legacy of an African shrub. Ann N Y Acad Sci 2000; 909:88.

779. McCracken KA, Bowen WD, Matsumoto RR. Novel sigma receptor ligands attenuate the locomotor stimulatory effects of cocaine. Eur J Pharmacol 1999; 365:35.

780. Pani L, Kuzmin A, Martellotta MC, et al. The calcium antagonist PN-200-110 inhibits the reinforcing properties of cocaine. Brain Res Bull 1991; 26:445.

781. Malcolm R, Brady KT, Moore J, Kajdasz D. Amlodipine treatment of cocaine dependence. J Psychoactive Drugs 1999; 31:117.

782. Gorelick DA. Enhancing cocaine metabolism with butyrylcholinesterase as a treatment strategy. Drug Alcohol Dep 1997; 48:159.

783. Kantak KM, Collins SL, Lipman EG, et al. Evaluation of anti-cocaine antibodies and a cocaine vaccine in a rat self-administration model. Psychopharmacology 2000; 148:251.

784. Carrera MR, Ashley JA, Zhou B, et al. Cocaine vaccines: antibody protection against relapse in a rat model. Proc Natl Acad Sci USA 2000; 97:6202.

785. Landry DW. Immunotherapy for cocaine addiction. Sci Am 1997; 276:42.

786. Landry DW, Zhao K, Yang G X-Q, et al. Antibody catalyzed degradation of cocaine. Science 1993; 259:1899.

787. Avants SK, Margolin A, Holford TR, Kosten TR. A randomized controlled trial of auricular acupuncture for cocaine dependence. Arch Intern Med 2000; 160:2305.

788. Bullock ML, Kiresuk TJ, Pheley AM, et al. Auricular acupuncture in the treatment of cocaine abuse. A study of efficacy and dosing. J Subst Abuse Treat 1999; 16:31.

789. Rounsaville BJ, Anton SF, Carroll K, et al. Psychiatric diagnosis of treatment-seeking cocaine abusers. Arch Gen Psychiatry 1991; 48:43.

790. Giannini AJ, Malone DA, Giannini MC, et al. Treatment of depression in chronic cocaine and phencyclidine abuse with desipramine. J Clin Pharmacol 1986; 26:211.

791. Weiss RD, Pope HS, Mirin SM. Treatment of chronic cocaine abuse and attention deficit disorder, residual type, with magnesium pemoline. Drug Alcohol Depend 1985; 15:69.

792. Concores JA, Davies RK, Mueller PS, Gold MS. Cocaine abuse and adult attention deficit disorder. J Clin Psychiatry 1987; 48:376.

793. Nunes EV, McGrath PJ, Wager S, Quitkin FM. Lithium treatment for cocaine abusers with bipolar spectrum disorders. Am J Psychiatry 1990; 147:655.

794. Levin FR, Evans SM, McDowell DM, Kleber HD. Methylphenidate treatment for cocaine abusers with attention-deficit/hyperactivity disorder: a pilot study. J Clin Psychiatry 1998; 59:300.

795. Castaneda R, Levy R, Hardy M, Trujillo M. Long-acting stimulants for the treatment of attention-deficit hyperactivity disorder in cocaine-dependent adults. Psychiatr Serv 2000; 51:169.

796. Levin FR, Evans SM, Coomaraswammy S, et al. Flupenthixol treatment for cocaine abusers with schizophrenia: a pilot study. Am J Drug Alcohol Abuse 1998; 24:343.

797. Satel SL, Gawin FH. Seasonal cocaine abuse. Am J Psychiatry 1989; 146:534.

798. Jonas JM, Gold MS, Sweeney D, Pottash AL. Eating disorders and cocaine abuse: a survey of 259 cocaine abusers. J Clin Psychiatry 1987; 48:47.

799. Walfish S, Massey R, Krone A. MMPI profiles of cocaine-addicted individuals in residential treatment: implications for practical treatment planning. J Subst Abuse Treat 1990; 7:151.

800. Weiss RD, Mirin SM. Subtypes of cocaine abusers. Psychiatr Clin North Am 1986; 9:491.

801. Hall GW, Carriero NJ, Takushi RY, et al. Pathological gambling among cocaine-dependent outpatients. Am J Psychiatry 2000; 157:1127.

802. Rutherford MJ, Cacciola JS, Alterman AI. Antisocial personality disorder and psychopathy in cocaine-dependent women. Am J Psychiatry 1999; 156:849.

803. Kang SY, Kleinman PH, Woody GE, et al. Outcomes for cocaine abusers after once-a-week psychosocial therapy. Am J Psychiatry 1991; 148:630.

804. O'Brien CP, Childress AR, Arndt ID, et al. Pharmacological and behavioral treatments of cocaine dependence: controlled studies. J Clin Psychiatry 1988; 49 (Suppl):17.

805. Crits-Cristoph P, Siqueland L, Blaine J, et al. Psychosocial treatments for cocaine dependence: National Institute on Drug Abuse Collaborative Cocaine Treatment Study. Arch Gen Psychiatry 1999; 56:493.

806. Simpson DD, Joe GW, Fletcher BW, et al. A national evaluation of treatment outcomes for cocaine dependence. Arch Gen Psychiatry 1999; 56:507.

807. Hser YI, Joshi V, Anglin MD, Fletcher B. Predicting post-treatment cocaine abstinence for first-time admissions and treatment repeaters. Am J Public Health 1999; 89:666.

Chapter 6

Barbiturates and Other Hypnotics and Sedatives

Nor all the drowsy syrups of the world
Shall ever medicine thee to that sweet sleep
Which thou ow'dst yesterday.
—William Shakespeare, *Othello*

There was a pill for everything—for tranquility, for sleep, for death.
—Barbara Gordon

They got the President to stop taking Halcion. That was the year's bright spot for the war on drugs.
—Unnamed U.S. drug enforcement official, 1992

A hypnotic drug "… produces drowsiness and facilitates the onset and maintenance of a state of sleep that resembles natural sleep in its electroencephalographic characteristics and from which the recipient can be aroused easily."[1] A sedative drug "… decreases activity, moderates excitement, and calms the recipient." In high enough doses, most sedative or hypnotic drugs—benzodiazepines are an exception—induce general anesthesia, and a broad classification would include alcohols and volatile anesthetics. This chapter addresses commercially available substituted barbituric acid compounds and nonbarbituric hypnotics and sedatives.

Pharmacology and Animal Studies

GABA and its receptors

Barbiturates and benzodiazepines potentiate the effects of γ-aminobutyric acid (GABA), an inhibitory neurotransmitter that acts by facilitating chloride conductance. Stereospecific receptors for GABA, barbiturates, and benzodiazepines form parts of a supramolecular GABA$_A$–benzodiazepine–chloride ion channel complex, which consists of pentameric membrane proteins assembled from at least 18 subunits (α 1-6, β 1-3, γ 1-3, δ, ε, θ, ρ 1-3). Most GABA$_A$ receptors are composed of α, β, and γ subunits. (GABA$_B$ receptors do not have a chloride channel but rather are G-protein-coupled and unaffected by barbiturates or benzodiazepines.) The GABA binding site resides on the β subunit of the complex and the benzodiazepine receptor on the α subunit. The barbiturate recognition site is at or close to the chloride channel. The different receptors are allosterically coupled, and the molecular composition of their subunits varies with different brain regions. Benzodiazepines enhance GABA binding, GABA enhances benzodiazepine binding, and barbiturates increase the binding of both GABA and benzodiazepines in a chloride-dependent manner. The convulsant bicuculline antagonizes GABA, perhaps by competing with it at its receptor.

The convulsant picrotoxin also antagonizes GABA but acts at the barbiturate site. The effects of GABA, benzodiazepines, and barbiturates on each other's receptors and ultimately on chloride channels appear to be through allosteric modification.[2–4]

Barbiturate Pharmacology

Barbiturates in high enough doses "… depress the activity of all excitable tissues."[1] In sedative or hypnotic doses, their actions are largely confined to the central nervous system (CNS), and certain barbiturates have selective anticonvulsant properties at even lower doses. This dissociation between sedative and anticonvulsant properties is the result of barbiturates' dual actions—indirect and direct—at inhibitory synapses: they not only potentiate GABA, but also have their own direct effects on chloride channels, the latter antagonized by picrotoxin. Barbiturates also antagonize glutamate excitatory postsynaptic transmission. Selectively anticonvulsant barbiturates (e.g., phenobarbital) modulate GABA and glutamate responses at doses too low to cause direct inhibitory actions, whereas anesthetic barbiturates (e.g., pentobarbital) at low doses are both modulatory and directly inhibitory.[4,5] Barbiturates facilitate chloride conductance by prolonging the duration of channel openings rather than by increasing their frequency.[6]

Barbiturates are strongly reinforcing in dogs and monkeys, which self-inject them to the point of unconsciousness.[7] By inducing their own metabolism through stimulation of cytochrome P450, barbiturates produce pharmacokinetic tolerance that peaks within a few days.[1] More important is pharmacodynamic tolerance, which continues to develop over weeks or months. Tolerance is greater to sedative than to anticonvulsant effects, and cross-tolerance (albeit incomplete) exists between barbiturates and other sedatives, including benzodiazepines and ethanol.[8]

Benzodiazepine Pharmacology

In contrast to barbiturates, benzodiazepines are not general neuronal depressants. Acting at the CNS, they produce sedation, sleep, decreased anxiety, anterograde amnesia, and muscle relaxation, and they are anticonvulsant.[9] Benzodiazepines occupy stereospecific receptors on the GABA–benzodiazepine macromolecular complex and exert their effects on chloride conductance only indirectly—by allosterically influencing GABA receptor binding. They increase the frequency rather than the duration of chloride channel openings.[6] Although benzodiazepine agonists do not affect chloride conductance in the absence of GABA, they do have other actions, including enhancement of calcium-dependent potassium conductance and inhibition of certain sodium and calcium channels.[10] It is possible that these effects are secondary to benzodiazepine inhibition of adenosine uptake.[11]

Compounds that bind to the benzodiazepine receptor produce a continuum of effects.[12] Partial agonists produce more limited effects than full agonists, compete with full agonists for receptor binding, and thereby antagonize their actions. By contrast, full and partial inverse agonists—among which are a variety of nonbenzodiazepine beta-carboline compounds—produce effects opposite to those of benzodiazepines: inhibition of GABA-induced chloride currents, proconflict behavior, and seizures.[13,14] Full antagonists—for example, flumazenil—block the actions of both agonists and inverse agonists and have little biological activity of their own.[15]

In animal models, low concentrations of benzodiazepine agonists are anxiolytic, and this action seems to be at least partly independent of GABA. (Interestingly, benzodiazepine withdrawal anxiety in a rat model is blocked by pretreatment with the calcium channel blocker verapamil.[16]) Higher benzodiazepine concentrations, acting through GABA, are anticonvulsant. Still higher concentrations produce sedation and then muscle relaxation.[12,17] Signs of benzodiazepine withdrawal—anxiety, seizures—resemble the effects of inverse agonists, suggesting a shift in the set-point of the receptor toward inverse agonism. Such a rearrangement might also explain the observations that the activity of flumazenil then changes from antagonist to weak inverse agonist and that pretreatment with flumazenil reduces the severity of benzodiazepine withdrawal.[18]

To bind GABA, the receptors must have combinations of α and β subunits. To bind benzodiazepines, the receptors must have α and γ subunits, and the α subunits must be types 1, 2, 3, or 5. The major subtype of $GABA_A$ receptor (60% of all

GABA$_A$ receptors) contains α1 subunits and is present in most regions of the brain. Less abundant are those containing α2 subunits (15–20% of GABA$_A$ receptors and present especially in cerebral cortex and hippocampal dentate gyrus) and those containing α3 subunits (10–15% of GABA$_A$ receptors and present especially in layers V and VI of cerebral cortex, brainstem and thalamic reticular formation, hippocampal hilar cells, and cerebellar Golgi cells).[3,19]

Animal studies using knock-in point mutations have identified molecular specificities for the various pharmacological effects of benzodiazepines. It appears that GABA$_A$ receptors containing α1 subunits mediate sedative, amnestic, and anticonvulsant actions. Receptors containing α2 subunits mediate anxiolytic and muscle relaxant actions.[19–22]

Consistent with these observation is the classification of GABA$_A$ receptors as either benzodiazepine type I or benzodiazepine type II. Type I receptors have α_1 subunits and bind both benzodiazepines and the nonbenzodiazepine sedative drug zolpidem. Type II receptors have α_2, α_3, or α_5 subunits, bind benzodiazepines, but have less or no affinity for zolpidem.[23]

A very different peripheral benzodiazepine receptor is found on the outer mitochondrial membrane in various tissues, including adrenal, testis, and ovary. Present in low concentrations in brain, peripheral benzodiazepine receptors are most concentrated in proliferating glia. Their function is unknown.[24]

Stereospecific benzodiazepine receptors imply the existence of endogenous ligands, analogous to endorphins. One candidate is a polypeptide called diazepam binding inhibitor (DBI).[25] Injected intraventricularly into animals, DBI blocks the anticonflict actions of diazepam and by itself elicits proconflict behavior, an effect antagonized by flumazenil. A fragment of DBI, octadecaneuropeptide (ODN), has similar actions, suggesting that DBI is a precursor molecule. DBI's distribution in brain overlaps but is not identical to that of GABA. Cerebral DBI expression significantly increases in the brains of mice dependent on ethanol, morphine, or nicotine, and it increases further during abrupt withdrawal.[26]

Other possible benzodiazepine receptor ligands include beta-carboline compounds isolated from mammalian CNS and having pharmacological and behavioral effects similar to those of DBI.[17] Still another possible ligand is tribulin, an endogenous monoamine oxidase (MAO) inhibitor and benzodiazepine receptor ligand found in the urine of patients with panic attacks and the urine of rats subjected to stress.[17] A true benzodiazepine, *N*-desmethyldiazepam (an agonist and active metabolite of diazepam), has also been identified in animal and human brain, and subsequent reports describe nanogram concentrations of diazepam, oxazepam, and lorazepam in brain and serum.[27,28]

It is thus possible that there are both anxiogenic and anxiolytic endogenous ligands for benzodiazepine receptors, serving the biological role of adjusting vigilance/alertness homeostasis.[17,29]

Animals self-administer benzodiazepines but much less vigorously than barbiturates, psychostimulants, or opioids.[30] Orally administered benzodiazepines have little if any reinforcing effects in rats or monkeys. Intravenous administration is modestly reinforcing, with short-acting drugs such as triazolam or midazolam preferred over longer-acting agents such as diazepam or chlordiazepoxide.[31]

In contrast to barbiturates, benzodiazepines do not induce their own enzymatic metabolism, and the tolerance that develops to their effects is entirely pharmacodynamic. It is controversial whether different benzodiazepine actions have different degrees of tolerance. The widespread clinical impression—emphasized by the pharmaceutical industry—that tolerance develops to sedative but not to anxiolytic effects is supported by rather sparse animal data. As with other drugs, the basis of tolerance is unclear. It seems to require benzodiazepine receptor binding—flumazenil blocks it—and may involve receptor down-regulation through changes in gene expression, but it is independent of duration or dose.[32–34] (Interestingly, chronic exposure to inverse agonists causes receptor up-regulation.[35]) Benzodiazepines are cross-tolerant with other sedatives and with ethanol, and in mice chronic ethanol administration causes decreased benzodiazepine-receptor binding.[36]

Diazepam and related agents are 1,4-benzodiazepines, so named for the location of two nitrogen atoms on a seven-membered diazepine ring. Structurally different are 2,3-benzodiazepines, some of which have anxiolytic properties. Their binding sites, present in the striatum and the nucleus accumbens, have not been identified; they are not located on the GABA–benzodiazepine complex. 2,3-Benzodiazepines may act by altering the phosphorylation of proteins involved in signal transduction. They augment morphine-induced analgesia apparently without producing tolerance or dependence.[37,38]

Barbiturates

Historical Background and Epidemiology

In 1900, the only commercially available hypnotic-sedatives were bromides, chloral hydrate, paraldehyde, urethan, and sulfonal, and reports of abuse of bromide, chloral hydrate, and paraldehyde had already appeared.[1,39,39a,39b] Barbital was introduced in 1903, and a report of abuse appeared a year later.[40] Phenobarbital appeared in 1912, followed by a large number of long-acting, short-acting, and ultra–short-acting preparations (Table 6–1; Figure 6–1).

It was soon recognized that tolerance develops rapidly to sedation induced by barbiturates,

rendering them ineffective as long-term sleeping pills,[41] and that chronic use could lead to severe abstinence symptoms.[42] Nonetheless, by 1962 over a million pounds of barbiturates were sold yearly in the United States, equivalent to 24 100 mg doses for every man, woman, and child in the country.[43] Although legitimate use of barbiturates subsequently declined with the emergence of benzodiazepines,[44] abuse and overdose today are by no means rare. A 1995 survey found that 7.4% of U.S. high school students had used barbiturates, and 0.1% reported daily use. Barbiturates are abused by patients who obtain them through physician prescription and by street users who procure them illegally. In either setting, barbiturates—"goof balls," "purple hearts," "gorilla pills," "F-40s," "pink ladies," "downers," "barbs," "red devils" (secobarbital), "yellow-jackets," "Mexican yellows" (pentobarbital), "blue angels," "blue birds," "blue devils" (amobarbital), "rainbows" (Tuinal)—are usually taken orally, but street addicts also administer them intravenously or intramuscularly.[45] The abuse potential is greatest for short-acting agents,

Table 6–1. Barbiturates Currently or Recently Available in the United States

Barbiturate	Plasma Half-life (hours)	Duration of Action
Long-acting		
Phenobarbital (Luminal, and in mixtures, e.g., Bellergal, Donnatol, Gustase, Kinesed, Primatene, Quadrinal, Tedral)	80–120	6–12
Mephobarbital (Mebaral)	11–67	6–12
Barbital	5–6	6–12
Primidone (Mysoline)	3–2	6–12
Intermediate-acting		
Amobarbital (Amytal, and in Tuinal)	8–42	3–6
Aprobarbital (Alurate)	14–34	3–6
Butabarbital (Butisol)	34–42	3–6
Butalbital (only in mixtures, e.g., Essgic, Fiorinal, Fioricet, Medigesic, Pacaps, Phrenilin, Repan, Sedapap, Tencet, Tencon)	35–88	3–6
Short-acting		
Hexobarbital	5–6	3
Pentobarbital (Nembutal)	15–48	3
Secobarbital (Seconal)	15–40	3
Ultra-short-acting		
Methohexital (Brevital)	3–6	0.3
Thiamylal (Surital)	–	0.3
Thiopental (Pentothal)	6–46	0.3

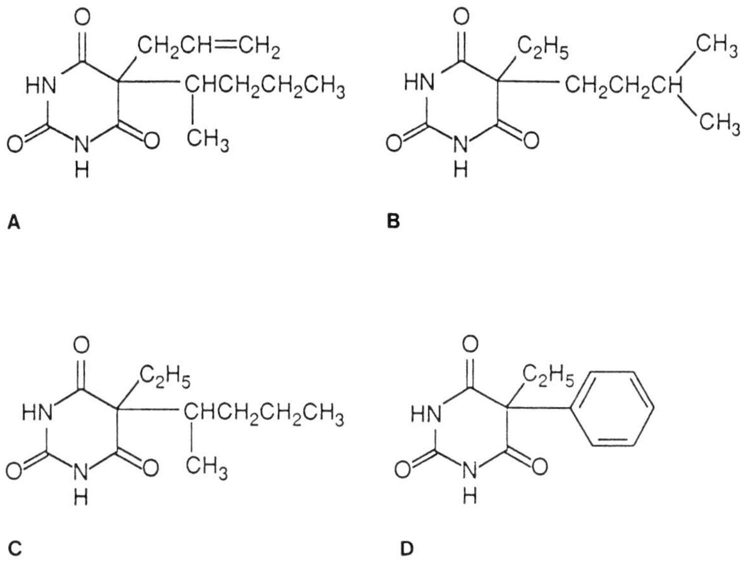

Figure 6–1. Secobarbital (A), Amobarbital (B), Pentobarbital (C), and Phenobarbital (D).

but none is exempt; abuse and symptomatic withdrawal have even been reported for the analgesic preparations Fiorinal and Fioricet, tablets of which contain butalbital.[46,46a,46b] Barbiturate addicts are often physically dependent on opioids and ethanol as well.[47]

Acute Effects

The acute effects of barbiturates are similar to those of ethanol.[48] A single dose of 200–400 mg secobarbital or 200–600 mg amobarbital in a novice produces a few hours of light-headedness, euphoria, distortion of time sense, decreased attention and intellectual performance, sedation, ataxia, slurred speech, nystagmus, and diplopia.[49] There may be excitement, particularly as the sedative effect wears off. Marked variations in response occur in subjects taking the same dose repeatedly, with either euphoria, depression, or hostility. There is decrease in the amount of sleep spent in the rapid eye movement (REM) phase. The electroencephalogram shows increased fast activity (15–35 Hz), most prominent frontally. Higher doses cause respiratory depression; carbon dioxide-sensitive areas of the medulla are more affected than oxygen receptors in the aortic and carotid bodies.

Duration of action of barbiturates (and benzodiazepines) depends on absorption, redistribution, and the presence or absence of active metabolites. It does not correlate well with biological half-lives, especially after single doses.[50]

Barbiturate poisoning follows suicide attempts, accidental ingestion by children, and overdose by addicts. Drug automatism, unwitting repetition of hypnotic doses because of impaired memory, is probably infrequent.[2] Ethanol often aggravates symptoms; fatalities have occurred with combined blood concentrations of only 0.5 mg/dL for secobarbital and 100 mg/dL for ethanol.[50] Severe poisoning causes coma and respiratory depression. In milder cases, respirations may be rapid and shallow or of Cheyne–Stokes type. Hypotension is secondary to hypoxia, venous vasodilation, and hypovolemia from vomiting, diarrhea, or dehydration during prolonged coma. Very high doses of barbiturates directly depress the myocardium and brainstem vasomotor centers. Hypothermia, sometimes marked, can lead to dangerous cardiac arrhythmias.[51] Tendon reflexes may be depressed, and flexor or extensor posturing occurs.[52] Bullous skin eruptions result from a direct toxic action of barbiturates on the epidermis.[50] Deep vein thrombosis follows sustained immobility. Aspiration pneumonia is common. Very severe barbiturate poisoning can result in absent pupillary and other brainstem reflexes and an isoelectric (flat-line) electroencephalogram—the clinical picture of brain death—yet such patients may fully recover.

Treatment of barbiturate overdose begins with assessment of cardiorespiratory status, endotracheal intubation, oxygen, and intravenous fluids.[50,51,53] Because barbiturates decrease gastrointestinal motility, the stomach is evacuated by emesis or lavage, followed by activated charcoal and a cathartic. Artificial ventilation and blood pressure support may be necessary. Fluid replacement is preferable to pressors, which aggravate hypotension by reducing cardiac output. If shock persists despite normal central venous pressure, dopamine or dobutamine can be given. For long-acting barbiturates (e.g., phenobarbital), forced diuresis with mannitol and urinary alkalinization are instituted unless there is anuria secondary to shock. Hemodialysis works faster than peritoneal dialysis and is more effective for long-acting agents. CNS stimulant drugs are contraindicated.

Tolerance to barbiturate sedation develops rapidly (in fact, can be seen after a single dose) and reaches a maximum level that varies among individuals. Although tolerance has allowed physically dependent subjects to ingest 2.5 g of short-acting barbiturates daily, there is, in contrast to opioids or amphetamines, much less tolerance to lethal doses, and someone with little intoxication on a high fixed daily dose of barbiturate may become severely symptomatic with an additional small increment.[43,45] As in animals, degrees of cross-tolerance exist between barbiturates, other hypnotic-sedatives, and ethanol.

Dependence and Withdrawal

Physical dependence is manifested by withdrawal symptoms similar to ethanol's: insomnia, anxiety, tremor, hyperreflexia, weakness, anorexia, nausea, vomiting, abdominal cramps, mydriasis, postural hypotension, tachypnea, and tachycardia. Rebound REM sleep produces frequent dreaming and nightmares.[53] Hallucinations occur, often auditory (and persecutory), less often visual; they usually clear within 1 or 2 weeks but can persist longer. Seizures are most likely to occur on the second or third day following withdrawal of short-acting agents. Symptoms resembling delirium tremens, with

confusion, disorientation, delusions, hallucinations, hyperthermia, and cardiovascular instability, begin on the second to fifth day and last from 1 day to several weeks. Electroencephalographic slowing and paroxysmal discharges occur during the first few days of withdrawal and are provoked (with myoclonic jerks) for much longer with photic stimulation.[42]

Abrupt withdrawal from oral pentobarbital or secobarbital taken in a daily dose of 400 mg for several months produced paroxysmal electroencephalographic changes without symptoms in one-third of subjects. Withdrawal from 600 mg/day caused minor symptoms in half the subjects and a seizure in 10%. Of those taking 900 mg or more daily, three-fourths had seizures and two-thirds delirium tremens.[54]

Treatment or prevention of barbiturate withdrawal can be accomplished with short-acting barbiturates (e.g., pentobarbital) given in doses (preferably oral) of 200–400 mg every 4 to 6 hours until mild signs of intoxication appear. After 2 or 3 days of stabilization at this dose, the drug is slowly withdrawn at a rate of no more than 100 mg daily. If abstinence symptoms appear, withdrawal is stopped until they subside; it is then resumed at the same or a slower rate. If the initial 200 mg dose of pentobarbital produces gross signs of intoxication, it is unlikely that the subject is physically dependent on barbiturates. Severe withdrawal symptoms call for higher doses and more rapid stabilization. Some investigators believe that phenobarbital produces smoother withdrawal with less risk of overdose and recommend substituting 30 mg phenobarbital for each "equivalent" 100 mg amobarbital, secobarbital, or pentobarbital (up to 500 mg phenobarbital per day).[55] As with ethanol withdrawal, delirium tremens is a medical emergency requiring intensive sedation and supportive therapy and carrying substantial mortality; once such symptoms appear, they are not readily reversible with barbiturate administration[47] (see Chapter 12).

A neonatal withdrawal syndrome affects infants of mothers taking barbiturates, sometimes at customary hypnotic or anticonvulsant doses.[56] Symptoms resemble those of neonatal opioid abstinence but occur later than with heroin (up to a week after delivery) and can last several months. Low birth weight has not been an associated feature.

Other Medical and Neurological Complications

Stroke

Cerebral infarction can follow barbiturate overdose and decreased brain perfusion, but occlusive or hemorrhagic strokes have not otherwise been convincingly demonstrated. Coma with right hemiplegia occurred in a 20-year-old man taking orally a combination of secobarbital and strychnine ("M and M's"). Cerebral angiography suggested arteritis, but he had been taking other drugs as well for at least 10 years.[57] Radiographic evidence of cerebral vasculitis was found in four other barbiturate abusers, two of whom also abused chlorpromazine and a third other unidentified drugs.[58] Monkeys receiving dissolved secobarbital capsules 1.5 mg/kg intravenously three times weekly for a year had widespread narrowing of cerebral arteries at angiography, and histologically there were scattered talc crystals in brain capillaries without cellular reaction. Frontal lobe microinfarction was seen in one animal.[59]

Cognitive Impairment

Chronic barbiturate abuse leads to psychological and social deterioration, with "poor grooming, lying, bizarre and paranoid thought processes, and erratic and suicidal behavior."[53] Volunteers and epileptics receiving phenobarbital demonstrate impaired concentration and short-term memory.[60] In contrast to alcoholics, barbiturate-dependent subjects do not have abnormal computed tomography (CT) scans.[61] Barbiturates do reduce cerebral glucose metabolism, however.[62]

Fetal Effects

Of obvious importance is whether barbiturate exposure in utero or early in life causes long-lasting cognitive or behavioral alteration.[63] Such effects have been observed in some[64–66] but not all[67] studies of children receiving phenobarbital for febrile seizures; in one report, the mean IQ of children receiving phenobarbital was several points lower than the group receiving placebo 6 months after discontinuation of the drug.[68] A Danish study of adult men exposed in utero to phenobarbital found significantly lower verbal intelligence scores compared with controls. Exposure that included the last trimester was the most detrimental, and the adverse effect was greatest in subjects from lower socioeconomic backgrounds.[69] Phenobarbital caused morphological abnormalities in neurons in culture and impaired brain growth and learning in animals exposed prenatally or postnatally.[70–72] Long-term abnormalities are found in neurons of the cerebellum, hippocampus, olfactory bulbs, and cerebral cortex of exposed rodents.[73]

Enzyme Induction and Drug Interactions

The effects of barbiturates on cytochrome P450 induces a wide array of enzymes. Induction of δ-aminolevulinic acid synthase causes dangerous exacerbations of acute intermittent or variegate porphyria. Enzyme induction accelerates the metabolism of vitamins D and K, steroid hormones (including oral contraceptives), digoxin, anticoagulants, guanidine, cyclic antidepressants, phenothiazines, and phenytoin.[1,50]

Benzodiazepines

Historical Background and Epidemiology

The first available benzodiazepine was chlordiazepoxide in 1960, followed a year later by diazepam. Marketed as anti-anxiety agents or tranquilizers, they soon became the most widely prescribed drugs in the United States. In the 1970s, flurazepam was marketed as a hypnotic and replaced barbiturates as the most-prescribed sleeping pill in the United States. In the 1980s, the shorter-acting triazolam became the most popular hypnotic. By the 1990s, eight benzodiazepines were promoted in the United States as tranquilizers, and five as hypnotics (Table 6–2; Figure 6–2). Clonazepam is used mainly as an anticonvulsant and for panic disorder, and midazolam is used for anesthesia induction.[9] Nitrazepam is available as both a hypnotic and an anticonvulsant in Europe. As with barbiturates, reports of abuse of individual benzodiazepines appeared within a few years of their introduction.[74–87] In 1981, a household survey found that 2% of adult Americans had used tranquilizers without appropriate prescription during the previous year.[31] Tranquilizer use among American high school

Table 6–2. Benzodiazepines

	Plasma Half-life (hours)
Promoted as Tranquilizers	
Alprazolam (Xanax)	12
Chlorazepate (Tranxene)	1–3
Chlordiazepoxide (Librium, others)	5–30
Diazepam (Valium, others)	20–70
Halazepam (Paxipam)	10–20
Lorazepam (Ativan)	9–19
Oxazepam (Serax, Zaxopam)	23–29
Prazepam (Centrax)	0.6–2
Promoted as Hypnotics	
Estazolam (Prosom)	8–31
Flurazepam (Dalmane)	2–3
Quazepam (Doral)	25–41
Temazepam (Restoril)	10–16
Triazolam (Halcion)	1.5–5.5
Promoted as Anticonvulsants	
Clonazepam (Klonopin)	18–50
Promoted for Anesthesia Induction	
Midazolam (Versed)	2–5

seniors peaked in 1977 (10.8% within the previous year, 4.6% within the previous month), falling to 6.1% and 2.1% by 1985.[88] In 1991, a survey of American resident physicians and senior medical students revealed that of 11 drugs (including tobacco and ethanol), only benzodiazepines and ethanol (and, in the case of the medical students, "psychedelics other then LSD [lysergic acid diethylamide]") were taken more often than by national age-related comparison groups.[89,90]

The addictive liability of benzodiazepines is much less than that of barbiturates; there is slower onset of action, less euphoria, and a greater difference between a therapeutic dose and a dose producing physical dependence.[91] Although choice tests in sedative and ethanol abusers indicate a preference for benzodiazepines over placebo, similar tests in either normal or anxious subjects with no history of sedative abuse show no such preference.[92–94] Such findings are consistent with animal studies.[95] Drug-seeking behavior—obtaining prescriptions from several physicians or purchasing the drug on the street—and dosage escalation are therefore rarely encountered among the millions of current users.[93,96] In fact, in the surveys described

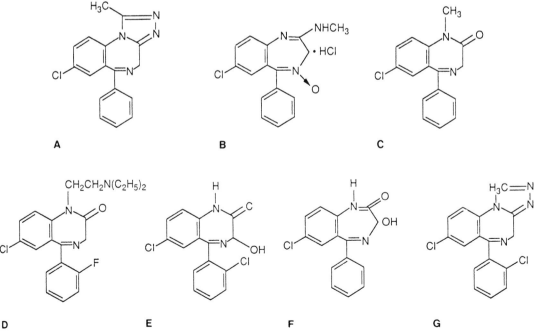

Figure 6–2. Alprazolam (A), Chlordiazepoxide (B), Diazepam (C), Flurazepam (D), Lorazepam (E), Oxazepam (F), and Triazolam (G).

here, although 2% of Americans took tranquilizers without proper prescription, only 0.1% did so for 30 days or more during the previous year, and the great majority of medical students and residents who used benzodiazepines did so for self-treatment rather than recreation.[89,90]

Although widespread overprescribing of benzodiazepines has been claimed, epidemiological studies reveal that in the vast majority of instances they are prescribed and taken appropriately.[31,97–100] In fact, surveys indicate that most patients tend to take less than prescribed and for shorter periods.[93] About 15% of benzodiazepine users take the drug on a long-term basis and appear to benefit from doing so, again without dosage escalation or abuse. Abstinence symptoms are more likely to develop when treatment is abruptly discontinued in such patients, but as with opioids physical dependence is not the same as addiction or abuse. Patients with a prior history of substance abuse who receive benzodiazepines for anxiety disorder are at no greater risk than others to abuse benzodiazepines, and benzodiazepines do not trigger relapse of substance abuse in such patients.[100a]

Despite these considerations, the New York State Department of Health in 1989 decreed that benzodiazepines (which are Schedule IV drugs) be prescribed on triplicate prescriptions for a maximum of 30 days, with each patient's, physician's, and pharmacist's name entered into a database.[101] The result was predictable. Because patients were required to return every 30 days for refills and physicians were reluctant to have their names on a computerized blacklist, needed treatment was denied. Moreover, although benzodiazepine prescribing did decline substantially, prescriptions for less effective and often more dangerous sedatives (meprobamate, methyprylon, ethchlorvynol, butalbital, chloral hydrate, hydroxyzine) rose sharply (even as their use was decreasing nationally). Whether the reduced prescribing of benzodiazepines led to decreased street diversion is uncertain.[102,103]

Nearly all recreational benzodiazepine users also use other psychoactive drugs, especially ethanol.[31,104–108] Agents with rapid onset of action (e.g., diazepam) are more popular than agents with slower onset (e.g., oxazepam).[109] Parenteral use is rare.[110] Illicit use is especially frequent among patients in methadone maintenance programs,[31,111–113] perhaps reflecting drug interactions that enhance subjective opioid effects.[114] In the UK intravenous administration of the liquid content of temazepam capsules became popular during the 1990s.[115] Inadvertent intra-arterial injection led to cases of limb ischemia, myoglobinuria, and renal failure. Temazepam is now available only as a tablet.[116–118]

Co-abuse of opioids and benzodiazepines (orally or intravenously) is reportedly common in Ireland,[119] France,[120] and Australia.[121]

During the 1990s, widespread oral abuse of flunitrazepam (Rohypnol) was reported among American adolescents and young adults, especially in Florida and Texas. Known as "roofies," "R-2s," and "Roches Do," the drug received much media attention for its association with amnesia and sexual assault ("date-rape pill").[122,123] Flunitrazepam is 7 to 10 times as potent a sedative as diazepam, with a rapid (15–20 minutes) onset of action. Banned in the United States, it is still manufactured legally in Europe and both legally and illegally in Mexico.[124] In Sweden during 1992–1998, 641 fatalities were attributed to flunitrazepam intoxication, most in combination with other drugs or ethanol.[125]

Acute Effects

Although some benzodiazepines are marketed as anxiolytics and others as hypnotics, the differences are "possibly insignificant."[9] Their effectiveness as muscle relaxants in usual oral doses has also been questioned. Differences exist among benzodiazepines in rapidity of absorption after oral administration and in duration of action. For example, oxazepam requires hours to reach peak plasma concentrations, whereas diazepam reaches peak concentrations in about an hour; alprazolam, lorazepam, and chlordiazepoxide have intermediate rates of absorption. One reason triazolam replaced flurazepam as the nation's most popular prescription hypnotic was its shorter biological half-life, reducing the likelihood of drowsiness (and traffic accidents) the following day. Some benzodiazepines such as diazepam have biologically active metabolites, and this feature, plus the redistribution pattern of lipophilic benzodiazepines after they enter the brain, means that as with barbiturates, clinical effects often do not correlate with serum half-lives.[9] Of available benzodiazepines, only lorazepam is predictably absorbed after intramuscular injection.

The greatest advantage of benzodiazepines over barbiturates is safety in overdose. Benzodiazepines are implicated in about 20% of Drug Abuse Warning Network (DAWN) reports and 15% of toxicological fatalities, but in the vast majority, additional drugs—usually other sedatives or ethanol—have been taken.[31] Benzodiazepines alone seldom produce respiratory depression, and patients who have taken benzodiazepines with barbiturates are no more likely to have depressed respiration than patients who have taken barbiturates alone.[126] In mice, diazepam did not increase the LD-50 of ethanol.[127] It is extremely difficult to commit suicide with benzodiazepines. A review of 1239 deaths in which diazepam was implicated found that in only two was diazepam taken alone.[128] Even very large doses of benzodiazepines are more likely to produce somnolence, ataxia, and dysarthria than coma and respiratory depression. In a report of 60 cases of chlordiazepoxide poisoning, coma did not occur even with blood levels over 60 μg/mL; therapeutic doses of chlordiazepoxide usually produce levels of 0.5–3 μg/mL.[129]

When benzodiazepines are contributing to coma, the general management is the same as for barbiturate or ethanol poisoning. Overdose of benzodiazepines alone seldom requires ventilatory or blood pressure support, and hemodialysis is ineffective.[50,130] Intravenous flumazenil, a specific benzodiazepine antagonist, quickly reverses stupor or coma when benzodiazepines have been taken alone, but because its duration of action is brief (20 to 45 minutes), it often must be given in repeated boluses or by continuous infusion.[15,131] Benzodiazepine overdose, moreover, rarely causes morbidity or mortality. Flumazenil can precipitate seizures in long-term benzodiazepine users and cardiac arrhythmia in patients who have taken tricyclic antidepressants.[132] Flumazenil is also contraindicated in patients who have received theophylline, carbamazepine, chloral hydrate, chloroquine, or chlorinated hydrocarbons.[133]

Benzodiazepines produce troublesome and potentially dangerous effects in addition to lethargy, especially in the elderly.[133a,133b] Psychomotor performance is impaired in a manner that mimics the effects of old age itself: muscle strength and coordination are decreased, and impaired memory and confusion occur.[134] Older subjects taking benzodiazepines are at increased risk for falls and fractures, especially with agents such as nitrazepam or flurazepam, which are not only long-acting themselves, but also have long-acting metabolites.[135] The risk is further increased when benzodiazepines are taken with ethanol, which enhances their absorption and has additive sedative and ataxic effects.[136] In a randomized clinical trial, tapering and stopping psychotropic medications, including benzodiazepines, other hypnotics, neuroleptic drugs, and antidepressants over a 14-week period reduced falls by 39%.[137]

Although tolerance develops rapidly to sedation and incoordination, it is less evident for anterograde amnesia,[138] a desirable feature when benzodiazepines are used for anesthesia induction but decidedly undesirable for travelers who take benzodiazepines to sleep on airplanes.[139–141] The mechanisms underlying amnesia are unclear. Diazepam produces little amnesia when given orally and rapid but brief amnesia when given intravenously; lorazepam, by contrast, produces more delayed but longer lasting amnesia when given orally or intravenously.[31]

Dependence and Withdrawal

Physical dependence does develop to benzodiazepines, and severe abstinence signs have been observed in rats, dogs, and baboons.[142–145] Rebound insomnia follows abrupt cessation of benzodiazepine hypnotics, and early morning awakening and daytime anxiety can emerge in chronic users of short-acting agents.[146,147] Similarly, withdrawal symptoms in patients taking benzodiazepine tranquilizers can either follow cessation of therapeutic doses[107,143,148–153] or emerge during chronic use (reflecting tolerance).[135]

Withdrawal symptoms usually occur 3 to 10 days after stopping long-acting agents and within 24 hours with short-acting agents.[154] The principal symptom, anxiety, can be difficult to distinguish from the patient's predrug state, but there may also be headache, muscle stiffness, tachycardia, sweating, anorexia, diarrhea, tremor, paresthesias, psychosis, hallucinations, delirium, and seizures.[155–160] Unusual perceptual disturbances, with a false sense of movement and hypersensitivity to sensory stimuli—light, sound, and touch—are particularly characteristic of the benzodiazepine abstinence syndrome, which can last 1 to 6 weeks.[96] In a double-blind, placebo-controlled study, patients who abruptly discontinued therapeutic doses of benzodiazepines after at least 9 months of use developed symptoms that were clearly distinct from pretreatment anxiety, including tinnitus, muscle twitching, paresthesias, visual disturbances, and confusion; none had seizures, disorientation, or psychosis.[150] Withdrawal symptoms have also occurred in patients taking benzodiazepines for nonpsychiatric reasons such as muscle spasm.[145] Symptoms are most severe with short-acting agents and can be minimized by short treatment courses, low or intermittent flexible daily doses, and gradual dosage reduction.[96,159–161] The high doses of alprazolam recommended for panic attacks made long-term users especially vulnerable to physical dependence. Propranolol, carbamazepine, and sedative and antidepressant drugs have reportedly relieved benzodiazepine withdrawal symptoms.[149,156,162]

Other Medical and Neurological Complications

Paradoxical Reactions and Amnesia

Benzodiazepines cause paradoxical reactions that suggest withdrawal: anxiety, hyperactivity, irritability, hostility, agitation, depression, rage attacks, panic, delirium, hallucinations, and increased seizure frequency.[163,164] Aimless wandering and bizarre behavior lasting hours have affected patients who later had no recollection of the experience. Such symptoms are especially common with triazolam.[165] Data from the Food and Drug Administration (FDA) revealed that hyperexcitability, cognitive disturbance, "confusion," hallucinations, and depression occurred much more often with triazolam than with flurazepam or temazepam. In addition, triazolam was nearly as likely as flurazepam, and much more likely than temazepam, to cause daytime sedation. It was also more likely to cause withdrawal symptoms including seizures, and it was the only drug among the three to cause amnesia.[166] Similarly, a controlled study found "next-day amnesia" in 40% of triazolam users and 0 temazepam users.[167]

That study has been criticized on the grounds that equivalent doses were not compared, and the FDA spontaneous reporting system has been criticized as anecdotal.[168,169] Media attention, however, led to the withdrawal of triazolam from the market in the Netherlands and Britain.[146,170–172]

Dystonia

A report from Philadelphia described six patients who developed acute dystonia after ingesting "Street Xanax" that the sellers claimed was alprazolam but which turned out to be haloperidol.[173]

Infection

Abiotrophia sepsis and a subclavian artery mycotic aneurysm developed in a man who injected crushed lorazepam tablets.[173a]

Effects on Cognition

Long-term benzodiazepine treatment, with or without physical dependence, appears to be without permanent consequence.[31] Reports of psychological or cognitive impairment in long-term users are rare and, as with many other drugs, difficult to interpret.[174–176] Elderly subjects reportedly had verbal memory impairment 6–10 days after discontinuing chronic benzodiazepine use; they had become benzodiazepine dependent, however, most taking at least 40 mg diazepam equivalent daily and withdrawing over less than 10 days.[176a] Other investigators found no significant cognitive morbidity associated with long-term benzodiazepine use in healthy older adults.[176b,176c,176d]

Fetal Effects

Descriptions of alleged fetal effects are few and anecdotal. A report from Sweden described dysmorphism, mental retardation, Dandy–Walker malformation, Moebius syndrome, seizures, or hemiplegia in several infants born to mothers taking benzodiazepines. The dysmorphism was considered similar but not identical to the fetal alcohol syndrome.[177] Animal studies showed lowered threshold to bicuculline-induced but not pentylenetetrazol-induced seizures following in utero diazepam exposure.[178]

Nonbarbiturate, Nonbenzodiazepine Sedative-Hypnotics

A number of nonbarbiturate sedatives—ethinamate, ethchlorvynol, glutethimide, meprobamate, methaqualone, methyprylon—came on the market in the 1950s, each followed in short order by reports of abuse.[179–185] Although some of these agents have since been withdrawn, others are still widely sold (Table 6–3).[186]

Despite their chemical dissimilarity, nonbarbiturate, nonbenzodiazepine sedative-hypnotics produce symptoms of intoxication and withdrawal similar to those of barbiturates.

Methaqualone

In the 1970s, methaqualone abuse became widespread among young people in the United States, West Germany, Japan, and Britain.[187] (A British commercial preparation, Mandrax, contains antihistamine.) Methaqualone—"Canadian blues," "quacks," "sopars," "ludes"—was often taken with wine or soft drinks in "juice bars" ("luding out") and was popular as a "downer" among cocaine

Table 6–3. Nonbarbiturate, Nonbenzodiazepine Sedative-Hypnotics

---

Bromide
Buspirone (Buspar)
Chloral hydrate (Noctec, others)
Chlormezanone (Trancopal)
Diphenhydramine (Benadryl, and in over-the-counter sleeping pills, e.g., Miles Nervine, Nyrol, Sleep-eze, Sominex, Compoz)
Ethchlorvynol (Placidyl)
Ethinamate (Valmid, no longer produced in the U.S.)
Glutethimide (Doriden, after 1991 available only as generic)
Hydroxyzine (Vistaril, Atarax, others)
Meprobamate (Miltown, Equanil; in Equagesic with aspirin; in Deprol with benactyzine)
Methaqualone (Quaalude, Sopar, no longer produced in the U.S.)
Methyprylon (Nodular, no longer produced in the U.S.)
Paraldehyde
Triclofos (Triclos, no longer produced in the U.S.)
Zaleplon (Sonata)
Zolpidem (Ambien, Stilnox, Niotal)

---

users.[188,189] Poisoning causes delirium, hallucinations, hypertonicity, myoclonus, seizures, papilledema, coma, and death.[190–194] A tendency to congestive heart failure contraindicates forced diuresis.[193] There may be elevated prothrombin time and bleeding, and peripheral neuropathy has been reported.[195,196]

In the early 1970s, overdose accounted for most methaqualone fatalities; a decade later, as methaqualone abuse was becoming a nationwide epidemic, traumatic deaths (especially vehicular accidents) were more common.[197,198] "Counterfeit" methaqualone pills sold on the street contain unpredictable amounts of drug plus other agents, including phencyclidine, barbiturates, or diazepam.[198] A man had seizures and coma after taking methaqualone with diphenhydramine; methaqualone blood levels were much lower than usually associated with coma, suggesting potentiation by the antihistamine.[199]

In the 1980s, production and distribution of methaqualone became illegal in the United States, and abuse subsequently declined. Illegally manufactured and imported methaqualone remains available, however.[200]

Glutethimide

Of the sedatives discussed in this chapter, glutethimide probably has the least to recommend it. Its addiction liability is as great as the barbiturates, and its plasma half-life is as high as 100 hours following overdose, which is especially difficult to treat. Acute effects are barbiturate-like; overdose, however, causes less respiratory depression and more severe circulatory failure. There is also fever, muscle spasm, twitching, and even seizures. Coma can be prolonged with unpredictable fluctuations in depth.[201–204] Anticholinergic actions cause dilated unreactive pupils, xerostomia, ileus, and atonic bladder; in one report, pupillary dilation was unilateral.[205] In addition to its own prolonged half-life, glutethimide has active metabolites that accumulate with chronic use or after overdose. Management is supportive, as with barbiturates. Hemodialysis can shorten coma.

As a drug of abuse, glutethimide in the 1980s was often injected parenterally combined with codeine ("hits," "loads"), and numerous fatalities were reported (see Chapter 3).[206,207] Glutethimide abstinence symptoms, including seizures, occur in abusers taking large daily doses (0.5–3 g).[1] Glutethimide addicts have reportedly developed lasting peripheral neuropathy, cerebellar ataxia, and altered mentation.[208–210] Symptomatic hypocalcemia with elevated parathormone levels developed in a young man who had abused glutethimide for 15 years.[211]

Methyprylon

Methyprylon has barbiturate-like effects, and its plasma half-life is increased following overdose.[1,50] As with glutethimide, methyprylon poisoning is less likely than barbiturates to cause respiratory depression and more likely to cause hypotension. Coma can last days and is shortened by hemodialysis. Methyprylon addiction produces an abstinence syndrome similar to that of barbiturates.

Ethchlorvynol

Acute effects of ethchlorvynol include dizziness, syncope, nausea, vomiting, facial numbness, and hypotension. Overdose causes severe respiratory depression with bradycardia and pulmonary edema. Hypothermia, nystagmus, and disconjugate eye movements are common, and coma tends to be deep, nonfluctuating, and prolonged.[212,213] Severe peripheral neuropathy, hemolysis, and thrombocytopenia are reported.[213–215] Treatment includes forced diuresis, peritoneal dialysis, exchange transfusion, hemodialysis, and hemoperfusion with activated charcoal or amberlite resin.[213,216–218]

Meprobamate

Similar to benzodiazepines, meprobamate does not produce general anesthesia, and it is uncertain if it has dissociable sedative and anxiolytic effects. Although its legitimate use declined markedly with the advent of benzodiazepines, it is still abused, and studies reveal preference for meprobamate over benzodiazepines.[219–221] Overdose causes respiratory depression, hypotension, congestive heart failure, and pulmonary edema.[222] A tendency to relapse after apparent clearing of coma is a common feature

of meprobamate overdose, perhaps the result of gastric hypomotility, undissolved tablets, and delayed absorption. Charcoal or resin filter hemoperfusion is more effective than hemodialysis in treating severe overdose.[223–226] Meprabromate withdrawal frequently produces hallucinations and seizures.[1]

Paraldehyde

Paraldehyde is no longer produced in the United States, but dependence sometimes occurred in alcoholics who received it during withdrawal and then developed a preference for it. It can deteriorate in the bottle to acetic acid, producing metabolic acidosis; it also causes hemorrhagic gastritis and pulmonary damage.[227]

Chloral Hydrate

A popular drug of abuse in the 19th century, chloral hydrate is seldom taken illicitly today. Following absorption, it is rapidly metabolized to trichloroethanol, which is entirely responsible for chloral hydrate's hypnotic effects. It is widely believed (but difficult to prove) that chloral hydrate and ethanol are synergistic ("Mickey Finn"), perhaps because chloral hydrate inhibits ethanol metabolism, whereas ethanol enhances chloral hydrate metabolism. Many clinicians also believe that elderly subjects tolerate chloral hydrate better than barbiturates. Acute intoxication, which resembles barbiturate poisoning, sometimes produces pinpoint pupils. Withdrawal can cause seizures, delirium, and death. Survivors often have liver and kidney damage with jaundice and proteinuria, and chronic users may develop acute toxicity because of impaired hepatic detoxification.[1,50]

Bromides

Bromide salts are no longer present in over-the-counter headache remedies and sedatives in the United States. Signs of chronic bromide intoxication include lethargy, inattentiveness, impaired memory, ataxia, dysarthria, and tremor; high doses cause delusions, delirium, hallucinations, and coma.[228,229] A rash (acneiform, nodular, or bullous) occurs in about one-third of intoxicated subjects. Serum bromide concentration is usually more than 19 mEq/L but may be lower. Serum chloride is correspondingly reduced, but if laboratory "chloride" determinations are actually for total halide, levels appear normal.[230] Treatment is with sodium chloride, 2 g three times daily, plus diuresis.[50]

Antihistamines

The antihistamine/anticholinergic hydroxyzine is used as an anxiolytic, and diphenhydramine or other antihistamines are the principal ingredients in many over-the-counter sleeping pills (in some products replacing bromide or scopolamine). Their abuse potential is low, in part because of dose-related side effects (confusion, forgetfulness, anxiety, tremor, dizziness, dry mouth, paresthesias, muscle cramps). Case reports describe cough syrup abuse by polydrug abusers, and tripelennamine combined with pentazocine ("T's and blues") was widely abused in the United States during the 1980s (see Chapter 3). In a study of volunteer sedative abusers, subjects frequently identified diphenhydramine as a barbiturate, benzodiazepine, or other hypnotic and at doses below 600 mg gave it favorable subjective ratings.[231]

Buspirone

Concerns about abuse and dependence and a desire for nonsedative anxiolytic agents led to the development of a novel class of nonbenzodiazepine drugs that act selectively at serotonin 5-HT$_{1A}$ receptors (which are especially prominent in limbic areas).[232] Buspirone, gepirone, and ipsapirone in several trials were as effective as benzodiazepines in relieving anxiety yet did not cause sedation, motor incoordination, or impaired judgment and did not interact with ethanol.[232–234] Moreover, animal and human studies suggest that neither tolerance nor physical dependence develops and that addiction liability is minimal.[233–238]

The lexicon of abused drugs is of course replete with agents initially touted as nonaddicting (e.g., heroin and meperidine), but as of the early 2000s there were no reports of buspirone abuse. Perhaps related to actions at dopamine receptors, buspirone in high doses causes akathisia, tremor, rigidity,

orofacial dyskinesia, myoclonus, and dystonia. In one case, dystonia persisted for several months after buspirone was discontinued.[239]

Zolpidem

Zolpidem is a non-benzodiazepine drug that binds to Type I benzodiazepine receptors. It is thus a sedative, not an anxiolytic, and as such is the most widely prescribed sleeping pill in the United States. Sensory distortion, hallucinations, and psychosis are reported, usually but not always in association with excessive dosage.[240–242,242a,242b] As with benzodiazepines, zolpidem overdose is rarely fatal unless it is taken with other CNS depressants. Tolerance and physical dependence to zolpidem have been produced in baboons and, infrequently, described in humans.[241–248] A review of 15 cases reported up to 2000 noted that six of the patients had been dependent on "other drugs or alcohol" before switching to zolpidem.[249] Withdrawal signs include tremor, agitation, and seizures. In one case withdrawal signs were not suppressed by chlordrazepoxide but promptly ceased with tapering doses of zolpidem.[250] Abuse of the similar nonbenzodiazepine zoplicone, with escalating doses producing euphoria, was described in a 59-year-old German woman without any prior substance abuse or other psychiatric disorder.[251] As of 2002 no cases of abuse or dependence had been reported involving another similar agent, zaleplon.[252] Baboons self-administer zolpidem and zaleplon.[253]

2,3-Benzodiazepines

Tofisopam (Grandaxin), a 2,3-benzodiazepine, is commercially available as an anxiolytic in Japan and parts of Europe. 2,3-Benzodiazepines augment opioid signal transduction without producing tolerance or dependence; they might thereby be useful in the treatment of opioid addiction. Recreational use has not been described.[253a]

Valerian

In the United States more than US$3 billion are spent annually on "herbal supplements," and among the most popular is valerian. The term describes nearly 200 plants of the *Valeriana* genus which have been used worldwide for millennia to treat insomnia and other disorders. Multiple constituents, including valeptriates, valeranone, valerenal, and valerenic acid have sedating effects and act at $GABA_A$ receptors but not at benzodiazepine receptors.[254] Controlled trials (difficult to assess because of valerian's strong odor) suggest efficacy in insomnia with much less likelihood, compared with benzodiazepines, of "hangover."[255] Tolerance and dependence have not been described.

γ-*Hydroxybutyric acid,* γ-*Butyrolactone,* *1,4-Butanediol*

Present in normal brain, γ-hydroxybutyric acid (GHB) is a metabolite of GABA. It binds to $GABA_B$ receptors as well as to its own high-affinity receptors and seems to be involved in sleep cycle and temperature regulation, memory, emotional control, growth hormone release, and glucose metabolism. GHB inhibits dopamine release at low doses and stimulates it at high doses.[256–259]

GHB became commercially available in the United States during the 1980s with claims to body builders that it could increase muscle mass without exercise. Adverse effects led the FDA in 1990 to ban over-the-counter sales. The drug quickly became popular as a euphoriant, however, and during the 1990s became a fixture at "rave" parties. Its reputation as a "date rape" drug, with reports of fatalities, led to its classification in 1999 as a Schedule I drug.[260] In 2003 the classification was changed to Schedule III, allowing GHB therapy for narcoleptic cataplexy. In Europe GHB is also used to treat narcolepsy.[256,261] Imports carry such brand names as "Gamma-OH" and "Somsanit." Street products from clandestine laboratories carry a wide array of labels (Table 6–4). Products are sold as either a liquid, a powder, or a gel. Mail order kits and Internet websites offer instructions for home manufacture. Two precursors of GHB, γ-butyrolactone (GBL) and 1,4-butanediol (1,4-BD), are readily available in the United States as "dietary supplements," "cleaners," or "solvents," thereby exempting them from FDA regulation. Health food stores sell GBL and 1,4-BD under numerous brand names (see Table 6–4).[262,263]

In 2000 the National Institute of Drug Abuse reported that since 1990 over 7000 GHB/GBL/1,4-BD overdoses had been reported in 45 U.S. states, including 65 GHB-related deaths and 30 GHB-related sexual assaults. In 1998 DAWN reported 1343 emergency room encounters involving GHB, compared with 20 in 1992.[263]

Table 6–4. Products containing γ-Hydroxybutyric acid, γ-Butyrolactone, or 1,4-Butanediol

γ-Hydroxybutyric acid products illegally imported:
    Alcover, Gamma-OH, Somatomax-PM, Somsanit, Anectamine, Natural Sleep 500
γ-Hydroxybutyric acid street names:
    G, GHB, Scoop, Easy Lay, Great Hormones at Bedtime, Georgia Home Boy, Grievous Bodily Harm, GBH,
    Liquid Ecstasy, Liquid E Liquid X, GH Beers, Growth Hormone Booster, Soap, Salty Water, G-Riffick, Cherry Meth,
    Organic Quaalude
γ-Butyrolactone dietary supplements:
    Gamma Ram, Furanone, Nu-Life, RenewTrient, Renewsolvent, Revivarant G, Jolt, Verve, Verve 5.0, GH Gold,
    Eclipse 4.0, Furan, G3, V3, Gen X, Remedy GH, ReActive, Rest-Eze, Beta-Tech, Thunder, Furomax, Blue Nitro,
    Blue Nitro Vitality, Invigorate, Insom X, GH Revitalizer, Gamma G, Reinforce, Firewater, Revivarant, Regenerize
γ-Butyrolactone "cleaners" and "solvents": Verve, Verve 5.0, Miracle Cleaning
1,4-Butanediol dietary supplements:
    Rejuv@Nite, Ultradiol, Enliven, N-Force, Liquid Gold, Zen, Soma Solutions, Blue Raine, Thunder, Serenity, NRG3,
    Thunder Nectar, Inner G, Somato Pro, Weight Belt Cleaner, X-12, Rest-Q, Biocopia PM, Dormir, Amino Flex,
    Cherry fx, Bombs, Lemon fx Drops, Orange fx Rush, Revitalize Plus, GHRE
1, 4-Butanedial "cleaners" and "solvents":
    Blue Raine, Thunder, Serenity II, Mystik, Midnight, Miracle Cleaning Products

---

Modified from Zvosec D, Smith SW, McCutcheon JR, et al. Adverse events, including death, associated with the use of 1,4-butanediol. N Engl J Med 2001; 344:87.

Animals self-administer GHB, and human addiction occurs.[264] In addition to producing a euphoric high, GHB causes sedation and respiratory depression. Effects appear 15 to 20 minutes after oral ingestion and last for up to 10 hours. GBL is absorbed even more rapidly and has a longer duration of action. GHB, GBL, and 1,4-BD are often taken with ethanol, which potentiates their effects, and because 1,4-BD and ethanol are both metabolized by alcohol dehydrogenase, each markedly prolongs the effects of the other.[265] Symptoms of GHB/GBL/1,4-BD intoxication include combative and self-injurious behavior, vomiting, dyspnea, insomnia, hallucinations, dizziness, tremor, ataxia, amnesia, hypothermia, sweating, incontinence, hypotonia, myoclonus, seizures, and coma. Stimulation can provoke agitation and combativeness even in patients with severe respiratory depression.[266] Bradycardia, hypotension, and metabolic acidosis occur.[267] Bundle-branch block and other electrocardiographic abnormalities are described in children.[263] A young man developed somnolence alternating with agitation, incomprehensible speech, and incontinence after ingesting ethanol plus laser printer toner-cartridge cleaner, which contains 1,4-BD.[267a]

In a report of 88 consecutive cases of GHB overdose seen at San Francisco General Hospital, 39% involved co-ingestion of ethanol and 28% co-ingestion of other drugs, including amphetamine, methylenedioxymethamphetamine ("Ecstasy"), cocaine, another sedative, marijuana, and LSD. Among 11 patients requiring mechanical ventilation, recovery time ranged from 161 to 439 hours.[268]

Relevant to its use as a "date rape" drug, GHB, usually added surreptitiously to ethanol, reportedly causes "drop attacks," in which the victim loses muscular control and drops to the floor, maintaining consciousness but unable to resist attack. Moreover, anterograde amnesia may block the victim's recall of the assault.[124]

Treatment of overdose includes respiratory support, atropine for bradycardia, and benzodiazepines for seizures. Anecdotal reports describe reversal of coma following physostigmine or neostigmine.[256] For 1,4-BD poisoning the alcohol dehydrogenase inhibitor 4-methylpyrazole (fomepizole) has been recommended.[267a] Specific GABA-receptor and GHB-receptor antagonists have been deveoped, but their use is restricted to the laboratory.[268a] Vomiting

sometimes lasts for hours after sedation has cleared.[124] Diagnosis depends on history. Gas chromatography/mass spectroscopy can detect GHB/GBL/1,4-BD in blood and urine but is unavailable in most centers.[269]

Withdrawal symptoms in chronic users include sympathetic hyperactivity and acute psychosis.[262,270–273] When ethanol withdrawal is also present, symptoms can be severe and protracted. A young woman addicted to GHB (she took it every 2 hours and had made numerous attempts to stop) also took heavy ethanol to counter GHB-induced tremor, insomnia, and paranoia and developed thiamine-responsive Wernicke–Korsakoff syndrome.[274]

GHB has been used to treat ethanol withdrawal, and it relieved symptoms in a man with ethanol-sensitive myoclonus/dystonia syndrome.[275,276]

References

1. Charney DS, Mihic SJ, Harris RA. Hypnotics and sedatives. In: Hardman JG, Limbird LE, eds. Goodman and Gilman's The Pharmacological Basis of Therapeutics, 10th edition. New York: McGraw-Hill, 2001; 399.
2. Ito T, Suzuki T, Wellman SE, et al. Pharmacology of barbiturate tolerance/dependence: GABA$_A$ receptors and molecular aspects. Life Sci 1996; 59:169.
3. Weinberger DR. Anxiety at the frontier of molecular medicine. N Engl J Med 2001; 344:1247.
4. Hevers W, Luddens H. The diversity of GABA$_A$ receptors. Pharmacological and electrophysiological properties of GABA$_A$ channel subtypes. Mol Neurobiol 1998; 18:35.
5. MacDonald RL, McLain MJ. Anticonvulsant drugs: mechanisms of action. Adv Neurol 1986; 44:713.
6. Twyman RE, Rogers CJ, MacDonald RL. Differential regulation of gamma-aminobutyric acid receptor channels by diazepam and phenobarbital. Ann Neurol 1989; 25:213.
7. Fraser HF, Jasinski DR. The assessment of the abuse potentiality of sedative/hypnotics (depressants): methods used in animals and man. In: Martin WR, ed. Drug Addiction. New York: Springer-Verlag, 1977; 589.
8. Saunders PA, Ito Y, Baker ML, et al. Pentobarbital tolerance and withdrawal: correlation with effects on the GABA-A receptor. Pharmacol Biochem Behav 1990; 37:343.
9. Baldessarini RJ. Drugs and the treatment of psychiatric disorders. Depression and anxiety disorders. In: Hardman JG, Limbird LE, eds. Goodman and Gilman's

The Pharmacological Basis of Therapeutics, 10th edition. New York: McGraw-Hill, 2001; 447.

10. Rampe D, Triggle DJ. Benzodiazepines and calcium channel function. Trends Pharmacol Sci 1986; 7:461.

11. Phillis JW, O'Regan MH. Benzodiazepine interaction with adenosine systems explains some anomalies in GABA hypothesis. Trends Pharmacol Sci 1988; 9:153.

12. Gardner CR. Functional in vivo correlates of the benzodiazepine agonist–inverse agonist continuum. Prog Neurobiol 1988; 31:425.

13. Ninan PT, Insel TM, Cohen RM, et al. Benzodiazepine receptor-mediated experimental "anxiety" in primates. Science 1982; 218:1332.

14. Braestrup C, Schmiechen R, Neef G, et al. Interaction of convulsive ligands with benzodiazepine receptors. Science 1982; 216:1241.

15. Amrein R, Leishman B, Bentzinger C, Roncari G. Flumazenil in benzodiazepine antagonism. Med Toxicol 1987; 2:411.

16. Little HJ. The benzodiazepines: anxiolytic and withdrawal effects. Neuropeptides 1991; 19:11.

17. Polc P. Electrophysiology of benzodiazepine receptor ligands: multiple mechanisms and sites of action. Prog Neurobiol 1988; 31:349.

18. Nutt DJ. Pharmacological mechanisms of benzodiazepine withdrawal. J Psychiat Res 1990; 24:105.

19. Mohler H, Fritschy JM, Rudolf U. A new benzodiazepine pharmacology. J Pharmacol Exp Ther 2002; 300:2.

20. Rudolf U, Crestani F, Mohler H. GABA$_A$ receptor subtypes: dissecting their pharmacological function. Trends Pharmacol Sci 2001; 22:188.

21. Low K, Crestani F, Keist R, et al. Molecular and neuronal substrate for the selective attenuation of anxiety. Science 2000; 290:131.

22. McKernan RM, Rosahl TW, Reynolds DS, et al. Sedative but not anxiolytic properties of benzodiazepines are mediated by the GABA$_A$ receptor γ_1 subtype. Nat Neurosci 2000; 3:587.

23. Smith TAD. Type A gamma-aminobutyric acid (GABA$_A$) receptor subunits and benzodiazepine binding: significance to clinical syndromes and their treatment. Br J Biomed Sci 2001; 58:111.

24. Verma A, Snyder SH. Peripheral type benzodiazepine receptors. Annu Rev Pharmacol Toxicol 1989; 29:307.

25. Costa E, Guidotti A. Diazepam binding inhibitor (DBI): a peptide with multiple biological actions. Life Sci 1991; 49:325.

26. Ohkuma S, Katsura M, Tsujimura A. Alterations in cerebral diazepam binding inhibitor expression in drug dependence: a possible biochemical alteration common to drug dependence. Life Sci 2001; 68:1215.

27. Sangameswaran L, Fales HM, Friedrich P, DeBlas AL. Purification of a benzodiazepine from bovine brain and detection of benzodiazepine-like immunoreactivity in human brain. Proc Natl Acad Sci USA 1986; 83:9236.

28. Sand P, Kavvadias D, Feineis D, et al. Naturally occurring benzodiazepines: current status of research and clinical implications. Eur Arch Psychiatr Clin Neurosci 2000; 250:194.

29. Teuber L, Watjens F, Jensen LH. Ligands for the benzodiazepine binding site—a survey. Curr Pharmaceut Design 1999; 5:317.

30. Griffiths RR, Weerts EM. Benzodiazepine self administration in humans and laboratory animals—implications for problems of long-term use and abuse. Psychopharmacology 1997; 134:1.

31. Woods JH, Katz JL, Winger G. Abuse liability of benzodiazepines. Pharmacol Rev 1987; 39:254.

32. File SE. Tolerance to the behavioral actions of benzodiazepines. Neurosci Biobehav Rev 1985; 9:113.

33. Kang I, Miller LG. Decreased GABA-A receptor sub-unit mRNA concentrations following lorazepam administration. Br J Pharmacol 1991; 103:1285.

34. Miller LG. Chronic benzodiazepine administration: from the patient to the gene. J Clin Pharmacol 1991; 31:492.

35. Pritchard GA, Galpern WR, Lumpkin M, Miller LG. Chronic benzodiazepine administration. VIII. Receptor upregulation produced by chronic exposure to the inverse agonist FG-7142. J Pharmacol Exp Ther 1991; 258:280.

36. Barnhill JG, Ciraulo DA, Greenblatt DJ, et al. Benzodiazepine response and receptor binding after chronic ethanol ingestion in a mouse model. J Pharmacol Exp Ther 1991; 258:812.

37. Helmuth L. A possible target for better benzodiazepines. Science 2000; 290:23.

38. Horvath EJ, Horvath K, Hamari T, et al. Anxiolytic 2,3-benzodiazepines, their specific binding to the basal ganglia. Prog Neurobiol 2000; 60:309.

39. Krafft-Ebbing RV. Ueber Paraldehyde-Gebrauch und Missbrauch nebst einem Falle von Paraldehyde-Delirium. Z Ther 1887; 7:244.

39a. Kelp H. Chloral-wirkung in grossen dosen. Allg Z Psychiatr Ihre Grenzeb 1875; 31:389.

39b. Seguin EC. The abuse and use of bromides. J Nerv Ment Dis 1877; 4:445.

40. Fernandez G, Clarke M. A case of "Veronal" poisoning. Lancet 1904; I:223.

41. Kales A, Kales JD, Bixler EO, Scharf MB. Effectiveness of hypnotic drugs with prolonged use: flurazepam and pentobarbital. Clin Pharmacol Ther 1975; 18:356.

42. Wulff MH. The barbiturate withdrawal syndrome: a clinical and electrophysiologic study. Electroencephalogr Clin Neurophysiol 1959; 14 (Suppl):1.

43. AMA Committee on Alcoholism and Addiction and Council on Mental Health. Dependence on barbiturates and other sedative drugs. JAMA 1965; 193:673.

44. Wysowski DK, Baum C. Outpatient use of prescription sedative-hypnotic drugs in the United States, 1970 through 1989. Arch Intern Med 1991; 151:1779.

45. Coupey SM. Barbiturates. Pediatr Rev 1997; 18: 260-264.

46. Preskorn S, Schwin RL, McKuelly WV. Analgesic abuse and the barbiturate abstinence syndrome. JAMA 1980; 244:369.

46a. Raja M, Altavista MC, Azzoni A, et al. Severe barbiturate withdrawal syndrome in migrainous patients. Headache 1996; 36:119.

46b. Young WB, Siow HC. Should butalbital-containing analgesics be banned? Yes. Curr Pain Headache Rep 2002; 6:151.

47. O'Brien CP. Drug addiction and drug abuse. In: Hardman JG, Limbird LE, eds. Goodman and Gilman's The Pharmacological Basis of Therapeutics, 9th edition. New York: McGraw-Hill, 1996; 557.

48. Guarino J, Roache JD, Kirk WT, Griffiths RR. Comparison of the behavioral effects and abuse liability of ethanol and pentobarbital in recreational sedative abusers. NIDA Res Monogr 1990; 95:453.

49. Mendelson WB. The Use and Misuse of Sleeping Pills. New York: Plenum Press, 1980.

50. Osborn H. Sedative-hypnotic agents. In: Goldfrank LR, Flomenbaum NE, Lewin NA, et al, eds. Toxicologic Emergencies, 6th edition. Stamford, CT: Appleton & Lange, 1998; 1001.

51. Gary NE, Tresznewsky O. Barbiturates and a potpourri of other sedatives, hypnotics, and tranquilizers. Heart Lung 1983; 12:122.

52. Simon RP. Decorticate and decerebrate posturing in sedative drug-induced coma. Neurology 1982; 32:448.

53. Khantzian EJ, McKenna GJ. Acute toxic and withdrawal reactions associated with drug use and abuse. Ann Intern Med 1979; 90:361.

54. Fraser HF, Wikler A, Essig CF, Isbell H. Degree of physical dependence induced by secobarbital or pentobarbital. JAMA 1958; 166:126.

55. Smith DE, Wesson DR. Phenobarbital technique for treatment of barbiturate dependence. Arch Gen Psychiatry 1971; 24:56.

56. Kandall SR. Treatment strategies for drug-exposed neonates. Clin Perinatol 1999; 26:231.

57. Rumbaugh CL, Fang HCH. The effects of drug abuse on the brain. Medical Times, March 1980:37s.

58. Rumbaugh CL, Bergeron RT, Fang HCH, McCormick R. Cerebral angiographic changes in the drug abuse patient. Radiology 1971; 101:335.

59. Rumbaugh CL, Fang HCH, Higgins RE, et al. Cerebral microvascular injury in experimental drug abuse. Invest Radiol 1976; 11:282.

60. MacLeod CM, Dekaban AS, Hunt E. Memory impairment in epileptic patients: selective effects of phenobarbital on concentration. Science 1978; 202:1102.

61. Allgulander C, Borg S, Vikander B. A 4–6 year follow-up of 50 patients with primary dependence on sedative and hypnotic drugs. Am J Psychiatry 1984; 141:1580.

62. Theodore WA, DiChiro G, Margolin R, et al. Barbiturates reduce human cerebral glucose metabolism. Neurology 1986; 36:60.

63. Fishman RHB, Yanai J. Long-lasting effects of early barbiturates on central nervous system and behavior. Neurosci Biobehav Rev 1983; 7:19.

64. Camfield CS, Chaplin S, Doyle AB, et al. Side-effects of phenobarbital in toddlers: behavioral and cognitive aspects. J Pediatr 1979; 95:361.

65. Wolf SM, Forsythe A. Behavioral disturbance, phenobarbital, and febrile seizures. Pediatrics 1978; 61:728.

66. Vining EP, Mellits ED, Dorsen MM, et al. Psychologic and behavioral effects of antiepileptic drugs in children: a double-blind comparison between phenobarbital and valproic acid. Pediatrics 1987; 80:165.

67. Wolf SM, Forsythe A, Stunden AA, et al. Long-term effect of phenobarbital on cognitive function in children with febrile convulsions. Pediatrics 1981; 68:820.

68. Farwell JR, Lee YJ, Hirtz DG, et al. Phenobarbital for febrile seizures—effects on intelligence and on seizure recurrence. N Engl J Med 1990; 322:364.

69. Reinisch JM, Sanders SA, Mortensen EL, et al. In utero exposure to phenobarbital and intelligence deficits in adult men. JAMA 1995; 274:1518.

70. Bergey GKK, Swaiman KF, Schrier BK, et al. Adverse effects of phenobarbital on morphological and biochemical development of fetal mouse spinal cord neurons in culture. Ann Neurol 1981; 9:584.

71. Diaz J, Schain RJ, Bailey BG. Phenobarbital-induced brain growth retardation in artificially reared rat pups. Biol Neonate 1977; 32:77

72. Reinisch JM, Sanders SA. Early barbiturate exposure: the brain, sexually dimorphic behavior and learning. Neurosci Biobehav Rev 1982; 6:311.

73. Maytal J, Shinnar S. Barbiturates. In: Spencer PS, Schaumburg HH, eds. Experimental and Clinical Neurotoxicology, 2nd edition. New York: Oxford University Press, 2000:219.

74. Guile LA. Rapid habituation to chlordiazepoxide "Librium." Med J Aust 1963; 2:56.

75. Czerwenka-Wenkstetten H, Hofman G, Krypsin-Exner K. Ein Fall von Valium-Entzugsdelir. Wien Med Wochenschr 1965; 47:994.

76. Selig JW. A possible oxazepam abstinence syndrome. JAMA 1966; 198:279.

77. Johnson L, Clift AD. Dependence on hypnotic drugs in general practice. BMJ 1968; IV:613.

78. Parry HJ, Butler MB, Mellinger GD, et al. National patterns of psychotherapeutic drug use. Arch Gen Psychiatry 1973; 28:769.

79. Swanson DW, Weddige RL, Morse RM. Abuse of prescription drugs. Mayo Clin Proc 1973; 48:359.

80. Rucker TD. Drug use: data, sources, and limitations. JAMA 1974; 230:888.

81. Korsgaard S. Misbrug av lorazepam. Vgeschrift for Laeger 1976; 135:164.

82. Lader M. Benzodiazepines: the opium of the masses? Neuroscience 1978; 3:159.

83. Allgulander C, Borg S. Case report: a delirious abstinence syndrome associated with chlorazepate "Tranxilen." Br J Addict 1978; 73:175.

84. Stark L, Sykes R, Mullin P. Temazepam abuse. Lancet 1987; II:802.

85. Farrell M, Strang J. Misuse of temazepam. BMJ 1988; 297:1402.

86. Juergens S, Morse R. Alprazolam dependence in seven patients. Am J Psychiatry 1988; 145:625.

87. Schmauss C, Apelt S, Emrich HM. Preference for alprazolam over diazepam. Am J Psychiatry 1989; 146:408.

88. Johnston LD, O'Malley PM, Bachman JG. Drug use among American high school students, college students, and other young adults: national trends through 1985. Rockville, MD: DHHS Publication (ADM) 86-1450, 1986.

89. Baldwin DC, Hughes PH, Conard SE, et al. Substance use among senior medical students. JAMA 1991; 265:2074.

90. Hughes PH, Conard SSE, Baldwin DC, et al. Resident physician substance use in the United States. JAMA 1991; 265:2069.

91. Ladewig D. Dependence liability of the benzodiazepines. Drug Alcohol Depend 1984; 13:139.

92. American Psychiatric Association Task Force on Benzodiazepine Dependency. Benzodiazepine dependency, abuse. Washington, DC: APA, 1990.

93. Woods JH, Katz JL, Winger G. Use and abuse of benzodiazepines. Issues relevant to prescribing. JAMA 1988; 260:3476.

94. Ciraulo DA, Barnhill JG, Greenblatt DJ, et al. Abuse liability and clinical pharmacokinetics of alprazolam in alcoholic men. J Clin Psychiatry 1988; 49:333.

95. Griffiths RR, Ator NA, Lukas SE, et al. Experimental abuse liability assessment of benzodiazepines. In: Usdin E, Skolnick P, Tallman JF, et al., eds. Pharmacology of Benzodiazepines. London: Macmillan, 1982:609.

96. Tyrer PJ. Benzodiazepines on trial. BMJ 1984; 288:1101.

97. Ballenger JC. Psychopharmacology of the anxiety disorders. Psychiatr Clin North Am 1984; 7:757.

98. Tennant FS, Pumphrey EA. Benzodiazepine dependence of several years duration: clinical profile and therapeutics. In: Harris LS, ed. Problems of Drug Dependence 1984. Washington, DC: NIDA Res Monogr 1984; 55:211.

99. Ellis P, Carney MW. Benzodiazepine abuse and management of anxiety in the community. Int J Addict 1988; 23:1083.

100. Warneke LB. Benzodiazepines: abuse and new use. Can J Psychiatry 1991; 36:194.

100a. Posternak MA, Mueller TI. Assessing the risks and benefits of benzodiazepines for anxiety disorders in patients with a history of substance abuse or dependence. Am J Addict 2001; 10:48.

101. Reidenberg MM. Effect of the requirement for triplicate prescriptions for benzodiazepines in New York State. Clin Pharmacol Ther 1991; 50:129.

102. Weintraub M, Singh S, Byrne L, et al. Consequences of the 1989 New York State triplicate benzodiazepine prescription regulations. JAMA 1991; 266:2392.

103. Glass RM. Benzodiazepine prescription regulation. Autonomy and outcome. JAMA 1991; 266:2431.

104. Abuse of benzodiazepines: the problems and solutions. A report of a Committee of the Institute for Behavior and Health, Inc. Am J Drug Alcohol Abuse 1988; 14 (Suppl 1):1.

105. Busto U, Sellers EM, Sisson B, Segal R. Benzodiazepine use and abuse in alcoholics. Clin Pharmacol Ther 1982; 31:207.

106. Chan AWK. Effects of combined alcohol and benzodiazepine: a review. Drug Alcohol Depend 1984; 13:315.

107. DuPont RL. A practical approach to benzodiazepine discontinuation. J Psychiatr Res 1990; 24 (Suppl 2):81.

108. Cole JO, Chiarello RJ. The benzodiazepines as drugs of abuse. J Psychiatr Res 1990; 24 (Suppl 2):135.

109. Griffiths RR, Wolf B. Relative abuse liability of different benzodiazepines in drug abusers. J Clin Psychopharmacol 1990; 10:237.

110. Kaminer Y, Modai I. Parenteral abuse of diazepam: a case report. Drug Alcohol Depend 1984; 14:63.

111. Magura S, Goldsmith D, Casriel C, et al. The validity of methadone clients' self-reported drug use. Int J Addict 1987; 22:727.

112. Weddington WA, Carney A. Alprazolam abuse during methadone maintenance therapy. JAMA 1987; 257: 3363.

113. Fraser A. Alprazolam abuse and methadone maintenance. JAMA 1987; 258:2061.

114. Preston KL, Griffiths RR, Stitzer ML, et al. Diazepam and methadone interactions in methadone maintenance. Clin Pharmacol Ther 1984; 36:534.

115. Lavelle TL, Hammersley R, Forsyth A. The use of buprenorphine and temazepam by drug injectors. J Addict Dis 1991; 10:5.

116. Blair SD, Holcombe C, Coombes EN, et al. Leg ischaemia secondary to non-medical injection of temazepam. Lancet 1991; 338:1393.

117. Jenkinson DF, Pusey CD. Rhabdomyolysis and renal failure after intro-arterial temazepam. Nephrol Dial Transplant 1994: 9:1334.

118. Deighan CJ, Wong KM, McLaughlin KJ, et al. Rhabdomyolysis and acute renal failure resulting from alcohol and drug abuse. Q J Med 2000; 93:29.

119. Rooney S, Kelly G, Bamford L, et al. Co-abuse of opiates and benzodiazepines. Irish J Med Sci 1999; 168:36.

120. Salvaggio J, Jacob C, Schmitt C, et al. Abuse of flunitrazepam in opioid addicts. Ann Med Interne 2000; 151 (Suppl A):A6.

121. Ross J, Darke S. The nature of benzodiazepine dependence among heroin users in Sydney, Australia. Addiction 2000; 95:1785.

122. Rome ES. It's a rave new world: rave culture and illicit drug use in the young. Cleveland Clin J Med 2001; 68:541.

123. Waltzman ML. Flunitrazepam: a review of "roofies." Pediatr Emerg Care 1999; 15:59.

124. Schwartz RH, Milteer R. Drug-facilitated sexual assault ("date rape"). South Med J 2000; 93:558.

125. Druid H, Holmgren P, Ahlner J. Flunitrazepam: an evaluation of use, abuse, and toxicity. Forensic Sci Int 2001; 122:136.

126. Greenblatt DJ, Allen MD, Noel BJ, Shader RI. Acute overdosage with benzodiazepine derivatives. Clin Pharmacol 1977; 21:497.

127. Vapaatalo H, Karppanen H. Combined toxicity of ethanol with chlorpromazine, diazepam, chlormethiazole, or pentobarbital in mice. Agents Actions 1969; 1:43.

128. Finkle BS, McClosky KL, Goodman LS. Diazepam and drug-associated deaths: a survey in the United States and Canada. JAMA 1979; 242:429.

129. Cate JC, Jatlow PI. Chlordiazepoxide overdose: interpretation of serum drug concentrations. Clin Toxicol 1973; 6:553.

130. Gaudreault P, Guay J, Thivierge RL, Verdy I. Benzodiazepine poisoning. Clinical and pharmacological considerations and treatment. Drug Safety 1991; 6:247.

131. Geller E, Crome P, Schaller MD, et al. Risks and benefits of therapy with flumazenil (Anexate) in mixed drug intoxications. Eur Neurol 1991; 31:241.

132. Weinbroum AA, Flaishon R, Sorkine P, et al. A risk-benefit assessment of flumazenil in the management of benzodiazepine overdose. Drug Sol 1997; 17:181.

133. Howland MA. Flumazenil. In: Goldfrank LR, Flomenbaum NE, Lewin NA, et al., eds. Goldfrank's Toxicologic Emergencies, 6th edition. Stamford, CT: Appleton & Lange, 1998:1017.

133a. Prinz PN, Vitiello MV, Raskind MA, Thorpy MJ. Geriatrics: sleep disorders and aging. N Engl J Med 1990; 323:520.

133b. Greenblatt DJ, Harmatz JS, Shapiro L, et al. Sensitivity to triazolam in the elderly. N Engl J Med 1991; 324:1691.

134. Larson EB, Kukull WA, Buchner D, Reifler BV. Adverse drug reactions associated with global cognitive impairment in elderly persons. Ann Intern Med 1987; 107:169.

135. Tinetti ME. Preventing falls in elderly persons. N Engl J Med 2003; 348:42.

136. Hayes SL, Pablo G, Radomski T, Palmer RF. Ethanol and oral diazepam absorption. N Engl J Med 1977; 296:186.

137. Campbell AJ, Robertson MC, Gardner MM, et al. Psychotropic medication withdrawal and a home-based exercise program to prevent falls: a randomized controlled trial. J Am Geriatr Soc 1999; 47:850.

138. Lucki I, Rickels K, Geller AM. Chronic use of benzodiazepines and psychomotor and cognitive test performance. Psychopharmacology 1986; 88:426.

139. Juhl RP, Daugherty VM, Kroboth PD. Incidence of next-day anterograde amnesia caused by flurazepam hydrochloride and triazolam. J Clin Psychopharmacol 1984; 3:622.

140. Shader RI, Greenblatt DJ. Triazolam and anterograde amnesia: all is not well in the Z-zone. J Clin Psychopharmacol 1983; 3:273.

141. Morris HH, Estes ML. Traveler's amnesia. Transient global amnesia secondary to triazolam. JAMA 1987; 258:945.

142. McNicholas LF, Martin WR, Cherian S. Physical dependence on diazepam and lorazepam in the dog. J Pharmacol Exp Ther 1983; 226:783.

143. Owen RT, Tyrer P. Benzodiazepine dependence: a review of the evidence. Drugs 1983; 25:385.

144. Ryan GP, Boisse NR. Experimental induction of benzodiazepine tolerance and physical dependence. J Pharmacol Exp Ther 1983; 226:100.

145. Lader M, File S. The biological basis of benzodiazepine dependence. Psychol Med 1987; 17:539.

146. Griffiths RR, Lamb RJ, Ator NA, et al. Relative abuse liability of triazolam: experimental assessment in animals and humans. Neurosci Biobehav Rev 1985; 9:133.

147. Kales A, Scharf MB, Kales JD, Soldatos CR. Rebound insomnia: a potential hazard following withdrawal of certain benzodiazepines. JAMA 1979; 241:1692.

148. Rickels K, Case WG, Downing RW, Winokur A. Long-term diazepam therapy and clinical outcome. JAMA 1983; 250:767.

149. Tyrer PJ, Seivewright N. Identification and management of benzodiazepine dependence. Postgrad Med J 1984; 60 (Suppl 2):41.

150. Busto U, Sellers EM, Naranjo CA, et al. Withdrawal reaction after long-term therapeutic use of benzodiazepines. N Engl J Med 1986; 315:854.

151. Nutt D. Benzodiazepine dependence in the clinic: reason for anxiety? Trends Pharmacol Sci 1986; 7:457.

152. Schmauss C, Apelt S, Emrich HM. Characterization of benzodiazepine withdrawal in high- and low-dose dependent psychiatric inpatients. Brain Res Bull 1987; 19:393.

153. Dickinson B, Rush PA, Radcliffe AB. Alprazolam use and dependence. A retrospective analysis of 30 cases of withdrawal. West J Med 1990; 152:604.

154. Committee on the Review of Medicines. Systematic review of the benzodiazepines. BMJ 1980; 1:910.

155. Einarson TR. Lorazepam withdrawal seizures. Lancet 1980; I:151.

156. Abernathy DR, Greenblatt DJ, Shader RI. Treatment of diazepam withdrawal syndrome with propranolol. Ann Intern Med 1981; 94:354.

157. Fialip J, Aumaitre O, Eschalier A, et al. Benzo-diazepine withdrawal seizures. Analysis of 48 case reports. Clin Neuropharmacol 1987; 10:538.

158. Roy-Byrne PP, Hommer D. Benzodiazepine withdrawal: an overview and implications for the treatment of anxiety. Am J Med 1988; 84:1041.

159. Greenblatt DJ, Miller LG, Shader RI. Benzodiazepine discontinuation syndromes. J Psychiatr Res 1990; 24:73.

160. Harrison M, Busto U, Naranjo CA, et al. Diazepam tapering in detoxification for high-dose benzodiazepine abuse. Clin Pharmacol Ther 1984; 36:527.

161. Greenblatt DJ, Harmatz JS, Zinny MA, Shader RI. Effect of gradual withdrawal on the rebound sleep disorder after discontinuation of triazolam. N Engl J Med 1987; 317:722.

162. Klein E, Uhde TW, Post RM. Preliminary evidence for the utility of carbamazepine in alprazolam withdrawal. Am J Psychiatry 1986; 143:235.

163. Karch FE. Rage reaction associated with chlorazepate dipotassium. Ann Intern Med 1979; 91:62.

164. Fouilladieu J-L, D'Engert J, Conseiller C. Benzodiazepines. N Engl J Med 1984; 310:464.

165. Oswald I. Triazolam syndrome 10 years on. Lancet 1989; II:451.

166. Bixler EO, Kales A, Brubaker BH, Kales JD. Adverse reactions to benzodiazepine hypnotics: spontaneous reporting system. Pharmacology 1987; 35:286.

167. Bixler EO, Kales A, Manfredi RL, et al. Next-day memory impairment with triazolam use. Lancet 1991; 337:827.

168. Gillin JC. The long and short of sleeping pills. N Engl J Med 1991; 324:1735.

169. Greenblatt DJ, Shader RI, Harmatz JS. Triazolam in the elderly. N Engl J Med 1991; 325:1744.

170. Trappler B, Bezeredi T. Triazolam intoxication. Can Med Assoc J 1982; 126:893.

171. van der Kroef C. Reactions to triazolam. Lancet 1979; II: 526.

172. Gabe J. Benzodiazepines as a social problem: the case of Halcion. Subst Use Misuse 2001; 36:1233.

173. Hendrickson RG, Morocco AP, Greenberg MI. Acute dystonic reactions to "Street Xanax." N Engl J Med 2002; 346:1753.

173a. Leonard MK, Pox CP, Stephens DS. *Abiotrophia* species bacteremia and a mycotic aneurysm in an intravenous drug abuser. N Engl J Med 2001; 344:233.

174. Brooker AE, Wiens AN, Wiens DA. Impaired brain functions due to diazepam and meprobamate abuse in a 53-year-old male. J Nerv Ment Dis 1984; 142:498.

175. Golombok S, Moodley P, Lader M. Cognitive impairment in long-term benzodiazepine users. Psychol Med 1988; 18:365.

176. Bergman H, Borg S, Engelbrektson K, et al. Dependence on sedative-hypnotics: neuropsychological impairment, field dependence and clinical course in a 5-year follow-up study. Br J Addict 1989; 84:547.

176a. Rummans TA, Davis LJ, Morse RM, et al. Learning and memory impairment in older, detoxified, benzodiazepine-dependent patients. Mayo Clin Proc 1993; 68:731.

176b. Rickels K, Lucki I, Schweizer E, et al. Psychomotor performance of long-term benzodiazepine users before, during and after benzodiazepine discontinuation. J Clin Psychopharmacol 1999; 19:107.

176c. Vignola A, Lamoureux C, Bastian CH, et al. Effects of chronic insomnia and use of benzodiazepines on daytime performance in older adults. J Gerontol Psychol Sci 2000; 55B:54.

176d. McAndrews MP, Weiss RT, Sandor P: Cognitive effects of long-term benzodiazepine use in older adults. Hum Psychopharmacol Clin Exp 2003; 18:51.

177. Laegreid L, Olegard R, Wahlstrom J, Conradi N. Abnormalities in children exposed to benzodiazepines in utero. Lancet 1987; I:108.

178. Bitran D, Primus RJ, Kellogg CK. Gestational exposure to diazepam increases sensitivity to convulsants that act at the GABA/benzodiazepine receptor complex. Eur J Pharmacol 1991; 196:223.

179. Lemere F. Habit-forming properties of meprobamate. Arch Neurol Psychiatry 1956; 76:205.

180. Brouschek R, Feuerlein M. Valamin als Suchtmittel. Nervenarzt 1956; 27:115.

181. Battegay R. Sucht nach Abusus von Doriden. Praxis 1957; 46:991.

182. Cahn CH. Intoxication to ethchlorvynol (Placidyl). Can Med Assoc J 1959; 81:733.

183. Jensen GR. Addiction to "Noludar." N Z Med J 1960; 59:431.

184. Tengblad K-F. Heminevrin-enformani. Lahartidingen 1961; 58:1936.

185. Ewart RBL, Priest RG. Methaqualone addiction and delirium tremens. BMJ 1967; III:92.

186. Gillin JC, Byerley WF. The diagnosis and management of insomnia. N Engl J Med 1990; 322:239.

187. Falco M. Methaqualone misuse: foreign experience and United States drug control policy. Int J Addict 1976; 11:597.

188. Fishburne PM, Abelson HI, Cisin I. National Survey on Drug Abuse: main findings: 1979. Washington, DC: DHHS Publication No. (ADM) 80-976, 1980.

189. Inaba DS, Gay GR, Newmeyer JA, Whitehead C. Methaqualone abuse. "Luding out." JAMA 1973; 224:1505.

190. Sanderson JH, Cowdell RH, Higgins G. Fatal poisoning with methaqualone and diphenhydramine. Lancet 1966; II:803.

191. Wallace MR, Allen E. Recovery after massive overdose of diphenhydramine and methaqualone. Lancet 1968; II:1247.

192. Gerald MC, Schwirian PM. Non-medical use of methaqualone. Arch Gen Psychiatry 1973; 28:627.

193. Pascarelli EF. Methaqualone abuse, the quiet epidemic. JAMA 1973; 224:1512.

194. Abboud RT, Freedman MT, Rogers RM, Daniele RP. Methaqualone with muscular hyperactivity necessitating the use of curare. Chest 1974; 65:204.

195. Marks P. Methaqualone and peripheral neuropathy. Practitioner 1974; 212:721.

196. Hoaken PCS. Adverse effects of methaqualone. Can Med Assoc J 1975; 112:685.

197. Anon. Methaqualone abuse implicated in injuries and death nationwide. JAMA 1981; 246:813.

198. Wetli CV. Changing patterns of methaqualone abuse. JAMA 1983; 249:621.

199. Coleman JR, Barone JA. Abuse potential of methaqualone–diphenhydramine combination. Am J Hosp Pharm 1981; 38:160.

200. O'Malley PM, Bachman JG, Johnson LD. Period, age, and cohort effects on substance use among young Americans: a decade of change, 1976-86. Am J Public Health 1988; 78:1315.

201. Mayer JF, Schreiner GE, Westervelt FB. Acute glutethimide intoxication. Am J Med 1962; 33:70.

202. Caplan JL. Recovery in severe glutethimide poisoning. Postgrad Med J 1967; 43:611.

203. Myers RR, Stockard JJ. Neurologic and electroencephalographic correlates in glutethimide intoxication. Clin Pharmacol Ther 1975; 17:212.

204. Hansen AR, Kennedy KA, Ambre JJ, Fischer LJ. Glutethimide poisoning. N Engl J Med 1975; 292:250.

205. Brown DG, Hammill JF. Glutethimide poisoning: unilateral pupillary abnormalities. N Engl J Med 1971; 285:806.

206. Feuer E, French J. Descriptive epidemiology of mortality in New Jersey due to combinations of codeine and glutethimide. Am J Epidemiol 1984; 119:202.

207. Bender FH, Cooper JV, Dreyfus R. Fatalities associated with an acute overdose of glutethimide (Doriden) and codeine. Vet Hum Toxicol 1988; 30:332.

208. Lingl FA. Irreversible effects of glutethimide addiction. Am J Psychiatry 1966; 123:349.

209. Nover R. Persistent neuropathy following chronic use of glutethimide. Clin Pharmacol Ther 1967; 8:283.

210. Haas DC, Marassigan A. Neurological effects of glutethimide. J Neurol Neurosurg Psychiatry 1968; 31:561.

211. Ober RP, Hennessy JF, Hellman RM. Severe hypocalcemia associated with chronic glutethimide addiction. A case report. Am J Psychiatry 1981; 138:1239.

212. Westervelt FB. Ethchlorvynol (Placidyl) intoxication. Ann Intern Med 1966; 64:1229.

213. Teehan BP, Maher JF, Carey JJH, et al. Acute ethchlorvynol (Placidyl) intoxication. Ann Intern Med 1970; 72:875.

214. Ogilvie RI, Douglas DE, Lochead JR, et al. Ethchlorvynol (Placidyl) intoxication and its treatment by hemodialysis. Can Med Assoc J 1966; 95:954.

215. Klock JC. Hemolysis and pancytopenia in ethchlorvynol overdose. Ann Intern Med 1974; 81:131.

216. Hyde JS, Lawrence GI, Moles JB. Ethchlorvynol intoxication: successful treatment by exchange transfusion and peritoneal dialysis. Clin Pediatr 1968; 4:739.

217. Tozer TN, Witt LD, Gee L, et al. Evaluation of hemodialysis for ethchlorvynol (Placidyl) overdose. Am J Hosp Pharm 1974; 31:986.

218. Lynn RI, Honig CL, Jatlow PI, Kliger AS. Resin hemoperfusion for treatment of ethchlorvynol overdose. Ann Intern Med 1979; 91:549.

219. Essig CF, Ainslie JD. Addiction to meprobamate. JAMA 1957; 164:1382.

220. Haizlip TM, Ewing JA. Meprobamate habituation: a controlled clinical study. N Engl J Med 1958; 258:1181.

221. Roache JD, Griffiths RR. Lorazepam and meprobamate dose effects in humans: behavioral effects and abuse liability. J Pharmacol Exp Ther 1987; 243:978.

222. Kintz P, Tracqui A, Mangin P, Lugnier AA. Fatal meprobamate self-poisoning. Am J Forens Med Pathol 1988; 9:139.

223. Maddock RK, Bloomer HA. Meprobamate overdosage, evaluation of its severity and methods of treatment. JAMA 1967; 201:999.

224. Jenis EH, Payne RJ, Goldbaum LR. Acute meprobamate poisoning. A fatal case following a lucid interval. JAMA 1969; 207:361.

225. Hoy WE, Rivero A, Marin MG, Rieders F. Resin hemoperfusion for treatment of a massive meprobamate overdose. Ann Intern Med 1980; 93:455.

226. Jacobsen D, Wiik-Larson E, Saltvedt E, Bredesen JE. Meprobamate kinetics during and after terminated hemoperfusion in acute intoxications. Clin Toxicol 1987; 25:317.

227. Hayward JN, Boshell BR. Paraldehyde intoxication with metabolic acidosis. Am J Med 1957; 23:965.

228. Kunze U. Chronic bromide intoxication with a severe neurological deficit. J Neurol 1976; 213:149.

229. Trump DL, Hochberg MC. Bromide intoxication. Johns Hopkins Med J 1976; 138:119.

230. Palatucci DM. Paradoxical levels in bromide intoxication. Neurology 1978; 28:1189.

231. Wolf B, Guarino JJ, Preston KL, Griffiths RR. Abuse liability of diphenhydramine in sedative abusers. In: Harris L, ed. Problems of Drug Dependence 1989. Rockville, MD: NIDA Res Monogr 1990; 95:486.

232. Traber J, Glaser T. 5-HT$_{1A}$ receptor-related anxiolytics. Trends Pharmacol Sci 1987; 8:432.

233. Smiley A, Moskowitz H. Effects of long-term administration of buspirone and diazepam on driver steering control. Am J Med 1986; 80:22.

234. Taylor DP, Moon SL. Buspirone and related compounds as alternative anxiolytics. Neuropeptides 1991; 19 (Suppl):15.

235. File SE. The search for novel anxiolytics. Trends Neurosci 1987; 10:461.

236. Griffith JD, Jasinski DR, Casten GP, McKinney GR. Investigation of the abuse liability of buspirone in alcohol-dependent subjects. Am J Med 1986; 80:30.

237. Schnabel T. Evaluation of the safety and side-effects of antianxiety agents. Am J Med 1987; 82:7.

238. Lader M. Assessing the potential for buspirone dependence or abuse and effects of its withdrawal. Am J Med 1987; 82:20.

239. Boylan K. Persistent dystonia associated with buspirone. Neurology 1990; 40:1904.

240. Markowitz JS, Brewerton TD. Zolpidem-induced psychosis. Ann Clin Psychiatry 1996; 8:89.

241. Cavallaro R, Regazzetti MG, Covelli G, et al. Tolerance and withdrawal with zolpidem. Lancet 1993; 342:374.

242. Brodeur MR, Stirling AL. Delirium associated with zolpidem. Ann Pharmacol 2001; 35:1562.

242a. Morselli PL. Zolpidem side-effects. Lancet 1993; 342:868.

242b. Toner LC, Tsambras BM, Catalano G, et al. Central nervous system side effects associated with zolpidem treatment. Clin Neuropharmacol 2000; 23:54.

243. Barrero-Hernandez FJ, Ruiz-Veguilla M, Lopez-Lopez MI, et al. Epileptic seizures as a sign of abstinence from chronic consumption of zolpidem. Revist Neurol 2002; 34:1.

244. Aragona M. Abuse, dependence, and epileptic seizures after zolpidem withdrawal; review and case report. Clin Neuropharmacol 2000; 23:281.

245. Vartzopoulos D, Bozikas V, Phocas C, et al. Dependence on zolpidem in high dose. Int Clin Psychopharmacol 2000; 15:181.

246. Goder R, Treskov V, Burmester J, et al. Zolpidem: the risk of tolerance and dependence according to case reports, systematic studies and recent molecular biological data. Fortschr Neurol Psychiatr 2001; 69:592.

247. Golden SA, Vagnoni C. Zolpidem dependence and prescription fraud. Am J Addict 2000; 9:96.

248. Correas Lauffer J, Braquehais Conesa D, Barbado Del Cura E, et al. Abuse, tolerance and dependence of zolpidem: three case reports. Acta Espanol Psiquiatr 2002; 30:259.

249. Soyka M, Bottlender R, Möller H-J. Epidemiological evidence for a low abuse potential of zolpidem. Pharmacopsychiatry 2000; 33:138.

250. Madrak LN, Rosenberg M. Zolpidem abuse. Am J Psychiatry 2001; 158:1330.

251. Kahlert I, Brune M. A case of primary zoplicone dependence. Dtsch Med Wochenschr 2001; 126:653.

252. Isreal AG, Kramer JA. Safety of zaleplon in the treatment of insomnia. Ann Pharmacol 2002; 36:852.

253. Ator NA. Zaleplon and triazolam: drug discrimination, plasma levels, and self-administration in baboons. Drug Alcohol Dep 2000; 61:58.

253a. Horvath EJ, Horvath K, Hámori T, et al. Anxiolytic 2,3-benzodiazepines, their specific binding to the basal ganglia. Prog Neurobiol 2000; 60:309.

254. Houghton PJ. The scientific basis for the reputed activity of Valerian. J Pharm Pharmacol 1999; 51:505.

255. Donath F, Quispe S, Diefenbach K, et al. Critical evaluation of the effect of valerian extract on sleep structure and sleep quality. Pharmacopsychiatry 2000; 33:47.

256. Li J, Stokes SA, Woeckener A. A tale of novel intoxication: a review of the effects of gamma-hydroxybutyric acid with recommendations for management. Ann Emerg Med 1998; 31:729.

257. Ito Y, Ishige K, Zaitsu E, et al. Gamma-hydroxybutyric acid increases intracellular Ca^{2+} concentration and nuclear cyclic-AMP-responsive element- and activator protein 1 DNA-binding activities through $GABA_B$ receptor in cultured cerebellar granule cells. J Neurochem 1995; 65:75.

258. Tunnicliff G. Sites of action of gamma-hydroxybutyrate (GHB)—a neuroactive drug with abuse potential. J Toxicol Clin Toxicol 1997; 35:581.

259. Maitre M, Andriamampandry C, Kemmel V, et al. Gamma-hydroxybutyric acid as a signaling molecule in brain. Alcohol 2000; 20:277.

260. Bradsher K. 3 guilty of manslaughter in slipping drug to girl. NY Times, March 15, 2000.

261. Moncini M, Masini E, Gambassi F, et al. Gamma-hydroxybutyric acid and alcohol-related syndromes. Alcohol 2000; 20:285.

262. Zvosec D, Smith SW, McCutcheon JR, et al. Adverse events, including death, associated with the use of 1,4-butanediol. N Engl J Med 2001; 344:87.

263. Shannon M, Ruand L. Gamma-hydroxybutyrate, gamma-butyrolactone, and 1,4-butanediol: a case report and review of the literature. Pediatr Emerg Care 2000; 16:435.

264. Fattore L, Martellotta MC, Cossu G, et al. Gamma-hydroxybutyric acid: an evaluation of its rewarding properties in rats and mice. Alcohol 2000; 20:247.

265. Schneidereit T, Burkhart K, Donovan JW, et al. Butanediol toxicity delayed by preingestion of ethanol. Int J Med Toxicol 2000; 3:1.

266. Li J, Stokes SA, Woeckener A. A tale of novel intoxication: seven cases of gamma-hydroxybutyric acid overdose. Ann Emerg Med 1998; 31:723.

267. Anon. Acute reactions to drugs of abuse. Med Lett 2002; 44:21.

267a. Case Records of the Massachusetts General Hospital: a 21-year-old man with sudden alteration of mental status. N Engl J Med 2003; 349:1267.

268. Chin RL, Sporer KA, Cullison B, et al. Clinical course of gamma-hydroxybutyrate overdose. Ann Emerg Med 1998; 31:716.

268a. Quang LS, Desai MC, Kraner JC, et al. Enzyme and receptor antagonists for preventing toxicity from the gamma-hydroxybutyric acid precursor 1,4-butanediol in CD-1 mice. Ann N Y Acad Sci 2002; 965:1.

269. Kohrs FP, Porter WH. Gamma-hydroxybutyrate intoxication and overdose. Ann Emerg Med 1999; 33:475.

270. Galloway GP, Frederick SL, Staggers FE, et al. Gamma-hydroxybutyrate: an emerging drug of abuse that causes physical dependence. Addiction 1997; 92:82.

271. Dyer JE, Roth B, Huma BA. GHB withdrawal syndrome: eight cases. J Toxicol Clin Toxicol 1999; 37:650.

272. Bowles TM, Sommi RW, Amiri M. Successful management of prolonged gamma-hydroxybutyrate and alcohol withdrawal. Pharmacotherapy 2001; 21:254.

273. Greene T, Dougherty T, Rodi A. Gamma-butyrolactone (GBL) withdrawal presenting as acute psychosis. J Toxicol 1999; 37:651.

273a. Mycyk MB, Wilemon C, Aks SE. Two cases of withdrawal from 1,4-butanediol use. Ann Emerg Med 2001; 38:345.

274. Friedman J, Westlake R, Furman M. "Grievous bodily harm": gamma hydroxybutyrate abuse leading to a Wernicke–Korsakoff syndrome. Neurology 1996; 46:469.

275. Gallimberti L, Gentile N, Cibin M, et al: Gamma-hydroxybutyric acid for the treatment of alcohol withdrawal syndrome. Lancet 1989; 2:787.

276. Priori A, Bertolasi L, Pesenti A, et al: Gamma-hydroxybutyric acid for alcohol-sensitive myoclonus with dystonia. Neurology 2000; 54:1706.

Chapter 7
Marijuana

"This will be deducted from your share in paradise," he said, as he handed me my portion.
—Theophile Gautier

La cucaracha, la cucaracha
Ya no puede caminar
Porque no tiene, porque no tiene
Marijuana que fumar.
—Pancho Villa marching song

Man, they can say what they want about us vipers, but you just dig them lushhounds
with their old antique jive ... that come uptown juiced to the gills, crackin' out of line
and passin' out in anybody's hallway. Don't nobody come up thataway when he picks
upon some good grass.
—Mezz Mezzrow

If they really wanted to stop people from smoking pot, they should legalize medical
marijuana. Under this country's healthcare system, nobody would be able to get it.
—Marlon Edwards

Marijuana is derived from the hemp plant, *Cannabis sativa.* A resin covering the flowers and leaves of the female plant contains the active substances. Preparations made mainly from this resin—called "hashish" in the Middle East and "charas" in India—are several times more potent than marijuana, which is made from cut tops and leaves or whole plants and called "bhang," "kif," "dagga" (low resin content), or "ghanja" (high resin content).[1,2] The resin protects the plant from heat and dryness and is most abundant in plants grown in tropical climates; for that reason, marijuana from Latin America or Southeast Asia is likely to be more potent than marijuana from the continental United States. It weakens with aging. Among the plant's many cannabinoid compounds (cannabinols) are several isomers of tetrahydrocannabinol (THC), of which δ-9-THC is the principal psychoactive agent (Figure 7–1). Delta-8-THC has similar effects but is present in only minute amounts. Cannabinol and cannabidiol are anticonvulsant, but cannibinol is only mildly psychoactive, and cannabidiol is not psychoactive at all. 9-β-hydroxyhexahydrocannabinol

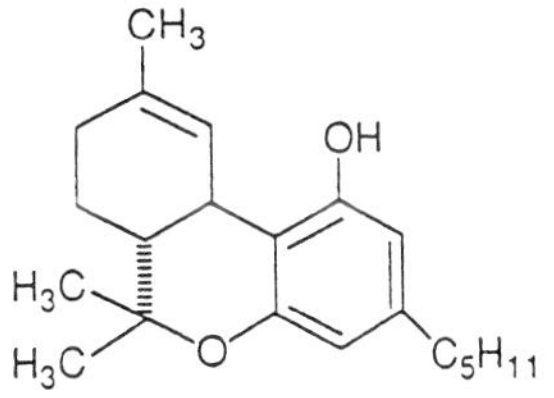

Figure 7–1. Tetrahydrocannabinol.

225

is a potent analgesic, and cannabidolic acid has both sedative and antimicrobial actions. The 11-hydroxy metabolites of δ-9-THC and δ-8-THC are as psychically active as their parent compounds.[3]

Pharmacology and Animal Studies

Acute Effects in Animals

Psychoactive cannabinoids, as exemplified by δ-9-THC, have unique effects in animals. In mice, low doses produce simultaneous depression and stimulation termed the *popcorn effect*.[1,2] The animals appear sedated until one mouse is stimulated, causing it to jump hyperreflexly; as it falls on another mouse, that animal then jumps, and the subsequent chain reaction throughout the cage resembles corn popping in a pan. Higher doses of δ-9-THC produce more typical sedation, as do both low and high doses of nonpsychoactive cannabinoids. In contrast to barbiturates and ethanol, however, even high doses of cannabinoids do not produce general anesthesia.[2] Accompanying the stimulatory effect of δ-9-THC is increased aggressiveness in rodents (an observation that is not predictive of its effect on humans).

Perhaps paralleling combined stimulatory and sedative effects, δ-9-THC in animals can be proconvulsant at low doses with tolerance developing to its anticonvulsant effects. By contrast, cannabidiol is more consistently anticonvulsant at both low and high doses.[1,2,4] The proconvulsant and anticonvulsant actions of cannabinoids vary with species, seizure model, and route of administration.[5–8] Delta-9-THC protected chickens from photic-induced but not pentylenetetrazol-induced seizures.[9] In mice, δ-9-THC was anticonvulsant for maximal electroshock seizures but proconvulsant for pentylenetetrazol-induced and strychnine-induced seizures.[10] In cats, δ-9-THC prevented kindled amygdaloid seizures if given early but not if given after seizures were developed.[11] In baboons, δ-9-THC blocked established kindled amygdaloid seizures but not photic-induced seizures.[12] In seizure-prone gerbils, δ-9-THC was anticonvulsant.[13] A strain of New Zealand rabbits is uniquely susceptible to seizures induced by psychoactive cannabinoids in doses equivalent to these consumed by humans, and these seizures are blocked by pretreatment with cannabidiol.[14,15] In studies of transcallosal cortical-evoked responses in rats and spinal monosynaptic reflexes in cats, low doses of δ-9-THC enhanced synaptic transmission, whereas higher doses of δ-9-THC and all doses of cannabidiol caused only depression.[16] In rats, cannabidiol was anticonvulsant for both maximal electroshock and audiogenic seizures and enhanced the anticonvulsant potency of phenytoin (although it antagonized that of ethosuximide, clonazepam, and trimethadione).[17] Although cannabidiol and phenytoin are effective against similar types of seizures, electrophysiological studies suggest they have different mechanisms of action.[18]

In some animal models, δ-9-THC and other psychoactive cannabinoids have been as potently analgesic as morphine. Other workers have not found comparable analgesic efficacy. As with actions on seizures, cannabinoid analgesia varies with the particular agent, species, pain model, and route of administration.[4,19]

Cannabinoid Pharmacology

Receptors and Ligands

A mouse behavioral assay reliably correlates a tetrad of signs—reduced motility, catalepsy, analgesia, and reduced body temperature—with the psychoactivity of cannabinoids in humans.[20] The major psychoactive cannabinoid in marijuana, δ-9-THC, was isolated in 1964 and found to decrease levels of cyclic adenosine monophosphate (cAMP) in cultured neurons. This observation led to the identification of stereospecific cannabinoid receptors, which are G-protein-coupled and consist of seven transmembrane domains with an extracellular N-terminal tail and an intracellular C-terminal tail.[21,22] Two cannabinoid receptors are recognized. CB$_1$ receptors are expressed by neurons in both the central and peripheral nervous system. CB$_2$ receptors are expressed by cells of the immune system.[22a] Cannabinoid receptors are found in all vertebrates studied; rat and human cannabinoid receptors display 97.3% sequence conservation.[23] In humans the gene for the CB$_1$ receptor resides on the short arm of chromosome 6. Cannabinoid receptors are not found in *Drosophila* or *Caenorhabditis elegans*.[24]

During the 1990s two endogenous cannabinoid ligands ("endocannabinoids") were identified in mammalian brain: arachidonylethanolamide (known as "anandamide," the Sanskrit word for bliss) and 2-arachidonylglycerol (2-AG).[25] These ligands bind to both CB_1 and CB_2 receptors. A third ligand, termed "noladin," is present only in the brain and binds only to CB_1 receptors.[26] Oleamide, a lipid found in the cerebrospinal fluid of sleep-deprived cats, binds to CB_1 and CB_2 receptors and induces sleep, suppresses immune responses, facilitates memory extinction, and reduces body temperature and pain perception; it does not, however, affect locomotion, a marker for reinforcement.[27] A number of synthetic CB_1 and CB_2 synthetic agonists and antagonists have been developed. Studies with those agents and with gene knockout animals suggests the existence of one or more non-CB_1/non-CB_2 receptors, but the vast majority of cannabinoid receptors are either CB_1 or CB_2, with variable distributions of CB_1 receptors in different regions of the CNS.[28–30]

CB_1 receptors are located at presynaptic axons and terminals of all neurons on which they are expressed. They cause inhibition of transmitter release (glutamate, γ-aminobutyric acid [GABA], acetylcholine, norepinephrine, dopamine, serotonin) by shortening the duration of presynaptic action potentials.[22,31,32] The mechanism is twofold. First, G-protein-coupled reduction in cAMP causes decreased phosphorylation of potassium channels by cAMP-dependent protein kinase A (PKA), resulting in activation of these channels and enhanced rectifying potassium currents.[33,34] Second, through a non-cAMP-mediated mechanism, a direct G-protein-mediated inhibition of calcium channel proteins results in reduced calcium currents.[28] Although 2-AG is nearly 200 times as abundant as anandamide in brain, only anandamide appears to participate in intercellular signaling; 2-AG might be involved in intracellular signaling.

Unlike other neurotransmitters anandamide does not reside in vesicles but rather is synthesized from a phospholipid precursor (*N*-arachidoylyl-phosphatidylethanolamine, or NAPE) situated within the lipid bilayer of the neuronal membrane. Depolorazation of the membrane leads to calcium accumulation, which in turn causes hydrolytic cleavage of NAPE by phospholipase D (PLD) to produce anandamide. 2-AG is formed by a similar mechanism. Anandamide functions as a retrograde synaptic messenger molecule.[28,35–38] Arising within the postsynaptic membranes of depolarized neurons it diffuses into the synaptic cleft and binds to presynaptic CB_1 receptors, activating them. G-protein-coupled effects on potassium and calcium currents result in inhibition of neurotransmitter release from presynaptic terminals. Inhibition of inhibitory neurotransmitter release is called *depolarization-induced suppression of inhibition* (DSI). Inhibition of excitatory neurotransmitter release is called *depolarization-induced suppression of excitation* (DSE). Both DSI and DSE persist for tens of seconds.[22] Anandamide then dissociates from CB_1 receptors and following reuptake into the postsynaptic neuron is hydrolyzed intracellularly by fatty acid amide hydrolase (FAAH). The product of hydrolysis by FAAH—arachidonic acid—is then reincorporated into membrane lipids.[39]

In addition to their actions on potassium and calcium channels CB_1 receptor agonists, via G proteins, stimulate production of mitogen-activated protein (MAP) kinase and, independently of G proteins, stimulate generation of the lipid second messenger ceramide. Through MAP kinase cannabinoids may play a role in neurodevelopment.[40] Through ceramide they may induce apoptosis.[24,32,41,42] Cannabinoids induce apoptosis of cultured glioma cells and regression of malignant gliomas in vivo.[43] Delta-9-THC induced apoptosis in hippocampal slices and cultured neurons, raising the possibility that its detrimental effects on memory might be the result of neurotoxicity as well as attenuated long-term potentiation[44] (see below).

Administration of the CB_1 receptor antagonist to neonatal mice caused growth stunting and death within several days.[45] CB_1 knockout mice, however, remain viable.[46]

Functional Role of Endocannabinoids

The relative abundance of CB_1 receptors in different regions of the brain implies that endocannabinoids play a role in a number of nervous system activities. CB_1 receptors are prominent within the olfactory system, and while cannabis does not seem to affect olfaction in humans, endocannabinoids might be of importance to olfaction in lower animals such as rodents.[20]

In the hippocampus CB_1 receptors are abundant presynaptically on GABAergic and glutamatergic neurons. Inhibition of glutamate release inhibits induction of long-term potentiation (LTP) and long-term depression (LTD), with impaired memory; this effect appears to override a similar inhibition of GABA release.[20,47,48] CB_1 knockout mice have enhanced LTP and improved memory.[49,50] They are also impaired in memory extinction (i.e., normal forgetting), an active suppression of previously learned associations, lack of which could masquerade as memory acquisition/consolidation.[51,52] (Studies are not entirely consistent, however. In some, the selective CB_1-receptor antagonist rimonabant [SR141716A] had no effect on LTP or on learning.[22])

In the basal ganglia abundant CB_1 receptors on both GABAergic and glutamatergic neurons probably account for the complex effects of cannabinoids on movement—e.g., decreased locomotor activity followed at higher doses by catalepsy.[53] Anandamide is released in the striatum by activation of dopamine D_2 receptors.[54] In the cerebellum CB_1 receptors are found on glutamatergic parallel fiber terminals and GABAergic basket cell terminals, both synapsing onto Purkinje cells.[55] In the cerebral cortex they are found especially in GABAergic neurons within layers II, III, V, and VI.[22] Relevant to the analgesic effects of cannabinoids, CB_1 receptors are prominent in the periaqueductal gray (PAG) of the midbrain, the rostral ventrolateral medulla, the dorsal horn of the spinal cord, and the dorsal root ganglia.[56] CB_2 receptors on mast cells, which release inflammatory mediators that activate nociceptive neurons, may also play a role in analgesia, and in mice both CB_1 and CB_2 receptor agonists have peripheral analgesic effects which are additive. Without administration of an agonist, CB_1 or CB_2 receptor antagonists produce hyperalgesia, suggesting tonic release of CB_2 and CB_2 agonists.[57,58] In the hypothalamus endocannabinoids interact with the anorexigenic peptide leptin and the orexigenic peptide neuropeptide Y to regulate food intake.[59]

Antiemetic effects of cannabinoids are likely related to the abundance of CB_1 receptors in the area postrema, solitary nucleus, and dorsal nucleus of the vagus.[60] CB_1 receptors are also present on peripheral autonomic nerve endings, probably related to cannabinoid-associated bradycardia and hypotension.[61]

In a number of models—e.g., glutamate-induced death of cultured rat hippocampal neurons, ischemic injury in rats, closed head injury in rats—cannabinoids are neuroprotective, but it is unclear whether the effect is CB_1 receptor-mediated.[62] In some cases it is blocked by CB_1 receptor antagonists and in others it is not. The psychoactive CB_1 receptor agonist δ-9-THC is neuroprotective.[62a] So are cannabidiol, a non-psychoactive cannabinoid present in marijuana, and HU-211, a synthetic drug with a cannabinoid structure; neither of these drugs binds to CB_1 receptors. Following brain trauma 2-AG brain levels are increased in mice, whereas anandamide levels are increased in rats.[62b] Proposed mechanisms of neuroprotection include N-methyl-D-aspartate antagonism, reduction of tumor necrosis factor alpha (TNF-α) levels, and antioxidant properties.[26,62b,62c]

Some investigators, in contrast, describe *increased* excitotoxicity in animals receiving CB_1 agonists, with reduced damage when CB_1 receptors are blocked.[62d,62e] A possible explanation is that cannabinoids (including endocannabinoids) are protective when they block glutamate release and damaging when they block GABA release.[22a] Also contributing may be specific local actions that vary across different brain regions.[62c]

Through actions in the hypothalamus cannabinoid agonists increase blood levels of adrenocorticotropic hormone, follicle stimulating hormone (FSH), growth hormone, prolactin, and thyrotropin. Hypothermia results from actions in both hypothalamus and caudal brainstem.[63]

In rats cannabinoid receptors and ligands appear early in embryogenesis. Suggesting a role for the cannabinoid system in brain development, the distribution of CB_1 receptors in the early fetus—e.g., in elongating axons of white matter—is very different from their distribution in the adult brain.[64] CB_1 agonists induced migration of human embryonic kidney cells transfected with CB_1 receptor gene, and the effect was blocked by inhibitors of either CB_1 receptors or MAP kinase.[65]

Reinforcement, Tolerance, and Dependence

A long-standing controversy is whether cannabinoids are reinforcing in animals. Animals do not readily self-administer cannabinoids, and the physical properties of the drugs—gummy and water insoluble—make injectable preparations difficult. (Probably for that reason, they are hardly ever abused parenterally by humans.) The use of synthetic cannabinoids in classical experimental settings (e.g., drug discrimination, conditioned place preference, intracranial self-stimulation, intravenous self-administration; see Chapter 2) has shown that cannabinoids are both reinforcing and capable of producing physical dependence.[66]

In drug discrimination studies non-cannabinoid drugs do not substitute for δ-9-THC. (An exception is partial substitution by diazepam, suggesting involvement of GABA.[67]) Substitution of cannabinoids by each other is blocked by the CB_1 receptor antagonist SR141716A. Interestingly, δ-9-THC does not fully substitute for anandamide.[68]

In conditioned place preference (CPP) studies high doses of δ-9-THC and other cannabinoids produce aversion. Low doses produce aversion in naive animals and CPP in pre-exposed animals.[69] Aversion is dependent on both CB_1 receptors and endogenous dynorphin transmission. CPP, on the other hand, requires μ-opioid receptors.[70] It is also dependent on CB_1 receptor activation of the MAP kinase pathway.[71] Conversely, the CB_1 receptor antagonist rimonabant blocks morphine CPP.[66]

Low doses of THC lower the threshold for intracranial self-stimulation (ICSS). CB_1 receptor blockade and naloxone each reduce this effect.[72]

The disinclination of rodents to self-administer δ-9-THC has been used polemically by those who believe marijuana is less "addicting" than other recreational drugs. Monkeys do self-administer δ-9-THC, however, an effect blocked by CB_1 antagonism,[73] and rats self-administer the synthetic CB_1 agonists HU-210, CP55940, and WIN55212-2.[74,75,75a,75b] Delta-9-THC is most readily self-administered in animals that have previously self-administered other drugs, suggesting an effect of sensitization.[75a] Naloxone blocks cannabinoid self-administration, and morphine self-administration is absent in CB_1 receptor knockout mice.[75,76]

Delta-9-THC and other cannabinoid agonists increase the firing of dopaminergic (DA) cells in the ventral tegmental area (VTA) and increase dopamine efflux in the nucleus accumbens (NA). Cannabinoid-induced dopamine release is blocked by naloxone; cannabinoid-induced VTA dopaminergic cell firing is not.[66] Repeated cannabinoid exposure induces behavioral sensitization as well as cross-sensitization to psychomotor stimulants and opioids.[77,78] In rats rimonabant blocked relapse to cocaine-seeking triggered by cocaine-associated cues or by cocaine itself but not relapse triggered by exposure to stress.[79] Pre-treatment with δ-9-THC in rats increased the rewarding properties of heroin and amphetamine.[80] In rodents nicotine administration facilitated pharmacological and biochemical responses, tolerance, and physical dependence induced by δ-9-THC,[81] and CB_1 receptor knockout abolished the rewarding effects of nicotine.[82] In mice and rats rimonabant blocked voluntary ethanol intake.[83]

Rapid tolerance develops to most of the effects of CB_1-receptor agonists, including analgesia, locomotion, hypothermia, cataplexy, suppression of operant behavior, gastrointestinal transit, body weight, cardiovascular actions, ataxia, anticonvulsant actions, and corticosterone release.[66,84] Chronic tolerance is associated with reduction of G-protein mRNA levels and desensitization of CB_1 receptors.[66,85] Cross-tolerance is seen between cannabinoids and opioids for a number of effects, especially analgesia. Knockout mice lacking the pre-proenkephalin gene develop less tolerance to δ-9-THC analgesia and hypolocomotion.[86]

Even very high doses of δ-9-THC fail to produce somatic signs of spontaneous withdrawal in many species including primates. Spontaneous abstinence signs do follow abrupt cessation of chronic administration of the CB_1-receptor agonist WIN55212-2, and the CB1-receptor antagonist rimonabant precipitates withdrawal signs in animals chronically receiving δ-9-THC. These include, in rodents, wet dog shakes, head shakes, face rubbing, tremor, ataxia, hunched posture, piloerection, hyperlocomotion, mastication, and scratching.[87,88] In dogs there is salivation, vomiting, diarrhea, tremor, and restless asocial behavior.[47] In CB_1-receptor knockout mice δ-9-THC fails to produce signs of abstinence.[76] Interactions with opioids are again observed. Naloxone precipitates withdrawal in cannabinoid-dependent rats, rimonabant precipitates withdrawal in morphine-dependent rats, the severity of withdrawal is reduced in knockout mice lacking either the pre-proenkephalin gene or μ-opiate receptors, and the severity of morphine withdrawal is reduced in knockout mice lacking CB_1-receptors.[89,90] The endocannabinoid 2-AG attenuated naloxone-precipitated withdrawal signs in morphine-dependent mice.[91] Interestingly, lithium prevented cannabinoid withdrawal signs in rats; the effect was accompanied by increased levels of oxytocin in the paraventricular and supraoptic nuclei of the hypothalamus and blocked by pretreatment with an oxytocin antagonist.[92]

Similar to the withdrawal syndromes of other drugs, cannabinoid withdrawal is associated with reduced mesolimbic dopaminergic activity, elevated corticotropin releasing factor levels, and enhanced Fos immunoreactivity in the central nucleus of the amygdala.[93] During cannabinoid withdrawal adenylyl cyclase activity is increased especially in the cerebellum.[94]

Historical Background and Epidemiology

Marijuana was described in China in the third millennium BC.[95] The hemp fiber was used for clothing, bowstrings, and paper, and although recreational intoxication was frowned on in the Taoist culture, marijuana was used medicinally and in religious and magical rites. As an intoxicant, marijuana played a more prominent role in ancient India; according to the Hindu *Vedas*, the god Siva discovered cannabis and concocted the liquid refreshment from it called *bhang* (which additionally contains poppy seeds, ginger, cloves, cardamom, nutmeg, and milk). A more potent brew made from the flowers and upper leaves is called *ganja,* and an even stronger concoction made with high resin content is called *charas.* For at least 3000 years, marijuana, ingested or smoked, has been as popular in India as ethanol is in the West.

In the 5th century BC, Herodotus described the Scythian Cult of the Dead: Hemp was placed on red-hot stones in a closed room producing an intoxicating vapor.[96] Pliny and Dioscorides also described marijuana intoxication, and possible Old Testament references include the "honeycomb" of the Song of Solomon and the "honeywood" of I Samuel.[97]

In the Middle East during the 11th century, members of the Sufi Islamic sect used hashish—comparable in potency to charas and either eaten as a paste or mixed with sesame and chewed like gum—to achieve religious ecstasy.[95] The association of cannabis with this despised and economically downtrodden minority launched the drug's false reputation as an inspirer of violence. The Arab reference to hashish users as *ashishin* became transcribed during the Crusades to the word *assassin.*

Introduced into Europe, cannabis was cultivated for its fiber. (In the 16th century, Rabelais described many marvelous uses of cannabis—he called it "pantagruelian"—but intoxication was not one of them.[98]) During this time, it was used as a folk medicine (including seizure prevention); nonmedicinal ingestion was largely restricted to religious cults.[95]

Marijuana smoking has long been popular in Africa; Dutch settlers observed the custom among the Hottentots, who called the cannabis plant *dagga.* Napoleon's invasion of Egypt familiarized a new generation of Europeans with hashish, and in mid-19th-century Paris, the celebrated "Club des Hachichins" included among its members Theophile Gautier, Victor Hugo, Alexandre Dumas, Eugene Delacroix, and Charles Baudelaire.[99]

In the United States during the 18th century, cannabis was also grown for its fiber. In the mid-19th century, it was listed in the U.S. Dispensatory for treating "neuralgia, gout, tetanus, hydrophobia, epidemic cholera, convulsions, chorea, hysteria, mental depression, insanity, and uterine hemorrhage." William Osler considered marijuana the treatment of choice for migraine.[100] In 1905, cannabis was offered by Sears, Roebuck as a cure for morphine addiction. Unrecognized as a euphoriant, cannabis was not included in the Harrison Narcotics Act of 1914. Its use among Mexicans, however, led to popular associations with disreputable behavior, and just as America's anti-opioid attitudes arose out of fear and distrust of Chinese immigrants, by the 1920s several western states had passed anti-marijuana laws. During this time, cannabis continued to be present in both prescription and over-the-counter pharmaceuticals, and smoked "reefers" became popular with the Black urban jazz culture (inspiring such works as Louis Armstrong's "Muggles," Cab Calloway's "Reefer Man," and Fats Waller's "Viper's Drag"). To what extent racism contributed to the Marijuana Tax Act of 1937 is still debated, but that federal legislation—vigorously opposed by the American Medical Association on the grounds that serious ill effects of cannabis had never been demonstrated—banned its nonmedicinal possession or sale.[101]

Draconian state laws soon followed: penalties included life imprisonment for first-offense selling (Utah) and death for selling to minors (Missouri).[97]

Despite such measures, marijuana became—and remains—the most widely used illicit drug in the United States. As use steadily rose during the 1960s, federal attempts to reduce importation escalated—e.g., "Operation Intercept," President Nixon's program to stop the flow of marijuana from Mexico by military interdiction and spraying of Mexican crops with the herbicide paraquat. In 1971 a National Commission on Marijuana and Drug Abuse recommended a "policy of discouragement"—not legalization as with alcohol and tobacco, but "decriminalization" of possession. The Commission was concerned about the thousands of arrests that were occurring annually for marijuana use as well as the likelihood that marijuana's illegality made it a "gateway" drug by bringing street purchasers into contact with cocaine or heroin purveyors. This report was rejected by federal authorities.[102]

Prior to 1970 80% of marijuana sold in the United States came from Mexico. Today much comes from other Latin American countries, Jamaica, Southeast Asia, and Nigeria. Domestic production has increased as well, and indoor hydroponic cultivation of plant varieties with high δ-9-THC content (e.g., Sinsemilla and Netherwood) produces marijuana of considerably higher potency than formerly available.[103] (The average content of δ-9-THC in marijuana plants ranges from 0.3% to 4.0% based on soil, climate, growing conditions, and handling after harvest. With modern technology content of up to 20% can be achieved.[104]) Today marijuana is America's biggest cash crop, with annual gross sales of US\$32 billion (compared with US\$14 billion for corn and US\$11 billion for soybeans).

Marijuana use in the United States peaked during the 1970s, fell during the 1980s, then rose again during the 1990s.[105–108] Today two-thirds of Americans have tried marijuana, and 40% of them have used it more than 100 times. About 7 million Americans use marijuana at least weekly.[109,110] During 2000, 15.6% of U.S. eighth graders, 32.2% of tenth graders, and 36.5% of twelfth graders reported using marijuana during the previous year, and 20% of twelfth grade users used it daily.[111]

Federal penalties remain draconian. Possession of 100 plants results in 5 to 40 years imprisonment without parole, and cultivation of 60,000 plants carries the death penalty. (By contrast, the average time spent in jail for murder in the United States is 9 years.) In 1997 there were 695,000 arrests for marijuana offenses; 85% were for personal possession.[102] State laws vary widely. In Alaska it is legal to grow marijuana for one's own use. In Oklahoma cultivating any amount results in life imprisonment. Today dozens, and perhaps hundreds, of Americans are serving life sentences for possession of marijuana.[112]

The high cost of potent marijuana—10 pounds carries a potential street value of US\$50,000—has carried with it an increase in violent crimes among its traffickers.[113] Reminiscent of the earlier "crack" cocaine epidemic, murders in New York City have involved territorial disputes between rival Jamaican gangs ("posses").[114]

The efficacy of marijuana decriminalization was put to the test in the Netherlands, which in 1976 adopted a policy of non-enforcement for violations involving possession or sale of up to 30 g of cannabis. (This was later lowered to 5 g.) It was sold in coffee shops, and the rules forbade advertising, sales to minors, and "hard drug" sales on the premises. In 1999 approximately 1200 coffee shops in the Netherlands were selling marijuana. The available evidence suggests that cannabis use in the Netherlands did not increase as a result of this policy. Similar experiences in other countries (Spain, Italy, Portugal, Luxembourg, Belgium, Australia) support this conclusion.[112,115] In 2003 both the United Kingdom and Canada decriminalized the possession of small amounts of marijuana.[112]

American marijuana users come from all age groups, socioeconomic classes, and geographic regions. The major period of risk for initiation to marijuana use—similar to tobacco and ethanol—is before age 20 years, and those who have not experimented with it by then are unlikely to do so. Similar to ethanol, but in contrast to tobacco, the prevalence of marijuana use declines after age 21 years.[116,117] On the other hand, of those who try marijuana more than once, about one-third will subsequently use marijuana regularly,[103] and 2.2% will meet DSM-IV criteria for dependence.[118] Other surveys give more ominous figures, e.g., that 10% to 15% of those who have ever tried marijuana will become psychologically dependent, with some manifesting physical withdrawal signs.[119–122]

Acute Effects

Intended Effects and Physiological Alterations

In the United States, marijuana ("grass," "pot," "tea," "reefer," "weed," "hash," "skunk," "skunkweed," "sens," "Mary Jane," "MJ," "Colombian gold," "Acapulcan gold," "Panama red," "Thai sticks," "Cambodian red," "chronic," "chocolate," "hydro," "bubble gum") is usually smoked. Marijuana rolled into cigarette paper creates a "joint," "bone," or "nail." An increasingly popular form of delivery is a hollowed-out cigar or cigar wrapping filled with marijuana ("blunts"). Marijuana or hashish can also be smoked using a pipe or water pipe ("bong"). "Shotgunning" refers to inhaling smoke and then exhaling it into another person's mouth. As with other psychoactive agents, effects vary not only with dose, but also with social setting and expectation. An average cigarette delivers 2.5–5 mg δ-9-THC, but, as noted, current preparations of marijuana are considerably more potent. Hashish is more potent than marijuana itself, and hashish oil, a fluid distilled from hashish, is more potent still.[103] Effects begin within 10 to 20 minutes and last 2 to 3 hours. Ingested marijuana is only about one-third as potent, but the effects last up to 12 hours.[123]

During the first few minutes, smoked marijuana may produce jitteriness, anxiety, or fear. There then ensues a relaxed, dreamy euphoria ("stoned"), often with jocularity or silliness. If a user is alone, sleepiness is more likely. There is disinhibition or depersonalization, subjective slowing of time, and a sensation of altered body proportion.[124–126] In contrast to the dulled thinking associated with ethanol, users report increased awareness of events or stimuli; objective testing, however, reveals decreased auditory signal detection, impaired visual acuity for detecting small moving targets or discriminating colors, and no change in cutaneous sensitivity.[127–130] Familiar objects or relationships may appear novel or profound, yet there are decreased empathy and perception of the emotions of others.[131] Paranoid feelings are common but usually of minor concern.[132] The limbs feel numb, weak, or floating, and there is a sensation of pressure in the head or dizziness. Speech may be rapid or flighty. At high doses, memory and problem solving are impaired.[133,134] A case report described

transient global amnesia triggered by acute marijuana use.[134a] There is also difficulty in digit repetition, serial subtraction, concept formation, reading comprehension, and coherent speaking.[135–137] Although subjective effects and tachycardia resolve within a few hours of use, impaired performance on cognitive tasks can last for more than 24 hours.[138] Balance and hand steadiness are also impaired, compromising complex motor tasks such as driving.[139,140] In contrast to ethanol, however, there is rarely gross ataxia or nystagmus.[125]

Marijuana causes conjunctival injection, decreased salivation, urinary frequency, tachycardia, and increased systolic blood pressure and urinary epinephrine; it also causes postural hypotension and faintness (Table 7–1).[116,141] Propranolol prevents tachycardia induced by marijuana, but not its subjective or behavioral effects.[142] Alpha-methyltyrosine, which reduces brain dopamine and norepinephrine, similarly does not prevent marijuana-induced psychological effects.[143] Marijuana reduces urinary methoxyhydroxyphenylglycol levels and increases homovanillic acid, consistent with altered turnover of norepinephrine and dopamine.[144]

Appetite and thirst increase. There is decreased intraocular pressure, long-lasting bronchodilation, and analgesia to both traumatic and experimental pain.[127,145] If sleep occurs, there is less time spent

Table 7–1. Marijuana: Acute Effects

Anxiety, jitteriness, paranoia
Euphoria, relaxation, jocularity
Depersonalization
Subjective time-slowing
Dizziness, sensation of floating
Impaired memory and problem solving
Impaired balance and hand steadiness
Conjunctival injection
Decreased salivation
Urinary frequency
Tachycardia
Systolic hypertension with postural hypotension
Increased appetite and thirst
Decreased intraocular pressure
Analgesia
Auditory and visual illusions and hallucinations
Psychotic excitement or depression
Bradycardia, hypotension
Acute dysphoria, panic

in the rapid eye movement phase, and the subject awakens with little sense of "hangover."[146]

Except for a slight shift toward slower alpha frequencies, the electroencephalogram in humans shows no gross changes during a conventional "high."[147] Visual, auditory, and somatosensory evoked response amplitudes are depressed.[148] While smoking marijuana, a patient with implanted brain electrodes developed euphoria and high-voltage δ waves in the septal region but not in other areas, including the amygdala, thalamus, hippocampus, or caudate.[149] Similar changes in monkeys persisted after the drug was stopped.[150]

Positron emission tomography in experienced users revealed that mean global cerebral blood flow (CBF) was unchanged during marijuana smoking. Regional CBF, however, decreased in temporal lobe auditory regions, visual cortex, frontoparietal lobe, and thalamus and increased in orbital and medial frontal lobes, insula, temporal poles, anterior cingulate, and cerebellum. The findings are consistent with marijuana's effects on perception, cognition, and emotion.[151]

Not surprisingly, in human volunteers the CB_1 receptor antagonist SR141716 blocked the acute psychological and physiological effects of smoked marijuana.[152]

Effects of Higher Doses; Adverse Reactions

High doses of cannabis cause auditory and visual illusions or hallucinations that consist of flashes of light or color, geometric figures, human faces, or complex pictures.[153] Bizarre illusions include loss of depth perception, a "strobe light effect" (seeing a moving object as if it were a series of still pictures), the appearance of people talking with their mouths and voices unsynchronized, and "streaking" (moving light sources in a dark environment becoming long streaks as in a time-exposed photograph).[154] Fantastic complex hallucinations with extraordinary dilation of subjective time were vividly described by 19th-century users.[155] Anecdotal reports suggest that marijuana improves night vision.[156]

Still higher doses cause confusion, disorientation, markedly impaired memory, anxiety, and psychotic depression or excitement.[153] Bradycardia and hypotension occur.[157] Fatal overdose has not been documented. A 23-year-old was found dead

from no apparent cause, and cannabinoids were identified in the urine.[158] A man attempted suicide by smoking hashish and was comatose for 4 days.[159] A small child after ingesting 1.5 g cannabis resin had hypothermia, alternating stupor and excitement, ataxia, and decreased respiratory rate; recovery occurred after several hours.[160] Coma in two small children followed accidental ingestion of cannabis cookies.[161] A young man smuggled Moroccan hashish oil into the United States by swallowing drug-filled balloons; he developed euphoria and then 48 hours of sleepiness, tachycardia, disorientation to place, and, unexpectedly, anisocoria.[162]

Without other signs of toxicity, marijuana sometimes causes acute adverse reactions consisting of intense emotional upset, confusion, paranoia, delusions, depression, or panic ("freaking out"). Such symptoms can last hours or days.[153,163–165] They are rare, usually follow first use, and are more often associated with ingestion than smoking—probably because the effects of smoked marijuana are so short-lived, and doses of 20–70 mg δ-9-THC are required.[125,166] Especially vulnerable to anxiety or psychosis are subjects whose ingestion has been inadvertent—for example, unknowingly eating laced brownies or cookies. Claims of "acute cannabis psychosis" lasting 6 weeks or longer were not confirmed in several field studies.[167,168] Marijuana has been reported to trigger psychosis in people with previous psychotic histories or hallucinogenic drug use (see later), and acute dysphoric reactions are more common in patients with chronic pain and depression. They can occur, however, in otherwise normal users.[165,169–171] Two small children repeatedly given oral marijuana by their parents developed manic psychosis requiring antipsychotic medication; they eventually recovered.[172] Mania, paranoia, and auditory hallucinations also affected several Jamaican adults who increased their usual dose.[173] Manic psychosis developed in a marijuana user who was also taking fluoxetine.[174] Three American users developed "Koro" (an acute panic reaction with the illusion of penile retraction heretofore considered a cultural phenomenon restricted to the Indian subcontinent).[175] In this and other similar reports, recovery was complete with abstinence,[176,177] although in one case a young man, who also used amphetamines, self-enucleated his right eye.[178]

"Flashbacks" refer to the spontaneous experience weeks to months after using marijuana of hallucinations or other feelings associated with the original use.[178–180] However—despite the claim that marijuana is an independent risk factor for the development of schizophrenia[181]—there is little evidence that it causes lasting violent or psychotic behavior. (For a taste of anti-marijuana propaganda at its most droll, the interested reader is recommended the 1930s cult film classic, *Reefer Madness*.) Acute marijuana panic states and toxic psychoses can usually be managed with calm reassurance. Benzodiazepines or haloperidol relieve severe symptoms.[125,182,183]

Metabolism and Elimination

Within a few minutes of smoking a marijuana cigarette, plasma levels of δ-9-THC reach about 100 ng/mL, falling to 10 ng/mL at 1 hour, 1 ng/mL at 4 hours and 0.1 ng/mL at 24 hours.[125,184] The rapid drop in plasma concentrations is the result of tissue distribution and accounts for the relatively short subjective effects compared with the elimination half-life, which averages 59 hours in novices and 28 hours in chronic smokers.[185] Absorption of oral δ-9-THC is slow and erratic, with peak plasma levels after 1 hour.[184] Ingested δ-9-THC results in higher plasma levels of the active metabolite 11-hydroxy-THC than of the parent compound; smoked marijuana produces barely detectable levels of this metabolite. In first-time or irregular users, cannabinoid metabolites are detectable in urine for several days.[4] Frequent users accumulate δ-9-THC and continue to shed metabolites for more than a week; an incarcerated heavy user had a positive urine sample for 2 months.[186]

Hemp Seed Oil

Hemp seed oil, legally available in "health food" stores, rarely contains psychoactive cannabinoids, and its metabolites are unlikely to be confused on urine toxicological assays with those of marijuana.[187] Some products do contain δ-9-THC, however, and psychological effects were described after eating salad prepared with hemp seed oil.[188]

Tolerance

Tolerance develops to marijuana's cardiovascular, motor, and psychic effects and is more pharmacodynamic than pharmacokinetic.[157,189] Very high doses are taken in many countries, and American soldiers in Germany consumed up to 2000 mg hashish daily.[190] The possibility of reverse tolerance to stimulatory effects is controversial. In a study of human volunteers, experienced marijuana smokers obtained a "high" more readily than did novices,[124] but alternative explanations include greater skill at efficiently inhaling marijuana smoke and a conditioned placebo effect based on expectation.[191] In favor of dissociative tolerance—unmasking of stimulant effects by the development of tolerance to depressant effects—are chronic users who are not as functionally impaired as novices yet report a subjective "high."[124]

Genetics

Studies on genetic propensity to marijuana use are limited, but evidence exists, including twin studies, that genetic influences interact with environmental factors.[192–196,196a] The genetic influence appears to be mediated through subjective responses to the drug. An association of marijuana use and conduct disorder appears to be due largely to shared environmental influences.[194]

Provocative are reports in humans that particular polymorphisms at the CB_1 receptor confer susceptibility not only to dependence on marijuana but to cocaine and amphetamine dependence as well.[195] A polymorphism of the gene encoding fatty acid amide hydrolase (which inactivates endocannabinoids; see above) also confers risk for abuse of illicit drugs or ethanol.[195a]

Dependence and Withdrawal

The question of physical dependence on marijuana is controversial. As described above, withdrawal signs can be provoked in animals: irritability, aggression, yawning, tremor, photophobia, piloerection, and penile erections.[197] Similarly, humans withdrawing from several weeks of high-dose marijuana have displayed various combinations of emotional liability, anxiety, restlessness, insomnia, anorexia, nausea, vomiting, diarrhea, tremor, hyperreflexia, sweating, and salivation.[197a–201a] Such symptoms are infrequent, however, and most chronic users, if they have symptoms at all, describe simply jitteriness, anorexia, headache, sleep disturbance, and mild gastrointestinal upset.[202] Aggressive behavior has been observed.[203] Of 54 marijuana users seeking treatment for dependence, over half had withdrawal symptoms.[120] Some consider such symptoms indicative of physical withdrawal.[204] Others, noting that they tend to occur within a few hours of abstinence and clear within a few days, whereas the biological half-life of cannabinoids in chronic users is 20 to 30 hours, consider cannabis withdrawal symptoms psychological in origin.[205] There is consensus, however, that addictive craving is common.

Marijuana and Other Drugs

Street preparations of marijuana may be contaminated with oregano, stramonium leaves, lysergic acid diethylamide (LSD), methamphetamine, or other agents, and marijuana is often deliberately taken with other drugs such as heroin, cocaine, or phencyclidine ("supergrass").[206–208] Barbiturates or ethanol and marijuana have additive or synergistic subjective and psychomotor effects.[209,210] In humans, marijuana does not potentiate opioid effects,[211] and naltrexone does not attenuate the subjective effects of δ-9-THC.[212] On the other hand, behavioral signs of rimonabant-induced withdrawal in rats receiving δ-9-THC are mimicked by giving naloxone, withdrawal signs precipitated by naloxone in morphine-dependent mice are attenuated by administering δ-9-THC, CB_1 receptor knockout mice have greatly reduced morphine self-administration, and μ-opioid receptor knockout mice receiving δ-9-THC have attenuated withdrawal signs after receiving rimonabant.[22]

Increasingly popular during the 1990s was marijuana soaked in embalming fluid ("happy sticks," "wet," "illie," "dank," "amp," "therm," "hydro," "fry," "boat," "skerm"). Preparations often contain phencyclidine as well. Despite marketing to the contrary, some products contain phencyclidine but no embalming fluid; others contain mint, phencyclidine, and embalming fluid but no marijuana. The purpose of embalming fluid is to create more uniform distribution of phencyclidine throughout the cigarette.[213] The psychotic reactions associated with this form of marijuana are more readily attributable to phencyclidine than to embalming fluid.[214]

In rodents, pretreatment with either δ-9-THC or the nonpsychoactive cannabinoid cannabidiol increases brain levels of other drugs, including cocaine and phencyclidine. The mechanism is unclear, but it might contribute to the popularity of using marijuana in conjunction with other agents.[215]

The degree to which marijuana serves as a "gateway" drug to "harder" agents is controversial.[216,217] Most users of heroin or cocaine have used marijuana, but most marijuana users do not go on to use heroin or cocaine. The National Household Survey on Drug Abuse found that during the 1990s youthful marijuana use increased while progression to "hard drug" use declined.[216]

A study of monozygotic and dizygotic twins found that marijuana use before age 17 years did increase the risk of later ethanol and "hard drug" use and dependence; the authors concluded that the association between early marijuana use and later drug use or dependence could not be solely explained by common predisposing genetic or shared environmental factors.[218] The findings might reflect pharmacological mechanisms—e.g., cross-sensitization between δ-9-THC and other drugs.[80] They might also reflect the fact that marijuana's illegality brings users into contact with purveyors of other illicit drugs.

Medical and Neurological Complications

Cognition

Whether marijuana use produces lasting mental abnormalities is controversial, and since the 1960s more than 50 studies have addressed the subject.[219,220] Reports from India and Morocco were the first to describe personality change with chronic cannabis use, an antimotivational syndrome consisting of diminished drive and ambition, apathy and flat affect, decreased attentiveness, and impaired recent memory.[190,221,222] Such symptoms were reported in Americans taking chronic high doses, and cerebral atrophy was observed by pneumoencephalography.[223] Others were unable to confirm these reports. Studies with computed tomography (CT) showed normal cerebral ventricular size in users, and several studies failed to demonstrate neuropsychological differences between cannabis users and controls.[224?233]

In Jamaica, where marijuana is smoked, chewed, added to food, and used as a medicinal in tea from early childhood, a National Institute of Mental Health study found no evidence of antimotivational syndrome and no significant physical abnormalities.[167] That study, however, included only 30 daily cannabis users, and many of the controls sometimes used cannabis tea. Moreover, subjects were farmers and laborers, and so subtle intellectual impairment could have gone undetected.

In Costa Rica, where marijuana is widely used, no differences on physical examination, neuropsychological assessment, or laboratory testing were evident between 80 users and 80 nonusers.[232] A later study from Costa Rica, however, found impaired working memory, short-term memory, and attentional skills in older long-term cannabis users compared with younger short-term users.[233a] By contrast, a study from Baltimore found gradual decline in Mini-Mental State scores among middle-aged adults over a 12-year period, but the degree of decline was not associated with marijuana use.[233b] In Greece, 47 hashish users were compared with 40 nonusers, and no differences in cognitive function were observed.[147]

In a study with volunteers, high doses (210 mg) of δ-9-THC were given daily for 30 days. The most striking finding was the rapid development of tolerance and lack of psychotomimetic effects.[234] Similarly, volunteers who smoked 35–198 mg δ-9-THC daily for 78 days had no untoward mental effects.[235] An Egyptian study found impaired psychomotor and visual-motor performance and impaired memory for designs in cannabis users compared with controls.[236] Other studies found decreased work output among cannabis smokers,[237–239] and the Greek study found that hashish users were more likely than nonusers to have personality disorders.[147] There appears to be no relation between marijuana use and crime independent of the drug's illegality.[240]

Early neuropsychological studies comparing heavy marijuana users with nonusers have been confounded by the absence of any measure of intellectual functioning before drug use. One study that provided such data found no adverse effects of chronic marijuana use.[226] Another found impairments in verbal expression and mathematical skills but only in very heavy users.[241] A study comparing "cannabis-dependent" adolescents with occasional users and nonusers found abnormal visual and verbal memory in the heavy users, with "significant improvement" after 6 weeks of abstinence.[242]

A study of college undergraduates compared heavy users (who smoked marijuana most days) and light users (who smoked every several days); all were abstinent for at least 19 hours before testing. Heavy users were significantly more impaired in tests of attention and executive function but not in tests of recall memory. The authors were unable to say whether the impairment was due to residual drug in the brain, to drug withdrawal, or to a neurotoxic effect of the drug.[243] In another report, the same investigators compared heavy users (who had smoked marijuana at least 5000 times in their lives and were currently smoking daily), former heavy users (who had smoked fewer than 12 times in the last month), and control subjects. A monitored washout period of 28 days preceded testing. At days 0, 1, and 7 current heavy users were significantly more impaired than control subjects on recall of word lists; by day 28, however, there were no differences between the three groups on any test results.[244]

In a longitudinal study of adolescents, IQ scores were determined at age 9 to 12 years and again at 17 to 20 years, and correlations were sought between decline and marijuana use. A detrimental effect was found in current users who smoked at least five times per week but not in former heavy users.[245]

A study of U.S. high school seniors, matched for IQ in the fourth grade, found deficits in mathematical skills, verbal expression, and memory in heavy users of marijuana compared with light users and non-users. Subjects were abstinent for only 24 hours prior to testing, however.[246] In another study, long-term cannabis users (mean 24 years) were significantly impaired on tests of attention and memory compared with shorter-term users (mean 10 years) and non-users; testing followed at least 12 hours of abstinence, and the results were not affected by how recently the subjects had last used marijuana.[247] A critique of this study pointed out potential confounders, for example that users were seeking treatment for cannabis dependence whereas controls were recruited by advertisement from the general population, that subjects with depression, anxiety, or other psychiatric conditions were not excluded, and that 47% of long-term cannabis users had a history of regular use, dependence on, or treatment for ethanol or other drugs.[248] A similar study found impaired visual scanning relative to controls in adults who had begun marijuana use before age 15 years but not in those who began use after age 15 years.[249]

In response to those who attribute the detrimental psychological effects of cannabis to lingering acute toxicity, several studies found little or no influence of acute marijuana administration on cognitive functioning in experienced users.[250,251]

A study of adolescents and young adults matched for age and IQ found a dose-related negative effect of heavy cannabis use on tests of memory, executive functioning, psychomotor speed, and manual dexterity. Testing followed 28 days of abstinence, and subjects with ethanol or other drug dependence or other psychiatric disorders were excluded. Duration of use did not affect performance.[252] Addressing confounders, this study persuasively demonstrated persistent detrimental effects of heavy marijuana use on human cognition.[253]

Other studies in human cannabis users have found abnormalities in brain event-related potentials[254] and altered blood flow and metabolism in the prefrontal cortex and cerebellum.[255–257,257a] In rodents, δ-9-THC caused impaired learning and memory that persisted after several months of abstinence,[219,258] and δ-9-THC as well as a synthetic cannabinoid, WIN 55212-2, produced morphological changes in the hippocampus.[259] In rats δ-9-THC caused changes in CB_1 receptors in the hippocampus that correlated with selective deficits in working memory.[260] Others, however, were unable to demonstrate lasting alterations in CB_1 receptors following chronic δ-9-THC administration in either rats or monkeys.[261]

Psychiatric Illness

An extensive literature has explored the association of cannabis use and psychiatric illness, including schizophrenia and depression.[262,263] Causality is claimed in both directions.

In several longitudinal cohort studies, subjects with no baseline depressive symptoms who used cannabis were significantly more likely than nonusers to develop depression.[264–266] In one report, cannabis use among adolescents predicted later depression, but depression did not predict cannabis use.[266] Both the CB_1 receptor gene and a susceptibility locus for bipolar disorder are located on chromosome 6q, but a polymorphism in the promotor region of the CB_1 receptor gene did not correlate with mood disorders or psychosis.[267]

Cannabis use provokes relapse in schizophrenia and can aggravate existing symptoms.[262,262a,262b] Increased dopamine release would be a plausible mechanism.[268] As with depression, longitudinal studies of psychosis-free subjects found cannabis use a risk factor for the development of schizophrenia.[269-272] Patients with pre-existing schizophrenia, however, often use marijuana to counter distressing symptoms;[272] this pattern seems to be more common among adolescents than adults.[273] Polymorphism within the CB_1 gene was associated with substance-abusing versus non-substance-abusing schizophrenics.[274] In an autoradiographic study using a radiolabeled CB_1 ligand, increased density of ligand binding to CB_1 receptors in the dorsolateral prefrontal cortex was found in schizophrenic subjects independent of recent cannabis use.[275]

Although depression or schizophrenia can appear in cannabis users lacking evidence of these disorders at the time of first use, it is more plausible that cannabis precipitates symptoms among vulnerable individuals than that it *causes* these disorders.[276]

Respiratory Tract

Marijuana causes bronchial and laryngeal damage, with hoarseness, cough, and impaired pulmonary function.[277–279] Pneumomediastinum, subcutaneous emphysema, and even pneumorachis (epidural pneumatosis) have followed marijuana smoking with expiration against resistance.[280] Altered alveolar macrophage function predisposes to pulmonary infection.[278] Hydrocarbon tars in marijuana smoke are more carcinogenic than those in tobacco smoke,[281,282] and users are at risk for cancer of the mouth, larynx, and lung.[283–288] Compared with tobacco smoking, marijuana is associated with nearly fivefold greater increments in blood carboxyhemoglobin levels.[289] Digital clubbing has been observed in hashish users without other evidence of pulmonary disease.[290] Contamination of cannabis plants with the herbicide paraquat adds further potential danger to the respiratory system,[291] as does the presence in most marijuana samples of pathogenic inhalable *Aspergillus*, a particular risk to users infected with human immunodeficiency virus (HIV).[292,293] In the United States a multistate outbreak of *Salmonella* enteritis was traced to contamination of marijuana samples.[294] Four Puerto Rican policemen assigned to uprooting illegally cultivated marijuana developed acute pulmonary histoplasmosis.[295]

Allergy, Cirrhosis, Peripheral Vascular Disease

Anaphylactic reaction to marijuana has been reported;[296] acute uvulitis and upper airway obstruction in a smoker required emergency antihistamines and corticosteroids.[297] Less convincingly, marijuana has been linked to cirrhosis[298] and gastroenteritis.[299] Obliterative arteritis of the arms and legs is anecdotally described.[300] In a report from France, 10 young men developed subacute distal limb ischemia resulting in necrosis and gangrene; pathology resembled Buerger's disease. All patients were "moderate" tobacco smokers and "regular" cannabis users.[301]

Immunosuppression

Reported abnormalities of cellular immunity include inhibition of phytohemagglutinin-stimulated lymphocyte blastogenesis, decreased numbers of T lymphocytes, impaired macrophage function, reduced cytokine secretion, altered killer cell activity, delayed allogenic skin graft rejection, and enhanced susceptibility of mice to gram-negative bacterial infection.[199,302–304] Some workers, while confirming marijuana's effects on T cell function, found such abnormalities to be transitory. Others, studying skin tests for cellular immunity or cultured lymphocyte responses to mitogens, did not detect abnormalities attributable to marijuana

smoking.[199] Marijuana users, in contrast to heavy ethanol users, do not seem to be especially vulnerable to infection independent of direct contamination; in particular, marijuana has not hastened the development of acquired immunodeficiency syndrome (AIDS) in HIV-infected users.[305–307] Frequent marijuana use is a risk factor for sexually transmitted disease.[308] In Australia several outbreaks of hepatitis A virus infection were traced to shared implements for smoking marijuana.[309]

Endocrine Effects

Marijuana inhibits secretion of luteinizing hormone (LH), follicle stimulating hormone (FSH), and testosterone. In men, there is decreased sperm count, gynecomastia, and impotence and in women menstrual irregularity and anovulatory menstrual cycles.[199,308,309] These changes are reversible; permanently impaired potency or fertility have not been reported in chronic marijuana users. A 16-year-old boy who had smoked marijuana since age 11 years had pubertal arrest; with abstinence, growth resumed, and testosterone levels became normal.[310]

In humans, marijuana depresses growth hormone and cortisol response to insulin hypoglycemia.[311] In animals, it depresses thyroid gland function and plasma prolactin levels and raises levels of plasma adrenocorticotropic hormone (ACTH) and adrenocortical steroids.[312] Tolerance develops to these hormone changes. In rats, δ-9-THC suppression of LH was attributed to blocked release of LH-releasing hormone, whereas suppression of growth hormone release was secondary to stimulation of somatostatin release.[313] One report, cautioning against too readily extrapolating animal endocrine effects to humans, found no change in plasma prolactin levels among marijuana-smoking men. Another study found no effects of moderate short-term marijuana use on plasma prolactin, ACTH, cortisol, LH, and testosterone in men.[314] In other reports, moderate short-term marijuana use had no effect on plasma prolactin, ACTH, cortisol, LH, and testosterone,[315] and chronic marijuana use had no effect on blood levels of testosterone, LH, FSH, prolactin, or cortisol.[316]

Cardiovascular Effects

In subjects with angina pectoris, marijuana decreases exercise performance by increasing myocardial oxygen demand and decreasing myocardial oxygen delivery.[317] Anecdotal reports describe acute myocardial infarction in young people during or soon after cannabis use,[318,318a] and in a case–control study the risk of myocardial infarction was increased nearly fivefold during the 60 minutes after marijuana smoking.[319] Myocardial infarction followed the combined recreational use of cannabis and sildenafil (Viagra); by inhibiting cytochrome P450, cannabis probably potentiated the effects of sudenafil, which include systemic vasodilation.[320] In a report from India a young man with rheumatic heart disease died after ingesting a large dose of bhang.[321] Paroxysmal atrial fibrillation has occurred in healthy children and young adults in association with cannabis use.[322,323] Renal infarction occurred in a heavy cannabis user.[324]

Stroke

A number of reports describe ischemic stroke in young marijuana users.[325–338,338a,338b] Some are more convincing than others. In two young men, the only abnormality was conjugate deviation of the eyes for days or weeks after marijuana use.[325,328] Another young man awoke with hemiparesis and dysarthria the morning after smoking marijuana.[328] Imaging studies were not performed in these patients. Better documented were two young men—both hypertensive cigarette smokers—who developed hemiparesis during marijuana smoking and whose CT scans demonstrated cerebral infarction.[329] A proposed mechanism was drug-induced hypotension. A 30-year-old chronic smoker of marijuana and tobacco had three episodes suggestive of transient ischemia and then a striatocapsular infarct with hemiparesis and aphasia.[331]

While smoking marijuana, a 22-year-old man had transient ischemic attacks consisting of either aphasia or left hemiparesis and then developed permanent left hemiplegia.[332] A 15-year-old boy who had been continuously smoking marijuana for several days had a large cerebellar infarct while still smoking.[333] A young man who smoked marijuana heavily had a posterior cerebral artery territory infarction during an episode of coital headache.[334] Occipital infarction occurred in an adolescent daily marijuana smoker who was heterozygous for factor V Leiden mutation.[335] A young man had several brief episodes of left-sided numbness while smoking marijuana and then, during an alcohol binge, infarction in the right middle cerebral artery territory.[336] A young man had a cerebral infarct attributed to the additive effects of cannabis and cisplatin chemotherapy.[337] Three young men without other stroke risk factors or other evident drug use had transient ischemic attacks temporally associated with smoking marijuana; in all three magnetic resonance imaging (MRI) showed cerebral white matter signals consistent with small vessel leukoencephalopathy.[338]

After smoking high-potency marijuana ("superskunk"), a healthy 40-year-old man developed transient global amnesia unusual in its severity —retrograde amnesia went back 20 years, and the episode lasted four days. A mechanism, vascular or otherwise, was not determined.[339]

As noted above, cannabis causes tachycardia, increased systolic blood pressure, and orthostatic hypotension.[116,141] Effects on CBF vary.[151,255,256,340] In one study inexperienced marijuana smokers had increased anxiety and decreased CBF after use, whereas experienced smokers had reduced anxiety and increased CBF.[341] Reduced cerebral blood volume (with marked dizziness) during orthostatic hypotension suggests impaired cerebral autoregulation.[342] Studies with transcranial Doppler sonography in young abstinent marijuana users revealed increased cerebrovascular resistance "similar to that of 60-year-old individuals."[343] In rats δ-9-THC has vasoconstrictor actions.[344]

Trauma

Marijuana smokers are overrepresented in highway fatalities.[291,345] Studies with volunteers confirm impairment in driving ability for up to 150 minutes after smoking enough marijuana to achieve a "high."[346]

Seizures

Anecdotal reports of seizures associated with marijuana are rare.[347] Whether marijuana use or withdrawal can trigger seizures in epileptics is uncertain.[348] Patients with petit mal absence may be susceptible.[46] For most users, however, marijuana may be anticonvulsant.[349] As noted above, different cannabinoid compounds are either proconvulsant or anticonvulsant in different animal models. (For a discussion of cannabinoids as potential anticonvulsant drugs in humans, see below.)

Heat Stroke

Heat stroke, with delirium and temperature of 41.7°C, occurred in a man who smoked marijuana while jogging.[350]

Cranial and Peripheral Nerves

Trochlear nerve dysfunction, with superior oblique muscle paresis, was reported in 20 "medium to heavy" marijuana users; if the drug was causal, the mechanism is obscure.[351] Electromyographic studies of peripheral nerves in cannabis users have shown no abnormalities.[352]

Parenteral Marijuana

Rarely water infusions of cannabis plant material have been injected intravenously; complications seem to be from the crude plant material rather than from cannabinoid effects and include gastroenteritis, hypoalbuminemia, hepatitis, hypovolemia, renal insufficiency, thrombocytopenia, and rhabdomyolysis.[353–355]

Obstetric and Pediatric Aspects

In the United States, marijuana is used by up to one-third of pregnant women.[356] Studies of effects on offspring are conflicting, in part because use is often underreported.[357–365] In a study that performed urine assays—without which 16% of marijuana users would have been unidentified—marijuana smoking during pregnancy was associated with decreased birth weight and length.[366] The newborns had reduced nonfat mass and normal fat stores, similar to what is found in the offspring of tobacco smokers and implicating hypoxia or other nonnutritional causes of impaired fetal growth. Cannabinoids easily cross the placenta, especially early in gestation, and fetal abnormalities could be the consequence of direct toxicity, abnormal maternal ventilation-perfusion, or inhalation of carbon monoxide.[367]

Whether these changes lead to neurobehavioral abnormalities is uncertain. Offspring of moderate to heavy marijuana users have reportedly had tremor, decreased responsiveness to stimuli during sleep, abnormally high-pitched cries, altered sleep patterns, and impulsivity.[368–371a] Others have found no such abnormalities. Neurobehavioral development was normal among 1-year-olds and 2-year-olds exposed prenatally to marijuana,[371] yet at age 4 years the same children performed poorly on verbal and memory tests.[372] In a longitudinal study of several hundred children prenatal marijuana exposure was associated at age 10 years with impaired learning and memory and with impulsivity, even when other risk factors, including ethanol, were controlled.[373] Compared with controls, 1-month-old infants exposed in utero to marijuana had lower arousal, poor "self-regulation," hypertonia, and excitability.[374] A literature review concluded that fetal cannabis exposure is not associated with reduction of "global IQ," but rather with impaired executive function—e.g., attentional behavior and "visual analysis/hypothesis testing."[375]

Third-trimester exposure to marijuana was associated with abnormally prolonged visual evoked potential latencies at 18 months of age in the absence of neonatal behavioral disturbances.[376] Interactions of endocannabinoids with opioid and other neurotransmitter/neuromodulator systems raises the possibility that in utero exposure to marijuana might increase the risk of later dependence on other drugs. In animals, however, prenatal exposure to δ-9-THC did not increase the reinforcing properties of morphine.[377]

Sudden infant death syndrome was associated with *paternal* marijuana use during periods of conception, pregnancy, and postnatally.[378] Infants exposed to marijuana through breastfeeding had delayed motor development compared with controls.[379] As with other drugs, the effects of marijuana on fetal and later development are difficult to separate from confounding variables such as maternal nutrition, other substance abuse, and home environment.

In human lymphocytes, cannabinoids reportedly prevented normal chromosome segregation and induced chromosomal breakage.[380,381] Not all workers were able to confirm such effects.[382] In rodents, cannabinoids caused morphologically abnormal ova, fetal wastage, and increased mortality at birth, especially among female offspring.[361,383–385] Also reported are liver, kidney, and vascular abnormalities; hydrocephalus; and delayed postnatal growth and brain protein synthesis.[385–389] In a study with rats, maternal exposure to cannabinoids altered the development of nigrostriatal, mesolimbic, and tuberoinfundibular dopaminergic neurons.[390] Other workers could not confirm cannabinoid effects on either protein synthesis or development.[391]

As with humans, neurobehavioral abnormalities in animals have been elusive, especially in properly controlled studies.[392,393] When pair-fed controls and surrogate fostering were employed, there were neither short-term nor long-term effects of marijuana on nipple attachment, locomotion, activity level, avoidance, water maze learning, or auditory startle.[394–396]

A case–control study of abruptio placentae in humans revealed that weekly use of marijuana during pregnancy carried a risk ratio of 2.8.[397]

Therapeutic Uses

Historical Background

Cannabis has been used for millennia to treat medical illness.[46,398–400] Pen Ts'ao, a Chinese herbal compendium of the third millennium BCE, recommended it for constipation, gout, malaria, rheumatism, pain, and menstrual problems. In India the Athera Veda of the second millennium BCE recommended it for sedation and fever reduction, and it is still used by Ayurvedic practitioners as a decongestant, astringent, appetite stimulator, anesthetic, and aphrodisiac. During the 19th century William O'Shaughnessy of the English East India Company conducted experiments on marijuana's efficacy in seizures, tetanus, rabies, and pain relief, and in England it was used for insomnia, asthma, opium withdrawal, and childbirth analgesia. (A recipient for the latter use was Queen Victoria.) In France it was used to treat insanity. Wier Mitchell, William Gowers, and William Osler each recommended marijuana for the symptomatic and preventive treatment of migraine. In 1941, 4 years after cannabis became illegal in the United States, it was dropped from the U.S. Pharmacopeia, yet the following year the editor of the *Journal of the American Medical Association*, Morris Fishbein, continued to recommend oral preparations of marijuana for the treatment of catamenial migraine. Today marijuana has advocates for the treatment of pain, nausea, anorexia, asthma, glaucoma, spasticity, and epilepsy. A 1991 survey of 1000 American oncologists found that many would recommend marijuana to their patients.

Delta-9-THC, marketed as a dronabinol (Marinol), is approved by the Food and Drug Administration (FDA) in the United States for chemotherapy-induced nausea and vomiting and for wasting in AIDS. (Surveys indicate that dronabinol is neither abused nor diverted to a street market.[400a]) A synthetic cannabinoid, nabilone (Cesamet), is available in Europe. Whether smoked marijuana itself should be available to treat such conditions, however, has engendered a debate as contentious as that concerning blanket legalization. The reason is that the two issues are difficult to separate.

Marijuana is a Schedule I drug—i.e., lacking any medical usefulness and carrying considerable dependence liability. Despite a federal appeals court decision in 1991 that the U.S. Drug Enforcement Agency was illogical in the rigidity of its position, the FDA refused to reconsider. In 1996 California passed the "Compassionate Use Act" ("Proposition 215") which allowed any seriously ill person to obtain marijuana upon recommendation of a physician. Since then eight additional states—Alaska, Arizona, Colorado, Hawaii, Maine, Nevada, Oregon, and Washington—have passed similar legislation, and in 2001 it became legal in Canada for patients with specific medical conditions to buy, grow, and use marijuana on a physician's recommendation.[399] In California, marijuana, available in "Cannabis buyers' clubs," was dispensed mostly to patients with AIDS, but also to some with cancer, chronic pain, or multiple sclerosis.[401] The response of the director of the White House Office of National Drug Control Policy (Barry McCaffrey, a general) was to threaten any practitioner who prescribed or even *recommended* marijuana with revocation of the practitioner's DEA registration, exclusion from Medicare and Medicaid, and criminal prosecution.[402] The editor of the *New England Journal of Medicine* denounced this federal policy as "misguided, heavy-handed, and inhumane" and called for Schedule II reclassification.[403] (Dronabinol is Schedule III.) A California court granted injunction against federal "gagging," declaring that the First Amendment protects physician–patient communication. Federal authorities responded to the ruling by closing down a number of California buyers' clubs.[404,405]

In 1999 the Institute of Medicine recommended that research on cannabinoid drugs should include clinical trials for symptom management and assessment of psychological effects and health risks. The report endorsed the use of smoked marijuana when other interventions failed, but under the supervision of an investigational review panel.[406]

In a comparable report the American Medical Association recommended scientific study of smoked marijuana in selected conditions (AIDS wasting syndrome, severe chemotherapy-induced emesis, multiple sclerosis, spinal cord injury, dystonia, and neuropathic pain) and retention of its Schedule I status pending the outcome of such studies.[407] Opponents of medical marijuana cite the lack of efficacy and safety studies required for FDA-approved prescription drugs and the impossibility of regulating the content of smoked leaves (ignoring, however, the entirely unregulated availability of "herbal" medicines and food "supplements"). They also believe that the movement to legalize marijuana for medicinal purposes is largely driven by those who would legalize it for recreational purposes.[408]

In 2001 the U.S. Supreme Court overturned an Appeals Court ruling that medical necessity offered a defense against federal prosecution for using marijuana. In his opinion, Justice Clarence Thomas declared, "Marijuana has no medical benefits worthy of an exception" to marijuana's Schedule I classification.[409] The ruling did not overturn Proposition 215, however, and in 2002 a federal appeals court in California ruled that the federal government may not revoke the licenses of doctors who recommend marijuana to their patients.[410] The following year the U.S. Supreme Court let stand that ruling, although it remained illegal for physicians to write prescriptions (or their equivalent) for marijuana.[410a,410b]

Amidst such alarums and excursions what is the evidence for the medicinal efficacy of δ-9-THC, other cannabinoids, or cannabis itself?

Pain Control

As noted above, δ-9-THC has considerable analgesic efficacy in animals, and the endogenous cannabinoid and opioid systems interact in complex ways.[56,411] CB$_1$ receptors are prominent in the descending pain-modulatory system that includes the midbrain periaqueductal gray, the rostroventral medulla, and the dorsal horns of the spinal cord. Many patients with chronic pain report benefit from smoked marijuana, and it reportedly is antinociceptive in human experiments.[412–414] Randomized controlled trials, however, have assessed only oral δ-9-THC or synthetic cannabinoids; a meta-analysis of nine such studies, which addressed cancer pain, "non-malignant pain," and postoperative pain, found analgesic efficacy no better than with codeine 50–120 mg.[415] In one study of cancer pain, 20 mg of oral δ-9-THC produced mild analgesia, but side effects included somnolence, ataxia, blurred vision, slurred speech, and disorientation.[416] Interestingly, a number of nonpsychoactive cannabinoids that do not bind to CB$_1$ receptors demonstrate analgesic efficacy in preliminary human clinical trials.[411,417,417a] Even more experimental are agents that perturb the endocannabinoid system, for example by blocking fatty acid amide hydrolase, the enzyme that degrades anandamide.[418]

Anorexia, Nausea, and Vomiting

A meta-analysis of 30 randomized trials concluded that oral (dronabinol or nabilone) or intramuscular (levonantradol) cannabinoids were superior to prochlorperazine, metoclopromide, or domperidone in the treatment of chemotherapy-induced nausea and vomiting.[419] Mood elevation was considered a "positive" side effect, but patients often had to discontinue the cannabinoid drug because of dysphoria, depression, paranoia, or hallucinations. Patients overwhelmingly preferred cannabinoids for future chemotherapy. There were no studies using smoked marijuana and no studies comparing cannabinoids with 5-HT$_3$ receptor antagonists (currently the drugs of choice). Smoked marijuana is the preference for many cancer and AIDS patients with anorexia, nausea, vomiting, and weight loss;[420,421] 80% of the 10,000 patients served by the San Francisco Cultivators Club had AIDS.[406] Comparisons of smoked marijuana and 5-HT$_3$ receptor antagonists have not been performed.

Asthma

Delta-9-THC reduces pulmonary airway resistance, but smoked marijuana would be an impractical means of treating asthma. A δ-9-THC aerosol delivery system has had limited application.[46]

Glaucoma

Delta-9-THC and other psychoactive cannabinoids lower intraocular pressure by acting at CB$_1$ receptors within the eye. Controlled studies reveal a short duration of action and unacceptable side effects; the Institute of Medicine report concluded that chronic therapy with cannabinoids for glaucoma is impractical.[406] Anecdotal reports, however, describe benefit from marijuana smoking after all else failed.[422,423]

Multiple Sclerosis

In a survey of 112 patients with multiple sclerosis in the United States and the United Kingdom who smoked marijuana, over 90% reported improvement in spasticity, muscle pain, tremor, and depression, and a majority reported improvement in depression, weakness, imbalance, visual symptoms, bowel and bladder dysfunction, paresthesias, trigeminal neuralgia, and tiredness.[424] Placebo responses are common in multiple sclerosis, however. In a randomized double-blind placebo-controlled study of postural response and spasticity in multiple sclerosis, patients perceived themselves as clinically improved after smoking marijuana, yet examiners found an increase in tracking errors.[425] Three placebo-controlled studies of oral δ-9-THC (or δ-9-THC plus cannabidiol) in the treatment of spasticity in multiple sclerosis found either short-lived or no benefit and unacceptable side effects.[426–428] A randomized, placebo-controlled trial in the U.K., using a marijuana extract containing mostly δ-9-THC and cannabidiol, found little benefit on objective measures of spasticity yet significant benefit from the subjective standpoint of the patients.[428a] Anecdotal case reports describe dramatic objective improvement following oral δ-9-THC or nabilone in individual multiple sclerosis patients with tremor or spasticity.[429,430] Delta-9-THC also reportedly reduced spasticity following spinal cord trauma.[431] Marijuana smoking suppressed pendular nystagmus in a patient with multiple sclerosis.[432]

In mice with chronic relapsing experimental autoimmune encephalomyelitis (EAE, an animal model for multiple sclerosis) cannabinoids not only relieved spasticity but favorably altered the course of the disease.[433] Knockout mice lacking CB$_1$ receptors had increased central nervous system damage when subjected to EAE, and exogenous CB$_1$ agonists reduced damage in an experimental model of allergic uveitis.[433a] Such observations suggest that cannabinoids might not only acutely reduce symptoms in some patients with multiple sclerosis but might also, by immunomodulatory or neuroprotective mechanisms, slow the course of the illness.

In 2004 a liquid extract from marijuana, to be sprayed sublingually, was introduced in the U.K. for treating multiple sclerosis.[433b]

Epilepsy

In a case–control study from Harlem Hospital Center, marijuana use was protective against new-onset seizures in men; use was significantly less for cases than controls (28.9% versus 40.6%), and the protective effect persisted after controlling in multivariate analysis for heroin, ethanol, and other confounders (Table 7–2).[349] Among women, a smaller nonsignificant difference existed in the same direction (11.7% versus 15.2%). Frequency and duration of marijuana use was similar among cases and controls. About one-third were daily users, and two-thirds were weekly users; 70% had

Table 7–2. Adjusted Odds Ratio of Marijuana Use and New-onset Seizures

	Men: Odds Ratio (95% Confidence Interval)	Women: Odds Ratio (95% Confidence Interval)
Unprovoked seizures		
Marijuana use ever	0.42 (0.22–0.82)	1.09 (0.35–3.40)
Marijuana use within 3 months of admission	0.36 (0.18–0.74)	1.87 (0.56–6.20)
Provoked seizures		
Marijuana use ever	1.03 (0.36–2.89)	0.79 (0.14–4.37)
Marijuana use within 3 months of admission	0.18 (0.04–0.84)	1.08 (0.12–9.79)

Source: Ng SKC, et al. Illicit drug use and the risk of new onset seizures. Am J Epidemiol 1990; 132:47.

used marijuana for at least 2 years and 50% for at least 5 years. Of special interest is that although marijuana smoked within 90 days conferred maximal protection, the risk was reduced for unprovoked seizures (unaccompanied by an additional potential precipitant such as metabolic derangement or head trauma) even in those who had last smoked it more remotely.

These findings are consistent with animal studies demonstrating the anticonvulsant properties of some cannabinoids. Marijuana was recommended for the treatment of epilepsy as far back as the 15th century,[434] yet few trials have been conducted in humans.[435–443] Five mentally retarded, poorly controlled epileptic children were switched from conventional anticonvulsants to "isomeric homologs of THC"; three responded "at least as well as to previous therapy," one was much improved, and one became entirely seizure-free.[438] In a single case report, marijuana smoking was necessary for seizure control.[435] A New Mexico survey of 42 epileptics under age 30 years found that 29% used marijuana; one subject reported that marijuana decreased seizures and another that it "caused" them.[440] In another case report, intravenous cannabidiol did not alter (and may be even increased) the electroencephalographic spike and wave abnormalities of a young man with well-controlled "tonic-clonic seizures."[442] A young man who abused ethanol and smoked marijuana daily developed episodic olfactory hallucinations, confusion, urinary incontinence, and electroencephalographic temporal lobe spikes when he stopped using marijuana; symptoms cleared with resumption and recurred when he again discontinued the drug.[444]

There has been only one prospectively designed treatment study, a double-masked, placebo-controlled trial of patients refractory to other drugs.

Cannabidiol, given to eight of the 16 patients, acutely exacerbated electroencephalographic but not behavioral seizures. After 4 to 5 months, however, seven of eight patients receiving cannabidiol were electroencephalographically and behaviorally seizure-free compared with one of eight controls. The only sign of toxicity was somnolence.[443] These observations imply that marijuana's cannabinoid compounds include potentially useful anticonvulsant drugs.

Movement Disorder

Anecdotal reports suggest cannabinoids are useful in treating a variety of movement disorders. Eleven of 13 patients with Tourette syndrome reported "marked improvement" in symptoms after smoking marijuana, and in a randomized placebo-controlled crossover trial, oral δ-9-THC produced significant improvement of tics and obsessive-compulsive behavior that correlated with plasma cannabinoid concentration.[445,446]

Anecdotal descriptions of marijuana benefiting dystonia[432] were not borne out in a randomized trial using nabilone.[447] In an open trial marijuana had no effect on parkinsonian tremor.[448] In a randomized, double-masked placebo-controlled trial, nabilone significantly reduced levodopa-induced dyskinesia in patients with Parkinson's disease.[449]

A patient with AIDS and intractable hiccups obtained relief by smoking marijuana.[450]

Migraine

Abrupt cessation of chronic marijuana smoking can precipitate migraine attacks.[451] Although marijuana has been used to treat migraine for centuries, evidence for its efficacy is strictly anecdotal.[398,452]

Neuroprotection

As noted above, cannabinoids are neuroprotective in animals with central nervous system ischemic or excitotoxic injury.[26,62b,453] Cannabidiol and HU211, cannabinoids with little affinity for CB_1 receptors, are as effective as δ-9-THC, suggesting a non-CB_1-receptor-mediated mechanism.[22,432,452] Studies in humans are awaited.

Immunosuppression/Anti-Inflammation

In a mouse model of immune-mediated arthritis cannabidiol had a potent anti-arthritic effect.[454]

Substance Abuse Treatment

Delta-9-THC and anandamide share considerable cross-tolerance with ethanol, and the pharmacological and behavioral effects of ethanol could be mediated through CB_1-receptor signal transduction.[455] In ethanol-preferring rodents the CB_1-receptor antagonist rimonabant reduced ethanol consumption.[456] CB1-receptor agonists show cross-sensitization with both opioids and psychostimulants. In rats the agonist HU-210 precipitated relapse to cocaine-seeking, whereas rimonabant blocked relapse induced by either cocaine itself or cocaine-associated cues.[457] Trials of cannabinoid receptor antagonists in drug-dependent humans are awaited.

Long-term Treatment

The silliness of U.S. marijuana policy does not negate the potentially harmful consequences of its use, including addiction, cognitive impairment, and fetal damage. Of the more than 10 million current users in the United States, more than a million are psychologically dependent—that is, addicted—and many seek treatment.[103,458-460] In 1999, 220,000 marijuana users were admitted to publicly funded substance abuse treatment programs in the United States.[218] The vast majority of marijuana-dependent

subjects use other drugs as well, especially cocaine, ethanol, and tobacco. In contrast to heroin, no effective pharmacotherapy for marijuana dependence exists. Analogous to methadone maintenance therapy for heroin addiction, oral δ-9-THC was tried in marijuana smokers; there was neither reduction in marijuana smoking nor alteration in the effects of smoked marijuana on psychomotor tasks.[461] Of 110 adults who received intensive group therapy over 12 weeks, only 30% reported complete abstinence from marijuana during the month following treatment.[458] Such an outcome practically defines addiction.

References

1. Dewey WL. Cannabinoid pharmacology. Pharmacol Rev 1986; 38:151.
2. Pertwee RG. The central neuropharmacology of psychotropic cannabinoids. Pharmacol Ther 1988; 36:189.
3. Perez-Reyes M, Timmons MC, Lipton MA, et al. Intravenous injection in man of delta-9-tetrahydrocannabinol and 11-hydroxy-delta-9-tetrahydrocannabinol. Science 1972; 177:633.
4. Seth R, Sinha S. Chemistry and pharmacology of cannabis. Prog Drug Res 1991; 36:71.
5. Colasanti BK, Lindamood C, Craig CR. Effects of marijuana cannabinoids on seizure activity in cobalt-epileptic rats. Pharmacol Biochem Behav 1982; 16:573.
6. Karler R, Turkanis SA. Subacute cannabinoid treatment: anticonvulsant activity and withdrawal excitability in mice. Br J Pharmacol 1980; 68:479.
7. Consroe P, Benedito MA, Leite JR, et al. Effects of cannabidiol on behavioral seizures caused by convulsant drugs or current in mice. Eur J Pharmacol 1982; 83:293.
8. Consroe P, Martin A, Singh V. Antiepileptic potential of cannabidiol. J Clin Pharmacol 1981; 21 (Suppl):428S.
9. Johnson DD, McNeill JR, Crawford RD, Wilcox WC. Epileptiform seizures in domestic fowl. V. The anticonvulsant activity of delta-9-tetrahydrocannabinol. Can J Physiol Pharmacol 1975; 53:1007.
10. Sofia RD, Solomon TA, Barry H. Anticonvulsant activity of delta-9-tetrahydrocannabinol compared with three other drugs. Eur J Pharmacol 1976; 35:7.
11. Wada JA, Wake A, Sato M, Corcoran ME. Antiepileptic and prophylactic effects of tetrahydrocannabinols in amygdaloid kindled rats. Epilepsia 1975; 16:503.
12. Wada JA, Osawa T, Corcoran ME. Effects of tetrahydrocannabinols on kindled amygdaloid seizures in Senegalese baboons, *Papio papio*. Epilepsia 1975; 16:439.

13. Ten-harn M, Laskota WJ, Lumak P. Acute and chronic effects of beta-9-tetrahydrocannabinol on seizures in the gerbil. Eur J Pharmacol 1975; 31:148.

14. Consroe P, Fish BS. Rabbit behavioral model of marijuana psychoactivity in humans. Med Hypotheses 1981; 7:1079.

15. Consroe P, Martin P, Eisenstein D. Anticonvulsant drug antagonism of delta-9-tetrahydrocannabinol-induced seizures in rabbits. Res Commun Chem Pathol Pharmacol 1977; 16:1.

16. Turkanis SA, Karler R. Electrophysiologic properties of the cannabinoids. J Clin Pharmacol 1981; 21 (Suppl):449S.

17. Consroe P, Wolkin A. Cannabidiol-antiepileptic drug comparisons and interactions in experimentally induced seizures in rats. J Pharmacol Exp Ther 1977; 20:26.

18. Karler R, Turkanis SA. The cannabinoids as potential antiepileptics. J Clin Pharmacol 1981; 21:4375.

19. Martin BR. Structural requirements for cannabinoid-induced anti-nociceptive activity in mice. Life Sci 1985; 36:1523.

20. Elphick MR, Egertová M. The neurobiology and evolution of cannabinoid signaling. Phil Trans R Soc Lond 2001; 356:381.

21. Pertwee RG. Pharmacology of cannabinoid CB1 and CB2 receptors. Pharmacol Ther 1997; 74:129.

22. Iverson L. Cannabis and the brain. Brain 2003; 126:1252.

22a. Howlett AC, Barth F, Bonner TI, et al. International Union of Pharmacology. XXVII. Classification of cannabinoid receptors. Pharmacol Rev 2002; 54:161.

23. Gerard CM, Mollcreau C, Brownstein MJ, et al. Molecular cloning of a human cannabinoid receptor which is also expressed in testis. Biochem J 1991; 279:129.

24. Onaivi ES, Leonard CM, Ishiguro H, et al. Endocannabinoids and cannabinoid receptor genetics. Prog Neurobiol 2002; 66:307.

25. Felder CC, Glass M. Cannabinoid receptors and their endogenous agonists. Annu Rev Pharmacol Toxicol 1998; 38:179.

26. Mechoulam R. Discovery of endocannabinoids and some random thoughts on their possible roles in neuroprotection and aggression. Prostagland Leukotriene Essential Fatty Acids 2002; 66:93.

27. Murillo-Rodriguez E, Giordano M, Cabeza R, et al. Oleamide modulates memory in rats. Neurosci Lett 2001; 313:61.

28. Wilson RI, Nicoll RA. Endocannabinoid signaling in the brain. Science 2002; 296:678.

29. Fride E. Endocannabinoids in the central nervous system–an overview. Prostagland Leukotriene Essential Fatty Acids 2002; 66:221.

30. Chaperon F, Thiebot MH. Behavioral effects of cannabinoid agents in animals. Crit Rev Neurobiol 1999; 13:243.

31. Schlicker E, Kathmann M. Modulation of transmitter release via presynaptic cannabinoid receptors. Trends Pharmacol Sci 2001; 22:565.

32. McAllister SD, Glass M. CB1 and CB2 receptor-mediated signaling: a focus on endocannabinoids. Prostagland Leukotriene Essential Fatty Acids 2002; 66:161.

33. Ameri A. The effects of cannabinoids on the brain. Prog Neurobiol 1999; 58:315.

34. Deadwyler SA, Hampson RE, Mu J, et al. Cannabinoids modulate voltage-sensitive potassium in A-current in hippocampal-neurons via a cAMO-dependent process. J Pharmacol Exp Ther 1995; 273:734.

35. Wilson RI, Nicoll RA. Endogenous cannabinoids mediate retrograde signaling at hippocampal synapses. Nature 2001; 410:588.

36. Christie MJ, Vaughan CW. Cannabinoids act backwards. Nature 2001; 410:527.

37. Ohno-Shosaku T, Maejima T, Kano M. Endogenous cannabinoids mediate retrograde signals from depolarized postsynaptic neurons to presynaptic terminals. Neuron 2001; 29:729.

38. Maejima T, Ohno-Shosaku T, Kano M. Endogenous cannabinoid as a retrograde messenger from depolarized postsynaptic neurons to presynaptic terminals. Neurosci Res 2001; 40:205.

39. Bracey MH, Hanson MA, Masuda KR, et al. Structural adaptations in a membrane enzyme that terminates endocannabinoid signaling. Science 2002; 298:1793.

40. Fernandez-Ruiz J, Bercendero F, Hernandez ML, et al. The endogenous cannabinoid system and brain development. Trends Neurosci 2000; 23:14.

41. Guzmán M, Galve-Roperh I, Sánchez C. Ceramide: a new second messenger of cannabinoid action. Trends Pharmacol Sci 2001; 22:19.

42. Downer E, Boland B, Fogarty M, et al. Delta-9-tetrahydrocannabinol induces the apoptotic pathway in cultured cortical neurons via activation of the CB1 receptor. Neuroreport 2001; 12:3973.

43. Guzman M, Sanchez C, Galve-Roperh I. Control of the cell survival/death decision by cannabinoids. J Mol Med 2001; 78:613.

44. Chan GC, Hinds TR, Impey S, et al. Hippocampal neurotoxicity of delta-9-tetrahydrocannabinol. J Neurosci 1998; 18:5322.

45. Fride E, Ginzburg Y, Brever A, et al. Critical role of the endogenous cannabinoid system in mouse pup suckling and growth. Eur J Pharmacol 2001; 419:207.

46. Iversen LL. The Science of Marijuana. Oxford: Oxford University Press, 2000.

47. Lichtman AH, Varvel SA, Martin BR. Endocannabinoids in cognition and dependence. Prostagland Leukotriene Essential Fatty Acids 2002; 66:269.

48. Hampson RE, Deadwyler SA. Role of cannabinoid receptors in memory storage. Neurobiol Dis 1998; 5:474.

49. Reibaud M, Obinu MC, Ledent C, et al. Enhancement of memory in cannabinoid CB1 receptor knockout mice. Eur J Pharmacol 1999; 379:R1.

50. Bohme GA, Laville M, Ledent C, et al. Enhanced long-term potentiation in mice lacking cannabinoid CB1 receptors. Neuroscience 2000; 95:5.

51. Marsicano G, Wotjak CT, Azad SC. The endogenous cannabinoid system controls extinction of aversive memories. Nature 2002; 418:530.

52. Varvel SA, Lichtman AH. Evaluation of CB1 receptor knockout mice in the Morris water maze. J Pharmacol Exp Ther 2002; 301:915.

53. Rodriguez de Fonseca F, Del Acco I, Martin-Calderón, et al. Role of the endogenous cannabinoid system in the regulation of motor activity. Neurobiol Dis 1998; 5:483.

54. Giuffrida A, Parsons LH, Kerr TM, et al. Dopamine activation of endogenous cannabinoid signaling in dorsal striatum. Nature Neurosci 1999; 2:358.

55. Kreitzer AC, Regehr WG. Retrograde inhibition of presynaptic calcium influx by endogenous cannabinoids at excitatory synapses onto Purkinje cells. Neuron 2001; 29:717.

56. Meng ID, Manning BH, Martin WJ, et al. An analgesia circuit activated by cannabinoids. Nature 1998; 395:381.

57. Calignano A, LaRana G, Giuffrida A, et al. Control of pain initiation by endogenous cannabinoids. Nature 1998; 394:227.

58. Fields HL, Meng ID. Watching the pot boil. Nat Med 1998; 4:1008.

59. DiMarzo V, Goparaju SK, Wang L, et al. Leptin-regulated endocannabinoids are involved in maintaining food intake. Nature 2001; 410:822.

60. Van Sickel MD, Oland LD, Ho W, et al. Cannabinoids inhibit emesis through CB, receptors in the brainstem of the ferret. Gastroenterology 2001; 121:767.

61. Hillard CJ. Endocannabinoids and vascular function. J Pharmacol Exp Ther 2000; 294:27.

62. Porter AC, Felder CC. The endocannabinoid nervous system: unique opportunities for therapeutic intervention. Pharmacol Ther 2001; 90:45.

62a. van der Stelt M, Velduis WB, Bar PR, et al. Neuroprotection by delta-9-tetrahydrocannabinol, the main active compound in marijuana, against ouabain-induced in vivo excitotoxicity. J Neurosci 2001; 21:6475.

62b. Marsicano G, Goodenough S, Monory K, et al. CB1 cannabinoid receptors and on-demand defense against excitotoxicity. Science 2003; 302:84. J Neurosci 2003; 302:84.

62c. Mechoulam R, Lichtman AH. Stout guards of the central nervous system. Science 2003; 302:65.

62d. Clement AB, Hawkins EG, Lichtman AH, et al. Increased seizure susceptibility and proconvulsant activity of anandamide in mice lacking fatty acid amide hydrolase. J Neuro Sci 2003; 23:3916

62e. Hansen HH, Azcoita I, Pons S, et al. Blockade of cannabinoid CB(1) receptor function protects against in vivo disseminating brain damage following NMDA-induced excitotoxicity. J Neurochem 2002; 82:154.

63. Breivogel CS, Childers SR. The functional neuroanatomy of brain cannabinoid receptors. Neurobiol Dis 1998; 5:417.

64. Fernandez-Ruiz J, Berrendero F, Hernández M, et al. The endogenous cannabinoid system and brain development. Trends Neurosci 2000; 23:14.

65. Song Z-H, Zhong M. CB1 cannabinoid receptor-mediated cell migration. J Pharmacol Exp Ther 2000; 294:204.

66. Maldonado R, Rodriguez de Fonseca F. Cannabinoid addiction: behavioral models and neural correlates. J Neurosci 2002; 22:3326.

67. Wiley JL, Martin BR. Effects of SR141716A on diazepam substitution for δ-9-tetrahydrocannabinol in rat drug discrimination. Pharmacol Biochem Behav 1999; 64:519.

68. Wiley JL. Cannabis: discrimination of "internal bliss." Pharmacol Biochem Behav 1999; 64:257.

69. Valjent E, Maldanado R. A behavioral model to reveal place preference to delta-9-tetrahydrocannabinol in mice. Psychopharmacology 2000; 147:436.

70. Ghozland S, Mathews H, Simonin F, et al. Motivational effects of cannabinoids are mediated by μ- and κ-opioid receptors. J Neurosci 2002; 22:1146.

71. Valjent E, Maldonado R. A behavioral model to reveal place preference to delta-9-tetrahydrocannabinol in mice. Psychopharmacology 2000; 147:436.

72. Gardner EL, Vorel ER. Cannabinoid transmission and reward-related events. Neurobiol Dis 1998; 5:502.

73. Tanda G, Munzar P, Goldberg SR. Self-administration behavior is maintained by the psychoactive ingredient of marijuana in squirrel monkeys. Nat Neurosci 2000; 3:1073.

74. Navarro M, Carrera MR, Fratta W, et al. Functional interaction between opioid and cannabinoid receptors in drug self-administration. J Neurosci 2001; 21:5344.

75. Fattore L, Cossu G, Martellotta CM, et al. Intravenous self-administration of the cannabinoid CB1 receptor agonist WIN55212-2 in rats. Psychopharmacology 2001; 156:410.

75a. Maldonado R: Study of cannabinoid dependence in animals. Pharmacol Ther 2002; 95:153.

75b. Justinova Z, Tanda G, Redhi GH, et al: Self-administration of delta-9-tetrahydrocannabinol (THC) by drug naïve squirrel monkeys. Psychopharmacology 2003; 169:135.

76. Ledent C, Valverde O, Cossu G, et al. Unresponsiveness to cannabinoids and reduced addictive effects of opiates in CB1 receptor knockout mice. Science 1999; 283:401.

77. Cadoni C, Pisanu A, Solinas M, et al. Behavioral sensitization after repeated exposure to delta-(9)-tetrahydrocannabinol and cross-sensitization with morphine. Psychopharmacology 2001; 158:259.

78. Pontieri FE, Monnazzi P, Scontrini A, et al. Behavioral sensitization to heroin by cannabinoid pretreatment in the rat. Eur J Pharmacol 2001; 421:R1.

79. DeVries TJ, Shaham Y, Homberg JR, et al. A cannabinoid mechanism in relapse to cocaine-seeking. Nat Med 2001; 7:1151.

80. Lamarque S, Taghzouti K, Simon H. Chronic treatment with delta-(9)-tetrahydrocannabinol enhances the locomotor response to amphetamine and heroin. Implications for vulnerability to drug addiction. Neuropharmacology 2001; 41:118.

81. Valjent E, Mitchell JM, Besson MJ, et al. Behavioral and biochemical evidence for interactions between delta-9-tetrahydrocannabinol and nicotine. Br J Pharmacol 2002; 135:564.

82. Castane A, Valjent E, Ledent C, et al. Lack of CB1 cannabinoid receptors modifies nicotine behavioral responses, but not nicotine abstinence. Neuropharmacology 2002; 43:857.

83. Hungund BL, Basavarajappa BS. Are anandamide and cannabinoid receptors involved in ethanol tolerance? A review of the evidence. Alcohol Alcoholism 2000; 35:126.

84. Bass CE, Martin BR. Time course for the induction and maintenance of tolerance to delta-9-tetrahydrocannabinol in mice. Drug Alcohol Depend 2000; 60:113.

85. Rubino T, Patrini G, Parenti G, et al. Chronic treatment with a synthetic cannabinoid CP55940 alters G-protein expression in the rat central nervous system. Mol Brain Res 1997; 44:191.

86. Valverde O, Maldonado R, Valjent E, et al. Cannabinoid withdrawal syndrome is reduced in pre-proenkephalin knock-out mice. J Neurosci 2000; 20:9284.

87. Aceto MD, Scates SM, Lowe JA, et al. Spontaneous and precipitated withdrawal with a synthetic cannabinoid, WIN55212-2. Eur J Pharmacol 2001; 416:75.

88. Aceto MD, Scates SM, Lowe JA, et al. Dependence on delta-9-tetrahydrocannabinol: studies on precipitated and abrupt withdrawal. J Pharmacol Exp Ther 1996; 278:1290.

89. Navarro M, Chowen J, Carrera MRA, et al. CB1 cannabinoid receptor antagonist-induced opiate withdrawal in morphine-dependent rats. Neuroreport 1998; 9:3397.

90. Litchtman AH, Sheikh HH, Loh SM, et al. Opioid and cannabinoid modulation of precipitated withdrawal in delta-tetrahydrocannabinol and morphine-dependent mice. J Pharmacol Exp Ther 2001; 298:1007.

91. Yamaguchi T, Hagiwara Y, Tanaka H, et al. Endogenous cannabinoid, 2-arachonoylglycerol, attenuates naloxone-precipitated withdrawal signs in morphine-dependent mice. Brain Res 2001; 909:121

92. Cui SS, Bowen RC, Gu GB, et al. Prevention of cannabinoid withdrawal syndrome by lithium: involvement of oxytocinergic neuronal activation. J Neurosci 2001; 21:9867.

93. Rodriguez de Fonseca F, Carrera MRA, Navarro M, et al. Activation of corticotropin-releasing factor in the limbic system during cannabinoid withdrawal. Science 1997; 276:2050.

94. Tzavara ET, Valjent E, Firmo C, et al. Cannabinoid withdrawal is dependent upon PKA activation in the cerebellum. Eur J Neurosci 2000; 12:1038.

95. Abel EL. Marijuana, The First Twelve Thousand Years. New York: Plenum Press, 1980.

96. Herodotus. The Histories. Book Four. Harmondsworth, UK: Penguin Books, 1954.

97. Brecher EM. Licit and Illicit Drugs. Boston: Little, Brown, 1972.

98. Rabelais F. The Histories of Gargantua and Pantagruel, Book Three. Harmondsworth, UK: Penguin Books, 1955.

99. Gautier T. Hachich. Revue des Deux Mondes, February 1, 1846. Reprinted in: Ebin D, ed. The Drug Experience. New York: Orion Press, 1961; 1.

100. Osler W, MacCrae T. Principles and Practice of Medicine, 8th edition. New York: D. Appleton, 1916; 1089.

101. Federal regulation of the medicinal use of cannabis (edit.). JAMA 1937; 108:1543.

102. Ungerleider JT. Marijuana: still a "signal of misunderstanding." Proc Assoc Am Phys 1999; 111:173.

103. Gruber AJ, Pope HG. Marijuana use among adolescents. Pediatr Clin North Am 2002; 49:389.

104. Smith DE, Heilig S, Seymour RB. Marijuana at the millennium: medical and social implications. J Psychoactive Drugs 1998; 30:123.

105. O'Malley PM, Bachman JG, Johnson LD. Period, age, and cohort effects on substance use among young Americans: a decade of change, 1976-86. Am J Public Health 1988; 78:1315.

106. Alcohol and other drug use among high school students—United States, 1990. MMWR 1991; 40:776.

107. Bachman JG, Wallace, JM, O'Malley PM, et al. Racial/ethnic differences in smoking, drinking, and illicit drug use among American high school seniors, 1976-89. Am J Public Health 1991; 81:372.

108. Bachman JG, Johnson LD, O'Malley PM. Explaining recent increases in students' marijuana use: impacts of perceived risks and disapproval, 1976 through 1996. Am J Public Health 1998; 88:887.

109. U.S. Department of Health and Human Services Substance Abuse and Mental Health Services Administration Office of Applied Studies. National Household Survey on Drug Abuse. U.S. Government Printing Office, 1999.

110. Johnson RA, Gerstein DR. Initiation of use of alcohol, cigarettes, marijuana, cocaine, and other substances in U.S. birth cohorts since 1919. Am J Public Health 1998; 88:27.

111. Johnston LD, O'Malley PM, Bachman JG. Monitoring the future national results on adolescent drug use: overview of key findings, 2000. NIH Publication No. 01-4923. Bethesda, MD: National Institute on Drug Abuse, 2001.

112. Schlosser E. The U.S. bucks a trend on marijuana laws. NY Times June 1, 2003.

113. Flynn K. Violent crimes undercut marijuana's mellow image. NY Times, May 19, 2001.

114. Friedman AS, Glassman K, Terras BA. Violent behavior as related to use of marijuana and other drugs. J Addict Dis 2001; 20:49.

115. MacCoun R, Reuter P. Evaluating alternative cannabis regimes. Br J Psychiatry 2001; 178:123.

116. Marijuana and Health. Ninth Annual Report to the U.S. Congress from the Secretary of Health and Human Services. Rockville, MD: NIDA, DHHS Publication No. (ADM) 82-1216, 1982.

117. Kandel DB, Logan JA. Patterns of drug use from adolescence to young adulthood. I. Periods of risk for initiation, continued use, and discontinuation. Am J Public Health 1984; 74:660.

118. Von Sydow K, Lieb R, Pfister H, et al. The natural course of cannabis use, abuse, and dependence over four years: a longitudinal community study of adolescents and young adults. Drug Alcohol Depend 2001; 64:347.

119. Anthony JC, Warner LA, Kessler RC. Comparative epidemiology of dependence on tobacco, alcohol, controlled substances, and inhalants: basic findings from the National Comorbidity Study. Clin Exp Psychopharmacol 1994; 2:244.

120. Budney AJ, Novy PL, Hughes JR. Marijuana withdrawal among adults seeking treatment for marijuana dependence. Addiction 1999; 94:1311.

121. Swift W, Copeland J, Hall W. Choosing a diagnostic cutoff for cannabis dependence. Addiction 1998; 93:1681.

122. Swift W, Hall W, Copeland J. One-year follow-up of cannabis dependence among long-term users in Sydney, Australia. Drug Alcohol Depend 2000; 59:309.

123. Lieberman CM, Lieberman BW. Marihuana-a medical review. N Engl J Med 1971; 284:88.

124. Weil AT, Zineberg NE, Nelsen JM. Clinical and psychological effects of marijuana in man. Science 1968; 162:1234.

125. Otten EJ. Marijuana. In: Goldfrank LR, Flomenbaum NE, Lewin NA, et al., eds. Goldfrank's Toxicologic Emergencies, 6th edition. Stamford, CT: Appleton Lange, 1998; 1121.

126. Borg J, Gershon S. Dose effects of smoked marihuana on human cognitive and motor functions. Psychopharmacologia 1975; 42:211.

127. Milstein SL, MacCannell KL, Karr G, Clark S. Marijuana-produced changes in cutaneous sensitivity and affect: users and non-users. Pharmacol Biochem Behav 1974; 2:367.

128. Moskowitz H, McGlothlin W. Effects of marijuana on auditory signal detection. Psychopharmacologia 1974; 40:137.

129. Adams AJ, Brown B, Flom MC, et al. Alcohol and marijuana effects on static visual acuity. Am J Optom Physiol Opt 1975; 52:729.

130. Brown B, Adams AJ, Hagerstrom-Portnoy G, et al. Effects of alcohol and marijuana on dynamic

visual acuity. I. Threshold measurements. Percept Psychophysiol 1975; 18:441.

131. Clopton PL, Janowsky DS, Clopton JM, et al. Marihuana and the perception of affect. Psychopharmacology 1979; 61:203.

132. Keeler MH, Moore E. Paranoid reactions while using marijuana. Dis Nerv Syst 1974; 35:535.

133. Sharma S, Moskowitz H. Effects of two levels of attention demand on vigilance performance under marijuana. Percept Motor Skills 1974; 38:967.

134. Roth WT, Rosenbloom M J, Darley CF, et al. Marijuana effects on TAT form and content. Psychopharmacologia 1975; 43:261.

134a. Stracciari A, Guarino M, Crespi C, et al. Transient amnesia triggered by acute marijuana intoxication. Eur J Neurol 1999; 66:521.

135. Belmore SM, Miller LL. Levels of processing acute effects of marijuana on memory. Pharmacol Biochem Behav 1980; 13:199.

136. Melges FT, Tinklenberg JR, Hollister LE, Gillespie HK. Marijuana and the temporal span of awareness. Arch Gen Psychiatry 1971; 24:564.

137. Klonhoff H, Low M, Marcus A. Neuropsychological effects of marijuana. Can Med Assoc J 1973; 108:150.

138. Heishman SJ, Huestis MA, Henningfield JE, Cone EJ. Acute and residual effects of marijuana: profiles of plasma THC levels, physiological, subjective and performance measures. Pharmacol Biochem Behav 1990; 37:561.

139. Janowsky DS, Meacham MP, Blaine JD, et al. Marijuana effects on simulated flying ability. Am J Psychiatry 1976; 133:384.

140. Kvalseth TO. Effects of marijuana on human reaction time and motor control. Percept Motor Skills 1977; 45:935.

141. Schaefer CF, Cunn CG, Dubowski KM. Marihuana dosage control through heart rate. N Engl J Med 1975; 293:101.

142. Bachman JA, Benowitz NL, Herning RI, Jones RT. Dissociation of autonomic and cognitive effects of THC in man. Psychopharmacology 1979; 61:171.

143. Hollister LE. Interactions in man of delta-9-tetrahydrocannabinol. I. Alphamethylparatyrosine. Clin Pharmacol Ther 1974; 15:18.

144. Markianos M, Vakis A. Effects of acute cannabis use on urinary neurotransmitter metabolites and cyclic nucleotides in man. Drug Alcohol Depend 1984; 14:175.

145. Tashkin DP, Soares JR, Hepler RS, et al. Cannabis, 1977. Ann Intern Med 1978; 89:539.

146. Tassinari CA, Peraita-Adrados MR, Ambrosetto G, Gastaut H. Effects of marijuana and delta-9-THC at high doses in man. A polygraphic study. Electroencephalogr Clin Neurophysiol 1974; 36:94.

147. Fink M, Volavka J, Panagiotopoulos CP, Stafanis C. Quantitative EEG studies of marijuana, delta-9-THC and hashish in man. In: Braude MC, Szara S, eds.

Pharmacology of Marijuana. New York: Raven Press, 1976:383.

148. Herning RI, Jones RT, Peltzman DJ. Changes in human event related potentials with prolonged delta-9-tetrahydrocannabinol (THC) use. Electroencephalogr Clin Neurophysiol 1979; 47:556.

149. Heath RG. Marijuana effects on deep and surface electroencephalographs of man. Arch Gen Psychiatry 1972; 26:577.

150. Heath RG. Marihuana and delta-9-THC: acute and chronic effects on brain function of monkeys. In: Braude M, Szara S, eds. Pharmacology of Marihuana. New York: Raven Press, 1976; 345.

151. O'Leary DS, Block RI, Koeppel JA, et al. Effects of smoking marijuana on brain perfusion and cognition. Neuropsychopharmacology 2002; 26:802.

152. Huestis MA, Gorelick DA, Heishman SJ, et al. Blockade of effects of smoked marijuana by the CB1-selective cannabinoid receptor antagonist SR141716. Arch Gen Psychiatry 2001; 58:30.

153. Bromberg W. Marijuana intoxication. Am J Psychiatry 1934; 91:303.

154. Levi L, Miller NR. Visual illusions associated with previous drug abuse. J Clin Neuroophthalmol 1990; 10:103.

155. Ludlow F. The Hasheesh Eater: Being Passages from the Life of a Pythagorean, 1857. Reprinted in: Ebin D, ed. The Drug Experience. New York: Orion Press, 1961.

156. West ME. Cannabis and night vision. Nature 1991; 351:703

157. Benowitz NL, Jones RT. Cardiovascular effects of prolonged delta-9-tetrahydrocannabinol ingestion. Clin Pharmacol Ther 1975; 18:287.

158. Heyndrickx A, Scheiris C, Schepens P. Toxicological study of a fatal intoxication in man due to cannabis smoking. J Pharm Belg 1970; 24:37.

159. Gourves J, Viallard C, LeLuan D, et al. Case of coma due to Cannabis sativa. Presse Med 1971; 79:1389.

160. Bro P, Shou J, Topp G. Cannabis poisoning with analytical verification. N Engl J Med 1975; 293:1049.

161. Boros CA, Parsons DW, Zoanetti GD, et al. Cannabis cookies: a cause of coma. J Pediatr Child Health 1996; 32:194.

162. Lopez HH, Goldman SM, Liberman II, Barnes DT. Cannabis-accidental peroral intoxication. JAMA 1974; 227:1041.

163. Weil AT. Adverse reactions to marijuana: classification and suggested treatment. N Engl J Med 1970; 282:997.

164. Imade AG, Ebie JC. A retrospective study of symptom patterns of cannabis-induced psychosis. Acta Psychiatr Scand 1991; 83:134.

165. Wylie AS, Scott RTA, Burnett SJ. Psychosis due to "skunk." BMJ 1995; 311:125.

166. Thacore VR, Shukla SRP. Cannabis psychosis and paranoid schizophrenia. Arch Gen Psychiatry 1976; 33:383.

167. Rubin V, Comitas L. Ganja in Jamaica: A Medical Anthropological Study of Chronic Marijuana Use. The Hague: Mouton, 1975.

168. Thornicroft G. Cannabis and psychosis. Is there epidemiological evidence for an association? Br J Psychiatry 1990; 157:25.

169. Treffert DA. Marijuana use in schizophrenia: a clear hazard. Am J Psychiatry 1978; 135:1213.

170. Ablon SL, Goodwin FK. High frequency of dysphoric reactions to tetrahydrocannabinol among depressed patients. Am J Psychiatry 1974; 131:448.

171. Knudson P, Vilmar T. Cannabis and neuroleptic agents in schizophrenia. Acta Psychiatr Scand 1984; 69:162.

172. Binitie A. Psychosis following ingestion of hemp in children. Psychopharmacologia 1975; 44:301.

173. Harding T, Knight F. Marijuana-modified mania. Arch Gen Psychiatry 1973; 29:635.

174. Stoll AL, Cole JO, Lukas SF. A case of mania as a result of fluoxetine–marijuana interaction. J Clin Psychiatry 1991; 52:280.

175. Earlywine M. Cannabis-induced Koro in Americans. Addiction 2001; 96:1663.

176. Rottanburg D, Robins AH, Ben-Arie O, et al. Cannabis-associated behavior with hypomanic features. Lancet 1982; II:1364.

177. Palsson A, Thulin SO, Tunving KK. Cannabis psychosis in South Sweden. Acta Psychiatr Scand 1982; 66:311.

178. Keeler M, Reifler CB, Lipzin MB. Spontaneous recurrence of marijuana effect. Am J Psychiatry 1968; 125:384.

179. Stanton MD, Mintz J, Franklin RM. Drug flashbacks. II. Some additional findings. Int J Addict 1976; 11:53.

180. Niveau G. Cannabis-related flash-back, a medico-legal case. Encephale 2002; 28:77.

181. Andreasson S, Allebeck P, Eugstrom A, Rydberg U. Cannabis and schizophrenia: a longitudinal study of Swedish conscripts. Lancet 1987; II:1483.

182. Khantzian EJ, McKenna GJ. Acute toxic and withdrawal reactions associated with drug use and abuse. Ann Intern Med 1979; 90:361.

183. Chaudry HR, Moss HB, Bashir A, Suliman T. Cannabis psychosis following bhang ingestion. Br J Addict 1991; 86:1075.

184. Agurell S, Halldin M, Lindgren J-E, et al. Pharmacokinetics and metabolism of delta-1-tetrahydrocannabinol and other cannabinoids with emphasis on man. Pharmacol Rev 1986; 38:21.

185. Busto U, Bendayan R, Sellers EM. Clinical pharmacokinetics of non-opiate abused drugs. Clin Pharmacokinet 1989; 16:1.

186. Morgan JP. Marijuana metabolism in the context of urine testing for cannabinoid metabolites. J Psychoactive Drugs 1988; 20:107.

187. Tormey WP. Consequences of using legal hemp products. Clin Toxicol 1999; 37:899.

188. Meier H, Vonesch HJ. Cannabis poisoning after eating salad. Schweiz Med Wochenschr 1997; 127:214.

189. Jones RT, Benowitz N. The 30-day trip-clinical studies of cannabis tolerance and dependence. In: Braude MC, Szara S, eds. Pharmacology of Marihuana. New York: Raven Press, 1976; 627.

190. Tennant FS, Groesback CJ. Psychiatric effects of hashish. Arch Gen Psychiatry 1972; 27:133.

191. Jones RT. Marijuana-induced "high": influence of expectation, setting, and previous drug experience. Pharmacol Rev 1971; 23:359.

192. Tsuang MT, Harley RM, et al. The Harvard Twin Study of Substance Abuse: what we have learned. Harvard Rev Psychiatry 2001, 9:267.

193. Kendler KS, Neale MC, Thornton LM, et al. Cannabis use in the last year in a U.S. national sample of twin and sibling pairs. Psychol Med 2002; 32:551.

194. Miles DR, van den Bree MB, Pickens RW. Sex differences in shared genetic and environmental influences between conduct disorder symptoms and marijuana use in adolescents. Am J Med Genet 2002; 114:159.

195. Comings DE, Muhleman D, Gade R, et al. Cannabinoid receptor gene (CNR1): association with i.v. drug use. Mol Psychiatry 1997; 2:161.

195a. Sipe JC, Chiang K, Gerber AL, et al. A missense mutation in human fatty acid amide hydrolase associated with problem drug use. Proc Natl Acad Sci USA 2002; 99:8394.

196. Tsuang MT, Lyons MJ, Meyer JM, et al. Co-occurrence of abuse of different drugs in men: the role of drug-specific and shared vulnerabilities. Arch Gen Psychiatry 1998; 55:967.

196a. Bierut LJ, Dinwiddie SH, Begleiter H, et al. Familial transmission of substance dependence: alcohol, marijuana, cocaine, and habitual smoking. A report from the Collaborative Study on the Genetics of Alcoholism. Arch Gen Psychiatry 1998; 55:982.

197. Kaymakcalan S. Tolerance to and dependence on cannabis. Bull Narc 1973; 25:39.

197a. Bensusan SD. Marijuana withdrawal symptoms. BMJ 1971; I:112.

198. Mendelson JH, Mello NK, Lex BW, Bavli S. Marijuana withdrawal syndrome in a woman. Am J Psychiatry 1984; 141:1289.

199. Hollister LE. Health aspects of cannabis. Pharmacol Rev 1986; 38:1.

200. Wiesbeck GA, Schukit MA, Kalmign JA, et al. An evaluation of the history of a marijuana withdrawal syndrome in a large population. Addiction 1996; 91:1469.

201. Stephens RS, Roffman RA, Simpson EE. Adult marijuana users seeking treatment. J Consult Clin Psychol 1993; 61:1100.

201a. Budney AJ, Hughes JR, Moore BA, et al. Marijuana abstinence effects in marijuana smokers maintained in their home environment. Arch Gen Psychiatry 2001; 58:917.

202. Haney M, Ward AS, Comer SD, et al. Abstinence symptoms following smoked marijuana in humans. Psychopharmacology 1999; 141:385.

203. Kouri EM, Pope HG, Lukas SE. Changes in aggressive behavior during withdrawal from long-term marijuana use. Psychopharmacology 1999; 143:302.

204. Ashton CH. Pharmacology and effects of cannabis: a brief review. Br J Psychiatry 2001; 178:101.

205. Smith NT. A review of the published literature into cannabis withdrawal symptoms in human users. Addiction 2002; 97:621.

206. Miller NS, Klahr AL, Gold MS, et al. The prevalence of marijuana (cannabis) use and dependence in cocaine dependence. N Y State J Med 1990; 90:491.

207. Saxon AJ, Calsyn DA, Blaes PA, et al. Marijuana use by methadone maintenance patients. In: Harris L, ed. Problems of Drug Dependence 1990. NIDA Res Monogr 1991; 105:306.

208. Miller NS, Giannini AJ. Drug misuse in alcoholics. Int J Addict 1991; 26:851.

209. MacAvoy MG, Marks DF. Divided attention performance of cannabis users and non-users following cannabis and alcohol. Psychopharmacologia 1975; 44:147.

210. Dalton WS, Martz R, Lemberger L, et al. Effects of marijuana combined with secobarbital. Clin Pharmacol Ther 1975; 18:298.

211. Johnstone RE, Lief PL, Kulp RA, Smith TC. Combination of delta-9-tetrahydrocannabinol with oxymorphone or pentobarbital: effects on ventilatory control and cardiovascular dynamics. Anesthesiology 1974; 42:674.

212. Wachtel SR, deWit H. Naltrexone does not block the subjective effects of oral delta(9)-tetrahydrocannabinol in humans. Drug Alcohol Depend 2000; 59:251.

213. Weiner AL. Emerging drugs of abuse in Connecticut. Conn Med 2000; 64:19.

214. Holland JA, Nelson L, Ravikumar PR, et al. Embalming fluid-soaked marijuana: new high or new guise for PCP? J Psychoactive Drugs 1998; 30:215.

215. Reid MJ, Bornheim LM. Cannabinoid-induced alterations in brain disposition of drugs of abuse. Biochem Pharmacol 2001; 61:1357.

216. Golub A, Johnson BD. Variation in youthful risks of progression from alcohol and tobacco to marijuana and to hard drugs across generations. Am J Public Health 2001; 91:225.

217. Kandel DB. Does marijuana use cause the use of other drugs? JAMA 2003; 289:482.

218. Lynskey MT, Heath AC, Bucholz KK, et al. Escalation of drug use in early-onset cannabis users vs co-twin controls. JAMA 2003; 289:427.

219. Weinrieb RM, O'Brien CP. Persistent cognitive deficits attributed to substance abuse. In: Brust JCM, ed. Neurological Complications of Drug and Alcohol Abuse. Neurol Clin 1993; 11:66.

220. Pope HG, Gruber AJ, Yurgelun-Todd D. The residual neuropsychological effects of cannabis: the current status of research. Drug Alcohol Depend 1995; 38:25.

221. Kolansky H, Moore WT. Marijuana: can it hurt you? JAMA 1975; 232:923.

222. Cohen S. Adverse effects of marijuana: selected issues. Ann N Y Acad Sci 1981; 362:119.

223. Campbell AMG, Evans M, Thomson JLG, Williams MJ. Cerebral atrophy in young cannabis smokers. Lancet 1971; II:1219.

224. Mendelson J, Meyere R. Behavioral and biological concomitants of chronic marijuana use by heavy and casual users. In: National Commission on Marijuana and Drug Abuse: Marijuana: A Signal of Misunderstanding, Appendix, Vol 1. Washington, DC: U.S. Government Printing Office, 1972:68.

225. Beaubrun MH, Knight F. Psychiatric assessment of 30 chronic users of cannabis and 30 matched controls. Am J Psychiatry 1973; 130:309.

226. Culver CM, King FW. Neuropsychological assessment of undergraduate marijuana and LSD users. Arch Gen Psychiatry 1974; 31:707.

227. Connell PH, Dorn N, eds. Cannabis and Man. New York: Churchill Livingstone, 1975.

228. Bruhn P, Maage N. Intellectual and neuropsychological functions in young men with heavy and long-term patterns of drug abuse. Am J Psychiatry 1975; 132:397.

229. Satz R, Fletcher JM, Sutker L. Neuropsychological, intellectual, and personality correlates of marijuana use in native Costa Ricans. Ann N Y Acad Sci 1976; 282:266.

230. Co BT, Goodwin DW, Gado M, et al. Absence of cerebral atrophy in chronic cannabis users by computerized transaxial tomography. JAMA 1977; 237:1299.

231. Kuchnle J, Mendelson JH, Davis KR, New PFJ. Computerized tomographic examination of heavy marijuana smokers. JAMA 1977; 237:1231.

232. Carter WE. Cannabis in Costa Rica. Philadelphia: ISHI Press, 1980.

233. Hannertz J, Hinmarsh T. Neurological and neuroradiological examination of chronic cannabis smokers. Ann Neurol 1983; 13:207.

233a. Fletcher JM, Page JB, Francis DJ, et al. Cognitive correlates of long-term cannabis use in Costa Rican men. Arch Gen Psychiatry 1996; 53:1051.

233b. Lyketsos CG, Garreett E, Liang K-Y, et al. Cannabis use and cognitive decline in persons under 65 years of age. Am J Epidemiol 1999; 149:794.

234. Kolansky H, Moore WT. Toxic effects of chronic marijuana use. JAMA 1972; 222:35.

235. Cohen S, Lessin PJ, Hahn PM, Tyrell ED. A 94-day cannabis study. In: Braude MC, Szara S, eds. Pharmacology of Marihuana. New York: Raven Press, 1976:621.

236. Soueif MI. Chronic cannabis users: further analysis of objective test results. Bull Narc 1975; 27:1.

237. Miles CG, Congreve GRS, Gibbins RJ, et al. An experimental study of the effects of daily cannabis smoking on behavior patterns. Acta Pharmacol Toxicol 1974; 34 (Suppl 1):l.

238. Sharma BP. Cannabis and its users in Nepal. Br J Psychiatry 1975; 127:550.

239. Mendelson JH, Koehnle JC, Greenberg I, Mello N. The effects of marijuana use on human operant behavior; individual data. In: Braude M, Szara S, eds. Pharmacology of Marihuana. New York: Raven Press, 1976:643.

240. Goode E. The criminogenics of marijuana. Addict Dis 1974; 1:279.

241. Block RI, Farnham S, Braverman K, et al. Long-term marijuana use and subsequent effects on learning and cognitive functions related to school achievement: preliminary study. NIDA Res Monogr 1990;101:96.

242. Schwartz RH, Gruenewald PJ, Klitzner M, Fedio P. Short-term memory impairment in cannabis-dependent adolescents. Am J Dis Child 1989; 143:1214.

243. Pope HG, Yurgelun-Todd D. The residual cognitive effects of heavy marijuana use in college students. JAMA 1996; 275:521.

244. Pope HG, Gruber AJ, Hudson JI, et al. Neuropsychological performance in long-term cannabis users. Arch Gen Psychiatry 2001; 5:909.

245. Fried P, Watkinson B, James D, Gray R. Current and former marijuana use: preliminary findings in a longitudinal study of effects on IQ in young adults. Can Med Assoc J 2002; 166:887.

246. Block RI, Ghoneim MM. Effects of chronic marijuana use on human cognition. Psychopharmacology 1993; 110:219.

247. Solowij N, Stephens RS, Roffman RA, et al. Cognitive functioning of long-term heavy cannabis users seeking treatment. JAMA 2002; 287:1123.

248. Pope HG. Cannabis, cognition, and residual confounding. JAMA 2002; 287:1172.

249. Ehrenreich H, Rinn T, Kunert JH, et al. Specific attentional dysfunction in adults following early start of cannabis use. Psychopharmacology 1999; 142:295.

250. Hart CL, Gorp W, Haney M, et al: Effects of acute smoked marijuana on complex cognitive performance. Neuropsychopharmacology 2001; 25:757.

251. Chait LD. Subjective and behavioral effects of marijuana the morning after smoking. Psychopharmacology 1990; 100:328.

252. Bolla KI, Brown K, Eldreth D, et al. Dose-related neurocognitive effects of marijuana use. Neurology 2002; 59:1337.

253. Koppel BS. Heavy marijuana use: the price of getting high. Neurology 2002; 59:1295.

254. Solowij N, Michie PT, Fox AM. Effects of long term cannabis use on selective attention: an event-related potential study. Pharmacol Biochem Behav 1991; 40:683.

255. Loeber RT, Yurgelun-Todd DA. Human neuroimaging of acute and chronic marijuana use: implications for frontocerebellar dysfunction. Hum Psychopharmacol Clin Exp 1999; 14:291.

256. Block RI, O'Leary DS, Hichwa RD, et al. Cerebellar hypoactivity in frequent marijuana users. Neuroreport 2000; 11:749.

257. Wilson W, Mathew R, Turkington T, et al. Brain morphological changes and early marijuana use: a magnetic resonance and positron emission tomography study. J Addict Dis 2000; 19:1.

257a. Block RI, O'Leary DS, Augustinack JC, et al. Effects of frequent marijuana use on attention related regional cerebral blood flow. Abstr Soc Neurosci 2000; 26:2080.

258. Presburger G, Robinson JK. Spatial signal detection in rats is differentially disrupted by delta-9-tetrahydrocannabinol, scopolamine, and MK-801. Behav Brain Res 1999; 99:27.

259. Lawston J, Borella A, Robinson JK, et al. Changes in hippocampal morphology following chronic treatment with the synthetic cannabinoid WIN 55, 212-2. Brain Res 2000; 877:407.

260. Varvel SA, Hamm RJ, Martin BR, et al. Differential effects of delta-9-THC on spatial reference and working memory in mice. Psychopharmacology 2001; 157:147.

261. Westlake TM, Howlett AC, Ali SF, et al. Chronic exposure to delta-9-tetrahydrocannabinol fails to irreversibly alter brain cannabinoid receptors. Brain Res 1991; 544:145.

262. Johns A. Psychiatric effects of cannabis. Br J Psychiatry 2001; 178:116.

262a. Verdoux H, Gindre C, Sorbara F, et al. Effects of cannabis and psychosis vulnerability in daily life: an experience sampling test study. Psychol Med 2003; 33:23.

262b. Fergusson DM, Horwood LJ, Swain-Campbell NR. Cannabis dependence and psychotic symptoms in young people. Psychol Med 2003; 33:15.

263. Roy JM, Tennant CC. Cannabis and mental health. More evidence establishes clear link between use of cannabis and psychiatric illness. BMJ 2002; 325:1183.

264. Bovasso GB. Cannabis abuse as a risk factor for depressive symptoms. Am J Psychiatry 2001; 158:2033.

265. Brook DW, Brook JS, Zhang C, et al. Drug use and the risk of major depressive disorder, alcohol dependence, and substance use disorders. Arch Gen Psychiatry 2002; 59:1039.

266. Patton GC, Caffey C, Carlin JB, et al. Cannabis use and mental health in young people: cohort study. BMJ 2002; 325:1195.

267. Tsai SJ, Wang YC, Hong CJ. Association study between cannabinoid receptor gene (CNR-1) and pathogenesis and psychotic symptoms of mood disorders. Am J Med Genet 2001; 105:219.

268. Voruganti LN, Slomka P, Zabel P, et al. Cannabis-induced dopamine release: an in-vivo SPECT study. Psychiatry Res 2001; 107:173.

269. Arseneault L, Cannon M, Poulton R, et al. Cannabis use in adolescence and risk for adult psychosis: longitudinal prospective study. BMJ 2002; 325:1212.

270. Zammit S, Allebeck P, Andreasson S, et al. Self-reported cannabis use as a risk factor for schizophrenia in Swedish conscripts of 1969; historical cohort study. BMJ 2002; 325:1199.

271. van Os J, Bak M, Hanssen M, et al: Cannabis use and psychosis: a longitudinal population-based study. Am J Epidemiol 2002; 156:319.

272. Bersani G, Orlandi V, Kotzalidis GD, et al. Cannabis and schizophrenia: impact on onset, course, psychopathology and outcomes. Eur Arch Psychiatry Clin Neurosci 2002; 252:86.

273. McGee R, Williams S, Poulton R, et al. A longitudinal study of cannabis use and mental health from adolescence to early adulthood. Addiction 2000; 95:491.

274. Leroy S, Griffon N, Bourdel MC, et al. Schizophrenia and the cannabinoid receptor type 1 (CB1): association study using single-base polymorphism in coding exon 1. Am J Med Genet 2001; 105:749.

275. Dean B, Sundram S, Bradbury R, et al. Studies on [3H]CP-55940 binding in the human central nervous system: regional specific changes in density of cannabinoid-1 receptors associated with schizophrenia and cannabis use. Neuroscience 2001; 103:9.

276. Degenhardt L, Hall W. Cannabis and psychosis. Curr Psychiatry Rep 2002; 4:191.

277. Taylor DR, Ferguson DM, Milne BJ. A longitudinal study of the effects of tobacco and cannabis exposure on lung function in young adults. Addiction 2002; 97:1055.

278. Tashkin DP. Airway effects of marijuana, cocaine, and other inhaled illicit agents. Curr Opin Pulm Med 2001; 7:43.

279. Sparacino CM, Hyldburg PA, Hughes TJ. Chemical and biological analysis of marijuana smoke condensate. NIDA Res Monogr 1990; 99:121.

280. Hazovard E, Koninck JC, Attucci S, et al. Pneumorachis and pneumomediastinum caused by repeated Muller's maneuvers: complications of marijuana smoking. Ann Emerg Med 2001; 38:694.

281. World Health Organization Programme on Substance Abuse. Cannabis: a health perspective and research agenda. Geneva: WHO, 1997.

282. Hall W. The respiratory risks of cannabis smoking. Addiction 1998; 93:1461.

283. Fergeson RP. Metastatic lung cancer in a young marijuana smoker. JAMA 1989; 261:41.

284. Donald PJ. Advanced malignancy in the young marijuana smoker. Adv Exp Med Biol 1991; 288:33.

285. Almadori G, Palutetti G, Cerullo M, et al. Marijuana smoking as a possible cause of tongue carcinoma in young patients. J Laryngol Otol 1990; 104:896.

286. Hall W, MacPhee D. Cannabis and cancer: Addiction 2002; 97:243-247.

287. Mao Li, Oh Y. Does marijuana or crack cocaine cause cancer? J Natl Cancer Inst 1998; 90:1182.

288. Zhang ZF, Morgenstern H, Spitz MR, et al. Marijuana use and increased risk of squamous cell carcinoma of the head and neck. Cancer Epidemiol Biomark Prev 1999; 8:1071.

289. Wu T-C, Tashkin DP, Djahed B, Rose JE. Pulmonary hazards of smoking marijuana as compared with tobacco. N Engl J Med 1988; 318:347.

290. Baris YI, Tan E, Kalyoncu F, et al. Digital clubbing in hashish addicts. Chest 1990; 98:1545.

291. Nicholi AM. The nontherapeutic use of psychoactive drugs. A modern epidemic. N Engl J Med 1983; 308:925.

292. Levitz SM, Diamond RD. Aspergillosis and marijuana. Ann Intern Med 1991; 115:578.

293. Denning DW, Follansbee SE, Scolaro M, et al. Pulmonary aspergillosis in the acquired immunodeficiency syndrome. N Engl J Med 1991; 324:654.

294. Taylor DN, Wachsmuth IK, Shangkuan Y-H, et al. Salmonellosis associated with marijuana. N Engl J Med 1982; 306:1249.

295. Ramirez RJ. Acute pulmonary histoplasmosis: newly recognized hazard of marijuana plant hunters. Am J Med 1990; 88:60N.

296. Liskow B, Liss JL, Parker CW. Allergy to marijuana. Ann Intern Med 1971; 85:571.

297. Boyce SH, Quigley MA. Uvulitis and partial upper airway obstruction following cannabis inhalation. Emerg Med 2002; 14:106.

298. Kew MC, Bersohn L, Siew S. Possible hepatotoxicity of cannabis. Lancet 1969; I:578.

299. Tennant FS, Preble M, Prendergast TJ, Ventry P. Medical manifestations associated with hashish. JAMA 1971; 216:1965.

300. Sterne J, Ducasting C. Les arterites du cannabis indica. Arch Mal Coeur 1960; 53:143.

301. Disdier P, Granel B, Serratrice J, et al. Cannabis arteritis revisited–ten new case reports. Angiology 2001; 52:505.

302. Watzl B, Scuderi P, Watson RR. Influence of marijuana components (THC and CBD) on human mononuclear cell cytokine secretion in vitro. Adv Exp Med Biol 1991; 288:63.

303. Specter S, Lancz G. Effects of marijuana on human natural killer cell activity. Adv Exp Med Biol 1991; 288:47.

304. Klein TW, Friedman H, Specter S. Marijuana, immunity, and infection. J Neuroimmunol 1998; 83:102.

305. Coates RA, Farewell VT, Rabovd J, et al. Cofactors of progression to acquired immunodeficiency syndrome in a cohort of male sexual contacts of men with human immunodeficiency virus disease. Am J Epidemiol 1990; 132:717.

306. DiFranco MJ, Sheppard HW, Hunter DJ, et al. The lack of association of marijuana and other recreational drugs with progression to AIDS in the San Francisco Men's Health Study. Ann Epidemiol 1996; 6:283.

307. Hall W, Solowij N, Lemon J. The Health Consequences of Cannabis Use. National Drug Strategy Monograph Series No. 25. Canberra: Australian Government Publishing Service, 1994.

308. Bayer CB, Shafer MA, Teitle E, et al. Sexually transmitted diseases in a health maintenance organization teen clinic: associations of race, partner's age, and marijuana use. Arch Pediatr Adolesc Med 1999; 153:838.

309. Shaw DD, Whiteman DC, Merritt AD, et al. Hepatitis A outbreaks among illicit drug users and their contacts in Queensland, 1997. Med J Aust 1999; 170:584.

310. Copeland KC, Underwood LC, Van Wyk JJ. Marijuana smoking and pubertal arrest. J Pediatr 1980; 96:1079.

311. Benowitz NL, Jones RT, Lerner CB. Depression of growth hormone and cortisol response to insulin-induced hypoglycemia after prolonged oral delta-9-tetrahydrocannabinol administration in man. J Clin Endocrinol Metab 1976; 42:938.

312. Harclerode J. Endocrine effects of marijuana in the male: preclinical studies. In: Braude MC, Ludford JP, eds. Marijuana Effects on the Endocrine and Reproductive Systems. NIDA Res Monogr 1984; 44:46.

313. Rettori V, Aguila MC, Gimeno MF, et al. In vitro effect of delta-9-tetrahydrocannabinol to stimulate somatostatin release and block that of luteinizing hormone-releasing hormone by suppression of the release of prostaglandin E2. Proc Natl Acad Sci USA 1990; 87:10063.

314. Mendelson JH, Ellingboe J, Mello NK. Acute effects of natural and synthetic cannabis compounds on prolactin levels in human males. Pharmacol Biochem Behav 1984; 20:103.

315. Dax EM, Pilotte NS, Adler WH, et al. Short-term delta-9-tetrahydrocannabinol (THC) does not affect neuroendocrine or immune parameters. NIDA Res Monogr 1990: 105:567.

316. Block RI, Farinpour R, Schlechte JA. Effects of chronic marijuana use on testosterone, luteinizing hormone, follicle stimulating hormone, prolactin and cortisol in men and women. Drug Alcohol Depend 1991; 28:121.

317. Aronow WS, Cassidy J. Effect of smoking marijuana and of a high-nicotine cigarette on angina pectoris. Clin Pharmacol Ther 1975; 17:549.

318. MacInnes DC, Miller KM. Fatal coronary artery thrombosis associated with cannabis smoking. J R Coll Gen Pract 1984; 34:575.

318a. Bachs L, Marland H. Acute cardiovascular fatalities following cannabis use. Forensic Sci Int 2001; 124:200.

319. Mittleman MA, Lewis RA, Maclure M, et al. Triggering myocardial infarction by marijuana. Circulation 2001; 103:2805.

320. McLeod AL, McKenna CJ, Northridge DB. Myocardial infarction following the combined recreational use of Viagra and cannabis. Clin Cardiol 2002; 25:133.

321. Gupta BD, Jani CB, Shah PH. Fatal "Bhang" poisoning. Med Sci Law 2001; 41:349.

322. Singh GK. Atrial fibrillation associated with marijuana use. Pediatr Cardiol 2000; 21:284.

323. Kosier DA, Filipiak KJ, Stolarz P, et al. Paroxysmal atrial fibrillation following marijuana intoxication: two-case report of possible association. Int J Cardiol 2001; 78:183.

324. Lambrecht GL, Malbrain MC, Coremans P, et al. Acute renal infarction and heavy marijuana smoking. Nephron 1995; 70:494.

325. Mohan H, Sood GC. Conjugate deviation of the eyes after cannabis intoxication. Br J Ophthalmol 1964; 48:160.

326. Garrett CP, Braithwaite RA, Teale JD. Unusual case of tetrahydrocannabinol intoxication confirmed by radioimmunoassay. BMJ 1977; II:166.

327. Wilkins MR, Kendall MJ. Stroke affecting young men after alcoholic binges. BMJ 1985; 291:1392.

328. Cooles P. Stroke after heavy cannabis smoking. Postgrad Med J 1987; 63:511.

329. Zachariah SB. Stroke after heavy marijuana smoking. Stroke 1991; 22:406.

330. Mesec A, Rot U, Grad A. Cerebrovascular disease associated with marijuana abuse: a case report. cerebrovasc Dis 2001; 11:284.

331. Barnes D, Palace J, O'Brien MD. Stroke following marijuana smoking. Stroke 1992; 23:1381.

332. Lawson TM, Rees A. Stroke and transient ischaemic attacks in association with substance abuse in a young man. Postgrad Med J 1996; 72:692.

333. White D, Martin D, Geller T, et al. Stroke associated with marijuana abuse. Pediatr Neurosurg 2000; 32:92.

334. Alvaro LC, Iriondo I, Villaverde FJ. Sexual headache and stroke in a heavy cannabis smoker. Headache 2002; 42:224.

335. Marinella MA. Stroke after marijuana smoking in a teenager with factor V Leiden mutation. South Med Assoc J 2001; 94:1217.

336. McCarron MO, Thomas AM. Cannabis and alcohol in stroke. Postgrad Med J 1997; 73:448.

337. Russmann S, Winkler A, Lövblad KO, et al. Lethal ischemic stroke after cisplatin-based chemotherapy for testicular carcinoma and cannabis inhalation. Eur Neurol 2002; 48:178.

338. Mousak A, Agathos P, Kerezoudi E, et al. Transient ischemic attack in heavy cannabis smokers–how "safe" is it? Eur Neurol 2000; 44:42.

338a. Mesec A, Rot U, Grad A: Cerebrovascular disease associated with marijuana abuse: a case report: Cerebrovasc Dis 2001; 11:284.

338b. Moussouttas M: Cannabis use and cerebrovascular disease. Neurologist 2004; 10:47.

339. Straccieri A, Guarino M, Crespi C, et al. Transient amnesia triggered by acute marijuana intoxication. Eur J Neurol 1999; 6:521.

340. Mathew RJ, Wilson WH. Substance abuse and cerebral blood flow. Am J Psychiatry 1991; 148:292.

341. Mathew RJ, Wilson WH, Tant SR. Acute changes in cerebral blood flow associated with marijuana smoking. Acta Psychiatr Scand 1989; 79:118.

342. Matthew 0RJ, Wilson WH, Humphreys D, et al. Middle cerebral artery velocity during upright posture after marijuana smoking. Acta Psychiatr Scand 1992; 86:173.

343. Hernig RI, Better WE, Tate K, et al. Marijuana abusers are at increased risk for stroke. Preliminary evidence from cerebrovascular perfusion data. Ann N Y Acad Sci 2001; 939:413.

344. Adams MD, Earhardt JT, Dewey WL, Harris LS. Vasoconstrictor actions of delta-8 and delta-9-tetrahydrocannabinol in the rat. J Pharmacol Exp Ther 1976; 196:649.

345. Cimbura G, Lucas DM, Bennett RC, Donelson AC. Incidence and toxicological aspects of cannabis detected in 1394 fatally injured drivers and pedestrians in Ontario (1982-1984). J Forensic Sci 1990; 35:1035.

346. Hollister LE, Gillespie HK, Ohlsson A, et al. Do plasma concentrates of delta-9-tetrahydrocannabinol reflect the degree of intoxication? J Clin Pharmacol 1981; 21:1715.

347. Zagnoni PG, Albano C. Psychostimulants and epilepsy. Epilepsia 2002; 43 (Suppl 2):28.

348. Gordon E, Devinsky O. Alcohol and marijuana: effects on epilepsy and use by patients with epilepsy. Epilepsia 2001; 42:1266.

349. Ng SKC, Brust JCM, Hauser WA, Susser M. Illicit drug use and the risk of new onset seizures. Am J Epidemiol 1990; 132:47.

350. Walter FG, Bey TA, Ruschke DS, et al. Marijuana and hyperthermia. J Toxicol Clin Toxicol 1996; 34:217.

351. Coleman JH, Tacker HL, Evans WE, et al. Neurological manifestations of chronic marihuana intoxication. I. paresis of the fourth cranial nerve. Dis Nerv Syst 1976; 37:29.

352. DiBendetto M, McNammee HB, Kuchnle JC, Mendelson JH. Cannabis and the peripheral nervous system. Br J Psychiatry 1977; 131:361.

353. Lundberg GD, Adelson J, Prosnitz EH. Marijuana-induced hospitalization. JAMA 1971; 215:121.

354. Payne RJ, Brand SN. The toxicity of intravenously used marijuana. JAMA 1975; 233:351.

355. Farber SJ, Huertas VE. Intravenously injected marijuana syndrome. Arch Intern Med 1976; 136:337.

356. Zuckerman B, Bresnahan K. Developmental and behavioral consequences of prenatal drug and alcohol exposure. Pediatr Clin North Am 1991; 38:1387.

357. Hingson R, Alpert JJ, Day N, et al. Effects of maternal drinking and marijuana use on fetal growth and development. Pediatrics 1982; 70:539.

358. Linn S, Schoenbaum SC, Monson RR, et al. The association of marijuana use with outcome of pregnancy. Am J Public Health 1983; 73:1161.

359. Gibson GT, Bayhurst PA, Colley DP. Maternal alcohol, tobacco, and cannabis consumption on the outcome of pregnancy. Aust N Z Obstet Gynaecol 1983; 25:15.

360. Fried PA, Watkinson B, Willan A. Marijuana use during pregnancy and decreased length of gestation. Am J Obstet Gynecol 1984; 150:23.

361. Tennes K, Avitable N, Blackard A, et al. Marijuana: prenatal and postnatal exposure in the human infant. In: Pinkert TM, ed. Current Research on the Consequences of Maternal Drug Use. NIDA Res Monogr 1985; 59:48.

362. Hatch EE, Bracken MB. Effect of marijuana use in pregnancy on fetal growth. Am J Epidemiol 1986; 124:986.

363. Kline J, Stein Z, Hutzler M. Cigarettes, alcohol, and marijuana: varying associations with birthweight. Int J Epidemiol 1987; 16:44.

364. Fried PA. Marijuana use during pregnancy: consequences for the offspring. Semin Perinatol 1991; 15:280.

365. Hingson R, Zuckerman B, Amaro H, et al. Maternal marijuana use and neonatal outcome: uncertainty posed by self-reports. Am J Public Health 1986; 76:667.

366. Zuckerman B, Frank DA, Hingson R, et al. Effects of marijuana and cocaine use on fetal growth. N Engl J Med 1989; 320:762.

367. Frank DA, Bauchner H, Parker S, et al. Neonatal body proportionality and body composition after in utero exposure to cocaine and marijuana. J Pediatr 1990; 117:622.

368. Fried PA, Makin JE. Neonatal behavioral correlates of prenatal exposure to marijuana, cigarettes, and alcohol in a low risk population. Neurobehav Toxicol Teratol 1987; 9:1.

369. Lester BM, Dreher M. Effects of marijuana use during pregnancy on newborn cry. Child Dev 1989; 60:765.

370. Sher MS, Richardson GA, Coble PA, et al. The effects of prenatal alcohol and marijuana exposure: disturbances in neonatal sleepcycling and arousal. Pediatr Res 1988; 24:101.

371. Fried PA, Watkinson B. 12- and 24-month neurobehavioral follow-up of children prenatally exposed to marijuana, cigarettes, and alcohol. Neurotoxicol Teratol 1988; 10:305.

371a. Leech SL, Richardson GA, Goldschmidt L, et al. Prenatal substance exposure: effects on attention and impulsivity of 6-year-olds. Neurotoxicol Teratol 1999; 21:109.

372. Fried PA, Watkinson B. 36- and 48-month neurobehavioral follow-up of children prenatally exposed to marijuana, cigarettes, and alcohol. J Dev Behav Pediatr 1990; 11:49.

373. Richardson GA, Ryan C, Willford J, et al. Prenatal alcohol and marijuana exposure: effects on neuropsychological outcomes at 10 years. Neurotoxicol Teratol 2002; 24:309.

374. Lester BM, Tronick EZ, LaGasse L, et al. The maternal lifestyle study: effects of substance exposure during pregnancy on neurodevelopmental outcome in 1-month old infants. Pediatrics 2002; 110:1182.

375. Fried PA, Smith AM. A literature review of the consequences of prenatal marijuana exposure. An emerging theme of a deficiency in aspects of executive function. Neurotoxicol Teratol 2001; 23:1.

376. Scher MS, Richardson GA, Robles N, et al. Effects of prenatal substance exposure: altered maturation of visual evoked potentials. Pediatr Neurol 1998; 18:236.

377. Ambrosio E, Martin S, Garcia-Lecumberri C, et al. The neurobiology of cannabinoid dependence: sex differences and potential interactions between cannabinoid and opioid systems. Life Sci 1999; 65:687.

378. Klonoff-Cohen H, Lam-Kruglick P. Maternal and paternal recreational drug use and sudden infant death syndrome. Arch Pediatr Adolesc Med 2001; 155:765.

379. Astley SJ, Little RF. Maternal marijuana use during lactation and infant development at one year. Neurotoxicol Teratol 1990; 12:161.

380. Stenchever MA, Kunysz TJ, Allen MA. Chromosome breakage in users of marijuana. Am J Obstet Gynecol 1974; 118:106.

381. Zimmerman S, Zimmerman AM. Genetic effects of marijuana. Int J Addict 1990-91; 25:19.

382. Matsuyama SS, Jarvik LF, Fu TK, Yen FS. Chromosomal studies before and after supervised marijuana smoking. In: Braude MC, Szara S, eds. Pharmacology of Marihuana. New York: Raven Press, 1976:723.

383. Persaud TVN, Ellington AC. Cannabis in early pregnancy. Lancet 1967; II:1306.

384. Morishima A. Effects of cannabis and natural cannabinoids on chromosomes and ova. In: Braude MC, Ludford JP, eds. Marijuana Effects on the Endocrine and Reproductive Systems. NIDA Res Monogr 1984; 44:25.

385. Hutching DE, Morgan B, Brake SC, et al. Delta-9-tetrahydrocannabinol during pregnancy in the rat. I. Differential effects on maternal nutrition, embryotoxicity, and growth in the offspring. Neurotoxicol Teratol 1987; 9:39.

386. Wright PL, Smith SH, Keplinger ML, et al. Reproductive and teratological studies of delta-9-tetrahydrocannabinol and crude marijuana extract. Toxicol Appl Pharmacol 1976; 38:223.

387. Fried PA, Charlebois A. Effects upon rat offspring following cannabis inhalation before and/or after mating. Can J Psychol 1979; 33:125.

388. Hingson R, Alpert JJ, Day N, et al. Effects of maternal drinking and marijuana use on fetal growth and development. Pediatrics 1982; 70:539.

389. Morgan B, Brake SC, Hutchings DE, et al. Delta-9-tetrahydrocannabinol during pregnancy in the rat: effects on development of RNA, DNA, and protein in offspring brain. Pharmacol Biochem Behav 1988; 31:365.

390. Rodriguez-de-Fonseca F, Cabeira M, Fernandez-Ruiz JJ, et al. Effects of pre- and perinatal exposure to hashish extracts on the ontogeny of brain dopaminergic neurons. Neuroscience 1991; 43:713.

391. Fleischman RW, Hayden DW, Rosenkrantz H, Braude M. Teratologic evaluation of delta-9-tetrahydrocannabinol in mice, including a review of the literature. Teratology 1975; 12:47.

392. Hutchings DE, Brake SC, Morgan B. Animal studies of prenatal delta-9-tetrahydrocannabinol: female embryolethality and effects on somatic and brain growth. Ann N Y Acad Sci 1989; 562:133.

393. Abel EL, Rockwood GA, Riley EP. The effects of early marijuana exposure. In: Riley E, Vorhees C, eds. Handbook of Behavioral Teratology. New York: Plenum Press, 1986:267.

394. Brake S, Hutchings DE, Morgan B, et al. Delta-9-tetrahydrocannabinol during pregnancy in the rat. II. Effects on ontogeny of locomotor activity and nipple attachment in the offspring. Neurotoxicol Teratol 1987; 9:45.

395. Hutchings DE, Miller N, Gamagaris Z, Fico TA. The effects of prenatal exposure to delta-9-tetrahydrocannabinol on the rest-activity cycle of the preweanling rat. Neurotoxicol Teratol 1989; 11:353.

396. Hutchings DE, Brake SC, Banks AN, et al. Prenatal delta-9-tetrahydrocannabinol in the rat: effects on auditory startle in adulthood. Neurotoxicol Teratol 1991; 13:413.

397. Williams MA, Lieberman E, Mittendorf R, et al. Risk factors for abruptio placentae. Am J Epidemiol 1991; 134:965.

398. Russo E. Cannabis for migraine treatment: the once and future prescription? An historical and scientific review. Pain 1998; 76:3-8.

399. Kane B. Medical marijuana: the continuing story. Ann Intern Med 2001; 134:1159.

400. Voth EA, Schwartz RH. Medicinal applications of delta-9-tetrahydrocannabinol and marijuana. Ann Intern Med 1997; 126:791.

401. Feldman HW, Mandel J. Providing medical marijuana: the importance of cannabis clubs. J Psychoactive Drug 1998; 30:179.

400a. Calhoun SR, Galloway GP, Smith DE. Abuse potential of dronabinol (Marinol). J Psychoactive Drugs 1998; 30:187.

402. Mead A. Proposition 215: a dilemma. J Psychoactive Drugs 1998; 30:149.

403. Kassirer JP. Federal foolishness and marijuana. N Engl J Med 1997; 336:366.

404. Holland J. Breaking the law to ease the pain. NY Times, April 20, 2001.

405. Kent H. A step ahead of the law. "Compassion Club" sells marijuana to patients referred by MDs. Can Med Assoc J 1999; 161:1024.

406. Joy JE, Watson SJ, Benson JA, eds. Institute of Medicine. Marijuana and Medicine: Assessing the Science Base. Washington, DC: National Academy Press, 1999.

407. Smith DE. Review of the American Medical Association Council on Scientific Affairs Report on Medical Marijuana. J Psychoactive Drugs 1998; 30:127.

408. Dupont RL. Examining the debate on the use of medical marijuana. Proc Assoc Am Physician 1999; 111:166.

409. Greenhouse L. Justices set back use of marijuana to treat sickness. NY Times, May 15, 2001.

410. Liptak A. Medical marijuana wins a court victory. NY Times, October 30, 2002.

410a. Greenhouse L. Justices say doctors may not be punished for recommending marijuana. NY Times, October 15, 2003.

410b. Tuller D. Doctors tread thin line on marijuana. NY Times, October 28, 2003.

411. Holdcraft A, Patel P. Cannabinoids and pain relief. Expert Rev Neurother 2001; 1:92.

412. Randall RC, ed. Muscle Spasm, Pain, and Marijuana Therapy. Washington, DC: Galen Press, 1991.

413. Ware MA, Gamsa A, Persson J, et al. Cannabis for chronic pain: case series and implications for clinicians. Pain Res Management 2002; 7:95.

414. Greenwald MK, Stitzer ML. Antinociceptive, subjective and behavioral effects of smoked marijuana in humans. Drug Alcohol Depend 2000; 59:261.

415. Campbell FA, Tramer MR, Carroll D, et al. Are cannabinoids an effective and safe treatment option in the management of pain? A qualitative systematic review. BMJ 2001; 323:13.

416. Noyes R, Brunk F, Avery DH, et al. The analgesic properties of delta-9-tetrahydrocannabinol and codeine. Clin Pharmacol Ther 1976; 18:84.

417. Piomelli D, Giuffrida A, Calignano A, et al. The endocannabinoid system as a target for therapeutic drugs. Trends Pharmacol Sci 2000; 21:218.

417a. Karst M, Salim K, Burstein S, et al. Analgesic effect of the synthetic cannabinoid CT-3 on chronic neuropathic pain. A randomized controlled trial. JAMA 2003; 290:1757.

418. Cravatt BF, Demarest K, Patricelli MP, et al. Supersensitivity to anandamide and enhanced endogenous cannabinoid signaling in mice lacking fatty acid amide hydrolase. Proc Natl Acad Sci USA 2001; 98: 9371.

419. Tramer MR, Carroll D, Campbell FA, et al. Cannabinoids for control of chemotherapy induced nausea and vomiting: quantitative systematic review. BMJ 2001; 323:16.

420. Dansak DA. Medical use of recreational drugs by AIDS patients. J Addict Dis 1997; 16:25.

421. Hall W, MacPhee D. Cannabis use and cancer. Addiction 2002; 97:243.

422. Grinspoon L, Bakalar JB. Marihuana, the forbidden medicine. New Haven, CT: Yale University Press, 1997.

423. Porcella A, Maxia C, Gessa GL, et al. The synthetic cannabinoid WIN55212-2 decreases intraocular pressure in human glaucoma resistant to conventional therapies. Eur J Neurosci 2001; 13:409.

424. Consroe P, Musty R, Rein J, et al. The perceived effects of smoked cannabis on patients with multiple sclerosis. Eur Neurol 1997; 38:48.

425. Greenberg HS, Werness SAS, Pugh JE, et al. Short-term effects of smoking marijuana on balance in patients with multiple sclerosis. Lancet 1995; 345:579.

426. Petro DJ, Ellenberger C. Treatment of human spasticity with delta-9-tetrahydrocannabinol. J Clin Pharmacol 1981; 21 (Suppl 8–9): 413S.

427. Ungerleider JT, Andyrsiak T, Fairbanks L, et al. Delta-9-THC in the treatment of spasticity associated with multiple sclerosis. Adv Alcohol Subst Abuse 1987; 7:39.

428. Killestein J, Hoogervorst ELJ, Reif M, et al. Safety, tolerability, and efficacy of orally administered cannabinoids in MS. Neurology 2002; 58:1404.

428a. Zajicek J, Fox P, Sanders H, et al: Cannabinoids for treatment of spasticity and other symptoms related to multiple sclerosis (CAMS study): multicentre randomised placebo-controlled trial. Lancet 2003; 362:1517.

429. Clifford DB. Tetrahydrocannabinol for tremor in multiple sclerosis. Ann Neurol 1983; 13:669.

430. Martyn CN, Illis LS, Thom J. Nabilone in the treatment of multiple sclerosis. Lancet 1995; 345:579.

431. Consroe P. Brain cannabinoid systems as targets for the therapy of neurological disorders. Neurobiol Dis 1998; 5:534.

432. Dell'Osso LF. Suppression of pendular nystagmus by smoking cannabis in a patient with multiple sclerosis. Neurology 2000; 54:2190.

433. Baker D, Pryce G, Croxford JL, et al. Cannabinoids control spasticity and tremor in a multiple sclerosis model. Nature 2000; 404:84.

433a. Pryce G, Ahmed Z, Hankey DJR, et al. Cannabinoids inhibit neurodegeneration in models of multiple sclerosis. Brain 2003; 126:2191.

433b. Tuller D: Britain poised to approve medicine derived from marijuana. NY Times, January 27, 2004.

434. Mechoulam R, Carlini EA. Toward drugs derived from cannabis. Naturwissenschaften 1978; 65:174.

435. Consroe PF, Wood GC, Buchsbam H. Anticonvulsant nature of marijuana smoking. JAMA 1975; 234:306.

436. O'Shaughnessy WB. On the preparation of Indian hemp or ganja. Trans Med Phys Soc Bombay 1842; 8:421.

437. Reynolds JR. Therapeutic uses and toxic effects of *Cannabis indica*. Lancet 1980; I:637.

438. Davis JP, Ramsey HH. Antiepileptic actions of marijuana-active substances. Fed Proc 1949; 8:284.

439. Karler R, Turkanis SA. Cannabis and epilepsy. Adv Biosci 1978; 22-23:619.

440. Feeney DM. Marijuana use among epileptics. JAMA 1976; 235:1105.

441. Feeney DM. Marijuana and epilepsy: paradoxical anticonvulsant and convulsant effects. Adv Biosci 1978; 22-23:643.

442. Perez-Reyes M, Wingfield M. Cannabidiol and electroencephalographic epileptic activity. JAMA 1974; 230:1635.

443. Cunha JM, Carlini EA, Pereira AE, et al. Chronic administration of cannabidiol to healthy volunteers and epileptic patients. Pharmacology 1980; 21:175.

444. Ellison JM, Gelwan E, Ogletree J. Complex partial seizure symptoms affected by marijuana abuse. J Clin Psychiatry 1990; 51:439.

445. Muller-Vahl KR, Kolbe H, Dengler R. Gilles de la Tourette syndrome. Effect of nicotine, alcohol and marijuana on clinical symptoms. Nervenarzt 1997; 68:985.

446. Muller-Vahl KR, Schneider U, Koblenz A, et al. Treatment of Tourette's syndrome with delta-9-tetrahydrocannabinol: a randomized crossover trial. Pharmacopsychiatry 2002; 35:57.

447. Fox SH, Kellett M, Moore AP, et al. Randomized double-blind, placebo-controlled trial to assess the potential of cannabinoid receptor stimulation in the treatment of dystonia. Mov Disord 2002: 17:145.

448. Frankel JP, Hughes A, Lees AJ, et al. Marijuana for Parkinsonian tremor. J Neurol Neurosurg Psychiatry 1990; 53:436.

449. Sieradzan KA, Fox SH, Hill M, et al. Cannabinoids reduce levodopa-induced dyskinesia in Parkinson's disease: a pilot study. Neurology 2001; 57:2108.

450. Gilson I, Busalacchi M. Marijuana for intractable hiccups. Lancet 1998; 351:267.

451. El-Mallakh RF. Marijuana and migraine. Headache 1987; 27:442.

452. Porter AC, Felder CC. The endocannabinoids nervous system: unique opportunities for therapeutic intervention. Pharmacol Ther 2001; 90:45.

453. Panikashvili D, Simeonidou C, Ben-Shabat S, et al. An endogenous cannabinoid (2-AG) is neuroprotective after brain injury. Nature 2001; 413:527.

454. Malfait AM, Gallily R, Sumariwalla PF, et al. The nonpsychoactive cannabis constituent cannabidiol is an oral anti-arthritic therapeutic in murine collagen-induced arthritis. Proc Natl Acad Sci USA 2000; 97:9363.

455. Hungund BL, Basavarajappa BS. Are anandamide and cannabis receptors involved in ethanol tolerance? A review of the evidence. Alcohol Alcohol 2000; 35:126.

456. Colombo G, Agabio R, Fa M, et al. Reduction of voluntary ethanol intake in ethanol preferring sP rats by the cannabinoid antagonist SR-141716. Alcohol Alcohol 1998; 33:126.

457. Piomelli D. Cannabinoid activity curtails cocaine craving. Nat Med 2001; 10:1099.

458. Roffman RA, Stephens RS, Simpson EE, Whitaker DL. Treatment of marijuana dependence: preliminary results. J Psychoactive Drugs 1988; 20:129.

459. Zweben JE, O'Connell K. Strategies for breaking marijuana dependence. J Psychoactive Drugs 1988; 20:121.

460. Hser YI, Grella CE, Hubbard RL, et al. An evaluation of drug treatments for adolescents in 4 US cities. Arch Gen Psychiatry 2001; 58:689.

461. Hart CL, Haney M, Ward AS, et al. Effects of oral THC maintenance on smoked marijuana self-administration. Drug Alcohol Depend 2002; 67:301.

Chapter 8
Hallucinogens

. . . the visit to the World's Biggest Drug Store safely behind us, . . . I had returned to that reassuring but profoundly unsatisfactory state known as 'being in one's right mind.'
—Aldous Huxley

Picture yourself in a boat on a river
With tangerine trees and marmalade skies.
Somebody calls you, you answer quite slowly
A girl with kaleidoscope eyes.
—John Lennon

Tune in, turn on, drop out.
—Timothy Leary

Hallucinogens are chemicals that in low doses alter perception, thought, or mood, while preserving alertness, attentiveness, memory, and orientation. They cause auditory, visual, and tactile distortions and hallucinations—that is, dream-like episodes—in awake humans.[1] Also known as *psychedelics* ("mind revealing"), most of these agents are indole-containing ergot derivatives (e.g., lysergic acid diethylamide [LSD]), indolealkylamines (e.g., psilocybin), or phenylalkylamines (e.g., mescaline) (Table 8–1). Not classified as hallucinogens are marijuana, anticholinergics, bromides, phencyclidine, cocaine, and amphetamine, which produce confusion, delirium, or psychosis at hallucinogenic doses.

Pharmacology and Animal Studies

The study of hallucinogens poses special problems. LSD's Schedule I classification restricts human research,[2] and animal studies, which obviously require end points other than altered perception, cannot easily be extrapolated to human experience. LSD, mescaline, or psilocybin have caused hyperactivity in rats, catatonia in pigeons and salamanders, agitation in fish, aggressive behavior in ants,

Table 8–1. Hallucinogenic Compounds

Ergot-Derived
d-Lysergic acid diethylamide (LSD)

Indolealkylamines
Psilocybin
Psilocin
N,N-dimethyltryptamine (DMT)
N,N-diethyltryptamine (DET)

Phenylalkylamines
Mescaline
2,4-Dimethoxy-4-methylamphetamine (DOM)
4-Bromo-2,5-dimethoxyamphetamine (DOB)
2,5-Dimethoxy-4-ethylamphetamine (DOET)
3-Methoxy-4,5-methylenedioxyamphetamine (MMDA)
3,4-Methylenedioxyamphetamine (MDA; see Chapter 4)
3,4-Methylenedioxymethamphetamine (MDMA; see Chapter 4)
3,4-Methylenedioxyethamphetamine (MDEA; see Chapter 4)

disorganized web-spinning in spiders, aimless crawling in worms, surface detachment in snails, and status epilepticus in an elephant.[3–8]

As noted, "classical" hallucinogens either have a phenylalkylamine structure similar to amphetamine or contain an indole ring as found in serotonin. Phenylalkylamines are divided into phenylethylamines (e.g., mescaline) and phenylisopropylamines (e.g., 2,4-dimethoxy-4-methylamphetamine, DOM). Indolealkylamines are divided into N-substituted tryptamines (e.g., psilocybin), α-alkyltryptamines (e.g., 5-methoxy-α-methyltryptamine), ergolines (e.g., LSD), and β-carbolines (e.g., harmaline).[9] These agents all share two fundamental properties. First, animals trained to discriminate any one of them from saline will generalize to all the others. (Substitution of one agent for another is not always complete, however, and for the β-carbolines it is inconsistent enough that some workers question their designation as classical hallucinogens.[10]) Second, they all bind to 5-HT$_2$ serotonin receptors. Phenylalkylamine hallucinogens do not bind with high affinity to any population of receptors other than 5HT$_2$ receptors. Indolealkylamine hallucinogens, by contrast, bind to multiple populations of 5-HT receptors, and LSD binds to dopamine D$_1$- and D$_2$-receptors and adrenergic α-2 receptors as well.[11–13] Both phenylalkylamine and indolealkylamine hallucinogens bind to all three subpopulations of 5-HT$_2$ receptors (5-HT$_{2A}$, 5-HT$_{3B}$, 5-HT$_{2C}$). Studies with specific receptor antagonists suggest that the stimulus-discrimination and other effects of hallucinogens are mediated through 5-HT$_2$ receptors.[14,15] Such studies further suggest that 5-HT$_{2A}$ agonist activity is necessary but not sufficient to elicit hallucinations in humans, for compounds such as lisuride are strong 5-HT$_{2A}$ agonists and mimic LSD effects in animals but are not hallucinatory in humans.[16]

Structure–activity studies have identified a behavioral continuum among phenylalkylamine hallucinogens and other compounds that possess the same chemical skeleton as amphetamine. At one end are psychostimulants, such as amphetamine, which exert their actions primarily through dopaminergic mechanisms. At the other end are hallucinogens such as mescaline or DOM, which act through serotonergic pathways. Animals trained to discriminate amphetamine from saline do not generalize to DOM and vice versa. In the middle of the continuum are drugs such as 3,4-methylenedioxyamphetamine (MDA), which are both stimulatory and hallucinogenic. Animals trained to discriminate MDA from saline generalize to both amphetamine and DOM (see Chapter 4).[17,18]

5-HT$_2$ receptors are G-protein-coupled and enhance phosphatidylinositol intracellular signaling.[19] As with amphetamine and cocaine, the behavioral effects of LSD depend on dopamine- and adenosine 3′,5′-monophosphate (cAMP)-regulated phosphoprotein-32 (DARPP-32: see Chapter 2), although LSD and psychostimulants affect different phosphorylation sites on DARPP-32.[19a] 5-HT$_2$ receptors affect both γ-aminobutyric acid (GABA)ergic and glutamatergic neurotransmission. Studies show 5-HT$_{2A}$ receptor-mediated enhancement of glutamatergic excitatory postsynaptic potentials in apical dendrites of layer V cortical pyramidal cells,[20] and 5-HT$_{2A}$ agonists prevent the neurotoxicity induced by N-methyl-D-aspartate (NMDA) antagonists such as phencyclidine (PCP).[21] On the other hand, psilocybin and psilocin (as well as serotonin) suppressed glutamate transmission in rat hippocampal CA$_1$ pyramidal neurons.[22] In rats GABAergic interneurons in layer III of the piriform cortex are excited via G-HT$_{2A}$ receptors by serotonin, LSD, and the phenylethylamine hallucinogen 1-(2,5-dimethoxy-4-iodophenyl-2-aminopropane (DOI)); suggesting partial agonism, high doses of LSD and DOI blocked the 5HT excitation of these interneurons.[23] It has been proposed that LSD, DOM, and DOI block the neurotoxic and behavioral effects of NMDA antagonists by activating inhibitory 5-HT$_{2A}$ receptors on GABAergic interneurons that normally inhibit glutamatergic projections to cingulate cortex.[24] In rats LSD administration produces a several-fold increase in Fos-like immunoreactivity (an early gene, indicating neuronal activation) in medial frontal cortex, anterior cingulate cortex, and central nucleus of amygdala.[25] Unexpectedly, c-fos expression in the nucleus accumbens was much higher following LSD than following cocaine or morphine, drugs with considerably greater addictive potential.[26] In rabbits, LSD enhances classical conditioning, an effect blocked by a selective 5-HT$_{2A}$/5-HT$_{2C}$ receptor antagonist.[27]

Retinal as well as cortical actions may contribute to LSD and mescaline hallucinations. In rats, systemic LSD or mescaline suppresses the primary component of the flash-evoked cortical potential

(FEP), consistent with reduced conduction through the retinogeniculocortical system, and this suppression is blocked by the serotonin receptor antagonists cyproheptadine and methysergide. Intraocular mescaline or LSD also attenuates the FEP, and topical or intraocular atropine antagonizes the effects of systemic mescaline on the FEP.[28] In an alternative view, hallucinogenic drugs are considered to "disrupt thalamo-cortical gating of external and internal information to the cortex," resulting in "an overloading inundation of information and subsequent fragmentation and psychosis."[29]

Animals do not self-administer LSD, mescaline, or psilocybin.[30,31] LSD does produce a conditioned place preference, but only at very high doses.[32] Animals rapidly develop tolerance to these and other hallucinogens, with cross-tolerance between LSD, phenylalkylamines, and indolealkylamines, but withdrawal signs are not observed.[33]

Historical Background and Epidemiology

Of the world's more than 700,000 species of plants, nearly 100 have been identified as hallucinogenic (Table 8–2), and human ingestion, intentional and unintentional, goes back as far as recorded history.[1] The parasitic fungus ergot (*Claviceps* sp.) infests a variety of grains, especially rye, and contains a large number of pharmacologically active ergot alkaloids, including isoergine (lysergic acid amide), a hallucinogen about 10% as potent as LSD. Hallucinogenic ergot alkaloids may have been the source of the ancient Greek Mysteries of Eleusis, at which initiates sought a glimpse of the hereafter.[34] (Participants included Aeschylus, Sophocles, Plato, and Aristotle.) Similar plant ergots—especially the woodrose ololiuqui (*Rivea corymbosa*, closely related to the morning glory)—were used for religious purposes by the Aztecs, as was the indoleamine-containing mushroom Teonanacatl (*Psilocybe* sp.).[35,36] In fact, it has been argued that the religions of mankind began with neolithic exposure to mushroom-induced ecstasy.[37]

In medieval Europe (and in 1951 in France), accidental ingestion of the rye fungus *Claviceps purpurea* produced epidemics of gangrenous and convulsive ergotism with hallucinations ("St. Anthony's fire").[38] Similar poisoning may have accounted for outbreaks of "witchcraft" throughout the Middle Ages and, in 1692, in Salem, Massachusetts. The Salem tragedy, which resulted in the torture or hanging of at least 20 innocent people, began with the sudden appearance in the community of bizarre behavior, including terrifying hallucinations.[39]

For thousands of years, American Indians of Mexico and the southwestern United States have used the peyote cactus (*Lophophora williamsii*) and the San Pedro cactus (*Trichocercus pachanoi*) to induce visions in religious ceremonies.[39a] The psychoactive ingredient is mescaline (3,4,5-trihydroxy-phenylethylamine), named after the Mescalaro Apaches and present in much higher concentration in peyote than in the easier to find San Pedro cactus.[40,41] Either the raw peyote plant itself is eaten, or dried powdered cactus "buttons" are taken orally (or in enemas). Celebrated 19th-century users of mescaline were S. Weir Mitchell and Havelock Ellis. Each described the experience enthusiastically.

> Mitchell: "A white spear of grey stone grew up to huge height, and became a tall, richly finished Gothic tower of very elaborate and definite design. . . . Every projecting angle, cornice, and even the face of the stones . . . were covered or hung with clusters of what seemed to be huge precious stones. . . . These were green, purple, red, and orange. . . . All seemed to possess an interior light."[42,43]

Table 8–2. Miscellaneous Hallucinogenic Plants

Plant	Active Substances
Peyote cactus (*Lophophora williamsii*)	Mescaline
Psilocybe mushroom	Psilocybin, psilocin
Panaeolus mushroom	Psilocybin, psilocin
Gymnopilus mushroom	Psilocybin, psilocin
Amanita muscaria mushroom	Ibotenic acid
Morning glory (*Ipomoea* sp.)	*d*-Lysergic acid amide
Woodrose (*Rivea corymbosa*)	*d*-Lysergic acid amide
Nutmeg (*Myristica fragrans*)	Myristicin, elemicin
Periwinkle (*Catharanthus roseus*)	Indole alkaloids
Catnip (*Nepeta cataria*)	Nepetalactone
Yohimbe (*Corynanthe yohimbe*)	Yohimbine (see Chapter 4)
Juniper (*Juniperus macropoda*)	Unknown
Kava (*Piper methysticum*)	Unknown
Passion flower (*Passiflora caerulea*)	Harmine alkaloids
Virola (*Virola calophylla*)	Indolealkylamines
Iboga (*Tabernanthe iboga*)	Ibogaine

Ellis: "I would see thick glorious fields of jewels, solitary or clustered, sometimes brilliant and sparkling, sometimes with a dull rich glow. Then they would spring up into flower-like shapes, then seem to turn into gorgeous butterfly forms or endless fields of glistening, iridescent wings of wonderful insects."[44]

These descriptions led to an editorial in the *British Medical Journal* proclaiming that "… such eulogy for any drug is a danger to the public."[45] Peyote is still used sacramentally in the United States by members of the Native American Church,[46] and less orthodox users have recommended it as a means to self-transcendence and cosmic revelation.[47] (A less rhapsodic description of a mescaline experience, by a Professor of Eastern Religions and Ethics, referred to "transcendence into a world of farcical meaninglessness."[48])

Mexican Indians have worshipfully eaten hallucinogenic mushrooms, especially *Psilocybe mexicana* and other *Psilocybe* species, which contain the indoles psilocybin (4-phosphoryl-*N,N*-dimethyltryptamine) and psilocin (4-hydroxy-*N*, *N*-dimethyltryptamine).[46] Natives of Siberia and northwestern Canada have employed the mushroom *Amanita muscaria* (fly agaric) in shamanistic practices; active ingredients include ibotenic acid— a glutamate receptor agonist—and its metabolite muscimol—a GABA agonist.[36] There is evidence that *Amanita muscaria* was the original basis of the Rigveda deity Soma and the Greek god Dionysius (until geographic separation from the mushroom's northern source led to southern replacement by the fermented grape).[49]

Natives of the Orinoco and Amazon basins make hallucinogenic snuffs from a number of plants, including *Anadenanthera* seeds, which contain *N,N*-dimethyltryptamine (DMT), and *Virola* bark, which contains 5-methoxy-*N,N*-dimethyltryptamine.[1,50] The β-carbolines, harmine and harmaline, are present in seeds of *Peganum harmala*, which are chewed as intoxicants in India; the same hallucinogenic compounds are found in the vine *Banisteriopsis caapi*, used in psychotropic beverages and snuffs by Amazonian Indians.[46,51] A beverage known as ayahuasca in Brazil, yaje in Columbia, and natem in Ecuador is made from stalks of *Banisteriopsis* and leaves of *Psychotria viridis* or *Diplopterys cabrerana*, which contain DMT. DMT is psychologically inactive when ingested due to metabolism by monoamine oxidase (MAO), but

harmine and harmaline inhibit MAO, allowing access of DMT into the central nervous system.[52] West African natives chew the roots of *Tabernanthe iboga*, a shrub containing the hallucinogen ibogaine, and the bark of *Corynanthe yohimbe*, which contains yohimbine (see Chapter 4).[46] Other naturally occurring hallucinogenic agents include nepetalactone in *Nepeta cataria* ("catnip"), *d*-lysergic acid amide in several species of morning glory (*Ipomoea violacea*) or woodrose (*Rivea corymbosa*), and myristicin in seeds of *Myristica fragans* (nutmeg).[46,53]

Lysergic acid, the nucleus of psychoactive ergot alkaloids, is not hallucinogenic, but in 1943 it was discovered that a semisynthetic derivative, *d*-lysergic acid diethylamide (LSD), produced striking mental symptoms (Figure 8–1). Albert Hofmann, a pharmacologist at Sandoz Laboratories in Basel, was working with LSD when he developed "kaleidoscope-like" hallucinations. He then deliberately ingested 250 μg of LSD and experienced several hours of grotesque illusions and hallucinations accompanied by depersonalization and a sense of demonic possession. When his symptoms cleared, he felt well and had total recall of the experience.[54]

In the years that followed, LSD was studied as a possible model for schizophrenia[55] and as a psychotherapeutic agent.[56] Neither venture was successful, but the ensuing publicity soon led to recreational use. Referred to as "Acid," "Purple Haze," "Purple Hearts," "Window Pane," and "Sunshine," it was especially popular with American college students, and, associated with such cult figures as Timothy Leary, became a symbol of the counterculture of the 1960s. LSD and other hallucinogenic drugs were soon banned by federal statute. (In 1978, the American Indian Religious Freedom Act made an exception in the sacramental use of peyote, a First Amendment protection that lasted until

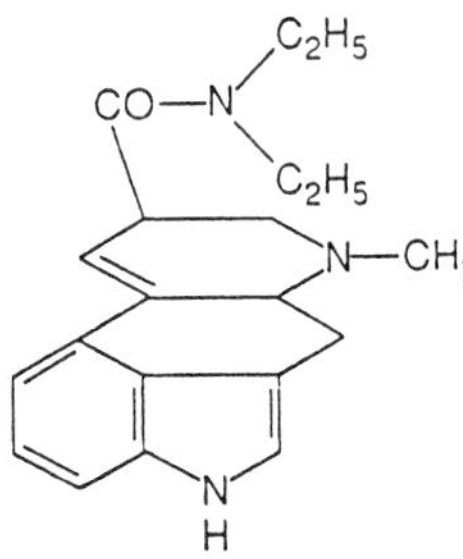

Figure 8–1. Lysergic Acid Diethylamide (LSD).

1990, when the U.S. Supreme Court ruled that states may prohibit use of peyote for religious purposes.[57,58])

In 1979, hallucinogenic drugs had been used by 25% of Americans aged 18 to 25 years, by 13% of American high school seniors, and by 7% of children aged 12 to 17 years.[59] Its popularity then declined, only to rise again during the 1990s, in both North America and Europe.[53,60–63] A 1993 survey of 50,000 U.S. teenagers found that LSD had been used by 3.5% of eighth graders, 6% of tenth graders, and 10% of twelfth graders. Of twelfth graders who had ever tried LSD, 20% had used it during the preceding 30 days.[62] Among American college students LSD use during the preceding 30 days rose from 1.03% in 1993 to 1.15% in 1997; it then fell back to 0.95% in 1999.[64] Typical users are Caucasian middle-class males; LSD tends to be avoided by African-Americans. As with marijuana, psychostimulants, and opioids, schizophrenics are overrepresented among users.[65] Along with methamphetamine and methylenedioxymethamphetamine (MDMA, "Ecstasy"), LSD is a popular feature of "rave" dance parties in North America and Europe.[53,66] (LSD and MDMA taken together are referred to as "candy-flipping."[67])

One of the cheapest illegal drugs, LSD sold during the 1990s at US$2 to US$3 for doses ranging from 20 to 100 μg, enough to produce effects lasting 8 to 12 hours.[68] (Doses were generally much larger during the 1960s.) When diluted with 750 ml of ethanol, 1 g of LSD provides 10,000 individual doses.[53] Available in impregnated blotting paper, sugar cubes, crackers, chewing gum, postage stamps, or squares of gelatin (known as "windowpane acid"), it is nearly always taken orally, but LSD-impregnated paper can be placed on the skin or in the conjunctival sac for absorption of the drug.[69] Tablet and liquid forms, once popular, are today seldom available.[53] Rarely LSD is snorted or injected.[70] Current street names for LSD include "The Hawk," "Yellow Dots," "25," "The Beast," "The Ghost," "Acid," "Blue Caps," "Blue Dots," "Microdots," and "Deeda."[69]

During the 1980s and 1990s, mushroom abuse also became increasingly popular in the United States and Europe.[71–75] In a 1985 survey of 1500 American college students, 15% had abused mushrooms compared with only 5% who had used LSD.[76] A 1986 survey of California high-school students

revealed that psilocybin-containing mushrooms had been eaten by 3.4% of seventh graders, 5.8% of ninth graders, and 8.8% of eleventh graders.[77] Among middle- to upper-class adolescents in a substance abuse program in Virginia during 1988, 26% had abused psilocybin-containing mushrooms.[77]

A 1997 survey of Canadian junior high and high-school students found that the only drugs with increased prevalence of use during the preceding 2 years were mescaline and psilocybin.[78] In Britain and Ireland abused mushrooms include *Psilocybe semilanceata* ("liberty cap," containing psilocybin), *Amanita muscaria* ("fly agaric," containing muscimol), and Teonanacatl (a Mexican mushroom containing mescaline).[79]

Acute Effects

Intended Effects

Hallucinogenic drugs produce three major kinds of effects: (1) perceptual (distortions or hallucinations), (2) psychological (depersonalization or altered mood), and (3) somatic (dizziness, paresthesias, or tremor).

Within a few minutes of ingestion, 0.5–3 μg/kg of LSD produces dizziness, sleepiness, weakness, blurred vision, paresthesias, chilliness, headache, nausea, and either euphoria or anxiety. In the second or third hour, visual illusions appear, including micropsia, macropsia, and altered body image. Hearing seems keener, afterimages are prolonged (palinopsia), and there may be synesthesias (stimuli in one modality producing perceptions in another; e.g., colors are heard). Somewhat later hallucinations occur, usually visual. They consist at first of brightly colored geometric designs and later of formed images—faces, animals, buildings, or landscapes, often elaborately beautiful or grotesque. Subjective time is prolonged. Familiar surroundings seem strange (derealization), and there are peculiar alterations of self-awareness (depersonalization), hypervigilance, or autistic withdrawal. Concentrating on inner feelings or the seemingly profound significance of trivial objects, the subject appears cataleptic. Memories intrude vividly, giving the sensation of events occurring in the wrong order. Mystical elation may alternate with anxiety or paranoia. Insight is usually but not always retained.[80,81]

The number and variety of symptoms are greater when the subject is alone, especially in the dark. Subjective effects usually last 6 to 12 hours, but fragments of the syndrome tend to recur spontaneously in "waves" of progressively shorter duration and diminished intensity for several hours longer.[82]

Hyperreflexia, fever, ataxia, tremor, pupillary dilation (with preserved light reflex), increased blood pressure, tachycardia, and piloerection parallel or precede the subjective symptoms.[83,84] Electroencephalographic changes consist of slightly increased alpha frequency and decreased alpha amount.[85] Initial insomnia is followed by sleep with enhanced rapid eye movement phase out of proportion to sleep deprivation.[86]

Symptoms and signs are dose-related between 1 and 16 µg/kg; pretreatment with reserpine enhances and prolongs an LSD response.[70,80] Tolerance develops rapidly to pupillary and psychic effects, and there is cross-tolerance to mescaline and psilocybin but not to amphetamine or delta-9-tetrahydrocannibinol.[70,87–90] Withdrawal symptoms do not occur after chronic use, which even among "acid heads" is infrequently more than weekly.[85,91]

LSD and its major metabolite 2-oxy-LSD are excreted in the urine for 12 to 36 hours after use, but most hospitals do not include LSD (or other classical hallucinogens) as part of standard drug screening.[53]

Unintended Effects

Adverse reactions ("bad trips") consist of intense depression, marked paranoia, or panic. They can occur with LSD doses as low as 25 µg and in users who have previously had only "good trips," and they can lead to homicide or suicide.[53,91–94] Ocular injuries include self-enucleation and retinal burns from staring at the sun.[95,96] Such symptoms usually clear within 24 hours and can be managed with "talking down"; if the patient is unmanageable, benzodiazepines are preferable to phenothiazines, which can cause paradoxical reactions.[80,97–100] There is sometimes prolonged depression, paranoia, or psychosis, and it is then uncertain if LSD was causal or simply exacerbated a pre-existing mental disturbance.[100–104] A case report described catatonia appearing 2 days after LSD ingestion and resolving

"dramatically" several days later following a single treatment of electroconvulsive therapy.[104a] Prolonged adverse reactions have occurred in apparently normal individuals, however, and although LSD has reportedly caused persistent polymodal hallucinosis in schizophrenic patients,[105] most schizophrenics are no more sensitive than others to LSD's psychotomimetic effects.[70,106]

Of a different nature are "flashbacks," which consist of spontaneous recurrence of LSD symptoms without taking the drug.[80,107] Their reported frequency ranges from 15% to 77% and increases with repeated LSD use, but they can occur after single exposure.[91,100,108,109] Precipitants include a dark environment, marijuana, fatigue, anxiety, ethanol, amphetamine, and intention.[110] Symptoms may last only a few seconds and are perceptual or emotional. Visual phenomena include heightened imagery, polyopia, palinopsia, perceptual distortions, illusions of movement, "streaking" (moving lights in a dark environment resembling long streaks as in a time-exposed photograph), "disjointed movements" (as with a strobe light), and geometric or formed hallucinations.[110–112] Flashbacks usually respond to sedatives and diminish in duration, intensity, and frequency over months or years.[100] Chlorpromazine can exacerbate them.[97,110]

Very high doses of LSD cause hypertension, respiratory depression, coma, and convulsions.[69,113,114] Hyperactivity following large doses of LSD can produce severe hyperthermia.[115,116] A violent patient restrained in a straightjacket developed a temperature of 41.6°C, hypotension, rhabdomyolysis, and fatal renal failure.[117] In animals, LSD causes dose-related hyperthermia independent of other behavioral responses.[118] Fatalities among LSD users are usually the result of accidents or suicide, however.[80]

Medical and Neurological Complications

Post-hallucinogen Perceptual Disorder

"Flashbacks," described above, may be part of a broader syndrome, "post-hallucinogen perceptual disorder." Some LSD users have visual disturbances which are continuous rather than paroxysmal and last many years. In addition to perceptual distortions and spontaneous imagery, subjects demonstrate abnormalities in visual acuity, flicker fusion thresholds, and dark adaptation.[119] Electroencephalographic changes suggest occipital cortex disinhibition in the processing of visual information.[120] Psychic alteration may accompany the visual symptoms; one patient described continuous euphoria interrupted by waves of panic.[121] Others describe anxiety, depression, depersonalization, or derealization. In one report, isolated palinopsia with no other visual or psychic symptoms persisted in three subjects for up to 3 years.[122] Benzodiazepines often reduce symptoms. Neuroleptics, including risperidone, tend to exacerbate them. Anecdotal reports describe both efficacy and exacerbation with serotonin reuptake inhibitors.[123,124] Case reports also describe benefit from either clonidine or naltrexone.[125,126] Interestingly, in volunteers chronic tricyclic antidepressants or lithium increased the physical, hallucinatory, and psychological responses to LSD, whereas serotonin reuptake inhibitors and monoamine oxidase inhibitors decreased the effects.[127]

Stroke

Many ergot agents are vasoconstrictors, and cerebral vessel strips undergo spasm when immersed in solution containing LSD, an effect blocked by methysergide.[128] Following ingestion of LSD, a 14-year-old boy developed seizures and, 4 days later, left hemiplegia; carotid angiography showed progressive narrowing of the internal carotid artery from its origin to the siphon, with occlusion at its bifurcation.[129] A young woman developed sudden left hemiplegia 1 day after using LSD; at angiography, there was marked vasoconstriction of the internal carotid artery at the siphon, which 9 days later was occluded.[130] A 19-year-old with acute aphasia and cerebral angiographic findings consistent with arteritis had used both LSD and heroin, but the temporal relationship of drug use to stroke was uncertain.[131] Another patient with angiographic evidence of "vasculitis" had used both LSD and "diet pills."[132]

Cognitive or Behavioral Change

Controversial is whether repeated LSD use causes permanent mental change, such as paranoia, depression, psychosis, or memory disturbance.

Passivity, tangential thinking, and a tendency to ascribe special significance to everyday events are described, and of 136 users who received treatment for an acute adverse reaction to LSD, 18 continued to have "psychotic residua" a year later.[119] As with other drugs, a causal relationship is difficult to establish, and the weight of evidence is against long-term damage to cognition or behavior.[91,100,133–137]

Hepatitis

Hepatitis has followed intravenous LSD use.[138]

Effects on Chromosomes

Chromosomal breakage was reported in human leukocytes incubated with LSD and in leukocytes from LSD users.[139,140]

Human spontaneous abortion and infant deformity were attributed to maternal LSD use, and teratogenicity was described in animals.[141–145] A number of investigators failed to find such association, however.[146–148] In one study, chromosomal aberrations disappeared within a few months of discontinuing LSD use; in other studies they were not found at all.[149–151] Chromosomal abnormalities were similarly absent in lymphocytes of Mexican Huichol Indians, generations of whom had used mescaline.[152] The absence of structural chromosomal abnormalities does not prove that LSD (or any other drug) is not mutagenic, and LSD is genotoxic in *Escherichia coli* and in barley.[152a] The weight of evidence is against such mutagenesis with doses taken by humans.

Lymphoma

A population-based case–control study in the United Kingdom found that LSD use increased the risk of developing non-Hodgkin's lymphoma.[153]

Retroperitoneal Fibrosis

Retroperitoneal fibrosis similar to that seen with methysergide overuse has occurred in chronic LSD users.[154]

Other Hallucinogenic Agents

Mescaline

Mescaline (Figure 8–2), infrequently abused as a street drug, is taken orally as peyote buttons ("tops," "moon," "cactus," "mesc," "the bad seed," "peyote," "p") or as mescaline powder in capsules or dissolved in water.[41] (Most alleged street mescaline powder is really LSD or phencyclidine.) Five milligrams per kilogram of mescaline is hallucinogenic, and 20–60 mg/kg causes bradycardia, hypotension, and respiratory depression.[36] One peyote button contains about 45 mg mescaline; synthetic mescaline usually comes in doses of 200–500 mg. As with LSD, side effects include nausea, vomiting, abdominal cramps, and diarrhea. There may also be flushing, sweating, and piloerection.[155] Psychic effects include olfactory, tactile, auditory, visual, or gustatory hallucinations; distortions of space and time; and paranoia, panic, or suicidal ideation. Symptoms last 6 to 12 hours.[36]

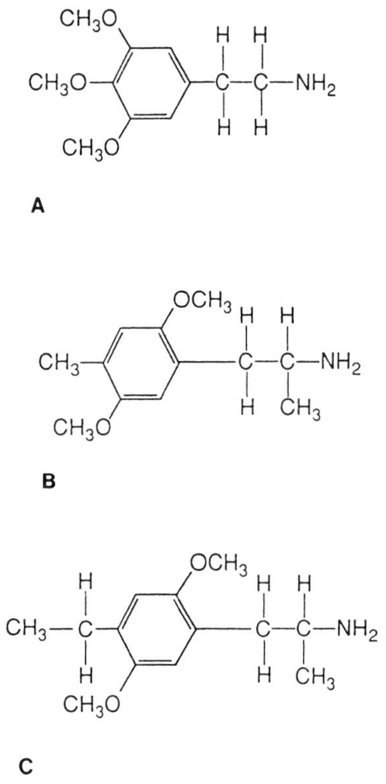

Three cases of botulism were reported in members of the Native American Church who ingested peyote from a communal jar during a ceremony.[156] Fatal Mallory–Weiss gastroesophageal lacerations and hemoaspiration occurred in an alcoholic man who developed vomiting after ingesting peyote.[157] Mescaline-induced delirium has resulted in fatal trauma.[158]

Psilocybin, Psilocin

Psilocybin and psilocin (Figure 8–3) are present in both Central American *Psilocybe* species of mushrooms ("magic mushrooms," "blue legs," "liberty caps") and in *Panaeolus* species native to the United States.[159–161] Other mushrooms containing psilocybin include *Conocybe cyanopus*, *Gymnopilus* (*Philiota*) *spectabilis*, and *Psathyrella foenisecii*.[162,163] Mushrooms are usually dried or frozen; even cooking does not destroy the hallucinogenic compounds. Mail-order kits of spores are available for home-growing.[162] Two to six mushrooms cause symptoms, and as many as 100 have been taken at one time. There is much variability in response: agitation and hallucinations have followed 10 mushrooms and gastritis without psychic effects has followed 200.[164] Other effects include anticholinergic symptoms and seizures.[165–169] Hallucinations usually last a few hours but have lasted several days. Positron emission tomographic (PET) studies of volunteers acutely taking psychotomimetic doses of psilocybin revealed frontal lobe changes in glucose metabolism similar to those found in schizophrenics during acute psychotic episodes.[170]

Figure 8–2. Mescaline (A), 2,5-Dimethoxy-4-Methylamphetamine (DOM) (B), 2,5-Dimethoxy-4-Ethylamphetamine (DOET) (C).

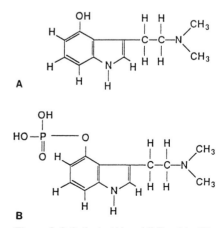

Figure 8–3. Psilocin (A) and Psilocybin (B).

Wolff–Parkinson–White syndrome, arrhythmia, and myocardial infarction occurred in an 18-year-old boy during psilocybin mushroom intoxication.[171]

Obsessive-compulsive disorder and body dysmorphic disorder have been anecdotally reported to benefit from use of psilocybin.[172,173]

Intravenous injection of mushroom extracts causes vomiting, cyanosis, fever, arthralgia, abnormal liver function, and methemoglobinemia.[165,174]

LSD, Mescaline, and Psilocybin Compared

LSD, mescaline, and psilocybin differ in potency, time to peak action, and duration of effects. One microgram LSD is equivalent to 5–6 mg mescaline and 150–200 μg psilocybin. LSD's hallucinogenic effects begin after 1 to 1.5 hours, mescaline's after 2 to 2.5 hours, and psilocybin's after 30 minutes. The psychic and physiological effects of the three drugs are indistinguishable even to experienced users.[80,84,175]

Amanita muscaria

Rarely abused in the United States is *Amanita muscaria*, which produces euphoria, mania, delirium, ataxia, and both Lilliputian and Brobdingnagian illusions. Less often there are frank visual hallucinations. Seizures, coma, and death can follow ingestion.[176] The mushroom contains ibotenic acid, which is glutamatergic, and its metabolite muscimol, which is GABAergic.[162]

Other Synthetic Hallucinogens

N,N-dimethyltryptamine (DMT) and *N,N*-diethyltryptamine (DET) are easily synthesized and available on the illicit street market. DMT is inactive orally and is therefore injected, smoked, or taken as a snuff. It produces LSD-like effects, including adverse reactions.[177,178] DMT is unique among classical hallucinogens in its inability to induce tolerance to its psychological effects, a feature perhaps related to its being an agonist at 5-HT$_{1A}$ as well as 5-HT$_2$ receptors.[179]

Also abused as street drugs are DOM (nicknamed "STP" after a commercial oil additive said to increase the power of automobile engines) (see Figure 8–2), 4-bromo-2,5-dimethoxyamphetamine (DOB), 2,5-dimethoxy-4-ethylamphetamine (DOET) (see Figure 8–2), 3,4,5-trimethoxyamphetamine (TMA), and 3-methoxy-4,5-methylenedioxyamphetamine (MMDA).[80,93,179–181] Panic, violent behavior, seizures, and death have followed abuse of DOB,[182] as have diffuse vascular spasm and limb ischemia, resulting in bilateral above-the-knee amputations.[183] As noted in Chapter 4, MDA and 3,4-methylenedioxymethamphetamine (MDMA, "Ecstasy") can be taken to induce hallucinations.[184]

Psychosis lasting 3 weeks occurred in an amateur chemist who snorted and injected isosafrole (4-propenyl-1,2-methylenedioxybenzene) because of its resemblance to MDA; such a reaction had not followed his use of amphetamine, marijuana, or LSD.[185]

Morning Glory

Seeds of the morning glory (*Ipomoea* sp.) or the related Mexican plant ololiuqui (*Rivea corymbosa*) are popular hallucinogens in the United States. In one case, emotional lability, fixed dilated pupils, and increased awareness of colors followed ingestion of 250 seeds.[186] In another case, ingestion of 300 seeds produced vivid visual and tactile hallucinations, fantasies, and depersonalization, and 3 weeks later suicide occurred during a flashback hallucinatory psychosis.[187] Other acute effects include nausea, vomiting, diarrhea, muscle tightness, and paresthesias of the limbs.[36] Ololiuqui is still used for religious purposes in Mexico, and teas made from morning glory seeds (e.g., "Panacea Tea") are available in American "health food" stores.[188] Of the many ergot alkaloids present in morning glory seeds, the most psychoactive appears to be *d*-lysergic acid amide (ergine).[189]

Nutmeg

In the United States, nutmeg abuse is common among prison inmates.[46,190] (It is so described in *The Autobiography of Malcolm X*.[191]) Effects are the result of several phenylalkylamines—myristicin, elemicin, eugenol, safrole, and borneal—and their active metabolites MMDA and TMA.[36,190,192] One to three nutmegs (5–30 g ground powder, or 1 to 4 tablespoons) produce psychic effects that resemble those of marijuana. After a delay of up to several hours, there is giddiness, anxiety, and excitement; euphoria; depersonalization; and distortions of space and time. Higher doses cause visual illusions and hallucinations. Fear of death or panic may ensue, followed by lethargy for more than 24 hours. Anticholinergic signs include flushing, tachycardia, and urinary retention, yet miosis is seen more often than mydriasis. Nausea, vomiting, abdominal pain, and hypotension limit nutmeg's popularity among the nonincarcerated.[193–198]

Kava

Kava (or kava-kava) is a beverage made by Pacific islanders from roots of the shrub *Piper methysticum*. Used both socially and in religious ceremonies, it induces sedation and euphoria without, apparently, interfering with "normal cognitive processes."[198a] High doses are hallucinogenic, and chronic users develop yellow skin discoloration, drowsiness, ataxia, liver damage, and malnutrition (the result of dysphagia secondary to oropharyngeal numbness caused by contact with the beverage). The pharmacological basis of kava's effects has not been identified. A number of compounds in kava are collectively referred to as kava lactones or kava pyrones and have variable actions at NMDA, serotonin, noradrenalin, dopamine and GABA receptors.[199] Herbal teas containing kava are sold in American "health food" stores, and toxicity has been reported.[200–204] Neurological manifestations of toxicity include dystonia, choreoathetosis, blepharospasm, tremor, and ataxia.[204a] Seizures are reported.[205] Saccadic dysmetria, saccadic slowing, and impaired visual attention without other cognitive impairment suggest cerebellar dysfunction. Liver enzymes are acutely elevated.[204a]

Ibogaine

During the 1990s ibogaine, from the West African plant *Tabernanthe iboga*, achieved considerable media attention because of claims that it was effective in treating addiction to cocaine or opioids. Containing an indole ring, ibogaine is capable of inducing hallucinations, yet it produces subjective effects quite different from those associated with LSD and classical hallucinogens.[206] Ibogaine at moderate doses produces an "oneirophrenic" state, with primary process thinking in the absence of psychotic symptoms—"a dream state without loss of consciousness." Higher doses produce frank hallucinations, usually visual, and often accompanied by severe anxiety, dysesthesias of the limbs, tremor, perspiration, mydriasis, dry mouth, tachycardia, and mild ataxia. Ibogaine does not bind to any known serotonin receptor subtype; rather, it and a metabolite have strong affinity for opioid κ receptors.[50,206] It may also act at sigma receptors and block glutamatergic transmission at NMDA receptors.

Salvinorin A

Salvia divinorum, a member of the mint family, has been used ritualistically for centuries by the Mazatec people of Oaxaca, Mexico. Powerfully hallucinogenic, its active ingredient is salvinorin A, which, like ibogaine, is an opioid κ-receptor agonist but does not bind to serotonin receptors. It can be eaten, chewed, or smoked, and during the 1990s it became widely available in the United States, largely through the Internet. As with other κ-agonists, undesired effects include feelings of unreality, depersonalization, impaired memory, and in higher doses unconsciousness.[207,208]

Herbal Teas

Other herbal teas sold in American "health food" stores often contain more than a dozen different types of leaves, seeds, and berries. Some, for example hydrangea or lobelia teas, are taken for psychostimulation and euphoria and do not cause hallucinations except in situations of obvious toxicity. Others, for example yohimbe bark or periwinkle teas, more readily produce hallucinations. Still others, such as those containing morning glory seeds, juniper, or catnip, are frankly sold for their hallucinogenic properties (see Table 8–2).[188,202]

Other Hallucinogenic Plants

Uncertain is the prevalence of abuse of many other native and imported hallucinogenic plants, any of which, in this era of easy travel, could produce confounding symptoms in patients brought to unsuspecting emergency rooms (see Table 8–2).

Toads

Bizarre even by the often rococo standards of substance abuse are "toad licking" and "toad skin smoking." Skin glands of the Australian cane toad (*Bufo alvarius*, in North America called the Colorado River toad) produce hallucinogenic secretions. As a consequence these creatures became popular pets in the United States.[209] (Toad-licking was depicted in a 1995 episode of the television show, "Beavis and Butt-Head."[210]) The hallucinogenic agent in *Bufo alvarius* was believed to be the serotonin-like compound bufotenine, which since 1967 has been a Schedule I drug. Human studies, however, suggested that the butofenine metabolite, 5-methoxydimethyltryptamine (5-MeO-DMT)—not bufotenine itself—is the responsible hallucinogen.[209,211] It was also shown that neither bufotenine nor 5-MeO-DMT is active orally, implying that toad-licking is a misplaced fad.[212] Subsequent work demonstrated that bufotenine by itself is blocked at the blood–brain barrier; in the presence of other bioactive ingredients in *Bufo* toad toxin, bufotenine (and, presumably, 5-MeO-DMT) do enter the brain. Whether bufotenine is hallucinogenic in the absence of 5-MeO-DMT remains uncertain. It is a powerful pressor.[213]

Reported side effects of toad-licking include sweating, salivation, palpitations, vomiting, and fecal incontinence.[214] Fifteen minutes after placing a toad in his mouth a 5-year-old boy developed profuse salivation and status epilepticus.[215]

References

1. Siegel RK. The natural history of hallucinogens. In: Jacobs BL, ed. Hallucinogens: Neurochemical, Behavioral, and Clinical Perspectives. New York: Raven Press, 1984; 1.
2. Strassman EJ. Human hallucinogenic drug research in the United States: a present-day history and review of the process. J Psychoactive Drugs 1991; 23:29.
3. Abramson HA, Evans LT. Lysergic acid diethylamide (LSD-25). II. Psychobiological effects on the Siamese fighting fish. Science 1954; 120:990.
4. Abramson HA, Jarvik ME. Lysergic acid diethylamide (LSD-25). IX. Effect on snails. J Psychol 1955; 40:337.
5. Witt PN. D-Lysergsäure-Diathylamid (LSD-25) im Spinnentest. Experientia 1951; 7:310.
6. West L, Pierce C, Thomas W. Lysergic acid diethylamide: its effect on a male Asiatic elephant. Science 1962; 138:1100.
7. Christiansen A, Baum R, Witt PN. Changes in spider webs brought about by mescaline, psilocybin, and an increase in body weight. J Pharmacol Exp Ther 1962; 136:31.
8. Siegel RK. Intoxication. Life in Pursuit of Artificial Paradise. New York: EP Dutton, 1989:57.
9. Glennon RA. Arylalkylamine drugs of abuse: an overview of drug discrimination studies. Pharmacol Biochem Behav 1999; 64:251.
10. Helsley S, Fiorella D, Rabin RA, et al. A comparison of N,N-dimethyltryptamine, harmaline, and selected congeners in rats trained with LSD as a discriminative stimulus. Prog Neuropsychopharmacol Biol Psychiatry 1998; 22:649.
11. Watts VJ, Lawler CP, Fox DR, et al. LSD and structural analogs: pharmacological evaluation of D1 dopamine receptors. Psychopharmacologia 1995; 118:401.
12. Marona-Lewicka D, Nichols DE. Complex stimulus properties of LSD: a drug discrimination study with alpha 2-adrenoceptor agonists and antagonists. Psychopharmacologia 1995; 120:384.
13. Giacomelli S, Palmery M, Romanelli L, et al. Lysergic acid diethylamide (LSD) is a partial agonist of D_2 dopaminergic receptors and it potentiates dopamine prolactin secretion in lactotrophs in vitro. Life Sci 1998; 63:215.
14. Nelson DL, Lucaites VL, Wainscott DB. Comparisons of hallucinogenic phenylisopropylamine binding affinities at cloned human 5-HT2A, 5-HT2B, and 5-HT2C receptors. Naunyn-Schmiedebergs Arch Pharmacol 1999; 359:1.
15. Ouagazzal A, Grottick AJ, Moreau J, et al. Effect of LSD on prepulse inhibition and spontaneous behavior in the rat. A pharmacological analysis and comparison between two rat strains. Neuropsychopharmacology 2001; 25:565.
16. Fiorella D, Rabin RA, Winter JC. Role of 5-HT2A and 5-HT2C receptors in the stimulus effects of hallucinogenic drugs. II. Reassessment of LSD false positives. Psychopharmacologia 1995; 121:357.
17. Glennon RA. Phenylalkylamine stimulants, hallucinogens, and designer drugs. NIDA Res Monogr 1991; 105:154.

18. McKenna DJ, Guan XM, Shulgin AT. 3,4-Methylene-dioxyamphetamine (MDA) analogues exhibit differential effects on synaptosomal release of 3H-dopamine and 3H-5-hydroxytryptamine. Pharmacol Biochem Behav 1991; 38:505.

19. Barkstrom JR, Chang MS, Chu H, et al. Agonist-directed signaling of serotonin 5-HT2C receptors: differences between serotonin and lysergic acid diethylamide (LSD). Neuropsychopharmacology 1999; 21 (Suppl 2):77S.

19a. Svenningsson P, Tzavara ET, Carruthers R, et al. Diverse psychotomimetics act through a common signaling pathway. Science 2003; 302:1412.

20. Aghajanian GK, Marek GJ. Serotonin and hallucinogens. Neuropsychopharmacology 1999; 21 (Suppl 2):16S.

21. Farber NB, Hanslick J, Kirby C, et al. Serotonergic agents that activate 5HT2A receptors prevent NMDA antagonist neurotoxicity. Neuropsychopharmacology 1998; 18:57.

22. Moldavan MG, Grodzinskaya AA, Solomko EF. The effect of *Psilocybe cubensis* extract on hippocampal neurons in vitro. Fiziolog Zhornal 2001; 47:15.

23. Marek GJ, Aghajanian GK. LSD and the phenylethylamine hallucinogen DOI are potent partial agonists at 5-HT2A receptors on interneurons in rat pyriform cortex. J Pharmacol Exp Ther 1996; 278:1373.

24. West WB, Lou A, Pechersky K, et al. Antagonism of a PCP drug discrimination by hallucinogens and related drugs. Neuropsychopharmacology 2000; 22:618.

25. Gresch PJ, Strickland LV, Sanders-Bush E. Lysergic acid diethylamide-induced Fos expression in rat brain: role of serotonin-2A receptors. Neuroscience 2002; 114:707.

26. Erdtmann-Vourliotis M, Mayer P, Riechert U, et al. Acute ingestion of drugs with low addictive potential (delta(9)-tetrahydrocannabinol, 3,4-methyl-enedioxymethamphetamine, lysergic acid diamide) causes a much higher c-fos expression in limbic brain areas than highly addicting drugs (cocaine and morphine). Brain Res Mol Brain Res 1999; 71:313.

27. Welsh SE, Kachelries WJ, Romano AG, et al. Effects of LSD, ritanserin, 8-OH-DPAT, and lisuride on classical conditioning in the rabbit. Pharmacol Biochem Behav 1998; 59:469.

28. Eells JT, Wilkison DM. Effects of intraocular mescaline and LSD on visual-evoked responses in the rat. Pharmacol Biochem Behav 1989; 32:191.

29. Vollenweider FX, Geyer MA. A systems model of altered consciousness: integrating natural and drug-induced psychoses. Brain Res Bull 2001; 56:495.

30. Brady JV, Griffith RR, Heinz RD, et al. Assessing drugs for abuse liability and dependence potential in laboratory primates. In: Bozarth MA, ed. Methods of Assessing the Reinforcing Properties of Abused Drugs. New York: Springer-Verlag, 1987:47.

31. Yokel RA. Intravenous self-administration: response rates, the effects of pharmacological challenges, and drug preference. In: Bozarth MA, ed. Methods of Assessing the Reinforcing Properties of Abused Drugs. New York: Springer-Verlag, 1987; 1.

32. Parker LA. LSD produces place preference and flavor avoidance but does not produce flavor aversion in rats. Behav Neurosci 1996; 110:503.

33. Schlemmer RF, David JM. A primate model for the study of hallucinogens. Pharmacol Biochem Behav 1986; 24:381.

34. Wasson RG, Ruck CAP, Hofmann A. The Road to Eleusis. New York: Harcourt Brace Jovanovich, 1978.

35. Elferink JGR. Some little-known hallucinogenic plants of the Aztecs. J Psychoactive Drugs 1988; 20:427.

36. Spoerke DG, Hall AH. Plants and mushrooms of abuse. Emerg Med Clin North Am 1990; 8:579.

37. Wasson RG. Soma: Divine Mushroom of Immortality. New York: Harcourt Brace Jovanovich, 1968.

38. Fuller JG. The Day of St. Anthony's Fire. New York: Macmillan, 1968.

39. Caporael LR. Ergotism: the satan loosed in Salem? Science 1976; 192:21.

39a. Bruhn JG, DeSmet PAGM, El-Seedi HR, et al. Mescaline use for 5700 years. Lancet 2002; 359:1866.

40. Brecher EM. Licit and Illicit Drugs. Boston: Little, Brown, 1972.

41. Schwartz RH. Mescaline: a survey. Am Fam Physician 1988; 37:122.

42. Mitchell SW. Remarks on the effects of *Anhalonium lewinii* (the mescal button). BMJ 1896; II:1625.

43. Metzer WS. The experimentation of S. Weir Mitchell with mescal. Neurology 1989; 39:303.

44. Ellis H. Mescal: a new artificial paradise. Reprinted in: Ebin D, ed. The Drug Experience. New York: Orion Press, 1961:223.

45. Anon. Paradise or inferno (edit.). BMJ 1898; I:390.

46. Farnsworth NR. Hallucinogenic plants. Science 1968; 162:1086.

47. Huxley A. The Doors of Perception. New York: Harper & Row, 1954.

48. Zaehner RC. Mysticism, sacred and profane. Reprinted in: Ebin D, ed. The Drug Experience. New York: Orion Press, 1961; 275.

49. Wohlberg J. Haoma-Soma in the world of ancient Greece. J Psychoactive Drugs 1990; 22:333.

50. McKenna DJ. Plant hallucinogens: springboards for psychotherapeutic drug discovery. Behav Brain Res 1996; 73:109.

51. Sanchez-Ramos JR. Banisterine and Parkinson's disease. Clin Neuropharmacol 1991; 14:391.

52. Riba J, Rodriguez-Fornells A, Urbano G, et al. Subjective effects and tolerability of the South American psychoactive beverage Ayahuasca in healthy volunteers. Psychopharmacology 2001; 154:85.

53. Schwartz RH. LSD. Its rise, fall, and renewed popularity among high school students. Pediatr Clin North Am 1995; 42:403.

54. Hoffmann A. How LSD originated. J Psychedelic Drugs 1979; 11:53.

55. Osmond H. A review of the clinical effects of psychotomimetic agents. Ann N Y Acad Sci 1957; 66:418.

56. Abramson HA. The use of LSD as an adjunct to psychotherapy. Fact and fiction. In: Sankar DVS, ed. LSD: A Total Study. New York: PJD Publications, 1975.

57. Greenhouse L. Court is urged to rehear case on ritual drugs. NY Times, May 11, 1990.

58. Bullis RK. Swallowing the scroll: legal implications of the recent Supreme Court peyote cases. J Psychoactive Drugs 1990; 22:325.

59. Fishburne PM, Abelson HI, Cisin I. National Survey on Drug Abuse: Main Findings: 1979. Washington, DC: DHHS, Publ (ADM) 80-976, 1980.

60. Johnston LD, O'Malley PM, Bachman JG. National Survey Results on Drug Use from Monitoring the Future Study, 1975–1993. Vol II. College Students and Young Adults. Rockville, MD: NIDA, 1994.

61. Golub A, Johnson BD, Sifaneck SJ, et al. Is the U.S. experiencing an incipient epidemic of hallucinogen use? Subst Use Misuse 2001; 36:1699.

62. Johnston LD, O'Malley PM, Bachman JG. National Survey Results on Drug Use from Monitoring the Future Study, 1975–1993, Vol 1. Secondary Students. Rockville, MD: NIDA, 1994.

63. Schuster P, Lieb R, Lamertz C, et al. Is the use of ecstasy and hallucinogens increasing? Results from a community study. Eur Addict Res 1998; 4:75.

64. Gledhill-Hoyt J. Increased levels of drug use among college students. Addiction 2000; 95:1655.

65. Duke PJ, Pantelis C, McPhillips MA, et al. Comorbid non-alcohol substance misuse among people with schizophrenia: epidemiological study in central London. Br J Psychiatry 2001; 179:509.

66. Gross SR, Barrett SP, Shestowsky JS, et al. Ecstasy and drug consumption patterns: a Canadian rave population study. Can J Psychiatry 2002; 47:546.

67. Schechter MD. "Candyflipping": synergistic discriminative effect of LSD and MDMA. Eur J Pharmacol 1998; 34:131.

68. Gold MS, Schuchard K. LSD use among U.S. high school students. JAMA 1994; 271:426.

69. Blaho K, Merigian K, Winbery S, et al. Clinical pharmacology of lysergic acid diethylamide: case reports and review of the treatment of intoxication. Am J Therapeut 1997; 4:211.

70. Freedman DX. LSD: the bridge from human to animal. In: Jacobs BL, ed. Hallucinogens: Neurochemical, Behavioral, and Clinical Perspectives. New York: Raven Press, 1984; 203.

71. Hyde C, Glancy G, Omerod P, et al. Abuse of indigenous psilocybin mushrooms: a new fashion and some psychiatric complications. Br J Psychiatry 1978; 132:602.

72. Young RE, Milroy R, Hutchinson S, et al. The rising price of mushrooms. Lancet 1982; I:213.

73. Siegel RK. New trends in drug use among young in California. Bull Narc 1985; 37:7.

74. Pierrot M, Josse P, Raspiller MF, et al. Intoxications by hallucinogenic mushrooms. Ann Med Interne (Paris) 2000; 151 (Suppl B):B16.

75. Musshoff F, Madea B, Beike J. Hallucinogenic mushrooms on the German market–simple instructions for examination and identification. Forensic Sci Int 2000; 113:389.

76. Thompson JP, Anglin MD, Emboden W, et al. Mushroom use by college students. J Drug Educ 1985; 15:111.

77. Schwartz RH, Smith DE. Hallucinogenic mushrooms. Clin Pediatr 1988; 27:70.

78. Adlaf EM, Ivis FJ. Recent findings from the Ontario Student Drug Use Survey. Can Med Assoc J 1998; 159:451.

79. O'Shea B, Fagan J. Lysergic acid diethylamide. Irish Med J 2001; 94:217.

80. Hollister LE. Effects of hallucinogens in humans. In: Jacobs BL, ed. Hallucinogens: Neurochemical, Behavioral, and Clinical Perspectives. New York: Raven Press, 1984; 19.

81. Moser P. LSD. In: Ebin D, ed. The Drug Experience. New York: Orion Press, 1961; 353.

82. O'Brien CP. Drug addiction and drug abuse. In: Hardman JG, Limbird LE, eds. Goodman and Gilman's The Pharmacological Basis of Therapeutics, 10th edition. New York, McGraw-Hill, 2001; 621.

83. Isbell H, Belleville RE, Fraser HF, et al. Studies in lysergic acid diethylamide (LSD-25). I. Effects in former morphine addicts and development of tolerance during chronic administration. Arch Neurol Psychiatry 1956; 76:468.

84. Isbell H. Comparison of the reactions produced by psilocybin and LSD-25 in man. Psychopharmacologia 1959; 1:29.

85. Gastaut H, Ferrer S, Castells C. Action de la diethylamide de l'acide d-lysergique (LSD-25) sur les fonctions psychiques et l'electroencephalogramme. Confin Neurol 1953; 13:102.

86. Musio JN, Roffwarg HP, Kaufmann E. Alterations in the nocturnal sleep cycle resulting from LSD. Electroencephalogr Clin Neurophysiol 1966; 21:313.

87. Isbell H, Wolbach AB, Wikler A, Miner EJ. Cross tolerance between LSD and psilocybin. Psychopharmacologia 1961; 2:147.

88. Wolbach AB, Isbell H, Miner EJ. Cross tolerance between mescaline and LSD-25, with a comparison of the mescaline and LSD reactions. Psychopharmacologia 1962; 3:1.

89. Rosenberg DE, Wolbach AB, Miner EJ, Isbell H. Observations on direct and cross tolerance with LSD and d-amphetamine in man. Psychopharmacologia 1963; 5:1.

90. Isbell H, Jasinski DR. A comparison of LSD-25 with delta-9-tetrahydrocannabinol (THC) and attempted

cross-tolerance between LSD and THC. Psychopharmacologia 1969; 14:115.

91. McGlothlin WH, Arnold DO. LSD revisited: a ten-year followup of medical LSD use. Arch Gen Psychiatry 1971; 24:35.

92. Cohen S. A classification of LSD complications. Psychosomatics 1966; 7:182.

93. Ungerleider JT, Fisher DD, Goldsmith SR, et al. A statistical survey of adverse reactions to LSD in Los Angeles County. Am J Psychiatry 1968; 125:352.

94. Klepfisz A, Racy J. Homicide and LSD. JAMA 1973; 223:429.

95. Thomas R, Fuller D. Self-inflicted ocular injury associated with drug use. J SC Med Assoc 1972; 68:202.

96. Fuller D. Severe solar maculopathy associated with use of lysergic acid diethylamide. Am J Ophthalmol 1976; 81:413.

97. Schwarz C. Paradoxical responses to chlorpromazine after LSD. Psychosomatics 1967; 8:210.

98. Ungerleider J, Fisher D, Fuller M, Caldwell A. The "bad trip": the etiology of the adverse LSD reaction. Am J Psychiatry 1968; 124:41.

99. Barnett BEW. Diazepam treatment for LSD intoxication. Lancet 1977; II:270.

100. Strassman RJ. Adverse reactions to psychedelic drugs. J Nerv Ment Dis 1984; 172:577.

101. Frosh W, Robbins E, Stern M. Untoward reactions to lysergic acid diethylamide (LSD) resulting in hospitalization. N Engl J Med 1965; 273:1235.

102. Bewley T. Adverse reaction from the illicit use of lysergide. BMJ 1967; III:28.

103. Baker A. Hospital admissions due to lysergic acid diethylamide. Lancet 1970; I:714.

104. Decker W, Brandes W. LSD misadventures in middle age. J Forensic Sci 1978; 23:3.

104a. Perera KM, Ferraro A, Pinto MR. Catatonia LSD induced? Aust N Z J Psychiatry 1995; 29:324.

105. Scher M, Neppe V. Carbamazepine adjunct for nonresponsive psychosis with prior hallucinogenic abuse. J Nerv Ment Dis 1989; 177:755.

106. Hatrick J, Dewhurst K. Delayed psychoses due to LSD. Lancet 1970; II:742.

107. Jacobs D. Psychiatric symptoms and hallucinogenic compounds. BMJ 1979; II:49.

108. Nagitch M, Fenwick S. LSD flashbacks and ego functioning. J Abnorm Psychol 1977; 86:352.

109. Stanton M, Bardoni A. Drug flashbacks: reported frequency in a military population. Am J Psychiatry 1972; 129:751.

110. Abraham HD. Visual phenomenology of the LSD flashback. Arch Gen Psychiatry 1983; 40:884.

111. Levi L, Miller NR. Visual illusions associated with previous drug abuse. J Clin Neuroophthalmol 1990; 10:103.

112. ffytche DH, Howard RJ. The perceptual consequences of visual loss: "positive" pathologies of vision. Brain 1999; 122:1247.

113. Fisher D, Ungerleider J. Grand mal seizures following ingestion of LSD. Calif Med 1976; 106:210.

114. Stimmel B. Cardiovascular Effects of Mood-Altering Drugs. New York: Raven Press, 1979.

115. Friedman SA, Hirsch SE. Extreme hyperthermia after LSD ingestion. JAMA 1979; 217:1549.

116. Klock JC, Boerner V, Becker CE. Coma, hyperthermia, and bleeding associated with massive LSD overdose. A report of eight cases. West J Med 1973; 119:183.

117. Mercieca J, Brown EA. Acute renal failure due to rhabdomyolysis associated with use of a straightjacket in lysergide intoxication. BMJ 1984; 288:1949.

118. Horita A, Hamilton AE. Lysergic acid diethylamide: dissociation of its behavioral and hyperthermic actions by dl-alpha-methyl-paratyrosine. Science 1969; 164:78.

119. Abraham HD, Aldridge AM. Adverse consequences of lysergic acid diethylamide. Addiction 1993; 88:1327.

120. Abraham HD, Duffy H. EEG coherence in post-LSD visual hallucinations. Psychiatry Res 2001; 107:151.

121. Abraham HD, Mamen A. LSD-like panic from risperidone in post-LSD visual disorder. J Clin Psychopharmacol 1996; 16:238.

122. Kawasaki A, Purvin V. Persistent palinopsia following ingestion of lysergic acid diethylamide (LSD). Arch Ophthalmol 1996; 114:47.

123. Aldura G, Crayton JW. Improvement of hallucinogen-induced persistent perception disorder by treatment with a combination of fluoxetine and olanzapine: case report. J Clin Psychopharmacol 2001; 21:343.

124. Markel H, Lee A, Holmes RD, et al. LSD flashback syndrome exacerbated by selective serotonin reuptake inhibitor antidepressants in adolescents. J Pediatr 1994; 125:817.

125. Lerner AG, Finkel B, Oyffe I, et al. Clonidine treatment for hallucinogen persisting perception disorder. Am J Psychiatry 1998; 155:1460.

126. Lerner AG, Oyffe I, Isaac G, et al. Naltrexone treatment of hallucinogen persisting perception disorder. Am J Psychiatry 1997; 154:437.

127. Bonson KR, Murphy DL. Alterations in responses to LSD in humans associated with chronic administration of tricyclic antidepressants, monoamine oxidase inhibitors or lithium. Behav Brain Res 1996; 73:229.

128. Altura B, Altura BM. Phencyclidine, lysergic acid diethylamide, and mescaline: cerebral artery spasms and hallucinogenic activity. Science 1981; 212:1051.

129. Sobel J, Espinas OE, Friedman SA. Carotid artery obstruction following LSD capsule ingestion. Arch Intern Med 1971; 127:290.

130. Lieberman AN, Bloom W, Kishore PS, Lin JP. Carotid artery occlusion following ingestion of LSD. Stroke 1974; 5:213.

131. Lignelli GJ, Buchheit WA. Angiitis in drug abusers. N Engl J Med 1971; 284:112.

132. Rumbaugh CL, Bergeron RT, Fang HCH, McCormick R. Cerebral angiographic changes in the drug abuse patient. Radiology 1971; 101:335.

133. McWilliams SA, Tuttle R. Long-term psychological effects of LSD. Psychol Bull 1973; 79:341.

134. Blacker KH, Jones RT, Stone GC, Pfefferbaum D. Chronic users of LSD: the "acidheads." Am J Psychiatry 1968; 125:97.

135. Wright M, Hogan T. Repeated LSD ingestion and performance on neuropsychological tests. J Nerv Ment Dis 1972; 154:432.

136. Tucker GJ, Quinlan D, Harrow M. Chronic hallucinogenic drug use and thought disturbance. Arch Gen Psychiatry 1972; 27:443.

137. Vardy MM, Kay SR. LSD psychosis or LSD-induced schizophrenia? A multi-method inquiry. Arch Gen Psychiatry 1983; 40:877.

138. Materson BJ, Barrett-Conner E. LSD "mainlining": a new hazard to health. JAMA 1967; 200:202.

139. Cohen MM, Marinello MJ, Back N. Chromosomal damage in human leukocytes induced by lysergic acid diethylamide. Science 1967; 155:1417.

140. Irwin S, Egozcue J. Chromosomal abnormalities in leukocytes from LSD-users. Science 1967; 157:313.

141. Auerback R, Rugowski JA. Lysergic acid diethylamide: effects on embryos. Science 1967; 157:1325.

142. Skakkebaek NE, Philip J, Rafelsen OJ. LSD in mice: abnormalities in meiotic chromosomes. Science 1968; 160:1246.

143. Alexander GJ, Miles B, Gold GM, Alexander RB. LSD: ingestion early in pregnancy produces abnormalities in offspring in rats. Science 1967; 157:459.

144. Eller JL, Morton JM. Bizarre deformities in offspring of user of lysergic acid diethylamide. N Engl J Med 1970; 283:395.

145. Chan CC, Fishman M, Egbert PR. Multiple ocular anomalies associated with maternal LSD ingestion. Arch Ophthalmol 1978; 96:282.

146. Loughman WD, Sargent TW, Isrealstein DM. Leukocytes of humans exposed to lysergic acid diethylamide: lack of chromosomal damage. Science 1967; 508:1967.

147. Sparkes RS, Melnyk J, Bozzetti LP. Chromosomal effect in vivo of exposure to lysergic acid diethylamide. Science 1968; 160:1343.

148. Warkany J, Takacs E. Lysergic acid diethyltryptamide (LSD): no teratogenicity in rats. Science 1968; 159:731.

149. Bender L, Siva-Sanker DV. Chromosome damage not found in children when treated with LSD. Science 1968; 159:749.

150. Hungerford DA, Tagler KM, Shagass C, et al. Cytogenic effects of LSD-25 therapy in man. JAMA 1968; 206:2287.

151. Corey MJ, Andrews JC, McLeod MJ, et al. Chromosome studies on patients (in vivo) and cells (in vitro) treated with lysergic acid diethylamide. N Engl J Med 1970; 282:939.

152. Cohen MM, Shiloh Y. Genetic toxicology of lysergic acid diethylamide (LSD-25). Mutat Res 1977-1978; 47:183.

152a. Li J-H, Lin L-F. Genetic toxicology of abused drugs: a brief review. Mutagenesis 1998; 13:557.

153. Nelson RA, Levine AM, Marks G, et al. Alcohol, tobacco, and recreational drug use and the risk of non-Hodgkin's lymphoma. Br J Cancer 1997; 76:1532.

154. Berk SI, LeBlond RF, Hodges KB, et al. A mesenteric mass in a chronic LSD user. Am J Med 1999; 1007:188.

155. Teitelbaum DT, Wingeleth DC. Diagnosis and management of recreational mescaline self-poisoning. J Anal Toxicol 1977; 1:36.

156. Hashimoto H, Clyde VJ, Parko KL. Botulism from peyote. N Engl J Med 1998; 339:203.

157. Nolte KB, Zumwalt RE. Fatal peyote ingestion associated with Mallory–Weiss lacerations. West J Med 1999; 170:328.

158. Reynolds PC, Jindrich EJ. A mescaline associated fatality. J Anal Toxicol 1985; 9:183.

159. Jacobs KW. Hallucinogenic mushrooms in Mississippi. J Miss State Med Assoc 1975; 16:35.

160. Pollock SH. A novel experience with Panaeolus: a case study from Hawaii. J Psychedelic Drugs 1974; 6:85.

161. Pollock SH. *Psilocybian mycetismus* with special reference to Panaeolus. J Psychedelic Drugs 1976; 8:43.

162. Goldfrank LR. Mushrooms: toxic and hallucinogenic. In: Goldfrank LR, Flomenbaum NE, Lewin NA, et al., eds. Goldfrank's Toxicologic Emergencies, 6th edition. Stamford, CT: Appleton & Lange, 1998; 1207.

163. Buck RW. Psychedelic effect of *Philiota spectabilis*. N Engl J Med 1967; 276:391.

164. Francis J, Murray VSG. Review of inquiries made to the NPIS concerning *Psilocybe* mushroom ingestion, 1973-1981. Hum Toxicol 1983; 2:349.

165. Curry SC, Rose MC. Intravenous mushroom poisoning. Ann Emerg Med 1985; 14:900.

166. McCormick DJ, Aubel A J, Gibbons MC. Nonlethal mushroom poisoning. Ann Intern Med 1979; 90:332.

167. McCawley EL, Brummett RE, Dana GW. Convulsions from *Psilocybe* mushroom poisoning. Proc West Pharmacol Soc 1962; 5:27.

168. Harries AD, Evans V. Sequelae of a "magic mushroom banquet." Postgrad Med J 1981; 57:571.

169. Peden NR, Pringle SD, Crooks J. The problem of Psilocybin mushroom abuse. Hum Toxicol 1982; 1:417.

170. Vollenweider FX, Leenders KL, Scharfetter C, et al. Positron emission tomography and fluorodeoxyglucose studies of metabolic hyperfrontality and psychopathology in the psilocybin model of psychosis. Neuropsychopharmacology 1997; 16:357.

171. Borowiak KS, Ciechanowski K, Waloszyzyk P. Psilocybin mushroom (*Psilocybe semilanceata*) intoxication with myocardial infarction. J Toxicol Clin Toxicol 1998; 36:47.

172. Hanes KR. Serotonin, psilocybin, and body dysmorphic disorder: a case report. J Clin Psychopharmacol 1996; 16:188.

173. Moreno FA, Delgado PL. Hallucinogen relief of obsessions and compulsions. Am J Psychiatry 1997; 154:1037.

174. Sivyer C, Dorrington L. Intravenous injection of mushrooms. Med J Aust 1984; 140:182.
175. Wolbach AB, Miner EJ, Isbell H. Comparison of psilocin with psilocybin, mescaline, and LSD-25. Psychopharmacologia 1962; 3:219.
176. Spoerke DG, Spoerke SE, Jumack BH. Rocky Mountain high. Ann Emerg Med 1985; 14:162.
177. Szara S, Rochland LH, Rosenthal D, Handlon JH. Psychological effects and metabolism of *N,N*-dimethyltryptamine in man. Arch Gen Psychiatry 1966; 15:320.
178. Rubin D. Dimethyltryptamine, a do-it-yourself hallucinogenic drug. JAMA 1967; 201:157.
179. Strassman RJ. Human psychopharmacology of *N,N*-dimethyltryptamine. Behav Brain Res 1996; 73:121.
180. Snyder SH, Faillace LA, Weingartner H. DOM (STP), a new hallucinogenic drug, and DOET: effects in normal subjects. Am J Psychiatry 1968; 125:357.
181. Snyder SH, Weingartner H, Faillace LA. DOET (2,5-dimethoxy-4-ethylamphetamine), a new psychotropic drug. Arch Gen Psychiatry 1971; 24:50.
182. Winek CL, Collum WD, Bricker JD. A death due to 4-bromo-2,5-dimethoxyamphetamine. Clin Toxicol 1981; 18:267.
183. Bowen JS, Davis GB, Kearney TE, Bardin J. Diffuse vascular spasm associated with 4-bromo-2,5-dimethoxyamphetamine ingestion. JAMA 1983; 249:1477.
184. Seiden LS, Kleven MS. Methamphetamine and related drugs: toxicity and resulting behavioral changes in response to pharmacological probes. NIDA Res Monogr 1989; 94:146.
185. Keitner GI, Sabaawi M, Haier RJ. Isosafrole and schizophrenia-like psychosis. Am J Psychiatry 1984; 141:997.
186. Ingram AL. Morning glory seed reaction. JAMA 1964; 190:1133.
187. Cohen S. Suicide following morning glory seed ingestion. Am J Psychiatry 1964; 120:1024.
188. Lewin NA, Holland MA, Goldfrank LR, Flomenbaum NE. Herbal preparations. In: Goldfrank LR, Flomenbaum NE, Lewin NA, et al., eds. Toxicologic Emergencies, 4th edition. Norwalk, CT: Appleton & Lange, 1990; 587.
189. Rice WB, Genest K. Acute toxicity of extracts of morning glory seeds in mice. Nature 1965; 207:302.
190. Weil AT. Nutmeg as a psychoactive drug. In: Efron DH, Holmstedt V, Kline NS, eds. Ethnopharmacologic Search for Psychoactive Drugs. New York: Raven Press, 1967:188.
191. Malcolm X, Haley A. The Autobiography of Malcolm X. New York: Grove Press, 1964.
192. Truitt EB, Callaway E, Braude MC, et al. The pharmacology of myristicin: a contribution to the psychopharmacology of nutmeg. J Neuropsychol 1961; 2:205.
193. Venables GS, Evered D, Hall R. Nutmeg poisoning. BMJ 1976; I:96.

194. Payne RB. Nutmeg intoxication. N Engl J Med 1963; 269:36.
195. Shafran I. Nutmeg toxicology. N Engl J Med 1976; 294:849.
196. Painter JC, Shanor SP, Winek CL. Nutmeg poisoning-a case report. Clin Toxicol 1971; 4:1.
197. Lavy G. Nutmeg intoxication in pregnancy. A case report. J Reprod Med 1987; 32:63.
198. Green RC. Nutmeg poisoning. JAMA 1959; 171:1342.
198a. Cairney S, Maruff P, Clough AR. The neurobehavioral effects of kava. Aust N Z J Psychiatry 2002; 36:657.
199. Baum SS, Hill R, Rammelspacher H. Effect of kava extract and individual kavapyrones on neurotransmitter levels in the nucleus accumbens of rats. Prog Neuropsychopharmacol Biol Psychiatry 1998; 22:1105.
200. Anon. Kava. Lancet 1988; II:258.
201. Cawte J. Psychoactive substances of the South Seas: betel, kava, and pituri. Aust N Z J Psychiatry 1985; 19:83.
202. Siegel RK. Herbal intoxication: psychoactive effects from herbal cigarettes, tea, and capsules. JAMA 1976; 236:473.
203. Brody JE. Americans gamble on herbs as medicine. NY Times, February 9, 1999.
204. Burros M. New questions about kava's safety. NY Times, January 16, 2002.
204a. Cairney S, Maruff P, Clough AR, et al. Saccade and cognitive impairment associated with kava intoxication. Hum Psychopharmacol Clin Exp 2003; 18:525.
205. Spillane PK, Fisher DA, Currie BJ. Neurological manifestations of kava intoxication. Med J Aust 1997; 167:172.
206. Popik P, Layer RT, Skolnick P. 100 years of ibogaine: neurochemical and pharmacological actions of a putative anti-addictive drug. Pharmacol Rev 1995; 47:235.
207. Jones RL. New cautions over a plant with a buzz. NY Times, July 9, 2001.
208. Roth BL, Baner K, Westkaemper R, et al. Salvinorin A: a potent naturally occurring non-nitrogenous κ opioid selective agonist. Proc Natl Acad Sci USA 2002; 99:11934.
209. Lyttle T, Goldstein D, Gartz J. *Bufo* toads and bufotenine: fact and fiction surrounding an alleged psychedelic. J Psychoactive Drugs 1996; 28:267.
210. Wishnia: Dances with toads. High Times, January 21, 1995.
211. Fabing HD, Hawkins JR. Intravenous bufotenine injection in the human being. Science 1956; 123:886.
212. Horgan J. *Bufo* abuse-a toxic toad get licked, boiled, tee'd up and tanned. Sci Am 1990; 263:26.
213. McBride MC. Bufotenine: toward an understanding of possible psychoactive mechanisms. J Psychoactive Drugs 2000; 32:321.
214. Howard R, Foerstl H. Toad-licker's psychosis–a warning. Br J Psychiatry 1990; 157:779.
215. Hitt M, Ettinger DD. Toad toxicity. N Engl J Med 1986; 314:1517.

Chapter 9
Inhalants

Oh, Tom! Such a gas has Davy discovered! . . . It made me laugh and tingle . . .
It made one strong, and so happy!
—Robert Southey

You're in outer space. You're Superman. You're floating in air, seeing double,
riding next to God. It's Kicksville.
—Anonymous juvenile glue sniffer

A strong smell of turpentine prevails throughout.
—Oliver Wendel Holmes, describing his vision of heaven while sniffing ether

Before they were recognized as general anesthetics, nitrous oxide and diethyl ether were used recreationally. Today volatile substance abuse is a worldwide problem.[1,2] The different products that are used often contain several psychically active compounds, yet the "highs" and "jags" produced are remarkably similar.

Pharmacology and Animal Studies

Among the several chemical classes of abused volatile compounds (Table 9–1), the aromatic hydrocarbon toluene and the halogenated hydrocarbon trichloroethane have been most extensively studied. Acute effects in animals are dose-related and similar to those of sedatives and ethanol: hyperactivity progresses to ataxia, sedation, coma, respiratory depression, and death.[3] In mice, toluene and xylene prevent pentylenetetrazol-induced seizures. In rats, toluene increases operant behavior that has been suppressed by electric shock.[4] In rodents and pigeons, low doses of toluene and xylene increase rates of operant responding, but high doses decrease them.[5,6] By contrast, halogenated hydrocarbons such as trichloroethane and ketones such as methyl-*n*-amylketone decrease response rates at both low and high doses.[3]

Animal evidence for the development of tolerance to these agents is equivocal. For toluene, it was found in rats but not in mice or monkeys.[7–9] For trichloroethane, it was not evident in mice.[10] Cross-tolerance has been demonstrated in mice between ethanol and several inhalational anesthetics, but such effects involving solvent compounds have not been reported.[3] Similarly, although mice develop withdrawal seizures following exposure to ethylene, diethyl ether, or cyclopropane and although chloroform can suppress the signs of barbiturate withdrawal, physical dependence to toluene, trichloroethane, or other solvent hydrocarbons has not been demonstrated in animals.[3]

Monkeys self-administer chloroform, diethyl ether, nitrous oxide, and toluene.[3,11,12] In drug discrimination studies, mice trained to identify barbiturate generalize to halothane, trichloroethane, and toluene.[13,14] In mice, ethanol enhances the behavioral and lethal effects of trichloroethane, and toluene and trichloroethane enhance the effects of

Table 9–1. Chemical Classification of Abused Volatile Compounds

Aliphatic hydrocarbons
n-Butane
Isobutane
n-Hexane
Propane
Pentane

Aromatic hydrocarbons
Toluene
Xylene
Benzene
Naphthalene
Paradichlorobenzene

Esters
Ethyl acetate

Ketones
Acetone
Butanone
Methylethylketone
Methyl-n-butylketone
Methylisobutylketone

Halogenated hydrocarbons
Chloroform
Halothane
Enflurane
Isoflurane
Trichloroethane
Dichloroethylene
Trichloroethylene
Tetrachloroethylene
Dichloromethane
Carbon tetrachloride
Dichlorodifluoromethane
Chlorodifluoromethane
Bromochlorodifluoromethane
Trichlorofluoromethane

Ethers
Diethyl ether

Anesthetic gases
Nitrous oxide

Nitrites
Butyl nitrite
Isobutyl nitrite
Amyl nitrite

ethanol and sedatives.[3,15] In an "elevated plus-maze" (a test used to predict antianxiety effects) toluene produced concentration-dependent effects similar to those produced by diazepam. By contrast, trichloroethane produced such effects only at doses that also increased locomotor activity.[16]

Like other self-administered drugs, toluene in rodents stimulates locomotor activity and enhances mesolimbic dopamine neurotransmission. The dopaminergic effect appears to be indirect, perhaps involving inhibition of N-methyl-D-aspartate (NMDA) neurotransmission and facilitation of γ-aminobutyric acid (GABA) neurotransmission.[17,18] The neural basis of inhalant abuse, however, is less understood than that of other recreational drugs. The recognition that ethanol effects are not simply the result of nonspecific "membrane perturbation" but rather involve specific interactions with a number of neurotransmitter receptors, especially glutamate and GABA (see Chapter 12), raises the possibility that general anesthetics, volatile solvents, and other abused vapors have similar receptor specificities.[19]

Historical Background and Epidemiology

The inhalation of vapors to achieve religious ecstasy pre-dates recorded history; substances have included cannabis and ergot hallucinogens (see Chapters 7 and 8). Evidence suggests that the prophetic trances of the ancient Greek Delphic oracles were induced by hydrocarbon gases (in particular, methane, ethane, and ethylene) seeping through fissures in the limestone floor of the temple.[19a] The discovery of diethyl ether in the 13th century added a secular element to such activity. In the 18th century, diethyl ether was marketed as a medicinal tonic called "Anodyne," and whether drunk or sniffed it quickly became a popular recreational drug in Britain— cheaper than heavily taxed alcoholic beverages and producing short-lived effects without hangover.[20] In the 19th century, diethyl ether was promoted as an alternative to ethanol in Ireland ("ether frolics"), and it was widely used by American students well before its demonstration as a surgical anesthetic by William Morton in 1846. Diethyl ether was drunk as an alcohol substitute during American Prohibition (1920–1933) and in Germany during World War II.

Nitrous oxide was discovered by Sir Joseph Priestley in 1776 and later synthesized by Sir Humphrey Davy, who personally described both its intoxicating effects and its addiction liability. Dubbed "laughing gas," nitrous oxide was inhaled recreationally by Davy's friends, including the poets Samuel Taylor Coleridge and Robert Southey and the thesaurist Peter Roget.[21,22] In the early

19th century, nitrous oxide sniffing was widespread in the United States; it was not until 1845 that the Connecticut dentist Horace Wells began using it as a general anesthetic.[22]

Chloroform, like diethyl ether, is a readily vaporized liquid. It was discovered in 1831, and recreational use quickly followed. Although a tendency to sudden death limited its popularity, 19th-century chloroform addicts were not rare; less odorous than diethyl ether or nitrous oxide, it was easily concealed, and users could sniff it throughout the day undetected. Horace Wells died a chloroform addict.[20]

In recent decades, inhalant abusers have turned to a wide variety of household products, especially glues, solvents, and fuels (Table 9–2).[23,24] The earliest reference to glue sniffing seems to have been a 1959 newspaper article describing children in several western American cities.[25] A national chorus of alarm followed, and as exaggerated warnings led to legislation and arrests, glue sniffing became a nationwide epidemic.[26] Diversification to other substances soon followed, and today volatile substance abuse involves children throughout the world.

In 1979, inhalants had been used by 17% of Americans aged 18 to 25 years and 10% of children aged 12 to 17 years.[27,28] Since then this prevalence has held steady. By the fourth grade 6% of U.S. children have tried inhalants, and sniffing by even younger children is not unusual. Reports include a 3-year-old gasoline addict.[29–31] Reported lifetime use peaks during the eighth grade at 21%, with 6% describing use within 30 days. Lifetime use reported by twelfth graders is 15%, with 2.5% describing use within 30 days. (The paradoxical drop in lifetime use with increasing age is perhaps explained by the tendency of inhalant users to drop out of school.) Today the first illicit drug to be used by children is more likely to be an inhalant than to be marijuana.[32,33]

In 1989, inhalant abuse in Britain accounted for 113 deaths, half in children 16 years old or

Table 9–2. Abused Products and Their Contents

Products	Contents
Aerosols (refrigerants, frying pan cleaners, antitussives, hair sprays, bronchodilators, shampoos, deodorants, antiseptics, pain killers)	Fluorinated hydrocarbons, propane, isobutane
Dry cleaning fluids, spot removers, furniture polish, degreasers	Chlorinated hydrocarbons, naphtha (gasoline hydrocarbons)
Glues, cements, rubber patching	Toluene, acetone, benzene, aliphatic acetates, n-hexane, cyclohexane, trichloroethylene, xylene, butyl alcohol, dichloroethylene, methylethylketone, methylethylisobutylketone, chloroform, ethanol, triorthocresyl phosphate
Lighter fluid	Aliphatic and aromatic hydrocarbons
Fire-extinguishing agents	Bromochlorodifluoromethane
Nail polish remover	Acetone, aliphatic acetates, benzene
Bottled fuel gas	Butane, propane
Typewriter correction fluid	Trichloroethane, trichloroethylene
Natural gas	Methane, ethane, propane, butane
Marker pens	Toluene, xylene
Mothballs	Naphthalene, paradichlorobenzene
Toilet deodorizers	Paradichlorobenzene
Paints, enamels, lacquers, lacquer and paint thinners	Toluene, methylene chloride, aliphatic acetates, benzene, ethanol
Petroleum (gasoline, naphtha gas, benzine)	Many aliphatic, aromatic, and other hydrocarbons (e.g., olefins, naphthanes), including butane, hexane, pentane, benzene, toluene, and xylene; tetraethyl lead
Anesthetics (surgical supply, whipped cream dispensers)	Nitrous oxide, diethyl ether, halothane, chloroform, enflurane, isoflurane, trichloroethylene
"Room odorizers"	Amyl, butyl, and isobutyl nitrite

younger.[34] The most common products used were gas fuels, especially butane for cigarette lighters (33%), antiperspirant or deodorant aerosols (21%), and glue (21%). (Many users had switched from glue because of its telltale odor, tendency to leave stains, and increasing scarcity on store shelves.) Similar experiences have been reported from other Western European countries, Hungary, Canada, Mexico, South America, Japan, South Africa, Israel, Australia, Singapore, Malaysia, and Nigeria.[35–48]

Among users in the United States, males outnumber females by 10:1. African-Americans are underrepresented.[32] In a report from a Virginia juvenile correctional facility 36% of white youths reported inhalant use compared with 1.4% of African-American youths. The most common substances used were gasoline, Freon, butane lighter fluid, glue, and nitrous oxide.[49] Inhalant abusers are usually not part of a drug subculture, although many take other drugs as well.[50] Regular users are most often children of low socioeconomic background, often neglected, abused, or from unstable homes.[30,51,51a] Similar to alcoholics, many carry a diagnosis of antisocial personality disorder.[52] Gasoline sniffing is particularly common among Native Americans in the United States and Canada; in one community, 50% of children age 4 to 18 years were chronic abusers.[23,53–55] Gasoline sniffing is also endemic in Australian Aboriginal communities.[38,56,57] During the 1990s, inhalant use by Native American adolescents fell relative to use by Latinos and non-Latino whites, probably a consequence of prevention programs in Native American communities.[58,59]

In the 1970s, it was discovered that fluorinated hydrocarbon propellants—which include the proprietary mixture Freon—adversely affect the earth's atmospheric ozone. A decline in abuse followed restrictions on their manufacture.[60]

In the United States, there are three main types of inhalant abusers: (1) inhalant-addicted adults, (2) adolescent polydrug users, and (3) younger inhalant users.[61] Most children eventually give up inhalants, but some become addicted and continue use through adulthood.[32,62] Overrepresented among adults are shoemakers and sandal makers, cabinetmakers, printers, painters, gas station attendants, automobile and bicycle repair shop workers, petroleum refinery workers, and workers in chemical plants.[63] Inhalant abuse is also common among military recruits and prison inmates.[30,64] The occupational risk of physicians and other medical workers for anesthesia abuse has been recognized for more than a century.[65]

Juvenile sniffers are not restricted to impoverished communities or broken homes; epidemics of solvent abuse have occurred in boarding schools. Obtaining products from home, school, grocery stores, hardware stores, or gas tanks, children sniff gasoline, glue, paint, lighter fluid, nail polish remover, marker pens, deodorants, kerosene, aerosols, typing correction fluid, school laboratory gas jets, nitrous oxide, lacquer thinner, transmission fluid, gun-cleaning solvents, and fire-extinguishing agents.[63]

Amidst this array are four major classes of inhalants: (1) volatile solvents such as glues, paint thinners, and gasoline; (2) aerosols such as hair sprays, deodorants, and spray paints; (3) volatile anesthetics such as diethyl ether or nitrous oxide; and (4) volatile nitrites.[66] Substances are usually sniffed (nasal) or "huffed" (oral inhalation) from a saturated rag (if liquid), a plastic bag (if viscous), or directly from a container.[28] A gently heated frying pan may be used. Sniffing can continue over hours, and chronic abusers might inhale 0.5 L daily for years. Infrequently the same substance is drunk, sometimes mixed with beer or chaser. Children have mixed nail polish remover with Coca-Cola.[41] Rarely volatile substances are injected intravenously.[67,68] A form of inhalant abuse carrying its own special hazard is propane or butane "fire breathing."[69]

Acute Effects

Whichever substance is used, the desired effects resemble ethanol intoxication: euphoria and relaxation with or without ataxia, diplopia, and slurred speech. As with ethanol, grandiosity and impulsiveness produce accidents and violence. There may be a feeling of "blankness" or "numbness," and consciousness may be briefly lost. Higher doses cause toxic psychosis. Delusions can lead to self-destructive behavior; during glue-sniffing, an 18-year-old enucleated his own eye.[70] Visual distortions or hallucinations can be either pleasant or terrifying—for example, savage animals, ghosts, or gory wounds.[30,71–73] The presence of hallucinations during intoxication is perhaps the symptom that most distinguishes inhalants from ethanol and sedatives.[41] High doses cause ataxia, nystagmus, dysarthria, and drowsiness progressing to coma and sometimes seizures.[74,75]

Dizziness, flushing, coughing, sneezing, increased salivation, nausea, and vomiting frequently accompany intoxication. Symptoms last only 15 to 30 minutes but can be sustained for hours by repeated use.[64,73] Except for occasional headache, most users do not experience "hangover."[76] Some have amnesia for the episode.[77]

Death occurs from vomiting and aspiration, suffocation by plastic bags, accidents, violence, or suddenly without apparent cause.[78–85] An epidemiological survey in Britain attributed death to direct toxic effects in 51%, asphyxia in 21%, aspiration of vomitus in 18%, and trauma in 11%.[86] Some substances—for example, trichloroethane, fluorinated hydrocarbons, and non-Freon aerosols such as isobutane and propane—cause cardiac arrhythmia, especially when there is hypoxia or exertion.[87] Directly spraying cold gases (e.g., butane or aerosol propellants) into the mouth stimulates the larynx and can lead to reflexic vagal cardiac depression.[88] Many inhalants depress myocardial contractility and increase the sensitivity of the heart to catecholamines.[89] Ventricular fibrillation followed toluene sniffing in a 16-year-old boy, and inhalant-related sudden death has occurred during sexual intercourse.[90] A 15-year-old boy was successfully resuscitated after being found in cardiorespiratory arrest following inhalation of a typewriter correction fluid containing trichloroethylene and trichloroethane.[91] Respiratory depression has followed inhalation of glue,[92] paint,[93] and gasoline.[94] A 15-year-old boy collapsed and died after inhaling bromochlorodifluoromethane from a fire extinguisher.[95] An 11-year-old boy was found dead after sniffing butane cigarette lighter fuel, and a 15-year-old boy died from pulmonary burns during propane "torch breathing."[96] Of 282 inhalant deaths in Britain, 17% were associated with deliberate sexual asphyxia.[86]

Clues to inhalant abuse are the smell of solvent on the breath (which may last hours after use) and, in those sniffing from plastic bags, a characteristic "glue-sniffer's rash" around the nose and mouth.[2,41] With the exception of gasoline, gas chromatography identifies most volatile compounds in the blood within 10 hours of exposure. Urinary metabolites can be detected for toluene, xylene, trichloroethylene, trichloroethane, and tetrachloroethylene. Breath analysis by mass spectrometry is also used.[35,97] Such technology is of little value, however, when inhalant abuse is unsuspected in the first place. A 38-year-old former alcoholic man had "seizures" consisting of episodic loss of consciousness followed by slurred speech, amnesia, and bizarre behavior; extensive investigations were non-diagnostic until his wife found him huffing trichloroethylene, which he had taken up after discontinuing ethanol.[98]

Because symptoms are so short-lived, inhalant intoxication infrequently requires treatment unless there are cardiorespiratory complications. Cardiac arrhythmia, however, remains a risk for several hours after intoxication has subsided.

In contrast to some animals, human inhalant abusers experience tolerance to acute effects.[30,99] Abrupt discontinuation can produce mild symptoms resembling ethanol withdrawal,[100] but chronic inhalant abuse does not seem to be associated with any consistent abstinence syndrome.[99,101–103] (Reports of delirium, hallucinations, or seizures are so exceptional as to invite skepticism.[63]) Psychic dependence—that is, addiction—is common, however.[41]

Medical and Neurological Complications

Systemic Organ Damage

Different volatile substances damage different organs. Fatal congestive heart failure occurred in a 24-year-old man who sniffed a shoe cleaning solvent containing trichloroethylene.[104] Massive pulmonary hemorrhages and cerebral edema were found at autopsy in a benzene sniffer.[80] Kidney, liver, and bone marrow damage follow exposure to many of these substances, especially benzene and chlorinated hydrocarbons.[105,106] (Because of its association with fatal liver, kidney, and cardiac disease, carbon tetrachloride is no longer present in household products, but it is still used in industry.[73]) Toluene causes metabolic acidosis with either a normal or increased anion gap; intoxication was reported in association with severe diabetic ketoacidosis.[107]

Fatal aplastic anemia affects glue sniffers.[108] Glue and solvent sniffers have developed emphysema and pulmonary hypertension.[109] A man mixed Vim and Ajax cleaning powders with water and deliberately sniffed the chlorine fumes produced; he developed reversible pulmonary insufficiency and cor pulmonale.[110]

Neuropsychiatric Damage

A number of studies found behavioral, cognitive, electroencephalographic, and computed tomographic (CT) abnormalities in inhalant abusers (as well as in occupationally exposed subjects).[111–120] The milder the impairment, the more difficult it is to infer causality. Methodological problems include small samples, lack of controls, lack of pre-exposure data, uncertainty regarding last use, and unmasked examiners. Certainly there are often other contributing factors, especially in emotionally deprived or physically abused children, and behavioral disturbance is as likely to be the cause of inhalant abuse as its result. Nonetheless, in some individuals, volatile substance abuse has devastating neuropsychiatric consequences.

Toluene

Persistent encephalopathy and cerebellar ataxia follow chronic toluene exposure.[121–131] Of 25 adults with symptomatic toluene poisoning from spray paint sniffing, nine had myopathic weakness, often severe and accompanied by hypokalemia, hypophosphatemia, and cardiac arrhythmia; six had gastrointestinal symptoms (nausea, vomiting, abdominal pain, hematemesis); and 10 had "neuropsychiatric syndromes."[132] Consistent with other reports,[133,134] renal tubular acidosis was common.

In a study of 20 young adults who had sniffed toluene-containing products for at least 2 years but had abstained for at least 4 weeks, 13 had neurological abnormalities, including cognitive (60%), pyramidal (50%), cerebellar (45%), and cranial nerve or brainstem (25%). Seven had disabling dementia, with apathy, poor concentration, memory loss, visuospatial dysfunction, and "impaired complex cognition." Oculomotor dysfunction included ocular flutter and opsoclonus. Four had anosmia, and two

had bilateral sensorineural deafness.[135] Magnetic resonance imaging in demented toluene abusers shows diffuse cerebral, cerebellar, and brainstem atrophy with loss of gray and white matter differentiation and, on T2-weighted images, increased signal in periventricular white matter and decreased signal in thalamus and basal ganglia.[136–140,140a] Autopsy in a demented patient revealed diffuse myelin pallor maximal in the cerebellar, periventricular, and deep cerebral white matter without neuronal loss, axonal swelling, or gliosis.[136] Autopsy on another toluene sniffer showed cerebral and cerebellar atrophy with degeneration and gliosis of long tracts.[129] In another autopsy report ultramicroscopic examination of macrophages showed trilaminar cytoplasmic inclusions similar to those found in adrenoleukodystrophy (ALD), and biochemical analysis of cerebral white matter showed increased amounts of very long chain fatty acids characteristic of ALD.[141]

A study of house painters exposed to solvents for decades revealed cognitive abnormalities but little or no evidence of brain atrophy on CT scans; however, cerebral blood flow was significantly reduced compared with controls.[117] Positron-emission tomographic studies of workers chronically exposed to tetrabromoethane showed cortical and subcortical hypometabolism,[142] and subjects occupationally exposed to toluene and trichloroethylene had abnormally reduced amplitudes of the N100 and P300 event-related potentials.[143]

In young rodents, toluene impairs learning, high-frequency hearing, and coordination and is concentrated in central nervous system (CNS) white matter.[144–148] Pathological CNS changes have not been observed, however.

Toluene abusers have developed irreversible optic atrophy,[126,149] and a young man who had sniffed glue for 5 years developed progressive optic neuropathy accompanied by severe sensorineural hearing loss.[150] More subtle but persistent visual abnormalities were described in 12 adolescent glue sniffers.[151] Two young paint sniffers with optic neuropathy, dementia, and cerebellar ataxia had abnormal brainstem auditory evoked potentials and CT evidence of pontomedullary atrophy.[152] Horizontal and vertical pendular nystagmus in four chronic glue sniffers was attributed to brainstem and cerebellar white matter damage; all four additionally had visual impairment, and two had optic atrophy.[153]

A 15-year-old boy developed status epilepticus while sniffing glue and thereafter had chronic epilepsy and behavioral problems.[154] A 22-year-old man who had sniffed lacquer thinner for nearly a decade developed hypokalemic periodic paralysis; attacks of weakness and hypokalemic hyperchloremic metabolic acidosis correlated temporally with toluene exposure.[155] Toluene probably does not cause peripheral neuropathy.[119,135]

Toluene Plus Methylene Chloride

Combined carbon monoxide and methanol poisoning affected a 17-year-old boy who sniffed a carburetor cleaner containing toluene and methylene chloride (which is metabolized to carbon dioxide and carbon monoxide); marked metabolic acidosis and elevated blood carboxyhemoglobin levels cleared with oxygen and ethanol treatment.[156]

Carbon Tetrachloride

In contrast to toluene, carbon tetrachloride causes delirium, cerebellar ataxia, seizures, and coma after brief exposure. Patients often have several days of headache and myalgia and then develop jaundice, renal failure, congestive heart failure, and CNS symptoms. Autopsies show Purkinje cell loss and perivenous hemorrhages most prominent in the cerebellum and basis pontis.[157–159]

Gasoline

Gasoline, which contains aliphatic and aromatic hydrocarbons, including toluene, also causes encephalopathy in chronic sniffers. Gasoline containing tetraethyl lead additionally causes lead encephalopathy.[57,160–166] An adolescent sniffer of leaded gasoline developed progressive dementia and ataxia, and died, and another 14-year-old gasoline sniffer died with dementia, chorea, peripheral neuropathy, myopathy, and hepatic and renal damage.[167,168] A 27-year-old gasoline sniffer developed generalized myoclonus, agitation, and hallucinations; erythrocytes had basophilic stippling, and blood lead level was 104 μg/dL.[169] More subtle neurological abnormalities are found in populations with a high prevalence of leaded gasoline abuse.[168] Symptomatic lead poisoning, with colic and anemia, occurred in a painter who ingested lead carbonate-containing paint deliberately to induce hallucinations.[170] In a report from Australia, leaded gasoline sniffers who had never been acutely encephalopathic had abnormalities of tandem gait, limb coordination, attention, recognition memory, and paired associate learning.[171] Peripheral neuropathy in some gasoline sniffers has been attributed to triorthocresylphosphate in the product.[172]

n-Hexane

Well studied is peripheral neuropathy in glue and lacquer-thinner sniffers.[119,173–181] Paresthesias in the feet are followed by ascending weakness and atrophy, leading to quadriplegia over a few weeks. Trophic changes are common, and cranial neuropathies occur. Cerebrospinal fluid is normal, or there is mildly elevated protein content. Nerve conduction velocities are reduced, and focal conduction block is described.[181a] Nerve biopsy reveals segmental distention of axons by masses of neurofilaments and secondary demyelination. Incomplete improvement occurs with abstinence, and the occasional presence of spasticity during recovery suggests that CNS damage also occurs but is masked by the peripheral signs. The responsible toxin is n-hexane, the metabolic product of which, 2,5-hexane-dione, is also the metabolite of methyl-n-butyl-ketone, a cause of peripheral neuropathy in industrial workers.[182] Both n-hexane and 2,3-hexane-dione cause peripheral nerve and CNS axonal degeneration in rats,[183,184] and n-hexane is also probably the responsible toxin in peripheral neuropathy associated with naphtha sniffing.[185] That additional substances in glue are neurotoxic is suggested by an epidemic of peripheral neuropathy among Berlin glue sniffers after methyl-ethyl-ketone was added to the n-hexane-containing product.[186] Severe polyneuropathy also affects sniffers of lacquer thinners containing n-heptane, and in other cases of solvent-related peripheral neuropathy trichloroethylene may contribute.[187,188] In the 1970s, oil of mustard, which irritates mucous membranes, was added to a number of glue products to discourage abuse.[189]

Parkinsonism followed years of occupational exposure to n-hexane in a middle-aged woman,[190] and rodents given *n*-hexane or 2,5-hexane-dione have reduced striatal levels of dopamine and homovanillic acid (but not norepinephrine or serotonin).[191] As with 1-methyl-4-phenyl-1,2,3, 6-tetrahydropyridine (MPTP) (see Chapter 3), the association has raised the possibility that human Parkinson's disease is related to similar environmental toxins.[192]

Trichloroethylene

Trichloroethylene, present in dry cleaning fluids, causes trigeminal neuropathy.[119,193] The mechanism is unclear, but the association led to its use earlier in this century to treat trigeminal neuralgia.

A 12-year-old habitual glue sniffer developed dense hemiparesis, and cerebral angiography showed occlusion of the middle cerebral artery. A proposed mechanism was vasospasm secondary to trichloroethylene-induced sensitization of vessel receptors to circulating catecholamines.[194] Radioisotope brain scan in a boy with status epilepticus after toluene sniffing showed several wedge-shaped areas of increased uptake in both cerebral hemispheres, consistent with infarcts.[195] Few studies in either animals or humans have addressed the effects of solvents on cerebral circulation. Chloroform, diethyl ether, and trichloroethylene are cerebral vasodilators, but chronic use leads to decreased cerebral blood flow.[196]

Nitrites

Popular among frequenters of disco-bars are amyl, butyl, and isobutyl nitrite ("snappers," "poppers," "pearls"). To circumvent Food and Drug Administration (FDA) regulations, butyl and isobutyl nitrite are sold in "head shops" as "room odorizers," "liquid aroma," or "liquid incense." Believed to enhance sexual pleasure, especially among homosexuals, they carry such trade names as "Rush," "Kick," "Vaporole," "Bullet," "Locker Room," "Heart On," "Bang," "Climax," and "Mama Poppers" and are often taken with ethanol, marijuana, or sedatives.[32,197] In 1986, 9% of American high school seniors reported having used alkyl nitrites at least once.[198] The euphoric "high" lasts only seconds to minutes. Cerebral vasodilation and

increased intracranial pressure accompany the euphoria; headache and nausea are frequent. There is also peripheral vasodilation, flushing, and a feeling of warmth.[197–199] Uncertain is whether the subjective effects of nitrites are the result simply of their vasodilatory actions or if they also have direct actions on the brain.[19]

Irritating to skin and mucous membranes, nitrites cause crusty perioral and nasal lesions and tracheobronchitis.[199] Nitrites also cause methemoglobinemia. Syncope tends to limit the dosage when they are inhaled, but symptomatic methemoglobinemia, with dyspnea, nausea, tachycardia, lethargy, stupor, seizures, cardiac arrhythmia, and circulatory failure, can follow inhalation.[200–204] Ingestion of nitrates has caused collapse, coma, and death despite treatment with methylene blue.[205–210]

Rupture of a basilar artery aneurysm occurred during sexual orgasm following nitrite inhalation in a 43-year-old man.[211]

A 15-year-old boy developed irreversible blindness and optic atrophy after inhaling amyl nitrite; an influenza-like illness prior to the episode offered an alternative mechanism, however.[212]

Nitrites are immunosuppressive,[213] and among their metabolites are carcinogenic nitrosoamines.[197,214] It is possible that nitrites carry independent risk either for acquiring human immunodeficiency virus (HIV) infection during homosexual intercourse or for developing Kaposi's sarcoma once infected.[198,214] Nitrite-induced production by macrophages of tumor necrosis factor-alpha (TNFα) directly stimulates HIV replication and the growth of Kaposi sarcoma cells.[215] In an epidemiological study of homosexual couples in Boston, the odds ratio (OR) for HIV infection was much greater among men who always used nitrites during unprotected receptive anal intercourse (OR = 31.8) than among men who sometimes (OR = 7.1) or never (OR = 9.0) used them.[215a] A study of homosexual HIV-infected men from Vancouver found nitrites an independent risk factor for Kaposi's sarcoma.[216] A similar study from San Francisco, however, did not.[217]

Nitrous Oxide

Not surprisingly, health care personnel are overrepresented among abusers of volatile anesthetics, especially nitrous oxide.[218–220] A survey at a leading American medical school revealed that up to 20% of medical and dental students used nitrous oxide recreationally, usually from whipped cream cans or cartridges, but sometimes from medical or commercial sources.[218] Comparable numbers were described among graduate students in New Zealand.[220a] Anoxic brain damage, sometimes fatal, has been reported in nitrous oxide abusers.[221–228] Pneumomediastinum has resulted from inhalation of pressurized nitrous oxide,[229] and acute pulmonary insufficiency followed inhalation of homemade nitrous oxide contaminated by nitrogen dioxide.[230]

Myeloneuropathy after prolonged exposure to nitrous oxide clinically resembles subacute combined degeneration secondary to cobalamin (vitamin B_{12}) deficiency. Patients have varying combinations of peripheral neuropathy, myelopathy, and altered mentation.[224–226,231–241] Electrophysiological studies reveal abnormal somatosensory evoked responses and visual evoked responses.[240] Anemia is conspicuously absent, and subtle hematological abnormalities—macrocytosis or neutrophil hypersegmentation—are infrequent. In 16 patients whose serum cobalamin was measured, it was normal in 13 and slightly decreased in 3.[231,232,236] Schilling tests have been normal except in one patient with a low normal serum cobalamin level and malabsorption consistent with pernicious anemia.[242]

A similar syndrome with typical pathological findings affects monkeys and fruit bats (but not mice or rats) exposed to nitrous oxide for prolonged periods.[243,244] Briefer heavy human exposure to nitrous oxide, moreover, causes megaloblastic bone marrow changes,[245] and both anemia and myeloneuropathy have been precipitated or exacerbated in cobalamin deficient patients undergoing nitrous oxide anesthesia.[246–248] Nitrous oxide oxidizes cobalamin, rendering inactive the vitamin B_{12}-dependent enzymes methionine synthetase[249] and methylmalonyl-CoA mutase,[250] and in a nitrous oxide abuser methylmalonic acid levels were increased in serum and, to an even greater degree, in cerebrospinal fluid.[242] Patients with nitrous oxide-induced myeloneuropathy should be treated with cyanocobalamin to replace their inactivated cobalamin. In nitrous oxide-exposed animals methionine protects against myelopathy,[251] and

methionine has been anecdotally reported to benefit exposed humans.[225]

Halothane, Chloroform

Fatal hepatitis and sudden death have occurred in hospital workers who deliberately inhaled, ingested, or injected halothane.[252–254] Among German adolescents, coma followed chloroform sniffing.[255]

Mothballs

Abuse of mothballs may involve sniffing, sucking, or chewing.[255a–d] Mothballs made of naphthalene cause headache, lethargy, vomiting, hemolysis, methemoglobinemia, hyperkalemia, fever, acute hepatic and renal failure, seizures, and coma. Mothballs made of paradichlorobenzene cause chronic kidney and liver disease. A 10-year-old boy who sniffed naphthalene mothballs for 8 hours nightly over 2 months developed progressive portal hypertension and died of liver failure.[255c] A 54-year-old woman who since her teens had sniffed or chewed naphthalene or paradichlorobenzene mothballs (or, alternatively, paradichlorobenzene-containing toilet deodorizers) developed end-state renal disease and progressive polyneuropathy with quadriparesis; she was also diabetic, but weakness improved with abstinence.[255d]

Salbutamol

Reports from England describe abuse of the antiasthmatic aerosol preparation of salbutamol, a beta-2-adrenergic agonist.[256–258] Probably both salbutamol itself (which has amphetamine-like effects) and fluorocarbons in the mixture contribute to addiction liability.[259,260]

Effects in Pregnancy

An estimated 12,000 pregnant women in the United States each year abuse inhalants.[261] Inhalant abuse before delivery causes neonatal depression.[62] Some inhalants appear to be teratogenic.[262]

Congenital cerebellar ataxia was reported in off-spring of mothers who abused toluene during pregnancy.[132,263] A "fetal solvent syndrome" is described, similar to the "fetal alcohol syndrome," with microcephaly, craniofacial anomalies, and retarded growth.[261,264–268] Of nine women giving birth to children with sacral agenesis, five had been exposed to xylene, trichloroethylene, methyl chloride, acetone, or gasoline.[269] Two case–control studies from Finland found an association between in utero solvent exposure and congenital CNS anomalies;[262,270] another Finnish case–control study did not.[271] In other studies, in utero solvent exposure was implicated in cleft palate[272] and cardiovascular malformations.[273] Other studies describe delayed growth and development, including cognition, speech, and motor skills, in children exposed in utero to toluene.[274,275] Severe mental retardation, hypotonia, and microcephaly with a prominent occiput were present in two children born to gasoline-sniffing parents.[276] In a cohort study from California, however, there was no difference in neurobehavioral development between children who were exposed in utero to solvents and those who were not.[277] The same study, however, found an association between solvent exposure and preeclampsia.[278] Renal tubular acidosis was present in an infant exposed in utero to toluene.[279]

An abstinence syndrome was described in neonates prenatally exposed to solvents. That study was not blinded, however.[280] In another study, trichloroethane and toluene did appear to produce neonatal signs similar to those produced by ethanol (and relieved by ethanol, barbiturates, and benzodiazepines).[281]

In a study of dental assistants, women exposed to high levels of nitrous oxide were less fertile than women who were unexposed or exposed only to low levels.[282]

A meta-analysis of studies involving occupational exposure to solvents during pregnancy (and thus less exposure than during deliberate sniffing or huffing) found an increased risk of fetal malformations and a trend toward increased rates of miscarriage.[282a] A prospective controlled study found that gestational exposure to organic solvents significantly increased the likelihood of major malformations (relative risk: 13); with one possible exception the risk was restricted to those who had temporary symptoms during exposure.[282b]

Animal studies confirm the teratogenicity of trichloroethane, toluene, and other inhalants. Animals exposed in utero to toluene had decreased fetal weight, retarded skeletal growth, and postnatal persistence of growth deficiency.[261,283–285] In exposed fetal mice, inhaled toluene was not associated with specific malformations,[286] but ingested toluene produced cleft palate.[287] In rats prenatal toluene exposure caused abnormal neurogenesis and migration in the somatosensory cortex and reduced volume of the dentate granule cell layer of the hippocampus.[288] Exposure of rats to large doses of nitrous oxide led to congenital malformations in offspring.[289] Exposure to small doses led to reduced fertility.[254]

Long-term Treatment

Long-term treatment of inhalant abuse has special difficulties. No effective pharmacotherapy exists (although anecdotal reports describe benefit from neuroleptics[290,291]). Addicts, whether juvenile or adult, tend to be social isolates lacking the cognitive capacity to participate in a rehabilitation program. Many also abuse ethanol and other drugs. Others deny that inhalant use is a form of drug abuse: "I don't do drugs, I just do tywol" (toluene).[292]

References

1. Brouette T, Anton R. Clinical review of inhalants. Am J Addict 2001; 10:79.
2. Henretig F. Inhalant abuse in children and adolescents. Pediatr Ann 1996; 25:47.
3. Evans EB, Balster RL. CNS depressant effects of volatile organic solvents. Neurosci Biochem Rev 1991; 15:233.
4. Glowa JR, Dews PB. Behavioral toxicology of volatile organic solvents. IV. Comparisons of the rate-decreasing effects of acetone, ethyl acetate, methyl ethyl ketone, toluene, and carbon disulfide on schedule-controlled behavior of mice. J Am Coll Toxicol 1987; 6:461.
5. Hinman DJ. Biphasic dose–response relationship for effects of toluene on locomotor activity. Pharmacol Biochem Behav 1987; 26:65.
6. Wood RW, Coleman JB, Schuler R, Cox C. Anticonvulsant and antipunishment effects of toluene. J Pharmacol Exp Ther 1984; 230:407.
7. Rees DC, Wood RW, Laties VG. Evidence of tolerance following repeated exposure to toluene in the rat. Pharmacol Biochem Behav 1989; 32:283.

8. Moser VC, Balster RL. The effects of acute and repeated toluene exposure on operant behavior in mice. Neurobehav Toxicol Teratol 1981; 3:471.

9. Taylor JD, Evans HL. Effects of toluene inhalation on behavior and expired carbon dioxide in macaque monkeys. Toxicol Appl Pharmacol 1985; 80:487.

10. Moser VC, Scimeca JA, Balster RL. Minimal tolerance to the effects of 1,1,1-trichloroethane on fixed ratio responding in mice. Neurotoxicology 1985; 6:35.

11. Yanagita T, Takahashi S, Ishida K, Fumamoto H. Voluntary inhalation of volatile anesthetics and organic solvents by monkeys. Jpn J Clin Pharmacol 1970; 1:13.

12. Wood RW, Grubman J, Weiss B. Nitrous oxide self-administration by the squirrel monkey. J Pharmacol Exp Ther 1977; 202:491.

13. Rees DC, Coggeshall E, Balster RL. Inhaled toluene produces pentobarbital-like discriminative stimulus effects in mice. Life Sci 1985; 37:1319.

14. Rees DC, Knisely JS, Balster RL, et al. Pentobarbital-like discriminative stimulus properties of halothane, 1,1,1-trichloroethane, isoamyl nitrite, flurothyl and oxazepam in mice. J Pharmacol Exp Ther 1987; 241:507.

15. Woolverton WL, Balster RL. Behavioral and lethal effects of combinations of oral ethanol and inhaled 1,1,1-trichloroethane in mice. Toxicol Appl Pharmacol 1981; 59:1.

16. Bowen SE, Wiley JL, Balster RL. The effects of abused inhalants on mouse behavior in an elevated plus-maze. Eur J Pharmacol 1996; 312:131.

17. Riegel AC, French ED. Abused inhalants and central reward pathways. Electrophysiological and behavioral studies in the rat. Ann N Y Acad Sci 2002; 965:281.

18. Cruz SL, Mirshaki T, Thomas B, et al. Effects of the abused solvent toluene on recombinant N-methyl-D-aspartate receptors expressed in Xenopus oocytes. J Pharmacol Exp Ther 1998; 286:334.

19. Balster RL. Neural basis of inhalant abuse. Drug Alcohol Depend 1998; 51:207.

19a. Hale JR, Zeilinga de Boer J, Chanton JP, et al. Questioning the Delphic Oracle. Sci Am 2003; 289:67.

20. Nagle DR. Anesthetic addiction and drunkenness: a contemporary and historical survey. Int J Addict 1968; 3:25.

21. Cartwright FF. The English Pioneers of Anesthesia. Bristol: John Wright, 1952.

22. Layzer RB. Nitrous oxide abuse. In: Eger EI, ed. Nitrous Oxide/N$_2$O. New York: Elsevier, 1985; 249.

23. Cohen S. Inhalant abuse: An overview of the problem. NIDA Res Monogr 1977; 15:2.

24. Kerner K. Current topics in inhalant abuse. NIDA Res Monogr 1988; 85:8.

25. Lenore R, Kupperstein LR, Susman RM. Bibliography of the inhalation of glue fumes and other toxic vapors. Int J Addict 1968; 3:177.

26. Brecher EM. Licit and Illicit Drugs. Boston: Little, Brown, 1972.

27. Fishburne PM, Abelson HL, Cisin I. National Survey on Drug Abuse: Main Findings 1979. Washington, DC: DHHS Publication No. (ADM) 80-976, 1980.

28. Barnes GE. Solvent abuse: a review. Int J Addict 1979; 14:1.

29. Easson WM. Gasoline addiction in children. Pediatrics 1962; 29:250.

30. Press E, Done AK. Solvent sniffing. Physiologic effects and community control measures for intoxication from the intentional inhalation of organic solvents. I. Pediatrics 1967; 39:451.

31. Beauvais F, Oetting ER. Inhalant abuse by young children. NIDA Res Monogr 1988; 85:30.

32. Edwards RW, Oetting ER. Inhalant use in the United States. NIDA Res Monogr 1995; 148:8.

33. Kurtzman TL, Otsuka KN, Wahl RA. Inhalant abuse by adolescents. J Adolescent Health 2001; 28:170.

34. Johns A. Volatile substance abuse and 963 deaths. Br J Addict 1991; 86:1053.

35. Ramsey J, Anderson HR, Bloor K, Flanagan RJ. An introduction to the practice, prevalence, and chemical toxicology of volatile substance abuse. Hum Toxicol 1989; 8:261.

36. Nicholi AM. The inhalants: an overview. Psychosomatics 1983; 24:914.

37. Moosa A, Loening WEK. Solvent abuse in black children in Natal. S Afr Med J 1981; 59:509.

38. Eastwell HD, Thomas BJ, Thomas BW. Skeletal lead burden in Aborigine petrol sniffing. Lancet 1983; II:524.

39. Davathasan G, Low D, Teoh PC, et al. Complications of chronic glue toluene abuse in adolescents. Aust N Z J Med 1984; 14:39.

40. Watson JM. Solvent abuse and adolescents. Practitioner 1984; 228:487.

41. Morton HG. Occurrence and treatment of solvent abuse in children and adolescents. Pharmacol Ther 1987; 33:449.

42. Tamura M. Japan: stimulant epidemics past and present. Bull Narc 1989; 41:83.

43. Lerner R, Ferrando D. Inhalants in Peru. NIDA Res Monogr 1995; 148:191.

44. Obot IS. Epidemiology of inhalant abuse in Nigeria. NIDA Res Monogr 1995; 148:175.

45. Medina-Mora ME, Berenzon S. Epidemiology of inhalant abuse in Mexico. NIDA Res Monogr 1995; 148:136.

46. Katona E. Inhalant abuse: a Hungarian review. NIDA Res Monogr 1995; 148:100.

47. Baldivieso LE. Inhalant abuse in Bolivia. NIDA Res Monogr 1995; 148:50.

48. Kin F, Navaratman V. An overview of inhalant abuse in selected countries of Asia and the Pacific Region. NIDA Res Monogr 1995; 148:29.

49. McGarvey EL, Clavet GJ, Mason W, et al. Adolescent inhalant abuse: environment of use. Am J Drug Alcohol Abuse 1999; 25:731.

50. Young SJ, Longstaffe S, Tenebein M. Inhalant abuse and the abuse of other drugs. Am J Drug Alcohol Abuse 1999; 25:371.

51. Bachrach KM, Sandler IN. A retrospective assessment of inhalant abuse in the barrio: implications for prevention. Int J Addict 1985; 20:1177.

51a. Fendrich M, Mackesy-Amiti ME, Wislar JS, et al. Childhood abuse and use of inhalants: differences by degree of use. Am J Public Health 1997; 87:765.

52. Dinwiddie SH, Reich T, Cloninger CR. The relationship of solvent use to other substance use. Am J Drug Alcohol Abuse 1991; 17:173.

53. Kaufman A. Gasoline sniffing among children in a Pueblo Indian village. Pediatrics 1973; 51:1060.

54. Seshia SS, Rajani KR, Boeckx RL, Chow PN. The neurological manifestations of chronic inhalation of leaded gasoline. Dev Med Child Neurol 1978; 20:323.

55. Remington G, Hoffman BF. Gas sniffing as a form of substance abuse. Can J Psychiatry 1984; 29:31.

56. MacLean SJ, d'Abbs PH. Petrol sniffing in Aboriginal communities: a review of interventions. Drug Alcohol Rev 2002; 21:65.

57. Cairney S, Maruff P, Burns C, et al. The neurobehavioral consequences of petrol (gasoline) sniffing. Neurosci Biobehav Rev 2002; 26:81.

58. Howard MO, Walker RD, Walker PS, et al. Inhalant use among urban American Indian youth. Addiction 1999; 94:83.

59. Beauvais F, Wayman JC, Jumper-Thurman P, et al. Inhalant abuse among American Indian, Mexican American, and non-Latino white adolescents. Am J Drug Alcohol Abuse 2002; 28:171.

60. Garriott JJ, Petty CS. Death from inhalant abuse: toxicological and pathological evaluation of 34 cases. Clin Toxicol 1980; 16:305.

61. Oetting ER, Edwards RW, Beauvais F. Social and psychological factors underlying inhalant abuse. NIDA Res Monogr 1988; 85:172.

62. Ashton CH. Solvent abuse. BMJ 1990; 300:135.

63. Westermeyer J. The psychiatrist and solvent-inhalant abuse: recognition, assessment, and treatment. Am J Psychiatry 1987; 144:903.

64. Press E, Done AK. Solvent sniffing. Physiologic effects and community control measures for intoxication from the intentional inhalation of organic solvents. II. Pediatrics 1967; 39:611.

65. Kerr N. Ether inebriety. JAMA 1891; 17:791.

66. Crider RA, Rouse BA. Inhalant overview. NIDA Res Monogr 1988; 85:1.

67. Ferguson CA. Chemical abuse in the north. Univ Manitoba Med J 1975; 45:129.

68. Storms WW. Chloroform parties. JAMA 1973; 225:160.

69. Marsh WW. Butane firebreathing in adolescents: a potentially dangerous practice. J Adolesc Health Care 1984; 5:59.

70. Jones NP. Self-enucleation and psychosis. Br J Ophthalmol 1990; 74:571.

71. Ackerly WC, Gibson G. Lighter fluid "sniffing." Am J Psychiatry 1964; 120:1056.

72. Tolan EJ, Lingl FA. "Model psychosis" produced by inhalation of gasoline fumes. Am J Psychiatry 1964; 120:757.

73. Meredith TJ, Ruprah M, Liddle A, Flanagan RJ. Diagnosis and treatment of acute poisoning with volatile substances. Hum Toxicol 1989; 8:277.

74. Watson JM. Solvent abuse and adolescents. Practitioner 1984; 228:487.

75. Meadows R, Verghese A. Medical complications of glue sniffing. South Med J 1996; 89:455.

76. Cohen S. The hallucinogens and the inhalants. Psychiatr Clin North Am 1984; 7:681.

77. Herzberg JL, Wolkind SN. Solvent sniffing in perspective. Br J Hosp Med 1983; 29:72.

78. Bass M. Sudden sniffing death. JAMA 1970; 212:2075.

79. Musclow CE, Awen CF. Glue-sniffing. Report of a fatal case. Can Med Assoc J 1971; 104:315.

80. Winek CL, Collom WD. Benzene and toluene fatalities. J Occup Med 1971; 13:259.

81. Cohen S. Inhalants. In: DuPont RI, Goldstein A, O'Donnell JJ, eds. Handbook on Drug Abuse. Washington, DC: US Government Printing Office, 1979; 213.

82. Edwards IR. Solvent abuse. N Z Med J 1982; 95:879.

83. Steadman C, Dorrington LC, Kay P, Stephens H. Abuse of a fire-extinguishing agent and sudden death in adolescents. Med J Aust 1984; 140:54.

84. McBride P, Busuttil A. A new trend in solvent abuse deaths? Med Sci Law 1990; 30:207.

85. Bowen SE, Daniel J, Balster RL. Deaths associated with inhalant abuse in Virginia from 1987 to 1996. Drug Alcohol Depend 1999; 53:239.

86. Anderson HR, Macnair RS, Ramsey JD. Deaths from abuse of volatile substances: a national epidemiological study. BMJ 1985; 290:304.

87. Wason S, Gibler B, Hassan M. Ventricular tachycardia associated with non-Freon aerosol propellants. JAMA 1986; 256:78.

88. Shepherd RT. Mechanism of sudden death associated with volatile substance abuse. Hum Toxicol 1989; 8:287.

89. Garb S, Chenoweth MB. Studies on hydrocarbon epinephrine induced ventricular fibrillation. J Pharmacol 1948; 94:12.

90. Cunningham SR, Dalyell GWN, McGirr P, Khan MM. Myocardial infarction and primary ventricular fibrillation after glue sniffing. BMJ 1987; 294:739.

91. Wodka RM, Jeong EWS. Cardiac effects of inhaled typewriter correction fluid. Ann Intern Med 1989; 110:91.

92. Cronk SL, Barkley DEH, Farrell MF. Respiratory arrest after solvent abuse. BMJ 1985; 290:897.

93. Chowdhury JK. Acute ventilatory failure from sniffing paint. Chest 1977; 71:687.

94. Carroll H, Abel G. Chronic gasoline inhalation. South Med J 1973; 66:1429.

95. Heath MJ. Solvent abuse using bromochlorodifluoromethane from a fire extinguisher. Med Sci Law 1986; 26:33.

96. Siegel E, Wason S. Sudden death caused by inhalation of butane and propane. N Engl J Med 1990; 323:1638.

97. Broussard LA. The role of the laboratory in detecting inhalant abuse. Clin Lab Sci 2000; 13:205.

98. Miller PW, Mycyck MB, Leikin JB, et al. An unusual presentation of inhalant abuse with dissociative amnesia. Vet Hum Toxicol 2002; 44:17.

99. Cohen S. Glue sniffing. JAMA 1975; 231:653.

100. Merry J, Zachariades N. Addiction to glue-sniffing. BMJ 1962; II:1448.

101. Crites J, Schukit MA. Solvent misuse in adolescents at a community alcohol center. J Clin Psychiatry 1979; 40:39.

102. Skuse D, Burrell S. A review of solvent abusers and their management by a child-psychiatric outpatient service. Hum Toxicol 1982; 1:321.

103. Sourindhrin I, Baird JA. Management of solvent misuse: a Glasgow community approach. Br J Addict 1984; 79:227.

104. Mee AS, Wright PL. Congestive (dilated) cardiomyopathy in association with solvent abuse. J R Soc Med 1980; 73:671.

105. Marjot R, McLeod AA. Chronic non-neurological toxicity from volatile substance abuse. Hum Toxicol 1989; 8:301.

106. Baerg RD, Kimberg DV. Centrolobular hepatic necrosis and acute renal failure in "solvent sniffers." Ann Intern Med 1970; 73:713.

107. Brown JH, Hadden DR, Hadden DS. Solvent abuse, toluene acidosis and diabetic ketoacidosis. Arch Emerg Med 1991; 8:65.

108. Powars D. Aplastic anemia secondary to glue sniffing. N Engl J Med 273; 700:1965.

109. Schikler KN, Lane EE, Seitz K, Collins WM. Solvent abuse associated with pulmonary abnormalities. Adv Alcohol Subst Abuse 1984; 3:75.

110. Rafferty P. Voluntary chlorine inhalation: a new form of self-abuse? BMJ 1980; 281:1178.

111. Chalupa B, Synkova J, Seveik M. The assessment of electroencephalographic changes and memory disturbances in acute intoxications with industrial poisons. Br J Indust Med 1960; 17:238.

112. Berry GJ. Neuropsychological assessment of solvent inhalants. In: Sharp CW, Carroll LT, eds. First International Symposium on Voluntary Inhalation of Industrial Solvents. Washington, DC: DHHS Publication No. (ADM) 79-779. US Government Printing Office, 1978.

113. Korman M, Matthews R, Lovitt R. Neuropsychological effects of abuse of inhalants. Percept Mot Skills 1981; 53:547.

114. Allison WM, Jerrom DW. Glue-sniffing: a pilot study of the cognitive effects of long-term use. Int J Addict 1984; 19:453.

115. Bigler ED. Neuropsychological evaluation of adolescent patients hospitalized with chronic inhalant abuse. Clin Neuropsychol 1979; 1:8.

116. Ron MA. Volatile substance abuse: a review of possible long-term neurological, intellectual, and psychiatric sequelae. Br J Psychiatry 1986; 148:235.

117. Arlien-Soborg P, Henriksen L, Gade A, et al. Cerebral blood flow in chronic toxic encephalopathy in house painters exposed to organic solvents. Acta Neurol Scand 1982; 66:34.

118. Chadwick OFD, Anderson HR. Neuropsychological consequences of volatile substance abuse: a review. Hum Toxicol 1989; 8:307.

119. Lolin Y. Chronic neurological toxicity associated with exposure to volatile substances. Hum Toxicol 1989; 8:293.

120. Zur J, Yule W. Chronic solvent abuse. 1. Cognitive sequelae. Child Care Health Dev 1990; 16:1.

121. Grabski D. Toluene sniffing producing cerebellar degeneration. Am J Psychiatry 1961; 118:461.

122. Satran R, Dodson VN. Toluene habituation: report of a case. N Engl J Med 1963; 268:719.

123. Knox JW, Nelson JR. Permanent encephalopathy from toluene inhalation. N Engl J Med 1966; 275:1494.

124. Kelly T. Prolonged cerebellar dysfunction associated with paint-sniffing. Pediatrics 1975; 56:605.

125. Procop LD. Neuropathy in an artist. Hosp Pract 1978; 13:89.

126. Fornazzari L, Wilkinson D, Kapur B, Carlen P. Cerebellar, cortical and functional impairment in toluene abuse. Acta Neurol Scand 1983; 67:319.

127. King MD. Neurological sequelae of toluene abuse. Hum Toxicol 1982; 1:281.

128. Boor JW, Hurtig HI. Persistent cerebellar ataxia after exposure to toluene. Ann Neurol 1977; 2:440.

129. Escobar A, Aruffo C. Chronic thinner intoxication: clinicopathologic report of a human case. J Neurol Neurosurg Psychiatry 1980; 43:986.

130. Malm G, Lying-Tunell V. Cerebellar dysfunction related to toluene sniffing. Acta Neurol Scand 1980; 62:188.

131. Lazar RB, Ho SU, Melen O, Daghestani AN. Multi-focal central nervous system damage caused by toluene abuse. Neurology 1983; 33:1337.

132. Streicher HZ, Gabow PA, Moss AH, et al. Syndromes of toluene sniffing in adults. Ann Intern Med 1981; 94:758.

133. Taher SM, Anderson RJ, McCartney R, et al. Renal tubular acidosis associated with toluene "sniffing." N Engl J Med 1974; 290:765.

134. Fischman CM, Oster JR. Toxic effects of toluene: a new cause of high anion gap metabolic acidosis. JAMA 1979; 241:1714.

135. Hormes JT, Filley CM, Rosenberg NL. Neurologic sequelae of chronic vapor abuse. Neurology 1986; 36:698.

136. Rosenberg NL, Kleinschmidt-DeMasters BK, Davis KA, et al. Toluene abuse causes diffuse central nervous system white matter changes. Ann Neurol 1988; 23:611.

137. Filley CM, Heaton RK, Rosenberg NL. White matter dementia in chronic toluene abuse. Neurology 1990; 40:532.

138. Caldemayer KS, Pascuzzi RM, Moran CC, et al. Toluene abuse causing reduced MR signal intensity in the brain. AJR Am J Roentgenol 1993; 161:1259.

139. Unger E, Alexander A, Fritz T, et al. Toluene abuse: physical basis for the hypointensity of the basal ganglia on T2-weighted images. Radiology 1994; 193:473.

140. Xiang L, Matthes JD, Li J, et al. MR imaging of "spray heads": toluene abuse via aerosol paint inhalation. AJNR Am J Neuroradiol 1993; 14:1195.

140a. Yamanouchi N, Okada S, Kodama K, et al. Effects of MRI abnormalities in WAIS-R performance in solvent abusers. Acta Neurol Scand 1997; 96:34.

141. Kornfeld M, Moser AB, Moser HW, et al. Solvent vapor abuse leukoencephalopathy. Comparisons to adrenoleukodystrophy. J Neuropathol Exp Neurol 1994; 53:389.

142. Morrow L, Callender T, Lottenberg S, et al. PET and neurobehavioral evidence of tetrabromoethane encephalopathy. J Neuropsychiatry Clin Neurosci 1990; 2:431.

143. Morrow L, Steinhauer SR, Hodgeson MJ. Delay in P300 latency in patients with organic solvent exposure. Arch Neurol 1992; 49:315.

144. Miyake H, Ikeda T, Maehara N, et al. Slow learning in rats due to long-term inhalation of toluene. Neurobehav Toxicol Teratol 1983; 5:541.

145. Lorenzana-Jiminez M, Salas M. Neonatal effects of toluene on motor behavior development of the rat. Neurobehav Toxicol Teratol 1983; 5:295.

146. Pryor GT, Dickinson J, Howd RA, Rebert CS. Neurobehavioral effects of subchronic exposure of weaning rats to toluene or hexane. Neurobehav Toxicol Teratol 1983; 5:47.

147. Pryor GT, Dickinson J, Howd RA, Rebert CS. Transient cognitive deficits and high-frequency hearing loss in weanling rats exposed to toluene. Neurobehav Toxicol Teratol 1983; 5:53.

148. Pryor GT. Persisting neurotoxic consequences of solvent abuse: a developing animal model for toluene-induced neurotoxicity. NIDA Res Monogr 1990; 101:156.

149. Keane JR. Toluene optic neuropathy. Ann Neurol 1978; 4:390.

150. Ehyai A, Freeman FR. Progressive optic neuropathy and sensorineural hearing loss due to chronic glue sniffing. J Neurol Neurosurg Psychiatry 1983; 46:349.

151. Cooper R, Newton P, Reed M. Neurophysiological signs of brain damage due to glue sniffing. Electroencephalogr Clin Neurophysiol 1985; 60:23.

152. Mettrick SA, Brenner RP. Abnormal brainstem auditory evoked potentials in chronic paint sniffers. Ann Neurol 1982; 12:553.

153. Maas FF, Ashe J, Spiegel P, et al. Acquired pendular nystagmus in toluene addiction. Neurology 1991; 41:282.

154. Allister C, Lush M, Oliver JS, Watson JM. Status epilepticus caused by solvent abuse. BMJ 1981; 283:1156.

155. Bennett RH, Forman HR. Hypokalemic periodic paralysis in chronic toluene exposure. Arch Neurol 1980; 37:673.

156. McCormick MJ, Mogabgab E, Adams SL. Methanol poisoning as a result of inhalational solvent abuse. Ann Emerg Med 1990; 19:639.

157. Cohen MM. Central nervous system in carbon tetrachloride intoxication. Neurology 1957; 7:238.

158. Luse SA, Wood WG. The brain in fatal carbon tetrachloride poisoning. Arch Neurol 1967; 17:304.

159. Johnson BP, Meredith TJ, Vale JA. Cerebellar dysfunction after acute carbon tetrachloride poisoning. Lancet 1983; II:968.

160. Boeckx RL, Postle B, Coodin FJ. Gasoline sniffing and tetraethyl lead poisoning in children. Pediatrics 1977; 60:140.

161. Fortenberry JD. Gasoline sniffing. Am J Med 1985; 79:740.

162. Coulehan JL, Hirsh W, Brillman J, et al. Gasoline sniffing and lead toxicity in Navajo adolescents. Pediatrics 1983; 71:113.

163. Young RSK, Grzyb SE, Crisman L. Recurrent cerebellar dysfunction as related to chronic gasoline sniffing in an adolescent girl. Clin Pediatr 1977; 16:706.

164. Procop LD, Karampelas D. Encephalopathy secondary to abusive gasoline inhalation. J Fla Med Assoc 1981; 68:823.

165. Tenenbein M. Leaded gasoline: the role of tetraethyl lead. Hum Exp Toxicol 1997; 16:217.

166. Goodheart RS, Dunne JW. Petrol sniffer's encephalopathy. A study of 25 patients. Med J Aust 1994; 160:178.

167. Robinson RO. Tetraethyl lead poisoning from gasoline sniffing. JAMA 1978; 240:1373.

168. Valpey R, Sumi S, Copass MK, Goble GJ. Acute and chronic progressive encephalopathy due to gasoline sniffing. Neurology 1978; 28:507.

169. Hansen KS, Sharp FR. Gasoline sniffing, lead poisoning, and myoclonus. JAMA 1978; 240:1375.

170. Chiba M, Toyada T, Inaba Y, et al. Acute lead poisoning in an adult from ingestion of paint. N Engl J Med 1980; 303:459.

171. Maruff P, Burns CB, Tyler P, et al. Neurological and cognitive abnormalities associated with chronic petrol sniffing. Brain 1998; 121:1903.

172. Karani V. Peripheral neuritis after addiction to petrol. BMJ 1966; II:216.

173. Gonzalez E, Downey J. Polyneuropathy in a glue sniffer. Arch Phys Med 1972; 53:333.

174. Matsumura M, Inoue N, Ohnishi A. Toxic polyneuropathy due to glue sniffing. Clin Neurol 1972; 12:290.

175. Goto I, Matsumura M, Inoue N, et al. Toxic polyneuropathy due to glue-sniffing. J Neurol Neurosurg Psychiatry 1974; 7:848.

176. Shirabe T, Tsuda T, Terao AA, Araki S. Toxic polyneuropathy due to glue sniffing: report of two cases with a light and electron microscopic study of the peripheral nerves and muscles. J Neurol Sci 1974; 21:101.

177. Procop LD, Alt M, Tison J. Huffer's neuropathy. JAMA 1974; 229:1083.

178. Korobkin R, Asbury AK, Sumner AJ, Nielsen SL. Glue-sniffing neuropathy. Arch Neurol 1975; 32:158.

179. Oh S, Kim J. Giant axonal swelling in "huffer's neuropathy." Arch Neurol 1976; 33:583.

180. Means ED, Procop LD, Hooper GS. Pathology of lacquer thinner-induced neuropathy. Ann Clin Lab Sci 1976; 6:240.

181. Means ED, Tison J, Procop LD. Experimental lacquer thinner neuropathy. Neurology 1978; 28:333.

181a. Pastore C, Izura V, Marhuenda D, et al: Partial conduction blocks in N-hexane neuropathy. Muscle Nerve 2002; 26:132.

182. Mendell J, Saida K, Ganansi M. Toxic polyneuropathy produced by methyl-*n*-butyl ketone. Science 1974; 185:787.

183. Schaumburg H, Spencer P. Degeneration in central and peripheral nervous systems produced by pure *n*-hexane: an experimental study. Brain 1976; 99:183.

184. Spencer P, Schaumburg H. Experimental neuropathy produced by 2,5-hexanedione—a major metabolite of the neurotoxic industrial solvent methyl-*n*-butyl ketone. J Neurol Neurosurg Psychiatry 1975; 38:771.

185. Tenenbein M, DeGroot W, Rajamo KR. Peripheral neuropathy following intentional inhalation of naphtha. Can Med Assoc J 1984; 131:1077.

186. Altenkirch H, Mager J, Stoltenburg G, Helmbrecht J. Toxic polyneuropathies after sniffing a glue thinner. J Neurol 1977; 214:137.

187. Bruchner JV, Petersen RG. Toxicology of aliphatic and aromatic hydrocarbons. NIDA Res Monogr 1977; 15:124.

188. Hayden J, Comstock E, Comstock B. The clinical toxicology of solvent abuse. Clin Toxicol 1976; 9:169.

189. Procop L. Neurotoxic volatile substances. Neurology 1979; 29:862.

190. Pezzoli G, Ferrante C, Barbieri S, et al. Parkinsonism due to *n*-hexane exposure. Lancet 1989; II:874.

191. Pezzoli G, Ricciardi S, Masotto C, et al. *n*-Hexane induces parkinsonism in rodents. Brain Res 1990; 531:355.

192. Pezzoli G, Perbellini L, Zecchinelli A, et al. *n*-Hexane and parkinsonism. Neurology 1992; 42 (Suppl 3):283.

193. Mitchell ABS, Parsons-Smith BG. Trichloroethylene neuropathy. BMJ 1969; I:422.

194. Parker MJ, Tarlow MJ, Milne-Anderson J. Glue sniffing and cerebral infarction. Arch Dis Child 1984; 59:675.

195. Lamont CM, Adams FG. Glue-sniffing as a cause of a positive radio-isotope brain scan. Eur J Nucl Med 1982; 7:387.

196. Mathew RJ, Wilson WH. Substance abuse and cerebral blood flow. Am J Psychiatry 1991; 148:292.

197. Sharp CW, Stillman RC. Blush not with nitrites. Ann Intern Med 1980; 92:700.

198. Newell GR, Spitz MR, Wilson MB. Nitrite inhalants: historical perspective. NIDA Res Monogr 1988; 83:1.

199. Wood RW. The acute toxicity of nitrite inhalants. NIDA Res Monogr 1988; 83:28.

200. Madarai B, Kapadia YK, Kerins M, et al. Methylene blue: a treatment for severe methaemoglobinaemia secondary to misuse of amyl nitrite. Emerg Med J 2002; 19:2700.

201. Stambach T, Haire K, Soni N, et al. Saturday night blue—a case of near fatal poisoning from the abuse of amyl nitrite. J Accid Emerg Med 1997; 14:339.

202. Malhotra R, Hughes G. Methaemoglobinaemia presenting with status epilepticus. J Accid Emerg Med 1995; 13:427.

203. Coleman MD, Coleman NA. Drug-induced methaemoglobinaemia. Treatment issues. Drug Saf 1996; 14:394.

204. Machabert R, Testud F, Descotes J. Methaemoglobinaemia due to amyl nitrite inhalation: a case report. Hum Exp Toxicol 1994; 13:313.

205. Horne MK, Waterman MR, Simon LM, et al. Methemoglobinemia from sniffing butyl nitrite. Ann Intern Med 1979; 91:417.

206. Haley TJ. Review of the physiological effects of amyl, butyl, and isobutyl nitrites. Clin Toxicol 1980; 16:317.

207. Shesser RS, Dixon D, Allen Y, et al. Fatal methemoglobinemia from butyl nitrite ingestion. Ann Intern Med 1980; 92:131.

208. Wason S, Detsky AS, Platt OS, Lovejoy FH. Isobutyl nitrite toxicity by ingestion. Ann Intern Med 1980; 92:637.

209. Dixon DS, Reisch RF, Santinga PH. Fatal methemoglobinemia resulting from ingestion of isobutyl nitrite, a "room odorizer" widely used for recreational purposes. J Forensic Sci 1981; 26:587.

210. Laaban JP, Bodenan P, Rochemaure J. Amyl nitrite poppers and methemoglobinemia. Ann Intern Med 1985; 103:804.

211. Nudelman RW, Salcman M. The birth of the blues. II. Blue movie. JAMA 1987; 257:3230.

212. Fledelius HC. Irreversible blindness after amyl nitrite inhalation. Acta Ophthalmol Scand 1999; 77:719.

213. Soderberg LS, Barnett JB. Exposure to inhaled isobutyl nitrite reduces T cell blastogenesis and antibody responsiveness. Fundam Appl Toxicol 1991; 17:821.

214. Haverkos HW. The search for cofactors in AIDS, including an analysis of the association of nitrite

inhalant abuse and Kaposi's sarcoma. Prog Clin Biol Res 1990; 325:93.

215. Soderberg LS. Immunomodulation by nitrate inhalants may predispose abusers to AIDS and Kaposi's sarcoma. J Neuroimmunol 1998; 83:157.

215a. Seage GR, Mayer KH, Horsburgh CR, et al. The relation between nitrite inhalants, unprotected receptive anal intercourse, and the risk of human immunodeficiency virus infection. Am J Epidemiol 1992; 135:1.

216. Archibald CP, Schechter MT, Craib KJ, et al. Risk factors for Kaposi's sarcoma in the Vancouver Lymphadenopathy-AIDS Study. J AIDS 1990; 3 (Suppl 1):S18.

217. Lifson AR, Darrow WW, Hessol NA, et al. Kaposi's sarcoma among homosexual and bisexual men enrolled in the San Francisco City Clinic Cohort Study. J AIDS 1990; 3 (Suppl 1):S32.

218. Rosenberg H, Orkin FK, Springstead J. Abuse of nitrous oxide. Anesth Analg 1979; 58:104.

219. Nitrous oxide hazards. FDA Drug Bull 1980; 10:15.

220. Aston R. Drug abuse. Its relationship to dental practice. Dent Clin North Am 1984; 28:595.

220a. Ng J, O' Grady G, Pettit T, et al: Nitrous oxide use in first-year students at Auckland University. Lancet 2003; 361:1349.

221. Brillant L. Nitrous oxide as a psychedelic drug. N Engl J Med 1970; 283:1522.

222. DiMaio VJM, Garriott JC. Four deaths resulting from abuse of nitrous oxide. J Forensic Sci 1978; 23:169.

223. Schwartz RH, Calihan M. Nitrous oxide: a potentially lethal euphoriant inhalant. Am Fam Phys 1984; 30:171.

224. Brett A. Myeloneuropathy from whipped cream bulbs presenting as a conversion disorder. Aust N Z J Psychiatry 1997; 31:131.

225. Butzkueven H, King JO. Nitrous oxide myelopathy in an abuser of whipped cream bulbs. J Clin Neurosci 2000; 7:73.

226. Iwata K, O'Keefe GB, Karanas A. Neurologic problems associated with chronic nitrous oxide abuse in a non-healthcase worker. Am J Med Sci 2001; 322:173.

227. Winek CL, Wahba WW, Rozin L. Accidental death by nitrous oxide inhalation. Forensic Sci Int 1995; 73:139.

228. Temple WA, Beasley DM, Baker DJ. Nitrous oxide abuse from whipped cream dispenser changers. N Z Med J 1997; 110:322.

229. LiPuma JP, Wellman J, Stern HP. Nitrous oxide abuse: a new cause for pneumomediastinum. Radiology 1982; 145:602.

230. Messina FV, Wynne JW. Homemade nitrous oxide: no laughing matter. Ann Intern Med 1982; 96:333.

231. Layzer R, Fishman R, Schafer J. Neuropathy following abuse of nitrous oxide. Neurology 1976; 28:504.

232. Sahenk Z, Mendell JR, Couri D, Nachtman J. Polyneuropathy from inhalation of N_2O cartridges through a whipped-cream dispenser. Neurology 1978; 28:485.

233. Layzer RB. Myeloneuropathy after prolonged exposure to nitrous oxide. Lancet 1978; II:1227.

234. Paulson GW. "Recreational" misuse of nitrous oxide. J Am Dent Assoc 1979; 98:410.

235. Gutmann L, Farrell B, Crosby TW, Johnson D. Nitrous oxide-induced myelopathy-neuropathy: potential for chronic misuse by dentists. J Am Dent Assoc 1979; 98:58.

236. Nevins MA. Neuropathy after nitrous oxide abuse. JAMA 1980; 244:2264.

237. Gutmann L, Johnsen D. Nitrous oxide-induced myeloneuropathy: report of cases. J Am Dent Assoc 1981; 103:239.

238. Sterman AB, Coyle PK. Subacute toxic delirium following nitrous oxide abuse. Arch Neurol 1983; 40:446.

239. Blanco G, Peters HA. Myeloneuropathy and macrocytosis associated with nitrous oxide abuse. Arch Neurol 1983; 40:416.

240. Heyer EJ, Simpson DM, Bodis-Wollner I, Diamond SP. Nitrous oxide: clinical and electrophysiologic investigation of neurologic complications. Neurology 1986; 36:1618.

241. Stabler SP, Allen RH, Barrett RE, Savage DG, Lindenbaum J. Cerebrospinal fluid methylmalonic acid levels in normal subjects and patients with cobalamin deficiency. Neurology 1991; 41:1627.

242. Pema PJ, Horak HA, Wyatt RH. Myelopathy caused by nitrous oxide toxicity. AJNR Am J Neuroradiol 1998; 19:994.

243. Dinn JJ, McCann S, Wilson P, et al. Animal model for subacute combined degeneration. Lancet 1978; II:1154.

244. van der Westhuyzen J, Fernandes-Costa F, Metz J. Cobalamin inactivation by nitrous oxide produces severe neurological impairment in fruit bats: protection by methionine and aggravation by folate. Life Sci 1982; 31:2001.

245. Amess JAC, Burman JF, Rees GM, et al. Megaloblastic hemopoiesis in patients receiving nitrous oxide. Lancet 1978; II:1023.

246. Schilling RF. Is nitrous oxide a dangerous anesthetic for vitamin B_{12}-deficient subjects? JAMA 1986; 255:1605.

247. Berger JJ, Modell JH, Sypert GW. Megaloblastic anemia and brief exposure to nitrous oxide—a causal relationship? Anesth Analg 1988; 67:197.

248. Holloway KL, Alberico AM. Postoperative myeloneuropathy: a preventable complication in patients with B_{12} deficiency. J Neurosurg 1990; 72:732.

249. Deacon R, Perry J, Lamb M, et al. Selective inactivation of vitamin B_{12} in rats by nitrous oxide. Lancet 1978; II:1023.

250. Kondo H, Osborne ML, Kolhouse JF, et al. Nitrous oxide has multiple deleterious effects on cobalamin metabolism and causes decreases in activities of both mammalian cobalamin-dependent enzymes in rats. J Clin Invest 1981; 67:1270.

251. Van der Westhuyzen J, Van Tonder S, Gibson JE, et al. Plasma amino acids and tissue methionine levels in fruit bats (*Rousettus aegyptiacus*) with nitrous oxide-induced vitamin B_{12} deficiency. Br J Nutr 1984; 53:657.

252. Spencer JD, Raasch FO, Trefny FA. Halothane abuse in hospital personnel. JAMA 1976; 235:1034.

253. Kaplan HG, Bakken J, Quadracci L, Schubach W. Hepatitis caused by halothane sniffing. Ann Intern Med 1979; 90:797.

254. Yamashita M, Matsuki A, Oyama T. Illicit use of modern volatile anesthetics. Can Anaesth Soc 1984; 31:76.

255. Beer J, Heer G, Schlup P. Chloroform sniffing: a new variant of substance abuse. Schweiz Med Wochenschr 1984; 114:1538.

255a. Zinham WH, Childs B. A defect of glutathione metabolism in erythrocytes from patients with a naphthalene-induced anemia. Lab Invest 1984; 50:10P.

255b. Anziulewicz JA, Herman JD, Chiarulli EE. Transplacental naphthalene poisoning. Am J Obstet Gynecol 1959; 78:519.

255c. Pysher T, Olson A, Drederick D, et al. Fatal hepatopathy due to chronic inhalation of naphthalene. Lab Invest 1984; 50:10P.

255d. Weintraub E, Gandhi D, Robinson C. Medical complications due to mothball abuse. South Med J 2000; 93:427.

256. Edwards JG, Holgate ST. Dependency on salbutamol inhalers. Br J Psychiatry 1979; 134:624.

257. Pratt HF. Abuse of salbutamol inhalers in young people. Clin Allergy 1982; 12:203.

258. Raine JM. Addiction to aerosol treatment. BMJ 1984; 288:241.

259. Brennan PO. Addiction to aerosol treatment. BMJ 1983; 287:1877.

260. Thompson PJ, Dhillan P, Cole P. Addiction to aerosol treatment: the asthmatic alternative to glue sniffing. BMJ 1983; 287:1515.

261. Jones HE, Balster RL. Inhalant abuse in pregnancy. Obstet Gynecol Clin North Am 1998; 25:153.

262. Holmberg PC. Central nervous system defects in children born to mothers exposed to organic solvents during pregnancy. Lancet 1979; II:177.

263. Goodwin JM, Gail C, Grodner B, Metrick S. Inhalant abuse, pregnancy, and neglected children. Am J Psychiatry 1981; 138:1126.

264. Toutant C, Lippmann S. Fetal solvent syndrome. Lancet 1979; I:1356.

265. Hersh JH, Podruch PE, Rogers G, Weisskopf B. Toluene embryopathy. J Pediatr 1985; 106:922.

266. Hersh JH. Toluene embryopathy: two new cases. J Med Genet 1989; 26:333.

267. Goodwin TM. Toluene abuse and renal tubular acidosis in pregnancy. Obstet Gynecol 1988; 71:715.

268. Fabro S, Brown NA, Scialli AR. Is there a fetal solvent syndrome? Reprod Toxicol Med Lett 1983; 2:17.

269. Kucera J. Exposure to fat solvents: a possible cause of sacral agenesis in man. J Pediatr 1969; 72:857.

270. Holmberg PC, Nurminen M. Congenital defects of the central nervous system and occupational factors during pregnancy. Am J Ind Med 1980; 1:167.

271. Rantala K, Riala R, Nurminen T. Screening for occupational exposures and congenital malformations. Scand J Work Environ Health 1983; 9:89.

272. Holmberg PC, Hernberg S, Kurppa K, et al. Oral clefts and organic solvent exposure during pregnancy. Int Arch Occup Environ Health 1982; 50:371.

273. Tikkanen J, Heinonen OP. Cardiovascular malformations and organic solvent exposure during pregnancy in Finland. Am J Ind Med 1988; 14:1.

274. Wilkins-Haug L, Gabow PA. Toluene abuse during pregnancy: obstetric complications and perinatal outcomes. Obstet Gynecol 1991; 7:504.

275. Arnold GL, Kirby RS, Langendoerfer S, et al. Toluene-embryopathy: clinical delineation and developmental follow-up. Pediatrics 1994; 93:216.

276. Hunter AG, Thompson D, Evans JA. Is there a fetal gasoline syndrome? Teratology 1979; 20:75.

277. Eskenazi B, Gaylord L, Bracken MB, Brown D. In utero exposure to organic solvents and human neurodevelopment. Dev Med Child Neurol 1988; 30:492.

278. Eskenazi B, Bracken MB, Holford TR, Crady J. Exposure to organic solvents and hypertensive disorders of pregnancy. Am J Ind Med 1988; 14:177.

279. Erramouspe J, Galvez R, Fischel DR. Newborn renal tubular acidosis associated with prenatal maternal toluene sniffing. J Psychoactive Drugs 1996; 28:201.

280. Tenenbein M, Casiro O, Seshia MM, et al. Neonatal withdrawal from maternal volatile substance abuse. Arch Dis Child 1996; 74: F204.

281. Evans EB, Balster RL. Inhaled 1,1,1-trichloroethane-produced physical dependence in mice: effects of drugs and vapors on withdrawal. J Pharmacol Exp Ther 1993; 264:726.

282. Rowland AS, Baird DD, Weinberg CR, et al. Reduced fertility among women employed as dental assistants exposed to high levels of nitrous oxide. N Engl J Med 1992; 327:993.

282a. McMartin KI, Liau M, Kopecky E, et al. Pregnancy outcome following maternal organic solvent exposure: a meta-analysis of epidemiological studies. Am J Ind Med 1998; 34:288.

282b. Khattak S, K-Moghtader G, McMartin K, et al. Pregnancy outcome following gestational exposure to organic solvents. A prospective controlled study. JAMA 1999; 281:1106.

283. Hudak A, Rodics K, Stuber I, et al. The effects of toluene inhalation on pregnant CFY rats and their offspring. Orz Munka-Uzemegeszegugui Intez Munkavedelm 1977; 23 (Suppl):25.

284. Jones HE, Balster RL. Neurobehavioral consequences of intermittent prenatal exposure to high concentrations of toluene. Neurotoxicol Teratol 1997; 19:305.

285. Wilkins-Haug L. Teratogen update: toluene. Teratology 1997; 55:145.

286. Hudak A, Ungvary G. Embryotoxic effects of benzene and its methyl derivatives: toluene, xylene. Toxicology 1978; 11:53.

287. Nawrot PS, Staples RE. Embryofetal toxicity and teratogenicity of benzene and toluene in the mouse. Teratology 1979; 19:41A.

288. Gospe SM, Zhou SS. Prenatal exposure to toluene results in abnormal neurogenesis and migration in rat somatosensory cortex. Pediatr Res 2000; 47:362.

289. Mazze RI, Fujinaga M, Baden JM. Reproductive and teratogenic effects of nitrous oxide, fentanyl, and their combination in Sprague-Dawley rats. Br J Anaesth 1987; 59:1291.

290. Hernandez-Avila CA, Ortega-Soto HA, Jasso A, et al. Treatment of inhalant-induced psychotic disorder with carbamazepine versus haloperidol. Psychiatr Serv 1998; 49:812.

291. Misra LK, Kofoed L, Fuller W. Treatment of inhalant abuse with risperidone. J Clin Psychiatry 1999; 60:620.

292. McSherry TM. Program experiences with the solvent abuser in Philadelphia. NIDA Res Monogr 1988; 85:106.

Chapter 10
Phencyclidine

"Amoeba," "Amp," "Angel Dust," "Bobbies," "Busy Bee," "Cadillac," "Crystal Joints," "CJ," "Cyclones," "Dank," "Devil's Dust," "Dippies," "DOA," "Dog," "Elephant Tranquilizer," "Embalming Fluid," "Goon," "Gorilla Tab," "Haze," "Hog," "Horse Tranquilizer," "Hydro," "Illie," "Kapow," "Love Boat," "Mr. Lovely," "Monkey Dust," "Peace Pill," "Pig Killer," "Purple Haze," "Rocket Fuel," "Scuffle," "Sherm," "Soma Surfer," "Superweed," "Water," "Wet," "Whack," "Window Pane," "Wobble Weed," "Worm," "Zombie."
—Street names for phencyclidine

That 22-minute journey to becoming the intelligence at the heart of the universe remains the most powerful and cosmic experience of my life.
—Ketamine user

Arylcyclohexylamine compounds, which include phencyclidine (1-(1-phenylcyclohexyl)piperidine, or PCP) and ketamine, have central nervous system (CNS) stimulant, depressant, hallucinogenic, and analgesic properties (Figure 10–1). They are termed *dissociative anesthetics* because in cats they produce dissociation of electroencephalographic activity between thalamoneocortical and limbic areas.[1] Humans anesthetized with these agents tend to keep their eyes open and seem "disconnected" from the environment; profound analgesia and amnesia can occur without loss of consciousness, a kind of catalepsy. These agents thus appear to be categorically separable from other psychotomimetic drugs, including hallucinogens.

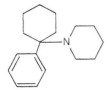

Figure 10–1. Phencyclidine.

Pharmacology and Animal Studies

Acute Effects

In mice and rats PCP elicits amphetamine-like behavior: with low doses there is increased locomotion and with higher doses stereotypic movements—repetitive head weaving, sniffing, rearing, and circling. In contrast to amphetamine, however, higher doses cause marked ataxia.[1–4] In monkeys low doses produce mild ataxia and calming. With higher doses there is nystagmus and catalepsy: the eyes remain open, and there is no respiratory depression, but the animal is immobile and unresponsive to the environment. Pigeons receiving PCP are also rendered cataleptic.

Neurotransmitter Systems

PCP affects a number of neurotransmitter systems, including dopamine, serotonin, norepinephrine, acetylcholine, and opioids.[5–9] Its principal actions, however, involve *N*-methyl-D-aspartate (NMDA) receptors and sigma receptors.

Receptors for the amino acid neurotransmitter glutamate are classified as either metabotropic or inotropic. Metabotropic receptors are coupled to G-proteins and signal transduction cascades. Inotropic receptors transmit their signals by altering membrane permeability to Na^+ and Ca^{2+} ions. Based on their preferential affinities for particular ligands, inotropic receptors are classified as NMDA receptors, α-amino-3-hydroxy-5-methyl-4-isoxazolproprionate (AMPA) receptors, and kainite receptors. AMPA and kainite receptors mainly allow influx of monovalent ions. NMDA receptors allow influx of both Na^+ and Ca^{2+}. To transmit a signal, NMDA receptors require the presence not only of glutamate but also of a co-agonist, glycine, each at its own recognition site. Signal transmission is also voltage-dependent; a depolarizing stimulus (provided by AMPA/kainite receptors) must be sufficient to remove Mg^{2+} from the ion channel, allowing Ca^{2+} to pass through. NMDA receptors contain additional modulatory sites for zinc (which inhibits ion channel opening), polyamines (which enhance ion channel opening) and, within the ion channel, PCP and other arylcyclohexylamines. The PCP binding site—termed the *PCP receptor*—within the ion channel is "use-dependent"; that is, it requires an open channel to provide access to the receptor. PCP then blocks ion flux, either through conformational changes or by plugging the channel. PCP inhibits NMDA agonists noncompetitively, that is, regardless of the concentration of agonist ligands. Other drugs that bind to the PCP receptor include dizocilpine (MK-801) and ketamine, as well as the so-called sigma opioids (e.g., cyclazocine and norme-trazocine), the "morphinans" (e.g., dextromethorphan and dextrorphan), and the 1-aminoadmantanes (e.g., amantadine and memantine).[10] (Competitive antagonists, which act at the NMDA receptor itself, include 2-amino-5-phosphonopentanoate [AP5] and 2-amino-7-phosphonoheptanoate [AP7].) NMDA receptors are most numerous in hippocampus, amygdala, thalamus, caudate, entorhinal cortex, and layers I and II of the somatosensory and motor cortex.[3,11–13]

As with psychostimulants the effects of PCP critically depend upon dopamine- and adenosine-3′,5′-monophosphate (cAMP)-regulated phosphoprotein-32 (DARPP-32; see Chapter 2). PCP modulates DARPP phosphorylation through distinct actions within glutamatergic systems.[13a]

PCP also binds to so-called sigma receptors, which were originally considered an opioid receptor subtype.[14] Sigma receptor ligands include the benzomorphan class of opioid mixed agonist-antagonists, such as cyclazocine and pentazocine, psychotomimetic effects of which are not blocked by naloxone. Sigma binding sites are most dense in the hippocampus, hypothalamus, limbic forebrain, midbrain, cerebellum, and brainstem. PCP has much greater affinity for PCP receptors than sigma receptors, and different agents have varying degrees of affinity for the two receptor types. Dizocilpine, which has high affinity for PCP receptors, binds hardly at all to sigma receptors.[15]

The function of sigma receptors is unknown, and the diversity of agents that bind to them implies receptor subtypes.[14,16] It is also unclear to what degree the behavioral effects of PCP are mediated by either sigma receptors or PCP receptors. Biological and behavioral effects in animals more readily correlate with PCP receptor binding than with sigma receptor binding,[17,18] and in human volunteers the analgesic potency of PCP analogs similarly correlates with PCP receptor affinity.[19] Dizocilpine, which binds to PCP receptors but not to sigma receptors, produces PCP-like behavior in rats, pigeons, and monkeys[20] yet in human volunteers is not psychotomimetic (see later).[21,22] In animals, PCP-like behavior is also produced by the competitive NMDA antagonists AP5 and AP7.[2]

PCP stimulates striatal tyrosine hydroxylase activity, inhibits dopamine reuptake, and facilitates dopamine release.[23] 6-Hydroxydopamine lesions of the nucleus accumbens (NA) block PCP-induced locomotor activity, and PCP bimodally increases and then decreases neuronal firing rates in the ventral tegmental area (VTA).[24] The mechanism of PCP's effects on dopamine neurotransmission are uncertain. Dopamine release in the prefrontal cortex induced by NMDA receptor antagonists appears to be secondary to *increased* release of glutamate and activation of AMPA and kainite receptors on dopaminergic nerve endings.[25] Although arylcyclohexylamines are NMDA receptor antagonists, they increase release of glutamate, which can then activate non-NMDA receptors.[26] Ketamine-induced release of dopamine in the prefrontal cortex as well as ketamine-induced impairment on prefrontal-dependent cognitive tasks, were blocked by AMPA/kainite receptor antagonists. A similar effect was observed with a group II metabotropic glutamate receptor agonist, which blocked PCP-induced cortical glutamate efflux and attenuated PCP's disruptive effects on working memory, stereo-typy, and locomotion. In that experiment, behavioral reversal occurred even though dopamine hyperactivity persisted, indicating involvement of non-dopaminergic pathways.[27]

NMDA antagonists also affect serotonin neurotransmission. NMDA inhibits neural activity in brainstem raphe nuclei, and PCP increases serotonin output in medial prefrontal cortex and hippocampus. A $5-HT_{2A}$ antagonist attenuated the locomotor activity and other behaviors induced by NMDA antagonists.[4,28]

In monkeys, cats, and rats, PCP and related agents impair learning at doses too low to cause gross motor disruption.[29] Such an effect might be related to inhibition of NMDA-receptor-dependent long-term potentiation in the hippocampus.[12]

In drug discrimination studies, dizocilpine and ketamine substitute for PCP.[30] Substitution is not always consistent, however, and competitive NMDA antagonists substitute for PCP even less consistently, indicating that NMDA antagonism per se is insufficient to account for PCP discrimination.[31,32] Substitution of potent sigma ligands for PCP is also inconsistent; animals trained to discriminate pentazocine generalize completely to the sigma receptor agonist N-allylnorametazocine (NANM) but only partially to PCP,[33] and although haloperidol blocks NANM discrimination, animals trained to discriminate NANM do not generalize to the potent sigma agonist (+)-3-(3-hydroxyphenyl)-N-(1-propyl) piperidine (3-PPP).[34] Animals trained to discriminate PCP do not generalize to dopaminergic, serotonergic, cholinergic, γ-aminobutyric acid (GABA)ergic, or opioid drugs.[3,24] Animals do generalize from PCP, dizocilpine, and ketamine to ethanol (which also antagonizes glutamate neurotransmission at NMDA receptors; see Chapter 12).[35]

Reinforcement, Tolerance, Dependence

Rats, dogs, monkeys, and baboons self-administer PCP, ketamine, and other PCP receptor ligands.[1,36–39] In studies using long interval schedules, monkeys responded up to 157 times per minute for an hour to receive a single dose.[40] Ketamine is less reinforcing,[39] and neither drug is as reinforcing as cocaine.[41] The reinforcing properties of dizocilpine are complex: it is self-administered by monkeys that have recently self-administered PCP or ketamine but, in contrast to PCP, not by monkeys that have recently self-administered cocaine.[42] Dizocilpine does facilitate intracranial self-stimulation,[43] and PCP receptor ligands—but not sigma receptor ligands—increase punished responding (reward seeking in the face of aversive stimuli).[44] Competitive NMDA antagonists are much less consistently self-administered by animals.[29]

Animals develop tolerance to some but not all of PCP's behavioral effects, for example, motor incoordination; locomotor activity, by contrast, is enhanced with repeated administration of the drug, and this sensitized response persists for up to 60 days after administration.[4,24] As with a number of other addicting drugs—for example, amphetamine, cocaine, tetrahydrocannabinol, caffeine, and nicotine—signs of physical dependence are not easily identified.[45,46] Rats given PCP for 7 days developed twofold tolerance and on abrupt withdrawal had piloerection, increased susceptibility to audiogenic seizures, transient weight loss, and reduced exploratory activity and rotorod performance.[47] Monkeys receiving large daily intravenous doses of PCP for several weeks developed an abstinence syndrome consisting of tremor, diarrhea, motor and oculomotor hyperactivity, bruxism, priapism, and, in some, convulsions. Naloxone failed to precipitate these signs, which seemed to require blood levels higher than can be achieved in humans on a long-term basis.[45,48] Monkeys and rats withdrawing from smaller doses demonstrated disruption of food-maintained operant performance without other behavioral abnormalities.[49] In rats the $5-HT_{1A}$ receptor antagonist buspirone blocked signs of PCP withdrawal.[23]

Antiepileptic Properties

Both noncompetitive and competitive NMDA receptor antagonists are antiepileptic. In animal models of focal seizures, PCP, ketamine, and dizocilpine do not affect interictal epileptiform activity but prevent generalization, and they prevent the development of kindled electrical and behavioral seizures. They are ineffective in models of petit mal epilepsy, perhaps because blockade of glutamatergic neurotransmission in the brainstem disinhibits inhibitory circuits involved in control of primary generalized seizures.[10] In high doses NMDA receptor blockers elicit epileptiform cortical discharges.

Neuroprotective Properties

Noncompetitive and competitive NMDA receptor antagonists are also neuroprotective in animal models of focal or global cerebral ischemia. To be effective they must be given within 1 to 2 hours of the insult. They also counteract rigidity and akinesia in animal models of parkinsonism.[10,50]

Analgesic Properties

NMDA receptor blockers are powerfully analgesic, and they potentiate the analgesia induced by μ-opioids.[10] Analgesia induced by NMDA receptor blockers is not reversed by the μ-opioid antagonist naloxone. It is inhibited, however, by the serotonin antagonist methysergide.[51]

Neuronal Injury

In a dose- and time-related fashion, noncompetitive and competitive NMDA receptor blockers in rats cause intracytoplasmic vacuolation in neurons of the posterior cingulate and retrosplenial cortex.[10] Two hours after receiving single doses of PCP, dizocilpine, 1-[1-(2-thienyl)cyclohexyl]piperidine (TCP), or ketamine, rats demonstrated cytoplasmic vacuolization in neurons of these regions. Within 24 hours the reaction subsided, and repeated low doses did not produce a cumulative effect.[52] Higher doses, however, caused irreversible neuronal necrosis.[53,54] Other reports describe damage to olfactory areas and the hippocampus.[55] The order of potency in producing these changes paralleled binding affinity to the PCP receptor: dizocilpine > PCP > TCP > ketamine. The competitive NMDA inhibitor AP5 was also neurotoxic. The mechanism of injury is uncertain. PCP-induced damage is potentiated by pretreatment with the cholinergic agonist pilocarpine and attenuated by coadministration of scopolamine.

Haloperidol and clozapine are also protective. Diazepam provides partial protection, and barbiturates completely protect. The nonbarbiturate anesthetic halothane is not protective.[56] A proposed mechanism for the damage is that NMDA receptor antagonists at the level of the thalamus block excitatory receptors on GABAergic inhibitory neurons. Reduced GABAergic inhibition of glutamatergic neurons projecting to the cerebral cortex results in excitotoxicity via unblocked AMPA or kainite receptors. AMPA/kainite receptor blockers protect against injury. Barbiturates might prevent injury by increasing GABAergic inhibition in thalamus and cortex. Haloperidol and clozapine might be protective by blocking the inhibitory effects of dopamine on GABAergic neurons.[25]

Endogenous Ligands

The presence of PCP-binding sites has led to a search for endogenous PCP receptor ligands. A peptide isolated from porcine brain, termed alpha-endopsychosin, inhibited PCP binding but not haloperidol binding; its distribution paralleled PCP receptors, with highest concentration in the hippocampus.[57] Another endogenous NMDA receptor blocker is N-acetyl-aspartyl-glutamate, the physiological role of which might be to protect neurons from excitotoxic damage.[58] An endogenous ligand for the sigma receptor (beta-endopsychosin) has also been reported.[2]

Historical Background and Epidemiology

PCP and Analogs

Phencyclidine was developed as an anesthetic agent in the 1950s (Sernyl), but postoperative delirium and psychosis prevented its use except in animals (Sernylan).[59] It was first used as a drug of abuse during the 1960s in California, where it became known as *PeaCe Pill*.[60] By the mid-1970s, perhaps related to restricted heroin supplies, its use had spread epidemically across the United States.[61] Sernylan was withdrawn from the market in 1978, and is currently classified as a schedule II drug.

PCP is easily manufactured by kitchen chemists, and in 1979, 15% of Americans aged 18 to 25 years,

4% of children aged 12 to 17 years, and 13% of high school seniors had tried it at least once.[62] During the 1980s, use declined among high school students, perhaps because of the drug's bad reputation as well as increasing availability of cocaine. In a 1987 survey of middle-class and upper-middle-class adolescents in a drug rehabilitation program, 56% had tried PCP, 21% used it once a month to once a week, 16% used it several times a week, and 8% considered PCP their "best drug experience."[63] In a 1988 study of 74 adolescent marijuana users, 24% had PCP in their urine, and it appeared that most of them had taken PCP without knowing it.[64] In 1999, however, lifetime use of PCP was reported by only 3.4% of U.S. high school seniors and 2.3% of young adults.[65]

Reports from the Drug Abuse Warning Network (DAWN) reflect wide variations in PCP use among DAWN's 27 metropolitan areas.[65] In 1987, PCP-related emergency room encounters in Washington, DC totaled 4235, with 103 deaths—41% of all American PCP-related deaths reported that year. Los Angeles was a distant second with 1589 encounters; New York City reported only 523. In 1976–1977, 51% of PCP encounters involved adolescents, and 24% of users were black. In 1987 only 15% were adolescent, and 60% were black. In 2003 an upsurge in PCP use was reported in Hartford and New Haven, Connecticut, and its use was on the rise in the New York City nightclub scene.[65a]

PCP can be eaten, snorted, or injected, and it has been taken rectally and in eye drops. It is most often smoked, sprinkled on tobacco, parsley, or marijuana, and is commonly substituted for or mixed with what is sold as lysergic acid diethylamide (LSD), mescaline, cannabis, amphetamine, or other drugs.[61] Street products include powders, pastes, capsules, tablets, and "leaf mixtures" containing mint, oregano, parsley, or, for added hallucinogenic effect, catnip.[60,66,67]

A number of PCP analogs have also appeared as street drugs, including phenylcyclohexylpyrrolidine (PHP), phenylcyclohexylethylamine (PCE), piperidinocyclohexanecarbonitrile (PCC), and thienylcyclohexylpiperidine (TCP).[60,68–72]

Ketamine

Ketamine, invented in the 1960s, soon entered the psychedelic underground as "rockmese."[73] Shorter acting and less toxic than PCP, it was approved for human use by the U.S. Food and Drug Administration (FDA) in 1970. Marketed as Ketalar (and, for animal anesthesia, Ketaset), it is a Schedule III drug. Recreational use initially involved mostly New Age spiritualists and health care professionals, but by the 1980s ketamine was a fixture of the rave culture, often combined with other stimulants. Users consider the drug a psychedelic ("mind-revealing": see Chapter 8) because of its alleged ability to increase empathy and insight, revive old memories, and provide religious ecstasy. It is also used as a date-rape drug.[73,74] Ketamine—"green," "jet," "K," "superacid," "supergrass" (if used with marijuana)—is sold as capsules, tablets, crystals, powder, or in solution and taken intramuscularly, intravenously, intranasally, or by smoking.[67,75–76a]

Dextromethorphan

Cough syrups containing dextromethorphan are widely available; more than 140 over-the-counter products are marketed. Like morphine, dextromethorphan and its active metabolite dextrorphan depresses cough centers in the medulla, but unlike morphine they do not cause respiratory depression. In fact, the principal actions of dextromethorphan and dextrorphan, like PCPs, are to block NMDA receptors and bind to sigma receptors. They also block reuptake of serotonin. Dextromethorphan abuse among adolescents and young adults is well-recognized.[77–79] Street names include "DM," "DKM," "DMX," "skittles," "Vitamin D," "Dex," "Tussin," and "Robo." Corocidin HBP Cough and Cold is known as "C-C-C" or "triple Cs." Doses are sometimes more than 100 times the recommended dose. Dextromethorphan often makes an appearance at "rave" parties, where it may be combined with methylenedioxymethamphetamine ("Ecstasy"). Psychic effects of dextromethorphan depend on its enzymatic conversion to detrorphan; "poor metabolizers" are relatively protected from the drug's psychotomimetic effects.[79]

Patterns of Use

Most PCP users take it about once a week, often in social groups, but some engage in amphetamine-like "runs" lasting 2 to 3 days. A cigarette containing PCP delivers 1–100 mg; chronic users may take 1 g daily. Nearly all PCP users take other drugs as well, especially marijuana ("whack," "whacky weed"), ethanol, amphetamine, and hallucinogens.[60] PCP is sometimes smoked with alkaloidal cocaine ("space-base").[80] Marijuana soaked in embalming fluid, a popular fad of the 1990s (see Chapter 7), often contained PCP.[81]

Acute Effects

PCP

The effects of PCP are highly variable, and attempts to separate symptoms and signs according to dose oversimplify (Table 10–1).[67,82–85] In general, low doses (1–5 mg) cause euphoria or dysphoria, emotional lability, a sense of time-slowing, and a feeling of numbness. Desired subjective states include mood elevation, heightened sensitivity to

Table 10–1. Phencyclidine Poisoning: Approximate Order of Symptoms with Increasing Dose

Relaxation, euphoria
Anxiety, emotional lability, dysphoria, paranoia
Subjective time-slowing
Decreased sensory perception
Altered body image, sensory illusions
Amnesia
Agitation, bizarre or violent behavior
Analgesia
Synesthesias
Nystagmus
Miosis
Tachycardia, hypertension
Hyperpnea
Fever
Hypersalivation, sweating
Dysarthria, ataxia, vertigo
Psychosis: paranoid or catatonic
Hallucinations
Dystonia, opisthotonus
Myoclonus
Rhabdomyolysis
Seizures
Stupor or coma with blank stare
Extensor posturing
Respiratory depression
Hypotension

stimuli, increased sociability, relaxation, and "hallucinations," although, in contrast to LSD, PCP is more likely to cause sensory distortions and altered body image than a true visual hallucination. Some subjects at the same low dose experience anxiety, hyperirritability, paranoia, disorientation, confusion, and amnesia. At 5–15 mg, confusion and agitation, bizarre behavior (for which there is often amnesia), body distortion, synesthesias, decreased sensory perception, and analgesia occur. Higher doses produce frank psychosis mimicking stuporous or excited catatonia or paranoid schizophrenia with persecutory auditory hallucinations. The electroencephalogram shows slowing, sometimes with paroxysmal sharp waves.[86]

Ketamine

The effects of ketamine, less toxic than PCP, are more often described in psychedelic terms—a sense of merging with another person or group, or becoming an animal, plant, or inanimate matter. "Awareness may seem to expand to include the entire universe."[73] Out-of-body and near-death experiences are recounted, as are states of non-thinking pure emotion and of a total loss of time sense. In a double-blind, placebo-controlled study of volunteers, ketamine produced dose-related psychedelic effects, including feelings of unreality, alteration in the passage of time, change in the size, depth, or shape of surrounding objects, difficulty controlling one's thoughts, changes in the intensity of sound, and feeling "high." Less often experienced were anxiety or suspiciousness. Very high doses of ketamine can cause psychosis or delirium, however.[87]

Overdose

Toxicity from PCP and related drugs causes tachycardia, hypertension, fever, hyperpnea, flushing, sweating, miosis (rarely mydriasis), hypersalivation, vertigo, ataxia, grimacing, choreoathetosis, torticollis, tortipelvis, myoclonus, and burst-like horizontal, vertical, or rotatory nystagmus.[88] Anesthetic doses (1 mg/kg or more) produce seizures (including status epilepticus), coma with extensor posturing yet open staring eyes, respiratory depression, and hypotension.[89–92] Fever as high as 42.2°C has been recorded, sometimes rising hours after admission;[93] malignant hyperthermia causes liver necrosis.[93] Myoglobinuria, possibly from muscle overactivity, causes renal failure,[68,78,79] and there may be hyperkalemia and metabolic acidosis.[79,94–97] Uric acid nephropathy also occurs.[98] Abdominal cramps and hematemesis have been attributed to contaminants. Death may be directly from overdose, but is more often the result of violence, including homicide, suicide, and accidents.[48,89–91,99–103] A special feature of NMDA receptor blockers is painless self-injury.[101] During recovery, which can take days, any stimulus may provoke agitation or psychotic behavior. Nystagmus often outlasts behavioral abnormalities.

PCP-intoxicated infants and small children are less likely than adults to display agitation or aggression but more likely to have choreoathetosis or seizures.[88] A report of seven such patients described decreased response to tactile and verbal stimuli and "stupor associated with a blank expressionless stare." Nystagmus was present in only 57%.[104] Small children have been poisoned by PCP after accidental ingestion, inhalation of smoke in an automobile, or following deliberate exposure by siblings or babysitters.[105]

The biological half-life of PCP for most people is around 21 hours but ranges from 11 to 51 hours. About 10% of the drug is excreted unchanged, and the rest is converted in the liver to hydroxyl and glucuronide metabolites. Renal excretion is increased by urinary acidification. Cerebrospinal fluid levels are several times higher than blood levels, and this "trapping" of the drug by the CNS accounts for its prolonged duration of action and positive blood and urine toxicology for days or even weeks in chronic users.[88,106] In fact, blood levels may continue to rise for several days after large overdoses.[107] Urine toxic screening can be falsely positive for PCP in persons taking ketamine or dextromethorphan.[108,109] Conversely, screening can be negative in users of street congeners such as PHP.[88]

Treatment of Overdose

Treatment of PCP intoxication begins with a calm environment (Table 10–2). Delirium and psychosis may be present from the outset or emerge as the

Table 10–2. Treatment of Phencyclidine Poisoning

Calm environment; do not try to "talk the patient down"
Safe restraints for violent patients
Consider continuous gastric suctioning
Activated charcoal (1 g/kg every 2–4 hours)
Forced diuresis; do not acidify urine
Tracheal suctioning
Cooling
Antihypertensives
Anticonvulsants
Diazepam intravenously or lorazepam intramuscularly, titered
Consider haloperidol, 2–5 mg, for frank psychosis
Close monitoring of cardiorespiratory status, fluid and electrolyte balance, and renal function (myoglobinuria)

patient awakens from coma. "Talking down" is ineffectual in such a setting and may aggravate symptoms. Violent patients must be safely restrained—self-injury is the most common cause of morbidity and mortality.[88]

Because of gastroenteric recirculation, continuous gastric suctioning can shorten PCP's half-life but is difficult in delirious patients, and fluid and electrolyte alterations must then be closely monitored.[110,111] Repeated doses of activated charcoal (1 g/kg every 2 to 4 hours) and forced diuresis with furosemide hasten nonrenal and renal clearance. Acidification of the urine—recommended by some[112]—is either useless or dangerous. Because only 10% of PCP is excreted unchanged by the kidneys, the increased drug clearance is clinically insignificant, and the frequent presence of myoglobinuria sets the stage for renal shutdown.[88] PCP's large volume of distribution, protein binding, and lipid solubility limit the benefit of hemoperfusion or hemodialysis.[88]

Hypersalivation requires frequent suctioning, and there may be need for cooling blankets and ice baths, antihypertensive therapy, or ventilatory support.[91,110,113] Extremely high fever may require gastric or rectal ice water lavage or paralysis with pancuronium.[93] Seizures, which are infrequent, can be treated with diazepam or phenytoin. Agitation is appropriately treated with a parenterally administered benzodiazepine in titrated doses every 5 to 10 minutes. Unlike diazepam, lorazepam is reliably absorbed intramuscularly. Neuroleptics are best avoided. Phenothiazines and haloperidol are epileptogenic and can potentiate hypotension, aggravate dystonia, or cause a malignant neuroleptic syndrome with exacerbation of myoglobinuria. Anticholinergic effects of phenothiazines can aggravate psychosis or delirium.[83]

Anecdotally verapamil has been recommended for PCP intoxication.[114,115] In rats, however, verapamil, nimodipine, and diltiazem potentiate PCP's behavioral effects.[116,117]

PCP's duration of action is dose-related, and symptoms are aggravated by concurrent use of other drugs, such as ethanol and marijuana.[118] In some patients, psychosis requiring neuroleptics (or resistant to them) can last several weeks.[119]

Tolerance and Withdrawal

Tolerance develops to PCP's effects in humans.[39] Although craving occurs with abstinence, withdrawal symptoms are usually limited to nervousness, "cold sweats," upset stomach, and tremor.[48,84] Of 37 adult men who had used PCP at least weekly (38% daily) for an average of 7 years, none developed withdrawal symptoms with abstinence.[120] Only 11% remained abstinent for a year, however, consistent with animal studies showing that PCP is reinforcing. Psychic dependence—craving—is also well recognized in ketamine users, who often take the drug in a pattern that resembles a cocaine binge.[105]

Withdrawal signs are frequently encountered in neonates exposed in utero to PCP. Irritability, jitteriness, poor cry, hypertonicity, vomiting, and diarrhea begin within 24 hours of delivery and can be treated with benzodiazepines, barbiturates, or paregoric.[121]

PCP and Schizophrenia

Considerable attention has focused on the resemblance of PCP psychosis to schizophrenia. Traditional approaches to schizophrenia divided symptoms into "positive" (paranoia, hostility, agitation, delusions, and hallucinations) and "negative" (alogia, affective flattening, attentional impairment, anhedonia, asociality, avolition, and apathy). Some investigators classify schizophrenic symptoms into three independent clusters, namely, reality distortion (hallucinations, delusions), psychomotor poverty (flat affect, social withdrawal), and disorganization (inappropriate affect, thought disorder).[122] Other workers classify symptoms as positive, negative, or cognitive, the latter including abnormalities of attention, working memory, and executive functions.[123] Whichever system is adopted, it is generally acknowledged that psychostimulants such as amphetamine induces only positive symptoms in otherwise normal users and tends to exacerbate only positive symptoms in schizophrenic subjects. PCP, by contrast, can induce a full schizophrenic syndrome in normal users and exacerbates the full gamut of symptoms in schizophrenic subjects.[122,124] Volunteers receiving subanesthetic doses of PCP (0.05–0.1 mg/kg intravenously) display negativism, withdrawal, and autism, and some develop catatonic posturing, concrete or bizarre responses to proverb interpretation and projective testing, and impoverished speech and thinking. Neuropsychological testing reveals impaired attention, perception, and symbolic thinking similar to that encountered in schizophrenics. Schizophrenics often have elevated thresholds for pain perception, a striking feature of PCP intoxication. Moreover, CNS abnormalities found in schizophrenics—decreased frontal lobe metabolism and impaired event-related evoked potentials—are induced by PCP but not amphetamine.[52,125–127] Increased binding of the radiolabeled PCP receptor ligand 1-[1-(2-thienyl)cyclohexyl]piperidine (TCP) was reported in schizophrenic brains.[128]

The dopamine D_2 antagonist haloperidol attenuates positive but not negative symptoms in both schizophrenia and PCP psychosis. The atypical antipsychotic clozapine attenuates both positive and negative symptoms of schizophrenia, including those induced by ketamine.[129] In rodents, chronic administration of PCP results in diminished dopaminergic neurotransmission in the prefrontal cortex and increased dopaminergic neurotransmission in subcortical mesolimbic pathways.[130,131] Such a pattern is found in schizophrenia, and it has been proposed that a prefrontal hypodopaminergic state underlies cognitive disturbance and negative symptoms, whereas a mesolimbic hyperdopaminergic state underlies positive symptoms.[123]

Such observations have generated an "NMDA receptor hypofunction hypothesis of schizophrenia,[4,132–134] and putative animal models of schizophrenia have been developed using PCP and other NMDA receptor antagonists.[135–139] In such models atypical antipsychotics such as clozapine and olanzapine are more effective than typical antipsychotics such as haloperidol in blocking the effects of NMDA antagonists.[4] The added efficacy of atypical antipsychotics might relate to their actions at indirectly perturbed serotonin receptors.[130,140]

An alternative view is that the psychotomimetic properties of PCP and related drugs correlate with their affinities to sigma receptors rather than to PCP receptors. As noted above, in animals PCP and dizocilpine appear to produce their behavioral effects by acting at PCP receptors. In fact, dizocilpine binds more avidly to PCP receptors than PCP does. In humans, however, PCP causes psychosis and dizocilpine does not. Dizocilpine, unlike PCP, does not bind to sigma receptors.[24] Typical and atypical antipsychotics bind to sigma receptors but are devoid of activity at PCP receptors.[15,24]

Psychotic symptoms can last days or weeks after single doses of PCP, and many chronic users demonstrate persistent behavioral and cognitive abnormalities.[61,83,84,119,141–143] As with other drugs, causality is difficult to establish.[144] Pre-existing schizophrenia is overrepresented among users with persistent psychosis, but the majority have no history of earlier psychiatric problems.[119] In monkeys receiving PCP daily for 2 weeks behavioral and prefrontal dopamine dysfunction persisted for several weeks after the drug was stopped.[130] In humans chronic PCP and ketamine use are associated with not only long-lasting flattened affect, depersonalization, and dissociative thought disorder, but also persisting memory impairment.[55]

Of obvious relevance to cognitive or psychiatric disturbance is the observation that in rodents PCP and related drugs cause pathological changes in the CNS[52,55] (see above). Risk of damage is proportionate to affinity for the PCP receptor, i.e., dizocilpine > PCP > ketamine, and primate brain, including human, is more resistant to damage than rat pathological brain. These findings prevented the development of dizocilpine as a neuroprotective agent, however. Whether subtle but qualitatively similar abnormalities contribute to long-lasting neuropsychiatric abnormalities in PCP users (or in schizophrenics) is uncertain.

Hypertension and Stroke

The duration of PCP-induced hypertension parallels the mental changes, lasting hours or days.[60,82,90,96] Although hypertension might be related to enhanced catecholamine or serotonin action,[145] contractile responses to PCP of isolated basilar and middle cerebral arteries were not prevented by methysergide, phentolamine, atropine, diphenhydramine, or indomethacin, suggesting the presence of PCP receptors on cerebral vessels.[146] The nature of such receptors is unclear; NMDA receptor agonists *constrict* rat pial arterioles.[147]

Hypertensive encephalopathy followed PCP ingestion in a young woman with systemic lupus erythematosus and a history of migraine.[148] A 13-year-old boy became comatose after taking PCP; blood pressure was normal on admission, and he became alert but 3 days later deteriorated with a blood pressure of 230/130 mmHg. At autopsy there was intracerebral hemorrhage.[113] Urine contained PCP in a 6-year-old with seizures and right hemiparesis. Computed tomography demonstrated parieto-occipital lucency and vessel enhancement, suggesting a vascular malformation. He recovered, and cerebral angiography was not done.[149] Subarachnoid hemorrhage has followed PCP use on at least three occasions.[150–152] Two involved adolescents,[150,151] in one of whom autopsy revealed perforation of the ventral surface of the basilar artery without aneurysm or vasculitis.[150] The third was a 33-year-old woman with an anterior communicating artery aneurysm.[152] Cerebral infarction followed PCP smoking in a 56-year-old man with atrial fibrillation; it was suspected that PCP cardiac stimulation caused dislodgment of clot from the heart.[152] A 45-year-old hypertensive diabetic man with coronary artery disease and a 3 pack-year history of smoking cigarettes had two episodes of transient monocular blindness within a few hours of smoking PCP.[153] Single-photon emission computed tomographic (SPECT) studies on several PCP users revealed asymmetric perfusion abnormalities in the cerebral cortex; each subject also used other drugs, however, including cocaine and ethanol.[154]

A 15-month-old girl became unresponsive with staring, upward rolling of the eyes, head turning to the left, and episodic stiffening of the limbs lasting a few minutes. Neuroleptic-induced dystonia was suspected, but signs did not abate with diphenhydramine administration. Urine was positive for PCP. She recovered completely over 24 hours.[155]

Immunosuppression

PCP specifically binds to lymphocytes and depresses both humoral and cellular immune responses.[156] The lymphocyte receptors are sigma in type and also bind several steroids, including progesterone, testosterone, and deoxycorticosterone.[157] It is uncertain if PCP lymphocyte binding is clinically important or if sigma receptors contribute to steroid-induced mental changes or immunosuppression.

Effects on Pregnancy

In addition to withdrawal signs, infants exposed in utero to PCP have had abnormal behavior; irregular ventilatory patterns during sleep; hydrocephalus; microcephaly; and anomalies of the heart, lungs, urinary or musculoskeletal systems, cerebellum, cerebral commissures, and optic chiasm.[158–164] These anomalies could, of course, be the result of other drugs or poor prenatal care although in one report multiple regression techniques pointed to PCP as specifically responsible for abnormalities of attention, tendon reflexes, and grasp and rooting reflexes.[161] In a study of 12 infants exposed in utero to PCP, there was no increase in congenital defects, but two-thirds had serious neonatal medical problems, usually respiratory; several infants were still irritable at 6 months of age and at 18 months had mild to severe abnormalities of language, behavior, and fine motor coordination.[121] In another report nine infants exposed to PCP throughout pregnancy had normal psychomotor development at 2 years of age.[163]

NMDA receptor stimulation is critical for neuronal survival and differentiation during early development of the central nervous system, and animal studies confirm that in utero exposure to NMDA receptor antagonists is harmful. Lasting abnormalities are described in electroencephalographic power spectra, monoamine metabolism, hippocampal physiology, electrical kindling threshold, spatial learning, brain and body weight, myelination, dopamine receptor sensitivity, lateral geniculate nucleus morphology, synaptic pruning, and neuronal migration.[165,166]

References

1. Balster RL, Chait LD. The behavioral effects of phencyclidine in animals. NIDA Res Monogr 1978; 21:53.
2. Contreras PC, Monahan JB, Lanthorn TH, et al. Phencyclidine. Physiological actions, interactions with excitatory amino acids, and endogenous ligands. Mol Neurobiol 1987; 1:191.
3. Johnson KM, Jones SM. Neuropharmacology of phencyclidine: basic mechanisms and therapeutic potential. Annu Rev Pharmacol Toxicol 1990; 30:707.
4. Breese GR, Knapp DJ, Moy SS. Integrative role for serotonergic and glutamatergic receptor mechanisms in the action of NMDA antagonists: potential relationships to antipsychotic drug actions on NMDA antagonist responsiveness. Neurosci Biobehav Rev 2002; 26:441.
5. Bowyer JF, Spuhler KP, Weiner N. Effects of phencyclidine, amphetamine, and related compounds on dopamine release from uptake into striatal synaptosomes. J Pharmacol Exp Ther 1984; 229:671.
6. French ED, Dilapil C, Quiron R. Phencyclidine binding sites in the nucleus accumbens and phencyclidine-induced hyperactivity are decreased following lesions of the mesolimbic dopamine system. Eur J Pharmacol 1985; 116:1.
7. Vargas HM, Pechnick RN. Binding affinity and anti-muscarinic activity of sigma and phencyclidine receptor ligands. Eur J Pharmacol 1991; 195:151.
8. Rasmussen K, Fuller RW, Stockton ME, et al. NMDA receptor antagonists suppress behaviors but not norepinephrine turnover or locus coeruleus unit activity induced by opiate withdrawal. Eur J Pharmacol 1991; 197:9.
9. Fryer JD, Lukes RJ. Noncompetitive functional inhibition at diverse, human nicotinic acetylcholine receptor subtypes by bupropion, phencyclidine, and ibogaine. J Pharmacol Exp Ther 1999; 288:88.
10. Sagratella S. NMDA antagonists: antiepileptic-neuroprotective drugs with diversified neuropharmacological profiles. Pharmacol Res 1995; 32:1.
11. Zukin SR, Javitt DC. Mechanisms of phencyclidine (PCP)-N-methyl-D-aspartate (NMDA) receptor interaction: implications for drug abuse research. NIDA Res Monogr 1990; 95:247.
12. Lodge D, Johnson KM. Noncompetitive excitatory amino acid receptor antagonists. Trends Pharmacol Sci 1990; 11:81.

13. Reynolds IJ, Miller RJ. Allosteric modulation of N-methyl-D-aspartate receptors. Adv Pharmacol 1990; 21:101.

13a. Svenningsson P, Tzavara ET, Carruthers R, et al. Diverse psychotomimetics act through a common signaling pathway. Science 2003; 302:1412.

14. Su TP. Sigma receptors. Putative links between nervous, endocrine and immune systems. Eur J Biochem 1991; 200:633.

15. Quiron R, Clicheportiche R, Contreras PC, et al. Classification and nomenclature of phencyclidine and sigma receptor sites. Trends Neurosci 1987; 10:444.

16. Itzhak Y, Stein I, Zhang SH, et al. Binding of sigma-ligands to C57BL/6 mouse brain membranes: effects of monoamine oxidase inhibitors and subcellular distribution studies suggest the existence of sigma-receptor subtypes. J Pharmacol Exp Ther 1991; 257:141.

17. Connick J, Fox P, Nicholson D. Psychotomimetic effects and sigma ligands. Trends Pharmacol Sci 1990; 11:274.

18. Boyce S, Rupniak NM, Steventon MJ, et al. Psychomotor activity and cognitive disruption attributable to NMDA, but not sigma, interactions in primates. Behav Brain Res 1991; 42:115.

19. Klepstad P, Maurset A, Moberg ER, Oye I. Evidence of a role for NMDA receptors in pain perception. Eur J Pharmacol 1990; 187:513.

20. Koek W, Woods JH, Winger GD. MK-801, a proposed noncompetitive antagonist of excitatory amino acid neurotransmission, produces phencyclidine-like behavioral effects in pigeons, rats, and rhesus monkeys. J Pharmacol Exp Ther 1988; 245:969.

21. Troupin AS, Mendius JR, Cheng F, Risinger MW. MK801. In: Meldrum BS, Porter RS, eds. Current Problems in Epilepsy. 4. New Anticonvulsant Drugs. London: John Libby, 1986; 191.

22. Sonders MS, Keana JFW, Weber E. Phencyclidine and psychomimetic sigma opiates: recent insights into their biochemical and physiological sites of action. Trends Neurosci 1988; 11:37.

23. Nabeshima T, Kitaichi K, Noda Y. Functional changes in neuronal systems induced by phencyclidine administration. N Y Acad Sci 1996; 801:29.

24. Steinpreis RE. The behavioral and neurochemical effects of phencyclidine in humans and animals: some implications for modeling psychosis. Behav Brain Res 1996; 74:45.

25. Anand A, Charney DS, Oren DA, et al. Attenuation of the neuropsychiatric effects of ketamine and lamotrigine: support for hyperglutamatergic effects of N-methyl-D-aspartate receptor antagonists. Arch Gen Psychiatry 2000; 57:270.

26. Moghaddam B, Adams B, Verma A, et al. Activation of glutamatergic neurotransmission by ketamine: a novel step in the pathway from NMDA receptor blockade to dopaminergic and cognitive disruptions associated with the prefrontal cortex. J Neurosci 1997; 17:2921.

27. Moghaddam B, Adams BW. Reversal of phencyclidine effects by a group II metabotropic glutamate receptor agonists in rats. Science 1998; 281:1349.

28. Ninan I, Kulkarni SK. 5HT2A receptor antagonists block MK-801-induced stereotypy and hyperlocomotion. Eur J Pharmacol 1998; 358:111.

29. Willetts J, Balster RL, Leander JD. The behavioral pharmacology of NMDA receptor antagonists. Trends Pharmacol Sci 1990; 11:423.

30. Klein M, Calderon S, Hayes B. Abuse liability assessment of neuroprotectants. Ann N Y Acad Sci 1999; 890:515.

31. Mansbach RS, Balster RL. Pharmacological specificity of the phencyclidine discriminative stimulus in rats. Pharmacol Biochem Behav 1991; 39:971.

32. France CP, Moerschbaecher JM, Woods JH. MK801 and related compounds in monkeys: discriminative stimulus effects on a conditional discrimination. J Pharmacol Exp Ther 1991; 257:727.

33. Steinfels GF, Alberici CP, Tam SW, Cook L. Biochemical, behavioral, and electrophysiologic actions of the selective sigma receptor ligand (+)pentazocine. Neuropsychopharmacology 1988; 1:321.

34. Balster RL. Substitution and antagonism in rats trained to discriminate (+)-N-allylnormetazocine from saline. J Pharmacol Exp Ther 1989; 249:749.

35. Krystal JH, Petrakis IL, Webb E, et al. Drug-related ethanol-like effects of the NMDA antagonist, ketamine, in recently detoxified alcoholics. Arch Gen Psychiatry 1998; 55:354.

36. Moreton JE, Meisch RA, Stark L, Thompson T. Ketamine self-administration by the rhesus monkey. J Pharmacol Exp Ther 1977; 203:303.

37. Risner ME. Intravenous self-administration of phencyclidine and related compounds in the dog. J Pharmacol Exp Ther 1982; 221:637.

38. Lukas SE, Griffiths RR, Brady JV, Wurster RM. Phencyclidine-analogue self-injection by the baboon. Psychopharmacology 1984; 83:316.

39. Carroll ME. PCP and hallucinogens. Adv Alcohol Subst Abuse 1990; 9:167.

40. Carroll ME. Performance maintained by orally delivered phencyclidine under second-order, tandem, and fixed interval schedules in food satiated and food deprived rhesus monkeys. J Pharmacol Exp Ther 1985; 232:351.

41. Marquis KL, Moreton JE. Animal models of intravenous phencyclidine self-administration. Pharmacol Biochem Behav 1987; 27:385.

42. Beardsley PM, Hayes BA, Balster RL. The self-administration of MK801 can depend on drug-reinforcement history, and its discriminative stimulus properties are phencyclidine-like in rhesus monkeys. J Pharmacol Exp Ther 1990; 252:953.

43. Corbett D. Possible abuse potential of the NMDA antagonist MK801. Behav Brain Res 1989; 34:239.

44. McMillan DE, Hardwick WC, deCosta BR, Rice KC. Effects of drugs that bind to PCP and sigma receptors on punished responding. J Pharmacol Exp Ther 1991; 258:1015.

45. Balster RL. Disruption of schedule-controlled behavior during abstinence from phencyclidine and tetrahydrocannabinol. NIDA Res Monogr 1990; 95:124.

46. Wessinger WD, Owens SM. Phencyclidine dependence: the relationship of dose and serum concentrations to operant behavioral effects. J Pharmacol Exp Ther 1991; 258:207.

47. Spain JW, Klingman GI. Continuous intravenous infusion of phencyclidine in unrestrained rats results in the rapid induction of tolerance and physical dependence. J Pharmacol Exp Ther 1985; 234:415.

48. Pradhan SN. Phencyclidine (PCP): some human studies. Neurosci Biobehav Rev 1984; 8:493.

49. Beardsley PM, Balster RL. Behavioral dependence upon phencyclidine and ketamine in the rat. J Pharmacol Exp Ther 1987; 242:203.

50. Kornhuber J, Weller M. Psychotogenicity and N-methyl-D-aspartate receptor antagonism: implications for neuroprotective pharmacotherapy. Biol Psychiatry 1997; 41:135.

51. Kohrs R, Durieux ME. Ketamine: teaching an old drug new tricks. Anesth Analg 1998; 87:1186.

52. Olney JW, Labruyere J, Price MT. Pathological changes induced in cerebrocortical neurons by phencyclidine and related drugs. Science 1989; 244:1360.

53. Allen HL, Iversen LL. Phencyclidine, dizocilpine, and cerebrocortical neurons. Science 1990; 247:221.

54. Sharp FR, Jasper P, Hall J, et al. MK801 and ketamine induce heat shock protein HSP72 in injured neurons in posterior cingulate and retrosplenial cortex. Ann Neurol 1991; 30:801.

55. Ellison G. The N-methyl-D-aspartate antagonists phencyclidine, ketamine and dizocilpine as both behavioral and anatomical models of the dementias. Brain Res Brain Res Rev 1995; 20:250.

56. Olney JW, Labruyere J, Wang G, et al. NMDA antagonist neurotoxicity: mechanism and prevention. Science 1991; 254:1515.

57. DiMaggio DA, Contreras PC, Quirion R, O'Donohue TL. Isolation and identification of an endogenous ligand for the phencyclidine receptor. NIDA Res Monogr 1986; 64:24.

58. Coyle JT. The nagging question of the function of N-acetylaspartyl glutamate. Neurobiol Dis 1997; 4:231.

59. Luby ED, Cohen BD, Rosenbaum C, et al. Study of a new schizophrenomimetic drug-Sernyl. Arch Neurol 1959; 81:363.

60. Lerner SE, Burns RS. Phencyclidine use among youth: history, epidemiology, and acute and chronic intoxication. NIDA Res Monogr 1978; 21:66.

61. Young I, Lawson GW, Gacono CB. Clinical aspects of phencyclidine (PCP). Int J Addict 1987; 22:1.

62. Fishburne PM, Abelson HI, Cisin I. National Survey on Drug Abuse: Main Findings: 1979. Washington, DC: DHHS Publication No. (ADM) 80-976, 1980.

63. Schwartz RH, Hoffman NG, Smith D, et al. Use of phencyclidine among adolescents attending a suburban drug treatment facility. J Pediatr 1987; 110:322.

64. Silber TJ, Josefsohn M, Hicks JM, et al. Prevalence of PCP use among adolescent marijuana users. J Pediatr 1988; 112:827.

65. Johnston LD, O'Malley PM, Bachman JG. Monitoring the Future: National Survey Results on Drug Use, 1975–1999, Vol. 1, 2-2000. Washington, DC: NIDA.

65a. Dewan SK. A drug feared in the '70s is tied to suspect in killings. NY Times, April 6, 2003.

66. Lundberg GD, Gupta RL, Montgomery SH. Phencyclidine patterns seen in street drug analysis. Clin Toxicol 1976; 9:503.

67. Siegel RK. Phencyclidine and ketamine intoxication: a study of four populations of recreational users. NIDA Res Monogr 1978; 21:119.

68. Shulgin AT, MacLean D. Illicit synthesis of phencyclidine (PCP) and several of its analogs. Clin Toxicol 1976; 9:553.

69. Budd RD. PHP, a new drug of abuse. N Engl J Med 1980; 303:588.

70. Gianini AJ, Price WA, Losielle RH, Malone DW. Treatment of phenylcyclohexylpyrrolidine (PHP) psychosis with haloperidol. J Toxicol Clin Toxicol 1985; 23:185.

71. Smialek J, Monforte J, Gault R, Spitz W. Cyclohexamine ("rocket fuel")-phencyclidine's potent analog. J Anal Toxicol 1979; 3:209.

72. Jerrard DA. "Designer drugs"— a current perspective. J Emerg Med 1990; 8:733.

73. Jansen KLR. A review of the nonmedical use of ketamine: use, users, and consequences. J Psychoactive Drugs 2000; 32:419.

74. Smith KM, Larive LL, Romanelli F. Club drugs: methylenedioxymethamphetamine, flunitrazepam, ketamine hydrochloride, and gamma-hydroxybutyrate. Am J Health-Syst Pharm 2002; 59:1067.

75. Anon. Ketamine abuse. FDA Drug Bull 1979; 9:24.

76. Ahmed SN, Petchkovsky L. Abuse of ketamine. Br J Psychiatry 1980; 137:303.

76a. Jansen KLR, Darracot-Cankovic R. The nonmedical use of ketamine. II. A review of problem use and dependence. J Psychoactive Drugs 2001; 33:151.

77. Nordt SP. "DXM": a new drug of abuse? Ann Emerg Med 1998; 31:794.

78. Wolfe TR, Caravati EM. Massive dextromethorphan ingestion and abuse. Am J Emerg Med 1995; 13:174.

79. Bobo WC, Miller SC, Jackson JC. Dextromethorphan as a drug of abuse. In: Graham AW, Schultz TK, Mayo-Smith MF, et al., eds. Principles of Addiction Medicine, 3rd edition. Chevy Chase, MD: American Society of Addiction Medicine, 2003:154.

80. Giannini AJ, Loiselle RH, Giannini MC. Space-base abstinence: alleviation of withdrawal symptoms in combinative cocaine–phencyclidine abuse. J Toxicol Clin Toxicol 1987; 25:493.

81. Holland JA, Nelson L, Ravikumar PR, et al. Embalming fluid-soaked marijuana: new high or new guise for PCP? J Psychoactive Drugs 1998; 30:215.

82. McCarron MM, Schultze BW, Thompson GA, et al. Acute phencyclidine intoxication: incidence of clinical findings in 1000 cases. Ann Emerg Med 1981; 10:237.

83. Allen RM, Young SJ. Phencyclidine-induced psychosis. Am J Psychiatry 1978; 135:1081.

84. Fauman MA, Fauman BJ. The psychiatric aspects of chronic phencyclidine use: a study of chronic PCP users. NIDA Res Monogr 1978; 21:18.

85. McCarron MM, Schulze BW, Thompson GA, et al. Acute phencyclidine intoxication: clinical patterns, complications, and treatment. Ann Emerg Med 1981; 10:290.

86. Stockard JJ, Werner SS, Albers JA, Chiappa KH. Electroencephalographic findings in phencyclidine intoxication. Arch Neurol 1976; 33:200.

87. Bowdle TA, Radant AD, Cowley DS, et al. Psychedelic effects of ketamine in healthy volunteers: relationship to steady-state plasma concentrations. Anesthesiology 1998; 88:82.

88. Goldfrank LR, Lewin NA. Phencyclidine. In: Goldfrank LR, Flomenbaum NE, Lewin NA, et al., eds. Toxicologic Emergencies, 6th edition. Stamford, CT: Appleton & Lange, 1998; 1105.

89. Kessler GF, Demers LM, Brennan RW. Phencyclidine and fatal status epilepticus. N Engl J Med 1974; 291:979.

90. Burns RS, Lerner SE. Perspectives: acute phencyclidine intoxication. Clin Toxicol 1976; 9:477.

91. Rappolt RT, Gay GR, Farris RD. Phencyclidine (PCP) intoxication: diagnosis in stages and algorithms of treatment. Clin Toxicol 1980; 16:509.

92. Alldredge BK, Lowenstein DH, Simon RP. Seizures associated with recreational drug abuse. Neurology 1989; 39:1037.

93. Rosenberg J, Pentel P, Pond S, et al. Hyperthermia associated with drug intoxication. Crit Care Med 1986; 14:964.

94. Armen R, Kanel G, Reynolds T. Phencyclidine-induced malignant hyperthermia causing submassive liver necrosis. Am J Med 1984; 77:167.

95. Cogen FC, Rigg G, Simmons JL, Domino EF. Phencyclidine-associated acute rhabdomyolysis. Ann Intern Med 1978; 88:210.

96. Richards JR. Rhabdomyolysis and drugs of abuse. J Emerg Med 2000; 19:51.

97. Patel R, Das M, Palazzolo M, et al. Myoglobinuric acute renal failure in phencyclidine overdose: report of observations in eight cases. Ann Emerg Med 1980; 9:549.

98. Patel R. Acute uric acid nephropathy: a complication of phencyclidine intoxication. Postgrad Med J 1982; 58:783.

99. Noguchi TT, Nakamura GR. Phencyclidine-related deaths in Los Angeles County, 1976. J Forensic Sci 1978; 23:503.

100. Fauman MA, Fauman BJ. Violence associated with phencyclidine abuse. Am J Psychiatry 1979; 136:1584.

101. Grove VE. Painless self-injury after ingestion of "angel dust." JAMA 1979; 242:655.

102. Lowry PW, Hassig SE, Gunn RA, Mathison JB. Homicide victims in New Orleans: recent trends. Am J Epidemiol 1988; 128:1130.

103. Poklis A, Graham M, Maginn D, et al. Phencyclidine and violent deaths in St. Louis, Missouri: a survey of medical examiners' cases from 1977 through 1986. Am J Drug Alcohol Abuse 1990; 16:265.

104. Schwartz RH, Einhorn A. PCP intoxication in seven young children. Pediatr Emerg Care 1986; 2:238.

105. Schwartz RH. Passive inhalation of marijuana, phencyclidine, and free base cocaine ("crack") by infants. Am J Dis Child 1989; 143:644.

106. Gorelick DA, Wilkins JN. Inpatient treatment of PCP abusers and users. Am J Drug Alcohol Abuse 1989; 15:1.

107. Jackson JE. Phencyclidine pharmacokinetics after a massive overdose. Ann Intern Med 1989; 111:613.

108. Shannon M. Recent ketamine administration can produce a urine toxic screen which is falsely positive for phencyclidine. Pediatr Emerg Care 1998; 14:180.

109. Budai B, Iskandar H. Dextromethorphan can produce false positive phencyclidine testing with HPLC. Am J Emerg Med 2002; 20:61.

110. Aronow R, Done A. Phencyclidine overdose: an emergency concept of management. J Am Coll Emerg Phys 1978; 7:56.

111. Done AK, Aronow R, Miceli JN. The pharmacokinetics of phencyclidine in overdosage and its treatment. NIDA Res Monogr 1978; 21:210.

112. Giannini AJ, Loiselle RHD, DiMarzio LR, Giannini MC. Augmentation of haloperidol by ascorbic acid in phencyclidine intoxication. Am J Psychiatry 1987; 144:1207.

113. Eastman JW, Cohen SN. Hypertensive crisis and death associated with phencyclidine poisoning. JAMA 1975; 231:1270.

114. Montgomery PT, Mueller ME. Treatment of PCP intoxication with verapamil. Am J Psychiatry 1985; 142:882.

115. Price WA, Giannini AJ. Management of acute PCP intoxication with verapamil. Clin Toxicol 1986; 24:85.

116. McCann DJ, Winter J.C. Effects of phencyclidine, N-alkyl-N-normetazocine (SKF 10047), and verapamil on performance in a radial maze. Pharmacol Biochem Behav 1986; 24:187.

117. Popoli P, Bendedetti M, Scotti-de-Carolis A. Influence of nimodipine and diltiazem, alone and in combination,

on phencyclidine-induced effects in rats: an EEG and behavioral study. Eur J Pharmacol 1990; 191:141.

118. Godley PJ, Moore ES, Woodworth JR, Fineg J. Effects of ethanol and delta-9-tetrahydrocannabinol on phencyclidine disposition in dogs. Biopharm Drugs Dispos 1991; 12:189.

119. Luisada PV. The phencyclidine psychosis. NIDA Res Monogr 1978; 21:241.

120. Gorelick DA, Wilkins JN, Wong C. Outpatient treatment of PCP abusers. Am J Drug Alcohol Abuse 1989; 15:367.

121. Howard J, Kropenske V, Tyler R. The long-term effects on neurodevelopment in infants exposed prenatally to PCP. NIDA Res Monogr 1986; 64:237.

122. Ellenbrook BA, Cools AR. Animal models for the negative symptoms of schizophrenia. Behav Pharmacol 2000; 11:223.

123. Tsai G, Coyle JT. Glutamatergic mechanisms in schizophrenia. Annu Rev Pharmacol Toxicol 2002; 42:165.

124. Javitt DC, Zukin SR. Recent advances in the phencyclidine model of schizophrenia. Am J Psychiatry 1991; 148:1301.

125. Pfefferbaum A, Ford JM, White PM, Roth WT. P3 in schizophrenia is affected by stimulus modality, response requirements, medication status, and negative symptoms. Arch Gen Psychiatry 1989; 46:1035.

126. Weinberger DR, Berman KF. Speculation on the meaning of metabolic "hypofrontality" in schizophrenia. Schizophr Bull 1988; 14:157.

127. Javitt DC, Schroeder CS, Arezzo JC, Vaughan HG. Selective inhibition of processing-contingent auditory event-related potential components by the PCP-like agent MK801. Electroencephalogr Clin Neurophysiol 1991; 79:65P.

128. Simpson MD, Sister P, Royston MC, Deakin JF. Alterations in phencyclidine and sigma binding sites in schizophrenic brains. Effects of disease process and neuroleptic medication. Schizophr Res 1991; 6:41.

129. Malhotra AK, Adler CM, Kennison SD, et al. Clozapine blunts N-methyl-D-aspartate antagonist psychosis: a study with ketamine. Biol Psychiatry 1997; 42:664.

130. Jentsch JD, Redmond DE, Elsworth JD, et al. Enduring cognitive deficits and cortical dopamine dysfunction in monkeys after long-term administration of phencyclidine. Science 1997; 277:953.

131. Svensson TH. Dysfunctional brain dopamine systems induced by psychotomimetic NMDA-receptor antagonists and the effects of antipsychotic drugs. Brain Res Brain Rev 2000; 31:320.

132. Jentsch JD, Roth RH. The neuropsychopharmacology of phencyclidine: from NMDA receptor hypofunction to the dopamine hypothesis of schizophrenia. Neuropsychopharmacology 1999; 20:201.

133. Carlsson A, Waters N, Holm-Waters S, et al. Interactions between monoamines, glutamate, and GABA in schizophrenia: new evidence. Annu Rev Pharmacol Toxicol 2001; 41:237.

134. Olney JW, Newcomer JW, Farber NB. NMDA receptor hypofunction of schizophrenia. J Psychiatric Res 1999; 33:523.

135. Sams-Dodd F. Phencyclidine in the social interaction test: an animal model of schizophrenia with face and predictive validity. Rev Neurosci 1999; 10:59.

136. Bakshi VP, Tricklebank M, Neijt HC, et al. Disruption of prepulse inhibition and increases in locomotor activity by competitive N-methyl-D-aspartate receptor antagonist in rats. J Pharmacol Exp Ther 1999; 222:643.

137. Curzon P, Decker MW. Effects of phencyclidine (PCP) and (+)MK-801 on sensorimotor gating in CD-1 mice. Prog NeuroPsychopharmacol Biol Psychiatry 1998; 22:129.

138. Thaker GK, Carpenter WT. Advances in schizophrenia. Nat Med 2001; 7:667.

139. Sharp FR, Tomitaka M, Bernaudin M, et al. Psychosis: pathological activation of limbic thalamocortical circuits by psychotomimetics and schizophrenia? Trends Neurosci 2001; 24:330.

140. Aghajanian GK, Marek GJ. Serotonin model of schizophrenia: emerging role of glutamate mechanisms. Brain Res Brain Res Rev 2000; 31:302.

141. Rainey JM, Crowder MK. Prolonged psychosis attributed to phencyclidine: report of three cases. Am J Psychiatry 1975; 132:1076.

142. Fauman B, Aldinger G, Fauman M. Psychiatric sequelae of phencyclidine abuse. Clin Toxicol 1976; 9:529.

143. Stillman R, Petersen RC. The paradox of phencyclidine (PCP) abuse. Ann Intern Med 1979; 90:428.

144. Weinrieb RM, O'Brien CP. Persistent cognitive deficits attributed to substance abuse. In: Brust JCM, ed. Neurologic Complications of Drug and Alcohol Abuse. Neurol Clin 1993, 11:663.

145. Illett KF, Jarott B, O'Donnell SR, Watstall JC. Mechanism of cardiovascular actions of 1-(phenylcyclohexyl)-piperidine hydrochloride (phencyclidine). Br J Pharmacol Chemother 1966; 28:73.

146. Altura B, Altura BM. Phencyclidine, lysergic acid diethylamide, and mescaline: cerebral artery spasm and hallucinogenic activity. Science 1981; 212:1051.

147. Altura BM, Huang Q-F, Gebrewold A, et al. Evidence for involvement of the N-methyl-D-aspartate receptor complex in regulation of pial microvasculature. Stroke 1992; 23:153.

148. Burns RS, Lerner SE. The effects of phencyclidine in man: a review. In: Domino EF, ed. PCP (Phencyclidine): Historical and Current Perspectives. Ann Arbor, MI: NPP Books, 1981; 449.

149. Crosley CJ, Binet EP. Cerebrovascular complications in phencyclidine intoxication. J Pediatr 1979; 94:316.

150. Boyko OB, Burger PC, Heinz ER. Pathological and radiological correlation of subarachnoid hemorrhage in phencyclidine abuse. Case report. J Neurosurg 1987; 67:446.

151. Besson HA. Intracranial hemorrhage associated with phencyclidine abuse. JAMA 1982; 248:585.

152. Sloan MA, Kittner SJ, Rigamonti D, Price TR. Occurrence of stroke associated with use/abuse of drugs. Neurology 1991; 41:1358.

153. Ubogu EE. Amaurosis fugax associated with phencyclidine inhalation. Eur Neurol 2001; 46:98.

154. Hertzman M, Reba RC, Kotlyarov EV. Single photon emission computed tomography in phencyclidine and related drug abuse. Am J Psychiatry 1990; 147:255.

155. Piecuch S, Thomas U, Shah BR. Acute dystonic reactions that fail to respond to diphenhydramine: think of PCP. J Emerg Med 1999; 17:527.

156. Khansari N, Whitten HD, Fudenberg HH. Phencyclidine-induced immunodepression. Science 1984; 225:76.

157. Su T-P, London ED, Jaffe JH. Steroid binding at sigma receptors suggests a link between endocrine, nervous, and immune systems. Science 1988; 240:219.

158. Golden NL, Sokol RJ, Rubin IL. Angel dust: possible effects on the fetus. Pediatrics 1980; 65:18.

159. Michaud J, Mizrahi EM, Urich H. Agenesis of the vermis with fusion of the cerebellar hemispheres, septo-optic dysplasia, and associated anomalies. Report of a case. Acta Neuropathol 1982; 56:161.

160. Ward SL, Schuetz S, Kirshna V, et al. Abnormal sleeping ventilatory pattern in infants of substance abusing mothers. Am J Dis Child 1986; 140:1015.

161. Golden NL, Kuhnert BR, Sokol RJ, et al. Neonatal manifestations of maternal phencyclidine exposure. J Perinat Med 1987; 15:185.

162. Wachsman L, Schuetz S, Chan LS, Wingert WA. What happens to babies exposed to phencyclidine (PCP) in utero? Am J Drug Alcohol Abuse 1989; 15:31.

163. Chasnoff IJ, Burns KA, Burns WJ, Scholl SH. Prenatal drug exposure: effects on neonatal and infant growth and development. Neurobehav Toxicol Teratol 1986; 8:357.

164. Tabor BL, Smith-Wallace T, Yonekura ML. Perinatal outcome associated with PCP versus cocaine use. Am J Drug Alcohol Abuse 1990; 16:337.

165. Deutsch SI, Mastropaolo J, Rosse RB. Neurodevelopmental consequences of early exposure to phencyclidine and related drugs. Clin Neuropharmacol 1998; 21:320.

166. Abdel-Rahman MS, Ismail EE. Teratogenic effect of ketamine and cocaine in CF-1 mice. Teratology 2000; 61:291.

Chapter 11
Anticholinergics

Your cup with numbing drops of night and evil, stilled of all remorse, she will infuse to charm your sight.
—Homer, *The Odyssey*

Upon my secure hour thy uncle stole
With juice of cursed hebona in a vial,
And in the pouches of my ears did pour
The leprous distillment, whose effect
Holds such an enmity with blood of man.
—William Shakespeare, *Hamlet*

Or have we eaten on the insane root that takes the reason prisoner?
—William Shakespeare, *Macbeth*

Ha, ha. Give me to drink mandragora.
—William Shakespeare, *Antony and Cleopatra*

A number of plants of the Solanaceae night-shade family contain the belladonna alkaloids atropine (hyoscyamine) and scopolamine (hyoscine), most concentrated in seeds and roots (Table 11–1, Figure 11–1).[1,2] One of these, *Datura stramonium*, grows throughout the United States and is widely used recreationally.

Pharmacology

Atropine and scopolamine are competitive inhibitors of cholinergic muscarinic receptors, located on tissues innervated by postganglionic cholinergic nerves. Except in extremely high doses they are ineffective at autonomic ganglia or the neuromuscular junction. Central nervous system (CNS) cholinergic transmission is mainly nicotinic in the spinal cord and both muscarinic and nicotinic in the brain.[3]

Selective antagonists have defined at least five muscarinic receptor subtypes. M_1 receptors are present in ganglia and secretory glands, M_2 receptors in myocardium and smooth muscle, and M_3 and M_4 receptors in secretory glands and smooth muscle; all five subtypes are present in the CNS. Muscarinic receptors interact with G-proteins. M_1, M_3, and M_5 receptors activate G_q, which stimulates phospholipase C. M_2 and M_4 receptors activate G_i and G_o, which inhibit adenyl cyclase and activate K^+ channels. In contrast to nicotinic receptors, which are ligand-gated ion channels activation of which produces a fast excitatory postsynaptic potential, muscarinic receptors produce slower responses that can be either excitatory or inhibitory.[3–5]

Table 11–1. Plants Containing Belladonna Alkaloids

Latin Name	Common Name	Toxin
Atropa belladonna	Belladonna, deadly nightshade	Atropine
Hyoscyamus niger	Henbane, black henbane	Atropine, scopolamine
Mandragora officinarum	Mandrake, Satan's apple	Atropine, scopolamine
Lycium halimifolium	Matrimony vine	Atropine
Lobelia inflata	Lobelia	Atropine, scopolamine, lobeline
Datura stramonium	Jimson weed, sacred	Atropine, scopolamine
	Datura, devil's weed, devil's apple, stink apple, loco weed, thorn apple, malpitte, green dragon	
Datura (or *Brugmansia*) *sauveolens*	Angel's trumpet	Atropine, scopolamine

In doses used clinically, atropine has little CNS action, and its peripheral effects are dose-related. Toxic doses cause CNS excitation, with restlessness, delirium, or hallucinations, followed by coma, respiratory failure, and circulatory collapse. By contrast, low doses of scopolamine—probably because it more readily crosses the blood–brain barrier—cause euphoria, drowsiness, amnesia, and non-rapid eye movement sleep. Higher doses (or sometimes low doses in the presence of pain) produce excitation.[3]

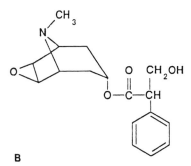

Figure 11-1. Atropine (A) and Scopolamine (B).

Historical Background and Epidemiology

Medicinal use of belladonna preparations dates back to ancient Hindu physicians. The ability of anticholinergic plants to induce hallucinations was recognized by the Egyptians and Greeks, who used them to foretell the future. In 38 AD, Mark Antony's troops ate *Datura* as they retreated from Parthia, resulting in delirium, stupor, and fatalities.[1] During the Middle Ages, anticholinergic plants were used by satanic cults to communicate with demons; participating "witches" used brooms as vaginal applicators.[6] The popularity of nightshade as a poison led Linnaeus to name the plant *Atropa belladonna*, after Atropos, the Fate who cuts the thread of life.[3,6a]

In 1676, bizarre behavior in the Jamestown colony was traced to ingestion of *Datura stramonium*, since then known as Jamestown or jimson weed. Thoreau described its use, and it has been suggested that Arthur Dimmesdale's symptoms in *The Scarlet Letter* were the result of atropine poisoning inflicted by Roger Chillingworth (a physician).[7] Today *Datura* species are used ritualistically by Amazonian natives in a beverage called *yage*, and they have been implicated in the creation of Haitian "zombies" rendered amnestic and submissive and used as slaves.[8] In South America (and sometimes in the United States) scopolamine and extracts from *Datura* or *Brugmansia* species are employed for less flamboyant criminal purposes; victims unwittingly ingest proffered candy or beverage, become docile, and are robbed with no later recollection of the circumstances.[9,10]

In the United States jimson weed and angel's trumpet became popular agents of abuse among adolescents during the 1960s, and widespread use has continued since then.[11–18] In the fall the plants' white trumpet-shaped flowers become thorny capsules filled with dark seeds, which weigh approximately 10 mg and contain 4% belladonna alkaloid.[1] Most often seeds are ingested; sometimes flowers are eaten, dried leaves are smoked, roots are chewed, or teas are drunk.[18a] Seeds, powders, teas, capsules, and "herbal cigarettes" are also available in "health food" stores, as is "Asthmador," an inhalant preparation cynically promoted as an asthma medication.[19,20] (In France antiasthmatic *Datura* cigarettes are marketed.[21,22]) Also abused in Midwestern and southeastern states is *Datura sauveolens* (angel's trumpet),[23,24] which caused intoxication in a 76-year-old man who ingested "moonflower" wine made from it.[25] Fourteen adolescents in Ohio became intoxicated after ingesting seeds or drinking teas made from seeds of *Datura inoxia*, also colloquially referred to as "moonflower."[25a] Different *Datura* species are popular in other countries, with reports from Belgium,[26] the Netherlands,[27] France,[28,29] Norway,[30] Germany,[31] Hungary,[32] Spain,[33] Poland,[34] Israel,[35] Australia,[36] Tunisia,[37] and Niger.[38] Henbane abuse has been reported in Germany and Turkey.[39,40]

Belladonna alkaloids are sometimes added to other street drugs or products.[41] Atropine poisoning affected two women who drank a commercial preparation of "burdock root tea"; burdocks do not themselves contain anticholinergic compounds.[42–44]

Anticholinergic poisoning has followed ingestion of Chinese herbal medicines (including *Panax ginseng*) adulterated with *Datura* species or *Mandragora officinarum*.[45,46] Toxic symptoms developed in a Brazilian woman who used toothpaste mixed with the leaves and flowers of *Datura* species: absorption was apparently mucosal.[47] Anticholinergic poisoning affected 15 people in Venezuela who ingested honey from wasp nests near *Datura* plants; two patients died from heatstroke.[48] A report from Sweden described seven people who developed sudden unilateral mydriasis after inadvertent ocular exposure to sap from angel's trumpet.[49]

During the mid-1990s poison centers in several eastern U.S. cities reported 370 cases of anticholinergic poisoning in heroin users whose drug mixture had been adulterated with scopolamine. In one-third the drugs were sniffed. Over half the patients presented with signs of heroin toxicity, but agitation and other typical anticholinergic signs emerged after naloxone was given.[50,51]

Anticholinergic poisoning has also been described in users of cocaine adulterated with either atropine or scopolamine.[52–54]

Less often abused are antiparkinsonian anticholinergics.[55–60] Of 21 trihexyphenidyl abusers from New Zealand, most were young and used additional drugs recreationally, but abuse is also well recognized among prisoners and among schizophrenics receiving anticholinergics for extrapyramidal symptoms, who sometimes escalate dosage when they discover the drug's euphorigenic properties.[58]

To what degree amitriptyline abuse is related to its anticholinergic properties—it also has dopaminergic actions—is uncertain, but amitriptyline overdose produces prominent anticholinergic symptoms and signs.[61,62] Anticholinergic toxicity occurred in users of cocaine adulterated with amitriptyline.[54] Many H_1-antihistamines have anticholinergic activity, and recreational use occurs.[63] Tripelennamine is abused parenterally in combination with pentazocine ("T's and blues") (see Chapter 3). Although phenothiazine neuroleptics have anticholinergic actions, they are not abused as street drugs. Scopolamine patches (Transderm) for motion sickness can cause disorientation, memory loss, restlessness, and hallucinations, but deliberate abuse of this product has not been reported.[64] Abuse of cyclopentolate eye drops ("Cyclogel")— instilled topically with absorption likely in the nasal mucosa—has been described in several patients.[65,66]

Acute Effects and Treatment

Datura contains more atropine than scopolamine, and so although scopolamine is chiefly responsible for the mental effects, systemic anticholinergic toxicity is a predictable accompaniment (Table 11–2).[67–71] Within 2 to 6 hours of seed ingestion there is euphoria and then, with sufficient dosage, excitement, delirium, or psychosis with hallucinations that are usually visual and often terrifying—for example, monsters, devils, or "buildings melting and pulsating";[23,72] insight as to their reality is often lost. (Although hallucinations are often a desired effect, they do not—in contrast to lysergic acid diethylamide (LSD) hallucinations— occur in the absence of excitement or delirium.) Vision is blurred; pupils are dilated and unreactive;

Table 11–2. Dose-related Effects of Atropine

Dose (mg)	Effects
0.5	Slight bradycardia; dryness of mouth; decreased sweating
1.0	Thirst; tachycardia; mild pupillary dilation
2.0	Tachycardia, palpitations; marked dryness of mouth; dilated pupils; blurring of near vision
5.0	All symptoms above marked; dysarthria; dysphagia; restlessness; fatigue; headache; dry, hot skin; difficulty with micturition; decreased intestinal peristalsis
10.0 or more	Above symptoms more marked; rapid, weak pulse; extreme mydriasis; very blurred vision; skin flushed, hot, dry; ataxia; delirium, hallucinations; coma

Source: Modified from Brown JH, Taylor P. Muscarinic receptor agonists and antagonists. In: Hardman JG, Limbird LE, eds. Goodman and Gilman's The Pharmacological Basis of Therapeutics, 9th edition. New York: McGraw Hill, 2001; 155, with permission of the publisher.

Table 11–3. Treatment of Anticholinergic Poisoning

Ipecac or gastric lavage
Activated charcoal, magnesium sulfate
Physostigmine, 0.5–3 mg intravenously every 30 min to 2 hours as needed
Aspirin, cooling blanket, ice bags, alcohol sponges, or bypass cooling
Bladder catheterization
Cardiac, respiratory, and blood pressure monitoring
Diazepam and phenytoin for seizures
Avoid neuroleptics

and there is dysphagia, urinary retention, dry flushed skin, high fever, hypertension, tachypnea, and tachycardia.[9,72–75] Agitation may alternate with relative calm. The most prominent signs have been summarized as, "hot as a hare, red as a beet, dry as a bone, blind as a bat, and mad as a hatter."

Sometimes seen are nystagmus, hyperreflexia, Babinski signs, extensor posturing, myoclonus, grand mal seizures, coma, circulatory collapse, respiratory failure, and death.[73,76,77] Delusions and hallucinations can lead to fatal accidents.[72] In a report of 10 cases of "angel's trumpet psychosis," flaccid paralysis was reported in subjects ingesting more than six flowers—enough to deliver at least 1.2 mg of atropine and 3.9 mg of scopolamine; in one case death was attributed to drowning after falling paralyzed into a puddle 3 inches deep.[23] The electroencephalogram shows diffuse slowing and paroxysmal sharp forms.[74] Hallucinations may be most prominent during recovery. Symptoms last hours to days, and survivors are unlikely to have neurological residua, although pupillary dilation can outlast other symptoms by days.[14,17,72,73]

Anticholinergic poisoning is seldom directly fatal, but lethality varies markedly among individuals. Survival has followed 500 mg of scopolamine and 1000 mg of atropine, yet children have died

after less than 10 mg of either drug. Alarming idiosyncratic reactions are more common with scopolamine.[3]

Belladonna alkaloids are not detected by routine drug screens, but they can be identified in urine using gas chromatography–mass spectrometry.[78]

The diagnosis of anticholinergic poisoning can be confirmed by giving an intramuscular injection of 1.0 mg physostigmine; a patient intoxicated by anticholinergics fails to develop salivation, sweating, or intestinal hyperactivity, and symptoms may improve within minutes.[3] Treatment then follows (Table 11–3): Ipecac or gastric lavage are employed even if ingestion occurred hours earlier—anticholinergics slow gastrointestinal motility. Activated charcoal and magnesium sulfate are then given. Physostigmine is used in patients with seizures, high fever, severe hypertension, severe agitation or hallucinations, coma, or life-threatening arrhythmias.[1] The dose is 0.5–3 mg, given intravenously over 2 minutes and repeated as needed every 30 minutes to 2 hours; it is metabolized much more rapidly than atropine or scopolamine and so may have to be repeated, in severe cases for 18 hours or more.[30] Physostigmine should not be used in mildly symptomatic patients, as it can itself precipitate seizures or cardiac arrhythmia.[76] Fever may require aspirin, a cooling blanket, ice bags, alcohol sponges, or bypass cooling. The bladder is catheterized, and fluids are given. Seizures are treated as necessary with diazepam and phenytoin.[1] Phenothiazines, because of their anticholinergic activity, are contraindicated, and sedatives should be used cautiously.[72,73]

Tricyclic antidepressant poisoning causes additional problems, notably hypotension, heart block, bradydysrhythmia, ventricular dysrhythmia, or asystole. Seizures and coma are common, and sodium bicarbonate is given if the electrocardiogram shows a QRS duration of more than 100 milliseconds or a terminal right axis deviation of more than 120 degrees.[78a]

Long-Term Effects

Few anticholinergic abusers take the drug on a daily basis. When they do, they develop tolerance to anticholinergic effects (including euphoria and sedation) and signs of physical dependence. A schizophrenic man who had formerly abused trihexyphenidyl began taking diphenhydramine (in over-the-counter Sominex) and gradually escalated the dose to 1600 mg daily; with abstinence he developed irritability, increased blinking, increased defecation, and craving.[63] A woman who abused cyclopentolate eye drops had withdrawal nausea, vomiting, weakness, and tremor.[66]

Chronic scopolamine administration increases the number of muscarinic receptors in the hippocampus of rats.[79] Animals fed *Datura stramonium* for several weeks had weight loss, decreased serum albumin and calcium levels, and increased blood urea nitrogen and alkaline phosphatase levels.[80] *Datura stramonium* also contains γ-L-glutamyl-L-aspartate, which inhibits glutamate binding in mouse hippocampus and impairs learning.[81] Rats chronically given *Datura* seeds also have decreased brain content of protein, DNA, and RNA.[82] The relevance of these observations to human use is unknown.

References

1. Shih RD, Goldfrank LR. Plants. In: Goldfrank LR, Flomenbaum NE, Lewin NA, et al., eds. Toxicologic Emergencies, 6th edition. Stamford, CT: Appleton & Lange, 1998; 1243.
2. Hung OL, Lewin NA, Howland MA. Herbal preparations. In: Goldfrank LR, Flomenbaum NE, Lewin NA, et al., eds. Toxicologic Emergencies, 6th edition. Stamford, CT: Appleton & Lange, 1998; 1221.
3. Brown JH, Taylor P. Muscarinic receptor agonists and antagonists. In: Hardman JG, Limbird LE, eds. Goodman and Gilman's The Pharmacological Basis of Therapeutics, 10th edition. New York: McGraw-Hill, 2001; 155.
4. Caulfield MP. Muscarinic receptors—characterization, coupling, and function. Pharmacol Ther 1993; 58:319.
5. Siegelbaum SA, Schwartz JH, Kandel ER. Modulation of synaptic transmission: second messengers. In: Kandel ER, Schwartz JH, Jessell TM, eds. Principles of Neural Science, 4th edition. New York: McGraw-Hill, 2000; 229.
6. Siegel RK. The natural history of hallucinogens. In: Jacobs BL, ed. Hallucinogens: Neurochemical, Behavioral, and Clinical Perspectives. New York: Raven Press, 1984:1.
6a. Holzman RS. The legacy of Atropos, the fate who cut the thread of life. Anesthesiology 1998; 89:241.
7. Khan JA. Atropine poisoning in Hawthorne's *The Scarlet Letter.* N Engl J Med 1984; 311:414.
8. Davis W. Passage to the Darkness. The Ethnobiology of the Haitian Zombie. Chapel Hill, NC: University of North Carolina Press, 1988.
9. Brizer DA, Manning DW. Delirium induced by poisoning with anticholinergic agents. Am J Psychiatry 1982; 139:1343.
10. Ardila A, Moreno C. Scopolamine intoxication as a model of transient global amnesia. Brain Cogn 1991; 15:236.
11. Keeler MH, Kane FJ. The use of hyoscyamine as a hallucinogen and intoxicant. Am J Psychiatry 1967; 124:852.
12. Muller DJ. Unpublicized hallucinogens. JAMA 1967; 202:650.
13. Gabel MC. Purposeful ingestion of belladonna for hallucinatory effects. J Pediatr 1968; 72:864.
14. Cummins BM, Obetz SW, Wilson MR. Belladonna poisoning as a facet of psychedelia. JAMA 1968; 204:1011.
15. Teitelbaum DT. Stramonium poisoning in "teenyboppers." Ann Intern Med 1968; 68:174.
16. DeYoung C, Cross EG. Stramonium psychedelia. Can Anaesth Soc J 1969; 16:429.
17. Levy R. Jimson seed poisoning: a new hallucinogen on the horizon. J Am Coll Emerg Physic 1977; 6:58.
18. Mahler DA. The jimson-weed high. JAMA 1975; 231:138.
18a. Greene JS, Patterson SG, Warner E. Ingestion of angel's trumpet: an increasingly common source of toxicity. South Med J 1996; 89:365.
19. Siegel RK. Herbal intoxication. Psychoactive effects from herbal cigarettes, tea, and capsules. JAMA 1976; 236:473.
20. Jacobs KW. Asthmador: a legal hallucinogen. Int J Addict 1974; 9:503.
21. Ballantyne A, Lippiett D, Park J. Herbal cigarettes for kicks. BMJ 1976; II:1539.
22. Larcan A. Conduites toxicomaniaques utilisant des cigarettes antiasthmatiques à base de *Datura.* Bull Acad Natl Med 1984; 168:455.
23. Hall RCW, Popkin MK, McHenry LE. Angel's trumpet psychosis: a central nervous system anticholinergic syndrome. Am J Psychiatry 1977; 134:312.

24. Hayman J. *Datura* poisoning: the Angel's Trumpet. Pathology 1985; 17:465.

25. Smith EA, Meloan CE, Pickell JA, Oehme FW. Scopolamine poisoning from home made "moon flower" wine. J Anal Toxicol 1991; 15:216.

25a. Goetz R, Siegel E, Scaglione J. Suspected moonflower intoxication-Ohio 2002. MMWR 2003; 52:788.

26. Coremans P, Lambrecht G, Schepens P, et al. Anticholinergic intoxication with commercially available thorn apple tea. J Toxicol Clin Toxicol 1994; 32:589.

27. Koevoets PF, van Harten PN. Thorn apple poisoning. Ned Tijdschr Geneeskd 1997; 141:888.

28. Strobel M, Chevalier J, DeLavarelle B. Coma febrile avec polynucleose du à une intoxication par *Datura stramonium*. Presse Med 1991; 20:2214.

29. Birmes P, Chounet V, Mazerolles M, et al. Self-poisoning with *Datura stramonium*. 3 case reports. Presse Med 2002; 31:69.

30. Amlo H, Haugeng KL, Wickstrom E, et al. Poisoning with Jimson weed. Five cases treated with physostigmine. Tidsskr Norsk Laegeforen 1997; 117:2610.

31. Mobus U, Felscher D, Schulz K. Nightshade plants act almost like LSD. Poisoning cases are on the rise. MMW Fortschr Med 1999; 141:46.

32. Osvath P, Nagy A, Fekete S, et al. A case of *Datura stramonium* poisoning—general problems of differential diagnosis. Orvosi Hetil 2000; 141:133.

33. Castanon Lopez L, Martinez Badas JP, Lapena Lopez DA, et al. *Datura stramonium* poisoning. Anal Esp Pediatr 2000; 53:53.

34. Groszek B, Gawlikowski T, Szkolnicka B. Self-poisoning with *Datura stramonium*. Przeglad Lakarski 2000; 57:577.

35. Kurzbaum A, Simsolo C, Kvasha L, et al. Toxic delirium due to *Datura stramonium*. Isr Med Assoc J 2001; 3:538.

36. Francis PD, Clarke CF. Angel trumpet lily poisoning in five adolescents: clinical findings and management. J Pediatr Child Health 1999; 35:93.

37. Thabet H, Brahmi N, Amomou M, et al. *Datura stramonium* poisonings in humans. Vet Hum Toxicol 1999; 41:320.

38. Djibo A, Boouzou SB. Acute intoxication with "sobi-lobi" (*Datura*). Four cases in Níger. Bull Soc Pathol Exot 2000; 93:294.

39. Betz P, Janzen J, Roider G, Penning R. Psychopathologische Befunde nach oraler Aufnahme von Inhaltsstoffen heimischer Nachtschattengewachse. Arch Kriminol 1991; 188:175.

40. Tugrul L. Abuse of henbane by children in Turkey. Bull Narc 1985; 37:75.

41. Harrison G. The abuse of anticholinergic drugs by adolescents. Br J Psychiatry 1980; 137:495.

42. Bryson PD, Watanabe AS, Rumack BH, Murphy RC. Burdock root tea poisoning. Case report involving a commercial preparation. JAMA 1978; 239:2157.

43. Bryson PD. Burdock root poisoning. JAMA 1978; 240:1586.

44. Rhoads PM, Tong TG, Banner W, Anderson R. Anticholinergic poisonings associated with commercial burdock. J Toxicol Clin Toxicol 1984–1985; 22:581.

45. But PP. Herbal poisoning caused by adulterants or erroneous substitutes. J Trop Med Hyg 1994; 97:371.

46. Chan TY. Anticholinergic poisoning due to Chinese herbal medicines. Vet Hum Toxicol 1995; 37:156.

47. Pereira CA, Nishioka SD. Poisoning by the use of *Datura* leaves in a homemade toothpaste. J Toxicol Clin Toxicol 1994; 32:329.

48. Ramirez M, Rivera E, Ereu C. Fifteen cases of atropine poisoning after honey ingestion. Vet Hum Toxicol 1999; 41:19.

49. Havelius U, Asman P. Accidental mydriasis from exposure to Angel's trumpet (*Datura sauveolens*) Acta Ophthalmol Scand 2002; 80:332.

50. Perrone J, Shaw L, DeRoos F. Laboratory confirmation of scopolamine co-intoxication in patients using tainted heroin. J Toxicol Clin Toxicol 1999; 37:491.

51. Hamilton RJ, Perrone J, Hoffman R, et al. A descriptive study of an epidemic of poisoning caused by heroin adulterated with scopolamine. J Toxicol Clin Toxicol 2000; 38:597.

52. Quandt CM, Sommi RW, Pipkin T, et al. Differentiation of cocaine toxicity. Role of the toxicology drug screen. Drug Intell Clin Pharm 1988; 22:582.

53. Nogue S, Sanz P, Munne P. Acute scopolamine poisoning after sniffing adulterated cocaine. Drug Alcohol Depend 1991; 27:115.

54. Weiner AL, Bayer MJ, McKay CA, et al. Anticholinergic poisoning with adulterated intranasal cocaine. Am J Emerg Med 1998; 16:517.

55. Pakes GE. Abuse of trihexyphenidyl. JAMA 1978; 240:2434.

56. Goggin DA, Solomon GF. Trihexyphenidyl abuse for euphorigenic effect. Am J Psychiatry 1979; 136:459.

57. Kaminer Y, Munitz H, Wijsenbeck H. Trihexyphenidyl (Artane) abuse: euphoriant and anxiolytic. Br J Psychiatry 1982; 140:473.

58. McInnis M, Petursson H. Trihexyphenidyl dependence. Acta Psychiatr Scand 1984; 69:538.

59. Crawshaw JA, Mullen PE. A study of benzhexol abuse. Br J Psychiatry 1984; 145:300

60. Wells BG, Marken PA, Rickman LA, et al. Characterizing anticholinergic abuse in community mental health. J Clin Psychopharmacol 1989; 9:431.

61. Cohen MJ, Hanbury R, Stimmell B. Abuse of amitriptyline. JAMA 1978; 240:1372.

62. Callahan M, Kassel D. Epidemiology of fatal tricyclic antidepressant ingestion: implications for management. Ann Emerg Med 1985; 14:1.

63. Feldman MD, Behar M. A case of massive diphenhydramine abuse and withdrawal from use of the drug. JAMA 1986; 225:3119.

64. Johnson P, Hansen D, Matarazzo D, et al. Transderm Scop patches for prevention of motion sickness. N Engl J Med 1984; 311:468.

65. Ostler HB. Cycloplegics and mydriatics: tolerance, habituation, and addiction to topical administration. J Paediatr Child Health 1990; 26:106.

66. Sato EH, deFreitas D, Foster CS. Abuse of cyclopentolate hydrochloride (Cyclogyl) drops. N Engl J Med 1992; 326:1363.

67. Arena JM. Atropine poisoning: a report of two cases from jimson weed. Clin Pediatr 1963; 2:182.

68. Farnsworth NR. Hallucinogenic plants. Science 1968; 162:1086.

69. Dewitt MS, Swain R, Gibson LPB. The dangers of jimson weed and its abuse by teenagers in the Kanawha Valley of West Virginia. West Virginia Med J 1997; 93:182.

70. Sopchak CA, Stork CM, Cantor RM, et al. Central anticholinergic syndrome due to Jimson weed. Physostigmine therapy revisited? J Toxicol Clin Toxicol 1998; 36:43.

71. Fussell K, Kirjis JN. A 21-year-old man with mental status changes. Tenn Med 1998; 91:151.

72. Gowdy JM. Stramonium intoxication. Review of symptomatology in 112 cases. JAMA 1972; 221:585.

73. Mikolich JR, Paulson GW, Cross CJ. Acute anticholinergic syndrome due to jimson seed ingestion. Ann Intern Med 1975; 83:321.

74. Mikolich JR, Paulson GW, Cross CJ, Calhoun R. Neurologic and electroencephalographic effects of jimsonweed intoxication. Clin Electroencephalogr 1976; 7:49.

75. Klein-Schwartz W, Oderda GM. Jimsonweed intoxication in adolescents and young adults. Am J Dis Child 1984; 138:737.

76. Oberndorfer S, Grisold W, Hinterholzer G, et al. Coma with focal neurological signs caused by *Datura stramonium* intoxication in a young man. J Neurol Neurosurg Psychiatry 2002; 73:458.

77. Giuhelli D, Contri L, Bott A, et al. Atropine poisoning: importance of the clinical diagnosis. Minerva Anestesiol 1998; 64:567.

78. Nogue S, Pujol L, Sanz P, et al. *Datura stramonium* poisoning. Identification of tropane alkaloids in urine by gas chromatography–mass spectrometry. J Int Med Res 1995; 23:132.

78a. Glauser J. Tricyclic antidepressant poisoning. Cleveland Clin J Med 2000; 67:709.

79. Ben-Barak J, Dudai Y. Scopolamine induces an increase in muscarinic receptor level in rat hippocampus. Brain Res 1980; 193:309.

80. Dugan GM, Gumbmann MR, Friedman M. Toxicological evaluation of jimson weed (*Datura stramonium*) seed. Food Chem Toxicol 1989; 27:501.

81. Ungerer A, Schmitz-Bourgeois M, Melan C, et al. Gamma-L-glutamyl-L-aspartate induces specific deficits in long-term memory and inhibits [³H]glutamate binding on hippocampal membranes. Brain Res 1988; 446:205.

82. Hasan SS, Kushwaha AK. Chronic effect of *Datura* (seed) extract on the brain of albino rats. Jpn J Pharmacol 1987; 44:1.

Chapter 12
Ethanol

Drink wine, not tears—the sage has said,
"Wine is the antidote for sorrow's poison."
—The Ruba'iat of Omar Khayyam

Oh! John Barleycorn is a wizard dopester. Brain and body, scorched and jangled
and poisoned, return to be tuned up by the very poison that caused the damage.
—Jack London

What must become of an infant who is conceived in gin with a poisonous distillation
of which it is nourished both in the womb and at the breast?
—Henry Fielding

History and Epidemiology

In metabolizing sugar to produce energy, yeast creates ethanol as a by-product. Tens of thousands of years ago paleolithic people began ingesting meads or wines made from the natural fermentation of honey, dates, or sap. With the development of agriculture in Eastern Turkey, Mesopotamia, and Egypt, beers were made from fermented barley and wheat, and wines were made from grapes cultivated for high sugar content. During the next several thousand years the scarcity of pure uncontaminated water—especially in urban centers—led to the widespread use of beer and wine as safe substitutes. Hippocrates remarked on the danger of drinking water other than from springs or deep wells, and during the Middle Ages alcohol became known as aqua vitae—the water of life.[1,2,2a] (In Asia the use of alcoholic beverages was less widespread, for the practice of boiling water allowed non-alcoholic teas as an alternative. Another disincentive to drinking ethanol was, and is, the genetic inability of many Japanese and Chinese to completely metabolize ethanol (see later).

Yeasts produce ethanol concentrations of only about 16%. Around 700 AD Arab alchemists took advantage of the different boiling points of ethanol and water (78°C vs. 100°C) to invent distillation. (In fact, the word "alcohol" is derived from the Arabic "al kohl," referring to a material's basic essence.) The result was distilled spirits of high ethanol content, the use of which spread across Europe after 1100 AD.[1,2] (Today 6 oz. of wine, 12 oz. of beer, and 1.5 oz. of 90 proof spirits contains roughly 12 g of ethanol.)

During the past three centuries in both Europe and the United States periods of heavy ethanol use have alternated with eras of temperance. The London "gin epidemic" of 1710–1750, vividly depicted in the engravings of William Hogarth, led physicians at the College of Physicians of London to express fear that parental use of ethanol caused brain damage in offspring.[3,4] In the United States during the 1790s the average annual consumption of ethanol in equivalent gallons per adult was 5.8 gallons; it was during this period that Dr. Benjamin Rush wrote "An Inquiry into the Effects of Ardent Spirits upon the Human Mind and Body," advocating abstinence from distilled spirits while acknowledging the beneficial effects of beer and wine. By 1830 average annual American consumption had risen to 7.1 gallons; two decades later, amidst a spreading temperance movement, it had fallen to 2.1 gallons. Except for brief surges during the 1860s and the first decade of the 20th century, it remained at that level until World War I. During this period a number of states, responding to pressure from groups such as the Women's Christian Temperance Union, adopted legal prohibition, but such statutes were often overturned by the courts. The emergence of the Anti-Saloon League in the early 20th century, however, ultimately led to national Prohibition in the form of the 18th Amendment to the Constitution. Although overall a colossal societal fiasco, Prohibition did result in a fall in average ethanol consumption to 0.9 gallons and a drop in the incidence of liver cirrhosis to half its 1907 peak. Following repeal of Prohibition in 1933 average annual consumption of ethanol rose gradually over the next 50 years, peaking at 2.76 gallons in 1980. During the 1980s a new temperance movement arose; Mothers Against Drunk Driving (MADD) was founded, every state raised the drinking age to 21 years, and warning labels appeared on alcoholic beverages. Since 1980 ethanol use has steadily fallen, especially the consumption of distilled spirits.[5,6] A 1992 study found that 44% of U.S. adults were current drinkers, 22% were former drinkers, and 34% were lifetime abstainers.[7]

Nonetheless, ethanol still causes more than 100,000 American deaths annually, amounting to nearly 5% of total mortality.[6,8–11] The downward trend in American ethanol consumption holds for whites but not for African-Americans or Hispanics.[12] Moreover, from 1985 to 2000 ethanol use by American adolescents did not change. The average age of beginning ethanol use is now 12 years; in 1998, 74% of high school seniors and 44% of eighth graders reported using ethanol during the past year, and one-third of high school seniors reported being drunk in the preceding month. Adolescents who begin drinking before age 15 years are 4 times as likely to develop alcoholism than those beginning after age 21 years (40% vs. 10%).[13]

A 1994 National Alcohol Survey found that the influence of drinking ethanol on mortality displays a J-shaped association for men but an insignificant relation for women. Light-to-moderate male drinkers had lower mortality than abstainers, consistent with physicians' impressions since Hippocrates as well as with other surveys.[14,15] Within this group, however, pattern of drinking was important; light-to-moderate drinkers who reported occasionally heavy drinking had higher mortality risks.[14]

In 1990, the cost of ethanol-related problems in the United States—including illness and lost productivity—was estimated at US$136 billion.[8–11] A decade later the figure was US$185 billion.[16] Mortality estimates, from the Centers for Disease Control, are based on the relative risk alcohol carries for diseases such as esophageal cancer, cirrhosis, pancreatitis, and stroke, and for automobile accidents, homicide, and suicide (Tables 12–1, 12–2). Each death represents, on average, 26 "years of potential life lost."[10]

How many Americans are alcoholics? According to the National Institute on Alcoholism and Alcohol Abuse, the answer is 10.4 million: 7.1 million men and 3.3 million women.[17] Such figures are both logistically and definitionally problematic. Screening questionnaires[18,19] tend to underestimate use, and most so-called laboratory markers are both insensitive and nonspecific (Table 12–3).[20–32] (There is evidence that blood levels of carbohydrate-deficient transferrin and γ-glutamyl transferase do reflect drinking intensity, although not drinking frequency.[32a]) Moreover, there is no consensus on what constitutes *alcoholism*. The term usually refers to a pattern of drinking, either episodic or continuous, that interferes with health, work, home, or social functioning. Americans who drink occupy a continuum of severity from infrequent to obsessive, and no point clearly separates alcoholics from nonalcoholics. The term *problem drinker* includes both ethanol addicts—that is, psychologically dependent but not necessarily physically dependent—and those who, even if abstinent most of the time, get into trouble when they drink (e.g., impaired job performance or arrests). The American Psychiatric Association's Diagnostic and Statistical Manual (DSM-IV) defines *alcohol abuse* in terms of impaired occupational or social functioning and *alcohol dependence* in terms of such impairment plus evidence of tolerance or withdrawal symptoms (see Chapter 1).[33]

It is estimated that 19 million Americans 18 years of age or older—or 7% of American adults and

Table 12–1. Centers for Disease Control Estimates of Alcohol-attributable Fractions, Total Estimated Mortality, and Estimated Alcohol-related Mortality, by Sex and Diagnosis—United States, 1987

Diagnosis	AAFs	MALE		FEMALE	
		Deaths	ARM	Deaths	ARM
Malignant neoplasms					
Cancer of the lip/oral cavity/pharynx	0.50	5259	2630	2622	1049
Cancer of the esophagus	0.75	6705	5029	2365	1774
Cancer of the stomach	0.20	8178	1636	5428	1086
Cancer of liver/intrahepatic bile ducts	0.15	4215	632	2831	425
Cancer of the larynx	0.50	2968	1484	690	276
Mental disorders					
Alcoholic psychoses	1.00	302	302	80	80
Alcohol dependence syndrome	1.00	3353	3353	908	908
Alcohol abuse	1.00	537	537	136	136
Cardiovascular disease					
Essential hypertension	0.08	1663	126	2368	180
Alcoholic cardiomyopathy	1.00	688	688	109	109
Cerebrovascular disease	0.07	58,302	3790	90,068	5854
Respiratory diseases					
Respiratory tuberculosis	0.25	911	228	396	99
Pneumonia and influenza	0.05	32,379	1619	34,852	1743
Digestive diseases					
Diseases of esophagus/stomach/duodenum	0.10	4545	455	4520	452
Alcoholic gastritis	1.00	60	60	13	13
Alcoholic fatty liver	1.00	672	672	242	242
Acute alcoholic hepatitis	1.00	518	518	276	276
Alcoholic cirrhosis of the liver	1.00	5517	5517	1991	1991
Alcoholic liver damage, unspecified	1.00	1514	1514	535	535
Other cirrhosis of the liver	0.50	7508	3754	5097	2549
Acute pancreatitis	0.42	1117	469	1005	422
Chronic pancreatitis	0.60	121	73	74	44
Unintentional injuries					
Motor vehicle accidents	0.42	33,904	14,240	14,386	6042
Other road vehicle accidents	0.20	159	32	72	14
Water transport accidents	0.20	853	171	95	19
Air/space transport accidents	0.16	1032	165	231	37
Alcohol poisonings	1.00	151	151	37	37
Accidental falls	0.35	6091	2132	5485	1920
Accidents caused by fires	0.45	2863	1288	1847	831
Accidental drownings	0.38	3529	1341	831	316
Other injuries	0.25	4469	1117	1410	353
Intentional injuries					
Suicide	0.28	24,073	6740	6472	1812
Homicide	0.46	15,007	6903	4792	2204
Metabolic disorder					
Diabetes mellitus	0.05	15,795	790	21,959	1098
Other alcohol-related diagnoses					
Alcoholic polyneuropathy	1.00	4	4	0	0
Excess blood alcohol level	1.00	9	9	2	2
Total			70,168		34,927

AAFs, Alcohol-attributable fractions; ARM, alcohol-related mortality.

Source: Modified from Alcohol-related mortality and years of potential life lost—United States, 1987. MMWR 1990; 39:173.

Table 12–2. Centers for Disease Control Estimates of Alcohol-related Mortality and Male to Female Ratio, by Sex and Diagnostic Category—United States, 1987

Diagnostic Category Deaths (%)	Male Deaths (%)		Female Deaths (%)		Total	
Malignant neoplasms	11,410	(16.3)	4609	(13.2)	16,019	(15.2)
Mental disorders	4192	(6.0)	1124	(3.2)	5316	(5.1)
Cardiovascular diseases	4604	(6.6)	6143	(17.6)	10,747	(10.2)
Respiratory diseases	1847	(2.6)	1842	(5.3)	3688	(3.5)
Digestive diseases	13,032	(18.6)	6524	(18.7)	19,556	(18.7)
Unintentional injuries	20,637	(29.4)	9569	(27.4)	30,205	(28.7)
Intentional injuries	13,644	(19.4)	4016	(11.5)	17,660	(16.8)
Other alcohol-related diagnoses	803	(1.1)	1100	(3.1)	1903	(1.8)
Total	70,160	(100.0)	34,927	(100.0)	105,094	(100.0)

Source: Modified from Alcohol-related mortality and years of potential life lost—United States, 1987. MMWR 1990; 39:173.

19% of American adolescents—are problem drinkers.[9] Applying DSM criteria, estimates of lifetime prevalence for ethanol abuse and dependence in the United States range from 13.7% to 23.5%.[7] In one study, lifetime prevalence for ethanol dependence was 20.1% in men and 8.2% in women.[34] A 1988 survey in Wisconsin revealed that 25% of adults were binge drinkers (five or more drinks at least once during the previous month), 8.6% consumed more than 60 drinks per month, and 6.2% had recently driven while intoxicated.[35] A national telephone survey of U.S. adults aged 18 years or older estimated that between 1993 and 2001 the number of binge-drinking episodes per year increased by 17% (from 6.3% to 7.4%); rates of binge-drinking were highest among subjects aged 18 to 25 years, yet two-thirds of binge-drinkers were aged 25 years or older.[36] A survey of U.S. college students found

Table 12–3. Laboratory Tests to Identify Alcoholics

Acetaldehyde binding to erythrocytes[20]
Transferrin carbohydrate content (Carbohydrate-deficient transferrin, DCT)[21,32,32a]
Gamma-glutamyl transferase levels[22]
Platelet monoamine oxidase levels[23]
Plasma dopamine beta-hydroxylase levels[23]
Erythrocyte and skeletal muscle Na,K-ATPase activity[24]
Blood dolichol concentration[25]
Serum beta-hexosaminidase levels[26]
Serum methanol levels[27]
Plasma carnitine levels[28]
Auditory evoked potentials[30]

that 40% had a binge-drinking episode within the prior 2 weeks.[37] So-called skid row alcoholics constitute fewer than 5% of problem drinkers, the great majority of whom are middle-class blue-collar or white-collar workers or housewives.[38] Estimated lifetime rates of ethanol abuse among American physicians range from 4% to 14%.[39,40]

Information from several national data sets led to an assertion that underage drinkers (12 to 20 years) account for 20% of the total ethanol consumed in the United States and that adult excessive drinkers account for 30%.[41] This report has been challenged on methodological grounds, including the definition of "excessive" as more than 2 drinks per day for men and one drink per day for women.[16,42]

At Harlem Hospital Center in New York City, 47% of 118 patients consecutively admitted to the general medical service were deemed alcoholic.[43] At the Johns Hopkins Hospital in Baltimore, alcoholism was diagnosed in 25% of inpatients from the Medicine Service, 30% from Psychiatry, 19% from Neurology, 12.5% from Obstetrics/Gynecology, and 23% from Surgery.[44] Twelve percent of American health care expenditure for adults is for alcohol abuse.[35] (Relevant to such figures is that the great majority of alcoholics are also heavy smokers.[45,46])

Ethanol consumption in several European countries, especially Ireland, France, and Germany, exceeds that in the United States. In the United Kingdom and Denmark wine consumption by children less than 16 years of age doubled between 1993 and 2003.[46a]

$$CH_3CH_2OH + NAD \xrightarrow{\quad\text{alcohol}\quad\atop\text{dehdrogenase}} CH_3CHO + NADH + H^+$$

ethanol   acetaldehyde

$$CH_3CHO + NAD + H_2O \xrightarrow{\quad\text{aldehyde}\quad\atop\text{dehydrogenase}} CH_3COO^- + NADH + 2H^+$$

acetaldehyde   acetate

Figure 12–1. Metabolism of ethanol.

Ethanol Metabolism

Ingested ethanol is metabolized by more than one route.[47,48] Ninety percent is oxidized in the liver to acetaldehyde by cytosolic alcohol dehydrogenase (ADH). The enzymatic cofactor, nicotinamide adenine dinucleotide (NAD), is thereby reduced to NADH (Figure 12–1). ADH ordinarily acts on a variety of substrates, probably including steroids and fatty acids. Ethanol is also oxidized by a microsomal ethanol-oxidizing system (MEOS), which is induced by sustained ethanol ingestion. A third route of ethanol metabolism is by peroxisomal catalase. Very small amounts of ingested ethanol are excreted unchanged in the urine or through the lungs. ("Alcohol breath" is actually the odor of isoamylacetate, ethyl acetate, and other congeners present in different alcoholic beverages.[49])

In each of these three pathways ethanol is oxidized to acetaldehyde, which is then oxidized to acetate and then to acetyl-CoA by NAD-dependent aldehyde dehydrogenase (ALDH), present in liver mitochondria. Following ingestion of 14C-labeled ethanol, the tracer appears in cholesterol, glycerol, and fatty acids.

These biochemical reactions explain a number of ethanol's effects. Hydrogen equivalents produced by ethanol oxidation enter mitochondria and bypass the tricarboxylic acid cycle; fatty acid oxidation is thereby slowed, and much of the carbon skeleton of ethanol is incorporated into fatty acids via acetyl-CoA. The result is hepatic lipid accumulation. Depending on the amount and pattern of drinking, ethanol also affects body weight. One gram of ethanol releases 7 kcal of energy. Light to moderate amounts of ethanol, metabolized by ADH, reduce lipid oxidation and increase fatty acid synthesis,

favoring lipid storage and weight gain. Heavy ethanol intake stimulates the MEOS system, which generates only heat with consequent weight loss.[50,51] Other effects of ethanol are a consequence of shifts in the ratio of NAD to NADH. An increased NADH to NAD ratio slows metabolism of phosphoenolpyruvate to dihydroacetate and glucose-6-phosphate and of the latter to glycogen, preventing gluconeogenesis and setting the stage for hypoglycemia (Table 12–4).[52] An elevated NADH to NAD ratio also interferes with the conversion of lactate to pyruvate, contributing to metabolic acidosis.

The major enzyme of the MEOS system is a unique ethanol-inducible cytochrome, P4502E1 (also called CYP2E1), induction of which contributes to metabolic tolerance to ethanol as well as to other drugs, including barbiturates and benzodiazepines.[47,52,53] CYP2E1 also catalyzes fatty acid hydroxylations, contributing to lipid accumulation, and it converts a number of xenobiotics—including industrial solvents, volatile anesthetics, acetaminophen, isoniazid, and cocaine—to toxic metabolites.

Each of ethanol's three metabolic pathways potentially produces free radicals which stress antioxidant systems. Ethanol, hyperlacticacidemia,

Table 12–4. Contributions to Alcoholic Hypoglycemia

Starvation
Depletion of liver glycogen
Reduced NAD/NADH ratio, limiting gluconeogenesis
Reduced breakdown of fatty acids to acetyl-CoA, further limiting gluconeogenesis
Blunted response to growth hormone

Source: Lieber CS. Medical and Nutritional Complications of Alcoholism: Mechanisms and Management. New York, Plenum Press, 1992.

and elevated NADH each increase xanthine oxidase activity and the production of superoxide. CYP2E1 aggravates oxidative stress by generating reactive oxygen species and by impairing defense systems such as glutathione; lipid peroxidation and superoxide production correlate with the amount of CYP2E1 induced.[54,55] Catalase generates hydrogen peroxide.

Lowered NAD levels slow the oxidation of acetaldehyde, a more potent toxin than ethanol. In addition to interfering with tissue metabolism, including heart, liver, and brain, acetaldehyde might contribute to ethanol tolerance, dependence, and withdrawal. Some rats self-administer acetaldehyde but not ethanol intraventricularly,[56] and mice develop physical dependence to acetaldehyde, with ethanol and acetaldehyde each attenuating the other's withdrawal signs.[57] Although ethanol rarely produces pharmacologically significant blood acetaldehyde levels in naïve animals or humans, acetaldehyde accumulates in the brains of chronic drinkers, and higher blood levels are found in alcoholics.[58]

Acetaldehyde might have indirect effects by causing central nervous system (CNS) accumulation of a family of compounds called tetrahydroisoquinolines (TIQ). These are of two types. Alkyl-substituted TIQs form by condensation of acetaldehyde with norepinephrine to form 4,6,7-trihydroxy-TIQ or with dopamine to form salsolinol.[59] Benzyl-substituted TIQs form by condensation of catecholamines with certain of their own metabolites, present in abnormally high amounts because of competition by acetaldehyde for ALDH. For example, dopamine condenses with phenacetaldehyde to form tetrahydropapaveroline (THP). Acetaldehyde also condenses with indoles to form beta-carboline adducts. TIQs are precursors to morphine in the poppy, and they bind to opioid receptors in the brain. In animals, direct injection of acetaldehyde, TIQs, or beta-carbolines into brain produces addictive-like preference for ethanol, and this behavior is attenuated by naloxone or naltrexone.[60,61] The clinical relevance of these observations is uncertain; as noted below, ethanol itself interacts with opiate receptors and endorphins.

Neurobiology of Ethanol

Ethanol affects a large number of neurotransmitter and second messenger systems (Table 12–5), and a

Table 12–5. Neurochemical Effects of Ethanol

Glutamate:	Acutely inhibits NMDA receptor activation; modulates gene expression of NMDA receptors
γ-aminobutyric acid (GABA)	Acutely enhances GABA ionotropic receptor function and $GABA_B$ metabotropic function
Serotonin (5-HT)	Potentiates ionotropic $5-HT_3$ receptor function; conflicting reports on metabotropic 5-HT receptors
Voltage-dependent calcium channels	Acutely inhibits L-type and N-type channels
Calcium-activated potassium channels	Acutely enhances channel conductance
Dopamine	Acutely enhances firing of dopaminergic neurons in the ventral tegmental area and release of dopamine in the nucleus accumbens
Opioids	Acutely facilitates μ-receptor binding and inhibits δ-receptor binding, with no effect on κ-receptor binding
Acetylcholine (ACh)	Increases affinity of nicotinic ACh receptors for ACh
Adenosine	Inhibits transport of adenosine into cells
ATP receptors	Inhibits receptor function
Neuropeptide Y	Interacts with a particular receptor subtype

decade ago conventional wisdom held that these effects were secondary to ethanol actions on cell membrane lipids. Ethanol and other alcohols, as well as volatile anesthetics, disrupt the phospholipid bilayer of cell membranes, increasing membrane fluidization and decreasing neuronal membrane excitability.[62] Tolerance appeared to correlate with decreasing "fluidizability" (i.e., increased membrane "stiffness"), and physical dependence appeared to correlate with persistence of this "stiffness" following abstinence.[63] The increased stiffness with chronic ethanol intake was attributed to increased cholesterol and fatty acid content, which reduced the ability of ethanol to enter the membrane.[62] Effects on membrane proteins were considered secondary; a specific ethanol receptor was deemed unlikely.

It turned out, however, that ethanol's ability to decrease neuronal excitability by nonselectively altering the microfluidity of biological membranes holds true only for concentrations far higher than those encountered clinically.[64,65] Moreover, when alcohols of increasing chain length were compared, a biological "cut-off" was observed. For example, longer-chain alcohols had greater solubility in lipid membranes, yet, unlike shorter-chain alcohols, they did not inhibit *N*-methyl-D-aspartate (NMDA) receptor-activated ion currents,[66] and anesthetic agents with identical lipid solubility had different effects on particular membrane proteins.[64,67] It was further shown that ethanol inhibition of a nicotinic acetylcholine receptor involved the extracellular amino-terminal domain of the receptor, not an intramembrane site.[68] The evidence now indicates that although specific ethanol receptors comparable to opioid or serotonin receptors are unlikely, ethanol does interact directly with membrane proteins.

Glutamate Receptors

Ethanol inhibits NMDA receptor activation at intoxicating blood ethanol levels[69–72] and produces a discriminative stimulus effect similar to that produced by NMDA antagonists.[73] During early ethanol withdrawal NMDA receptor function is up-regulated, and in animals the frequency and severity of ethanol withdrawal seizures are reduced by NMDA receptor antagonists. In turn, NMDA-induced seizures in rats are prevented by ethanol. Neuropathological changes associated with chronic ethanol exposure are plausibly attributed to NMDA receptor up-regulation and glutamate excitotoxicity.[73,74]

Inhibition of NMDA-evoked neuronal activity in the brain varies from region to region. The reason is that ethanol differentially affects particular NMDA receptor subtypes. NMDA receptors consist of NR1 subunits, which have several isoforms generated by alternative splicing of a single gene, as well as four NR2 subunits coded by four different genes. NMDA receptor composition varies regionally in the brain. In studies involving recombinant NMDA receptor expression in oocytes or cell lines, ethanol preferentially affects receptors containing NR1-1a or NR1-1b splice variants and NR2A or NR2B subunits.[65,75] The site of ethanol's action at the NMDA receptor is not known. Ethanol does not directly influence the binding properties of NMDA receptor agonists, and it does not appear to interact at the glutamate, the glycine, or the polyamine site

or, within the channel, at the Mg^{2+} or the phencyclidine/dizocilpine site.[65] Ethanol probably interacts with an allosteric site that modulates the kinetics of channel gating, and the cut-off effect observed with alcohols of increasing chain length is consistent with binding to a discrete hydrophobic pocket within the receptor protein.[66,76,77]

Acute inhibition of NMDA receptors by ethanol results in reduced Ca^{2+} influx, reduced cyclic GMP accumulation, and wide-ranging effects on intracellular signal transduction pathways.[69] With chronic ethanol exposure these effects produce compensatory increases in NMDA receptor number and function. Glutamate (but not glycine) binding sites are increased, and depending on brain region (e.g., cortex vs. hippocampus vs. cerebellum) there is preferential up-regulation of particular receptor subunits. These adaptations plausibly underlie physical dependence.

Ethanol modulates gene expression of NMDA receptors both at the level of gene transcription in the nucleus and at the level of post-transcription and post-translation in the cytoplasm.[73] NR1 and NR2 subunits of NMDA receptors have sites for phosphorylation by kinases such as phosphokinase A (PKA), phosphokinase C (PKC), calcium/calmodulin-dependent kinase II (CaMKII), and tyrosine kinases. Through its effects on second messenger systems, ethanol can modulate phosphorylation of particular subunits in particular regions of the brain, thereby up-regulating or down-regulating their functional activity.[77,78] For example, ethanol given to mice increases phosphorylation of the NMDA receptor NR2B subunit by Fyn kinase. Fyn kinase-deficient mice are hypersensitive to ethanol's hypnotic effects and do not exhibit acute tolerance.[73]

Ethanol also inhibits AMPA/kainate receptors but at concentrations much higher than required for NMDA receptor inhibition, and AMPA/kainate receptors chronically exposed to ethanol do not undergo adaptation sufficient to produce physical dependence.[72,78,79] In cultured cerebellar Purkinje neurons, chronic ethanol exposure enhanced Ca^{2+} signals in response to AMPA. The effect was considered indirect; by depolarizing the cell membrane via Na^+ channel opening, AMPA receptors lowered the threshold for calcium entry through NMDA receptors and voltage-gated calcium channels.[80]

Gamma-aminobutyric acid (GABA) and Inhibitory Glycine Receptors

Intoxicating concentrations of ethanol enhance the function of ionotropic $GABA_A$ receptors.[81] $GABA_A$ agonists and uptake inhibitors increase behavioral responses to ethanol, whereas $GABA_A$ antagonists and synthesis inhibitors reduce ethanol-induced behaviors. Mice bred to be either hyper- or hypo-responsive to ethanol are similarly hyper- or hypo-responsive to GABAergic drugs. As with NMDA receptors, $GABA_A$ receptor subtypes differ in their sensitivity to ethanol, and the difference depends both on receptor subunit composition and post-translational processing, especially phosphorylation.[82] (At least 17 isoforms of $GABA_A$ receptor subunits have been identified, some existing in alternatively spliced forms, with different distributions throughout the brain.[77]) Illustrating the importance of both transcription-determined receptor subtypes and post-translational modifications are studies showing that $GABA_A$ sensitivity to ethanol requires the presence of a particular splice variant of the receptor's $\gamma2$ subunit, and that when this subunit is genetically altered so that it can no longer be phosphorylated by protein kinase C at a particular site, sensitivity to ethanol is lost.[83–85]

Also similar to NMDA receptors, $GABA_A$ receptors are affected by different alcohols and volatile anesthetics, and potency increases with increasing alcohol chain length until a "cut-off" is reached, consistent with a hydrophobic binding cavity of limited size. The location of this binding site is unknown; it does not appear to be at either the receptor's benzodiazepine or barbiturate-binding site.[77,86] It does seem to be near the extracellular site of a membrane-spanning portion of the receptor.[87]

Ethanol also facilitates metabotropic G-protein-coupled $GABA_B$ receptors, which through signal transduction effects on potassium and calcium channels inhibit neuronal firing. Ethanol facilitates inhibitory glycine receptors as well. In mice intracerebroventricular administration of glycine enhanced the behavioral effects of ethanol, and the enhancement was blocked by the glycine antagonist strychnine.[84]

With chronic ethanol exposure adaptive responses decrease $GABA_A$ receptor-mediated chloride channel function, and this change is associated with selective alterations of $GABA_A$ receptor subunits.[77] Decreased $GABA_A$ receptor function presumably contributes to tolerance and physical dependence.

In healthy humans, ethanol prolonged the duration of the cortical silent period induced by transcranial magnetic stimulation, and it enhanced intracortical inhibition after paired magnetic stimulation. The findings were consistent with potentiation of GABA receptor-mediated currents.[88]

GABA receptor complexes contain benzodiazepine binding sites. In cultured neurons the weak benzodiazepine inverse agonists, RO15-4513 (an imidazobenzodiazepine), inhibits ethanol-stimulated chloride flux.[89] In rats, RO15-4513 blocks mild ethanol intoxication without affecting behavioral changes induced by the GABAergic agent pentobarbital.[90,91] RO15-4513 induces seizures during ethanol withdrawal but does not itself cause seizures or withdrawal-like signs.[92] It does not reverse severe ethanol intoxication (i.e., coma).[93]

Recently detoxified human alcoholics had reduced distribution volume of benzodiazepine receptors in the frontal, anterior cingulate, and cerebellar cortices. It is unclear whether the abnormality represented a toxic effect of ethanol or a vulnerability factor for developing alcoholism.[94]

Serotonin (5-HT) Receptors

Conflicting reports of ethanol's effects on serotonergic (5-HT) systems are not surprising, for at least 14 5-HT receptor subtypes exist. Most activate G-protein-mediated signaling pathways, but the $5-HT_3$ receptor is ionotropic, with a ligand-gated channel through which cations depolarize the membrane. $5-HT_3$ antagonists reduce ethanol intake in animals,[95] and in humans $5-HT_3$ antagonists alter the subjective perception of intoxication and reduce drinking.[96,97] On the other hand, overexpression of the $5-HT_3$ receptor in transgenic mice also reduces ethanol intake.[98]

Ethanol potentiates $5-HT_3$ receptor function, and as with NMDA and $GABA_A$ receptors, other alcohols have similar effects, with a "cut-off" as chain length increases. A hydrophobic binding site is therefore presumed, possibly, as with GABA and glycine receptors (which share conserved portions of the $5-HT_3$ receptor), involving amino acids near the extracellular side of a membrane-spanning portion of the receptor.[99]

5-HT$_{1B}$ receptors are largely presynaptic and appear to inhibit neurotransmitter release.[100] Such receptors are found on GABAergic terminals projecting from the nucleus accumbens (NA) to the ventral tegmental area (VTA). Compared with wild-type mice, knockout mice lacking 5-HT$_{1B}$ receptors drank twice as much ethanol, were less sensitive to ethanol-induced ataxia, and developed ethanol tolerance more slowly, yet they showed equivalent degrees of physical dependence (e.g., withdrawal seizures).[101]

Voltage-dependent Calcium Channels

Acutely intoxicating concentrations of ethanol inhibit L-type, N-type, and possibly T-type voltage-gated calcium channels. Ethanol probably acts directly on channel proteins. It might also inhibit L-type channel function indirectly by interacting with G$_i$ G-proteins, and it might inhibit N- and PQ-type channels indirectly by activating protein kinase A.[102–104] With chronic exposure L-type calcium channels are up-regulated, and this compensatory response requires activation of protein kinase C. Acute inhibition of L-type channels correlates with ethanol-induced suppression of vasopressin release from the neurohypophysis.[104] Channel up-regulation possibly contributes to signs of physical dependence, including seizures.[105] L-type channel blockers attenuate withdrawal tremor and seizures in animals[106] and reduce ethanol consumption in ethanol-preferring rats.[107] Up-regulation of calcium channels is greater in mice bred for sensitivity to the acute behavioral effects of ethanol compared with less sensitive mice.[108] Up-regulation is also greater in mice bred for severe withdrawal seizures compared with mice with mild signs of withdrawal.[109]

Calcium-activated Potassium (CAK) Channels and Voltage-gated Potassium Channels

Highly selective for K$^+$, CAK channels are activated by increases in intracellular calcium concentration; K$^+$ efflux repolarizes or hyperpolarizes the cell membrane. At relevant pharmacological concentrations ethanol enhances CAK channel conductances, probably by directly interacting with the channel protein and increasing the duration of the open state.[110]

Of four different types of voltage-gated potassium channels cloned from *Drosophila* and expressed in oocytes, one was inhibited by ethanol and the other three were not.[111]

Dopamine

Acutely, ethanol increases the firing rate of dopaminergic neurons in the VTA and the release of dopamine in the NA.[71] In rats withdrawing from chronic ethanol there is decreased dopamine release in the NA, which persists beyond clinical signs of withdrawal; dopamine release is restored by readministration of ethanol.[112,113] Rats bred to prefer ethanol self-administer it directly into the VTA; in these rats a dopamine D$_2$ agonist reduces ethanol intake whereas a D$_2$ antagonist increases it.[114] Knockout mice lacking dopamine D$_1$- or D$_2$-receptors or DARPP-32 (see Chapter 2) consume less ethanol and show less ethanol conditioned place preference. Extracellular NA dopamine levels increase in rats exposed to environments associated with ethanol. How directly ethanol is involved with dopamine neurotransmission is unclear; dopamine release induced by ethanol is blocked by opioid and serotonin antagonists.[71,115]

Opioids

Chronic ethanol intake in the rat caused increased synthesis of beta-endorphin in the hypothalamus, decreased synthesis of beta-endorphin in the pituitary, and decreased brain levels of met-enkephalin.[116,117] Effects of ethanol on the biosynthesis and regulation of opioid peptides vary with species, brain region, and duration of exposure.[118]

Acutely, ethanol inhibits opioid binding to δ-opioid receptors; chronic ethanol exposure causes compensatory upregulation of δ receptors. By contrast, μ-receptor binding is facilitated by acute ethanol, and κ-receptor binding is unaffected.[119,120] In rodents and primates opioid receptor antagonists (naloxone or naltrexone) reduce ethanol self-administration.[115,121,122] Similar reduction was observed with naltriben, a selective δ2-opioid receptor antagonist.[123] Given with these opioid receptor antagonists, ethanol no longer induces dopamine release in the NA,[124] and ethanol inhibition of glutamatergic neurotransmission is reversed.[125] Such observations have led to new pharmacological approaches to the treatment of alcoholism (see later), but the precise manner in which ethanol and endogenous opioid systems interact is unknown.

Acetylcholine (ACh)

Neuronal nicotinic acetylcholine (nnACh) receptors are very different structurally from muscle nicotinic-ACh receptors. Members of a gene superfamily of ligand-gated ion channels that includes $GABA_A$, glycine, and $5-HT_3$ receptors, nnACh receptors have a pentameric structure composed of different subunits that vary across brain regions. Presynaptic nnACh receptors modulate the release of dopamine, norepinephrine, glutamate, GABA, and other neurotransmitters.[126]

Ethanol not only increases the affinity of nnACh receptors for ACh but does so at concentrations significantly lower than required for its actions at GABA, glutamate, $5-HT_3$, and voltage-gated calcium channels (100 μM to 10 mM vs. 30 to 200 mM).[127] Studies of hybrid receptors expressed in oocytes or embryonic cell cultures identified the $\alpha3\beta4$ subunit combination as the most sensitive to ethanol.[128]

In cultured cortical neurons acute ethanol inhibits muscarinic ACh receptor activation of phosphoinositide metabolism. Chronic ethanol exposure, by contrast, causes up-regulation of muscarinic ACh receptors and potentiation of cAMP production.[71] Unexpectedly, in a study involving hippocampal slices, clinically intoxicating concentrations of ethanol enhanced muscarinic ACh transmission.[129]

Adenosine Receptors and Transporters

Acting through adenosine A_1, A_2, and other receptor subtypes in neuronal cell membranes, adenosine is a global inhibitory neuromodulator interfering with release of excitatory neurotransmitters.[71] Adenosine is transported into cells by several types of transporters, one of which is acutely inhibited by ethanol.[130] The inhibition is indirect; ethanol potentiates receptor-activated cAMP production, which in turn results in PKA phosphorylation of the transporter (or a regulatory component).[131] Inhibition of the adenosine transporter leads to accumulation of extracellular adenosine, which then acts at adenosine receptors to inhibit excitatory neurotransmission. With chronic ethanol exposure there is reduced receptor-stimulated cAMP production, reduced adenosine transporter phosphorylation, and tolerance to the sensitivity of adenosine transporters to ethanol.[132]

Intoxicating effects of ethanol, especially ataxia, are prevented by adenosine receptor antagonists and exacerbated by adenosine receptor agonists and by drugs that interfere with adenosine uptake. There is cross-tolerance between adenosine agonists and ethanol after chronic exposure.[71] Like ethanol, adenosine stimulates the production of cAMP, and desensitization of this effect follows chronic exposure. In cultured neurons adenosine deaminase prevents both acute and chronic effects of ethanol on cAMP signal transduction.[133]

ATP (P2X) Receptors

Extracellular ATP gates ion channels within P2X receptors on neurons of both the central and peripheral nervous systems. Activation of these receptors is excitatory, and it is probable that ethanol inhibits them by binding to a particular circumscribed region of hydrophobic amino acids, resulting in an allosteric alteration that decreases agonist affinity.[134]

Neuropeptide Y

Widely distributed in brain, neuropeptide Y (NPY) is involved in the control of food intake. Knockout mice lacking NPY increase their voluntary consumption of ethanol; with overexpression of NPY, consumption is suppressed. Ethanol interacts directly with the Y1 NPY receptor subtype.[115,135]

Genetic Aspects

Ethnicity, ADH, and ALDH

Alcoholism develops in only a minority of those who drink. In fact, half the ethanol drunk in America is consumed by 10% of the population.[136] Patterns of ethanol use show striking ethnic and cultural differences. Probably genetic is the much lower incidence of alcoholism among Mongoloid Asians than whites or blacks. Probably nongenetic is the greater prevalence of abstention among American black women compared with white, yet the greater likelihood of black women who drink becoming alcoholic.[9]

Alcohol dehydrogenase (ADH), the rate-limiting enzyme of ethanol metabolism, consists of multiple isoenzymes, the result of five structural genes encoding five different polypeptide subunits. These isoenzymes differ in their reactivity toward ethanol and contribute to different rates of ethanol metabolism. Peak blood ethanol concentrations (BEC) thus can be very different after equivalent amounts of ethanol, even among individuals of similar age, weight, and prior drinking experience.[137,138]

Aldehyde dehydrogenase (ALDH) is also genetically polymorphous, and its different forms account for striking ethnic differences in response to ethanol.[137,138] Compared with whites, a greater percentage of Mongoloid Asians have acute adverse reactions to ethanol, consisting of facial flushing, tachycardia, abdominal warmth, and dysphoria. The cause is genetic deficiency of an isoenzyme of ALDH, leading to elevated tissue levels of acetaldehyde, which is more vasodilatory and sympathomimetic than ethanol.[139,140] Among the 40% of Chinese, Japanese, and South American Indians who have this isoenzyme deficiency, alcoholism is much less prevalent than among those who do not.[141]

Hereditary Clinical Subtypes

Comparable ALDH deficiency does not affect whites and blacks, yet genetic influences contribute to alcoholism in these groups as well.[142,143] There is a twofold higher concordance for alcoholism in identical than in fraternal twins, and adopted-away children of alcoholics have an increased risk of alcoholism even when raised by nonalcoholic adoptive parents.[144,145] On the basis of such studies, Cloninger postulated two major genetic subtypes of alcoholism (Table 12–6).[1,136] Type I alcoholics display the psychological characteristics of passive-dependent or anxious personalities: (1) high harm avoidance ("cautious, apprehensive, pessimistic, inhibited, shy, and susceptible to fatigue"); (2) high reward dependence ("eager to help others, emotionally dependent, warmly sympathetic, sentimental,

Table 12–6. Proposed Genetic Subtypes of Alcholism[1]

Type I
High harm avoidance and reward dependence, low novelty seeking
Loss of control when not abstinent
Alcoholism onset in late adulthood
Men and women both affected (*milieu limited*)

Type II
High novelty seeking, low harm avoidance and reward dependence
Inability to abstain
Alcoholism onset in adolescence or early adulthood, with antisocial behavior
Male predominance (*male-limited*)

sensitive to social cues, and persistent"); and (3) low novelty seeking ("rigid, reflective, loyal, orderly, and attentive to details"). By contrast, type II alcoholics have antisocial personalities: (1) low harm avoidance ("confident, relaxed, optimistic, uninhibited, carefree, and energetic"); (2) low reward dependence ("socially detached, emotionally cool, practical, tough-minded, and independently self-willed"); and (3) high novelty seeking ("impulsive, exploratory, excitable, disorderly, distractable"). The drinking pattern of type I alcoholics is one of "loss of control"—they can abstain from ethanol for long periods, but once they begin drinking they cannot stop. Their problems usually begin in late adulthood after many years of exposure to socially encouraged heavy drinking, and they are fearful and guilty about their drinking. Men and women are both affected. Both hereditary and environmental factors are necessary for alcoholism to develop in type I individuals (milieu limited). The drinking pattern of type II alcoholics is "inability to abstain entirely." Largely limited to men, their disorder begins in adolescence or early adulthood with antisocial behavior and is relatively independent of environmental influences (male-limited). There is also a high incidence of depression and suicide.[136,146]

Not every study supports the existence of Cloninger's alcoholism subtypes.[147] Of 456 boys followed to age 47 years, 116 became alcoholic, 18% before age 20 years and 45% after age 21 years; there was no correlation between age of onset and alcoholic parentage.[148] In a twin study, a strong genetic influence was evident for men with early-onset alcoholism but not for men with late-onset alcoholism or for women with onset at any age.[149] Another study found greater influence of biological parents for severe alcoholism compared with mild alcoholism.[150] Type II alcoholism may well be simply one manifestation of a broader psychiatric diagnosis—antisocial personality disorder—rather than a form of primary alcoholism.[151] Cloninger's subtypes probably oversimplify the nurture versus nature aspects of a polygenetic group of disorders (see Chapter 2) collectively termed alcohol abuse/dependence and manifesting a continuum, not a dichotomy, of symptoms and signs.

Animal Studies

Most animals dislike ethanol, and ingenious strategies (such as vaporized cages) have been employed to produce intoxication. Strains of mice and rats have been bred, however, which not only prefer ethanol to water but also seek it out and develop tolerance and physical dependence.[152–154] Ethanol-preferring rodents will self-administer ethanol to intoxication, either orally, by intragastric administration, or by direct infusion into the VTA. Other rodent strains show different physiological responses to ethanol.[155] For example, long-sleep (LS) mice are sensitive to ethanol's disruption of the righting reflex, depression of body temperature, elevation of plasma corticosterone, and inhibition of cerebellar Purkinje cell firing; short-sleep (SS) mice are more resistant to these effects and exhibit greater preference for drinking ethanol.[156] In oocytes injected with mRNA from LS mice, ethanol facilitated GABA responses, whereas in oocytes injected with mRNA from SS mice, ethanol was inhibitory.[157] These actions imply different biophysical properties of GABA receptors in LS and SS mice.[158] Such speculation is supported by observations in other mouse strains that a point mutation in the gene for the alpha-6 subunit of the $GABA_A$ receptor, specific to cerebellar granule cells, rendered the animals intolerant to both ethanol and benzodiazepines.[159]

Analogous to human type II alcoholics, other strains of ethanol-seeking mice demonstrate exploratory behavior with little fear; compared with ethanol-avoiding mice they have low basal levels of brain dopamine and increased dopamine turnover.[136] As noted earlier, some strains differ in their responses to serotonin manipulation. The P strain of alcohol-preferring rats has depressed levels of serotonin in several brain areas, including the NA;[160] ethanol consumption increases NA levels of serotonin, and serotonin uptake inhibitors such as fluoxetine block ethanol preference.[161] Ethanol reinforcement in this strain might involve facilitation of serotonergic neurons in the dorsal raphe nucleus. In another mouse strain, knockout of the $5-HT_{1B}$ receptor gene resulted in increased aggression and increased ethanol ingestion. The knockout mice were less sensitive than wild-types to ethanol-induced ataxia, and they developed tolerance more slowly.[162,163] By contrast, the AA strain of ethanol-preferring rats had elevated levels of brain serotonin, and destruction of the dorsal raphe nucleus had no effect on ethanol preference.[164]

Other strains of ethanol-preferring rats have higher densities of GABA-containing nerve terminals in the NA, and ethanol differentially alters brain levels of $GABA_A$ receptor subunit mRNAs in withdrawal seizure-prone compared with withdrawal seizure-resistant mice.[165,166] Some strains of rodents demonstrate differences in brain levels of met-enkephalin or beta-endorphin.[167,168]

Animal studies have not been limited to rodents. A nonhuman primate model revealed high rates of ethanol consumption that correlated with either Cloninger Type I alcoholism (anxiety-driven) or Type II alcoholism (impaired impulse control, expulsion from social groups at an early age); the latter tended to have low cerebrospinal fluid levels of the serotonin metabolite 5-hydroxy-indoleacetic acid (5-HIAA).[169]

The fruit fly *Drosophila* has also been studied. Placed in an "inebriometer" (a tank containing ethanol vapor), drunken and sober flies can be identified. Mutations in the genes "amnesiac" (coding for an adenylyl cyclase-activating protein) and "rutabaga" (coding for adenylyl cyclase itself) are associated with increased ethanol sensitivity in these flies.[170] Different forms of the ADH enzyme have also been identified in different species of *Drosophila*.[171]

Recognizing the polygenetic nature of ethanol dependence, investigators are currently using animal models to identify quantitative trait loci (QTLs) related to ethanol preference, ethanol sensitivity, or ethanol withdrawal severity[172–175] (see Chapter 2). Studies with congenic mouse strains have revealed four QTLs on chromosomes 1, 2, 11, and 15 that account for 60% of the genetic variance in sensitivity to ethanol-induced sedation. QTLs for ethanol preference have been identified on chromosomes 1 and 9, with the dopamine D_2 receptor and the $5-HT_{1B}$ receptor as possible candidate genes on chromosome 9. Three QTLs accounting for 68% of the genetic variance in ethanol withdrawal severity have been localized to chromosomes 1 and 11.[176]

Human Genetic Markers

Primary alcoholics (those without other underlying psychiatric illness) and their nonalcoholic children have been studied for possible genetic markers or predictors of disease.[29,177] Compared with sons of nonalcoholics, sons of alcoholics are less intoxicated (as measured by body sway and psychomotor performance) at equivalent blood ethanol concentrations.[144] Decreased reaction to ethanol could presumably make it harder for someone to learn when to stop drinking. (In the same subjects diazepam did not produce different responses, suggesting ethanol specificity.[178]) In a follow-up study, 227 adolescent sons of alcoholics were compared with 227 sons of nonalcoholics. Forty percent of the men at high risk for alcoholism and less than 10% of the control subjects demonstrated a low intensity of response to ethanol. Ten years later 56% of the sons of alcoholics with low response had become alcoholic compared with 14% of the sons of alcoholics with a more sensitive response. Neither family history of alcoholism nor response to ethanol predicted any other drug abuse or any other psychiatric diagnosis.[179] Once established, the pattern of alcoholism does not differ between low-responders and more sensitive responders.[180]

Compared with controls, alcoholics and their preadolescent sons have dampened amplitudes of the P300 event-related potential, less electroencephalographic (EEG) alpha activity before ethanol consumption, and a greater amount of EEG alpha activity after ethanol consumption.[144,181–183] Low platelet monoamine oxidase B activity has been observed in alcoholics (especially type I), persisting with abstinence; it is unclear if such changes occur in nonalcoholic offspring.[29,184] Diminished platelet adenylyl cyclase response to stimulants persists in abstinent alcoholics, and diminished lymphocyte adenylyl cyclase response to adenosine

persists after the cells are cultured for several generations in ethanol-free media.[185,186] Some children of alcoholics have low levels of platelet adenylyl cyclase even if they are not themselves drinkers.[11] Nonalcoholics at high or low risk have different pituitary beta-endorphin and adrenal cortisol responses to ethanol,[187] and high-risk nonalcoholics have lower plasma GABA-like activity.[188] Compared with controls, sons of familial alcoholics have higher peak serum thyrotropin levels after receiving thyrotropin-releasing hormone.[189] There have been claims of linkage between a genetic determinant of alcoholism and the genes for the MNS blood groups (chromosome 4) or for esterase-D (chromosome 13).[190,191]

Ethanol-dependent patients often have comorbid psychiatric diseases, including anxiety, panic disorder, schizophrenia, antisocial personality, depression, and attention deficit hyperactivity disorder.[192–196] Cohort studies suggest that among patients with depression and alcoholism, depression is more often the result of the alcoholism than its cause.[197,198]

Dopamine D_2 Receptors and the A1 Allele

In 1990 a study using a Taq 1 endonuclease and frozen brains identified an allele—called A1—downstream from the coding region of the dopamine D_2 receptor gene on chromosome 11. A1 was present in 64% of alcoholics but only 17% of controls, and among alcoholics its presence increased disease severity.[199] A decade of controversy followed. Although some studies were confirmatory,[200–204] others found no difference in the prevalence of the A1 allele between alcoholics and nonalcoholics and no linkage within families of the A1 allele to alcoholism.[205–212] In one study A1 polymorphism bore no relationship to age of onset of alcoholism.[213] In another report although the A1 allele did not segregate with alcoholism per se, within individual families it was associated with alcoholism and severe medical complications.[214] In still another report the A1 allele was significantly increased not only in patients with alcoholism (42.3% vs. 14.5% for nonalcoholic controls) but also in patients with Tourette syndrome (44.9%), attention deficit hyperactivity disorder (46.2%), and autism (54.5%).[215] Others found an association of the A1 allele with tobacco and cocaine use, substance abuse in young people committing violent crimes, obesity, and pathological gambling.[216–221] A meta-analysis of studies showed positive association with alcoholism only if studies by the original investigators were included, with no association when all other studies were analyzed.[222] A large family-based study—the Collaborative Study on Genetics of Alcoholism (COGA)—used linkage analysis and for each proband required at least two ethanol-dependent first-degree relatives and at least one unaffected parent; no association was found between the A1 allele and alcoholism.[223]

Autopsy and positron emission tomography (PET) studies (using D_2-receptor-labeled ligands) revealed reduced numbers of striatal D_2 dopamine receptors in subjects with the A1 allele compared with those without it.[218,224] There did not appear to be any alteration of receptor structure but rather of receptor expression. A subsequent study found decreased densities of both dopamine D_2 and D_3 receptors in the NA and amygdala of Type 1 alcoholics.[225] The A1 allele was also associated with reduced P300 amplitude in sons of alcoholic fathers and with reduced craving for alcohol among alcoholics receiving the D_2 agonist bromocriptine.[226] In another report, the A1 allele was significantly more prevalent among alcoholics with a family history of alcoholism than among those without a family history.[227]

In an analysis of complete dopamine receptor D_2 gene coding sequences no structural coding abnormalities were present in alcoholics.[228] The role, if any, of the A1 allele as a risk factor for alcoholism would therefore be indirect, perhaps involving epistasis (interaction among multiple genes) and consistent with its presence being neither necessary nor sufficient to cause alcoholism.[229]

Advocates of the importance of the A1 allele do not view the dopamine D_2 receptor gene as an "alcoholism gene" but rather as "a reinforcement or reward gene." In fact, they lump impulsive, compulsive, and addictive behaviors (including compulsive eating, gambling, and sex) under the rubric "reward deficiency syndrome," with substance abuse and other inappropriate behaviors serving to compensate for reduced functioning of the dopamine-driven reward circuit.[230] Studies that fail to show an association with alcoholism they criticize on the grounds that other reward deficiency

syndromes were not properly excluded from control groups or that populations studied included both severely affected alcoholics (in whom heredity would play a major role) and mildly affected alcoholics (in whom heredity would play a lesser role).[231] They further note (responding to the COGA study) that with polygenetic disorders, in which each of many genes plays only a modifying and often a small role, association studies (employing population controls) are more sensitive than linkage studies (requiring large families).[218,232]

Other Receptors and QTLs

In addition to its reported association with the dopamine D_2 receptor A1 allele, severe alcoholism has been associated with a polymorphism near the 5′ regulatory region of the D_2 receptor gene, an allele termed B2.[233] This allele, like A1, is associated with abuse of cocaine and other drugs as well.[218] Other alcohol-associated mutations within the dopamine D_2 receptor gene (intronic and exonic) have also been described, and a 7 repeat allele of the dopamine receptor D_4 gene occurred at significantly higher frequency in alcoholics with a family history than in those without.[227]

Binge-drinking alcoholics and those with comorbid impulsive or sociopathic behavior have demonstrated association with particular serotonin receptor or transporter genes.[234,235] In one report serotonergic dysfunction was associated with reduced ethanol-induced sedation and excessive ethanol intake.[236]

As with animals, the polygenetic nature of human alcoholism has led investigators to adopt QTL strategies in identifying genetic influences.[236a] In Finnish sib pairs, antisocial alcoholism was linked to the 5-HT$_{1B}$ autoreceptor on chromosome 6.[237] In a Southwestern American Indian population, ethanol dependence was linked to dopamine D_4 receptor and tyrosine hydroxylase genes on chromosome 11 and to a GABA$_A$ receptor subtype gene on chromosome 4.[238] In the COGA, suggestive susceptibility loci for alcoholism were found on chromosomes 1, 2, and 7, and a protective locus was identified on chromosome 4 near the alcohol dehydrogenase genes. No evidence was found for linkage on chromosome 11.[239]

Ethanol Intoxication

Symptoms and Signs

Ethanol intoxication is so common that physicians tend to forget that it can be fatal, especially when additional drugs have been taken (Table 12–7). Rapidly absorbed from the gastrointestinal tract, ethanol is distributed throughout body water.[240] About 50 g (roughly 2 oz) of 100% ethanol—corresponding to approximately 4 oz. of 90-proof spirits, 14 oz. of wine, or 48 oz. of beer—would produce a mildly intoxicating blood ethanol concentration (BEC) of 100 mg/dL in a 70-kg man. In nontolerant individuals, ethanol is metabolized at 70–150 mg/kg body weight per hour with a fall in BEC of 10–25 mg/dL per hour (average 16 mg/dL per hour). Most adults therefore require 6 hours to metabolize a 50 g dose. Drinking only an additional 8 g per hour maintains the BEC at 100 mg/dL; drinking more rapidly raises it. In women, lower activity of gastric ADH leads to higher BECs compared with men.[241,242]

Early saturation of ADH accounts for the constant rate (zero-order kinetics) of ethanol metabolism. Induction of the MEOS by ethanol (and also by other drugs, such as barbiturates) accounts in part for ethanol tolerance, most of which, however, is pharmacodynamic[243] (see Chapter 1). (Zero-order

Table 12–7. Correlation of Symptoms with Blood Ethanol Concentration

Blood Ethanol Concentration (mg/dL)	Symptoms
50–150	Euphoria or dysphoria, shyness or expansiveness, friendliness or argumentativeness
	Impaired concentration, judgment, and sexual inhibitions
150–250	Slurred speech and ataxic gait, diplopia, nausea, tachycardia, drowsiness, or labile mood with sudden bursts of anger or antisocial acts
300	Stupor alternating with combativeness or incoherent speech, heavy breathing, vomiting
400	Coma
500	Respiratory paralysis, death

kinetics breaks down at very high ethanol concentration—that is, elimination becomes more dependent on concentration; the mechanism is unclear but does not appear to involve MEOS.[244]) Food in the stomach delays ethanol absorption, and alcoholics learn to enhance intoxication by not eating. Aspirin, cimetidine, and ranitidine reduce gastric ADH activity and when taken with ethanol produce substantially higher blood levels.[245]

Clinically ethanol is a CNS depressant; euphoria and hyperactivity associated with intoxication are the result of cerebral disinhibition, not direct stimulation. At any BEC, intoxication is greater when the level is rising than when it is falling, when the level is reached rapidly, and when the level has been recently achieved.[8] These factors as well as an individual's degree of tolerance mean that a single BEC determination is an unreliable indicator of drunkenness; Table 12–7 offers broad generalizations.[246] (The National Council on Alcoholism defines tolerance as either a blood ethanol level greater than 150 mg without gross evidence of intoxication or daily consumption of at least one-fifth of a gallon of liquor—or equivalent wine or beer—in a 180-lb individual.) Coma, respiratory depression, and death would occur in 50% of subjects at a BEC of 500 mg/dL, but levels of less than 400 mg/dL have been fatal, and levels above 800 mg/dL have been documented in alert patients.[247–250] Most states define legal intoxication as a BEC of at least 100 mg/dL. Driving skills, however, are impaired at levels as low as 50 mg/dL.[251]

Slow saccadic eye movements and interrupted, jerky smooth pursuit, sometimes impairing visual acuity, accompany low to moderate BECs. At these levels, there is increased EEG beta activity ("beta buzz"). Higher concentrations cause nystagmus, esophoria or exophoria, and diplopia, with EEG slowing.[252,253] Ethanol suppresses the rapid eye movement (REM) stage of sleep, followed, as levels fall, by REM "rebound" (and sometimes vivid dreaming). Nighttime hypoxemia is common in alcoholics, who may be at increased risk for sleep apnea.[254] Both low and high BECs cause hypothermia; when, as is not unusual, drinkers are exposed to low environmental temperature, hypothermia can be marked—it averaged 84.5°F (29.2°C) in a report of 31 patients—with a danger of cardiac arrhythmia.[255,256]

"Positional alcohol nystagmus" refers to nystagmus and vertigo during ethanol intoxication. Ethanol's specific gravity is lower than that of endolymph or of fluid in the semicircular canals. As ethanol enters (preferentially) the semicircular canals at BECs above 40 mg/dL, the osmotic difference between the semicircular canals and the endolymph turns the canals into gravity-sensitive receptors. The result is vertigo and nystagmus beating toward the lower ear. Following an equilibrium period of a few hours, ethanol diffuses (preferentially) out of the semicircular canals, resulting in a return of vertigo, now with nystagmus beating toward the upper ear.[257]

Two forms of ethanol intoxication merit separate categorization. "Pathological intoxication," also called idiosyncratic intoxication or acute alcoholic paranoid state, consists of sudden extreme excitement, sometimes with delusions, hallucinations, and violent behavior, even homicide. After minutes to hours, there is sleep and amnesia for the episode. Some cases of pathological intoxication may represent psychological dissociative reactions; others may be the result of paradoxical excitation, such as occurs with barbiturates. Alcoholic "blackouts" consist of periods of drinking for which the subject has no recollection even though at the time alertness was preserved and behavior appeared normal. Although they are usually associated with frank alcoholism, blackouts also occur in moderate drinkers. The amnesia of pathological intoxication and blackouts is a direct effect of ethanol; BECs as low as 40 mg/dL cause memory impairment, which progresses as the BEC rises. Experimental studies have shown that the effect is on encoding, not consolidation or retrieval. In fact, if ethanol is taken after an event has been encoded, consolidation is enhanced.[258,259]

Ethanol can precipitate cardiac arrhythmia, including atrial fibrillation and ventricular tachycardia, in the absence of alcoholic cardiomyopathy or other cardiac disease ("holiday heart syndrome"). Ethanol releases catecholamines from the adrenal medulla and also directly affects cardiac conduction. A careful drinking history should be obtained in any patient with unexplained palpitations or "lone" atrial fibrillation.[260]

Ethanol intoxication frequently accompanies other serious illness and can intensify depressed consciousness from any cause. Stupor in someone with "alcoholic breath" and signs of vasodilatation (flushing, tachycardia, hypotension, and hypothermia) obviously suggests ethanol overdose; such signs, however, can mask the presence of subdural hematoma, meningitis, hepatic encephalopathy, hypoglycemia, ketoacidosis, or other drug poisoning.

For every 100 mg/dL BEC, serum osmolarity rises about 22 mOsm/L. This hyperosmolarity does not cause symptoms because ethanol freely crosses cell membranes without causing shifts of water, but comatose patients whose serum osmolarity is higher than that predicted by serum sodium, glucose, and urea should be suspected of ethanol poisoning. Ethanol suppresses antidiuretic hormone and with high water intake can cause symptomatic hyponatremia ("beer potomania").[261]

Treatment of Intoxication

The treatment of severe ethanol poisoning is similar to that of other depressant drugs (Table 12–8). Death is from respiratory depression, and so patients require artificial ventilation in an intensive care unit. Hypovolemia, acid–base or electrolyte imbalance, hypoglycemia, and abnormal temperature are often present; if the blood glucose level is not known, 50% dextrose is given intravenously with parenteral thiamine and multivitamins. Ethanol's rapid gastrointestinal absorption means that gastric

Table 12–8. Treatment of Acute Ethanol Intoxication

For obstreperous or violent patients
Isolation, calming environment, reassurance—avoid sedatives
Close observation

For stuporous or comatose patients
If hypoventilation, artificial respiration in an intensive care unit
If serum glucose in doubt, intravenous 50% glucose
Thiamine, 100 mg, and multivitamins, intramuscularly or intravenously
Careful monitoring of blood pressure; correction of hypovolemia or acid–base imbalance
Consider hemodialysis if patient severely acidotic, deeply comatose, or apneic
Avoid emetics or gastric lavage
Avoid analeptics
Do not forget other possible causes of coma in an alcoholic, as well as concomitant drug use

lavage is useful only if other drugs have been ingested. Sedatives or neuroleptics in obstreperous or violent patients can push them into coma and respiratory depression. A familiar feature of ethanol intoxication is a patient's tendency to appear awake during examination only to lapse into stupor and respiratory depression when left alone.

A BEC of 400 mg/dL in a nonhabitual drinker can take 20 hours to become zero. Ethanol metabolism is increased by fructose, which, however, causes gastrointestinal upset, lactic acidosis, hyperuricemia, and osmotic diuresis. Hemodialysis or peritoneal dialysis hastens ethanol elimination and should be considered in patients with very high BECs, severe acidosis, or additional drug ingestion (including methanol or ethylene glycol) and in severely intoxicated children. Analeptics, such as ethamivan, caffeine, or amphetamine, are of no value and can precipitate seizures or cardiac arrhythmia.[247]

Numerous other drugs have been studied in ethanol poisoning.[262] In mice low doses of propranolol reduced ethanol-induced depression, but higher doses augmented it, and in humans, propranolol increased ethanol inebriation ratings.[263] L-Dopa, aminophylline, and ephedrine reportedly reduced human ethanol intoxication, perhaps through norepinephrine pathways;[264] the dopamine agonist apomorphine, however, aggravated symptoms.[265] By unclear mechanisms naloxone seems to reverse ethanol-induced coma in a small subset of patients; responders are not identifiable before treatment, however, and they tend to relapse after only minutes.[266]

Not commercially available is the experimental imidazobenzodiazepine drug, RO15-4513, which in animals reverses symptoms of mild intoxication but not stupor or respiratory depression.[93]

Interactions with Other Drugs

Ethanol is often ingested with other drugs, either recreationally or in suicide attempts. Although ethanol and barbiturates are cross-tolerant, together the intoxicating or lethal dose for each may be strikingly lowered. Death from apnea followed a secobarbital blood level of 50 µg/mL and a BEC of 100 mg/dL.[267] Ethanol combined with chloral hydrate ("Mickey Finn") has a particularly notorious reputation.[268]

Such additive or synergistic effects also occur when ethanol is taken with sedating antihistamines; neuroleptics; and other sedatives or tranquilizers, such as methaqualone (now a Schedule I drug), meprobamate, or benzodiazepines (Table 12–9).[269,270] Diazepam and flurazepam have blood half-lives of more than 24 hours and contribute to intoxication when ethanol is taken the next day. Opioids and ethanol also aggravate each other's effects, and many heroin or methadone users are also alcoholic. Death has followed ethanol taken with propoxyphene. Tricyclic antidepressants can either antagonize or aggravate ethanol's effects.

Table 12–9. Some Ethanol–Drug Interactions[269–272]

Additive or supra-additive sedation (in some cases despite cross-tolerance)
General anesthetics
Barbiturates
Benzodiazepines
Nonbenzodiazepine, nonbarbiturate sedatives
  (e.g., chloral hydrate, glutethimide, meprobamate)
Antihistamines
Tricyclic antidepressants
Neuroleptics
Opioids

Metabolic effects
Phenytoin (acute ethanol decreases phenytoin metabolism; chronic ethanol increases it)
Warfarin (acute ethanol decreases warfarin metabolism; chronic ethanol increases it)
Aspirin, cimetidine, ranitidine (reduction of gastric alcohol dehydrogenase activity, producing higher blood ethanol levels)

Other additive effects
Antihypertensives (postural hypotension)
Insulin and oral hypoglycemics (hypoglycemia)
Neuroleptics (lowered seizure threshold, liver damage)
Chloral hydrate (vasodilatation)

Disulfiram-like reactions
Sulfonylurea hypoglycemics
Chloramphenicol
Griseofulvin
Isoniazid
Metronidazole
Quinacrine

Interactions with congeners
Monoamine oxidase inhibitors and tyramine in certain wines—e.g., Chianti—produce acute hypertensive crisis
Cobalt in beer produces cardiomyopathy—additive to direct ethanol cardiotoxicity?

Ethanol's cross-tolerance with general anesthetics such as diethyl ether, chloroform, or fluorinated agents slows sleep induction, but synergistic interaction then increases the depth and length of the anesthetic stage reached. The balance between cross-tolerance and synergistic effects is complex and unpredictable, and this uncertainty, coupled with decreased adrenocortical response to stress, impending withdrawal, and associated disease (especially cardiomyopathy), makes alcoholics high anesthetic and surgical risks.[271]

Ethanol interacts in different ways with many drugs (see Table 12–9).[272] For example, it initially retards and then accelerates phenytoin metabolism, producing either drug toxicity or inadequate seizure control. Ethanol inhibits warfarin metabolism. In patients taking antihypertensives, it aggravates postural hypotension. When ethanol is taken with sulfonylurea hypoglycemics, procarbazine, sulfonamides, chloramphenicol, griseofulvin, quinacrine, or metronidazole, a disulfiram-like reaction results (see later). When ethanol is taken with disulfiram itself, the reaction can be fatal.

Ethanol Withdrawal

Symptoms and Signs

"Hangover" Versus Physical Dependence

"Hangover," consisting of headache, malaise, fatigue, nausea, sweating, and tremulousness, does not require chronic drinking. It is not an entirely harmless condition, however. Studies of motor coordination (e.g., simulated driving or piloting performance) reveal impairment.[273] Although hangover severity is related to the amount of ethanol consumed, additional factors are probably contributory. Acetaldehyde is implicated, and congeners in dark liquors such as whiskey and brandy might account for their greater tendency to cause hangover compared with clear liquors such as vodka and gin.[274] Lack of food, insufficient sleep, and dehydration also aggravate symptoms. Levels of thromboxane B_2 are elevated during hangover, and a study with volunteers suggested that the prostaglandin inhibitor tolfenamic acid reduced symptoms when given prophylactically.[275] Prophylactic vitamin B_6 also reportedly relieved symptoms.[276]

Table 12–10. Ethanol Withdrawal Syndromes

Early
Tremulousness
Hallucinosis
Seizures
Late
Delirium tremens

More severe or prolonged symptoms indicate physical dependence. Ethanol withdrawal has traditionally been divided into early and late syndromes (Table 12–10).[253,277,278]

Tremor

The most common symptom of early ethanol withdrawal is gross tremor, which requires at least several days of heavy drinking and is promptly relieved by ethanol. With continued abstinence, it becomes more intense and is accompanied by easy startling, anxiety, insomnia, nystagmus, flushing, sweating, anorexia, nausea, vomiting, weakness, tachypnea, tachycardia, and systolic hypertension. Except for agitation and inattentiveness, mentation remains intact during early withdrawal; altered mentation suggests the presence of other disturbances, such as seizures, Wernicke–Korsakoff syndrome, meningitis, or subdural hematoma. Tremor is distal, coarse, irregular, rapid, and worse with movement, interfering with eating or even standing. Without treatment it usually subsides over several days, although some patients feel "shaky inside" for a few weeks.[277,279]

Hallucinosis

Perceptual disturbances occur in about one-fourth of these patients and include vivid dreams, nightmares, illusions, and hallucinations, which can be auditory, visual, tactile, olfactory, or a combination (alcoholic hallucinosis). Visual hallucinations are most common, with imagery of insects, animals, people, or disembodied heads. Sometimes occurring only with eye closure, they are mostly fragmentary and tend to last minutes at a time over several days. Insight varies, and there are often paranoid delusions.[277,280] Hallucinations sometimes occur during active drinking or after more than a week of abstinence.[281] Such patients have led some workers to propose that "alcoholic hallucinosis," with largely visual symptoms, clear sensorium, and no other signs of withdrawal, is a disorder separable from "alcohol withdrawal hallucinations," with largely auditory hallucinations and other signs such as fever, tachycardia, tremor, or altered sensorium.[282]

A Harlem Hospital patient, blind from bilateral eye injury, during ethanol withdrawal developed not only formed visual hallucinations, which he recognized as such (e.g., little orange people walking through walls), but also Anton syndrome—he believed his vision had returned and confabulated descriptions.[283] Withdrawal hallucinations have been restricted to the right visual hemifield in patients with left hemineglect, consistent with "inner representation" hypotheses of the neglect syndrome.[284]

Of 70 patients with alcoholic hallucinosis (auditory, visual, or both) 24 had no other symptoms, and the rest had varying combinations of tremor, seizures, and delusions; four later developed delirium tremens.[280] Consistent with other reports,[281] eight continued to have hallucinations for months or years, sometimes with ideas of reference, loose associations, and flat affect. Ethanol or its withdrawal might have precipitated schizophrenia in some of these patients, but in none was that diagnosis apparent before the first bout of hallucinosis.[280] Another study, using controls, found no increased incidence of schizophrenia either among patients before their hallucinosis or among their relatives.[285]

Parkinsonism, Chorea, Myoclonus, and Panic

Transient parkinsonism and transient chorea have each occurred during ethanol withdrawal.[279,286] Parkinsonism affects patients older than 50 years of age, beginning within a few days of the last drink or sometimes during drinking.[287] It tends to clear over days or weeks without treatment, and such patients have been followed for years without developing Parkinson's disease.[288] (A case–control study found no association between overall ethanol consumption and Parkinson's disease; moreover, an inverse correlation was found between alcoholism and Parkinson's disease [odds ratio: 0.41].[289]) Oral-lingual choreiform dyskinesias, sometimes spreading to neck or arm muscles, typically affect younger patients during the second week of

abstinence.[290] Acutely ethanol decreases striatal dopamine release, perhaps accounting for parkinsonism. Chorea might be secondary to dopamine receptor supersensitivity.[279,291] Neuroleptic-induced tardive dyskinesia is more common among drinkers than nondrinkers.[292]

Myoclonus distinguishable clinically and electroencephalographically from partial seizures and unresponsive to anticonvulsants was described in two patients during ethanol withdrawal. No other structural or metabolic abnormality was found.[293]

Panic disorder is unexpectedly prevalent among alcoholics, especially in those with repeated episodes of withdrawal.[294]

Seizures

Ethanol can precipitate seizures in known epileptics, but the amount required is uncertain.[295–297] In nondrinking epileptics, "social" amounts of vodka (10–30 g of ethanol) twice weekly for 16 weeks had no effect on seizure frequency, anticonvulsant blood levels, or EEG findings.[298] How much a nonalcoholic epileptic can safely drink is unknown.

By contrast, ethanol causes seizures in alcoholics whether or not they are epileptic.[299] A widely cited study of ethanol-related seizures reviewed 241 patients seen over 15 years with both alcoholism and seizures, either prevalent or incident.[300] This and subsequent studies reinforced the concept that otherwise unexplained seizures in alcoholics ("alcohol seizures," "rum fits") are the result of withdrawal.[301] Either a single major motor seizure or a cluster occurring over several hours typically begins between 6 and 48 hours after cessation of chronic drinking. Status epilepticus occurs in fewer than 10%, but in communities with high alcoholism prevalence, ethanol accounts for a substantial proportion of status epilepticus cases.[302–304] Focal features, not always attributable to previous head injury or other brain lesions, are seen in up to 25%.[300,302] Alcohol seizures sometimes occur in otherwise asymptomatic patients and sometimes accompany tremor or hallucinosis.

How much ethanol is required to provoke alcohol seizures? In a classic review, Victor and Adams[277] stated that such seizures "tend to affect alcoholics only after many years of excessive drinking." Isbell et al,[252] studying 10 opioid-dependent volunteers, observed seizures in two made abruptly abstinent after several weeks of continuous drinking; both had been alcoholic in the past, however, and one may have had previous ethanol-related seizures. A seizure prevalence of 20% during ethanol withdrawal, moreover, is unusually high; in one study of 1024 alcoholics detoxified without psychoactive drugs, only 1% had seizures during withdrawal.[305] In a case–control study of incident seizures at Harlem Hospital Center, chronic daily ingestion of 50 g ethanol raised the odds ratio above 1, and at 200 g daily it was 20, but the minimal duration of drinking that conferred increased risk of seizures could not be determined.[306,307] In that study statistical analysis failed to demonstrate a clear-cut temporal relationship between seizures and early abstinence; many seizures occurred either during active drinking or more than a week after stopping, and those who had recently increased their ethanol consumption tended to have seizures sooner after the last drink than those who had decreased their consumption.

Both animal and human studies have led to a general acceptance of the concept of alcohol withdrawal seizures.[301,308] Relative and protracted withdrawal have been invoked to explain seizures occurring outside the period of early abstinence. An alternative possibility is that ethanol causes seizures by more than one mechanism.[309] In the past, the diagnosis of alcohol withdrawal seizures has been made by exclusion in heavy drinkers. The Harlem Hospital study, suggesting that some seizures considered withdrawal are not necessarily so, is consistent with a trend in the literature: as diagnostic accuracy improved, fewer seizures in drinkers were presumptively attributed to withdrawal, from 88% in 1967[300] to 59% in 1976[302] and 31% in 1980.[310] Animal studies indicate that seizures during ethanol withdrawal are of more than one type, with different time courses, phenomenology, and presumed neuronal mechanisms.[311] For example, withdrawal seizures in rodents are readily triggered by sound (audiogenic seizures) and appear to be initiated in the inferior colliculus.[312]

An Italian multicenter case–control study compared 237 patients with new-onset seizures with 474 hospital controls. Results were remarkably similar to the Harlem Hospital study. An increased risk of seizures appeared only above 50 g daily absolute ethanol for men and 25 g daily for women and rose in a dose-dependent fashion to an odds ratio of 16.6 for those drinking more than 200 g daily. That study did not address temporal relationships between seizures and active drinking.[313]

In another study the same investigators reported that ethanol did not increase the risk of symptomatic new-onset seizures in patients with head trauma, stroke, or brain tumor.[314] The average ethanol intake for patients was only 39 g per day, however, and no patient drank more than 200 g per day, an amount that conferred risk for new-onset symptomatic seizures in the Harlem Hospital study.

Ethanol-related seizures often do occur in patients with previous brain injury, and periodic lateralizing epileptiform discharges (PLEDS) are sometimes observed during ethanol withdrawal.[315,316] Some studies found the risk of seizures to increase with repeated ethanol detoxification, compatible with a kindling phenomenon.[317–319] This observation led to speculation that repeated severe withdrawal symptoms, including seizures, could result in permanent synaptic alteration and the development of non-withdrawal alcoholic epilepsy.[296]

The diagnosis of alcohol seizures requires exclusion of other lesions. Even though the yield is low in the absence of focal neurological signs,[320] computed tomography (CT) scan or magnetic resonance imaging (MRI) is indicated when seizures are of new onset, and a spinal tap is necessary if meningitis or subarachnoid hemorrhage is suspected and imaging does not reveal intracranial blood. Previous alcohol seizures do not exclude the possibility that a recurrent seizure has a more ominous cause. The electroencephalogram in patients with alcohol seizures is usually normal; the claim[300] that photomyoclonic or photoconvulsive responses are common during early withdrawal—with or without seizures—was not borne out by subsequent studies,[319,321] including a prospective analysis of 49 untreated patients from Harlem Hospital Center in which photomyoclonic response occurred in only two (4%) and photoconvulsive response in none.[322]

Delirium Tremens

In contrast to tremor, hallucinosis, and seizures, delirium tremens typically begins 48 to 72 hours after the last drink. Because of the popular misconception that any alcoholic with tremor and hallucinations has delirium tremens, it is overdiagnosed. In fact, delirium tremens consists of not only tremor and disordered sensory perception (illusions or hallucinations) but also delirium (defined as extreme inattentiveness and apparent nonawareness of the environment, usually with agitation and sometimes with depressed alertness), autonomic overactivity, and frequently a fatal outcome. In one series the syndrome was present in fewer than 5% of hospitalized patients with symptomatic ethanol withdrawal.[277] About one-third of patients with early alcohol seizures develop delirium tremens, but seizures during delirium tremens are unusual and suggest an additional diagnosis such as meningitis.

Delirium tremens tends to begin and end abruptly, lasting hours to a few days. Inattentiveness and confusion may rapidly alternate with lucidity, or symptoms may subside gradually. Concurrent disease such as liver failure, pneumonia, or pancreatitis increases the severity of delirium tremens, and relapses can occur for up to several weeks.[315,323,324] Elderly patients have more severe symptoms.[325] A typical patient is agitated and grossly tremulous, with fever, tachycardia, and profuse sweating. Tremor may be so widespread as to involve the face, tongue, and pharynx.[279] The patient picks at the bedclothes or stares wildly about, shouting at hallucinated objects or trying to fend them off. Fluid loss can be marked, and heat stroke or myoglobinuria are occasional features.[324] Less readily diagnosed are patients with "quiet delirium" or those with a single predominant symptom such as confusion, hallucinations, or delusions. Patients otherwise calm may have striking misperceptions, believing that they are drinking in a bar or, with extreme suggestibility, claiming to see objects described by the examiner but not actually present. In contrast to patients with early hallucinosis, who later can describe their illusions or hallucinations, those with full-blown delirium tremens seldom recall the episode.

In some patients with delirium tremens, tremor and signs of autonomic hyperactivity clear after a few days, yet delirium persists for up to a few weeks. Such "protracted alcohol withdrawal delirium" is not well-understood.[326,327]

The level of severity that separates the early and late ethanol withdrawal syndromes is not easy to define. A patient with early tremor, hallucinations, and otherwise clear sensorium is easily distinguished from one with full-blown delirium tremens, but some patients seem to fall between these extremes,

with widely varying combinations of symptoms and signs (Table 12-11).[328] Ethanol withdrawal might be viewed as a continuum of severity, determined not only by the amount of recent drinking but, again analogous to kindling, by the total duration of drinking and the number of previous withdrawal episodes. Moreover, chronic alcoholics have at least a brief withdrawal period every day. Even in drinkers without previous overt withdrawal symptoms, a kindling model might explain the observation that delirium tremens occurs most often after at least 10 years of alcoholism.[329]

In the past, reported mortality for delirium tremens was as high as 15%, mostly attributable to associated disease such as pneumonia or sepsis;

Table 12–11. Symptoms and Signs of Ethanol Withdrawal

Mood/Affect
Anxiety
Restlessness
Irritability
Depression

Gastrointestinal disturbance
Anorexia
Nausea
Vomiting
Other gastrointestinal disturbance

Autonomic nervous system disturbance
Fever
Hypothermia
Sweating
Flushing
Tachycardia
Palpitations
Hypertension
Headache

Neurological disturbance
Tremor
Impaired coordination
Decreased concentration
Dizziness
Altered consciousness

Sleep disturbance
Insomnia
Other sleep disturbance

Psychotic features
Illusions
Hallucinations (visual, auditory, tactile)
Delusions

Seizures

patients with delirium tremens are often hospitalized for a different problem. Sometimes death follows unexplained shock or occurs suddenly without apparent cause. Fatalities are variably attributed to cardiac arrhythmia, fat emboli, and heat stroke. Modern intensive care has greatly reduced mortality in delirium tremens.

Pathophysiology of Ethanol Withdrawal

Numerous neurophysiological abnormalities undoubtedly contribute to the symptoms and signs of ethanol withdrawal. Dexamethasone-suppression and corticotropin-releasing hormone tests in alcoholics demonstrate exaggerated release of corticotropin and vasopressin during withdrawal.[330] Glutamatergic up-regulation stimulates the release of corticotropin releasing hormone itself.[331] Increased plasma renin and aldosterone levels occur, and in mice intracerebroventricular injection of atrial natriuretic peptide attenuated the severity of handling-induced convulsions.[332] In a study of Japanese alcoholic men with different withdrawal syndromes (either delirium tremens, seizures, or hallucinations), a particular polymorphism of the gene for neuropeptide Y was associated with withdrawal seizures.[333]

The principal determinant of ethanol withdrawal in its several forms is glutamate receptor up-regulation.[74] Concomitant down-regulation of GABA receptors likely contributes.[334] The period of up-regulated glutamate receptors (NMDA and AMPA) in the VTA, the locus ceruleus, and other structures coincides with the time course of withdrawal seizures and autonomic instability in animals during withdrawal, and the NMDA receptor blocker dizocilpine decreases the occurrence and severity of ethanol withdrawal seizures.[335] Neuronal excitotoxicity occurring during withdrawal would plausibly explain the kindling pattern of repeated withdrawal episodes, including the likelihood and severity of seizures.[336-338] Excitotoxicity might also set the stage for seizures in alcoholics that occur, as in the study from Harlem Hospital Center, in the absence of withdrawal.[74,306,339,340] (Excitotoxicity also probably plays a key role in the pathophysiology of both Wernicke–Korsakoff syndrome and alcoholic dementia: see later.)

Treatment of Ethanol Withdrawal

Principles of Treatment

Dozens of drugs have been studied in patients withdrawing from ethanol; unfortunately, most of the literature on treatment is useless. Controls are lacking, and it is seldom stated what in fact was the aim of therapy, for example, relief of tremor, prevention of delirium tremens, or management of delirium tremens.[247,341] Some workers believe that early treatment of ethanol withdrawal can prevent delirium tremens; others doubt that such intervention can either prevent it or reduce its mortality.

Some recommend that mildly symptomatic patients be managed nonpharmacologically with reassurance, reduced sensory stimuli, rest, hydration, and nutrition.[315,342,343] In addition to avoiding unnecessary medication, such patients might experience negatively reinforcing symptoms that would decrease the likelihood of later relapse.[315] Others recommend sedatives either to prevent or to relieve early mild withdrawal symptoms (Table 12–12).[344] Such is the usual practice at Harlem Hospital Center, an acute-care-oriented and understaffed institution with frequent admissions for ethanol-related

Table 12–12. Treatment of Ethanol Withdrawal

Prevention or reduction of early mild symptoms:
Chlordiazepoxide 25–100 mg or diazepam 5–20 mg orally every 8 hours for the first day, tapering over 3 to 6 days
Thiamine 100 mg and multivitamins

For more severe symptoms, including delirium tremens:
Diazepam 10 mg intravenously or lorazepam 2 mg intravenously or intramuscularly, repeated every 5 to 15 minutes until calming and normalization of vital signs. Maintenance doses every 1 to 4 hours as needed
If refractory to benzodiazepines, phenobarbital 260 mg intravenously repeated in 30 minutes as needed
If refractory to phenobarbital, pentobarbital 3–5 mg/kg intravenously, with endotracheal intubation and repeated doses to produce general anesthesia
Careful attention to fluid and electrolyte balance; several liters of saline per day, or even pressors, may be needed
Cooling blanket or alcohol sponges for high fever
Prevent or correct hypoglycemia
Thiamine and multivitamins
Consider coexisting illness, e.g., liver failure, pancreatitis, sepsis, meningitis, or subdural hematoma

illness. Obviously sedatives must be used cautiously in patients with liver disease, head injury, or chronic obstructive pulmonary disease; indeed, respiratory depression following sedation can cause hypoxic mental changes that are misdiagnosed as worsening withdrawal symptoms.[315]

Rational pharmacotherapy of ethanol withdrawal calls for an agent cross-tolerant with ethanol, and benzodiazepines have replaced paraldehyde and barbiturates as the drugs of choice.[282,345–347] For prevention or reduction of mild early symptoms a long-acting benzodiazepine such as chlordiazepoxide or diazepam can be given orally in tapering doses. For treatment of more severe symptoms parenteral therapy may be necessary, and opinions differ as to which benzodiazepine is preferable.[348,349] Diazepam's prolonged duration of action (half life 43 ± 13 hours, including that of its active metabolite desmethyldiazepam) means that infrequent doses are needed once patients are stabilized.[350] Intramuscular absorption of diazepam is unpredictable, however, whereas lorazepam is rapidly and completely absorbed from intramuscular sites, and its intermediate half-life (14 ± 5 hours) means that a steady state is reached in 36 to 48 hours without extensive accumulation.[282] Moreover, in contrast to diazepam, neither lorazepam nor the shorter-acting oxazepam (half-life 8 ± 2.4 hours) undergo hepatic oxidation.[347] Finally, although it is less likely to accumulate than diazepam, lorazepam's anticonvulsant actions are more prolonged.[351]

If a long-acting benzodiazepine is used, it can be given in either a loading-dose regimen or a tapered dose regimen. In a loading-dose regimen a large dose (e.g., diazepam 20 mg) is given orally every hour until the patient is mildly intoxicated (calming, dysarthria, ataxia, fine nystagmus); the drug is then stopped and not resumed unless withdrawal symptoms appear. In a tapered-dose regimen smaller doses (e.g., diazepam 5–10 mg) are given every few hours for one or more days and then tapered over the next several days.

Because large amounts of long-acting benzodiazepines accumulate, dosage must be carefully titrated to avoid either oversedation (including precipitation of hepatic encephalopathy) or reappearance of withdrawal signs. For patients with moderate-to-severe symptoms a symptom-triggered regimen might be employed.[352] For example,

lorazepam 2 mg or diazepam 10 mg can be given parenterally and repeated every 5 to 15 minutes until calming and normalization of vital signs, with maintenance doses every hour or more as needed.[353] Such a regimen reportedly decreased the occurrence of delirium tremens.[354] An alternative choice is a benzodiazepine with an even shorter half-life than lorazepam, for example, oxazepam. For critically ill patients the very short-acting midazolam has been recommended. Older patients and heavy smokers may require unusually high doses of benzodiazepines.[325]

Many patients with mild-to-moderate withdrawal symptoms can be effectively treated as outpatients, which substantially reduces costs. Such an approach is of course impractical in some communities; in one study more inpatients (95%) than outpatients (72%) completed detoxification.[355]

Early or Mild Symptoms

Reports are conflicting on the efficacy of neuroleptics in early hallucinosis. They are not cross-tolerant with ethanol; they lower seizure threshold; and they cause hypotension, liver damage, acute dystonia, skin rash, bone marrow suppression, and impaired thermoregulation. Several studies found an increased frequency of seizures, delirium tremens, and death in patients receiving phenothiazines compared with those given placebo.[356–358] Neuroleptics are appropriately considered in patients whose only symptoms are hallucinations (especially when accompanied by delusions) or in whom hallucinations have outlasted other withdrawal symptoms.[281]

Blood and urinary catecholamines and their metabolites are increased during ethanol withdrawal and probably contribute to symptoms.[359] Propranolol decreases tremor and cardiac arrhythmia[360,361] but is no more effective than benzodiazepines and in one study exacerbated hallucinations.[362] Some workers have reported favorable results with clonidine,[345,359,363] atenolol,[364-366] or lofexidine.[359,367,368] One study of clonidine, however, found high frequencies of hallucinations, seizures, orthostatic hypotension, and drowsiness.[369]

Anticonvulsants, including carbamazepine, valproate, gabapentin, and vigabatrin, have also been used to treat ethanol withdrawal whether or not seizures were present.[370] In controlled trials carbamazepine was superior to placebo and equal in efficacy to phenobarbital or oxazepam in patients with mild-to-moderate withdrawal symptoms. In abstinent humans carbamazepine reportedly prevented not only seizures but also tremor, sweating, gastrointestinal symptoms, irritability, and insomnia.[371] Controlled trials found valproate to be more effective than either placebo or carbamazepine in preventing both withdrawal seizures and other severe symptoms.[372]

It should be emphasized that while neuroleptics, beta-blockers, clonidine, or anticonvulsants might suppress certain manifestations of ethanol withdrawal, they do not—in contrast to drugs cross-tolerant with ethanol—treat the primary neurological derangement.[350]

In that regard, a seemingly logical approach to therapy would be ethanol itself, the treatment nonhospitalized patients choose for themselves. Parenteral ethanol, however, has a low therapeutic index and is potentially hazardous. Moreover, ethanol has direct organ toxicity, including the CNS. Even though most patients resume drinking on discharge, ethanol has no role in the prevention or treatment of withdrawal symptoms.

If increased glutamatergic neurotransmission is the fundamental abnormality in ethanol withdrawal, antiglutamatergic agents or drugs affecting membrane calcium flux should be beneficial. Favorable responses to calcium channel blockers are described,[373–375] and, as noted, dizocilpine prevents ethanol withdrawal seizures in animals.[335] Unlike GABAergic drugs such as benzodiazepines and barbiturates, glutamatergic blockers would theoretically prevent excitotoxicity and perhaps kindled withdrawal symptoms and other neurotoxic consequences of glutamatergic disinhibition.[74] Such agents are not yet available.

In animals, nitric oxide synthase inhibition enhances the acute depressant effects of ethanol and decreases signs of ethanol withdrawal.[376]

South African investigators found nitrous oxide beneficial during ethanol withdrawal in humans. Doses were used that preserved full alertness. A proposed mechanism related to nitrous oxide's alleged agonist effects on limbic opioid systems.[377]

In Scandinavia, electroconvulsant therapy has been recommended for patients with persistent delirium.[378]

Seizures

The use of short-term anticonvulsants for ethanol-related seizures is controversial. In animals and humans, phenytoin failed to prevent alcohol seizures.[379,380] In rats, valproate and carbamazepine prevented withdrawal seizures,[381] and, as noted above, carbamazepine and valproate each reportedly prevented seizures in abstinent humans.[371,372]

A randomized, double-masked study compared intravenous lorazepam (2 mg) with placebo in alcoholics seen in an emergency department after a generalized seizure.[382] Over the next 6 hours 3% of those receiving lorazepam had a second generalized seizure compared with 24% of those receiving placebo (odds ratio for placebo: 10.4; $P<0.001$). Of those not admitted (71% of the lorazepam group, 58% of the placebo group), one from the lorazepam group and seven from the placebo group had a second seizure within 48 hours. The study did not report how many in each group went on to develop delirium tremens.

The treatment of status epilepticus during ethanol withdrawal is conventional. Intravenous diazepam and phenobarbital have the advantage, compared with phenytoin, of preventing or reducing other withdrawal symptoms.

Long-term anticonvulsants are generally not indicated in patients with alcohol seizures. Abstainers do not need them, and drinkers do not take them. Of agents that can be taken once daily, phenytoin is probably ineffective and phenobarbital can cause synergistic CNS depression. Of safer agents with possible efficacy, valproate and carbamazepine require twice- or thrice-daily dosage, virtually ensuring noncompliance.

Minerals and Vitamins

Respiratory alkalosis and hypomagnesemia occur during early ethanol withdrawal and return to normal before the appearance of delirium tremens.[383] Hyperventilation may recur during delirium tremens, but hypomagnesemia does not.[253] Both intracellular shift and body loss probably contribute to hypomagnesemia.[384] Attempts to correlate hypomagnesemia with alcohol seizures failed to produce convincing evidence of cause and effect, but hypomagnesemia could be contributory, and so magnesium sulfate is given to hypomagnesemic patients in early withdrawal.[383] Hypokalemia and hypocalcemia may also be present, and the latter sometimes responds to treatment only after hypomagnesemia is corrected.[385]

Thiamine and multivitamins are indicated even if there are no clinical signs of their depletion, for glucose can precipitate Wernicke syndrome in patients with borderline thiamine deficiency. There is often impaired gastrointestinal absorption of thiamine, which is therefore given parenterally.

Delirium Tremens

In contrast to early ethanol withdrawal—or to withdrawal from other drugs such as opioids—delirium tremens once present cannot be abruptly reversed by any agent, including sedatives cross-tolerant with ethanol (see Table 12–12). The treatment of delirium tremens is an emergency, and its cornerstone is sedation. Patients vary greatly in the dosage of benzodiazepine necessary for effective sedation; huge amounts are often required—for example, more than 2500 mg diazepam in the first 48 hours.[282] In some patients benzodiazepines are simply ineffective; it is postulated that the previously coupled chloride channel and benzodiazepine receptor become "uncoupled." Such a situation calls for switching to an intravenous barbiturate.[350]

The major hazard of high-dose benzodiazepine or barbiturate treatment is hepatic encephalopathy; liver disease decreases the metabolism of diazepam, and brains of patients with liver failure are hypersensitive to sedatives. The result can be coma lasting days.

The treatment of delirium tremens calls for an intensive care unit. Patients should be prone or in lateral decubitus position and restrained as needed. Oral medications are avoided. Most patients are dehydrated, some severely so, and many require up to 10 liters of intravenous saline daily. Patients with liver disease, however, retain sodium and water. Hyponatremia must be treated cautiously to avoid central pontine myelinolysis, and hypokalemia can cause cardiac arrhythmia. Fever, with or without infection, is often marked, requiring alcohol sponges, a cooling blanket, or parenteral cooling. Hypoglycemia may be unrecognized, and possible coexisting illnesses include liver failure, pancreatitis, sepsis, meningitis, and subdural hematoma.

Indirect Effects of Ethanol: Nutritional

Wernicke–Korsakoff Syndrome

History and Definition

In 1881 Carl Wernicke described altered mentation, abnormal eye movements, and ataxic gait in three patients; two were alcoholic, and one had persistent vomiting. All died, and at autopsy there were hemorrhagic lesions adjacent to the third and fourth ventricles and the aqueduct of Sylvius.[386] A few years later, S. S. Korsakoff described mental disturbance and polyneuropathy in alcoholics and noted a particular vulnerability of recent memory.[387] Subsequent investigators concluded that Wernicke and Korsakoff syndromes share the same pathology and are caused by thiamine deficiency. The clinical and pathological spectra of 245 patients with Wernicke–Korsakoff syndrome are the subject of a classic monograph by Victor et al.[388]

Although pathologically similar, Wernicke and Korsakoff syndromes are clinically distinct. Fullblown Wernicke syndrome consists of abnormal mentation, eye movements, and gait. Korsakoff syndrome is a qualitatively different mental disturbance (Table 12–13).

Wernicke Syndrome

In acute Wernicke syndrome mental symptoms evolve over days or weeks to a "global confusional state,"[388] with varying degrees of lethargy, inattentiveness, abulia, decreased spontaneous speech, and impaired memory.[389] Disordered perception is common; a patient might identify the hospital room as his or her apartment or a bar. In fewer than 10% is mentation normal. Stupor and coma were unusual in Victor's series but were the main findings in patients reported from Norway[390] and New Zealand.[391] In fact, in the Norwegian series, only one of 22 cases of autopsy-verified Wernicke syndrome had been diagnosed clinically. Similarly, in Perth, Australia, Wernicke syndrome was present at 2.8% of autopsies but had been diagnosed clinically only one-fifth of the time.[392] Many patients with the neuropathology of Wernicke syndrome do not display the full clinical triad of symptoms.[393]

Abnormal eye movements include nystagmus (horizontal and less often vertical or rotatory),

Table 12–13. Major Nutritional Disturbances in Alcoholics

Disorder	Clinical Features	Deficiency
Wernicke syndrome	Dementia, with lethargy, inattentiveness, apathy, and amnesia Ophthalmoparesis Gait ataxia	Thiamine
Korsakoff syndrome	Dementia, mainly amnesia, with or without confabulation	Thiamine
Cerebellar degeneration	Gait ataxia; limb coordination relatively preserved	?
Polyneuropathy	Distal limb sensory loss and weakness; less often autonomic dysfunction	?
Amblyopia	Optic atrophy, decreased visual acuity, central scotomas; total blindness rare	?
Pellagra	Skin rash, vomiting and diarrhea, delirium or dementia	Nicotinic acid

lateral rectus palsy (bilateral but usually asymmetric), and conjugate gaze palsy (horizontal with or without vertical, usually upward).[394] Progression leads to complete ophthalmoplegia. Sluggish pupillary reflexes and mild anisocoria are common, but unreactivity to light and ptosis are rare. Pretectal syndrome—pupillary light-near dissociation, limited upgaze, and convergence-retraction nystagmus—is observed,[395] as are internuclear ophthalmoplegia and ocular bobbing.[396]

More than 80% of patients have truncal ataxia, sometimes of a severity that prevents standing or walking. Limb ataxia is infrequent, especially in the arms; so is dysarthria. Peripheral neuropathy is present in the great majority.[388] Abnormal caloric vestibular testing was found in 17 consecutive patients with acute Wernicke syndrome, gradually improving over several months.[397]

Patients with Wernicke syndrome frequently have signs of nutritional deficiency, such as skin changes, red tongue, and cheilosis. They also often have jaundice, ascites, or spider angiomas. Although beri-beri heart disease is rare, tachycardia, dyspnea on exertion, and postural hypotension (unexplained by hypovolemia) are common, and sudden circulatory collapse can follow mild exertion.[398] Hypothermia and thermolability are not unusual.[399] Fever usually indicates infection. Severe metabolic acidosis is described.[400,401] In an unusual case, dysphagia preceded other signs of Wernicke's encephalopathy by 4 weeks, clearing with treatment.[402]

The electroencephalogram during acute Wernicke syndrome may show diffuse slowing or be normal.[388] Cerebral blood flow and cerebral oxygen and glucose consumption are "strikingly reduced"

independently of the level of alertness or the EEG findings.[403] Cerebrospinal fluid is normal except for occasional mild protein elevation. Elevated blood pyruvate, falling with treatment, is nonspecific. Decreased blood transketolase activity (which requires thiamine pyrophosphate as a cofactor) more reliably indicates thiamine deficiency and in experimental animals falls after only 2 days of restriction.[388] CT scanning sometimes shows diencephalic periventricular low-density abnormalities.[404,405] MRI shows abnormal signals in the periaqueductal area, medial thalamus, and, less often, splenium of the corpus callosum as well as mammillary body atrophy, sometimes evolving after treatment has been given.[406,407] Diffusion-weighted MRI imaging (DWI) also produces characteristic midline signals and can be useful in identifying early lesions and in providing prognostic clues.[408–410,410a,410b] DWI hyperintensities coupled with reduced apparent diffusion coefficients suggest irreversible tissue damage,[411] yet such changes can resolve with appropriate therapy.[412]

Korsakoff Syndrome

In the great majority of cases the more purely amnesic syndrome of Korsakoff emerges as other mental symptoms of Wernicke syndrome respond to treatment. How often Korsakoff syndrome arises without preceding Wernicke syndrome and how often the mental abnormality is restricted to memory are important questions in the current controversy over alcoholic dementia (see later). It is possible that repeated episodes of thiamine deficiency and "subclinical Wernicke disease" can eventually result in clinically significant persistent cognitive dysfunction.[413] The amnesia of such patients is both anterograde, with inability to retain new information, and retrograde, with lost recall for events months or years old.[414] Alertness, attentiveness, and behavior are relatively preserved, but there tends to be a lack of spontaneous speech or activity. Confabulation is not invariable and if initially present tends gradually to disappear. Insight is usually impaired, and there may be flagrant anosognosia for the mental disturbance.

In patients with pathologically verified Korsakoff syndrome psychological testing reveals cognitive impairment not explained by pure memory loss,[388] and different investigators have considered the fundamental defect either a disorder of temporal sequencing, an inability to adopt a new "mental set" to a changing situation, or separable perceptual and mnemonic disturbances.[415] Some have found remote memory to be as impaired as recent,[416] whereas others have observed steep temporal gradients in the retrograde amnesia.[417,418] Many patients are as likely to scramble past information as to forget it, for example, producing a year and a President that do not match. Such temporal confusion may influence the content of confabulation, with the information proffered signifying temporal displacement rather than complete fabrication. In any event the combination of anterograde and retrograde disturbance indicates abnormalities of both memorization and retrieval. In contrast to patients with Alzheimer's disease, Korsakoff patients tend to have normal primary or working memory (retention over 30 seconds, e.g., digit span) and semantic memory (memory for facts, concepts, or language); their impairment is one of episodic memory—specific verbal and visuo-spatial learning and retrieval. Similar to patients with Alzheimer's disease, Korsakoff patients have normal procedural memory (skill learning).[419]

Pathology of Wernicke-Korsakoff Syndrome

The histopathological lesions of Wernicke-Korsakoff syndrome consist of variable degrees of neuronal, axonal, and myelin loss; prominent blood vessels (secondary to endothelial and adventitial thickening); reactive microglia, macrophages, and astrocytes; and, infrequently, small hemorrhages.[388] (Large brainstem and thalamic hemorrhages were found at autopsy in two patients who had Wernicke syndrome plus liver and kidney failure,[420] and in another report CT scan showed primary intraventricular hemorrhage.[421]) Nerve cells may be relatively preserved in the presence of extensive myelin destruction and gliosis, and chronically astrocytosis predominates. Patients with "active" (acute and subacute) disease are more likely than patients with "inactive" (chronic) disease to have swollen capillary endothelium, macrophage response, and reactive astrocytes, and less likely to have spongy tissue, gliosis, and hemosiderin-filled old macrophages.[422] Lesions affect the thalamus (especially the dorsomedial nucleus and the medial pulvinar), the hypothalamus (especially, and perhaps invariably, the mammillary bodies), the midbrain (especially the periaqueductal areas), and the pons and medulla (especially the abducens and medial vestibular nuclei). Some reports describe loss of GABA-containing neurons in the superior prefrontal cortex of alcoholics with Wernicke–Korsakoff syndrome but not in "uncomplicated alcoholics."[413,423] Also described is neuronal loss in the nucleus basalis of Meynert, the locus ceruleus, and the dorsal raphe nuclei of the brainstem. In the cerebellum, severe Purkinje cell loss with Bergmann astrocytosis accompanies lesser degrees of neuronal loss and gliosis in the molecular and granular layers. Such changes are usually limited to the anterior-superior vermis.[388]

Controversial is whether the hippocampus is damaged in Wernicke–Korsakoff syndrome. MRI studies have shown significant reductions in hippocampal volume,[424–426] and autopsies have shown loss of hippocampal white matter volume with[427] or without[428] neuronal loss.

Clinical-Pathological Correlation

Attempts to correlate the anatomical lesions with symptoms and signs are controversial. Blaming the memory loss of Korsakoff syndrome on mammillary body damage is tempting in view of that structure's extensive connections with the hippocampus. There are, however, examples of severe mammillary body damage without memory impairment, and in Victor's series amnesia correlated better with lesions of the dorsomedial thalamic nuclei.[388] In an autopsy study in which strict criteria were applied to identify alcoholics with and without Korsakoff syndrome and in which subjects with liver disease were excluded, neurodegeneration of the mammillary bodies and the dorsomedial thalamic nuclei were substantial in both amnesic and non-amnesic alcoholics with evidence of Wernicke syndrome; however, neuronal loss in the anterior thalamic nuclei was consistently present only in alcoholics with Korsakoff syndrome.[429] (The anterior thalamic nuclei receive major projections from the mammillary bodies—the mammillothalamic tracts—and their selective damage in animals and humans causes severe memory impairment.[429,430])

Correlation of anterograde amnesia with hippocampal volume loss has been claimed[424] and denied.[425]

The combination of severely impaired anterograde verbal and visuospatial learning and retrieval with preserved primary working memory, semantic memory, and procedural memory is compatible with cholinergic impairment—in fact, more so than the broader amnestic constellation of Alzheimer's disease. Indeed, thiamine depletion inhibits acetylcholine synthesis,[431] and, as noted above, cholinergic neurons in the basal forebrain are depleted in Korsakoff syndrome.[432] The global confusion of Wernicke syndrome, on the other hand, can occur without visible thalamic lesions and may be related to cerebral thiamine depletion.[388] Patients with either Korsakoff syndrome or Alzheimer's disease have a more temporally extensive retrograde amnesia than is usually found with traumatic amnesia, hippocampal ischemia, or transient global amnesia, and the extent of retrograde amnesia parallels psychometric frontal lobe dysfunction. These findings suggest that although diencephalic lesions may account for anterograde amnesia, additional cortical pathology contributes to retrograde amnesia as well as non-amnesic cognitive abnormalities.[433–435]

Periaqueductal and oculomotor or abducens nucleus lesions are often found in patients whose eye movements became normal before death.[388] Both cerebellar and vestibular lesions probably contribute to ataxia; avian thiamine deficiency causes peripheral labyrinthine degeneration.[436]

Thiamine and Wernicke–Korsakoff Syndrome

Experimental and clinical evidence supports the specific role of thiamine in the Wernicke–Korsakoff syndrome. Thiamine pyrophosphate (TPP), the active form of thiamine, is a cofactor for several enzymes involved in glucose metabolism, including transketolase, alpha-ketoglutarate dehydrogenase, pyruvate dehydrogenase, and branched-chain alpha-ketoacid dehydrogenase.[8] It may have direct actions on axonal conduction and synaptic transmission. The triphosphate ester of thiamine (TTP), present in brain, is involved in the modulation of chloride channels.[437] Thiamine deficiency rapidly leads to decreased cerebral glucose utilization, and increased lactate production precedes visible lesions in vulnerable brain areas, probably reflecting a shift from aerobic metabolism to anaerobic glycolysis.[438–440]

Alcoholics have several reasons to be thiamine deficient.[441] First, compared with other nutrients such as cobalamin, thiamine body stores are limited—only 30–100 mg—and malnutrition can produce clinically significant depletion within weeks.[442] Liver disease further reduces the body pool. Second, ethanol damages the intestinal mucosa and inhibits the active transport mechanism necessary for thiamine absorption. Third, ethanol inhibits the enzyme that converts thiamine to TPP and stimulates the enzymes that break down TPP; active thiamine can therefore be reduced in the brain even in the presence of adequate nutrition and absorption.[441,443]

Wernicke encephalopathy also follows thiamine deficiency in nonalcoholics, including starvation diets, anorexia nervosa, gastrointestinal disease, and acquired immunodeficiency syndrome (AIDS).[444,445] Such patients are less likely to progress to a chronic severe Korsakoff amnestic state, however, favoring a role for ethanol toxicity in alcoholics with chronic cognitive impairment[446] (see later). (It is noteworthy, however, that ethanol did not appear to play a role in 16 of Korsakoff's original 46 patients.[414]) Animal studies suggest synergism of thiamine deficiency and ethanol toxicity in producing neuronal damage.[447]

After an observation period, patients with acute Wernicke syndrome were given different vitamins, and improvement occurred only after thiamine.[448] Thiamine-deficient foxes, cats, pigeons, rats, and monkeys develop lesions similar to those of Wernicke–Korsakoff syndrome.[436,449] Thiamine deficiency in rhesus monkeys caused anorexia, apathy, lethargy, and lower extremity weakness, promptly relieved by thiamine; during subsequent episodes of thiamine deprivation, symptoms were more severe and included ataxia and abnormal eye movements; pair-fed controls remained asymptomatic.[450] In both rats and monkeys thiamine deficiency causes learning and memory impairment which correlates with neuronal loss in the diencephalon and cerebral cortex. Oscillations of thiamine levels, comparable to those that occur in alcoholic patients, may be worse than chronic low levels.[450]

Wernicke–Korsakoff syndrome occurs in only a small minority of alcoholic or otherwise malnourished people and seems particularly to affect whites, suggesting a genetic influence. At Harlem Hospital Center, where prior to the AIDS epidemic nearly half of medical admissions were ethanol-related, 12 cases of Wernicke–Korsakoff syndrome were seen during 1975 through 1979; by contrast, 90 cases were seen at the Boston City Hospital during 1950 through 1951 and 129 cases at the Massachusetts General Hospital during 1952 through 1961.[388] Autopsy findings from different countries reveal considerable differences in the prevalence of Wernicke–Korsakoff syndrome—from 0.4% in France to 2.8% in Australia—with little relationship to per capita ethanol consumption.[451] In Australia the incidence ratio of Wernicke–Korsakoff syndrome to beriberi (thiamine-induced peripheral neuropathy and cardiomyopathy) is 1:5; among Asian populations it is less than 1:1000.[452,453] Particular strains of animals have a hereditary predisposition to the neurological effects of thiamine deficiency,[454–456] and in humans hereditary reduced affinity of transketolase for its cofactor TPP genetically predisposes to Wernicke–Korsakoff syndrome.[457–459] Perhaps Wernicke–Korsakoff syndrome, similar to other inborn errors of metabolism (e.g., glucose-6-phosphate-dehydrogenase deficiency) is the result of a genetic fault that causes symptoms only in the presence of a particular environmental stress.

How thiamine deficiency causes brain damage is unclear and undoubtedly complex. A proposed mechanism begins with decreased α-ketoglutarate dehydrogenase activity due to lack of its TPP cofactor.[445] There follows decreased intracellular energy (ATP) levels, which in turn cause increased release and extracellular levels of glutamate, initiating a cascade of increased intracellular Ca^{2+} and excitotoxicity, with activation of proteases, lipases, and endonucleases, free radical generation, and mitochondrial damage.[442] Contributory factors include reduced extracellular Mg^{2+}, with decrease in the protective, voltage-dependent Mg^{2+} block of the NMDA receptor. Hypomagnesemia also reduces the activity of thiamine-dependent and other enzymes which require Mg^{2+} as a cofactor. Possibly contributing to the damage is increased histamine release in certain diencephalic structures (e.g., thalamus) caused by thiamine deficiency; excessive histamine enhances NMDA activity by antagonizing an outward K^+ current and by directly facilitating the NMDA receptor, perhaps acting at its polyamine site. Finally, decreased activity of thiamine-dependent transketolase results in decreased synthesis of NADPH reducing equivalents and impaired lipid synthesis and amino acid production and transport.[459] In support of this model is the ability of the NMDA blocker dizocilpine to prevent Wernicke–Korsakoff pathology in thiamine-deficient animals.[460] The calcium channel blocker nimodipine also reduces pathological changes in the thalamus in such animals.[461] Consistent with the model is the observation in both animals and humans that thiamine replacement in acute Wernicke syndrome is ineffective unless hypomagnesemia is also corrected.[462] The selective vulnerability of particular structures in the thalamus, hypothalamus, and cerebral cortex is perhaps related to their high energy demands.[463]

Course and Treatment

Untreated acute Wernicke–Korsakofff syndrome is fatal.[464] Mortality was 10% among Victor's treated patients, and the presence of liver failure, infection, and delirium tremens often made the cause of death unclear.[388] Postural hypotension and tachycardia call for strict bed rest; associated medical problems may require intensive care. Thiamine, 50–100 mg, is given daily until a normal diet can be taken. The intravenous route is preferred because of the impaired gastrointestinal absorption of thiamine in chronic alcoholics.[465] In fact, acute Wernicke's encephalopathy followed 12 days of intramuscular thiamine.[466] Alternatively, fat-soluble allithiamines (e.g., thiamine propyl disulfide or thiamine tetra-hydrofurfuryl disulfide) are well absorbed in alcoholic patients.[467] High, efficiently delivered thiamine doses are especially important in patients with genetic low-affinity transketolase.[468] Hypomagnesemia, which retards the response to thiamine, requires early correction, along with other vitamins.[469,470] Protein intake may have to be titrated against the patient's liver status. The likely role of glutamate excitotoxicity in Wernicke–Korsakoff syndrome favors clinical trials with NMDA receptor blockers or inhibitors of glutamate release, but such agents have yet to be proven effective.

Following thiamine treatment, ocular abnormalities, especially abducens and gaze palsies, begin to improve within a few hours and usually resolve within a week; horizontal nystagmus often persists indefinitely. Mentation begins to improve within hours or days, and most patients are alert and attentive within a month; amnesia is then present in more than 80% and eventually clears in fewer than a quarter of cases. Improvement in ataxia begins within a few days but is complete in less than half, and nearly a third show no improvement at all.[388,471]

Improvement in memory was reported in patients with Korsakoff syndrome who received the serotonin uptake inhibitor fluvoxamine.[472] The role of serotonin pathways in mnemonic performance is complex, and the efficacy of such agents requires confirmation. Clonidine (but not L-dopa or ephedrine) reportedly improved anterograde but not retrograde amnesia in patients with Korsakoff syndrome;[473] such benefit was not found by others, however.[474]

The best approach to Wernicke syndrome is preventive. Any alcoholic patient should receive thiamine, as should any patient receiving glucose for unexplained seizures or coma. Wernicke syndrome too often appears in patients hospitalized a few days earlier for some other problem.

On the assumption that 1200 patients with Korsakoff syndrome require institutionalization annually in the United States, with long-term stay in one-third, it was proposed that fortification of alcoholic beverages with thiamine would be cost-effective.[475]

Alcoholic Cerebellar Degeneration

Definition and Clinical Picture

A "restricted form of cerebellar cortical degeneration" occurs in nutritionally deficient alcoholics without other signs of Wernicke–Korsakoff syndrome[476,477] (see Table 12–13). Truncal instability is the major symptom, often with incoordination of individual leg movements. Arm ataxia is much less prominent, and nystagmus, dysarthria, hypotonia, and independent head tremor are rare. Symptoms evolve over years, weeks, or days and eventually stabilize, sometimes even with continued drinking and poor nutrition. Ataxia unassociated with Wernicke syndrome is less likely to appear abruptly or to improve.[388] Stabilization does not occur at the same level of severity in all patients, and in some, years of unchanging ataxia are interrupted by further progression.

Pathology and Pathogenesis

Pathologically the superior vermis is invariably involved, with nerve cell loss and gliosis in the molecular, granular, and especially Purkinje cell layers. There may be secondary degeneration of the olives and the fastigial, emboliform, globose, and vestibular nuclei.[477,478] Involvement of the cerebellar hemispheric cortex is exceptional and limited to the anterior lobes. Pathological evidence of Wernicke syndrome may coexist even though unsuspected clinically. CT and autopsies, moreover, have revealed cerebellar atrophy in alcoholics not clinically ataxic.[479–481] In ataxic patients, positron emission tomography reveals superior vermal hypometabolism, which correlates with symptoms better than does CT atrophy.[482]

Ethanol acutely inhibits Purkinje cell firing,[483] perhaps contributing to the ataxia of inebriation.[484] Alcoholic cerebellar degeneration, however, is probably both nutritional and toxic in origin. As evidence for a nutritional contribution, identical lesions were observed in a nonalcoholic man with intestinal obstruction and "protracted nutritional depletion."[485] Moreover, ataxia can begin in malnourished alcoholics after days or weeks of abstinence.[477] The clinical and pathological similarity of alcoholic cerebellar degeneration to the cerebellar component of Wernicke syndrome further suggests shared mechanisms.[388] The majority of patients with alcoholic cerebellar degeneration, however, do not have pathological evidence of Wernicke syndrome. Cerebellar degeneration occurs in heavy drinkers who are neither amnestic nor evidently under-nourished.[486,487] At Harlem Hospital Center, Wernicke syndrome is unusual, yet alcoholic cerebellar degeneration occurs often, clinically and pathologically. Some workers have demonstrated direct cerebellar neuronal toxicity by ethanol or acetaldehyde.[488,489] In rats, ethanol ingestion causes Purkinje cell dendritic abnormalities not found in paired controls.[490,491] Acutely, ethanol caused neuronal cell death of cultured cerebellar granule cells, an effect prevented by NMDA.[492] Chronic exposure of cultured cerebellar granule cells to ethanol, however, caused up-regulation of NMDA receptors and neuronal damage that was blocked by NMDA receptor antagonists.[493]

Alcoholic Polyneuropathy

Definition and Clinical Picture

Alcoholic polyneuropathy refers to progressive sensorimotor peripheral neuropathy, probably both toxic and nutritional in origin, which stabilizes or improves with abstinence and an adequate diet (see Table 12–13). Alcoholic polyneuropathy is present in most patients with Wernicke–Korsakoff syndrome but more often occurs alone. It tends to be underdiagnosed. Fewer than 10% of alcoholics in one series were said to have peripheral neuropathy (usually in association with Wernicke–Korsakoff syndrome),[324] yet clinical evidence of polyneuropathy was found in one-third of alcoholic patients at Harlem Hospital Center.[494] A careful neurological examination often elicits sensory loss, and nerve conduction and electromyographic abnormalities (especially slowing of the H-reflex) occur in alcoholics without symptoms or signs.[495,496] In several series of patients with alcoholic polyneuropathy, women were overrepresented.[277,497]

Paresthesias are usually the first symptom, progressing over days or weeks to numbness. Burning or lancinating pain and tenderness of the calves or soles can be severe. Mildly-to-moderately impaired vibratory sense is the earliest sign of neuropathy in the great majority of patients; proprioception is usually preserved until other sensory loss has become substantial.

Loss of ankle tendon reflexes is another early sign; eventually there is diffuse hyporeflexia or areflexia. Weakness appears at any time and can become severe after only a few days, resembling Guillain–Barré neuropathy.[498–500] Unlike true Guillain–Barré neuropathy, however, rapidly progressive alcoholic neuropathy with weakness usually causes marked sensory loss as well, cranial nerves and respiration are spared, and cerebrospinal fluid (CSF) protein is normal or only mildly elevated.

Acute axonal polyneuropathy with severe distal weakness occurred in three patients, two of whom were not alcoholic. Signs of Wernicke encephalopathy (and appropriate MRI signal abnormalities) were also present, and both encephalopathy and polyneuropathy rapidly improved with thiamine supplementation. (It was not stated if additional vitamins were given.)[500a]

In typical alcoholic polyneuropathy the distal legs are affected first, although in some patients proximal weakness is greater than distal.[501] Radiologically demonstrable neuropathic arthropathy of the feet is common, as is skin thinning, glossiness, reddening, cyanosis, and hyperhidrosis.[494] Peripheral autonomic involvement, although usually less prominent than in diabetic neuropathy, causes urinary and fecal incontinence, hypotension, hypothermia, cardiac arrhythmia, dysphagia, dysphonia,[501] impaired esophageal peristalsis,[502] altered sweat patterns, and abnormal Valsalva ratio.[503,504] Pupillary parasympathetic denervation is rare.[505] Autonomic signs are associated with increased mortality.[506] The CSF in alcoholic polyneuropathy is normal except for occasional mild elevation of protein.

In a report from Japan, three groups of patients with polyneuropathy were compared clinically and pathologically: those considered to have pure alcoholic neuropathy without thiamine deficiency (ALN), those with alcoholic neuropathy and thiamine deficiency (ALN-TD), and those with pure non-alcoholic thiamine deficiency neuropathy (TDN). It was concluded that ALN is sensory-dominant, slowly progressive, and painful, and that it impairs superficial sensation and causes predominantly small-fiber axonal loss. By contrast, TDN is motor-dominant and acutely progressive, impairs both superficial and deep sensation, and causes predominantly large-fiber axonal loss. ALN-TD produces a mixture of these two forms.[506a]

Pathology and Pathogenesis

Pathologically there is degeneration of both myelin and axons, and controversy exists over which occurs first.[495,497,507,508] Electron microscopic evidence suggests that the earliest changes occur in Schwann cells,[509] but electrophysiological and conventional pathological findings indicate an axonal neuropathy, with small myelinated and unmyelinated fibers more affected than large myelinated fibers.[510] Nerve root involvement causes secondary degeneration of the dorsal columns. Damage to the vagus nerves and the sympathetic trunks occurs in both humans and animals.[501,511]

The basis of alcoholic polyneuropathy has long been debated. Severe weight loss is common, improvement occurs with nutritional supplements despite continued drinking, and abstinent alcoholics receiving a vitamin B-free diet have progressive neuropathic symptoms.[512] Moreover, heavy ethanol consumption for 4 weeks, with adequate diet, failed to produce electromyographic evidence of peripheral nerve damage in three volunteers.[513] Deficiency of more than thiamine may be operative, for although thiamine alone corrects neuropathy in vitamin-deficient pigeons,[514] polyneuropathy is not a feature of experimental thiamine deprivation in mice,[515] cats,[516] pigs,[517] or monkeys,[518] and thiamine deficiency for months produced only mild symptoms and signs of peripheral neuropathy in human volunteers.[519] Polyneuropathy follows deficiency of pantothenic acid,[520,521] pyridoxine,[520,522] and riboflavin[523] in animals and humans. By contrast, mildly slowed nerve conduction velocities, markedly reduced sensory amplitudes, and histological axonal degeneration were observed in alcoholics with polyneuropathy, whereas patients malnourished following gastrectomy had electromyographic and histological abnormalities more consistent with segmental demyelination.[497] The alcoholic patients, moreover, had normal blood thiamine levels, and only a minority had clinical evidence of malnutrition, which did not correlate with severity of neuropathy. In a comparable study, 18 patients had slowly progressive painful sensory polyneuropathy, heavy ethanol consumption (more than 100 g daily for at least 10 years), "normal thiamine status" (whole blood levels and erythrocyte transketolase activity) and predominantly small-fiber loss. By contrast, the authors noted, beri-beri polyneuropathy affects large fibers, painful symptoms are unusual, and motor symptoms are frequent.[510] Ethanol directly impairs fast axonal transport.[524] Such observations, while demonstrating that ethanol is directly toxic to peripheral nerves,[525] do not exclude the possibility that nutritional deficiency is contributory. In any event thiamine and multivitamins should be given to any alcoholic.

Amblyopia

Optic atrophy is common in alcoholics, with progressive visual loss, central or centrocecal scotomas, and temporal disc pallor (see Table 12–13).[526] Optic atrophy is always bilateral, and, because disc pallor is often restricted to the temporal margins, it can be quite subtle. Red–green color blindness occurs.[527] Demyelination affects the optic nerves, chiasm, and tracts, with predilection for the maculopapular bundle; electrophysiological and MRI studies favor the retina as the primary site of pathology.[528,529] The condition used to be called tobacco–alcohol amblyopia and was thought to represent direct toxicity. Amblyopia improved, however, in 25 patients who received dietary supplements but continued to drink ethanol and to smoke. In five of these, the only supplement was thiamine.[530] Amblyopia, moreover, was common among prisoners-of-war during World War II. Such observations do not exclude a contributory role for ethanol or tobacco toxicity, the latter perhaps related to tobacco's cyanide content.

During 1991 through 1993 an epidemic of optic neuropathy and peripheral neuropathy (Strachan syndrome) affected more than 50,000 people in Cuba. Most improved after treatment with vitamins, but tobacco use increased the risk of optic neuropathy.[531] An additional, albeit infrequent, risk factor was mutation of mitochondrial genes encoding subunits of Complex I of the respiratory chain, i.e., subclinical Leber hereditary optic neuropathy.[532]

Acute permanent visual loss in an alcoholic man with mild optic atrophy followed blood loss from peptic ulceration.[533] It is rare, however, for amblyopia in alcoholics to progress to total blindness, and improvement, albeit incomplete, nearly always follows abstinence and nutritional replacement.[528]

Pellagra

Nicotinic acid deficiency in alcoholics produces clinical pellagra, with skin, gastrointestinal, and mental abnormalities[277,534–537] (see Table 12–13).

Stomatitis and enteritis can be severe, with nausea, vomiting, and diarrhea. CNS symptoms include headache, irritability, and insomnia progressing to impaired memory, delusions, hallucinations, dementia, or delirium. In a review of 22 cases, signs progressed over hours, days, or weeks before or during hospitalization; death in several instances followed administration of thiamine and pyridoxine.[535] Frequent were fluctuating "confusion" and "clouding of consciousness," marked oppositional hypertonus (*gegenhalten*), and startle myoclonus. Pathologically there was neuronal chromatolysis, prominent in the brainstem (especially the pontine nuclei) and the cerebellar dentate nuclei. Several patients also had clinical signs of peripheral neuropathy and pathological evidence of Wernicke–Korsakoff or Marchiafava–Bignami disease.

Treatment of pellagra is with nicotinic acid or nicotinamide, orally at a dose of 50 mg up to 10 times daily or intravenously 25 mg twice or three times daily; thiamine and multivitamins are also given. Response is usually rapid; delirium may clear within hours. As with Wernicke syndrome, prevention is preferable to treatment.

Nutritional Deficiency Anemia

Anemia in alcoholics may be microcytic owing to iron deficiency, sideroblastic owing to malnutrition, or megaloblastic owing to folate deficiency.[538] The latter can mask true vitamin B_{12} deficiency secondary to ethanol-induced malabsorption.[539]

Indirect Effects of Ethanol: Non-nutritional

Hepatic Encephalopathy

Cirrhosis of the liver, encountered most often in alcoholics, is a leading cause of death in the United States, particularly among 25- to 64-year-olds living in urban areas such as New York City.[540] In a survey of 14 western European countries cirrhosis mortality was proportionate to per capita ethanol consumption (with the strongest ethanol effect found in Sweden).[541] Alcoholic liver disease causes neurological symptoms and signs—hepatic encephalopathy—that can be masked by simultaneous intoxication, withdrawal, Wernicke–Korsakoff

syndrome, meningitis, subdural hematoma, hypoglycemia, or other ethanol-related diseases. The mechanisms underlying both alcoholic liver disease and hepatic encephalopathy are multiple and complex.

Mechanisms of Liver Damage

Alcoholic liver disease—steatosis, steatonecrosis (alcoholic hepatitis), and cirrhosis—is mainly the result of direct or indirect toxicity, not nutritional deficiency. In nonhuman primates, isoenergetic replacement of dietary carbohydrates with ethanol (but not with fat) produced steatosis and cirrhosis even when the diet was otherwise adequate.[47] Protein deficiency aggravated the effect of ethanol by reducing lipoprotein synthesis and increasing hepatic lipid accumulation.

A major contributor to hepatic damage is oxidative stress.[48,55,542] Metabolism of ethanol to acetaldehyde reduces NAD to NADH and overwhelms the hepatocyte's ability to maintain redox homeostasis. Ethanol itself inhibits production of the antioxidant glutathione, as does the MEOS enzyme CYP2E1, which also generates reactive oxygen species that cause injury by inactivating enzymes and peroxidizing lipids. Acetaldehyde further depletes glutathione and forms adducts with numerous proteins, altering the functions of microtubules (Mallory bodies), mitochondria, and repair enzymes.[543] The inflammatory nature of alcoholic hepatitis suggests additional immune factors, probably cytokine-mediated.[544] A particular role has been proposed for tissue necrosis factor-alpha (TNFα).[545] Hepatic Kupffer cells, which produce cytokines, are activated in alcoholic liver disease by endotoxin from gut flora.[544] Activation of stellate cells by ethanol increases production of collagen.[546] Cultured hepatic cells expressing CYP2E1 when treated with a glutathione inhibitor developed both apoptosis and necrosis; this effect was prevented by a CYP2E1 inhibitor as well as by cyclosporin A, an inhibitor of mitochondrial membrane permeability transition, suggesting damage to mitochondria by CYP2E1-derived reactive oxygen species.[547]

Additional risk factors for liver disease in heavy drinkers include certain polymorphisms of the enzyme alcohol dehydrogenase (a special risk for women) and obesity.[545]

Heavy ethanol use greatly increases the risk for cirrhosis and for hepatocellular carcinoma in patients with hepatitis C virus (HCV) infection,[548,549] who have higher serum levels of HCV RNA and poorer response to interferon when they consume more than 10 g ethanol daily.[550] Injection drug use is the major source of HCV among alcoholics. A study from Harlem Hospital Center found that the combination of ethanol abuse and HCV infection accounted for 46% of cases of chronic liver disease; alcohol abuse alone accounted for 29% and HCV alone for 12%.[551]

Alcoholics are also at increased risk for acetaminophen hepatotoxicity.[552] In addition to CYP2E1, the MEOS system includes ethanol-inducible CYP3A, which metabolizes acetaminophen to a toxic metabolite.[553] By similar mechanisms alcoholics are also more susceptible to liver disease from other hepatotoxins, including carbon tetrachloride, halothane, isoniazid, phenylbutazone, and cocaine.[554]

Several features of alcoholic liver disease remain unexplained by these mechanisms. Most heavy drinkers do not develop serious liver disease; in a study of alcoholics who had consumed an average of 160 g ethanol daily for more than 10 years, 40% to 50% had no histological evidence of hepatic necrosis or fibrosis.[554,555] Women are more vulnerable than men to alcoholic liver disease, which in most men requires more than 80 g ethanol daily compared with only 20 g daily in women.[556,557] Attempts to identify a genetic basis for these differences in susceptibility (e.g., collagen synthesis or histocompatibility antigens) have been conflicting.[558] Less gastric metabolism of ethanol in women means that larger amounts of ethanol are delivered to the liver after oral consumption.[559,560]

Symptoms and Signs

The clinical manifestations of alcoholic liver disease correlate poorly with hepatic histopathology and range from asymptomatic hepatomegaly to anorexia, malaise, fever, jaundice, ascites, variceal bleeding, and encephalopathy (Table 12–14). Neurological symptoms and signs comprise a characteristic (although nonspecific) syndrome. Altered mentation includes behavioral change progressing to psychosis, inattentiveness progressing to delirium, and lethargy progressing to coma. Symptoms

Table 12–14. Hepatic Encephalopathy—Symptoms and Signs

Systemic
Jaundice
Ascites
Spider angiomata
Fever
Hyperventilation
Fetor hepaticus

Neurological
Altered mentation
Behavioral change (psychosis)
Inattentiveness (delirium)
Decreased alertness (coma)
Asterixis
Dysarthria
Hyperreflexia
Extensor posturing
Grimacing
Downward eye deviation

emerge abruptly or gradually, often accompanied by hyperventilation and fever.[561,562] Asterixis—a fleeting, repetitive loss of voluntary posture holding—is most easily demonstrated in extended wrists and fingers but also occurs in dorsiflexed ankles, closed eyelids, lips, and tongue; in non-alert patients it can sometimes be elicited by pressing on the fingertips to cause dorsiflexion of the hand. In contrast to myoclonus, asterixis is the result of electrical lapses in contracted muscles. (Without electromyography, myoclonus is diagnosed by observing muscle jerks against gravity.) Myoclonus is rarely if ever the result of liver failure, and its presence should suggest alternate diagnoses such as uremia. Seizures are also an infrequent feature of hepatic encephalopathy; their occurrence probably reflects ethanol withdrawal.[561] Liver failure does cause tremor (fine, rapid, and distal), gegenhalten, dysarthria, hyperactive tendon reflexes, extensor ("decerebrate") posturing,[563] grimacing, and sucking. Abnormal eye movements include tonic downward deviation, skew, and ocular bobbing.[564] Focal neurological signs such as hemiparesis suggest structural brain lesions, although in one study eight of 34 patients with hepatic encephalopathy had hemiparesis or monoparesis and no evident structural lesion at CT or MRI; two of the eight patients had seizures. Signs cleared with recovery from hepatic encephalopathy.[565] Many patients with hepatic encephalopathy have a sweetish, musty odor on the breath, so-called fetor hepaticus.[561]

The diagnosis of hepatic encephalopathy is usually easy in patients with known liver disease or jaundice; it can be difficult if there are extrahepatic shunting and only mildly abnormal liver function tests. Encephalopathy is precipitated by a variety of insults (Table 12–15), and coma can then occur abruptly, often in previously stable patients hospitalized for other reasons. Precipitants act in different ways. For example, acetazolamide increases renal venous ammonia levels and decreases renal perfusion, causing azotemia. Metabolic alkalosis favors the formation of nonionized ammonia, which more easily enters the brain. Barbiturates and benzodiazepines precipitate hepatic encephalopathy by facilitating GABA receptors. The brain in such patients seems to be particularly vulnerable, for elevated serum drug levels secondary to decreased liver metabolism are often insufficient to explain the severity of symptoms. Hepatic coma frequently complicates benzodiazepine treatment of ethanol withdrawal.

Table 12–15. Precipitators of Hepatic Encephalopathy

Causing increased ammonia production or entry into CNS
Excess dietary protein
Infection (including bacterial peritonitis and sepsis)
Surgery
Gastrointestinal hemorrhage
Constipation
Blood transfusion
Azotemia
Hypokalemia
Diuretics
Systemic alkalosis

Causing activation of CNS GABA receptors
Barbiturates, benzodiazepines, and ethanol

Aggravating CNS depression
Phenothiazines, other CNS depressant drugs
Other metabolic encephalopathy

Reduced hepatic metabolism of toxins
Dehydration
Hypotension
Hypoxia
Anemia
Portosystemic shunts
Progressive hepatic damage
Hepatoma

Patients with cirrhosis are at increased risk for bacterial infection; in addition to the immunosuppression caused by ethanol itself, cirrhosis impairs the function of macrophages. Septicemia or bacterial peritonitis develops within 48 hours in half of severe cirrhotics who have gastrointestinal hemorrhage. The presence of advanced liver disease in an alcoholic with altered mentation makes it more, not less, likely that that patient has meningitis.[565,566]

Laboratory Abnormalities

Most—but not all—patients with hepatic encephalopathy have hyperammonemia.[567] Tourniquets produce artificial elevations of venous ammonia, and so arterial samples have been recommended.[562] A recent report, however, described good correlation of either venous or arterial ammonia levels and severity of hepatic encephalopathy when newer and more reliable enzymatic assays for ammonia were used.[568] Liver enzymes (aspartate aminotransferase and alanine aminotransferase) are usually elevated, but only modestly, and the degree of elevation correlates poorly with the severity of symptoms. CSF pressure and protein in hepatic encephalopathy are usually normal; xanthochromia is present when serum bilirubin reaches 6 mg/dL. Elevated levels of CSF glutamine are found in nearly all patients, and increased brain concentrations of glutamine can be detected in vivo using proton magnetic resonance spectroscopy.[569] The Electroencephalography characteristically shows synchronous, symmetric, high-voltage slow waves, especially frontally, at first intermixed with preserved alpha activity but eventually replacing it; such a pattern is non-specific.[561] Also frequently abnormal are evoked-response potentials.[570] Respiratory alkalosis reflects primary neurogenic drive. Severe hypoglycemia, common in alcoholics with liver disease, can be masked by hepatic encephalopathy, with catastrophic results. Conversely, high blood levels of ammonia stimulate glucagon secretion, and increased hepatic gluconeogenesis from amino acids leads to further ammonia production. Stimulation of insulin then causes increased muscle uptake and metabolism of branched-chain amino acids, resulting in decreased serum levels of valine, leucine, and isoleucine. Blood levels of other amino acids are elevated.[562] Serum vitamin A levels are often decreased, reflecting reduced concentrations in the liver.[571]

Pathology and Pathogenesis

The most striking neuropathological alterations in hepatic encephalopathy are swollen astrocytes in cerebral cortex and other gray structures, including thalamus, basal ganglia, pontine nuclei, and deep cerebellar nuclei. Neuronal damage is far less conspicuous.[561] Cerebral edema is a feature of acute fulminating hepatic failure but not of encephalopathy associated with chronic liver disease.[572] Theories of pathogenesis focus on a number of possible circulating toxins (Table 12–16).[573]

Ammonia Hypothesis. In liver failure the synthesis of urea from ammonia decreases and the latter accumulates. The most venerable explanations of hepatic encephalopathy have implicated ammonia, acting either directly as a neurotoxin; synergistically with fatty acids and mercaptans; or indirectly through accumulation of glutamine and alpha-ketoglutaramate or depletion of glutamate, aspartate, and branched-chain amino acids.[573a] Ammonia is directly neurotoxic; it interferes with neuronal chloride extrusion and causes both stupor and astrocytic hyperplasia experimentally.[574,575] In animals with portocaval shunts, cerebral blood flow increases without alteration of cerebral oxygen metabolism; ammonium acetate challenge then produces a fall in both, reflecting the sensitivity of a chronically hyperammonemic brain to additional ammonia.[574,576]

Although accurately measured blood ammonia levels do correlate with severity of hepatic encephalopathy,[568] the role of ammonia in the pathogenesis of hepatic encephalopathy remains controversial.[577] Its effects could be direct or indirect. Short-chain fatty acids and mercaptans

Table 12–16. Hepatic Encephalopathy— Candidate Toxins

Ammonia
Glutamine, alpha-ketoglutaramate
Short-chain fatty acids
Mercaptans
False neurotransmitters (octopamine, beta-phenylethanolamine)
Tryptophan, quinolinic acid
Gamma-aminobutyric acid
Benzodiazepine

---

accumulate in liver failure and cause coma in experimental animals. Mercaptans, which probably account for fetor hepaticus, enhance the toxicity of ammonia and fatty acids, and blood levels of ammonia, fatty acids, or mercaptans sufficient to cause coma in animals are much less when any two are given together. Phenols have also been implicated in such synergism.[578]

In the liver, ammonia is detoxified by the urea cycle. In the brain, however, ammonia combines with glutamate to form glutamine, which is further metabolized to alpha-ketoglutaramate.[579] The presence of glutamine synthetase in glia is possibly related to astrocytic hypertrophy in hepatic encephalopathy.[580,580a] Inhibition of glutamine synthetase (with methionine sulfoximine) protects mice against ammonia intoxication even though brain ammonia is further elevated.[581] Perfusion of alpha-ketoglutaramate into the ventricles of rats produced neurological signs (including myoclonus); a possible explanation is that alpha-ketoglutaramate competes for glutamate receptors in brain. Alternatively, diversion by ammonia of glutamate to glutamine would deplete both glutamate and aspartate; these excitatory neurotransmitters reportedly produced arousal in patients with hepatic encephalopathy.[579,582]

False Neurotransmitter Hypothesis. In contrast to hypotheses implicating ammonia, a "false neurotransmitter" hypothesis proposes that amines such as octopamine or beta-phenylethanolamine, absorbed from the gut and bypassing the liver, enter peripheral and central catecholamine nerve terminals and, in effect, inhibit them.[562,583] Possible precursors of such inhibitory false neurotransmitters are aromatic amino acids, increased brain uptake of which would occur if there were depressed blood levels of branched-chain amino acids.[584] Elevation of brain octopamine in experimental animals, however, failed to reproduce signs of hepatic encephalopathy.[585] Serum levels of tryptophan are elevated in hepatic encephalopathy, and ammonia facilitates the transport of tryptophan across the blood–brain barrier.[586] Raised levels of brain tryptophan lead to increases in brain and CSF quinolinic acid, a potentially toxic excitatory neurotransmitter.[587] Rats with portocaval shunts, but not normal rats, develop neuronal degeneration and astrocytic hypertrophy after tryptophan loading.[588]

GABA/Benzodiazepine Receptor Ligand Hypothesis. An alternative hypothesis proposes that the crucial neurotoxin is either GABA or an endogenous benzodiazepine acting at the GABA receptor complex. GABA produced by enteric bacteria is believed to cross an abnormally permeable blood–brain barrier, producing neuronal inhibition. In support of this mechanism are increased serum levels of GABA and increased densities of GABA receptors preceding overt encephalopathy in experimental animals. Additionally, an abnormal visual-evoked potential pattern in hepatic encephalopathy is identical to that associated with coma secondary to barbiturates, benzodiazepines, or GABA agonists and unlike that associated with coma secondary to ammonia or mercaptans.[589–592] GABA antagonists such as bicuculline and chloride channel blockers such as isopropylbicyclophosphate reverse the clinical and electrophysiological signs of hepatic encephalopathy in rabbits.[593] On the other hand, blood GABA levels correlate poorly with the encephalopathy, and normal brain levels of GABA are reported in encephalopathic animals and humans.[573a] It is claimed, moreover, that even increased blood–brain barrier permeability would not allow increased penetration of GABA, which would be metabolized at the barrier by GABA-transaminase.[594]

Increased GABAergic tone could be the basis of hepatic encephalopathy without GABA itself accumulating. Possibilities include a toxin acting agonistically at benzodiazepine receptors on the GABA receptor complex.[595,596] Behavioral and electrophysiological abnormalities in rats with liver failure are reversed by the benzodiazepine antagonist flumazenil.[597] Urine, blood, and CSF benzodiazepine receptor-binding activity was much higher in patients with hepatic encephalopathy than in controls (including uremic patients),[598] and elevated levels of benzodiazepines—identified by mass spectroscopy as diazepam and N-desmethyldiazepam—were found in the brains of patients dying with hepatic encephalopathy.[599] Flumazenil improves the clinical and electrophysiological signs of hepatic encephalopathy in some (but not all) patients.[600]

If a benzodiazepine agonist is indeed the encephalopathic toxin, its source is obscure.[598] Attempts to identify an endogenous benzodiazepine receptor ligand (e.g., beta-carboline, diazepam-binding inhibitor, or desmethyldiazepam) have

produced conflicting results (see Chapter 6). It is possible that in hepatic encephalopathy the source of such a ligand is enteric bacteria or food.

Increased GABAergic tone would explain better than ammonia toxicity some features of hepatic encephalopathy. Ammonia is proconvulsant, whereas GABA is anticonvulsant, and myoclonus and seizures are not features of hepatic encephalopathy. Increased GABAergic tone would also explain the marked sensitivity of such patients to barbiturates and benzodiazepines.[601]

Possibly linking the ammonia and GABAergic hypotheses are observations that hyperammonemia increases brain levels of "peripheral-type" benzodiazepine receptors (PTBRs), which are located predominantly on astrocytic mitochondria. Increased expression of PTBRs, by stimulating cholesterol transport across mitochondrial membranes, results in increased synthesis of brain neurosteroids with $GABA_A$ receptor agonist properties.[573a,601a]

Manganese Hypothesis. Some investigators believe manganese accumulates in the globus pallidus of patients with cirrhosis. T1-weighted magnetic resonance images are compatible with this hypothesis, and manganese intoxication and hepatic encephalopathy produce similar symptoms.[602] Correlation of symptoms with the degree of MRI signal abnormality is disputed, however, and the therapeutic effects of agents such as edetate calcium disulfide or sodium para-aminosalicylic acid remain to be determined.

Treatment of Hepatic Encephalopathy

Much of the treatment of hepatic encephalopathy is directed toward decreasing ammonia levels in blood and brain (Tables 12–17, 12–18).[567] Dietary protein restriction is an obviously two-edged sword in malnourished patients. Bowel cleansing and surgical colonic exclusion eliminate urease-producing bacteria. So does neomycin, which can be given orally, up to 6 g daily, or by enema as a 1% solution once or twice daily. Absorbed oral or rectal neomycin causes nephrotoxicity and ototoxicity, however, and in most patients the preferred agent is lactulose. This synthetic nonabsorbable disaccharide is metabolized by colonic bacteria to lactic, acetic, and formic acids, producing a gradient that converts ammonia to ammonium ion, which is then

Table 12–17. Treatment of Hepatic Encephalopathy

Identify and treat precipitating factor(s)

Adequate calories (with protein restriction): provide at least 1600 calories per day from carbohydrate, orally or intravenously

Eliminate protein initially and then after a few days increase by 10–20 g per day every few days, depending on symptoms

Bowel cleansing: enemas, colonic lavage. Colonic exclusion in severe, chronic cases

Lactulose, 50–150 mg orally daily in divided doses, or as enema, 300 mL in 700 mL water

Alternatively: neomycin, 2–4 g orally daily, or as enema, 1% solution once or twice daily

Benzodiazepine antagonists

Attention to accompanying medical problems: acid–base disturbance, hypertension or hypotension, coagulation abnormalities, gastrointestinal bleeding, acute pancreatitis, sepsis. Ethanol withdrawal, meningitis, hypoglycemia, and intracranial hematoma or abscess may be masked

---

Table 12–18. Results of Controlled Trials of Treatments for Hepatic Encephalopathy as a Complication of Chronic Liver Disease[a]

Ammonia hypothesis
Reduced ammonia production
  Dietary protein restriction (+)
  Vegetable protein diet (+)
  Carbohydrate enemas (+)
  Water enemas (−)
  Oral lactulose (+)
  Oral lactitol (+)
  Oral lactose in lactase deficiency (+)
  Oral antibiotics
  Neomycin (+)
  Metronidazole (+)
  Rifaximin (+)
Enterococcus faccium (+)
Lactobacillus acidophilus
  Alone (−)
  With neomycin (+)
Helicobacter pylori eradication (NP)
Increased ammonia metabolism
  Ornithine α-ketoglutarate (−)
  Ornithine aspartate (+)
  Sodium benzoate (+)
  Phenylacetate (+)
  Zinc supplementation (±)

False-neurotransmitter hypothesis
Branched-chain amino acids
  Enteral (±)
  Parenteral (±)
Keto analogs (±)
L-dopa (−)
Bromocriptine (−)

γ-Aminobutyric acid–benzodiazepine receptor ligand hypothesis
Flumazenil (±)

Manganese hypothesis
Edetate calcium disodium (NP)
Sodium para-aminosalicylic acid (NP)

Source: Riodan SM, Williams R. Treatment of hepatic encephalopathy. N Engl J Med 1997; 337:473.
[a]A plus sign indicates that controlled trials support the treatment; a plus-minus that results of controlled trials are conflicting; a minus sign that controlled trials do not support the treatment; and NP that controlled trials have not been performed.

---

trapped in the gut and not absorbed. Lactulose causes diarrhea, which can be a problem in dehydrated or hypotensive patients. The oral dose is therefore titrated (usually 30–60 g daily) to cause two or three soft stools per day with acidic pH.

A controlled study demonstrated that lactulose and neomycin were equally effective in hepatic encephalopathy.[603] Although the two treatments should be mutually exclusive (because neomycin eliminates the bacteria that allow lactulose to work), additive benefits were found in one report, suggesting lactulose acts by mechanisms not yet understood.[604]

An alternative nonabsorable disaccharide is lactilol (available in Europe), and alternative oral antibiotics include metronidazole and rifaximin. Studies support populating the colon with non-urease-producing bacteria such as *Lactobacillus acidophilus* or *Enterococcus faecium*. Eradication of urease-producing *Helicobacter pylori* is also recommended on theoretical grounds.[567]

Because ornithine and aspartate are substrates for the metabolic conversion of ammonia to urea and to glutamine, treatment with ornithine aspartate was studied, with favorable results. Phenylacetate, which reacts with glutamine to form phenacetylglutamine, and sodium benzoate, which reacts with glycine to form hippurate, also appear to be beneficial.[567]

Zinc deficiency is common in cirrhotic patients, and urea cycle metabolism of ammonia involves two zinc-dependent enzymes. Some (but not all) studies of zinc supplementation in hepatic encephalopathy have been promising.[567]

The false transmitter hypothesis led to trials with L-dopa or bromocriptine in hepatic encephalopathy.[562] Early anecdotal observations were promising, but subsequent controlled trials were negative.[605] Improved mentation was also claimed following treatment with keto-analogs of amino acids or with infusions high in branched-chain and low in aromatic amino acids. Not all controlled trials showed benefit, however.[567]

Reports of improvement in encephalopathic animals following GABA or benzodiazepine antagonists led to trials in humans. GABA and chloride channel antagonists are too epileptogenic to be practical. Early studies with benzodiazepine antagonists were promising.[600] In one report oral flumazenil successfully relieved symptoms, including episodic coma, in a patient with chronic intractable portal systemic encephalopathy.[606] Serious side effects were not observed.[607] Unfortunately, flumazenil is rapidly metabolized, and its duration of action in most people lasts for only minutes to a few hours.[607] Moreover, controlled trials, including one that monitored EEG findings, reveal that only a minority of patients with moderate-to-severe hepatic encephalopathy respond to flumazenil, including patients who recently received benzodiazepines.[608–610] A Cochrane meta-analysis of 12 randomized trials concluded that flumazenil favorably influenced short-term improvement in some patients with chronic liver disease and encephalopathy but that it could not be recommended for "routine clinical use."[610a]

More aggressive therapeutic approaches to hepatic encephalopathy include surgical colonic exclusion, cross-circulation with primates or irreversibly comatose donors, charcoal hemoperfusion, and liver transplantation.[562]

General medical management in hepatic encephalopathy can be complex. Patients are often very ill with acid–base disturbances, hyponatremia, hypernatremia, hypokalemia, edema, hypotension, renal failure, coagulation abnormalities, gastrointestinal bleeding, acute pancreatitis, or sepsis.[611,612] Ethanol withdrawal, meningitis, hypoglycemia, and subdural hematoma may be masked. Moreover, in one study, liver biopsy revealed a nonalcohol-related cause in 20% of alcoholics with liver disease.[613]

Chronic Hepatic Encephalopathy

In some cirrhotics neurological symptoms become chronic, and in alcoholics the clinical picture can be quite confusing. A group of patients with portacaval anastomoses developed progressive neuropsychiatric symptoms unlike those of acute hepatic encephalopathy.[614] They were usually noisy and hyperactive, and some appeared to be schizophrenic or hypomanic. In addition, they had variable combinations of slowly progressive paraparesis and spastic bladder, cerebellar ataxia, parkinsonism, seizures, myoclonus, and focal cortical signs. In one of the paraparetic patients, and in others subsequently reported,[615] autopsy revealed "widespread demyelination" in the spinal cord, not resembling multiple sclerosis. EEG slowing and elevated serum ammonia concentrations were usually present, yet only a few had previous episodes of acute hepatic encephalopathy. Symptomatic improvement after dietary restriction, neomycin, or colonic exclusion was infrequent.

Similar to such patients are those with acquired chronic hepatocerebral degeneration, a characteristic syndrome of dementia, dysarthria, ataxia, intention tremor, and choreoathetosis affecting especially cranial muscles.[616–618] Muscle rigidity, grasp reflexes, mild pyramidal signs, nystagmus, and asterixis are common. The electroencephalogram is diffusely abnormal. MRI signal abnormalities are seen in the basal ganglia.[617,619] Pathologically, astrocytosis and neuronal degeneration in the cerebrum, cerebellum, and diencephalon progress to laminar or pseudolaminar necrosis at corticomedullary junctions and microcavitation in the putamen. In the original description of this syndrome, 23 of 27 patients had previous bouts of hepatic coma, and although all had either elevated serum ammonia levels or abnormal responses to ammonium citrate challenge, lowering of serum ammonia produced no improvement.[620] Anecdotally, improvement was described after treatment with branched-chain amino acids and after liver transplantation.[617,621]

In addition to these florid and often progressive manifestations of hepatic encephalopathy are more subtle forms, with altered mentation sometimes identifiable only with psychometric testing. In fact, it is estimated that if such patients are included, hepatic encephalopathy is present in 50% to 70% of all patients with cirrhosis.[622] Although those with progressive debilitating syndromes are unlikely to respond to pharmacotherapy, gradual improvement was described after liver transplantation.[623]

Alcoholics have many reasons to be mentally impaired, including direct toxicity of ethanol on the brain (alcoholic dementia; see later). A possible contribution of mild hepatic encephalopathy in such patients must always be considered.

Hypoglycemia

Impaired insulin response and glucose intolerance are frequent in alcoholics.[624,625] More serious is episodic hypoglycemia (Table 12–19), which tends to occur after 6 to 36 hours of moderate to heavy drinking, albeit infrequently; a blood glucose level below 50 mg/dL was found in only one of 131 intoxicated subjects.[626]

During a 12-month prospective survey of the Harlem Hospital emergency room, there were 125 visits for symptomatic hypoglycemia (Table 12–19).[627] In 60, ethanol played a role, either alone or in association with diabetes mellitus or sepsis. Symptoms included dizziness and tremor, abnormal behavior, depressed sensorium, and seizures. Hemiparesis was common on recovery from seizures or coma and in three instances was the presenting symptom in otherwise alert patients. Blood glucose levels tended to be lowest in comatose patients, but there was considerable overlap between groups, and overall there was little correlation between cause, glucose levels, and symptoms. Hypothermia was especially common among alcoholics. Eight patients relapsed after either admission or discharge from the emergency room, demonstrating that treated hypoglycemic patients should not be prematurely sent home but should be admitted, preferably to an intensive care unit. Relapse is especially likely when sepsis or diabetes is present. Overall mortality was 11%, yet only one death was attributable to hypoglycemia per se, and only four survivors had focal neurological residua.

Consistent with other reports, these patients demonstrated that hypoglycemic coma is less dangerous than equivalent degrees of anoxic/ischemic coma. Pathological changes are also different. Although anoxia/ischemia usually damages vascular border zones and end zones of the cerebrum, diencephalon, and cerebellum, hypoglycemia affects the cerebrum and basal ganglia more diffusely and tends to spare the cerebellum.[628] In hypoglycemia, cerebral oxygen consumption does not fall to the same extent as cerebral glucose metabolism, implying as yet unidentified energy sources. Nonetheless, symptomatic hypoglycemia is a medical emergency, for neurological residua do occur, and subtle cognitive changes are undoubtedly underdetected.[629,630] (They would be particularly difficult to demonstrate in alcoholics.) Any patient, alcoholic or not, with unexplained behavioral change, seizures, or depressed alertness should receive glucose and thiamine; those with status epilepticus or coma should be treated intravenously.

Nonalcoholics are vulnerable to ethanol-induced hypoglycemia by a different mechanism. Ethanol stimulates intestinal secretin, which in turn increases the insulin response to glucose. The result can be severe reactive hypoglycemia after a few drinks and a small meal.[631] Coma and seizures occurred in a 3-year-old who became severely hypoglycemic after drinking brandy,[269] and at Harlem Hospital Center ethanol-induced reactive hypoglycemia accounts for more pediatric admissions than does uncomplicated stupor following accidental ethanol ingestion.

Table 12–19. Hypoglycemic Symptoms in 125 Consecutive Patients at Harlem Hospital Center (Alcoholism, Alone or Associated with Diabetes or Sepsis, in 60)

Depressed sensorium	
Coma	39
Stupor	16
Obtundation	10
Behavior change	
Confusion	24
Bizarre behavior	14
Dizziness, tremor	10
Seizures	9
Sudden hemiparesis	3

Source: Malouf R, Brust JCM. Hypoglycemia: causes, neurological manifestations, and outcome. Ann Neurol 1985; 17:421.

Other Endocrinological Effects

Ethanol's effects on sexual activity have long been recognized; it "…provokes the desire but takes away the performance."[632] In men, chronic ethanol decreases testosterone production and causes testicular atrophy, impotence, and gynecomastia,[633] and the presence of the alcohol dehydrogenase 2-1 allele increases susceptibility to this effect.[634] Increased estrogen levels associated with liver disease contribute to feminization. Alcoholic women develop hyperprolactinemia, amenorrhea, and uterine atrophy. They are more likely to be infertile and once pregnant to have spontaneous abortion.[635] Ethanol indirectly suppresses release of luteinizing hormone (LH) by blocking the release of LH releasing hormone by nitric oxide.[636]

Ethanol inhibits antidiuretic hormone release at the level of the hypothalamus; diuresis occurs when the blood ethanol concentration is rising but not when it is falling.[637]

Ethanol stimulates adrenocorticotropic hormone (ACTH) release from the pituitary.[638] Pseudo-Cushing's syndrome consists of characteristic signs, increased cortisol secretion, absent diurnal cortisol rhythm, and inadequate suppression of cortisol by dexamethasone.[639] Ethanol withdrawal also stimulates ACTH release, sometimes for weeks.[640] Cushingoid signs eventually clear with abstinence.

Although acutely ethanol induces dose-related increases in plasma ACTH, chronic exposure blunts the hypothalamic-pituitary-adrenal (HPA) axis response to stress or immune signals. ACTH production by ethanol requires the delivery of both corticotropin-releasing hormone and vasopressin to the pituitary, and the blunted response appears to be the consequence of loss of pituitary response to vasopressin.[641]

Acutely and chronically ethanol inhibits growth hormone, although in alcoholics with cirrhosis, levels may be elevated.[119]

Hypocalcemia is common in alcoholics. Hypoalbuminemia, poor nutrition, and increased urinary and intestinal loss each contribute; impaired intestinal calcium absorption is attributed to hypovitaminosis D, hypoparathyroidism, and parathormone resistance secondary to magnesium deficiency.[642] Osteoporosis is a frequent consequence.[643] In normal volunteers, short-term ethanol administration caused transient hypoparathyroidism with hypocalcemia, hypercalciuria, and hypermagnesuria.[644]

Temperature

Through actions on the hypothalamus, ethanol increases skin blood flow and sweating and lowers body temperature.[645] When environmental temperature is low, life-threatening hypothermia can occur. Ethanol increases mortality in hyperthermic mice; conversely, elevated body temperature increases ethanol toxicity.[646]

Sleep Disorders

A majority of ethanol-dependent patients describe insomnia, and ethanol is often used for sleep. After at least 2 weeks' abstinence, insomniac alcoholic patients still had worse polysomnographic measures of sleep continuity, and whether or not ethanol had been taken for sleep, insomnia was associated with more severe alcoholism and predicted relapse.[647]

In patients undergoing treatment for sleep disorders associated with psychiatric illness, even moderate ethanol use can interfere with therapy.[648]

Alcoholic Ketoacidosis

Acid–base disturbances in alcoholics are often difficult to interpret.[649] Respiratory alkalosis accompanies ethanol withdrawal or hepatic encephalopathy; metabolic alkalosis follows vomiting associated with gastritis or pancreatitis; and lactic acidosis results from seizures, infection, and gastrointestinal or traumatic hemorrhage. Ethanol prolongs lactic acidosis of any cause. By generating NADH at the expense of NAD, it decreases conversion of lactate to pyruvate; if thiamine deficiency is also present, pyruvate cannot enter the tricarboxylic acid cycle and lactate elimination is further impaired.[650] Different kinds of acid–base disturbance in alcoholics can of course coexist.

Alcoholic ketoacidosis refers to ketosis and an increased anion gap resulting from accumulation of acetoacetate and hydroxybutyrate.[649] Typical patients are young binge drinkers who stop drinking when overcome by anorexia or vomiting, sometimes owing to gastritis or pancreatitis. Acute starvation for several days is followed by confusion, obtundation, and Kussmaul respirations; depressed consciousness tends to be less than with a similar degree of diabetic ketoacidosis. There may be coexisting lactic acidosis and metabolic or respiratory alkalosis, with complex dissociations of serum pH, ketosis, and anion gap. When beta-hydroxybutyrate predominates over acetoacetate, the nitroprusside test (Acetest) can be negative. Starvation and impaired gluconeogenesis produce hypoglycemia, but more often blood glucose levels are normal or moderately elevated. Decreased renal excretion of urate causes hyperuricemia. Serum insulin levels are often low, and serum levels of growth hormone, epinephrine, glucagon, and cortisol are high, yet glucose intolerance usually clears without insulin and is inapparent on recovery. Ethanol is rarely detectable in the blood. Repeated attacks of alcoholic ketoacidosis are common.

The cause of the ketosis is increased lipolysis and impaired fatty acid oxidation. Starvation is a major factor, and the role of ethanol per se is uncertain. (Normal rat liver slices incubated with ethanol do not display increased ketogenesis; liver slices from rats fed ethanol do.[651]) Treatment begins with attention to coexisting serious illness. Ketosis usually responds promptly to intravenous glucose (given with thiamine). Insulin is unnecessary unless the patient is diabetic; alcoholic ketoacidosis cannot then be distinguished from diabetic ketoacidosis, and insulin is given.[649] Sodium bicarbonate is also seldom needed, but dehydration and potassium depletion require saline and potassium salts (including potassium phosphate). Hypocalcemia in excess of hypoalbuminemia may reflect hypomagnesemia, correctable with magnesium sulfate.

Electrolyte Disturbance

Whereas acutely ethanol has diuretic effects, chronic heavy ethanol ingestion causes salt and water retention and expansion of extracellular volume. Calcium, magnesium, and phosphate depletion can cause neurological symptoms. Heavy ethanol use is associated with hyperuricemia and attacks of gout.[652]

Infection

Over 200 years ago Benjamin Rush remarked on the susceptibility of alcoholics to infection, including pneumonia, tuberculosis, and yellow fever.[653]

Alcoholics have vacuolated white blood cells and granulocytopenia, depressed leukocyte migration, suppressed interferon systems, and decreased humoral and cell-mediated immunity.[653,654] Cirrhosis, by uncertain mechanisms, further predisposes to infection.[655] Twenty-nine percent of adults with pneumococcal meningitis at Harlem Hospital Center were alcoholic,[656] as were five of eight patients with nontraumatic gram-negative meningitis at the Detroit Medical Center.[657] Similar susceptibility to tuberculosis leads to meningitis, tuberculoma, and Pott's disease, and cure is difficult if alcoholism is not simultaneously treated.[658] Infectious meningitis must always be considered in alcoholics with seizures or altered mentation, even when the clinical picture seems fully explained by intoxication, withdrawal, thiamine deficiency, hepatic encephalopathy, or hypoglycemia. Alcoholics are at special risk for sepsis secondary to soft tissue infection and for spontaneous bacterial peritonitis. Endocarditis, especially prevalent in cirrhotics, is more likely to involve the aortic valve, raising the risk of brain emboli, brain abscess, and septic aneurysm. Bacteremia and endocarditis caused by *Bartonella quintana* (the cause of trench fever during World War I) affects inner-city homeless alcoholics,[659] and an epidemic of diphtheria occurred among homeless alcoholics in Seattle.[660] Whether alcoholics are at special risk for AIDS or early CNS involvement in human immunodeficiency virus (HIV) infection is controversial.[661–663]

Pulmonary Effects

For reasons that are unclear, epidemiological studies in Finland, Italy, and the Netherlands found a U-shaped relation of ethanol consumption and chronic obstructive pulmonary disease (COPD). That is, adjusted for tobacco smoking, light drinkers were protected from COPD compared with abstainers, whereas heavy drinkers were at increased risk.[664]

Gastrointestinal Effects

Ethanol causes esophagitis, esophageal spasm, Mallory–Weiss tear, acute and chronic gastritis, peptic ulcer, alcoholic diarrhea, and acute and chronic pancreatitis. Chronic ethanol abuse favors gastric colonization by *Helicobacter pylori*.[665] Malabsorption of folic acid, iron, and vitamins, including pyridoxine and cobalamin, aggravates dietary insufficiency and produces a variety of neurological symptoms.

Cancer

Alcoholics have increased risk for cancer of the mouth, pharynx, larynx, and esophagus.[666] Ethanol does not cause cancer in experimental animals and in humans may act as a cocarcinogen with tobacco.[667] Hepatoma in alcoholics is closely linked with cirrhosis. A suggestive association has been found for cancer of large bowel and breast. There appears to be no association with cancer of the stomach, pancreas, lung, urinary bladder, prostate, or ovary or for malignant melanoma.[668]

Possible mechanisms by which ethanol might increase cancer risk include generation of acetaldehyde and free radicals, which impede DNA repair mechanisms and trap glutathione. Nutritional deficiencies (including vitamin A, folate, pyridoxine, zinc, and selenium) and immune system deficiencies could contribute.[669] Ethanol consumption accompanied by low folate intake increased the risk of breast cancer in a prospective study of postmenopausal women.[670] Proposed mechanisms for breast cancer risk also include ethanol-induced stimulation of insulin-like growth factors and of estrogen.[671,672]

Trauma

Trauma can be an indicator of early ethanol abuse,[673,674] and ethanol intoxication makes serious injury more likely when trauma occurs.[675,676] More than half of all traffic fatalities involve either a drunk driver or a drunk pedestrian (see Table 12–1),[677] and in the United States more than a quarter of these accidents involved drivers who have previously been arrested for drunken driving.[678]

Approximately 40% of Americans will be involved in an ethanol-related automobile crash during their lifetime.[679] Ethanol also contributes heavily to aviation and boating accidents, falls, drownings, and fires.[680–682] In one-third of suicides the victims have been drinking and suicide among alcoholics ranges from 8% to 21%.[683] Ethanol is also a major contributor to assault and homicide.[679] In one report, half of murderers or their victims had been drinking at the time of the crime.[684]

Alcoholics bleed easily. Thrombocytopenia is both a direct effect of ethanol and a consequence of cirrhosis with hypersplenism.[538] Liver disease also alters clotting factors, and experimentally ethanol enhances blood–brain barrier leakage around areas of cerebral trauma.[685,686] In rats with spinal cord trauma, ethanol exacerbated the release of free fatty acids and excitatory amino acids and the reduction of tissue magnesium levels; mortality and neurological residua were increased in ethanol-treated rats compared with controls.[687] Up-regulation of NMDA receptors in chronic alcoholics increases the likelihood of excitotoxic damage.[688] Close observation is essential after even mild head trauma in intoxicated patients; altered mentation must not be dismissed as drunkenness.

Relevant to ethanol-related trauma is its effects on bone. Low-to-moderate ethanol intake increases bone density, but chronic ethanol abuse is a risk factor for osteoporosis.[689] Ethanol has both direct and indirect effects on bone cells, acting through gonadal and mineral regulating hormones and secretion of cytokines[690,691] (see above).

Peripheral Nerve Pressure Palsies

Radial and peroneal nerve palsies are common in alcoholics. Underlying polyneuropathy increases the vulnerability of peripheral nerves to compression injury, and intoxicated subjects tend to sleep deeply in unusual locations and positions. Recovery takes days or weeks; splints during this period can prevent contractures.

Central Pontine Myelinolysis

Central pontine myelinolysis (CPM) is an underdiagnosed disease characterized by demyelinating lesions in the central part of the basis pontis. It is not restricted to alcoholics and can be asymptomatic. Of the four original autopsy cases, three were chronic alcoholics with malnutrition and dehydration.[692] Two of these developed pseudobulbar palsy and quadriplegia over several days and died 2 to 4 weeks later. A single large symmetric demyelinating lesion occupied much of the basis pontis, affecting all fiber tracts but sparing all but the most central axons, neurons, and vessels. The third patient had similar but smaller lesions without having had apparent symptoms. CPM occurs in roughly 0.25% of autopsied adults. When severe, lesions extend into the pontine tegmentum, causing sensory loss, abnormal eye movements, and coma. Histologically similar lesions also occur in midbrain, cerebellum, diencephalon, and cerebrum, leading some clinicians to prefer the term "osmotic demyelination syndrome."[693–696] An alcoholic patient with extrapontine myelinolysis exhibited parkinsonism and dystonia.[697]

CPM most often affects patients with debilitating conditions such as liver disease, burns, amyloidosis, cerebral trauma, diabetes, kidney transplantation, brain tumor, and leukemia. It can coexist with pellagra and Wernicke–Korsakoff syndrome[698] and occurs in children.[699] MRI has improved diagnostic accuracy,[700] yet CPM is still identified more often at autopsy than during life, especially when the underlying disease also causes neurological symptoms and signs. Gadolinium enhancement occurs early, but MRI findings can lag behind clinical disease by days to weeks in CPM.[693] Clinical signs and MRI abnormalities then improve together.[701]

Although cases have occurred in association with hypoglycemia[702] or without any electrolyte derangement,[703] in most instances CPM is the result of overvigorous correction of hyponatremia, the basis pontis being particularly vulnerable because of its unique "anatomic grid structure."[693] Whether speed of correction or overcorrection to hypernatremia is more dangerous is disputed; animal studies suggest that rapid correction of chronic hyponatremia is especially hazardous.[704,705] In any case, CPM is most often a preventable iatrogenic disease.

No specific treatment exists once CPM occurs, although neurological signs occasionally remit with supportive therapy.[706] Prevention involves treating hyponatremia such that serum sodium levels do not exceed 130 mEq/L; free water restriction and small amounts of hypertonic saline are titrated to raise serum sodium levels no more rapidly than 0.55 mEq/L per hour or 12 mEq/L per day.[8,707–710]

Effects of Ethanol of Uncertain Cause

Myopathy

Alcoholic myopathy was first recognized as recurrent and sometimes fatal myoglobinuria.[711] Subsequent reports described chronic progressive weakness, and today alcoholic myopathy is classified, clinically and pathologically, as subclinical, chronic, or acute.[712–715] The subclinical variety consists of elevated serum creatine phosphokinase (CPK) levels and electromyographic abnormalities, sometimes with intermittent cramps, weakness, or dark urine. Blood lactate may fail to rise after ischemic exercise, suggesting abnormal muscle phosphorylase. Subclinical myopathy is common; electromyographic abnormalities are found in a majority of chronic alcoholics, and histological changes—fiber vacuolation and degeneration, macrophages, and increased interstitial fat—occur in nearly half.

Chronic myopathy causes progressive proximal weakness, muscle tenderness, and more pronounced pathological alterations. Acute rhabdomyolysis, often exertional, causes sudden severe weakness and muscle pain, sometimes superimposed on chronic weakness during a drinking binge. Only one limb or muscle group may be affected, and sometimes the face or pharynx is involved.[716] Tenderness and swelling suggest thrombophlebitis. Myoglobinuria causes renal shutdown, and potassium release and hyperkalemia predispose to fatal cardiac arrhythmia. The diagnosis of acute alcoholic myoglobinuria is usually easy; in myopathic patients denying heavy ethanol intake, an ethanol challenge to produce myalgia has been recommended.[717] To be kept in mind are other causes of proximal weakness in alcoholics, such as hypokalemia following diarrhea,[718] pseudo-Cushing's syndrome,[639] and atypical polyneuropathy.

Whether subclinical, chronic, or acute, alcoholic myopathy improves with abstinence.[719] Although subjects are often malnourished, ethanol toxicity is probably more important than nutritional deficiency.[720] Twenty-three of 50 alcoholic men had histological evidence of myopathy, which correlated better with the amount of ethanol consumed than with nutrition; it occurred only in those who for many years had drunk the equivalent of at least 12 oz of whiskey a day.[721] Nonalcoholic volunteers consuming ethanol with adequate diets developed, by electron microscopy, intracellular edema, lipid and glycogen accumulation, and abnormal mitochondria and sarcoplasmic reticulum.[722] The relevance of these structural alterations to the acute reversible effects of ethanol on muscle function is unclear.[723] For example, both ethanol and acetaldehyde inhibit sodium–potassium-ATPase, mitochondrial fatty acid oxidation, protein synthesis, and calcium binding to troponin.[724] In alcoholic humans nuclear magnetic resonance spectroscopy is consistent with impaired glycolysis, and in alcoholic rhabdomyolysis production of lactate and pyruvate is decreased.[725] In chronic alcoholic myopathy Type II fibers are selectively affected and plasma selenium, alpha-tocopherol, and carnisonase are reduced, consistent with oxidative damage.[726,727]

Hereditary recurrent rhabdomyolysis affected two brothers whose symptoms—muscle pain and myoglobinuria—were provoked by strenuous exercise or ethanol ingestion. Muscle biopsy revealed ragged red fibers with abnormal mitochondria, and polymerase chain reaction detected deletions of mitochondrial DNA. Ethanol sensitivity in these patients might have been related to impaired oxidation of NADH (generated by alcohol dehydrogenase) secondary to defective mitochondrial energy transduction.[728]

Cardiomyopathy

Ethanol also damages cardiac muscle, and alcoholic cardiomyopathy, a low-output state clearly distinguishable from beri-beri heart disease, is possibly "the major cause of cardiomyopathy … in the Western World."[723] Nearly 90% of autopsies on chronic alcoholics reveal cardiomegaly with fiber hypertrophy, fibrosis, lipid and glycogen accumulation, swollen mitochondria, and necrosis.[727,729] Congestive heart failure, pulmonary emboli, conduction defects, and arrhythmias are frequent;

heart disease accounts for up to 15% of alcoholic deaths. In symptomatic patients mortality is 80% within 3 years unless abstinence occurs.[730,731]

Atrial and ventricular arrhythmia following acute heavy ethanol consumption, so-called holiday heart, can cause sudden death in alcoholics.[732] Whether moderate ethanol consumption precipitates cardiac arrhythmia in otherwise healthy people is less certain, as is the contribution of cigarette smoking.[733] Acute congestive heart failure and arrhythmia have accompanied myoglobinuria after heavy drinking,[734] and in normal volunteers, acute ethanol ingestion causes myocardial depression.[735]

On a brighter note, a cohort study of elderly persons found that moderate ethanol consumption *decreased* the risk of congestive heart failure, and the benefit did not appear to be entirely mediated by reduced risk of myocardial infarction.[736]

Marchiafava–Bignami Disease

Although an autopsy incidence among alcoholics of 6% has been claimed, Marchiafava–Bignami disease is probably much rarer.[737,738] It is defined by characteristic demyelinating lesions in the corpus callosum; the clinical spectrum is uncertain. Specifically associated with alcoholism, Marchiafava–Bignami disease was originally described in Italian men addicted to red wine[739] but has since been reported in non-Italians drinking beer or whiskey.[740] Rare cases have occurred in nonalcoholics.[741,742] Early symptoms are typically mental and include psychotic mania, depression, paranoia, and dementia. Major motor seizures are common, and there may be fluctuating hemiparesis, aphasia, rigidity, abnormal movements, dysarthria, and astasia-abasia. A callosal disconnection syndrome has infrequently been described.[740,743,744] One reported patient had Balint syndrome.[745] There is usually progression to coma and death over a few months, although sometimes the course evolves acutely over days or chronically over years. A patient with apraxia, grasp reflexes, and gait ataxia improved spontaneously; following his death 3 years later from liver failure, autopsy revealed Marchiafava–Bignami disease.[746] In some cases clinical recovery is complete; in others there is residual cognitive impairment.[747,748] The callosal lesions can be detected with MRI, and in patients with clinical recovery, CT and MRI abnormalities regress.[749–755]

Histological changes resemble those of central pontine myelinolysis but are located, with sharp demarcation, in the medial zone of the corpus callosum, sparing the dorsal and ventral rims and spreading rostrocaudally. Severe lesions can be necrotic or hemorrhagic.[756] The anterior and posterior commissures as well as the subcortical white matter, centrum semiovale, basal ganglia, and middle cerebellar peduncles (but not the basis pontis) can also be affected, with striking symmetry.[757] The internal capsule is usually spared. In nearly half the cases, there are cortical lesions corresponding to "Morel's laminar sclerosis."[737,757] These lesions, originally believed to cause dementia in alcoholics, consist of neuronal loss and gliosis in the third cortical layer of the frontal and parietal convexities. They are sometimes found in the absence of callosal damage.[758] Although the histological similarity of central pontine myelinolysis and Marchiafava–Bignami disease suggests common mechanisms, rarely have the two diseases occurred together.[759]

The cause of Marchiafava–Bignami disease is unknown, and there is no explanation for such severe symptoms with such mild lesions. Similar pathology can be created experimentally with cyanide, apparently by damaging oligodendroglia,[760] but a relation of such toxicity to either ethanol or malnutrition is dubious.

Alcoholic Myelopathy

A 1984 report described five well-nourished alcoholics without prior portocaval shunting who developed paresthesias of the feet and then progressive spastic paraparesis. Investigations, not described in detail, allegedly excluded cobalamin and other vitamin deficiency, spinal cord compression, and multiple sclerosis. With abstinence symptoms stopped progressing but did not improve.[760a] The lack of subsequent similar reports makes "alcoholic myelopathy" a dubious syndrome.

Movement Disorders

Differing from ethanol withdrawal tremor is *tremor of chronic alcoholism*, which resembles essential tremor with a prominent 4–7 Hz peak and a smaller amplitude 9.5 Hz peak and postural triggering. Family history is usually negative, and tremor is rarely severe. Propranolol is more likely to decrease tremor of chronic alcoholism than essential tremor.[706b,760c]

Although parkinsonism is sometimes observed during withdrawal (see above), moderate amounts of ethanol consumption do not increase the risk for Parkinson's disease. Some studies noted a reduced risk for Parkinson's disease among beer drinkers but not wine or liquor drinkers, suggesting that the effect was related to components of beer other than ethanol.[760d]

Myoclonus-dystonia, an autosomal dominant disorder, is often associated with alcoholism. The reason is probably that ethanol tends to reduce symptoms of the disorder.[760e]

Alcoholics are susceptible to periodic limb movements during sleep.[790f] A case report described ethanol-triggered paroxysmal nonkinesogenic dyskinesia in a patient with pallidal ischemia.[760g]

Coronary Artery Disease

Although studies were not always corrected for possible confounders,[761,762] low-to-moderate amounts of ethanol very likely decrease the risk of coronary artery disease and myocardial infarction.[763–770] In fact, it is estimated that mortality and morbidity attributable to coronary artery disease are 40% to 60% lower among moderate drinkers than among abstainers[771] and that abstinence from ethanol by the entire US population would result in over 80,000 additional coronary artery disease deaths per year.[772] The "French paradox" refers to the observation that despite a high level of risk factors such as cholesterol, diabetes, hypertension, and enthusiastic intake of saturated fat, French men have the lowest mortality rate from cardiovascular disease in Western industrialized nations (36% lower than in the United States); risk reduction correlates with consumption of ethanol (average 48 g per day), especially in wine.[773] Such risk reduction, of course, is offset by the mortality associated with alcoholism, including an increased risk of coronary artery disease among alcoholics. Nonetheless, prospective studies demonstrate that moderate consumption of beer, spirits, or wine protects against coronary artery disease,[774–776] that when myocardial infarction occurs, moderate drinkers have lower mortality,[777] and that at all levels of drinking wine drinkers have a reduced risk of both coronary artery disease and death from all causes compared with drinkers of beer and spirits.[775]

Stroke

Epidemiology

Coronary artery disease in heavy drinkers carries an indirect risk for cardioembolic stroke secondary to cardiac wall hypokinesia or arrhythmia. Thromboembolism is also a prominent feature of alcoholic cardiomyopathy, with or without arrhythmia.[778,779] It appears, moreover, that depending on dose ethanol either increases or decreases the risk of stroke independent of its cardiac effects.

Finnish investigators reported an association between recent heavy ethanol ingestion and both occlusive and hemorrhagic stroke.[780–784] These studies were retrospective and used population prevalence data as controls; other similarly designed analyses either failed to identify such an association[785] or found it only for intracerebral hemorrhage.[786] Chicago investigators reported that an association between ethanol intoxication and stroke disappeared when corrected for cigarette smoking.[787,788] In a more recent study the same Finnish investigators found that among young adults more ischemic strokes occurred during weekends and holidays than were expected but that the association was stronger for young women than for young men, suggesting triggering factors other than ethanol.[789]

Numerous case–control and cohort studies have addressed the relationship of stroke to chronic ethanol use.[790–808] Such studies have differed in end-points selected (e.g., total stroke, occlusive stroke, hemorrhagic stroke, or stroke mortality), amount and duration of ethanol consumption, correction for other risk factors (e.g., hypertension and smoking), ethnicity, socioeconomics, and selection of controls. Drinkers are overrepresented among hospitalized controls, leading to the impression that ethanol is protective against stroke; they are underrepresented among community controls identified by a questionnaire, leading to the impression that ethanol is a risk factor for stroke.[809]

Among cohort studies, the Yugoslavia Cardio-vascular Disease Study found increased stroke mortality among drinkers, and although the association was especially strong for hypertensives, it persisted after adjustment for blood pressure.[810] A reduced risk was found for modest drinkers. In the Honolulu Heart Study, heavy drinkers had an increased risk of hemorrhagic stroke independent of other risk factors, including hypertension and smoking.[811–813] There was no comparable risk for occlusive stroke. The Framingham Study described lower than expected stroke incidence among "moderate" drinkers and higher rates in both heavy drinkers and nondrinkers.[814] The Nurses' Health Study, adjusting for smoking and hypertension, found an inverse association between modest drinking and occlusive stroke and an increased risk at higher intake; both modest and heavy drinkers had an increased risk of subarachnoid hemorrhage.[815] In the Lausanne Stroke Registry, severity of internal carotid artery stenosis inversely correlated with "light to moderate" drinking; there were too few patients to assess heavy intake.[816] The Japanese Hisayama Study found no independent association between ethanol and occlusive or hemorrhagic stroke.[817] A study of Japanese physicians found a positive association between stroke mortality and ethanol.[818] Other Japanese investigators reported variable risk for hemorrhagic or occlusive stroke among drinkers—e.g., independent association between ethanol and hemorrhagic but not occlusive stroke,[819] no association between ethanol and occlusive stroke,[820] and a "J-shaped" relationship between ethanol intake and occlusive stroke, with drinkers of less than 42 g/day showing a lower risk and heavy drinkers showing a higher risk than "never drinkers."[821]

In 1989 a review of 62 epidemiological studies that examined the relationship between stroke and "moderate" ethanol consumption (less than two drinks, or 1 oz. of ethanol, daily), concluded that ethnicity plays a decisive role.[822] Among whites moderate doses of ethanol protected against ischemic stroke, but higher doses increased risk. Among Japanese little association existed between ethanol and ischemic stroke. In both populations all doses of ethanol increased the risk of both intracerebral and subarachnoid hemorrhage. Some studies suggested that the risk of hemorrhagic stroke declines with abstinence. There was insufficient evidence to draw an association between stroke and recent intoxication per se.

During the past decade epidemiological studies of ethanol and stroke have continued to produce conflicting results. An Australian case–control study found that low doses of ethanol (<20 g/day) protected against "all strokes, all ischemic strokes, and primary intracerebral hemorrhage."[823] A British case–control study found that the protective effect of "light or moderate" drinking compared with non-drinking disappeared when corrected for obesity and exercise.[824] An Italian case–control study found that ethanol risk for stroke "was practically lost" after correction for previous stroke, hypertension, diabetes, hyperlipidemia, and obesity.[825] A Danish study found that moderate wine drinking reduced the likelihood of stroke, moderate drinking of "spirits" increased the likelihood, and moderate drinking of beer had no effect in either direction.[826] In another Danish study subjects who drank wine had a decreased risk of stroke (ischemic, hemorrhagic, or not specified) compared with those who never or rarely drank wine; those who drank wine weekly had a lower risk than those who drank wine either daily or monthly. No effect of drinking either beer or liquor on stroke risk was found.[827]

A Finnish study found that recent heavy drinking but not former heavy drinking increased the risk of embolic stroke in patients with a source of thrombus in the heart or the large cerebral vessels.[828] Another Finnish study found an increased risk for hemorrhagic stroke in binge-drinking young adults.[829] Other investigators found heavy ethanol use a risk factor for intracerebral hemorrhage,[830] subarachnoid hemorrhage,[831,832] or both.[833]

The Northern Manhattan Stroke Study compared 677 patients with ischemic stroke and 1139 controls. "Moderate" ethanol intake (two drinks per day) was protective (odds ratio: 0.51). The effect of two to five drinks daily was uncertain. More than five drinks daily increased risk, and at seven drinks daily the odds ration was 2.96. Benefit and risk were the same for younger and older subjects, for men and women, for whites, blacks, and Hispanics, and for wine, beer, and spirits.[834]

In the U.S. Physicians Health Study, 22,071 healthy male physicians aged 40 to 84 years were prospectively followed for 12 years, during which 679 strokes were reported. Nearly all participants were light-to-moderate drinkers, and risk of ischemic stroke was significantly reduced in those who drank more than one drink per week compared with those who drank less. There was no difference in risk reduction between those who had one drink per week and those who had one or more drinks per day.[835]

The Framingham Study found a protective effect of light-to-moderate drinking on ischemic stroke.[836] In that study the incidence rates for stroke were highest in former drinkers who had drunk most heavily, and this risk held for men but not women. Ethanol reduced the risk of ischemic stroke in subjects aged 60 to 69 years but not in those younger or older, and only wine, not beer or spirits, was protective. (No data were offered on red versus white wine.) In that study, former drinkers were older, smoked more than never-drinkers, and were more likely to have heart disease and hypertension. The significance of special risk in former drinkers is therefore uncertain.[837]

In 2003 a meta-analysis addressed the association of ethanol intake and stroke in 19 cohort studies[796,811,815,818,821,836,838–850] and 16 case–control studies [788,795,798,804,809,823–825,830,834,851–856] over a period of two decades.[856a] The 35 studies were selected from a total of 122 reports. To be included a study had to be a case–control or cohort study in which total stroke, ischemic stroke, or hemorrhagic stroke was an end-point. Relative risk or relative odds and their variance of stroke associated with ethanol had to be reported, ethanol consumption had to be quantified, and abstainers had to be used as the reference group. All studies controlled for important stroke risk factors such as hypertension or cigarette smoking. The results of this meta-analysis revealed that compared with abstention, consumption of less than 12 g per day of ethanol was associated with a reduced risk of total stroke (relative risk: 0.80); consumption of 12–24 g per day was associated with a reduced risk of ischemic stroke (relative risk: 0.72). Consumption of more than 60 g per day was associated with an increased risk of total stroke (relative risk: 1.64), ischemic stroke (relative risk: 1.69), and hemorrhagic stroke (relative risk: 2.18). Light-to-moderate ethanol intake did not reduce the risk of hemorrhagic stroke. Thus, as with a similar meta-analysis 14 years earlier,[822] a J-shaped association was found between ethanol consumption and the relative risk of total and ischemic stroke and a linear association was found between ethanol consumption and the relative risk of hemorrhagic stroke.

Angiography and duplex ultrasound demonstrate a positive association of heavy ethanol consumption with carotid atherosclerosis; low ethanol intake, by contrast, has a beneficial effect.[857–859] Although moderate drinking reportedly did not reduce the risk of arteriosclerosis in small intracerebral arteries,[860,861] a study using CT scanning found that one to five drinks daily reduced the risk of leukoaraiosis in stroke patients, whereas heavier ethanol consumption increased the risk.[862] The Japanese Hisayama study found ethanol to be an independent risk factor for "vascular dementia."[863]

In the U.S. Cardiovascular Health Study 3660 adults aged 65 years and older, and without a history of cerebrovascular disease, underwent MRI of the brain. A U-shaped relationship was found between ethanol consumption and white matter abnormalities, with one to seven drinks per week protective compared with abstention and more than 15 drinks per week increasing risk. Protection against frank infarction continued above 15 drinks per week, however, but heavier intake increased the risk of ventricular enlargement and sulcal widening.[864] Higher doses thus appear to produce competing effects, with uncertain overall effects on neurological function. In the Framingham and the National Heart, Lung, and Blood Institute Twin Study, moderate ethanol consumption appeared to improve cognitive performance,[865,866] and other studies have found a J-shaped relationship between ethanol consumption and cognitive performance.[867–870] In the Rotterdam Study, light-to-moderate drinking was especially effective in reducing the risk for "vascular dementia," and the effect did not depend on the type of alcoholic beverage.[871]

Most studies on the relation of ethanol to stroke risk have based consumption on self-reports, and critics have questioned the reliability of such data. A prospective study from Finland and Lithuania found no correlation of stroke with self-reported ethanol drinking but did find correlation of ischemic stroke with serum gamma-glutamyl transferase concentration, considered a biological marker for heavy ethanol consumption.[872]

Mechanisms of Protection and Risk

As with coronary artery disease, several mechanisms might explain the association between drinking and stroke.[873] Ethanol acutely and chronically causes hypertension,[874–882] perhaps by increasing adrenergic activity and raising blood levels of cortisol, renin, aldosterone, and vasopressin.[883] In rats ethanol stimulates the secretion of corticotropin-releasing hormone (CRH), and the intracerebroventricular administration of CRH increases blood pressure and stimulates sympathetic activity. Inhibition of CRH release by dexamethasone attenuates stress-induced sympathetic activation. In human volunteers ethanol increased blood pressure and sympathetic discharge, and this effect was blocked by dexamethasone, consistent with CNS mediation of ethanol-induced hypertension.[884] The systolic blood pressure decline during the first week following a stroke is greater in heavy drinkers than in light drinkers or abstainers.[885] It is estimated that above a daily ethanol intake of 30 g an increment of 10 g ethanol per day increases systolic blood pressure by roughly 1–2 mmHg and diastolic blood pressure by 1 mmHg.[886] With abstinence blood pressure sometimes returns to normal.[887]

Ethanol lowers blood levels of low-density lipoproteins (LDL) and elevates levels of high-density lipoproteins (HDL).[770,888–891] The relationship is uncertain, however, for ethanol may not raise blood levels of the more protective HDL$_2$-subfraction.[892,893] In the Northern Manhattan Stroke Study the association between moderate ethanol consumption and reduced stroke risk was independent of the HDL cholesterol level.[834] In the Framingham study, among men with the apolipoprotein E2 allele, LDL cholesterol was lower in drinkers than in nondrinkers, whereas in men with the E4 allele LDL cholesterol was higher in drinkers than in nondrinkers.[894]

Lp(a) lipoprotein levels, which correlate with the extent of carotid atherosclerosis, are reduced by ethanol intake.[895]

Acutely, ethanol reportedly decreases fibrinolytic activity, raises levels of factor VIII, increases platelet reactivity to adenosine diphosphate (ADP), and shortens bleeding time.[896–900] In other studies, however, moderate ethanol consumption increased levels of prostacyclin,[901,902] decreased platelet function,[903–910] decreased plasma fibrinogen levels,[911] stimulated release of endothelin from endothelial cells,[912] and increased plasma levels of endogenous tissue plasminogen activator.[909,913] Ethanol increases the deformability of erythrocytes and decreases their aggregation.[914] Alcoholics with liver disease have decreased levels of clotting factors, excessive fibrinolysis, and platelet abnormalities.[882,915] During ethanol withdrawal, "rebound thrombocytosis" and platelet hyperaggregability are observed.[916,917] In rats this rebound followed withdrawal in animals receiving pure ethanol or white wine but not in those receiving red wine, perhaps reflecting a protective effect of red wine tannins.[918] In a conflicting report, however, ethanol withdrawal was associated with decreased platelet response to activators.[919] In humans, withdrawal was associated with increased fibrinolytic activity as a result of decreased levels of tissue-type plasminogen activator inhibitor.[920]

Many investigators consider atherosclerosis an inflammatory disease, and elevated concentrations of C-reactive protein (CRP), an acute-phase reactant, are associated with risk of coronary artery disease and ischemic stroke. Paralleling the J-shaped relationship of ethanol consumption with myocardial infarction and ischemic stroke, nondrinkers and heavy drinkers have higher CRP levels than moderate drinkers.[921,921e]

Advanced glycation end products (AGEs) are circulating proteins bound to sugars. AGEs in turn bind to low-density lipoproteins and reduce their clearance from the blood. AGEs are thereby a risk for atherosclerosis. Diabetic rats fed ethanol have reduced AGE levels; a proposed mechanism is AGE binding by the ethanol metabolite acetaldehyde.[922]

Early reports indicated that acute ethanol intoxication causes cerebral vasodilatation[923,924] and blood–brain barrier leakage of albumin.[925] Increased cerebral blood flow was also observed during withdrawal, although dehydration during hangover can reduce cerebral perfusion.[926] Decreased cerebral blood flow associated with chronic drinking was attributed to reduced cerebral metabolism.[927] Ethanol-related hemoconcentration may also lower cerebral blood flow.[781,882]

In vitro, ethanol can cause *constriction* of both large and small cerebral vessels, and some investigators have observed decreased cerebral blood flow and impaired cerebrovascular autoregulation during acute intoxication.[928] In rats, low boluses of ethanol produced cerebral vasodilatation, whereas higher doses produced vasoconstriction; constant infusions of ethanol produced similar vasodilatation or vasoconstriction, and at high infusion rates vessel rupture was found at autopsy. These changes

were independent of blood pressure.[929] In living rats ethanol-induced vasoconstriction of cerebral arterioles was accompanied by blockade of the vasodilatation produced by acetylcholine, histamine, and ADP but not the vasodilatation produced by nitroglycerin or the vasoconstriction produced by a thromboxane analog.[930,931]

Elevation of magnesium ion concentration relaxes spasms of cerebral vessels induced by all known vasoactive-neurohumoral substances as well as by phencyclidine, cocaine, LSD, and ethanol. In cultured canine vascular smooth muscle cells, ethanol exposure caused depletion of intracellular magnesium ion.[932] Such an effect could exacerbate ethanol-induced cerebral vasospasm. It could also lead to an increased ratio of calcium to magnesium ions, resulting in intracellular calcium ion overload and cell death.[933] The threshold for glutamate excitotoxicity, which plays a major role in ischemic neuronal death, may be lowered in ethanol-related brain infarcts, especially those affecting ethanol abusers with up-regulated glutamate receptors.[934] Pretreatment of animals with magnesium ion prevented ethanol-induced strokes.[932]

In view of studies suggesting a special benefit of wine—especially red wine—in reducing risk for myocardial and cerebral ischemia, investigators have tried to identify responsible constituents. Red wine contains numerous phenolic acids, polyphenols, and flavonoids capable of scavenging free radicals and reducing oxidative damage to low-density lipoprotein, thereby reducing their potential atherogenicity.[935–938] Whether such an effect outweighs the pro-oxidant effects of ethanol itself, however, is uncertain.[939]

Hyperhomocysteinemia is a risk factor for both myocardial ischemia and ischemic stroke. Homocysteine is normally metabolized either to methionine in a folate- and cobalamin-dependent reaction or to cystathionine in a pyridoxine-dependent reaction. Elevated plasma levels of homocysteine in nutritionally deficient alcoholics therefore increase their risk for brain infarction.[940,941]

Ethanol-induced neck trauma can precipitate traumatic stroke.[942]

Of the three subunits that form alcohol dehydrogenase (ADH1, ADH2, ADH3), the ADH3 gene locus has variant polymorphisms in nearly half of white populations. The γ_1 isoenzyme of ADH3 metabolizes ethanol 2½ times as rapidly as the γ_2 isoenzyme, and in the Physicians' Health Study, although moderate ethanol consumption was associated with reduced risk of myocardial infarction in all three genotypes ($\gamma_1\gamma_1$, $\gamma_1\gamma_2$, $\gamma_2\gamma_2$), homozygosity for the γ_2 allele conferred significantly greater risk reduction. Such subjects also had higher serum HDL levels.[943]

Bilateral anterior cerebral artery occlusion occurred in a young alcoholic woman with sickle cell trait; platelets showed hyperaggregation to epinephrine, raising the possibility that ethanol-induced catecholamine release contributed to cerebral thrombosis.[944]

In most cases of sudden deafness no cause is found; some cases are probably vascular in origin. In a case–control study moderate-to-heavy ethanol consumption was a risk factor for idiopathic sudden deafness.[945]

"Caffeinol"

In an animal model of cerebral infarction, administration of low-dose ethanol plus caffeine ("caffeinol") within 2 hours of stroke onset significantly reduced infarct volume. Ethanol alone aggravated infarct volume, and caffeine alone was without effect. Prior daily exposure to ethanol eliminated the efficacy of acute caffeinol treatment.[946] A pilot study of caffeinol in humans with ischemic stroke demonstrated safety even when combined with plasminogen activator.[947]

Alcoholic Dementia

Historical Background

Is ethanol directly neurotoxic? Can it cause progressive mental decline in the absence of nutritional deficiency, hepatic failure, or other well-recognized forms of brain damage in alcoholism? For decades the concept of "alcoholic dementia" has been controversial.[948] That malnutrition might be overrated as a cause of chronic dementia in alcoholics is suggested by reports of impaired cognition, cerebral atrophy, and neurophysiological or neuropharmacological abnormalities in seemingly well-nourished alcoholics.[949,950] Conversely, as noted above, chronic dementia infre-

quently follows non-alcoholic Wernicke syndrome or beri-beri.[446] Early descriptions of histological changes in alcoholic brains,[951] however, were dismissed by others as artifacts,[952] and later descriptions of reduced neuronal number or size, decreased glucose metabolism, and cholinergic receptor loss in frontal or temporal cortex of alcoholics[953–957] were said to be confounded by coexisting Wernicke syndrome or cirrhosis.[952] Observations that many alcoholics developed progressive dementia without prior episodes of Wernicke syndrome were countered by descriptions of Korsakoff syndrome insidiously developing after repeated bouts of presumed "subclinical" Wernicke syndrome.[413] Observations that the dementia of many alcoholics was often more "global" than that encountered in those with the predominantly amnestic disorder of Korsakoff syndrome[958] were countered by descriptions of patients with pathologically proven Korsakoff syndrome who had intellectual and behavioral disturbances not explained by impaired memory.[952,959,960] Finally, the significance of radiographically demonstrated "cerebral" atrophy" was questioned in the face of inconsistent correlation with psychometric dysfunction[961–965] and reports that the "atrophy" improved with abstinence.[966–970] Nonetheless, animal and human studies over the past decade provide compelling evidence that ethanol does directly damage neurons and offer a plausible mechanism.

Animal Studies

Properly designed animal studies require pair-fed controls and a sufficient period of abstinence to discount the effects of acute withdrawal. Such animals demonstrate impaired learning that tends to be subtle and selective, affecting some tasks but not others.[971,972] In rodents, chronic ethanol administration results in hippocampal neuronal loss, specifically a reduced number of CA1 and CA3 pyramidal neurons, mossy fiber–CA3 synapses, dentate gyrus granule cells, and local circuit interneurons.[973–978] Loss ranges from 10% to 50% of the neurons.[441] Neuropathological changes are evident after only 3 days of high intoxicating doses of ethanol, and the time-course of development of hippocampal damage parallels cognitive impairment.[441] Ethanol also produces loss of cholinergic neurons in the basal forebrain, more pronounced in the medial septal nucleus (which projects to the hippocampus) than in the nucleus basalis (which projects to the neocortex).[979] Impaired memory accompanies these changes, and transplantation of cholinergic neurons into hippocampus or cerebral cortex corrects both the cholinergic deficit and the abnormal memory.[980] Ethanol-induced functional alterations in the hippocampus include depressed inhibitory postsynaptic potentials in dentate granule and CA1 pyramidal cells and impaired long-term potentiation (LTP).[981–983] In rats receiving chronic ethanol to maintain BEC at 80–120 mg/dL for 12 months there was loss of hippocampal granule and pyramidal cells yet preserved numbers of mossy fiber–CA3 synapses, suggesting new synapse formation; at 18 months, synapses were also decreased, suggesting collapse of this plastic response.[984]

Ethanol-induced loss of dendritic spines has also been observed in cerebellar Purkinje cells of rodents.[972,985,986] Findings in other brain areas are less consistent. In one study rat cerebral cortex neurons were unchanged after sufficient ethanol to cause apnea; others reported ethanol-induced pathological changes in cerebral cortex, hypothalamus, and brainstem.[986,987] In one report "adolescent" rats given ethanol had increased numbers of spines on apical dendrites of pyramidal neurons in the somatosensory cortex, probably reflecting impairment of the naturally occurring elimination of redundant synapses during youth.[988]

Neuronal damage correlates with the total amount of ethanol consumed, usually becoming evident after a few months of oral administration.[441] Damage can develop after only 1 month of intermittent intraperitoneal ethanol, however,[989] and was apparent after only a few days of forced intragastric administration of high doses at short intervals.[990] A binge pattern of drinking, producing very high BECs, reduces the total amount of ethanol needed to produce brain damage in young rats.[991] In some studies, loss of hippocampal granule cells began during chronic ethanol exposure and continued after withdrawal;[992,993] in other studies hippocampal cell loss began only after ethanol administration was stopped.[994] Others have similarly observed that one or more ethanol withdrawal periods are more harmful to neurons than is continuous ethanol exposure.[995]

Observations in Humans

Human studies do not allow pair-fed controls, and skepticism is appropriate when assessing reports of alcoholic dementia unrelated to nutritional status. Brains of alcoholics have reduced weight and volume affecting especially the white matter,[996] and abnormal white matter signals are seen on MRI, including diffusion-weighted images.[997] Ventricles are enlarged and sulci widened, and significant reversal of cortical sulcal and ventricular enlargement occurs in alcoholics who maintain abstinence,[769,998–1000] Reports that cognitive improvement accompanies morphological improvement are less consistent.[1001] In some studies alcoholic men and women were both at risk for brain shrinkage;[1002] in others women were at greater risk than men.[1003] (Possibly confounding reports of gender differences are normal variations between men and women in the volume of particular brain regions and in the pattern of brain atrophy with age.[996]) Brain shrinkage and its reversal are not the result of water loss and rehydration, and the white matter loss involves many structural elements, not a specific lipid component.[996] In a phosphorus magnetic resonance spectroscopy study of middle-aged heavy drinkers, cerebral white matter phospholipid damage was detected in the absence of white matter volume loss.[1004]

Neuronal loss in humans is reported in the cerebral cortex (especially frontal lobe), hypothalamus, and thalamus; reduced volume or cell loss has been less consistently reported in the cholinergic basal forebrain nuclei and the hippocampus.[424,1005–1009] In one report, there was no neuronal loss in any hippocampal subregion, and hippocampal volume reduction was attributable to white matter reduction, again reversible with abstinence.[1010] In another report, the entorhinal cortex of alcoholics contained neurons with reduced nuclear size.[1011]

Dose-related loss of hypothalamic vasopressin-containing neurons was found in heavy drinkers, perhaps contributing to fluid and electrolyte abnormalities in alcoholics.[1012] Loss of brainstem serotonergic neurons was described in an alcoholic with no pathological evidence of Wernicke–Korsakoff syndrome. Serotonin depletion increases ethanol intake in rats; such depletion in humans might therefore contribute to increased ethanol craving.[1013]

Addressing the inconsistent findings of different investigators, a review of published neuropathological studies stressed the need for careful selection and classification of alcoholics into those with and without evident nutritional deficiency, and for detailed quantitative analysis.[1014] It was concluded that "uncomplicated alcoholics" have brain shrinkage largely accounted for by loss of white matter and at least partly reversible. Neuronal loss has been documented in specific areas of the cerebral cortex (especially the superior frontal association cortex), hypothalamus (supraoptic and paraventricular nuclei), and cerebellum. Less consistent are reported changes in hippocampus, amygdala, and locus ceruleus. There appears to be no change in the basal ganglia, nucleus basalis, or brainstem serotonergic neurons. Dendritic, synaptic, receptor, and neurotransmitter changes probably explain cognitive impairments that precede obvious morphological changes. Many regions that are normal in uncomplicated alcoholics are damaged in those with Wernicke–Korsakoff syndrome. Finally, the pattern of ethanol-induced damage is species-specific in different animal models.[1014]

In an autopsy study using nonalcoholic controls, selective neuronal loss in the superior frontal association cortex of chronic alcoholics with or without prior evidence of Wernicke–Korsakoff syndrome appeared to be confined to non-GABAergic pyramidal neurons.[1015] In another autopsy study, which used cDNA microarrays to compare gene expression in the frontal cortices of heavy alcoholics and controls, multiple genetic alterations, usually reduction, were identified in the alcoholics. The most pronounced differences were found in myelin-related genes involved in protein trafficking. "Alcoholic cases with concomitant diseases" were excluded, but nutritional deficiency was not commented on.[1015a]

Magnetic resonance spectroscopy using the neuronal/axonal marker *N*-acetyl-aspartate (NAA) confirmed the special vulnerability of the frontal lobes in human alcoholics; frontal white matter NAA was reduced by 14.7%.[1016] Other studies correlated frontal lobe damage with particular cognitive or behavioral abnormalities, for example, difficulty planning, organizing, problem solving, and abstracting, as well as disinhibition, perseverative responding, lack of insight, and difficulty comprehending affective prosody.[441,1017,1018] Alcoholic subjects without Wernicke–Korsakoff syndrome reportedly have impaired working memory and executive function in the absence of clinical amnesia.[1019,1020]

Many alcoholics have impaired olfactory memory; they can identify familiar odors but not recently learned unfamiliar odors. In rats receiving ethanol in a "binge" pattern, there was neuronal damage in the olfactory bulbs and some of their projections, including the pyriform and entorhinal cortices and the dentate gyrus. The pattern differed from that produced by chronic lower doses of ethanol, which maximally affect the hippocampal CA region and the cerebellum. Excitotoxic kindling was the proposed mechanisms for the binge pattern.[995]

Genetic factors might influence the ability of ethanol to produce brain shrinkage. Studies have implicated allelic variation in the alcohol dehydrogenase gene[1021] and in the gene for tumor necrosis factor-β.[1022] The apolipoprotein Eε 4 (APOEε 4) allele was reportedly more prevalent in alcoholic Wernicke–Korsakoff patients with "global" intellectual impairment than in those with a more purely amnestic disorder.[1023]

The Role of Glutamate

Animal studies thus demonstrate that ethanol is directly toxic to mammalian brain neurons, and even if nutritional deficiency or other brain injury can seldom be excluded in cognitively impaired human alcoholics, it seems likely that direct toxicity plays more than a minor role. A plausible mechanism is glutamate excitotoxicity and oxidative stress.[1024–1027] As noted above, ethanol acutely inhibits glutamate neurotransmission, with rebound increased glutamatergic transmission during withdrawal. Animal studies in which repeated bouts of ethanol withdrawal carried particular risk for neuronal loss favor excitotoxicity as a mechanism. Moreover, as described above, glutamate toxicity may play a crucial role in pathogenesis of Wernicke–Korsakoff syndrome, raising the possibility that some (or maybe most) cases of "alcoholic dementia" represent additive (or synergistic) effects of both thiamine deficiency and ethanol toxicity.

Dose Relationships and Neuroprotection

If ethanol is a direct neurotoxin, it becomes imperative to define a safe dose threshold. Since 1986,

19 studies have investigated the effects of "sober social drinking" on cognitive function, event-related potentials, or both. A review of these studies concluded that people drinking five or six "U.S. standard drinks" per day over extended time periods manifest "cognitive inefficiencies." At seven to nine drinks per day there are "mild cognitive deficits," and at 10 or more drinks per day cognitive deficits are equivalent to those found in diagnosed alcoholics.[1028] In a study of 1432 "non-alcoholic subjects," "heavy" ethanol consumption (average 418 g ethanol/week) was a risk factor for reduced frontal lobe volume, whereas light (88 g/week) and moderate (181 g/week) consumption were not.[1029] In the U.S. Atherosclerosis Risk in Communities (ARIC) study, cerebral atrophy was associated with ethanol intake in a dose-related fashion.[1029a]

Despite pathological evidence of the neurotoxic effects of ethanol, a number of epidemiological studies failed to identify a relationship between ethanol intake and the risk of dementia.[1030–1033] In fact, in the Zutphen Study and the Honolulu Heart Program moderate ethanol intake was found to be protective.[1034,1035] In the French PAQUID Study dementia was less prevalent in wine-drinkers, raising the possibility of a protective effect of antioxidant flavonoids in wine, especially red wine.[1036,1037] (Few subjects in that study drank beer or spirits, however.) In another study the protective effect of ethanol was most evident in subjects carrying the APOEε 4 allele.[1038] Another study found that ethanol intake was associated with a reduced risk of cognitive dysfunction among subjects without an APOEε 4 allele but with an increased risk among those with an APOEε 4 allele.[1039]

In the Rotterdam Study, a prospective cohort study, 7983 nondemented subjects aged 55 years and older were followed for several years; 197 developed dementia (Alzheimer's 146, vascular 29, "other" 22). One to three drinks daily reduced the risk of any dementia (odds ratio: 0.58) and vascular dementia (odds ratio: 0.29). Protection did not depend on whether subjects drank wine, spirits, or beer. The effect was most evident in men, and there was no interaction between ethanol and smoking.[871] The protective effect of ethanol was greatest among subjects with an APOEε 4 allele.

In the Copenhagen City Heart Study, a nested case–control study, 1709 nondemented subjects aged 65 years or more were re-examined after 20 years. Over the two decades 83 became demented (40 Alzheimer's, 15 vascular, 11 "other"). Moderate intake of wine, but not of spirits or beer, significantly reduced the risk of dementia. Subgroup analysis of those with Alzheimer's dementia revealed a trend similar to the overall group but short of significance, perhaps because of insufficient numbers. There was no difference in the effect of ethanol between men and women.[1040]

In the Cardiovascular Health Study, a nested case–control study from four communities in the United States, 373 demented patients aged 65 years or older were compared with controls. Two hundred and fifty-eight had Alzheimer's disease alone, 44 vascular dementia alone, 54 Alzheimer's plus vascular dementia, and 17 "other." Light-to-moderate ethanol consumption reduced the risk of dementia (for weekly intake of less than one drink, odds ratio: 0.65; one–six drinks, odds ratio: 0.46; 7-13 drinks, odds ratio: 0.69; 14 or more drinks, odds ratio: 1.22). There was no difference between wine, spirits, or beer, and ethanol appeared to be equally protective against both Alzheimer's and vascular dementia. In contrast to the Rotterdam Study, protection was most pronounced for those without an APOEε 4 allele; among those who drank seven or more drinks per week, the risk of dementia was greatest in those with an APOEε 4 allele.[1041]

It thus appears that ethanol's effects on cognition, like its effects on ischemic vascular disease, follows a J-shaped curve, with low-to-moderate intake reducing the risk of dementia but heavy intake increasing it. Although the reduced risk of ischemic cerebrovascular disease may contribute to the favorable effects of low-to-moderate ethanol consumption on cognition, cerebrovascular effects do not appear sufficient to explain the benefit in nonvascular dementia. Mechanisms remains speculative.[1042] Flavonoid antioxidants might confer a special benefit to red wine, but ethanol itself has antioxidant properties. (Investigators in the Rotterdam Study speculated that the greater benefit of ethanol among subjects with an APOEε 4 allele might be the result of ethanol's ability to block oxidation of the apolipoprotein, thereby preventing it from binding to β-amyloid.) Reservatrol, a compound found in grapes and red wine, triggers the activity of a group of genes called sirtuins, which extend the life span of yeast and in human cells blunt the activity of the tumor suppressor gene p53, blocking apoptosis.[1042a] Benefit and risk might also be related to ethanol's effects on neurotransmitter systems. For example, in rats low concentrations of ethanol stimulate acetylcholine release in the hippocampus, whereas higher concentrations inhibit it.[1043]

Needless to say, these observations and speculations, like those relating to ethanol's effects on cardiovascular and cerebrovascular disease, hardly mean that physicians should urge their teetotaling patients to start drinking.[874]

Fetal Alcohol Syndrome

Observations in Humans

The "gin epidemic" in 18th-century England led to speculation that ethanol abuse caused feeblemindedness in offspring,[1044] and during the 19th century high prevalences of stillbirth and infant mortality were reported among children of alcoholic women.[1045] In 1968, French workers reported an association of maternal alcoholism with congenital malformations, delayed psychomotor development, and behavioral problems.[1046] Shortly thereafter pediatricians in Seattle, noting frequent failure to thrive in offspring of alcoholic mothers, defined the fetal alcohol syndrome (FAS) (Table 12–20).[1047,1048]

Major clinical features include CNS dysfunction, growth deficiency, and distinctive facies; less often there are abnormalities of the heart, skeleton, urogenital organs, skin, and muscles.[9,1049,1050] Microphthalmia, malformed retinal vessels, optic atrophy, and blindness are common.[1051] So are developmentally delayed auditory function, sensorineural hearing loss, conduction hearing loss resulting from recurrent serous otitis media, and central hearing loss; auditory impairment in turn contributes to speech and language difficulty.[1052–1054] Prospective controlled studies reveal that the FAS occurs independently of maternal malnutrition, smoking, caffeine, other drugs, and age.[1055] (That does not mean that other drug exposure or the quality of prenatal care are irrelevant.) Binge drinking that produces high ethanol levels at a critical fetal period may be more important than chronic exposure, and early gestation appears to be the most vulnerable period.[1049,1054]

Children of alcoholic mothers are often intellectually borderline or retarded without other features of the FAS;[1051,1055,1056] fetal effects of ethanol thus cover a broad spectrum. Stillbirths and attention deficit disorder are especially frequent among offspring of heavy drinkers,[1057] and each anomaly of the FAS can occur alone or in combination with others.[1058,1059] An association between maternal drinking and spasmus nutans has been reported.[1060] The face of a typical patient with the FAS is distinctive and, as in Down's syndrome, easily recognized at birth.[1061,1062] Irritability, tremulousness, poor suck, and apparent hyperacusis last weeks to months; some symptoms (e.g., seizures) suggest ethanol withdrawal.[1063] Eighty-five percent perform more than 2 standard deviations below the mean on psychometric tests, and it is rare for those not grossly retarded to have even average mental ability.[1047] In one series the average IQ was 65 with a range of 16 to 105, and the lowest IQs were in those with the most complete phenotype.[1064]

Older children are frequently hyperactive and clumsy, with hypotonia or hypertonia. A 10-year follow-up of 10 children with FAS revealed that two were dead and eight were still growth-deficient and dysmorphic; four were of borderline intelligence, and four were severely retarded.[1065] Several had eustachian tube abnormalities, chronic otitis media, and deafness. Even more dramatically, a 30-year follow-up of 105 French FAS victims (77 of whom were patients from the authors' original report) revealed facial dysmorphism (especially a long face and bulky nose and chin), persistent though less marked growth failure, and even more pronounced microcephaly, with mental retardation frequent, and abnormal behavior invariable; interestingly, several siblings without evident dysmorphism at birth also demonstrated psychological impairment.[1066]

A study of 12-year-olds exposed in utero to ethanol divided them into three groups—recognized cognitive and other deficits, physical growth restriction only, and "normal." The majority of subjects in each group had behavioral problems.[1067] Psychiatric diagnoses commonly encountered in adults with either FAS or fetal alcohol effects include ethanol or drug dependence, depression, psychotic disorders, and avoidant, antisocial, or dependent personality disorder.[1068] High rates are reported of trouble with the law, inappropriate

Table 12–20. Clinical Features of the Fetal Alcohol Syndrome

Feature	Majority	Minority
CNS	Mental retardation	
	Microcephaly	
	Hypotonia	
	Poor coordination	
	Hyperactivity	
Impaired growth	Prenatal and postnatal for length and weight	
	Diminished adipose tissue	
Abnormal face		
Eyes	Short palpebral fissures	Ptosis
		Strabismus
		Epicanthal folds
		Myopia
		Microophthalmia
		Blepharophimosis
		Cataracts
		Retinal pigmentary abnormalities
Nose	Short, upturned	
	Hypoplastic philtrum	
Mouth	Thin vermilion lip borders	Prominent lateral palatine ridges
	Retrognathia in infancy	Cleft lip or palate
	Micrognathia or prognathia in adolescence	Small teeth with faulty enamel
Maxilla	Hypoplastic	
Ears		Posteriorly rotated
		Poorly formed concha
Skeletal		Pectus excavatum or carinatum
		Syndactyly, clinodactyly, or camptodactyly
		Limited joint movements
		Nail hypoplasia
		Radiolunar synostosis
		Bifid xiphoid
		Scoliosis
		Klippel–Feil anomaly
Cardiac		Septal defects
		Great vessel anomalies
Cutaneous		Abnormal palmar creases
		Hemangiomas
		Infantile hirsutism
Muscular		Diaphragmatic, inguinal, or umbilical hernias
		Diastasis recti
Urogenital		Labial hypoplasia
		Hypospadias
		Small rotated kidneys
		Hydronephrosis

sexual behavior, failure to care for their own children, and suicide.[1069]

In an attempt to identify a "neurobehavioral profile" for prenatal ethanol exposure, ethanol-exposed children without dysmorphic features were compared with children exposed in utero to either cocaine or polychlorinated biphenyls (PCBs). In contrast to the cocaine and PCB groups, who demonstrated poor recognition memory, the ethanol group had normal recognition memory but impairment on a test of processing speed.[1070]

Neuropathological abnormalities in FAS include microcephaly, reduced volume of the basal ganglia, and abnormalities of the cerebellar vermis and corpus callosum.[1071] Partial or complete agenesis of the corpus callosum is common, but even more so is callosal displacement, with the posterior callosum lying abnormally anterior and inferior. Such changes are more obvious in FAS than in fetal alcohol effects and correlate with impaired verbal learning and defects in the interhemispheric transfer of somatosensory information.[1072,1072a] Reduced white matter volume in the parietal lobes accompanies these callosal abnormalities,[1073] and the frequency of callosal and cerebellar vermal abnormalities following in utero ethanol exposure suggests a particular vulnerability of midline structures to ethanol teratogenicity.[1074,1075] In subjects prenatally exposed to ethanol but without the facial features of FAS, neuropathological abnormalities are less prominent, but volume reductions in the basal ganglia and parietal lobe are described.[1076] Dysmorphology of the parietal lobes occurs above and beyond the overall microcephaly.[1077] Normal cerebral cortical asymmetries are less apparent, and during adolescence reduced brain growth is most evident in frontal and inferior parietal/perisylvian gray matter, consistent with the behavioral and cognitive disturbances characteristic of these victims.[1077a,1077b]

Studies in Animals

Ethanol toxicity is the cause of the FAS, which has been reproduced in carefully controlled animal models that include chickens, rodents, dogs, pigs, and primates.[1078–1083] Rats exposed to ethanol in utero exhibit bony changes in the face and limbs and microcephaly.[1084] Litter weight, not litter size, is decreased compared with pair-fed controls in rats exposed to ethanol in utero; with surrogate mothers after delivery, there is catch-up in the weight among animals that received low doses of ethanol but not among the high-dose group.[1085] Some exposed rats exhibit impaired mental ability without other physical signs.[1086] Fetal ethanol exposure in mice produces neurological, ocular, cardiac, and skeletal anomalies, including exencephaly, hydrocephalus, and microphthalmia.[1078] Although adult mice receiving chronic ethanol exhibit audiogenic seizures only transiently, prenatal and neonatal exposure causes long-lasting seizures.[1087] In dogs, high doses of ethanol prevent intrauterine tissue differentiation, moderate doses

cause spontaneous abortion, and low doses cause significant increases in stillbirths.[1088] In Macaque monkeys, exposure comparable to binge drinking causes craniofacial and nervous system abnormalities similar to the human FAS.[1082,1089] In mice, a single exposure to ethanol on the seventh day of pregnancy (corresponding to the third week of human pregnancy) also produces typical features of the FAS.[1090]

Although in humans with FAS the hippocampi are reportedly normal-sized, in rodents exposed in utero to ethanol the hippocampi display reduced numbers of neurons, lower dendritic spine density on pyramidal neurons, and decreased morphological plasticity after environmental enrichment. Electrophysiological studies reveal abnormal synaptic activity in hippocampal brain slices, and the animals are impaired in learning and memory tasks sensitive to hippocampal damage.[1091,1092]

Unexpectedly, monkeys prenatally exposed to ethanol had *increased* numbers of axons in the corpus callosum, especially frontally.[1093]

In rats, ethanol interferes with myelinogenesis and causes neuroglial heterotopias and abnormal astrogliogenesis. There is decreased synthesis of DNA, RNA, and protein, decreased numbers of mitotic cells, alteration of the content and distribution of cytoskeletal proteins, reduced capacity of astrocytes to secrete growth factors, and evidence of oxidative stress. Radial glial cells do not develop normally, and transcription of glial fibrillary acidic protein is reduced.[1094] Ethanol chronically activates protein kinase C by acting on regulatory proteins, and it either increases or decreases brain levels of protein kinase A depending on brain region and cell type.[1095]

Ethanol-exposed rats have endocrine abnormalities that persist into adulthood. Decreased testosterone levels lead to lasting female-like behavior among males, and increased secretion of adrenal corticosteroids leads to male-like behavior among females.[1096]

Both paternal and maternal ethanol consumption lead to increased susceptibility to infection in offspring.[1097]

Mechanisms

The mechanism of ethanol's teratogenicity is unknown. Easily crossing the placenta, ethanol maintains a fetal blood concentration considerably longer than the maternal level.[1098] Failure of neuronal and glial migration suggests effects early in pregnancy,[1047] but subtle alterations in sleep patterns suggest later effects.[1099] Maternal ethanol use during the third trimester, including its use to inhibit premature labor by suppressing oxytocin release, might carry additional hazards. Neonatal rats continuously ingesting ethanol are less likely to show histological brain damage than rats receiving smaller overall doses given over short periods (comparable to binge drinking).[1100] Ingested ethanol passes through the liver before reaching the systemic circulation, and continuous small doses are fully metabolized. Much of a single large dose, however, passes through the liver and reaches the brain.

Proposed mechanisms for ethanol teratogenicity (not mutually exclusive) include the following:

1. The special vulnerability of neurons in the CA1 region of the hippocampus and cerebellar Purkinje cells parallels vulnerability to neonatal asphyxia, lending support to the hypothesis that ethanol's teratogenicity is the result of vasospasm and CNS ischemia.[1101–1103] Consistent with such a mechanism are studies in sheep and monkey fetuses in which ethanol infusion caused metabolic and then mixed acidosis with EEG slowing and eventual isoelectricity.[1104,1105]

2. These regions are also damaged in adult alcoholics, possibly consequent to up-regulation of NMDA glutamate receptors during withdrawal and excitotoxicity (see above). In fetal brain, neurotransmission at NMDA receptors plays a critical role in neuronal differentiation, but whereas chronic ethanol administration in adult animals produces up-regulation of NMDA receptors, chronic administration in fetuses decreases receptor binding in the hippocampus for glutamate and other NMDA receptor agonists.[74,1106,1107] Prenatal ethanol exposure reduces inhibition of phosphoinositide hydrolysis by either NMDA-receptor or metabotropic-glutamate receptor stimulation.[1108] In rodent fetal cortical neurons ethanol has different effects on different NMDA receptor subunits.[1109]

3. The period of synaptogenesis ("brain growth spurt period") occurs postnatally in rats but during the last trimester of gestation in humans. Transient blockade of NMDA glutamate receptors during the period of synaptogenesis causes widespread apoptotic neurodegeneration in infant rat brain. Ethanol treatment in infant rats causes similar but more extensive neurodegeneration. The apoptotic response induced by ethanol depends on how rapidly the dose is administered and how long blood ethanol concentration (BEC) is maintained above a toxic threshold of 180–200 mg/dL; a minimum duration was 4 hours, with severity of damage proportional to duration of critical BEC. An apoptotic response did not follow exposure to agonists or antagonists at dopamine, kainic acid, or muscarinic cholinergic receptors or to blockers of voltage-gated ion channels, but apoptosis did follow exposure to GABAergic agonists (benzodiazepines, barbiturates). GABAergic-agonist-induced apoptosis had a pattern somewhat different from NMDA-antagonist-induced apoptosis, but when the two patterns were superimposed on one another, the result closely resembled that produced by ethanol (which, as an NMDA receptor antagonist and a $GABA_A$ agonist, serves as a pharmacological composite).[1110] The authors of this important study note that the human brain growth spurt spans not only the last trimester of pregnancy but several years after birth. A single exposure to ethanol during this period sufficient to produce 4 hours of at least 200 mg/dL BEC might be sufficient to trigger apoptotic neurodegeneration.

4. Newborns of alcoholic mothers have low blood levels of somatomedin C and high levels of growth hormone (GH),[1111] and ethanol's effects on fetal growth could be mediated through depressant actions on the growth hormone releasing hormone (GHRH)–GH–insulin-like growth factor (IGF-I, IGF-II) axis.[1112]

5. In rats, maternal adrenalectomy prevented growth retardation in ethanol-exposed offspring but adrenal demedullation did not, suggesting that the effects of ethanol on fetal growth are mediated by actions on the maternal adrenal cortex.[1113]

6. Among the G-protein second messenger systems inhibited by ethanol are those involving acetylcholine muscarinic receptors coupled to phospholipid metabolism. In the developing brain, activation of these receptors induces proliferation of glial cells and acts as a trophic factor in developing neurons by preventing apoptosis. Their inhibition by ethanol could lead to loss of glial cells and neurons, contributing to microcephaly.[1114]

7. A gene called L1 codes for a cell membrane adhesion molecule essential for neuronal migration and normal brain development. Mutation of L1 causes mental retardation and brain malformations such as are seen in FAS. In cultures of rat cerebellar neurons transfected with the human L1 gene, exposure to ethanol at concentrations equivalent to mildly intoxicating BEC, the adhesiveness of the L1 molecules was completely lost.[1115,1116] An active fragment of the glial-derived activity-dependent neuroprotective protein (ADNP, which protects neurons against a large number of toxins and insults) prevented ethanol-induced fetal wastage and growth retardation in mice and also antagonized ethanol inhibition of L1-mediated cell adhesion.[1116a]

8. The vitamin A metabolite, retinoic acid (RA), plays an important role in embryogenesis and differentiation, and both vitamin A toxicity and deficiency produce fetal malformations that resemble FAS. RA synthesis from retinol is catalyzed by ADH; ethanol administration to pregnant rats alters levels of RA and RA receptor binding in the fetus; in quail embryos ethanol exposure mimics vitamin A deficiency and RA prevents the adverse effects of ethanol; and in neuroblastoma cell cultures ethanol and RA block each other's effects.[1117]

9. Ethanol withdrawal may itself be specifically damaging to nervous tissue.[1118,1119] Prevention of withdrawal signs by tapering ethanol dosage did not prevent CNS damage in fetal rats, however.[1120]

10. Injections of acetaldehyde in pregnant mice led to delayed neural tube closure in fetuses.[1121] Acetaldehyde could be an additional teratogen in the FAS, although in this experiment its teratogenicity could have been the result of metabolism back to ethanol.

11. Ethanol inhibits nerve growth factor and neuronal process formation; by this mechanism it might selectively damage those neurons growing most rapidly at the time of exposure.[1100,1122] Ethanol may also be toxic to the placenta, interfering with uptake of essential nutrients.[1048,1123–1125]

12. Ingested by female mice at the time of conception, ethanol interferes with chromosomal segregation, and acetaldehyde interferes with mitotic spindle mechanisms and is clastogenic.[1126] Isochrome 9q abnormality was reported in a dysmorphic 2-year-old whose mother had drunk heavily during the first several weeks of pregnancy.[1127]

13. Exposure of male animals or humans to ethanol before conception may predispose their offspring to lower birth weight and decreased viability, but the data are tenuous.[1128]

14. Extrapolating from reports that aspirin and other prostaglandin inhibitors antagonize ethanol-induced sleep, hypothermia, and increased activity, investigators pretreated pregnant mice with aspirin before they received ethanol. Signs comparable to FAS developed in 25% of fetuses whose mothers received aspirin, compared with 50% of fetuses whose mothers did not.[1129]

15. Genetic differences likely influence individual susceptibility to FAS. The $ADH_{\beta3}$ isoenzyme, encoded by an allele unique to African-Americans, provides more rapid metabolism of ethanol than other ADH isoenzymes, and there is evidence that it is protective, although not to a large degree. Other genetic polymorphisms might similarly influence risk.[1130]

The Scope of the Problem

A 1991 Centers for Disease Control (CDC) National Maternal and Infant Health Survey (NMIHS) found that 45% of American women drank ethanol during the 3 months before they learned they were pregnant, 21% drank after learning they were pregnant, 17% drank three or fewer drinks during pregnancy, and 0.6% had six or more drinks per week during pregnancy. Those who drank at all were more likely to be "white non-Hispanic" and to have at least 16 years of education and annual income of at least US$40,000. Frequent drinking, however, was more likely in racial/ethnic groups other than white and with annual incomes less than US$10,000.[1131] During the 1990s overall rates of ethanol use during pregnancy rose from 12.4% in 1991 to 16.3% in 1995 and then fell to 12.8% in 1999. During the same decade binge drinking during pregnancy rose from 1% in 1991 to 2.9% in 1995 and remained at 2.7% in 1999.[1132]

According to the CDC's National Birth Defects Monitoring Program (BDMP), in 1979 FAS affected 1 in 10,000 newborns in the U.S.; by 1993 the number had risen to 6.7 per 10,000.[1133] The higher figures were believed to reflect a true increase, not simply more accurate detection. In fact, because facial feature and low birth weight can be mild or absent, the incidence of fetal alcohol effects (FAE; or, as it is also called, "fetal alcohol spectrum disorders [FASD]" and "alcohol-related neurodevelopmental disorder [ARND]") is probably underestimated.[1134,1135] (A marketed assay for the presence of fatty acid ethyl esters in meconium is available as a biological marker for gestational alcohol exposure.[1136]) In a review that combined data from Seattle WA, Cleveland OH, and Roubaix, France it was estimated that the combined incidence of FAS and ARND was at least 9.1/1000—nearly 1% of all live births.[1137]

Although the teratogenic risk of ethanol is established, a threshold of safety has not been defined.[1138] FAS may affect 1% of children whose mothers drink 1 oz of ethanol per day early in pregnancy and over 30% of the offspring of heavy drinkers.[1053] In one study, which corrected for confounding variables, including tobacco, reduced infant size correlated with drinking only 100 g of ethanol per week at the time of conception.[1139] In another report low birth weight and decreased head circumference and body length correlated with only one drink per day during the first 2 months of the first trimester.[1140] In another study dysmorphism in 4-year-olds was assessed without knowledge of maternal drinking patterns; it was found in 20.4% of children whose mothers had drunk at least 1 oz of ethanol daily early in pregnancy compared with 9.3% of those whose mothers had drunk less.[1141] "Social drinking" during pregnancy led to EEG abnormalities in offspring, more severe in infants of intermittent drinkers than of frank alcoholics.[1142]

In studies from Seattle and Canada, ethanol consumption as low as 0.1 oz daily carried risk for subtle neurological and behavioral effects, including slow habituating responses and delayed weak sucking.[1143–1145] Only 10 g ethanol daily during early pregnancy was associated with low birth weight,[1146] and in mice a single exposure to ethanol at a critical time caused craniofacial anomalies.[1147]

Considering that ethanol use during pregnancy tends to be underreported,[1148] these findings raise the worrisome possibility that very low doses can cause subtle cognitive changes—that in fact there may be no such thing as a safe dose.[1148a] They also imply that by the time a woman reaches the antenatal clinic, damage has already been done. Some investigators criticize the studies cited, claiming that when other risk factors are properly considered,

there is no hazard associated with one or two drinks a day.[1149–1153] The burden of proof, however, is on those who believe that there is a safe dose of what is probably the leading teratogenic cause of mental retardation in the western world.[1064]

Ethanol is detectable in breast milk of mothers who drink alcoholic beverages, and their nursing infants display altered feeding and sleeping behavior.[1154] Moreover, motor development was mildly delayed at 1 year in infants breast-fed by mothers who drank ethanol.[1155] An obvious problem in interpreting these findings is correcting for substandard maternal behavior.[1156,1157]

Ethanol Substitutes

Methanol

Methanol (methyl alcohol, wood alcohol) is present in industrial solvents, gasohol, carburetor fluid, duplicator fluid, shellac, antifreeze, solid canned fuels, and windshield washing solution.[1158,1159] Contamination of bootleg spirits has resulted in epidemics of methanol poisoning. In 1951, 323 poisonings—with 41 deaths—followed the distribution of contaminated bootleg whiskey in Atlanta, Georgia.[1160] A smaller outbreak involved the ingestion of duplicating fluid by inmates of a Michigan prison.[1161]

Although methanol is rapidly absorbed from the gastrointestinal tract, inebriation is not prominent, and symptoms usually appear only after 12 to 36 hours. Methanol's metabolic products are toxic to retinal ganglion cells, causing visual blurring, sometimes with yellow spots or central scotomas and described as "flashes" or a "snowstorm." Complete blindness follows, with unreactive pupils, optic disc hyperemia, engorged retinal veins, and later optic atrophy.[1159] Other symptoms include headache, dizziness, nausea, vomiting, and abdominal pain (often due to pancreatitis). Suggestive of early methanol poisoning—and in contrast to ethanol poisoning—is the triad of visual complaints, abdominal pain, and metabolic acidosis, with a clear sensorium or only mild inebriation and lack of "alcoholic breath."[1162] Without treatment, symptoms progress to delirium, seizures, and coma. Respirations become slow, shallow, and gasping. Bradycardia signifies a grave prognosis.[1159,1161]

Blindness can follow ingestion of only 15 ml of methanol. It nearly always precedes death, which is usually associated with doses of 70–100 ml. There is much individual variation in the lethal dose, however. Death followed ingestion of only 6 ml absolute methanol, and survival followed ingestion of more than 500 ml.[1158]

Methanol is metabolized by ADH to formaldehyde and then to formic acid, which is responsible for severe anion gap metabolic acidosis.[1163,1164] (If hypotension is present, lactic acid contributes.) Formate is an inhibitor of cytochrome oxidases c and aa_3, and acidosis inhibits both cellular respiration and formate metabolism.[1165] Pathologically there is demyelination of the optic nerve behind the lamina cribrosa; papilledema is secondary to compressive obstruction of orthograde axoplasmic flow.[1166]

Treatment begins with cardiovascular and respiratory support and gastric emptying. Sodium bicarbonate may be required for several days, as acidosis commonly recurs after seemingly successful treatment. Bicarbonate therapy itself causes hypokalemia. Ethanol is given, because the affinity of ethanol for ADH greatly exceeds that of methanol, and ethanol thereby blocks the conversion of methanol to toxic metabolites. Methanol, which is normally present in the blood in trace amounts (probably derived from microflora in the gastrointestinal tract), has a half-life of about 24 hours; in the presence of ethanol the half-life can increase to days. The aim is to achieve a blood ethanol concentration of 100 mg/dL. A usual loading dose is 7.6–10 mL/kg 10% ethanol in 5% dextrose intravenously (or 0.8–1.0 mL/kg 95% ethanol orally); maintenance dosage is then 1.4 mL/kg per hour of 10% ethanol by continuous intravenous drip (or 0.15 mL/kg 95% ethanol orally).[1158] Chronic alcoholics and patients receiving hemodialysis require more. Hemodialysis is recommended for any patient who is symptomatic, has significant metabolic acidosis, has a blood methanol level higher than 25 mg/dL, or has evidence of renal compromise. During hemodialysis the maintenance dose of ethanol needs to be increased.[1159] Folate is also given, as the oxidation of formic acid to carbon dioxide is folate dependent. 4-Methylpyrazole (fomepizole), which inhibits ADH, has been used successfully in animals but is not yet available for general use in the United States.[1167–1169]

Following treatment there may or may not be recovery of vision; prognosis for improvement is poor in patients with initial severe impairment, dilated unreactive pupils, or widespread retinal edema.[1159] Survivors of methanol poisoning sometimes have movement disorders, including parkinsonism and dystonia.[1170–1172] CT or MRI reveal putaminal infarction, sometimes hemorrhagic.[1173] Electromyography demonstrates denervation consistent with anterior horn cell damage. Autopsy shows putaminal necrosis and widespread neuronal damage in the cerebrum, cerebellum, brainstem, and spinal cord.[1174]

Ethylene Glycol

Found in antifreezes, windshield de-icers, and brake fluids, ethylene glycol is deliberately drunk as an ethanol substitute. In 1997, 4867 cases of ethylene glycol poisoning were reported in the United States, 21 ending fatally.[1175] Within a few hours, inebriation is followed by nausea, vomiting, ataxia, nystagmus, ophthalmoparesis, myoclonus, seizures, hypoactive tendon reflexes, and stupor or coma. There may be hypothermia or mild fever. Metabolic acidosis with a marked anion gap is the result of several ethylene glycol metabolites (glycolic acids), the most important of which, oxylate, chelates calcium and causes tetany and cardiac symptoms, including pulmonary edema.[1159,1168,1176] Calcium oxylate crystals are often (but not always) seen in the urine within a few hours of ingestion. Their precipitation leads to renal failure several days later.[1177] Survivors sometimes have lasting cranial neuropathies—especially facial paralysis—appearing up to 18 days after ethylene glycol ingestion; a possible mechanism is deposition of oxylate crystals.[1178]

Treatment begins with gastric emptying and respiratory support. Like methanol, ethylene glycol is metabolized by ADH, and so ethanol is given. As with methanol poisoning, hemodialysis is recommended for symptomatic patients with metabolic acidosis, ethylene glycol blood levels above 25 mg/dL, or renal failure.[1158,1159,1179] Forced diuresis can prevent oxalate crystal precipitation, and thiamine and pyridoxine might help to divert ethylene glycol metabolism to products other than oxylate. 4-Methylpyrazole (fomepizole) is effective in ethylene-glycol-poisoned animals and humans.[1180,1181]

A woman who ingested 720 mL of antifreeze became comatose with dilated unreactive pupils, absent tendon reflexes, arterial pH of 6.46, and serum ethylene glycol concentration of 2600 mg/L. Following hemodialysis, during which ethanol was added to the dialysate, she made a complete recovery.[1182]

Isopropanol

Isopropanol, contained in rubbing alcohol, household cements, glass cleaners, and windshield de-icers, is also an occasional ethanol substitute.[1158,1183] To discourage deliberate ingestion, blue dye is often added to rubbing alcohol—hence the nickname "Blue Heaven." Intoxication also occurs by inhalation and absorption through the skin, especially in children. Metabolized to acetone, isopropanol usually causes ketosis without lactic acidosis. Gastritis, abdominal pain, and vomiting are prominent, followed by ataxia, confusion, or coma. Miosis, decreased tendon reflexes, hypothermia, renal tubular necrosis, myopathy, and hemolytic anemia occur. Hypotension is secondary to direct cardiac depression. Treatment is supportive, beginning with continuous gastric lavage—isopropanol continues to be secreted into the stomach. Hemodialysis is used for hypotensive or comatose patients.[1158,1184] Because isopropanol itself is the major toxin, ethanol is not given.

Absinthe

Pliny the Elder in the first century CE described a wine fortified with extract from the wormwood plant (*Artemisia absinthium*). During the 19th century absinthe, a French liqueur distilled from wormwood, ethanol, anise, fennel, and other herbs, became popular among writers and artists, including Vincent van Gogh and Henri de Toulouse-Lautrec.[1185] Chronic ingestion of absinthe causes a syndrome of insomnia, auditory and visual hallucinations, agitation, psychosis, seizures, and rhabdomyolysis. Today absinthe is banned in the United States, France, and most other European countries. (A less potent form is available in the Czech Republic.) Oil of

wormwood, however, is commercially available through the Internet for use in "aromatherapy," and a near-fatal overdose was reported.[1186]

Wormwood extract contains alpha-thujone, a compound similar to pinene (in turpentine) and camphor (in moth balls). In studies with *Drosophila* and mice, alpha-thujone was found to block brain GABA receptors.[1187]

Treatment of Chronic Alcoholism

Making the Diagnosis

Despite the fact that 90% of adults seen by primary care physicians report using ethanol and up to 45% report abuse,[18] physicians frequently do not ask patients about drinking or advise them to cut back.[1188] Simple screening questionnaires can be an effective starting point. For example, CAGE scores of 1 to 4 (Table 12–21) carry probabilities for ethanol abuse of 7%, 46%, 72%, and 98%.[18] The CAGE questionnaire is more specific than sensitive, however. A study of over 5000 primary care patients older than 60 years found that 15% of men and 12% of women drank in excess of limits recommended by the National Institute of Alcohol and Alcoholism (more than 14 drinks per week for men and more than seven drinks per week for women). The CAGE questionnaire alone, however, identified only 9% of the men and 3% of the women as problem drinkers. The rest were identified by asking about the precise amount and frequency of drinking.[1189]

Heterogeneity of Patients and Therapies

In the voluminous literature on the treatment of alcoholism, strong opinions outweigh scientific data. Noteworthy are the diversity of the patients

Table 12–21. The CAGE Score

1. Have you ever felt you should *cut down* on your drinking?
2. Have people *annoyed* you by criticizing your drinking?
3. Have you ever felt bad or *guilty* about your drinking?
4. Have you ever had a drink first thing in the morning to steady your nerves or to get rid of a hangover (*eye-opener*)?

being treated.[1190] As discussed earlier, a problem drinker is not necessarily physically dependent; no personality type defines an alcoholic; and genetics, associated psychiatric illness, and social deprivation play varying roles. The vast majority of American alcoholics are employed and live with their families.[1191] In recent decades, however, alcoholics have increasingly abused other drugs. In a 1985 study additional drug abuse was found in 45% of male and 11% of female alcoholics,[1192] and in a report from the San Diego Veterans Administration Medical Center, 53% of primary alcoholics used marijuana; 23%, psychostimulants; 14%, cocaine; and 11%, sedatives.[1193] Coexisting psychiatric illness is also common. In one series 50% of female alcoholics had additional psychiatric diagnoses, including unipolar depression (24%), bipolar depression (4%), anxiety disorders (10%), and psychosis (6%).[1194] In another study of alcoholics, 18% of men and 38% of women were depressed, 15% of men and 29% of women had phobias, and 5% of men and 9% of women had panic attacks.[1192] Further complicating treatment are attitudinal differences. For example, the U.S. Veterans Administration defines *secondary alcoholism* ("secondary to and a manifestation of an acquired psychiatric disorder") as a disease qualifying for disability. *Primary alcoholism*, on the other hand, is defined as "willful misconduct."[1195] Finally, ethanol directly or indirectly causes disturbances of memory and cognition that are bound to interfere with treatment.[1196]

Such heterogeneity has led to a variety of treatment approaches: for example, psychotherapy, group psychotherapy, family or "social network" therapy, drug therapy, and behavioral (aversion) therapy. Settings also vary: for example, a general hospital, a halfway house, a vocational rehabilitation clinic, or Alcoholics Anonymous. Taken overall, outcome seems to be independent of the particular treatment given.[1197-1201] That does not mean that for an individual patient one treatment is not preferable to another (Table 12–22).

Tranquilizers and other GABAergic agents

The use of tranquilizing or sedating drugs is especially controversial.[1202,1203] Benzodiazepines and barbiturates are cross-tolerant with ethanol and might therefore have the same rationale for treating

Table 12–22. Chronic Alcoholism—Pharmacotherapy

Tranquilizers
Aldehyde dehydrogenase inhibitors
Lithium and carbamazepine
Serotonin-selective agents
Dopamine-selective agents
Opioid-selective agents
N-methyl-D-aspartate (NMDA) antagonists
Gamma-hydroxybutyric acid
Calcium channel antagonists
Kudzu
Neuropeptide Y
Cannabinoid receptor antagonists
LSD

alcoholism that methadone has in treating opioid addiction. Sedatives carry their own abuse potential, however; in fact, the vast majority of benzodiazepine abusers are also alcoholic.[1204] Despite their cross-tolerance, tranquilizers and sedatives can also interact synergistically with ethanol. Their use in chronic alcoholism must therefore be judicious and selective. A recent review of controlled studies, moreover, concluded that benzodiazepine treatment overall does not improve abstinence rate.[1205]

More selective approaches include use of benzodiazepines in type I but not type II alcoholics; impulsivity in the latter may be aggravated by such treatment. Type I alcoholics without other psychiatric disorder, however, may not benefit from any pharmacotherapy.[1203] Those with secondary alcoholism should be treated for the primary mental disorder. Panic attacks respond to monoamine oxidase inhibitors, tricyclic antidepressants, serotonin reuptake blockers, or benzodiazepines, including alprazolam, clonazepam, and lorazepam. Social phobias are more likely to respond to beta-adrenergic blockers and single phobias to behavioral therapy. For general anxiety, with or without depression, some favor imipramine or amitriptyline over benzodiazepines.[1206] Others prefer the 5-HT$_{1A}$ agonist buspirone.[1207,1208] (see below.) Similarly, although alprazolam can be effective in depression,[1209] tricyclic antidepressants and serotonin reuptake blockers are probably safer in alcoholics. Nearly half of schizophrenics abuse ethanol or other drugs; pharmacotherapy in such patients is especially daunting.[1210]

A benzodiazepine inverse agonist, RO19-4603, alone or in combination with a benzodiazepine antagonist, reduced consumption in ethanol-preferring rats.[1211,1212] Such an approach has not been applied to humans.

The anticonvulsant topiramate facilitates GABA transmission (and probably also inhibits glutamate transmission). In a randomized double-blind trial, topiramate was superior to placebo at 6 months in reducing drinks per day, drinks per drinking day, blood gamma-glutamyl transferase levels, and reported craving.[1212a]

Aldehyde Dehydrogenase Inhibitors

Disulfiram. By inhibiting ALDH, disulfiram (Antabuse) blocks the oxidation of acetaldehyde and produces a constellation of disagreeable symptoms. Within 5 to 10 minutes of ethanol ingestion there is warmth and flushing of the face and chest, throbbing headache, dyspnea, nausea, vomiting, sweating, thirst, chest pain, palpitations, hypotension, anxiety, confusion, weakness, vertigo, and blurred vision.[1213] Severity and duration depend on the amount of ethanol drunk. Small amounts cause mild symptoms followed by drowsiness, sleep, and recovery; severe reactions are potentially fatal and require hospitalization and careful management of hypotension, cardiac ischemia, or arrhythmia. In up to 25% of patients taking more than 500 mg per day, fatigue and confusion progress to toxic psychosis, stupor, or catatonia.[1214] Disulfiram reactions can occur within a week of the last dose; if there is liver disease, the interval is even longer.[1215]

Although 150,000 to 200,000 Americans are currently maintained on disulfiram, evidence of efficacy is limited. Taken in the morning when the urge to drink is least, 250 or 500 mg daily does not alter the taste for ethanol and so helps only those who strongly wish to abstain. Two questions then arise: (1) Is disulfiram of any benefit? (2) If so, is benefit based on true pharmacological aversion, or is it simply psychological? Nearly 100 studies attempting to answer the first question are invalid because of lack of controls or insufficient power.[1216] In two well-designed trials, male alcoholics were randomized to disulfiram, 250 mg; disulfiram 1 mg (i.e., placebo); or no drug. All groups received counseling.[1217,1218] In the first study at 6 months there was a small but significant increase in total abstinence among those taking disulfiram in either dosage; this finding suggests the effect was mainly due to the patients' fear. In the second study at 12 months there were no differences in total abstinence, time to first drink, or social stability, but those receiving the full disulfiram dose had fewer drinking days than those receiving placebo or no drug. This difference is consistent with true pharmacological aversion. In other studies disulfiram reduced drinking frequency after relapse but was no better than counseling alone in sustaining continuous abstinence. It seemed to be most effective in older, employed, socially stable patients.[1219–1221]

A European study comparing disulfiram implants (unavailable in the United States), placebo implants, and no implants found fewer drinking days in patients with either type of implant, again suggesting a behavioral rather than a pharmacological effect.[1222]

A more recent review of 24 studies of outcome following oral disulfiram and 14 following implanted disulfiram during the period 1967–1995 concluded that although methodological rigor of these studies was better than that of earlier studies, it was still generally poor. The authors concluded that efficacy for promoting abstinence was "surprisingly lacking" and that there was no good evidence in favor of implanting disulfiram tablets.[1223]

Side effects of disulfiram—in the absence of ethanol—are dose-related and include hypertension, drowsiness, forgetfulness, ataxia, dysarthria, and peripheral neuropathy.[1224,1225] It may be difficult to separate disulfiram's complications from the effects of ethanol itself. With disulfiram polyneuropathy, however, symptoms usually begin 2 to 6 months after beginning disulfiram and progress more rapidly than with alcoholic polyneuropathy. Distal paresthesias are followed by numbness and weakness, which spread proximally. Nerve biopsy reveals neurofilament accumulations in distended axons.[1226,1227]

Such side effects can occur in patients taking only 250 mg daily, and one-fourth of patients taking more than 500 mg daily develop fatigue, confusion, psychosis, or stupor.[1213] Generalized seizures and optic neuritis are reported.[1228] Fulminant polyneuritis followed overdose of both disulfiram and ethanol,[1229] and delirium with visual hallucinations but without major autonomic symptoms followed ethanol ingestion while taking disulfiram.[1230]

Acute hepatitis and dermatitis also occur and unlike neurological complications are idiosyncratic non-dose-related reactions.[1226,1227]

Anecdotal reports suggest teratogenicity when disulfiram is taken during the first trimester of pregnancy.[1231]

Calcium Carbamide.   Available in Europe and Canada, calcium carbamide is believed by some to produce a milder aversive reaction than disulfiram.[1213] It causes hypothyroidism in patients with already reduced thyroid function, a common occurrence in alcoholics. In contrast to disulfiram, calcium carbamide does not inhibit dopamine-beta-hydroxylase and is less likely to cause or exacerbate depression or psychosis.[1232]

As noted earlier, a number of other drugs produce disulfiram-like reactions after ethanol ingestion, but the effects are usually mild, and such agents are of no use in treating alcoholics. Patients taking disulfiram can have aversive reactions when exposed to occupational solvents (e.g., paint or ceramics)[1233] or to other medications containing ethanol (e.g., asthma elixirs).[1215,1234] Symptoms suggestive of disulfiram reactions can occur in patients who take ethanol with chloral hydrate or who take monoamine oxidase inhibitors with tyramine-containing alcoholic beverages, such as Chianti wine.[1215]

Lithium and Carbamazepine

The frequent mood swings of alcoholics led to a controlled trial with lithium, which demonstrated decreased need for hospitalization among treated subjects.[1235] Rats receiving lithium also had reduced ethanol preference.[1236] Subsequent human controlled trials, however, failed to demonstrate benefit in either depressed or nondepressed alcoholics.[1237,1238] Lithium would still be appropriate for patients with bipolar disorder and secondary alcoholism. As with disulfiram, compliance is a problem, and ethanol lowers the threshold for lithium toxicity.

A randomized double-blind trial found carbamazepine superior to placebo in reducing drinking in ethanol-dependent patients, but only 29 patients were studied.[1239]

Serotonin-selective Agents

As noted above, at least 14 different 5-HT receptors have been identified, with further division within each family (5-HT$_{1A}$, 5-HT$_{1B}$, etc). Given that alcoholic populations are also heterogeneous and that serotonin plays a major role in appetite, mood, arousal, impulse control, and other personality traits, it is not surprising that trials of selective and sub-selective serotonin agonists, antagonists, and reuptake inhibitors to treat alcoholism have produced inconsistent results.[1240]

In animals, ethanol acutely releases 5-HT in the nucleus accumbens (NA) but chronically causes decreased release.[1241] Ethanol-preferring rats have lower levels of 5-HT in the NA than do non-preferring rats.[1242] 5-HT$_{1A}$ agonists and 5-HT$_{2A}$ and 5-HT$_3$ antagonists reduce ethanol consumption in ethanol preferring rats,[1243] and selective serotonin reuptake inhibitors (SSRIs) reduce ethanol consumption in monkeys.[1244] In humans the 5-HT$_3$ antagonist ondansetron increases both the intoxicating effects and the aversive feelings of ethanol consumption.[1245] Patients with Cloninger Type II alcoholism (or in a similar classification, Baron Type B alcoholism), characterized by early onset and impulsive or sociopathic behavior, have low blood levels of the serotonin precursor tryptophan compared with controls, as do alcoholics with comorbid depression.[1246]

Selective Serotonin Reuptake Inhibitors.   Early studies of SSRIs (fluoxetine, zimelidine, citalopram, and viqualine) in "early stage problem drinking" (50 g ethanol daily) found decreased drinking but did not identify patient traits that would predict response.[1247–1249] It was also difficult to determine whether suppression of ethanol intake was due to reduced reinforcement or "generalized decreases in consumatory behavior."[1250] Of four subsequent placebo-controlled trials using fluoxetine,[1251–1254] only one showed benefit.[1254] Moreover, in one, although there was no advantage of fluoxetine over placebo, both groups reduced drinking by over 75%, suggesting efficacy for concomitant cognitive-behavioral psychotherapy.[1253]

SSRIs have been studied in patients with behavior suggestive of 5-HT dysregulation, namely, depression and impulsive behavior.[1254] A double-blind trial of fluoxetine in alcoholics with comorbid depression found fluoxetine superior to placebo in reducing both drinking and mood disorder.[1255] A study using citalopram divided alcoholics into groups corresponding to Cloninger Type I or Type II; citalopram was superior to placebo in reducing drinking, with equal benefit in each subgroup.[1256] In two other studies sertraline and fluoxetine were compared with placebo in Babor Type B alcoholics (corresponding to Cloninger Type II); in both studies patients receiving the SSRI drank *more* heavily than those receiving placebo.[1257,1258] In a study of Babor Type A alcoholics, on the other hand, patients receiving sertraline drank less than those receiving placebo.[1258] In another study sertraline unexpectedly reduced drinking in patients without comorbid depression but not in those with comorbid depression.[1259]

5-HT$_1$ Partial Agonists. The net effect of the 5-HT$_1$ partial agonist buspirone is to augment 5-HT function, for postsynaptic receptors are more sensitive than inhibitory autoreceptors. On theoretical grounds, therefore, buspirone should reduce ethanol consumption, and in some animal studies it did.[1250] Studies of buspirone in humans without comorbidity, however, were largely negative.[1260] Three studies compared buspirone with placebo in alcoholics with comorbid anxiety. Two reported benefit;[1261,1262] one did not.[1263] In another study, although alcoholism with early age of onset was associated with low CSF levels of the serotonin metabolite 5-hydroxyindoleacetic acid (5HIAA), buspirone was of no value regardless of age of onset.[1264]

5-HT$_2$ Antagonists. In animals the 5-HT$_2$ antagonists ritanserin and amperozide reduce ethanol consumption; amperoside reduces food consumption as well, however.[1250] Two placebo-controlled trials showed ritanserin to be without benefit in the treatment of alcoholism.[1265,1266]

5-HT$_3$ Antagonists. Ethanol potentiates 5-HT$_3$ receptor-mediated ion currents in cell cultures, and this action is blocked by 5-HT$_3$ receptor antagonists. 5-HT$_3$ receptors are present on terminals of mesocorticolimbic dopaminergic neurons, where they potentiate dopamine release. 5-HT$_3$ receptor blockade thus reduces dopaminergic activity and the rewarding effects of abused drugs.

In animals 5-HT$_3$ antagonists decrease ethanol consumption.[1250]

Several studies suggest efficacy of the 5-HT$_3$ antagonist ondansetron in human alcoholism. In one report ondansetron reduced both the desire to drink and the positive subjective effects induced by ethanol.[1267] In a double-blind, placebo-controlled study, 0.5 mg but not 4 mg daily doses of ondansetron produced a trend toward reduced ethanol consumption, raising the possibility of an inverted U-shaped dose–response curve.[1268] In a larger double-blind trial ondansetron in a wide range of doses was superior to placebo in reducing ethanol consumption among early-onset but not late-onset alcoholics.[1250]

Dopamine-selective Agents

The dopamine agonists apomorphine and bromocriptine reduce ethanol ingestion by rats. Paradoxically, so does the dopamine release suppressor dihydroergotoxine combined with the dopamine blocker thioridazine.[1269] In animals the DA$_2$/DA$_3$ receptor antagonists haloperidol and tiapride reduce ethanol-induced hyperactivity, and the DA$_1$/DA$_2$ receptor antagonist flupenthixol is modestly effective in reducing ethanol consumption.[1250,1270]

In humans, tiapride was superior to placebo in increasing abstinence, and this drug is now available in Europe for treating ethanol dependence.[1271] In a comparable study, however, patients receiving flupenthixol experienced either no benefit or higher relapse rates.[1272]

Opioid-specific Agents

Mu-Receptor Antagonists. The interaction of ethanol and endogenous opioid systems is complex (see above), and so seemingly paradoxical observations are probably to be expected. In rats ethanol consumption is suppressed by morphine, methadone, levorphanol, and inhibitors of enkephalinase, and these effects are blocked by naloxone.[1273] In other animal studies, low doses of morphine increased ethanol consumption, but higher doses decreased it.[1274] In the 19th century, alcoholics were frequently treated with opioids, and some studies suggest that opioids reduce craving for ethanol.[1275] Although alcoholism is common among patients receiving methadone maintenance treatment, methadone per se is more likely to reduce craving for ethanol than to increase it.[1276]

On the other hand, naloxone attenuates ethanol self-administration in ethanol-preferring rats,[1277] and naltrexone reduces ethanol drinking by monkeys.[1278] Decreased ethanol consumption is not maintained with chronic administration of these antagonists, however,[1279] and in some studies reduced ethanol consumption appears to be part of a nonspecific action of naltrexone on consumatory behaviors.[1250] In rats naltrexone reverses ethanol-induced dopamine release in the NA.[1280] Both alcoholic and nonalcoholic humans report less positive subjective effects of ethanol and less desire to drink when taking naltrexone.[1281–1283]

Two double-blind trials comparing naltrexone with placebo in ethanol-dependent subjects found fewer drinking days or higher abstinence rates in those receiving naltrexone.[1284,1285] Although the number of patients was small in each study (70 and 97) and the period of study was only 12 weeks, the U.S. Food and Drug Administration subsequently approved naltrexone for the treatment of alcoholism, the first drug to be approved for this purpose in the United States since disulfiram nearly a half-century earlier.

In one of these studies[1285] the benefit of naltrexone was evident in subjects receiving concomitant supportive psychotherapy but not in those receiving therapy intended to improve "coping skills;" furthermore, 5 months after naltrexone was discontinued there was no difference in abstinence between naltrexone and placebo groups.[1286]

Naltrexone was superior to placebo in a study involving "non-severely dependent, socially stable, and motivated alcoholics."[1287] Three other randomized trials found no advantage of naltrexone over placebo; apparent benefit during the first weeks wore off despite continued treatment.[1288–1290] Two of these studies involved patients also dependent on cocaine.[1289,1290] In another study high rates of nausea and vomiting affected subjects receiving naltrexone.[1291]

A large multicenter, double-blind, placebo-controlled study assigned 627 U.S. veterans to either 12 months of naltrexone, 3 months of naltrexone followed by 9 months of placebo, or 12 months of placebo.[1292] There were no differences between groups in delay or prevention of relapse to heavy drinking, number of drinking days, or amount of ethanol consumed during drinking, and outcomes were not influenced by duration of naltrexone administration, degree of compliance with medication, or participation in counseling or Alcoholics Anonymous. Patients were nearly all men, with an average age (49) 10 years older than in previous studies, with more severe ethanol dependence, and often with inadequate social support. It is possible, therefore, that naltrexone might still provide benefit in younger, less severe alcoholics.[1293]

A German multicenter trial similarly found naltrexone no better than placebo in reducing episodes of heavy drinking.[1293a] A study from Spain compared naltrexone and acomprosate over a 12-month period; the mean number of days to relapse was 63 with naltrexone and 42 with acomprosate.[1294] A study from Finland found that although naltrexone was no better than placebo in maintaining abstinence, it was superior to placebo in preventing binges.[1295] Similar findings emerged in another study from Spain.[1295a] A Cochrane meta-analysis of 19 controlled studies involving naltrexone found superiority to placebo at 3 months in number of drinking days but no difference at 6 months in completion of treatment.[1295b]

In a randomized, double-blind trial, naltrexone combined with the 5-HT$_3$ antagonist ondansetron was superior to placebo in reducing ethanol consumption as reflected in serum levels of carbohydrate-deficient transferrin.[1295c]

Another potential complication of naltrexone is hepatotoxicity.[1283] Nalmefene, a mu and kappa opiate antagonist, is less hepatotoxic, and in a 12-week trial nalmephine was more likely than placebo to produce abstinence.[1296]

Delta-receptor Antagonists. Animal studies suggest that the delta-receptor antagonists naltriben and maltrindole have potential benefit in suppressing ethanol consumption.[1250]

NMDA Antagonists

Acamprosate. Chronic ethanol consumption causes up-regulation of NMDA receptors. Acamprosate (calcium acetyl-homotaurine), a synthetic compound structurally similar to GABA, appears to act by restoring normal NMDA receptor tone in the glutamate system. Proposed mechanisms of action include agonism at GABA receptors, antagonism at NMDA receptors, and antagonism at voltage-gated calcium channels.[1250,1283]

Although only weakly antagonistic at NMDA receptors, acamprosate may have region-specific actions through it its ability to modulate the expression of particular NMDA receptor subunits.[1297,1297a] In rodents, acamprosate attenuates ethanol but not water or food consumption, and it suppresses conditioned cue responses to ethanol in animals previously dependent.[1298] In mice, acamprosate reduced the development of conditioned place preference to ethanol and cocaine but not morphine.[1298a]

Sixteen clinical trials involving 4500 patients were conducted in 11 European countries; in four, acamprosate conferred significant benefit compared with placebo as reflected in greater rate of treatment completion, time to first drink, abstinence rate, and cumulative abstinence duration.[1299] Side effects included diarrhea in 10% and headache in 20%. Although unavailable in the United States as of 2003, evidence favoring the efficacy of acamprosate is stronger than for either disulfiram or naltrexone.

Other NMDA-receptor Antagonists. In animals the NMDA-receptor antagonists phencyclidine (PCP) and dizocilpine substitute for ethanol in drug discrimination paradigms, and in human alcoholics the related drug ketamine produces ethanol-like (but not cocaine-like or marijuana-like) subjective effects without inducing craving.[1300] Consistent with these observations, agonists at the glycine modulatory site of the NMDA-receptor complex reduce ethanol effects in animals, and D-cycloserine, a partial agonist at the glycine site, exacerbates ethanol intoxication in humans.[1300] Whether practical drug development will emerge from these observations remains to be seen. Psychiatrists in St. Petersburg, Russia, reported higher abstinence rates in alcoholics receiving ketamine in addition to psychotherapy ("ketamine psychedelic therapy") compared with those receiving psychotherapy alone.[1301]

Gamma-hydroxybutyric acid

A natural constituent of the brain (see Chapter 5), gamma-hydroxybutyric acid (GHB) appears to act agonistically at $GABA_B$ receptors as well as at specific GHB receptors.[1302] GHB dampens the severity of ethanol withdrawal signs in rodents, and it reduces voluntary ethanol intake in ethanol-preferring rats.[1303]

In an Italian double-masked clinical trial, GHB reduced ethanol consumption, and the drug has been used in that country since 1991 for the treatment of ethanol dependence.[1304,1305] A problem with GHB therapy is that 10% to 15% of patients so treated become abusers of the drug, escalating dosage to achieve euphoria.[1305,1306]

Calcium Chann el Antagonists

Dihydropyridine-type calcium channel blockers reduce ethanol discrimination and ethanol intake in ethanol-preferring rodents.[1250] In humans, however, isradipine did not alter ethanol-induced positive subjective mood.[1307] Clinical trials in ethanol-dependent subjects have not been conducted.

Kudzu

The root of *Pueraria lobata* (kudzu) has been used by Chinese herbalists for millennia to treat fever, diarrhea, and other disorders. Its use in ethanol-related diseases was described in a Chinese pharmacopoeia in 600 CE. In ethanol-preferring Syrian golden hamsters and rats, kudzu extract suppresses ethanol intake. Two isoflavones in kudzu are responsible for this effect. Daidzin is an inhibitor of aldehyde dehydrogenase. Daidzein is an inhibitor of alcohol dehydrogenase. Actions on monaminergic systems have also been hypothesized. Still widely used in China to treat alcoholism, kudzu has not yet received scientific validation in human clinical trials.[1308,1309]

Neuropeptide Y

Ethanol-preferring rats have lower levels of neuropeptide Y in their hippocampi and amygdalae than do nonpreferring rats, and animal studies suggest that neuropeptide Y administration produces behavioral and physiological ethanol-like effects.[1310,1311] The hypothesis that neuropeptide Y can act as an endogenous ethanol substitute raises the possibility of its use in preventing withdrawal or in treating dependence. Human studies have not been conducted, however.

Cannabinoid-receptor Antagonists

In neuroblastoma cell cultures, chronic ethanol exposure increases levels of the endogenous cannabinoid anandamide, and in mice, chronic ethanol ingestion causes down-regulation of cannabinoid CB_1 receptors. In rats ethanol and tetrahydrocannabinol demonstrate cross-tolerance.[1312] In ethanol-preferring rodents a CB_1 receptor antagonist reduced consumption of ethanol. Comparable human studies have not been conducted.[1313–1315]

LSD

During the 1950s and 1960s a number of studies addressed the use of LSD in treating alcoholism. The theoretical basis was more behavioral than specifically pharmacological; a psychedelic experience would increase self-awareness and reduce inner-conflict.[1316] Few studies were controlled and those that were had additional serious methodological flaws.[1317] Moreover, studies tended to be based on repression and other aspects of psychoanalytic theory which today are largely discredited.

Combination Therapy

The diversity of pharmacological actions among drugs that affect ethanol consumption makes combination therapy theoretically sensible, and animal and human studies have been promising. For example, combining an SSRI with a blocker of presynaptic serotonin autoreceptors results in much higher levels of serotonin than seen with SSRIs alone, and this combination produced additive therapeutic effects in ethanol-preferring rats.[1318] Similar animal studies have used various combinations of naltrexone, ondansetron, calcium channel blockers, and SSRIs.[1319]

In human studies naltrexone has been combined with the SSRI sertraline and with ondansetron, and acamprosate has been combined with naltrexone and with disulfiram, in each case producing promising preliminary results.[1250,1320] Definitive clinical trials have not been conducted, however. Of course concomitant psychotherapeutic support is essential with any pharmacotherapy, tailored to the characteristics of individual patients. Special consideration must be given for comorbid psychiatric disorders.

Alcoholics Anonymous

Benjamin Rush was one of the first to propose that alcoholism is a disease and that alcoholics are unable by themselves to stop drinking.[1321] This concept of "powerlessness in the face of alcohol" is the basic ideology of Alcoholics Anonymous (AA), which, since its founding by "Bill W" and "Dr. Bob" in Akron, Ohio in 1935, has grown to more than a million members in the United States and Canada and 800,000 more worldwide.[1322] The "success rate" of AA is difficult to estimate because many drop out early and medical records are not kept.[1323–1325] Abstinence at 1 year is probably between 26% and 50%. Of 100 alcoholics who first received inpatient counseling and then attended AA meetings, 8-year follow-up revealed that 29% had achieved at least 3 years of stable abstinence, 24% drank intermittently, and 47% continued to be severely alcoholic.[1326] Ancillary self-help organizations include Al-Anon for families of alcoholics and Alateen for teenage children of alcoholics.

Acupuncture

In a randomized prospective trial severe recidivist alcoholics received acupuncture using either specific or nonspecific insertion points. "Treated" patients were more likely to complete the course of therapy.[1327] This study has been criticized for faulty design; moreover, the specificity of acupuncture insertion points in any condition is doubtful.[1328,1329]

Conclusion

Although the need for hospitalization has been questioned,[1330,1331] "current standard treatment" of alcoholism consists of detoxification followed by several weeks of inpatient rehabilitation, including psychotherapy and behavior modification.[1191] Referral is then made to an outpatient facility, often AA. Pharmacotherapy is given cautiously for associated psychiatric problems. In 1984, more than 540,000 Americans were in treatment programs for alcoholism or combined alcohol and other drug dependency. Eight percent were inpatients, 10% were in residential facilities, and 82% were active outpatients.[1332]

Especially controversial is whether an alcoholic can ever safely resume "social drinking." Some believe that with "successful life adjustment" alcoholics can drink again.[1333] Needless to say, many disagree, and there is considerable evidence that stable moderate drinking is rarely accomplished in physically dependent alcoholics.[1326,1334–1336] What is generally recognized is that treatment must be individualized for each patient and that trial and error must be anticipated. For psychotherapy and drug treatment, evidence of benefit is sparse; for more unorthodox measures, which include not only acupuncture but also such radical interventions as stereotactic cingulotomy[1337] or hypothalamotomy,[1338] meaningful data are nonexistent.

Relevant but beyond the bounds of this discussion are preventive measures, including taxation and price manipulation, advertising restrictions and counteradvertising, depiction in the public media, education programs, establishment of legal drinking ages, and laws on drunken driving. As with other drugs, workplace screening programs raise serious ethical questions.[1339] The failure of Prohibition does not exonerate society's role in establishing responsible public policies related to ethanol abuse. During 1987 there were more than 5 times as many American alcoholics as cocaine or crack users and 30 times as many as alcoholics as heroin users; two-thirds of Americans seeking treatment in substance abuse programs report alcoholism as their primary problem. Yet in 1990 100% of a proposed US$100 million increase for federal block-grant funding of state substance abuse programs was mandated for users of illegal drugs.[1340]

References

1. Devor EJ, Cloninger CR. Genetics of alcoholism. Annu Rev Genet 1989; 23:19.
2. Vallee BL. Alcohol in the western world. Sci Am June 1998; 278:80.
2a. McGovern P. Ancient Wine: The Search for the Origins of Viniculture. Princeton University Press, 2003.
3. Coffey TG. Beer Street, Gin Lane. Some views of 18th Century Drinking. Q J Stud Alcohol 1966; 27:669.
4. Warner J, Her M, Gmel G, Rehm J. Can legislation prevent debauchery? Mother Gin and public health in 18th-century England. Am J Public Health 2001; 91:375.
5. Musto DF. Alcohol in American history. Sci Am April 1996; 274:78.
6. Doyle R. Deaths caused by alcohol. Sci Am December 1996; 275:30.
7. O'Connor PG, Schottenfeld RS. Patients with alcohol problems. N Engl J Med 1998; 338:592.
8. Charness ME, Simon RP, Greenberg DA. Ethanol and the nervous system. N Engl J Med 1989; 321:442.
9. Seventh Special Report to the U.S. Congress on Alcohol and Health. Rockville, MD: DHHS, Publication No. (ADM)-281-88-0002NIAAA, 1990.
10. Alcohol-related mortality and years of potential life lost–United States, 1987. MMWR 1990; 39:173.
11. Samson HH, Harris RA. Neurobiology of alcohol abuse. Trends Pharmacol Sci 1992; 13:206.
12. Midanik LT, Clarke WB. The demographic distribution of U.S. drinking patterns in 1990: description and trends from 1984. Am J Public Health 1994; 84:927.
13. Hogan MJ. Diagnosis and treatment of teen drug use. Med Clin North Am 2000; 84:927.
14. Rehun J, Greenfield TK, Rogers JD. Average volume of alcohol consumption, patterns of drinking, and all-cause mortality: results from the U.S. National Alcohol Survey. Am J Epidemiol 2001; 153:64.
15. Thun, MJ, Peto R, Lopez AD, et al. Alcohol consumption and mortality among middle-aged and elderly U.S. adults. N Engl J Med 1997; 337:1705.
16. Hanson GR, Li T-K. Public health implications of excessive alcohol consumption. JAMA 2003; 289:1031.
17. Williams GD, Stinson FS, Parker DA, et al. Demographic trends, alcohol abuse and alcoholism, 1985-1995. Alcohol Health Res World 1987; 11:80.
18. Buchsbaum DG, Buchanan RG, Centor RM, et al. Screening for alcohol abuse using CAGE scores and likelihood ratios. Ann Intern Med 1991; 115:774.
19. Yersin B, Trisconi Y, Paccaud F, et al. Accuracy of the Michigan Alcoholism Screening Test for screening of alcoholism in patients of a medical department. Arch Intern Med 1989; 149:2071.
20. Hernandez-Munoz R, Baraona E, Blackberg I, Lieber CS. Characterization of the increased binding of acetaldehyde to red blood cells in alcoholics. Alcoholism 1989; 13:654.
21. Schellenberg F, Benard JY, Le Golf AM, et al. Evaluation of carbohydrate-deficient transferrin compared with TF index and other markers of alcohol use. Alcoholism 1989; 13:605.
22. Reynaud M, Schwan R, Loiseaux-Meunier MN, et al. Patients admitted to emergency services for drunkenness: moderate alcohol users or harmful drinkers? Am J Psychiatry 2001; 158:96.
23. Lykouras E, Markianos M, Moussas G. Platelet monoamine oxidase, plasma dopamine beta-hydroxylase activity, dementia and family history of alcoholism in chronic alcoholics. Acta Psychiatr Scand 1989; 80:487.
24. Johnson JH, Crider BP. Increase in Na,K-ATPase activity of erythrocytes and skeletal muscle after chronic

ethanol consumption: evidence for reduced efficiency of the enzyme. Proc Natl Acad Sci USA 1989; 86:7857.

25. Roine RP, Nykanen I, Ylikahri R, et al. Effects of alcohol on blood dolichol concentration. Alcoholism 1989; 13:519.

26. Karkkainen P, Poikolainen K, Salaspuro M. Serum beta-hexosaminidase as a marker of heavy drinking. Alcoholism 1990; 14:187.

27. Roine RP, Eriksson CJ, Ylikahri R, et al. Methanol as a marker of alcohol abuse. Alcoholism 1989; 13: 172.

28. Glass IB, Chalmers R, Bartlett B, Littleton J. Increased plasma carnitine in severe alcohol dependence. Br J Addict 1989; 84:689.

29. Crabbe DW. Biological markers for increased risk of alcoholism and for quantitation of alcohol consumption. J Clin Invest 1990; 85:311.

30. Diaz F, Cadaveira F, Grau C. Short- and middle-latency auditory-evoked potentials in abstinent chronic alcoholics: preliminary findings. Electroencephalogr Clin Neurophysiol 1990; 77:145.

31. Tabakoff B, Hoffman PL, Lee JM, et al. Differences in platelet enzyme activity between alcoholics and non-alcoholics. N Engl J Med 1988; 318:134.

32. Brathen G, Bjerve KS, Brodtkorb E, et al. Detection of alcohol abuse in neurological patients: variables of clinical relevance to the accuracy of the % CDT-TIA and CDTect methods. Alcohol Clin Exp Res 2001; 25:46.

32a. Anton RF, Stout RL, Roberts JS, et al. The effects of drinking intensity and frequency on serum carbohydrate-deficient transferrin and gamma-glutamyl transferase levels in outpatient alcoholics. Alcohol Clin Exp Res 1998; 22:1456.

33. American Psychiatric Association, Committee on Nomenclature and Statistics: Diagnostic and Statistical Manual of Mental Disorders, 3rd edition, revised (DSM-IV). Washington, DC: American Psychiatric Association, 1987.

34. Kessler RC, Crum, RM, Warner LA, et al. Lifetime co-occurrence of DSM III-R alcohol abuse and dependence with other psychiatric disorders in the national comorbidity survey. Arch Gen Psychiatry 1997; 54:313.

35. Alcohol-related disease impact-Wisconsin 1988. MMWR 1990; 39:178.

36. Naimi TS, Brewer RD, Mokdad A, et al. Binge drinking among U.S. adults. JAMA 2003; 289:70.

37. O'Malley PM, Johnston LD. Epidemiology of alcohol and other drug use among American college students. J Stud Alcohol 2002; Suppl 14:23.

38. Ashley MJ, Olin JS, LeRiche WH. Skid row alcoholism: a distinct sociomedical entity. Arch Intern Med 1976; 136:272.

39. Hughes PH, Brandenburg N, Baldwin DC, et al. Prevalence of substance use among US physicians. JAMA 1992; 267:2333.

40. O'Connor PG, Spickard A. Physician impairment by substance abuse. Med Clin North Am 1997; 81:1037.

41. Foster SE, Vaughn RD, Foster WA, et al. Alcohol consumption and expenditures for underage drinking and adult excessive drinking. JAMA 2003; 289:989.

42. McNeil DG. Liquor industry and scientists at odds over alcohol study. NY Times, February 26, 2003.

43. McClusker J, Cherubin CE, Zimberg S. Prevalence of alcoholism in general municipal hospital population. NY State J Med 1971; 71:751.

44. Moore RD, Bone LR, Geller G, et al. Prevalence, detection, and treatment of alcoholism in hospitalized patients. JAMA 1989; 261:403.

45. DiFranza JR, Guerrera MP. Alcoholism and smoking. J Stud Alcohol 1990; 51:130.

46. Miller NS, Gold MS. Comorbid cigarette and alcohol addiction: epidemiology and treatment. J Addict Dis 1998; 17:55.

46a. Holden C. Winos on the rise in Britain. Science 2003; 302:224.

47. Lieber CS. Alcohol: its metabolism and interaction with nutrients. Annu Rev Nutr 2000; 20:395.

48. Lieber CS. Hepatic, metabolic, and nutritional disorders of alcoholism: from pathogenesis to therapy. Crit Rev Clin Lab Sci 2000; 37:551.

49. Griezerstein HB. Tolerance to ethanol: effect of congeners present in bourbon. Psychopharmacology 1977; 53:201.

50. Suter PM, Schutz Y, Jequier E. The effect of ethanol on fat storage in healthy subjects. N Engl J Med 1992; 326:983.

51. Suter PM, Hasler E, Vetter W. Effects of alcohol on energy metabolism and body weight regulation: is alcohol a risk factor for obesity? Nutr Rev 1997; 55:157.

52. Lieber CS. Medical and Nutritional Complications of Alcoholism: Mechanisms and Management. New York: Plenum Press, 1992.

53. Salmela KS, Kessova IG, Tsyrlov IB, et al. Respective roles of human cytochrome P4502E1, 1A2, and 3A4 in the hepatic microsomal ethanol oxidizing system. Alcohol Clin Exp Res 1998; 22:2125.

54. Mari M, Wu D, Nieto N, Cederbaum AI. CYP2E1-dependent toxicity and up-regulation of antioxidant genes. J Biomed Sci 2001; 8:52.

55. Zima T, Fiabva L, Mestek O, et al. Oxidative stress, metabolism of ethanol and alcohol-related diseases. J Biomed Sci 2001; 8:59.

56. Brown ZW, Amit Z, Rockman GE. Intraventricular self-administration of acetaldehyde, but not ethanol, in naive laboratory rats. Psychopharmacology 1979; 64: 271.

57. Ortiz A, Griffiths PJ, Littleton JM. A comparison of the effects of chronic administration of ethanol and acetaldehyde to mice: evidence for a role of acetaldehyde in ethanol dependence. J Pharm Pharmacol 1974; 26:249.

58. Korsten MA, Matsuzaki S, Feinman L, et al. High blood acetaldehyde levels after ethanol administration.

Differences between alcoholic and non-alcoholic subjects. N Engl J Med 1975; 292:386.

59. Rahwan RG. Toxic effects of ethanol: possible role of acetaldehyde, tetrahydroisoquinolines, and tetrahydro-beta-carbolines. Toxicol Appl Pharmacol 1975; 34:3.

60. Myers RD. Isoquinolines, beta-carbolines and alcohol drinking: involvement of opioid and dopaminergic mechanisms. Experientia 1989; 45:436.

61. Tuomisto L, Airaksinen MM, Peura P, Eriksson CJP. Alcohol drinking in the rat: increases following intracerebroventricular treatment with tetrahydro-betacarbolines. Pharmacol Biochem Behav 1982; 17: 831.

62. Goldstein DB. Effect of alcohol on cellular membranes. Ann Emerg Med 1986; 15:1013.

63. Harris RA, Baxter DM, Mitchell MA, et al. Physical properties and lipid composition of brain membranes from ethanol tolerant-dependent mice. Mol Pharmacol 1984; 25:401.

64. Peoples RW, Li C, Weight FF. Lipid vs. protein theory of alcohol action in the nervous system. Annu Rev Pharmacol Toxicol 1996; 36:185.

65. Wirkner K, Poelchen W, Köles L. Ethanol-induced inhibition of NMDA receptor channels. Neurochem Int 1999; 35:153.

66. Peoples RW, Weight FF. Cutoff in potency implicates alcohol inhibition of N-methyl-D-aspartate receptors in alcohol intoxication. Proc Natl Acad Sci USA 1995; 92:2825.

67. Franks NP, Lieb WR. Molecular and cellular mechanisms of general anesthesia. Nature 1994; 367:607.

68. Yu D, Zhang L, Eisele JL, et al. Ethanol inhibition of nicotinic acetylcholine type $\alpha 7$ receptors involves the amino-terminal domain of the receptor. Mol Pharmacol 1996; 50:1010.

69. Dodd PR, Beckmann AM, Davidson MS, Wike PA. Glutamate-mediated transmission, alcohol, and alcoholism. Neurochem Int 2000; 37:509.

70. Lovinger DM, White G, Weight FF. Ethanol inhibits NMDA-activated ion current in hippocampal neurons. Science 1989; 253:1721.

71. Diamond I, Gordon AS. Cellular and molecular neuroscience of alcoholism. Physiol Rev 1997; 77:1.

72. Dahchour A, DeWitte P. Ethanol and amino acids in the central nervous system: assessment of the pharmacological actions of acamprosate. Prog Neurobiol 2000; 60:343.

73. Kumari M, Ticku MK. Regulation of NMDA receptors by ethanol. Prog Drug Res 2000; 54:152.

74. Tsai GC, Coyle JT. The role of glutaminergic neurotransmission in the pathophysiology of alcoholism. Annu Rev Med 1998; 49:173.

75. Sucher NJ, Awobuluyi M, Choi Y-B, Lipton SA. NMDA receptors: from genes to channels. Trends Pharmacol Sci 1996; 17:348.

76. Wright JM, Peoples RW, Weight FF. Single-channel and whole-cell analysis of ethanol inhibition of NMDA-activated currents in cultured mouse cortical and hippocampal neurons. Brain Res 1996; 738:249.

77. Davis KM, Wu J-Y. Role of glutamatergic and GABAergic systems in alcoholism. J Biomed Sci 2001; 8:7.

78. Woodward JJ. Ionotropic glutamate receptors as sites of action for ethanol in the brain. Neurochem Int 1999; 35:107.

79. Frye GD, Fincher A. Sustained ethanol inhibition of native AMPA receptors on medial septum/diagonal band (MS/DB) neurons. Br J Pharmacol 2000; 129:87.

80. Netzeband JG, Trotter C, Caguioa JN, Gruol DL. Chronic ethanol exposure enhances AMPA-elicited Ca^{2+} signals in the somatic and dendritic regions of cerebellar Purkinje neurons. Neurochem Int 1999; 35:163.

81. Harris RA. Ethanol actions on multiple ion channels: which are important? Alcohol Clin Exp Res 1999; 23:1563.

82. Weiner JL, Valenzuela CF, Watson PL, et al. Elevation of basal protein kinase C activity increases ethanol sensitivity of $GABA_A$ receptors in rat hippocampal CA1 pyramidal neurons. J Neurochem 1997; 68:1949.

83. Wafford KA, Whiting PJ. Ethanol potentiation of $GABA_A$ receptors requires phosphorylation of the alternatively spliced variant of the $\gamma 2$ subunit. FEBS Lett 1992; 313:113.

84. Mihic SJ. Acute effects of ethanol on $GABA_A$ and glycine receptor function. Neurochem Int 1999; 35:115.

85. Loh E-W, Ball D. Role of the $GABA_{A\beta 2}$, $GABA_{A\alpha 6}$, $GABA_{A\alpha 1}$, and $GABA_{A\gamma 2}$ receptor subunit genes cluster in drug responses and the development of alcohol dependence. Neurochem Int 2000; 37:413.

86. Macdonald RL. Ethanol, gamma-aminobutyrate type A receptors, and protein kinase C phosphorylation. Proc Natl Acad Sci USA 1995; 92:3633.

87. Mihic SJ, Ye Q, Wick MJ, et al. Sites of alcohol and volatile anesthetic action on GABAA and glycine receptors. Nature 1997; 389:385.

88. Ziemann V, Lönnecker S, Paulus W. Inhibition of human motor cortex by ethanol. A transcranial magnetic stimulation study. Brain 1995; 118:1437.

89. Mhatre M, Ticku MK. Chronic ethanol treatment selectively increases the binding of inverse agonists for benzodiazepine binding sites in cultured spinal cord neurons. J Pharmacol Exp Ther 1989; 251:164.

90. Suzdak PD, Glowa JR, Crawley JN, et al. A selective imidazobenzodiazepine antagonist of ethanol in the rat. Science 1986; 234:1243.

91. Britton KT, Ehlers CL, Koob GF. Is ethanol antagonist RO15-4513 selective for ethanol? Science 1988; 239:648.

92. Liste RG, Karanian JW. RO15-4513 induces seizures in DBA/2 mice undergoing ethanol withdrawal. Alcohol 1987; 4:409.

93. Lister RG, Nutt DJ. Is RO15-4513 a specific alcohol antagonist? Trends Neurosci 1987; 10:223.

94. Abi-Dargham A, Krystal JH, Anjilvel S, et al. Alterations of benzodiazepine receptors in Type II alcoholic subjects measured with SPECT and [^{123}I]Iomazenil. Am J Psychiatry 1998; 155:1550.

95. LeMarquand D, Pihl RO, Benkelfat C. Serotonin and alcohol intake, abuse, and dependence: findings of animal studies. Biol Psychiatry 1994; 36:395.

96. LeMarquand D, Pihl RO, Benkelfat C. Serotonin and alcohol intake, abuse, and dependence: clinical evidence. Biol Psychiatry 1994; 36:326.

97. Sellers EM, Toneatto T, Romach MK, et al. Clinical efficacy of the 5HT3 antagonist ondansetron in alcohol abuse and dependence. Alcoholism Clin Exp Res 1994; 18:879.

98. Engel SR, Lyons CR, Allan AM. 5HT3 receptor overexpression decreases ethanol self-administration in transgenic mice. Psychopharmacology 1998; 140:243.

99. Lovinger DM. 5HT3 receptors and the neural actions of alcohols: an increasingly exciting topic. Neurochem Int 1999; 35:125.

100. Boschert U, Amara DA, Segu L, Hen R. The mouse 5-hydroxytryptamine1B receptor is localized predominantly on axon terminals. Neuroscience 1994; 58:167.

101. Crabbe JC, Phillips TJ, Feller DJ, et al. Elevated alcohol consumption in null mutant mice lacking 5HT$_{1B}$ serotonin receptors. Nat Genet 1996; 14:98.

102. Wang X, Wang G, Lemos JR, Treistman SN. Ethanol directly modulates gating of a dihydropyridine-sensitive Ca^{2+} channel in neurohypophyseal terminals. J Neurosci 1994; 14:5453.

103. Mullikin-Kilpatric D, Treistman SN. Inhibition of dihydropyridine-sensitive Ca^{++} channels by ethanol in undifferentiated and nerve growth factor-treated PC12 cells: interaction with the inactivated state. J Pharmacol Exp Ther 1995; 272:489.

104. Walter HJ, Massing RO. Regulation of voltage-gated calcium channels by ethanol. Neurochem Int 1999; 35:95.

105. Messing RO, Carpenter CL, Diamond I, Greenberg DA. Ethanol regulates calcium channels in clonal neural cells. Proc Natl Acad Sci USA 1986; 83:6213.

106. Little HJ, Dolin SJ, Halsey MJ. Calcium channel antagonists decrease the ethanol withdrawal syndrome. Life Sci 1986; 39:2059.

107. DeBeun R, Schneider R, Klein A, et al. Effects of nimodipine and other calcium channel antagonists in alcohol-preferring AA rats. Alcohol 1996; 13:263.

108. Huang G-J, McArdle JJ. Chronic ingestion of ethanol increases the number of Ca^{2+} channels of hippocampal neurons of long-sleep but not short-sleep mice. Brain Res 1993; 615:328.

109. Guppy LJ, Crabbe JC, Littleton JM. Time course and genetic variation in the regulation of calcium channel antagonist binding sites in rodent tissues during the induction of ethanol physical dependence and withdrawal. Alcohol 1995; 30:607.

110. Dopico AM, Chu B, Lemos JR, Treistman SN. Alcohol modulation of calcium-activated potassium channels. Neurochem Int 1999; 35:103.

111. Covarrubias M, Vyas TB, Escobar L, Wei A. Alcohols inhibit a cloned potassium channel at a discrete saturable site. J Biol Chem 1995; 270:19408.

112. Diana M, Pistis M, Muntoni A, Gessa G. Mesolimbic dopaminergic reduction outlasts ethanol withdrawal syndrome: evidence of protracted abstinence. Neuroscience 1996; 71:411.

113. Weiss F, Parsons LH, Schulteis G, et al. Ethanol self-administration restores withdrawal-associated deficiencies in accumbal dopamine and 5-hydroxytryptamine release in dependent rats. J Neurosci 1996; 16:3474.

114. Dyr W, McBride WJ, Lumeng L, et al. Effects of D$_1$ and D$_2$ dopamine receptor agents on ethanol consumption in the high alcohol-drinking (HAD) line of rats. Alcohol 1993; 10:207.

115. Weiss F, Porrino LJ. Behavioral neurobiology of alcohol addiction: recent advances and challenges. J Neurosci 2002; 22:3332.

116. Seizinger BR, Bovermann K, Hollt V, Herz A. Enhanced activity of the beta-endorphinergic system in the anterior and neurointermediate lobe of the rat pituitary after chronic treatment with ethanol liquid diet. J Pharmacol Exp Ther 1984; 230:455.

117. Seizinger BR, Bovermann K, Maysinga D, et al. Differential effects of acute and chronic ethanol treatment on particular opioid peptide systems in discrete regions of rat brain and pituitary. Pharmacol Biochem Behav 1983; 18 (Suppl 1):361.

118. Gianoulakis C. The effect of ethanol on the biosynthesis and regulation of opioid peptides. Experientia 1989; 45:428.

119. Pohorecky LA, Brick J. Pharmacology of ethanol. Pharmacol Ther 1988; 36:335.

120. Charness ME. Ethanol and opioid receptor signaling. Experientia 1989; 45:418.

121. Myers RD, Borg S, Mossberg R. Antagonism by naltrexone of voluntary alcohol selection in the chronically drinking macaque monkey. Alcohol 1986; 3:383.

122. Gardell LR, Hubbell CL, Reid LD. Naltrexone persistently reduces rats' intake of a palatable alcoholic beverage. Alcohol Clin Exp Res 1996; 20:584.

123. Krishnan-Sarin S, Portoghese PS, Li TK, Froehlich J. The delta2-opioid receptor antagonist naltriben selectively attenuates alcohol intake in rats bred for alcohol preference. Pharmacol Biochem Behav 1995; 52:153.

124. Benjamin D, Grant ER, Pohorecky LA. Naltrexone reverses ethanol-induced dopamine release in the nucleus accumbens in awake, freely-moving rats. Brain Res 1993; 621:137.

125. Nie Z, Madamba SG, Siggins GR. Ethanol inhibits glutamatergic neurotransmission in nucleus accumbens

neurons by multiple mechanisms. J Pharmacol Exp Ther 1994; 271:1566.

126. Wonnacott S. Presynaptic nicotine ACh receptors. Trends Neurosci 1997; 20:92.

127. Narahashi T, Aistrup GL, Marszalec W. Nagata K. Neuronal nicotinic acetylcholine receptors: a new target site of ethanol. Neurochem Int 1999; 35:131.

128. Convernton PJO, Connolly JG. Differential modulation of rat neuronal nicotine receptor subtypes by acute application of ethanol. Br J Pharmacol 1997; 122:1661.

129. Madamba SG, Hsu M, Schweitzer P, Siggins GR. Ethanol enhances muscarinic cholinergic neurotransmission in rat hippocampus in vitro. Brain Res 1995; 685:21.

130. Krauss SW, Ghirnikar RB, Diamond I, Gordon AS. Inhibition of adenosine uptake by ethanol is specific for one class of nucleoside transporters. Mol Pharmacol 1993; 44:1021.

131. Nagy L, Diamond I, Gordon AS. cAMP-dependent protein kinase regulates inhibition of adenosine transport by ethanol. Mol Pharmacol 1991; 40:812.

132. Coe IR, Dohrman DP, Diamond I, Gordon AS. Activation of cAMP-dependent protein kinase reverses tolerance of the nucleoside transporter to ethanol. J Pharmacol Exp Ther 1995; 276:365.

133. Nagy LE, Diamond I, Collier K, et al. Adenosine is required for ethanol-induced heterologous desensitization. Mol Pharmacol 1989; 36:744.

134. Weight FF, Li C, Peoples RW. Alcohol action on membrane ion channels gated by extracellular ATP (P2X receptors). Neurochem Int 1999; 35:143.

135. Thiele TE, Koh MT, Pedrazzini T. Voluntary alcohol consumption is controlled via the neuropeptide Y Y1 receptor. J Neurosci 2002; 22:RC208 (1-6).

136. Cloninger CR. Neurogenetic adaptive mechanisms in alcoholism. Science 1987; 236:410.3.

137. Li T-K, Bosron WF. Genetic variability of enzymes of alcohol metabolism in human beings. Ann Emerg Med 1986; 15:997.

138. Bosron WF, Lumeng L, Li TK. Genetic polymorphism of enzymes of alcohol metabolism and susceptibility to alcoholic liver disease. Mol Aspects Med 1988; 10:147.

139. Agarwal DP, Goedde HW. Human aldehyde dehydrogenases: their role in alcoholism. Alcohol 1989; 6:517.

140. Goedde HW, Agarwal DP. Pharmacogenetics of aldehyde dehydrogenase (ALDH). Pharmacol Ther 1990; 45:345.

141. Okamoto K, Murawaki Y, Yuasa And K, Kawasaki H. Effect of ALDH2 and CYP2E1 gene polymorphisms on drinking behavior and alcoholic liver disease in Japanese male workers. Alcohol Clin Exp Res 2001; 25 (Suppl 6):19S.

142. Mullan M. Alcoholism and the "new genetics." Br J Addict 1989; 84:1433.

143. Wallace J. The new disease model of alcoholism. West J Med 1990; 152:502.

144. Schukit M. Genetic aspects of alcoholism. Ann Emerg Med 1986; 15:991.

145. Pickens RW, Svikis DS, McGue M, et al. Heterogeneity in the inheritance of alcoholism. Arch Gen Psychiatry 1991; 48:19.

146. Buydens-Branchey L, Branchey MH, Noumair D. Age of alcoholism onset. 1. Relationship to psychopathology. Arch Gen Psychiatry 1989; 46:225.

147. Schukit MA, Irwin M. An analysis of the clinical relevance of type 1 and type 2 alcoholics. Br J Addict 1989; 84:869.

148. Vaillant GE. The Natural History of Alcoholism. Cambridge, MA: Harvard University Press, 1983.

149. McGue M, Pickens RW, Svikis DS. Sex and age effects on the inheritance of alcohol problems: twin study. J Abnorm Psychol 1992; 101:3.

150. Johnson EO, Pickens RW. Familial transmission of alcoholism among nonalcoholics and mild, severe, and dissocial subtypes of alcoholism. Alcohol Clin Exp Res 2001; 25:661.

151. Irwin M, Schukit M, Smith TL. Clinical importance of age of onset in type 1 and type 2 primary alcoholics. Arch Gen Psychiatry 1990; 47:320.

152. Li TK, Lumeng L, McBride WJ, et al. Rodent lines selected for factors affecting alcohol consumption. Alcohol 1987; (Suppl 1):91.

153. Li T-K, Lumeng L, Doolittle DP. Selective breeding for alcohol preference and associated responses. Behav Genet 1993; 23:163.

154. McBride WJ, Li T-K. Animal models of alcoholism: neurobiology of high alcohol-drinking behavior in rodents. Crit Rev Neurobiol 1998; 12:339.

155. Deitrich RA. Selective breeding for initial sensitivity to ethanol. Behav Genet 1993; 23:153.

156. Phillips TJ, Feller DJ, Crabbe JC. Selected mouse lines, alcohol and behavior. Experientia 1989; 45:805.

157. Wafford KA, Burnett DM, Dunwiddie TV, Harris RA. Genetic differences in the ethanol sensitivity of GABA-A receptors expressed in *Xenopus* oocytes. Science 1990; 249:291.

158. McIntyre TD, Trullas R, Skonick P. Differences in biophysical properties of the benzodiazepine/gamma-aminobutyric acid receptor chloride channel complex in the long-sleep and short-sleep mouse lines. J Neurochem 1988; 51:642.

159. Korpi ER, Kleingoor C, Kettenmann H, Seeburg PH. Benzodiazepine-induced motor impairment linked to point mutation in cerebellar GABA-A receptor. Nature 1993; 361:356.

160. Wong DT, Threlkeld PG, Lumeng L, Li T-K. Higher density of serotonin-1A receptors in the hippocampus and cerebral cortex of alcohol-preferring rats. Life Sci 1990; 46:231.

161. McBride WJ, Murphy JM, Lumeng L, Li T-K. Serotonin and ethanol preference. Rec Dev Alcohol 1989; 7:187.

162. Crabbe JC, Phillips TJ, Feller DJ, et al. Elevated alcohol consumption in null mutant mice lacking 5HT1B serotonin receptors. Nat Genet 1996; 14:98.

163. Brunner D, Hen R. Insights into the neurobiology of impulsive behavior from serotonin receptor knockout mice. Ann N Y Acad Sci 1997; 836:81.

164. Sinclair JD, Le AD, Kiianmaa K. The AA and ANA rat lines, selected for differences in voluntary alcohol consumption. Experientia 1989; 45:798.

165. Buck KJ, Hahner L, Sikela J, Harris RA. Chronic ethanol treatment alters brain levels of gamma-aminobutyric acid-A receptor subunit in RNAs: relationship to genetic differences in ethanol withdrawal seizure severity. J Neurochem 1991; 57:1452.

166. Crabbe JC, Phillips TJ. Selective breeding for alcohol withdrawal severity. Behav Genet 1993; 23:171.

167. Blum K, Briggs AH, Wallace JE, et al. Regional brain [Met]-enkephalin in alcohol-preferring and non-alcohol preferring inbred strains of mice. Experientia 1986; 43:408.

168. Gianoulakis C, Gupta A. Inbred strains of mice with variable sensitivity to ethanol exhibit differences in the content and processing of beta-endorphin. Life Sci 1986; 39:2315.

169. Higley JD, Linnoila M. A nonhuman primate model of excessive alcohol intake. Personality and neurobiological parallels of Type I- and Type II-like alcoholism. Rec Dev Alcohol 1997; 13:191.

170. Bellin HJ. The fruit fly: a model organism to study the genetics of alcohol abuse and alcoholism? Cell 1998; 93:909.

171. Ashburner M. Speculations on the subject of alcohol dehydrogenase and its properties in *Drosophila* and other flies. Bioessays 1998; 20:949.

172. Crabbe JC, Belknap JK, Buck KJ. Genetic animal models of alcohol and drug abuse. Science 1994; 264:1715.

173. Goate AM, Edenberg HJ. The genetics of alcoholism. Curr Opin Genet Dev 1998; 8:282.

174. Tarentino LM, McClearn GE, Rodriguez LA, Plomin R. Confirmation of quantitative trait loci for alcohol preference in mice. Alcohol Clin Exp Res 1998; 22:1099.

175. Crabbe JC, Phillips TJ, Buck KJ, et al. Identifying genes for alcohol and drug sensitivity: recent progress and future directions. Trends Neurosci 1999; 22:173.

176. Bennett B. Congenic strains developed for alcohol- and drug-related phenotypes. Pharmacol Biochem Behav 2000; 67:671.

177. Fergeson RA, Goldberg DM. Genetic markers of alcohol abuse. Clin Chim Acta 1997; 257:199.

178. Holden C. Probing the complex genetics of alcoholism. Science 1991; 251:163.

179. Schuckit MA. Low level of response to alcohol as a predictor of future alcoholism. Am J Psychiatry 1994; 151:184.

180. Schukit MA, Smith TL. The clinical course of alcohol dependence associated with a low level of response to alcohol. Addiction 2001; 96:903.

181. Hill SY, Steinhauer S, Park J, Zubin J. Event-related potential characteristics in children of alcoholics from high density families. Alcoholism 1990; 14:6.

182. Ehlers CL, Schukit MA. EEG fast frequency activity in the sons of alcoholics. Biol Psychiatry 1990; 27:631.

183. Hesselbrock V, Begleiter H, Porjesz B, et al. P300 event-related potential amplitude as an endophenotype of alcoholism-evidence from the collaborative study on the genetics of alcoholism. J Biomed Sci 2001; 8:77.

184. Sullivan JL, Baenziger JC, Wagner DL, Rauscher FP. Platelet MAO in subtypes of alcoholism. Biol Psychiatry 1990; 27:911.

185. Gordis E, Tabakoff B, Goldman D, Berg K. Finding the gene(s) for alcoholism. JAMA 1990; 263:2094.

186. Tabakoff B, Hoffman PL, Lee JM, et al. Differences in platelet enzyme activity between alcoholics and non-alcoholics. N Engl J Med 1988; 318:134.

187. Gianoulakis C, Beliveau D, Angelogianni P, et al. Different pituitary beta-endorphin and adrenal cortical response to ethanol in individuals with high and low risk for future development of alcoholism. Life Sci 1989; 45:1097.

188. Moss HB, Yao J, Burns M, et al. Plasma GABA-like activity in response to ethanol challenge in men at high risk for alcoholism. Biol Psychiatry 1990; 27:617.

189. Moss HB, Guthrie S, Linnoila M. Enhanced thyrotropin response to thyrotropin releasing hormone in boys at risk for development of alcoholism. Arch Gen Psychiatry 1986; 43:1137.

190. Hill SY, Aston C, Rabin B. Suggestive evidence of genetic linkage between alcoholism and MNS blood group. Alcoholism 1988; 12:811.

191. Tanna VL, Wilson AF, Winokur G, Elston RC. Possible linkage between alcoholism and esterase-D. J Stud Alcohol 1988; 49:472.

192. Comings DE. Genetic factors in substance abuse based on studies of Tourette syndrome and ADHD probands and relatives. II. Alcohol abuse. Drug Alcohol Depend 1994; 35:17.

193. Marshall JR. Alcohol and substance abuse in panic disorder. J Clin Psychiatry 1997; 58 (Suppl 2):46.

194. Modesto-Lowe V, Kranzler HR. Diagnosis and treatment of alcohol-dependent patients with comorbid psychiatric disorders. Alcohol Res Health JNIAAA 1999; 23:144.

195. Cantor-Graae E, Nordstrum LG, McNeil TF. Substance abuse in schizophrenia: a review of the literature and a study of correlates in Sweden. Schiz Res 2001; 48:69.

196. Nurnberger JI, Foroud T, Flury L, et al. Evidence for a locus on chromosome 1 that influences vulnerability to alcoholism and affective disorder. Am J Psychiatry 2001; 158:718.

197. Schukit MA. A study of young men with alcoholic close relatives. Am J Psychiatry 1982; 139:791.

198. Harrington R, Fudge H, Rutter M, et al. Adult outcomes of childhood and adolescent depression. Arch Gen Psychiatry 1990; 47:465.

199. Blum K, Noble EP, Sheridan PJ, et al. Allelic association of human dopamine D-2 receptor gene in alcoholism. JAMA 1990; 263:2055.

200. Blum K, Noble EP, Sheridan P, et al. Association of the A1 allele of the D$_2$ dopamine receptor gene with severe alcoholism. Alcohol 1991; 8:409.

201. Amadeo S, Abbar M, Fourcade ML, et al. D$_2$ dopamine receptor gene and alcoholism. J Psychiatr Res 1993; 27:173.

202. Noble EP, Syndulko K, Fitch RJ, et al. D$_2$ dopamine receptor Taq1 A alleles in medically ill alcoholic and nonalcoholic patients. Alcohol 1994; 29:729.

203. Neiswanger K, Hill SY, Kaplan BB. Association and linkage studies of the Taq1 A allele of the dopamine D$_2$ receptor gene in samples of female and male alcoholics. Am J Med Genet 1995; 60:267.

204. Lawford BR, Young RM, Rowell JR, et al. Association of the D$_2$ dopamine receptor Al allele with alcoholism. Medical severity of alcoholism and type of controls. Biol Psychiatry 1997; 41:386.

205. Bolos AM, Dean M, Lucas-Derse S, et al. Population and pedigree studies reveal a lack of association between the dopamine D-2 receptor gene and alcoholism. JAMA 1990; 264:3156.

206. Gelernter J, O'Malley S, Risch N, et al. No association between an allele at the D$_2$ dopamine receptor gene (DRD2) and alcoholism. JAMA 1991; 266:1801.

207. Cook BL, Wang ZQ, Crowe RR, et al. Alcoholism and the D$_2$ receptor gene. Alcohol Clin Exp Res 1992; 4:806.

208. Goldman D, Dean M, Brown GL, et al. D$_2$ dopamine receptor genotype and cerebrospinal fluid homovanillic acid, 5-hydroxyindoleacetic acid, and 3-methoxy-4-hydroxyphenylglycol in Finland and the United States. Acta Psychiatr Scand 1992; 86:351-357.

209. Schwab S, Soyka M, Niederecker M, et al. Allelic association of human D$_2$-receptor DNA polymorphism ruled out in 45 alcoholics. Am J Hum Genet 1991; 49 (Suppl):203.

210. Geijer T, Neiman J, Rydberg U, et al. Dopamine D$_2$ receptor gene polymorphisms in Scandinavian chronic alcoholics. Eur Arch Psychiatry Clin Neurosci 1994; 244:26.

211. Heinz A, Sander T, Harms H, et al. Lack of allelic association of dopamine D$_1$ and D$_2$ (Taq1A) receptor gene polymorphisms with reduced dopaminergic sensitivity in alcoholism. Alcohol Clin Exp Res 1996; 20:1109.

212. Suarez BK, Parsian A, Hampe CL, et al. Linkage disequilibria and the D$_2$ dopamine receptor locus (DRD2) in alcoholics and controls. Genomics 1994; 19:12.

213. Anghelescu I, Germeyer S, Muller MJ, et al. No association between dopamine D$_2$ receptor taqA1 allele and earlier age of onset of alcohol dependence according to different specified criteria. Alcohol Clin Exp Res 2001; 25:805.

214. Parsian A, Todd RD, Devor EJ, et al. Alcoholism and alleles of the human dopamine D$_2$ receptor locus: studies of association and linkage. Arch Gen Psychiatry 1991; 48:655.

215. Comings DE, Comings BG, Muhleman D, et al. The dopamine D$_2$ receptor locus as a modifying gene in neuropsychiatric disorders. JAMA 1991; 266:1793.

216. Smith SS, O'Hara BF, Persico AM, et al. Genetic vulnerability in drug abuse: the dopamine D$_2$ receptor Taq1B RFLP is more frequent in polysubstance abusers. Arch Gen Psychiatry 1992; 49:723.

217. Persico AM, Bird G, Gabbay FH, et al. D$_2$ dopamine receptor gene TaqA1 and B1 restriction fragment length polymorphism: enhanced frequencies in psychostimulant-preferring polysubstance abusers. Biol Psychiatry 1996; 40:776.

218. Noble EP. The D$_2$ dopamine receptor gene: a review of association studies in alcoholism and phenotypes. Alcohol 1998; 16:33.

219. Noble EP, Blum K, Khalsa ME, et al. Allelic association of the D$_2$ dopamine receptor gene with cocaine dependence. Drug Alcohol Depend 1993; 33:271.

220. Comings DE, Muhleman D, Ahn C, et al. The dopamine D$_2$ receptor gene: a genetic risk factorin substance abuse. Drug Alcohol Depend 1994; 34: 175.

221. Lu RB, Lee JF, Ko HC, Lin WW. Dopamine D$_2$ receptor gene (DRD2) is associated with alcoholism with conduct disorder. Alcohol Clin Exp Res 2001; 25:177.

222. Gelernter J, Goldman D, Risch N. The A1 allele at the D$_2$ dopamine receptor gene and alcoholism. A reappraisal. JAMA 1993; 269:1673.

223. Edenberg HJ, Foroud T, Koller DL, et al. A family-based analysis of the association of the dopamine D$_2$ receptor (DRD2) with alcoholism. Alcohol Clin Exp Res 1998; 22:505.

224. Pohjalainen T, Rinne J, Nagren K, et al. Genetic determinant of human D$_2$ dopamine receptor binding characteristics in vivo. Am J Hum Genet 1996; 59 (Suppl 4):A387.

225. Tupala E, Hall A, Berstrom K, et al. Dopamine D$_2$/D$_3$-receptor and transporter densities in nucleus accumbens and amygdala of type 1 and 2 alcoholics. Mol Psychiatry 2001; 6:261.

226. Lawford BR, Young RM, Rowell JA, et al. Bromocriptine in the treatment of alcoholics with the D$_2$ dopamine receptor A1 allele. Nat Med 1995; 1:337.

227. Ovchinnikov IV, Druzina E, Ovtchinikova O. Polymorphisms of dopamine D$_2$ and D$_4$ receptor genes in Slavic-surnamed alcoholic patients. Addict Biol 1999; 4:399.

228. Gejman PV, Ram A, Gelernter J, et al. No structural mutation in the dopamine D$_2$ receptor gene in alcoholism or schizophrenia. Analysis using denaturing gradient gel electrophoresis. JAMA 1994; 271:204.

229. Cloninger CR. D$_2$ dopamine receptor gene is associated but not linked with alcoholism. JAMA 1991; 266:1833.

230. Blum K, Braverman ER, Holder JM, et al. Reward deficiency syndrome: a biogenetic model for the diagnosis and treatment of impulsive, addictive, and

compulsive behaviors. J Psychoactive Drugs 2000; 32 (Suppl):1.

231. Hill SY. Alternative strategies for uncovering genes contributing to alcoholism risk: unpredictable findings in a genetic wonderland. Alcohol 1998; 16:53.

232. Comings DE. Why different rules are required for polygenetic inheritance: lessons from studies of the DRD2 gene. Alcohol 1998; 16:61.

233. Blum K, Noble E, Sheriden PJ, et al. Genetic predisposition in alcoholism. Association of the D_2 dopamine receptor Taq B RFLP in severe alcoholics. Alcohol 1993; 10:59.

234. Matsushita S, Yoshino A, Murayama M, et al. Association study of serotonin transporter gene regulatory region polymorphism and alcoholism. Am J Med Genet 2001; 105:446.

235. Preuss UW, Koller G, Bondy B, et al. Impulsive traits and 5-HT$_{2A}$ receptor promoter polymorphism in alcohol dependents: possible association but no influence of personality disorders. Neuropsychobiology 2001; 43:186.

236. Heinz A, Mann K, Weinberger DR, Goldman D. Serotonergic dysfunction, negative mood states, and response to alcohol. Alcohol Clin Exp Res 2001; 25:487.

236a. Tarantino LM, McClearn GE, Rodriguez LA, et al. Confirmation of quantitative trait loci for alcohol preference in mice. Alcohol Clin Exp Res 1998; 22:1099.

237. Lappalainen J, Long JC, Eggert M, et al. Linkage of antisocial alcoholism to the serotonin 5-HT$_{1B}$ receptor gene in 2 populations. Arch Gen Psychiatry 1998; 55:989.

238. Long J, Knowler WC, Hanson RL, et al. Evidence for genetic linkage to alcohol dependence on chromosomes 4 and 11 from an autosome-wide scan in an American Indian population. Am J Med Genet (Neuropsychiatr Genet) 1998; 81:216.

239. Reich T, Edenberg HJ, Goate A, et al. Genome-wide search for genes affecting the risk for alcohol dependence. Am J Med Genet (Neuropsychiatr Genet) 1998; 81:207.

240. Hobbs WWR, Rall TW, Verdoorn TA. Hypnotics and sedatives; ethanol. In: Hardman JG, Limbird LE, eds. Goodman and Gilman's The Pharmacological Basics of Therapeutics, 9th edition. New York: McGraw-Hill, 1996:361.

241. Frezza M, diPadova C, Pozzato G, et al. High blood alcohol levels in women. The role of decreased alcohol dehydrogenase activity and first-pass metabolism. N Engl J Med 1990; 322:95.

242. Schenker S, Speeg KV. The risk of alcohol intake in men and women. N Engl J Med 1990; 322:127.

243. Tabakoff B, Cornell N, Hoffman PL. Alcohol tolerance. Ann Emerg Med 1986; 15:1005.

244. Holford NHG. Clinical pharmacokinetics of ethanol. Clin Pharmacokinet 1987; 13:273.

245. Roine R, Gentry T, Hernandez-Munoz R, et al. Aspirin increases blood alcohol concentrations in humans after ingestion of ethanol. JAMA 1990; 264:2406.

246. Minion GE, Slovis CM, Boutiette L. Severe alcohol intoxication: a study of 204 consecutive patients. J Toxicol Clin Toxicol 1989; 27:375.

247. Sellers EM, Kalant HL. Alcohol intoxication and withdrawal. N Engl J Med 1976; 294:757.

248. Davis AR, Lipson AH. Central nervous system depression and high blood ethanol levels. Lancet 1986; I:566.

249. Redmond AD. Central nervous system depression and high blood ethanol levels. Lancet 1986; I:805.

250. Johnson RA, Noll EC, Rodney WM. Survival after a serum ethanol concentration of $1\frac{1}{2}$%. Lancet 1982; II:1394.

251. AMA Council on Scientific Affairs. Alcohol and the driver. JAMA 1986; 255:522.

252. Isbell H, Fraser HF, Wikler A. An experimental study of the etiology of "rum fits" and delirium tremens. Q J Stud Alcohol 1955; 16:1.

253. Kalant H. Direct effects of ethanol on the nervous system. Fed Proc 1975; 34:1930.

254. Vitiello MV, Prinz PN, Personius JP, et al. Relationship of alcohol abuse history to nighttime hypoxemia in abstaining chronic alcoholic men. J Stud Alcohol 1990; 51:29.

255. Woodhouse P, Keatings WP, Coleshaw SR. Factors associated with hypothermia in patients admitted to a group of inner city hospitals. Lancet 1989; II:1201.

256. Weyman AE, Greenbaum DM, Grace WJ. Accidental hypothermia in an alcoholic population. Am J Med 1974; 56:13.

257. Fetter M, Haslwanter T, Bork M, Dichgans J. New insights into positional alcohol nystagmus using three-dimensional eye-movement analysis. Ann Neurol 1999; 45:216.

258. Sweeney DF. Alcoholic blackouts: legal implications. J Subst Abuse Treat 1990; 7:155.

259. Parker ES. Alcohol and cognition. Psychopharmacol Bull 1984; 20:494.

260. Editorial. Alcohol and atrial fibrillation. Lancet 1985; I:1374.

261. Harrow AS. Beer potomania syndrome in an alcoholic. Va Med 1989; 116:270.

262. Fraser AG. Pharmacokinetic interactions between alcohol and other drugs. Clin Pharmacokinet 1997; 33: 79.

263. Alkana RL, Parker ES, Cohen HB, et al. Reversal of ethanol intoxication in humans: an assessment of the efficacy of propranolol. Psychopharmacology 1976; 51:29.

264. Alkana RL, Parker ES, Cohen HB, et al. Reversal of ethanol intoxication in humans: an assessment of the efficacy of L-DOPA, aminophylline, and ephedrine. Psychopharmacology 1977; 55:203.

265. Alkana RL, Willingham TA, Cohen HB, et al. Apomorphine and amantadine: interaction with ethanol in humans. Fed Proc 1976; 36:331.

266. Ducobu J. Naloxone and alcohol intoxication. Ann Intern Med 1984; 100:617.

267. Gupta RC, Kofoed J. Toxicological statistics for barbiturates, other sedatives, and tranquilizers in Ontario: a 10-year survey. Can Med Assoc J 1966; 94:863.

268. Gessner PK. Effect of trichloroethanol and of chloral hydrate on the in vivo disappearance of ethanol in mice. Arch Int Pharmacodyn Ther 1973; 202:392.

269. Anon. Alcohol-drug interactions. FDA Drug Bull 1979; 9:10.

270. Tanaka E, Misawa S. Pharmacokinetic interactions between acute alcohol ingestion and single doses of benzodiazepines and tricyclic and tetracyclic antidepressants–an update. J Clin Pharm Ther 1998; 23:331.

271. Edwards R. Anesthesia and alcohol. BMJ 1985; 291:423.

272. Seixas FA. Alcohol and its drug interactions. Ann Intern Med 1975; 83:86.

273. Yesavage JA, Leirer VO. Hangover effects on aircraft pilots 14 hours after alcohol ingestion: a preliminary report. Am J Psychiatry 1986; 143:1546.

274. Wiese JG, Shlipak MG, Browner WS. The alcohol hangover. Ann Intern Med 2000; 132:897.

275. Kaivola S, Parantainen J, Osterman T, Timonen H. Hangover headache and prostaglandins; prophylactic treatment with tolfenamic acid. Cephalgia 1983; 3:31.

276. Khan MA, Jensen K, Krogh HJ. Alcohol-induced hangover: a double-blind comparison of pyritinol and placebo in preventing hangover symptoms. Q J Stud Alcohol 1973; 34:1195.

277. Victor M, Adams RD. The effect of alcohol on the nervous system. Res Publ Assoc Res Nerv Ment Dis 1953; 32:526.

278. Fox A, Kay J, Taylor A. The course of alcohol withdrawal in a general hospital. Q J Med 1997; 90:253.

279. Neiman J, Lang AE, Fornazarri L, Carlen PL. Movement disorders in alcoholism. A review. Neurology 1990; 40:741.

280. Victor M, Hope JM. The phenomenon of auditory hallucinations in chronic alcoholism. J Nerv Ment Dis 1958; 126:451.

281. Surawicz FG. Alcoholic hallucinosis: a missed diagnosis. Can J Psychiatry 1980; 25:57.

282. McMicken DB. Alcohol withdrawal syndromes. Emerg Med Clin North Am 1990; 8:805.

283. Schwarz BE, Brust JCM. Anton's syndrome accompanying withdrawal hallucinosis in a blind alcoholic. Neurology 1984; 34:969.

284. Chamorro AA, Sacco RL, Ciecierski K, et al. Visual hemineglect and hemihallucinations in a patient with a subcortical infarction. Neurology 1990; 40:1463.

285. Schukit MA, Winokur G. Alcoholic hallucinosis and schizophrenia. A negative study. Br J Psychiatry 1971; 119:549.

286. Shen WW. Extrapyramidal symptoms associated with alcohol withdrawal. Biol Psychiatry 1984; 19:1037.

287. Shandling M, Carlen PL, Lang AE. Parkinsonism in alcohol withdrawal: a follow-up study. Mov Disord 1990; 5:36.

288. Carlen PL, Lee MA, Jacob MA, Livshits O. Parkinsonism provoked by alcoholism. Ann Neurol 1981; 9:84.

289. Benedetti MG, Bower JH, Maraganore DM, et al. Smoking, alcohol, and coffee consumption preceding Parkinson's disease. A case-control study. Neurology 2000; 55:1350.

290. Fornazarri L, Carlen PL. Transient choreiform dyskinesias during alcohol withdrawal. Can J Neurol Sci 1982; 9:89.

291. Balldin J, Alling C, Gottfries CG, et al. Changes in dopamine receptor sensitivity in humans after heavy alcohol intake. Psychopharmacology 1985; 86:142.

292. Olivera AA, Kiefer MW, Manley NK. Tardive dyskinesia in psychiatric patients with substance use disorders. Am J Drug Alcohol Abuse 1990; 16:57.

293. Drake ME. Recurrent spontaneous myoclonus in alcohol withdrawal. South Med J 1983; 76:1040.

294. George DT, Nutt DJ, Dwyer BA, Linnoila M. Alcoholism and panic disorder: is the comorbidity more than coincidence? Acta Psychiatr Scand 1990; 81:97.

295. Heckmatt J, Shaikh AA, Swash M, Scott DF. Seizure induction by alcohol in patients with epilepsy: experience in two hospital clinics. J R Soc Med 1990; 83:6.

296. Chan AWK. Alcoholism and epilepsy. Epilepsia 1985; 26:223.

297. Simon RP. Alcohol and seizures. N Engl J Med 1988; 319:715.

298. Hoppener RJ, Kuyer A, van der Lugt PJM. Epilepsy and alcohol: the influence of social alcohol intake on seizures and treatment in epilepsy. Epilepsia 1983; 24:459.

299. Earnest MP. Seizures. In: Brust JCM, ed. Neurologic Complications of Drug and Alcohol Abuse. Neurol Clin 1993; 11:563.

300. Victor M, Brausch CC. The role of abstinence in the genesis of alcoholic epilepsy. Epilepsia 1967; 8:1.

301. Earnest MP, Feldman H, Marx JA, et al. Alcohol-related first seizures: the role of abstinence. Neurology 1989; 39 (Suppl):147.

302. Earnest MP, Yarnell PR. Seizure admissions to a city hospital: the role of alcohol. Epilepsia 1976; 17:387.

303. Pilke A, Partinen M, Kovanen J. Status epilepticus and alcohol abuse: analysis of 82 status epilepticus admissions. Acta Neurol Scand 1984; 70:443.

304. Lowenstein DH, Alldredge BK. Status epilepticus at an urban public hospital in the 1980s. Neurology 1993; 43:483.

305. Whitfield CL, Thompson G, Lamb A, et al. Detoxification of 1024 alcoholic patients without psychoactive drugs. JAMA 1978; 239:1409.

306. Ng SKC, Hauser WA, Brust JCM, Susser M. Alcohol consumption and withdrawal in new-onset seizures. N Engl J Med 1988; 319:666.

307. Ng SKC, Hauser WA, Brust JCM, Susser M. Alcohol consumption and withdrawal in new onset seizures. N Engl J Med 1989; 320:597.

308. Goldstein DB. The alcohol withdrawal syndrome. A view from the laboratory. Rec Dev Alcohol 1986; 4:213.

309. Hauser WA, Ng SKC, Brust JCM. Alcohol, seizures, and epilepsy. Epilepsia 1988; 29 (Suppl 2):S66.

310. Hillbom ME. Occurrence of cerebral seizures provoked by alcohol abuse. Epilepsia 1980; 21:459.

311. Gonzalez LP, Czachura JF, Brewer KW. Spontaneous versus elicited seizures following ethanol withdrawal: differential time course. Alcohol 1989; 6:481.

312. Faingold CL, N'Govemo P, Riaz A. Ethanol and neurotransmitter interactions–from molecular to integrative effects. Prog Neurobiol 1998; 55:509.

313. Leone M, Bottacchi E, Morgando E, et al. Alcohol use is a risk factor for a first generalized tonic-clonic seizure. Neurology 1997; 48:614.

314. Leone M, Tononi C, Bogliun G, et al. Chronic alcohol use and first symptomatic epileptic seizures. J Neurol Neurosurg Psychiatry 2002; 73:495.

315. Gorelick DA, Wilkins JN. Special aspects of human alcohol withdrawal. Rec Dev Alcohol 1986; 4:283.

316. Chu N-S. Periodic lateralized epileptiform discharges with pre-existing focal brain lesion. Role of alcohol withdrawal and anoxic encephalopathy. Arch Neurol 1980; 37:551.

317. Maier DM, Pohorecky LA. The effect of repeated withdrawal episodes on subsequent withdrawal severity in ethanol treated rats. Drug Alcohol Depend 1989; 23:103.

318. Brown ME, Anton RF, Malcolm R, Ballenger JC. Alcohol detoxification and withdrawal seizures: clinical support for a kindling hypothesis. Biol Psychiatry 1988; 23:507.

319. Lechtenberg R, Worner TM. Seizure risk with recurrent alcohol detoxification. Arch Neurol 1990; 47:535.

320. Feussner JR, Linfors EW, Blessing CL, Starmer CF. Computed tomography brain scanning in alcohol withdrawal seizures. Ann Intern Med 1981; 94:519.

321. Vossler DG, Browne TR. Rarity of EEG photoparoxysmal and photomyogenic responses following treated alcohol-related seizures. Neurology 1990; 40:723.

322. Fisch BJ, Hauser WA, Brust JCM, et al. The EEG response to diffuse and patterned photic stimulation during acute untreated alcohol withdrawal. Neurology 1989; 39:434.

323. Tavel ME, Davidson W, Baterton TD. A critical analysis of mortality associated with delirium tremens. Am J Med 1961; 242:18.

324. Thompson WL. Management of alcohol withdrawal syndromes. Arch Intern Med 1978; 138:278.

325. Liskow BI, Rinck C, Campbell J, DeSouza C. Alcohol withdrawal in the elderly. J Stud Alcohol 1989; 50:414.

326. Miller FT. Protracted alcohol withdrawal delirium. J Subst Abuse Treat 1994; 11:127.

327. Hersh D, Kranzler HR, Meyer RE. Persistent delirium following cessation of heavy alcohol consumption: diagnostic and treatment implications. Am J Psychiatry 1997; 154:846.

328. Williams D, Lewis J, McBride A. A comparison of rating scales for the alcohol withdrawal syndrome. Alcohol 2001; 36:104.

329. Ballenger JC, Post RM. Kindling as a model for alcohol withdrawal syndromes. Br J Psychiatry 1978; 133:1.

330. Hundt W, Zimmermann V, Pottig M, et al. The combined dexamethasone-suppression/CRH-stimulation test in alcoholics during and after acute withdrawal. Alcohol Clin Exp Res 2001; 25:687.

331. Service RF. Probing alcoholism's "dark side." Science 1999; 285:1473.

332. Kovacs GL. The role of atrial natriuretic peptide in alcohol withdrawal: a peripheral indicator and central modulator? Eur J Pharmacol 2000; 405:103.

333. Okubo T, Harada S. Polymorphism of the neuropeptide Y gene: an association study with alcohol withdrawal. Alcohol Clin Exp Res 2001; 25 (Suppl 6):59S.

334. Adinoff B. The alcohol withdrawal syndrome: neurobiology of treatment and toxicity. Am J Addict 1994; 3:277.

335. Grant KA, Valverius P, Hudspith M, Tabakoff B. Ethanol withdrawal seizures and the NMDA receptor complex. Eur J Pharmacol 1990; 176:289.

336. Becker HC, Hale RL. Repeated episodes of ethanol withdrawal potentiate the severity of subsequent withdrawal seizures: an animal model of alcohol withdrawal "kindling." Alcohol Clin Exp Res 1993; 17:94.

337. Warner TM. Relative kindling effect of readmissions in alcoholics. Alcohol Alcohol 1996; 31:375.

338. Ulrichsen J, Ebert B, Haughbol S, et al. Serotonin 1A receptor autoradiography during alcohol withdrawal kindling. Psychopharmacology 1997; 132:19.

339. Sullivan EV, Lim KO, Pfefferbaum A, et al. Relationship between AW seizures and temporal lobe white matter. Alcohol Clin Exp Res 1996; 2:348.

340. Bartolomei F, Barrie M, Gastaut JL, Sucket L. Alcoholic epilepsy: a unified and dynamic classification. Eur Neurol 1997; 37:13.

341. Moskowitz G, Chalmers TC, Sacks HS, et al. Deficiencies of clinical trials of alcohol withdrawal. Alcoholism 1983; 7:42.

342. Naranjo CA, Sellers EM. Clinical assessment and pharmacotherapy of the alcohol withdrawal syndrome. Rec Dev Alcohol 1986; 4:265.

343. Whitfield EL, Thompson G, Lamb A, et al. Detoxification of 1024 alcoholic patients without psychoactive drugs. JAMA 1978; 293:1409.

344. Devenyi P, Harrison ML. Prevention of alcohol withdrawal seizures with oral diazepam loading. Can Med Assoc J 1985; 132:798.

345. Guthrie SK. The treatment of alcohol withdrawal. Pharmacotherapy 1989; 9:131.

346. Romach MK, Sellers EM. Management of the alcohol withdrawal syndrome. Annu Rev Med 1991; 42:323.

347. Hall W, Zador D. The alcohol withdrawal syndrome. Lancet 1997; 349:1897.

348. Shaw GK. Detoxification: the use of benzodiazepines. Alcohol Alcohol 1995; 30:765.

349. Bird RD, Makela EH. Alcohol withdrawal: what is the benzodiazepine of choice? Ann Pharmacother 1994; 28:67.

350. Hamilton RJ. Substance withdrawal. In: Goldfrank LR, Flomenbaum NE, Lewin NA, et al, eds. Goldfrank's Toxicologic Emergencies, 6th edition. Stamford, CT: Appleton & Lange, 1998; 1127.

351. Ahmed S, Chadwick D, Walker RJ. The management of alcohol-related seizures: an overview. Hosp Med 2000; 61:793.

352. Saitz R, O'Malley SS. Pharmacotherapies for alcohol abuse. Withdrawal and treatment. Med Clin North Am 1997; 81:881.

353. Saitz R, Mayo-Smith MF, Roberts MS, et al. Individualized treatment for alcohol withdrawal: a randomized double-blind controlled trial. JAMA 1994; 272: 519-523.

354. Jaeger TM, Lohr RH, Pankratz VS. Symptom-triggered therapy for alcohol withdrawal syndrome in medical patients. Mayo Clin Proc 2001; 76:695.

355. Hayashida M, Alterman AI, McLellan AT, et al. Comparative effectiveness and costs of inpatient and outpatient detoxification of patients with mild-to-moderate alcohol withdrawal syndrome. N Engl J Med 1989; 320:358.

356. Goldbert TM, Sanz CJ, Rose HE, et al. Comparative evaluation of treatments of alcohol withdrawal syndromes. JAMA 1967; 201:99.

357. Kaim SC, Kett CJ, Rothfeld B. Treatment of the acute alcohol withdrawal state: a comparison of four drugs. Am J Psychiatry 1969; 125:1640.

358. Kaim SC, Klett CJ. Treatment of delirium tremens: a comparison of four drugs. Q J Stud Alcohol 1972; 33:1065.

359. Linnoila M, Mefford I, Nutt D, Adinoff B. Alcohol withdrawal and noradrenergic function. Ann Intern Med 1987; 107:875.

360. Zilm DH, Sellers EM, MacLeod SM, et al. Propranolol effect on tremor in alcohol withdrawal. Ann Intern Med 1975; 83:234.

361. Zilm DH, Jacob MS, MacLeod SM, et al. Propranolol and chlordiazepoxide effects on cardiac arrhythmias during alcohol withdrawal. Alcoholism Clin Exp Res 1980; 4:400.

362. Jacob MS, Zilm DH, MacLeod SM, et al. Propranolol-associated confused states during alcohol withdrawal. J Clin Psychopharmacol 1983; 3:185.

363. Wilkins AJ, Jenkins WJ, Steiner JA. Efficacy of clonidine in treatment of alcohol withdrawal state. Psychopharmacology 1983; 81:78.

364. Kraus ML, Gottlieb LD, Horwitz RI, Anscher M. Randomized clinical trial of atenolol in patients with alcohol withdrawal. N Engl J Med 1985; 313:905.

365. Horwitz RI, Gottlieb LD, Kraus ML. The efficacy of atenolol in the outpatient management of the alcohol withdrawal syndrome. Results of a randomized clinical trial. Arch Intern Med 1989; 149:1089.

366. Lerner WD, Fallon HJ. The alcohol withdrawal syndrome. N Engl J Med 1985; 313:951.

367. Cushman P, Sowers JP. Alcohol withdrawal syndrome: clinical and hormonal responses to alpha-2-adrenergic agonist treatment. Alcoholism 1989; 13:361.

368. Cushman P, Forbes R, Lerner W, Stewart M. Alcohol withdrawal syndromes: clinical management with lofexidine. Alcoholism 1985; 9:103.

369. Robinson BJ, Robinson GM, Maling TJ, Johnson RH. Is clonidine useful in the treatment of alcohol withdrawal? Alcoholism 1989; 13:95.

370. Malcolm R, Myrick H, Brady KT, Ballinger JC. Update on anticonvulsants for the treatment of alcohol withdrawal. Am J Addict 2001; 10 (Suppl):16.

371. Bjorkqvist SE, Isohanni M, Makela P, et al. Ambulant treatment of alcohol withdrawal symptoms with carbamazepine: a formal multicentre double-blind comparison with placebo. Acta Psychiatr Scand 1976; 53:333.

372. Kosten TR, O'Connor PG. Management of drug and alcohol withdrawal. N Engl J Med 2003; 348:1786.

373. Greenburg DA, Carpenter FL, Messing RO. Ethanol-induced component of 45Ca^{2+} uptake in PC 12 cells is sensitive to Ca^{2+} channel modulating drugs. Brain Res 1987; 410:143.

374. Little HJ, Dolin SJ, Halsley MJ. Calcium channel antagonists decrease the ethanol withdrawal syndrome. Life Sci 1986; 39:2059.

375. Koppi S, Eberhardt G, Haller R, Koig P. Calcium channel-blocking agent in the treatment of acute alcohol withdrawal-caroverine versus meprobamate in a randomized double-blind study. Neuropsychobiology 1987; 17:49.

376. Adams ML, Cicero TJ. Alcohol intoxication and withdrawal: the role of nitric oxide. Alcohol 1998; 16:153.

377. Lichtigfeld FJ, Gillman MA. Role of dopamine mesolimbic system in opioid action of psychotropic analgesic nitrous oxide (PAN) in alcohol and drug withdrawal. Clin Neuropharmacol 1996; 15:297.

378. Fink M. Delirium following cessation of alcohol consumption. Am J Psychiatry 1998; 155:1638.

379. Alldredge BK, Lowenstein DH, Simon RP. A placebo-controlled trial of intravenous diphenylhydantoin for the short-term treatment of alcohol withdrawal seizures. Am J Med 1989; 87:645.

380. Rathlev NK, D'Onofrio G, Fish SS, et al. The lack of efficacy of phenytoin in the prevention of recurrent alcohol-related seizures. Ann Emerg Med 1994; 23:513.

381. Stornebring B. Treatment of alcohol withdrawal seizures with carbamazepine and valproate. In: Porter RJ, Mattson RH, Cramer JA, et al, eds. Alcohol and Seizures. Basic Mechanisms and Clinical Concepts. Philadelphia: FA Davis, 1990; 315.

382. D'Onofrio G, Rathlev NK, Ulrich AS, et al. Lorazepam for the prevention of recurrent seizures related to alcohol. N Engl J Med 1999; 340:915.

383. Victor M. The role of hypomagnesemia and respiratory alkalosis in the genesis of alcohol-withdrawal symptoms. Ann N Y Acad Sci 1973; 215:235.

384. Flink EB. Magnesium deficiency in alcoholism. Alcoholism 1986; 10:590.

385. Meyer JG, Urban K. Electrolyte changes and acid–base balance after alcohol withdrawal, with special reference to rum fits and magnesium deficiency. J Neurol 1977; 215:135.

386. Wernicke C. Lehrbuch der Gehirnkrankheiten für Aertze und Studierende, Vol 2. Kassel: Theodore Fischer, 1881:229.

387. Victor M, Yakovlev PL. S.S. Korsakoff's psychic disorder in conjunction with peripheral neuritis. A translation of Korsakoff's original article with brief comments on the author and his contribution to clinical medicine. Neurology 1955; 5:394.

388. Victor M, Adams RD, Collins GH. The Wernicke–Korsakoff Syndrome, 2nd edition. Philadelphia: FA Davis, 1989.

389. Reuler JB, Girard DE, Cooney TG. Wernicke's encephalopathy. N Engl J Med 1985; 312:1035.

390. Torvik A, Lindboe CF, Rodge S. Brain lesions in alcoholics. A neuropathological study with clinical correlations. J Neurol Sci 1982; 56:233.

391. Wallis WE, Willoughby E, Baker P. Coma in the Wernicke–Korsakoff syndrome. Lancet 1978; II:400.

392. Harper C. The incidence of Wernicke's encephalopathy in Australia–a neuropathological study of 131 cases. J Neurol Neurosurg Psychiatry 1983; 46:593.

393. Caine D, Halliday GM, Kril JJ, Harper CG. Operational criteria for the classification of chronic alcoholics: identification of Wernicke's encephalopathy. J Neurol Neurosurg Psychiatry 1997; 62:51.

394. Sharma S, Sumich PM, Francis IC, et al. Wernicke's encephalopathy presenting with upbeating nystagmus. J Clin Neurosci 2002; 9:476.

395. Keane JR. The pretectal syndrome. 206 patients. Neurology 1990; 40:684.

396. Luda E. Le signe du bobbing oculaire dans l'encephalopathie de Wernicke. Rev Otoneuroophtalmol 1980; 52:123.

397. Ghez C. Vestibular paresis: a clinical feature of Wernicke's disease. J Neurol Neurosurg Psychiatry 1969; 32:134.

398. Birchfield RL. Postural hypotension in Wernicke's disease. A manifestation of autonomic nervous system involvement. Am J Med 1964; 36:404.

399. Lipton JM, Payne H, Garza HR, Rosenberg RN. Thermolability in Wernicke's encephalopathy. Arch Neurol 1978; 35:750.

400. Blanc P, Henriette K, Boussuges A. Severe metabolic acidosis and heart failure due to thiamine deficiency. Nutrition 2001; 18:118.

401. Chadda K, Raynard B, Antoun S, et al. Acute lactic acidosis with Wernicke's encephalopathy due to acute thiamine deficiency. Intensive Care Med 2002; 28:1499.

402. Truedsson M, Ohlsson B, Sjoberg K. Wernicke's encephalopathy presenting with severe dysphagia: a case report. Alcohol Alcohol 2002; 37:295.

403. Shimojyo S, Scheinberg P, Reinmuth O. Cerebral blood flow and metabolism in the Wernicke–Korsakoff syndrome. J Clin Invest 1967; 46:849.

404. Mensing JW, Hoogland PH, Sloof JL. Computed tomography in the diagnosis of Wernicke's encephalopathy: a radiological-neuropathological correlation. Ann Neurol 1984; 16:363.

405. Jacobson RR, Lishman WA. Cortical and diencephalic lesions in Korsakoff's syndrome: a clinical and CT scan study. Psychol Med 1990; 20:63.

406. Charness ME, DeLaPaz RL. Mamillary body atrophy in Wernicke's encephalopathy: antemortem identification using magnetic resonance imaging. Ann Neurol 1987; 22:595.

407. Park SH, Na DL, Lee SB, Myung HJ. MRI findings in Wernicke's encephalopathy: in the acute phase and follow-up. Neurology 1992; 42 (Suppl 3):278.

408. Doherty MJ, Watson NF, Uchino K, et al. Diffusion abnormalities in patients with Wernicke encephalopathy. Neurology 2002; 58:655.

409. Weidauer S, Nichtweiss M, Lanfermann H, et al. Wernicke encephalopathy: MR findings and clinical presentation. Eur Radiol 2003; 13:1001.

410. Park SH, Kim M, Na DL, et al. Magnetic resonance reflects the pathological evolution of Wernicke encephalopathy. J Neuroimaging 2001; 11:406.

410a. Rugilo CA, Roca U, Zurr MC, et al. Diffusion abnormalities and Wernicke encephalopathy. Neurology 2003; 60:727.

410b. Kashihara K, Irisawa M. Diffusion-weighted magnetic imaging in a case of acute Wernicke's encephalopathy. J Neurol Neurosurg Psychiatry 2002; 73:181.

411. Bergui M, Bradac GB, Zhang J. Diffusion abnormalities and Wernicke encephalopathy. Neurology 2003; 60:727.

412. Chu K, Kang DW, Kim HJ, et al. Diffusion-weighted imaging abnormalities in Wernicke encephalopathy: reversible cytotoxic edema? Arch Neurol 2002; 59:123.

413. Kril JJ. The contribution of alcohol, thiamine deficiency and cirrhosis of the liver to cerebral cortical damage in alcoholics. Metab Brain Dis 1995; 10:9.

414. Kopelman MD. The Korsakoff syndrome. Br J Psychiatry 1995; 166:154.

415. Victor M, Talland G, Adams RD. Psychological studies of Korsakoff's psychosis. I. General intellectual functions. J Nerv Ment Dis 1959; 128:528.

416. Sanders HI, Warrington EK. Memory for remote events in amnestic patients. Brain 1971; 94:661.

417. Albert MS, Butters N, Levin J. Temporal gradients in the retrograde amnesia of patients with alcoholic Korsakoff's disease. Arch Neurol 1979; 36:211.

418. Sacks O. The Man Who Mistook His Wife for a Hat and Other Clinical Tales. New York: Summit Books, 1985; 22.

419. Kopelman MD, Corn TH. Cholinergic "blockade" as a model for cholinergic depletion. A comparison of the memory deficits with those of Alzheimer-type dementia and the alcoholic Korsakoff syndrome. Brain 1988; 111:1079.

420. Rosenblum WI, Feigen I. The hemorrhagic component of Wernicke's encephalopathy. Arch Neurol 1965; 13:627.

421. Pfister HW, Von Rosen F, Bise K. Severe intraventricular hemorrhage shown by computed tomography as an unusual manifestation of Wernicke's encephalopathy. J Neurol Neurosurg Psychiatry 1995; 59:555.

422. Torvik A, Lindboe CF, Rogde S. Brain lesions in alcoholics. A neuropathological study with clinical correlations. J Neurol Sci 1982; 56:233.

423. Krill JJ, Halliday GM, Cartwright H, Svoboda M. Neuronal changes in the cerebral cortex of chronic alcoholics. Alcohol Clin Exp Res 1994; 18:35.

424. Jernigan TL, Butters N, DiTriaglia G, et al. Reduced cerebral grey matter observed in alcoholics using magnetic resonance imaging. Alcohol Clin Exp Res 1991; 15:418.

425. Visser P, Krabbendam L, Verhey F, et al. Brain correlates of memory dysfunction in alcoholic Korsakoff's syndrome. J Neurol Neurosurg Psychiatry 1999; 67:774.

426. Sullivan EV, Marsh L. Hippocampal volume deficits Korsakoff syndrome. Neurology 2003; 61:1716.

427. Mayes A, Meudell PR, Mann D, et al. Location of lesions in Korsakoff's syndrome: neuropsychological and neuropathological data on two patients. Cortex 1988; 24:367.

428. Harding AJ, Wong A, Svoboda M, et al. Chronic alcohol consumption does not cause hippocampal neuron loss in humans. Hippocampus 1997; 7:78.

429. Harding A, Halliday G, Caine D, Kril J. Degeneration of anterior thalamic nuclei differentiates alcoholics with amnesia. Brain 2000; 123:141.

430. Aggleton JP, Saunders RC. The relationships between temporal lobe and diencephalic structures implicated in anterograde amnesia. Memory 1997; 5:49.

431. Witt ED. Neuroanatomical consequences of thiamine deficiency: a comparative analysis. Alcohol Alcoholism 1985; 20:201.

432. Cullen KM, Halliday GM. Mechanisms of cell death in cholinergic basal forebrain neurons in chronic alcoholics. Metab Brain Dis 1995; 10:81.

433. Kopelman MD. Remote and autobiographical memory, temporal context memory, and frontal atrophy in Korsakoff and Alzheimer patients. Neuropsychologia 1989; 27:437.

434. Kopelman MD. Frontal dysfunction and memory deficits in the alcoholic Korsakoff syndrome and Alzheimer-type dementia. Brain 1991; 114:117.

435. Becker JT, Furman JMR, Panisset M, Smith C. Characteristics of the memory loss of a patient with Wernicke–Korsakoff's syndrome without alcoholism. Neuropsychologia 1990; 28:171.

436. Swank RL, Prados M. Avian thiamine deficiency. II. Pathologic changes in the brain and cranial nerves (especially the vestibular) and their relation to the clinical behavior. Arch Neurol Psychiatry 1942; 47:97.

437. Butterworth RF. Pathophysiology of alcoholic brain damage: synergistic effects of ethanol, thiamine deficiency and alcoholic liver disease. Metab Brain Dis 1995; 10:1.

438. Hakim AM, Pappius HM. Sequence of metabolic, clinical, and histological events in experimental thiamine deficiency. Ann Neurol 1983; 13:365.

439. Hakim AM. The induction and reversibility of cerebral acidosis in thiamine deficiency. Ann Neurol 1984; 16:673.

440. Singleton CK, Martin PR. Molecular mechanisms of thiamine utilization. Curr Mol Med 2001; 1:197.

441. Fadda F, Rossetti ZL. Chronic ethanol consumption: from neuroadaptations to neurodegeneration. Prog Neurobiol 1998; 56:385.

442. Wood B, Currie J. Presentation of acute Wernicke's encephalopathy and treatment with thiamine. Metab Brain Dis 1995; 10:57.

443. Lavoie J, Butterworth RF. Reduced activities of thiamine-dependent enzymes in brains of alcoholics in the absence of Wernicke's encephalopathy. Alcohol Clin Exp Res 1995; 19:1073.

444. Langlais PJ. Pathogenesis of diencephalic lesions in an experimental model of Wernicke's encephalopathy. Metab Brain Dis 1995; 10:31.

445. Butterworth RF, Gaudreau C, Vincelette J, et al. Thiamine deficiency and Wernicke's encephalopathy in AIDS. Metab Brain Dis 1991; 6:207.

446. Homewood J, Bond NW. Thiamin deficiency and Korsakoff's syndrome: failure to find memory impairments following nonalcoholic Wernicke's encephalopathy. Alcohol 1999; 19:75.

447. Kril JJ, Homewood J. Neuronal changes in the cerebral cortex of the rat following alcohol treatment and thiamin deficiency. J Neuropathol Exp Neurol 1993; 52:586.

448. Phillips GB, Victor M, Adams RD, et al. A study of the nutritional defect in Wernicke's syndrome: the effect of a purified diet, thiamine, and other vitamins on the clinical manifestations. J Clin Invest 1952; 31:859.

449. Dreyfus PM, Victor M. Effects of thiamine deficiency on the central nervous system. Am J Clin Nutr 1961; 9:414.

450. Mesulam M-M, Van Hoesen GW, Butters N. Clinical manifestations of chronic thiamine deficiency in the rhesus monkey. Neurology 1977; 27:239.

451. Harper C, Fornes P, Duyckaerts C, et al. An international perspective on the prevalence of the Wernicke–Korsakoff syndrome. Metab Brain Dis 1995; 10:17.

452. Nixon PF. Biochemical aspects of the pathogenesis of the Wernicke–Korsakoff syndrome. Aust Drug Alcohol Rev 1988; 7:75.

453. Price J, Mitchell S, Wiltshire B, et al. A follow-up study of patients with alcohol-related brain damage in the community. Aust Drug Alcohol Rev 1988; 7:83.

454. Lofland HB, Goodman HO, Clarkson TB, et al. Enzyme studies in thiamine deficient pigeons. J Nutr 1963; 79:188.

455. Impeduglia G, Martin PR, Kwast M, et al. The influence of thiamine deficiency on the response to ethanol in two inbred rat strains. J Pharmacol Exp Ther 1987; 240:754.

456. Savage LM, Langlais PJ. Differential outcomes attenuate memory impairments on matching-to-position following pyrithiamine-induced thiamine deficiency in rats. Psychobiology 1995; 23:153.

457. Blass JP, Gibson GE. Abnormality of a thiamine-requiring enzyme in patients with Wernicke–Korsakoff syndrome. N Engl J Med 1977; 297:1367.

458. Mukherjee AB, Svononos S, Ghazanfari A, et al. Transketolase abnormality in cultured fibroblasts from familial chronic alcoholic men and their male offspring. J Clin Invest 1987; 79:1039.

459. Martin PR, McCool BA, Singleton CK. Molecular genetics of transketolase in the pathogenesis of the Wernicke–Korsakoff syndrome. Metab Brain Dis 1995; 10:45.

460. Robinson JK, Mair RG. MK-801 prevents brain lesions and delayed-nonmatching-to-sample deficits produced by pyrithiamine-induced encephalopathy in rats. Behav Neurosci 1992; 106:623.

461. Vogel S, Hakim AM. Effect of nimodipine on the regional cerebral acidosis accompanying thiamine deficiency in the rat. J Neurochem 1988; 51:1102.

462. Dyckner T, Ek B, Nyhlin H, Wester PO. Aggravation of thiamine deficiency by magnesium depletion. Acta Med Scand 1985; 218:129.

463. Langlais PJ, Savage LM. Thiamine deficiency in rats produces cognitive and memory deficits on spatial tasks that correlate with tissue loss in diencephalon, cortex and white matter. Behav Brain Res 1995; 68:75.

464. Rosenbaum M, Merritt HH. Korsakoff's syndrome. Clinical study of the alcoholic form, with special regard to prognosis. Arch Neurol Psychiatry 1939; 41:978.

465. Thompson A, Baker H, Leevy CM. Thiamine absorption in alcoholism. Am J Clin Nutrition 1968; 21:537.

466. Harper CG, Giles M, Finlay-Jones R. Clinical signs in the Wernicke–Korsakoff complex: a retrospective analysis of 131 cases diagnosed at necropsy. J Neurol Neurosurg Psychiatry 1986; 49:341.

467. Thompson A, Frank O, Baker H, et al. Thiamine propyl disulfide: absorption and utilization. Ann Intern Med 1971; 74:529.

468. Jeyasingham MD, Pratt OE, Burns A, et al. The activation of red blood cell transketolase in groups of patients especially at risk from thiamine deficiency. Psychol Med 1987; 17:311.

469. Ross J, Birmingham CL. Wernicke's encephalopathy. N Engl J Med 1985; 313:637.

470. Flink EB. Role of magnesium depletion in Wernicke–Korsakoff syndrome. N Engl J Med 1978; 298:743.

471. Ambrose ML, Bowdon SC, Whelen G. Thiamin treatment and working memory function of alcohol-dependent people: preliminary findings. Alcohol Clin Exp Res 2001; 25:112.

472. McEntee WJ, Mair RG. Memory improvement in Korsakoff's disease with fluvoxamine. Arch Gen Psychiatry 1990; 47:978.

473. Mair RG, McEntee WJ. Cognitive enhancement in Korsakoff's psychosis by clonidine: a comparison with L-DOPA and ephedrine. Psychopharmacology 1986; 88:374.

474. Martin PR, Ebert MH, Gordon EK, et al. Catecholamine metabolism during clonidine withdrawal. Psychopharmacology 1984; 84:58.

475. Centerwall BS, Criqui MH. Prevention of the Wernicke–Korsakoff syndrome: a cost-benefit analysis. N Engl J Med 1978; 299:285.

476. Romano J, Michael M, Merritt HH. Alcoholic cerebellar degeneration. Arch Neurol Psychiatry 1940; 44:1230.

477. Victor M, Adams RD, Mancall EL. A restricted form of cerebellar cortical degeneration occurring in alcoholic patients. Arch Neurol 1959; 71:579.

478. Phillips SC, Harper CG, Kril J. A quantitative histological study of the cerebellar vermis in alcoholic patients. Brain 1987; 110:301.

479. Hillbom M, Muuronen A, Holm L, Lindmarsh T. The clinical versus radiological diagnosis of alcoholic cerebellar degeneration. J Neurol Sci 1986; 73:45.

480. Dano P, Le Guyade J. Atrophie cérébrale et alcoholisme chronique. Rev Neurol 1988; 144:202.

481. Melgaard B, Ahlgren P. Ataxia and cerebellar atrophy in chronic alcoholics. J Neurol 1986; 233:13.

482. Gilman S, Adams K, Koeppe RA, et al. Cerebellar and frontal hypometabolism in alcoholic cerebellar degeneration studied with positron emission tomography. Ann Neurol 1990; 28:775.

483. Eidelberg E, Bond ML, Kelter A. Effects of alcohol on cerebellar and vestibular neurons. Arch Int Pharmacodyn Ther 1973; 185:583.

484. Northrup LR. Additive effects of ethanol and Purkinje cell loss in the production of ataxia in mice. Psychopharmacology 1976; 48:189.

485. Mancall EL, McEntee WJ. Alterations of the cerebellar cortex-nutritional encephalopathy. Neurology 1965; 15:303.

486. Shear PK, Sullivan EV, Lane B, Pfefferbaum A. Mammillary body and cerebellar shrinkage in chronic

alcoholics with and without amnesia. Alcohol Clin Exp Res 1996; 20:1489.

487. Karhunen PJ, Erkinjuntti T, Laippala P. Moderate alcohol consumption and loss of Purkinje cells. BMJ 1994; 308:1663.

488. Tavares MA, Paula-Barbosa MM, Gray EG. A morphometric Golgi analysis of the Purkinje cell dendritic tree after long-term alcohol consumption in the adult rat. J Neurocytol 1983; 12:939.

489. Phillips SC. Qualitative and quantitative changes of mouse cerebellar synapses after chronic alcohol consumption and withdrawal. Exp Neurol 1985; 88:748.

490. Pentney RJ, Quackenbush LJ, O'Neill M. Length changes in dendritic networks of cerebellar Purkinje cells of old rats after chronic ethanol treatment. Alcoholism 1989; 13:413.

491. Dlugos CA, Pentney RJ. Morphometric evidence that the total number of synapses on Purkinje neurons of old F344 rats is reduced after long-term ethanol treatment and restores to control levels after recovery. Alcohol Alcohol 1997; 32:161.

492. Pantazis NJ, Dohrman DP, Thomas JD, et al. NMDA prevents alcohol-induced neuronal cell death of cerebellar granule cells in culture. Alcohol Clin Exp Res 1995; 19:846.

493. Hoffman PC. Glutamate receptors in alcohol withdrawal-induced neurotoxicity. Metab Brain Dis 1995; 10:73.

494. Thornhill HL, Richter RW, Shelton MV, et al. Neuropathic arthropathy (Charcot forefeet) in alcoholics. Orthop Clin North Am 1973; 4:7.

495. Guiheneuc P, Bathien N. Two patterns of results in polyneuropathies investigated with the H-reflex. J Neurol Sci 1976; 30:83.

496. Lefebvre D'Amour M, Shahani BT, Young RR, et al. The importance of studying sural nerve conduction and late responses in the evaluation of alcoholic subjects. Neurology 1979; 29:1600.

497. Behse F, Buchthal F. Alcoholic neuropathy: clinical, electrophysiological, and biopsy findings. Ann Neurol 1977; 2:95.

498. Vallet JM, Hugon J, Tabaraud F, et al. Acute or subacute alcoholic polyradiculoneuropathy: clinical, electrophysical, and histological findings in nine cases. Neurology 1988; 38 (Suppl 1):222.

499. Tabaraud F, Vallat JM, Hugan J, et al. Acute or subacute alcoholic neuropathy mimicking Guillain-Barré syndrome. J Neurol Sci 1990; 97:195.

500. Wöhrle JC, Spengos K, Steinke W, et al. Alcohol-related acute axonal polyneuropathy: a differential diagnosis of Guillain-Barré syndrome. Arch Neurol 1998; 55:1329.

500a. Ishibashi S, Yokota T, Shiojiri T, et al. Reversible acute axonal polyneuropathy associated with Wernicke–Korsakoff syndrome: impaired physiological nerve conduction due to thiamine deficiency? J Neurol Neurosurg Psychiatry 2003; 74:674.

501. Novak DJ, Victor M. The vagus and sympathetic nerves in alcoholic polyneuropathy. Arch Neurol 1974; 30:273.

502. Winship DH, Caflisch CR, Zboralske FF, et al. Deterioration of esophageal peristalsis in patients with alcoholic neuropathy. Gastroenterology 1968; 55:173.

503. Low PA, Walsh JC, Huang CY, et al. The sympathetic nervous system in alcoholic neuropathy–a clinical and pathological study. Brain 1975; 98:357.

504. Villalta J, Estruch R, Antunes E, et al. Vagal neuropathy in chronic alcoholics: relation to ethanol consumption. Alcohol Alcoholism 1989; 24:421.

505. Myers W, Willis K, Reeves A. Absence of parasympathetic denervation of the iris in alcoholics. J Neurol Neurosurg Psychiatry 1979; 42:1018.

506. Johnson RH, Robinson BJ. Mortality in alcoholics with autonomic neuropathy. J Neurol Neurosurg Psychiatry 1988; 51:476.

506a. Koike H, Iijima M, Sugiura M, et al. Alcoholic neuropathy is clinicopathologically distinct from thiamine-deficiency neuropathy. Ann Neurol 2003; 54:19.

507. Tackmann W, Minkenberg R, Strenge H. Correlation of electro-physiological and quantitative histological findings in the sural nerve of man. Studies on alcoholic neuropathy. J Neurol 1977; 216:289.

508. Said G, Landrieu P. Etude quantitative des fibres nerveuses isolée dans les polynevrites alcooliques. J Neurol Sci 1978; 35:317.

509. Juntunen J, Teravainen H, Eriksson K, et al. Experimental alcoholic neuropathy in the rat: histological and electrophysiological study on the myoneural junctions and the peripheral nerves. Acta Neuropathol 1978; 41:131.

510. Koike H, Morik, Misu K, et al. Painful alcoholic polyneuropathy with predominant small-fiber loss and normal thiamine status. Neurology 2001; 56:1727.

511. Rossi MA, Zucoloto S. Effect of alcohol on ganglion cells in the superior cervical ganglion of young rats. Beitr Pathol 1976; 157:183.

512. Strauss MB. The etiology of "alcoholic" polyneuritis. Am J Med Sci 1935; 189:378.

513. Mayer RF. Peripheral nerve conduction in alcoholics. Studies of the effects of acute and chronic intoxication. Psychosom Med 1966, 28:475.

514. Swank RL. Avian thiamine deficiency: correlation of pathology, and clinical behavior. J Exp Med 1940; 71:683.

515. Dunn TB, Morris HP, Dubnik CS. Lesions of chronic thiamine deficiency in mice. J Natl Cancer Inst 1947; 8:139.

516. Berry C, Neumann C, Hinsey JC. Nerve regeneration in cats on vitamin B_1 deficient diets. J Neurophysiol 1945; 8:315.

517. Wintrobe MM, Follis RH, Humphreys S, et al. Absence of nerve degeneration in chronic thiamine deficiency in pigs. J Nutr 1944; 28:283.

518. Rinehart JF, Friedman M, Greenberg LD. Effect of experimental thiamine deficiency on the nervous system of the rhesus monkey. Arch Pathol 1949; 48:129.

519. Williams RD, Mason HL, Power MH, et al. Induced thiamine (vitamin B$_1$) deficiency in man. Arch Intern Med 1943; 71:38.

520. Swank RL, Adams RD. Pyridoxine and pantothenic acid deficiency in swine. J Neuropathol Exp Neurol 1948; 7:274.

521. Bean WB, Hodges RE, Daum KE. Pantothenic acid deficiency induced in human beings. J Clin Invest 1955; 34:1073.

522. Vilter RW, Mueller JF, Glazer HS, et al. Effect of vitamin B$_6$ deficiency induced by desoxypyridoxine in human beings. J Lab Clin Med 1953; 42:335.

523. Lane M, Alfrey CP, Mengel CE, et al. The rapid induction of human riboflavin deficiency with galactoflavin. J Clin Invest 1964; 43:357.

524. McLane JA. Decreased axonal transport in rat nerve following acute and chronic ethanol exposure. Alcohol 1987; 4:385.

525. Monforte R, Estruch R, Valls-Solé J, et al. Autonomic and peripheral neuropathies in chronic alcoholics: a dose-related toxic effect of ethanol. Arch Neurol 1995; 52:45.

526. Victor M. Tobacco–alcohol amblyopia. A critique of current concepts of this disorder, with special reference to the role of nutritional deficiency in its causation. Arch Ophthalmol 1963; 70:313.

527. Sivyer G. Evidence of limited repair of brain damage in a patient with alcohol–tobacco amblyopia. Med J Aust 1989; 151:541.

528. Victor M, Dreyfus PM. Tobacco–alcohol amblyopia. Further comments on its pathology. Arch Ophthalmol 1965; 74:649.

529. Kermode AG, Plant GT, Miller DH, et al. Tobacco–alcohol amblyopia: magnetic resonance imaging findings. J Neurol Neurosurg Psychiatry 1989; 52:1447.

530. Carroll FD. The etiology and treatment of tobacco–alcohol amblyopia. Am J Ophthalmol 1944; 27:713.

531. The Cuba Neuropathy Field Investigation Team. Epidemic optic neuropathy in Cuba: clinical characterization and risk factors. N Engl J Med 1995; 333:1176.

532. Kerrison JB, Newman NJ. Clinical spectrum of Leber's hereditary optic neuropathy. Clin Neurosci 1997; 4:295.

533. Shimozono M, Townsend JC, Ilsen PD, Bright DC. Acute vision loss resulting from complications of ethanol abuse. J Am Optom Assoc 1998; 69:293.

534. Vannuci H, Moreno FS. Interaction of niacin and zinc metabolism in patients with alcoholic pellagra. Am J Clin Nutr 1989; 50:364.

535. Serdaru M, Hausser-Hauw C, LaPlane D, et al. The clinical spectrum of alcoholic pellagra encephalopathy. Brain 1988; 111:829.

536. Hauw J-J, deBaecque C, Hausser-Hauw C, Serdaru M, Chromatolysis in alcoholic encephalopathies. Pellagra-like changes in 22 cases. Brain 1988; 111:843.

537. Kertesz SG. Pellagra in two homeless men. Mayo Clinic Proc 2001; 76:315.

538. Lindenbaum J. Metabolic effects of alcohol on the blood and bone marrow. In: Lieber CS, ed. Metabolic Aspects of Alcoholism. Baltimore: University Park Press, 1977:215.

539. Lindenbaum J, Lieber CS. Alcohol-induced malabsorption of vitamin B$_{12}$ in man. Nature 1969; 224:806.

540. New York City. Summary of Vital Statistics 1984. New York: Department of Health, Bureau of Health Statistics and Analysis.

541. Ramstedt M. Per capita alcohol consumption and liver mortality in 14 European countries. Addiction 2001; 96 (Suppl 1):S19.

542. Hagymasi K, Blazovics A, Lengyel G, et al. Oxidative damage in alcoholic liver disease. Eur J Gastroenterol Hepatol 2001; 13:49.

543. Lieber CS. Microsomal ethanol-oxidizing system (MEOS): the first 30 years (1968–1998)—a review. Alcohol Clin Exp Res 1999; 23:991.

544. McLain CJ, Barve S, Deaciuc I, et al. Cytokines in alcoholic liver disease. Semin Liver Dis 1999; 19:205.

545. Tilg H, Diehl AM. Cytokines in alcoholic and nonalcoholic steatohepatitis. N Engl J Med 2000; 343:1467.

546. Crabb DW. Pathogenesis of alcoholic liver disease: newer mechanisms of injury. Keio J Med 1999; 48:184.

547. Wu D, Cederbaum AI. Removal of glutathione produces apoptosis and necrosis in HepG2 cells overexpressing CYP2E1. Alcohol Clin Exp Res 2001; 25:619.

548. Harris DR, Gonin R, Alter HJ, et al The relationship of acute transfusion-associated hepatitis to the development of cirrhosis in the presence of alcohol abuse. Ann Intern Med 2001; 134:120.

549. Degos F. Hepatitis C and alcohol. J Hepatol 1999; 31 (Suppl 1):113.

550. Schiff ER. Hepatitis C and alcohol. Hepatology 1997; 26 (Suppl 1):39S.

551. Friedan TR, Ozick L, McCord C, et al. Chronic liver disease in Central Harlem: the role of alcohol and viral hepatitis. Hepatology 1999; 29:883.

552. Johnston SC, Pelletier LL. Enhanced hepatoxicity of acetaminophen in the alcoholic patient. Two case reports and a review of the literature. Medicine 1997; 76:185.

553. Sinclair J, Jeffrey E, Wrighton S, et al Alcohol-mediated increases in acetaminophen hepatoxicity: role of CYP2E and CYP3A. Biochem Pharmacol 1998; 55:1557.

554. Diehl AM. Alcoholic liver disease. Med Clin North Am 1989; 73: 815.

555. Day CP. Who gets alcoholic liver disease: nature or nurture? J R Coll Physicians Lond 2000; 34:557.

556. Pares A, Caballeria J, Bruguera M, et al. Histological course of alcoholic hepatitis. Influence of abstinence, sex, and extent of hepatic damage. J Hepatol 1986; 2:33.

557. Sorensen TIA, Orholm M, Bensten KD, et al. Prospective evaluation of alcohol abuse and alcoholic liver disease in men as predictors of development of cirrhosis. Lancet 1984; I:241.

558. Montiero E, Alves MP, Santos ML, et al. Histocompatibility antigens: markers of susceptibility to and protection from alcoholic liver disease in a Portuguese population. Hepatology 1988; 8:455.

559. Saunders JB, Davis M, Williams R. Do women develop alcoholic liver disease more readily than men? BMJ 1981; 282:1140.

560. Baraona E, Abittan CS, Dohman K, et al. Gender differences in pharmacokinetics of alcohol. Alcohol Clin Exp Res 2001; 25:502.

561. Adams RD, Foley JM. The neurological disorder associated with liver disease. Res Publ Assoc Res Nerv Ment Dis 1953; 32:198.

562. Gammal SH, Jones EA. Hepatic encephalopathy. Med Clin North Am 1989; 73:793.

563. Conomy JP, Swash M. Reversible decerebrate and decorticate postures in hepatic coma. N Engl J Med 1968; 278:876.

564. Rai G, Buxton-Thomas M, Scanlon M. Ocular bobbing in hepatic encephalopathy. Br J Clin Pract 1976; 30:202.

565. Cadranel J-F, Lebiez E, Di Martino V, et al. Focal neurological signs in hepatic encephalopathy in cirrhotic patients: an underestimated entity? Am J Gastroenterol 2001; 92:515.

566. Gomez F, Ruiz P, Schreiber AD. Impaired function of macrophage Fcγ receptors and bacterial infection in alcoholic cirrhosis. N Engl J Med 1994; 331:1122.

567. Riodan SM, Williams R: Treatment of hepatic encephalopathy. N Engl J Med 1997; 337:473.

568. Ong JP, Aggerwal A, Easley KA, et al. Correlation between ammonia levels and the severity of hepatic encephalopathy. Am J Med 2003; 114:188.

569. Kreis R, Farrow N, Ross BD. Diagnosis of hepatic encephalopathy by proton magnetic resonance spectroscopy. Lancet 1990; 336:635.

570. Yang S-S, Chu N-S, Liaw Y-F. Somatosensory evoked potentials in hepatic encephalopathy. Gastroenterology 1985; 89:625.

571. Leo MA, Lieber CS. Hepatic vitamin A depletion in alcoholic liver injury. N Engl J Med 1982; 307:597.

572. Traber PG. Hepatic encephalopathy. N Engl J Med 1986; 314:786.

573. Butterworth RF. Neurotransmitter dysfunction in hepatic encephalopathy: new approaches and new findings. Metab Brain Dis 2001; 16:55.

573a. Felipo V, Butterworth RF. Neurobiology of ammonia. Prog Neurobiol 2002; 67:259.

574. Raabe W, Onsted G. Portacaval shunting changes neuronal tolerance to ammonia. Ann Neurol 1980; 8:106.

575. Cole M, Rutherford RB, Smith FO. Experimental ammonia encephalopathy in the primate. Arch Neurol 1972; 26:130.

576. Gjedde A, Lockwood AH, Duffy TE, et al. Cerebral blood flow and metabolism in chronically hyperammonemic rats: effect of acute ammonia challenge. Ann Neurol 1978; 3:325.

577. Wang V, Saab S. Ammonia levels and the severity of hepatic encephalopathy. Am J Med 2003, 114:237.

578. Zieve L, Brunner G. Encephalopathy due to mercaptans and phenols. In: McCandless DW, ed. Cerebral Energy Metabolism and Metabolic Encephalopathy. New York: Plenum, 1985:179.

579. Duffy TE, Vergara F, Plum F. Alpha-ketoglutaramate in hepatic encephalopathy. Res Publ Assoc Res Nerv Ment Dis 1974; 53:39.

580. Martinez-Hernandez A, Bell KP, Norenberg MD. Glutamine synthetase: glial localization in brain. Science 1977; 195:1356.

580a. Jalan R, Shawcross D, Davies N. The molecular pathogenesis of hepatic encephalopathy. Int J Biochem Cell Biol 2003; 35:1175.

581. Warren KS, Schenker S. Effect of an inhibitor of glutamine synthesis (methionine sulfoximine) on ammonia toxicity and metabolism. J Lab Clin Med 1964; 64:442.

582. Lockwood AH, McCandless DW. Hepatic encephalopathy. N Engl J Med 1986; 314:785.

583. Fischer JE, Baldessarini RJ. Neurotransmitter metabolism in hepatic encephalopathy. N Engl J Med 1975; 293:1152.

584. James JH, Ziparo V, Jepsson B, et al. Hyperammonemia, plasma amino acid imbalance, and blood–brain amino acid transport: a unified theory of portal systemic encephalopathy. Lancet 1979; II:772.

585. Anon. False neurotransmitters and liver failure. Lancet 1982; I:86.

586. Freese A, Swartz KJ, During MJ, Martin JB. Kynurenine metabolites of tryptophan: implications for neurologic diseases. Neurology 1990; 40:691.

587. Moroni F, Lombardi G, Carla V, et al. Increase in the content of quinolinic acid in cerebrospinal fluid and frontal cortex of patients with hepatic failure. J Neurochem 1986; 47:1667.

588. Bucci L, Ioppolo A, Chiavarelli R, Biogotti A. The central nervous system toxicity of long-term oral administration of L-tryptophan to porto-caval shunted rats. Br J Exp Pathol 1982; 63:235.

589. Jones EA, Schafer DF. Hepatic encephalopathy: a neurochemical disorder. Prog Liver Dis 1986; 8:525.

590. Pappas SC. Increased gamma-aminobutyric acid (GABA) receptors in the brain precedes hepatic encephalopathy in fulminant hepatic failure. Hepatology 1984; 4:1051.

591. Ferenci P, Schafer DF, Kleinberger G, et al. Serum levels of gamma-aminobutyric acid-like activity in acute and chronic hepatocellular disease. Lancet 1983; II:811.

592. Tran VT, Snyder SH, Major LF, et al. GABA receptors are increased in the brains of alcoholics. Ann Neurol 1981; 9:289.

593. Bassett ML, Mullen KD, Skolnick P, et al. Amelioration of hepatic encephalopathy by pharmacologic antagonism of the GABA-A/benzodiazepine receptor complex in a rabbit model of fulminant hepatic failure. Gastroenterology 1987; 93:1069.

594. Cooper AJL, Ehrlich ME, Plum F. Hepatic encephalopathy: GABA or ammonia? Lancet 1984; II:158.

595. Jones EA, Skolnick P, Gammal SH, et al. The gamma-aminobutyric acid A (GABA-A) receptor complex and hepatic encephalopathy. Some recent advances. Ann Intern Med 1989; 110:532.

596. Basile AS, Jones EA, Skolnick P. The pathogenesis and treatment of hepatic encephalopathy: evidence for the involvement of benzodiazepine ligands. Pharmacol Rev 1991; 43:28.

597. Bosman DK, van den Buijs CA, de Haan JG, et al. The effects of benzodiazepine antagonists and partial inverse agonists on acute hepatic encephalopathy in the rat. Gastroenterology 1991; 101:772.

598. Mullen KD, Szauter KM, Kaminsky-Ross K. "Endogenous" benzodiazepine activity in body fluids of patients with hepatic encephalopathy. Lancet 1990; 336:81.

599. Basile AS, Hughes RD, Harrison PM, et al. Elevated brain concentrations of 1,4-benzodiazepines in fulminant hepatic failure. N Engl J Med 1991; 325:473.

600. Ferenci P, Grimm G. Benzodiazepine antagonist in the treatment of human hepatic encephalopathy. Adv Exp Med Biol 1990; 272:255.

601. Bakti G, Fisch HV, Karlaganis G, et al. Mechanism of the excessive sedative response of cirrhotics to benzodiazepines: model experiments with triazolam. Hepatology 1987; 7:629.

601a. Desjardins P, Butterworth RF. The "peripheral-type" benzodiazepine (omega 3) receptor in hyperammonemic disorders. Neurochem Int 2002; 41:109.

602. Hoyumpa AM, Desmond PV, Avant GR, et al. Hepatic encephalopathy. Gastroenterology 1979; 76:184.

603. Conn HO, Leevy CM, Vlahcevic ZR, et al. Comparison of lactulose and neomycin in the treatment of chronic portal-systemic encephalopathy. Gastroenterology 1977; 72:573.

604. Pirotte J, Guffens JM, Devos J. Comparative study of basal arterial ammonemia and of orally-induced hyperammonemia in chronic portal-systemic encephalopathy, treated with neomycin and lactulose. Digestion 1974; 10:435.

605. Michel H, Cauvet G, Grainer PM, et al. Treatment of cirrhotic hepatic encephalopathy by L-DOPA: a double-blind study of 58 patients. Digestion 1977; 15:232.

606. Ferenci P, Grimm G, Meryn S, et al. Successful long-term treatment of portal-systemic encephalopathy by the benzodiazepine antagonist flumazenil. Gastroenterology 1989; 96:240.

607. Jones EA, Skolnick P. Benzodiazepine receptor ligands and the syndrome of hepatic encephalopathy. Prog Liver Dis 1990; 9:345.

608. Gyr K, Meier R, Häussler J, et al. Evaluation of the efficacy and safety of flumazenil in the treatment of portal systemic encephalopathy: a double blind, randomized, placebo controlled multicenter study. Gut 1996; 39:319.

609. Barbaro G, DiLorenzo G, Soldini M, et al. Flumazenil for hepatic encephalopathy Grade III and IVa in patients with cirrhosis: an Italian multicenter double-blind, placebo-controlled, cross-over study. Hepatology 1998; 28:374.

610. Groeneweg M, Gyr K, Amrein R, et al. Effect of flumazenil on the electro-encephalogram of patients with portosystemic encephalopathy: results of a double-blind, randomized, placebo-controlled multicentre trial. Electroencephalogr Clin Neurophysiol 1996; 98:29.

610a. Als-Neilsen B, Kjaergard LL, Gluud. Benzodiazepine receptor antagonists for acute and chronic hepatic encephalopathy. Cochrane Database of Systematic Reviews (4):CD002798, 2001.

611. Warren SE, Mitas JA, Swerdlin A. Hypernatremia in hepatic failure. JAMA 1980; 243:1257.

612. Nelson DC, McGrew WRG, Hoyumpa AM. Hypernatremia and lactulose therapy. JAMA 1983; 249:1295.

613. Levin DM, Baker AL, Rochman H, et al. Nonalcoholic liver disease: overlooked causes of liver injury in patients with heavy alcohol consumption. Am J Med 1979; 66:429.

614. Reade AE, Sherlock S, Laidlaw J, et al. The neuropsychiatric syndromes associated with chronic liver disease and an extensive portal-systemic collateral circulation. Q J Med 1967; 36:135.

615. Gauthier G, Wildi E. L'encephalo-myelopathie portosystèmique. Rev Neurol 1975; 131:319.

616. Jog MS, Lang AE. Chronic acquired hepatocerebral degeneration: case reports and new insights. Mov Disord 1995; 10:714.

617. Ueki Y, Isozaki E, Miyazaki Y, et al. Clinical and neuroradiological improvement in chronic acquired hepatocerebral degeneration after branched-chain amino acid therapy. Acta Neurol Scand 2002; 106:113.

618. Layargues GP. Movement dysfunction and hepatic encephalopathy. Metab Brain Dis 2001; 16:27.

619. Lee J, Lacomis D, Domu S, et al. Acquired hepatocerebral degeneration: MR and pathologic findings. AJNR Am J Neuroradiol 1998; 19:485.

620. Victor M, Adams RD, Cole M. The acquired (non-Wilsonian) type of chronic hepatocerebral degeneration. Medicine 1965; 44:345.

621. Stracciari A, Guarino M, Pazzaglia P, et al. Acquired hepatocerebral degeneration: full recovery after liver transplantation. J Neurol Neurosurg Psychiatry 2001; 70:136.

622. Gitlin N, Lewis DC, Hinkley L. The diagnosis and prevalence of subclinical hepatic encephalopathy in apparently healthy, ambulant, non-shunted patients with cirrhosis. J Hepatol 1986; 3:75.

623. Powell EE, Pender MP, Chalk JB, et al. Improvement in chronic hepatocerebral degeneration following liver transplantation. Gastroenterology 1990; 98:1079.

624. Bunout D, Petermann M, Bravo M, et al. Glucose turnover rate and peripheral insulin sensitivity in alcoholic patients without liver damage. Ann Nutr Metab 1989; 33:31.

625. Swade TF, Emanuele NV. Alcohol and diabetes. Comp Ther 1997; 23:135.

626. Kallas P, Sellers EM. Blood glucose in intoxicated chronic alcoholics. Can Med Assoc J 1975; 112:590.

627. Malouf R, Brust JCM. Hypoglycemia: causes, neurological manifestations, and outcome. Ann Neurol 1985; 17:421.

628. Kalimo H, Olsson Y. Effects of severe hypoglycemia on the human brain: neuropathological case reports. Acta Neurol Scand 1980; 62:345.

629. Bale RN. Brain damage in diabetes mellitus. Br J Psychiatry 1973; 122:337.

630. Haumont D, Dorchy H, Pele S. EEG abnormalities in diabetic children: influence of hypoglycemia and vascular complications. Clin Pediatr 1979; 18:750.

631. O'Keefe SJD, Marks V. Lunchtime gin and tonic as a cause of reactive hypoglycemia. Lancet 1977; I:1286.

632. Shakespeare W. Macbeth, Act II, Scene 3.

633. Van Thiel DH, Gavaler JS. Hypothalamic-pituitary-gonadal function in liver disease with particular attention to the endocrine effects of chronic alcohol abuse. Prog Liver Dis 1986; 8:273.

634. Yamauchi M, Takeda K, Sakamoto K, et al. Association of polymorphism in the alcohol dehydrogenase 2 gene with alcohol-induced testicular atrophy. Alcohol Clin Exp Res 2001; 25 (Suppl 6):16S.

635. Mello NK, Mendelson JH, Teoh SK. Neuroendocrine consequences of alcohol abuse in women. Ann N Y Acad Sci 1981; 562:211.

636. Rettori V, McCann SM. The mechanism of action of alcohol to suppress gonadotropin secretion. Mol Psychiatry 1997; 2:350.

637. Eisenhoffer G, Johnson RH. Effect of ethanol ingestion on plasma vasopressin and water balance in humans. Am J Physiol 1982; 242:R522.

638. Rivier C, Bruhn T, Vale W. Effect of ethanol on the hypothalamic-pituitary-adrenal axis in the rat. Role of corticotropin-releasing factor (CRF). J Pharmacol Exp Ther 1984; 229:127.

639. Lamberts SWJ, Klijn JGM, deJong FH, et al. Hormone secretion in alcohol-induced pseudo-Cushing's syndrome. Differential diagnosis with Cushing's disease. JAMA 1979; 242:1640.

640. Willenbring ML, Morley JE, Niewoehner CB, et al. Adrenocortical hyperactivity in newly admitted alcoholics. Prevalence, course, and associated variables. Psychoneuroendocrinology 1984; 9:415.

641. Ogilvie K, Lee S, Weiss B, Rivier C. Mechanisms mediating the influence of alcohol on the hypothalamic-pituitary-adrenal axis responses to immune and nonimmune signals. Alcohol Clin Exp Res 1998; 22 (Suppl 5):243S.

642. Bjorneboe GE, Bjorneboe A, Johnson J, et al. Calcium status and calcium-regulating hormones in alcoholics. Alcoholism 1988; 12:229.

643. Spencer H, Rubio N, Rubio E, et al. Chronic alcoholism: frequently overlooked cause of osteoporosis in men. Am J Med 1986; 80:393.

644. Laitinen KK, Lamberg-Allardt C, Tunninen R, et al. Transient hypoparathyroidism during acute alcohol intoxication. N Engl J Med 1991; 324:721.

645. Moore JA, Kakihana R. Ethanol-induced hypothermia in mice: influence of genotype on the development of tolerance. Life Sci 1978; 23:2331.

646. Dinh TKH, Gailis L. Effect of body temperature on acute ethanol toxicity. Life Sci 1979; 25:547.

647. Brower KJ, Aldrich MS, Robinson EA, et al. Insomnia, self-medication, and relapse to alcoholism. Am J Psychiatry 2001; 158:399.

648. Castaneda R. Sussman N, Levy R, et al. A review of the effects of moderate alcohol intake on psychiatric and sleep disorders. Rec Dev Alcohol 1998; 14:197.

649. Osborn HH. Ethanol. In: Goldfrank LR, Flomenbaum NE, Lewin NA, et al, eds. Goldfrank's Toxicologic Emergencies, 6th edition. Stamford, CT: Appleton & Lange, 1998;1023.

650. Lein D, Mader TJ. Survival from profound alcohol-related lactic acidosis. J Emerg Med 1999; 17:841.

651. Lefevre A, Adler H, Lieber CS. Effect of ethanol on ketone metabolism. J Clin Invest 1970; 49:1775.

652. Vamvakas S, Teschner M, Bahner U, Heidland A. Alcohol abuse: potential role in electrolyte disturbances and kidney diseases. Clin Nephrol 1998; 49:205.

653. Sternbach GL. Infections in alcoholic patients. Emerg Med Clin North Am 1990; 8:793.

654. Cook RT. Alcohol abuse, alcoholism and damage to the immune system—a review. Alcohol Clin Exp Res 1998; 22:1927.

655. Anderson BR. Host factors causing increased susceptibility to infection in patients with Laennec's cirrhosis. Ann N Y Acad Sci 1975; 252:348.

656. Richter RW, Brust JCM. Pneumococcal meningitis at Harlem Hospital. N Y State J Med 1971; 71:2747.

657. Crane LR, Lerner AM. Non-traumatic gram-negative bacillary meningitis in the Detroit Medical Center, 1964–1974 (with special mention of cases due to *Escherichia coli*). Medicine 1978; 57:197.

658. Hudolin V. Tuberculosis and alcoholism. Ann N Y Acad Sci 1975; 252:353.

659. Spach DH, Kanter AS, Dougherty MJ, et al. Bartonella (*Rochalimaea*) *quintana* bacteremia in inner-city patients with chronic alcoholism. N Engl J Med 1995; 332:424.

660. Harnisch JP, Tronca E, Nolan CM, et al. Diphtheria among alcoholic urban adults. A decade of experience in Seattle. Ann Intern Med 1989; 111:71.

661. Kaslow RA, Blackwelder WC, Ostrow DG, et al. No evidence for a role of alcohol or other psychoactive drugs in accelerating immunodeficiency in HIV-1-positive individuals. A report from the multicenter AIDS Cohort Study. JAMA 1989; 261:3424.

662. McManus TJ, Weatherburn P. Alcohol, AIDS and immunity. Br Med Bull 1994; 50:115.

663. Dingle GA, Oei TP. Is alcohol a cofactor of HIV and AIDS? Evidence from immunological and behavioral studies. Psychol Bull 1997; 122:56.

664. Tabak C, Smit HA, Rasanen L, et al. Alcohol consumption in relation to 20-year COPD mortality and pulmonary function in middle-aged men from three European countries. Epidemiology 2001; 12:239.

665. Lieber CS. Gastric ethanol metabolism and gastritis: interactions with other drugs, *Helicobacter pylori*, and antibiotic therapy—a review. Alcohol Clin Exp Res 1997; 21:1360.

666. Garro AJ, Lieber CS. Alcohol and cancer. Annu Rev Pharmacol Toxicol 1990; 30:219.

667. McCoy GD, Napier K. Alcohol and tobacco consumption as risk factors for cancer. Alcohol Health Res World 1986; 10:28.

668. Rinborg V. Alcohol and the risk of cancer. Alcohol Clin Exp Res 1998; 22 (Suppl 7):323S.

669. Seitz HK, Poschl G, Simanowski VA. Alcohol and cancer. Rec Dev Alcohol 1998; 14:67.

670. Sellers TA, Kushi LH, Cerhan JR, et al. Dietary folate intake, alcohol, and risk of breast cancer in a prospective study of postmenopausal women. Epidemiology 2001; 12:420.

671. Yu H, Berkel J. Do insulin-like growth factors mediate the effect of alcohol on breast cancer risk? Med Hypotheses 1999; 52:491.

672. Dorgan JF, Baer DJ, Albert PS, et al. Serum hormones and the alcohol–breast cancer association in postmenopausal women. J Natl Cancer Inst 2001; 93:710.

673. Rudzinski M, Stankaitis JA. Recognizing the alcoholic patient. N Engl J Med 1989; 320:125.

674. Rivara FP, Koepsell TD, Jurkovich GJ, et al. The effects of alcohol abuse on readmission for trauma. JAMA 1993; 270:1962.

675. Luna GK, Maier RV, Swoder L, et al. The influence of ethanol intoxication on outcome of injured motorcyclists. J Trauma 1984; 24:695.

676. Fabbri A, Marchesini G, Morselli-Labate AM, et al. Blood alcohol concentration and management of road trauma patients in the emergency department. J Trauma Injury Infect Crit Care 2001; 50:521.

677. Epidemiology. In: Hurley J, Horowitz J, eds. Alcohol and Health. DHHS. New York: Hemisphere Publishing, 1987:1.

678. Brewer RD, Marries PD, Cole TB, et al. The risk of dying in alcohol-related automobile crashes among habitual drunk drivers. N Engl J Med 1994; 331:513.

679. Leads from the Morbidity and Mortality Weekly Report. JAMA 1994; 271:100.

680. Abel EL, Zeidenberg P. Age, alcohol and violent death: a postmortem study. J Stud Alcohol 1985; 46:228.

681. Modell JG, Mountz JM. Drinking and flying—the problem of alcohol use by pilots. N Engl J Med 1990; 323:455.

682. Anon. Drowning. MMWR 2001; 50:413.

683. Berglund M. Suicide in alcoholism. Arch Gen Psychiatry 1984; 41:888.

684. Combs-Orme T, Taylor JR, Scott EB, Holmes SJ. Violent deaths among alcoholics: a descriptive study. J Stud Alcohol 1983; 44:938.

685. Rosengren L, Persson L, Johansson B. Enhanced blood–brain barrier leakage to Evans blue-labeled albumin after air embolism in ethanol-intoxicated rats. Acta Neuropathol (Berlin) 1977; 38:149.

686. Flamm ES, Demopoulos HB, Seligman ML, et al. Ethanol potentiation of CNS trauma. J Neurosurg 1977; 46:328.

687. Halt PS, Swanson RA, Faden AI. Alcohol exacerbates behavioral and neurochemical effects of rat spinal cord trauma. Arch Neurol 1992; 49:1178.

688. Crews Ft, Steck JC, Chandler LJ, et al. Ethanol, stroke, brain damage, and excitotoxicity. Pharmacol Biochem Behav 1998; 59:981.

689. Turner RT. Skeletal response to alcohol. Alcohol Clin Exp Res 2000; 24:1693.

690. Kimble RB. Alcohol, cytokines, and estrogen in the control of bone remodeling. Alcohol Clin Exp Res 1997; 21:385.

691. Sampson HW. Alcohol, osteoporosis, and bone-regulating hormones. Alcohol Clin Exp Res 1997; 21:400.

692. Adams RD, Victor M, Mancall EL. Central pontine myelinolysis. A hitherto undescribed disease occurring in alcoholic and malnourished subjects. Arch Neurol Psychiatr 1959; 81:154.

693. Calakos N, Fischbein N, Baringer R, Jay C. Cortical MRI findings associated with rapid correction of hyponatremia. Neurology 2000; 55:1048.

694. Bourgouin PM, Chalk C, Richardson J, et al. Subcortical white matter lesions in osmotic demyelination syndrome. AJNR Am J Neuroradiol 1995; 16:1495.

695. Lebrun C, Thomas P, Chatel M, et al. Cortical sclerosis presenting with dementia as a sequel of rapid correction of hyponatremia. J Neurol Neurosurg Psychiatry 1999; 66:685.

696. Wright DG, Laureno R, Victor M. Pontine and extrapontine myelinolysis. Brain 1979; 102:361.

697. Seiser A, Schwartz S, Aichinger-Steiner MM, et al. Parkinsonism and dystonia in central pontine and extrapontine myelinolysis. J Neurol Neurosurg Psychiatry 1998; 65:119.

698. Cole M, Richardson EP, Segarra JM. Central pontine myelinolysis: further evidence relating the lesion to malnutrition. Neurology 1964; 14:165.

699. Valsamis MP, Peress NE, Wright LD. Central pontine myelinolysis in childhood. Arch Neurol 1971; 25:307.

700. Miller GM, Baker HL, Okasaki H, Whisnant JP. Central pontine myelinolysis and its imitators: MR findings. Radiology 1988; 168:795.

701. Bernsen HJ, Prick MJ. Improvement of central pontine myelinolysis as demonstrated by repeated magnetic resonance imaging in a patient without evidence of hyponatremia. Acta Neurol Belg 1999; 99:189.

702. Rajbhandari SM, Powell T, Davies-Jones GA, Ward JD. Central pontine myelinolysis and ataxia: an unusual manifestation of hypoglycemia. Diabet Med 1998; 15:259.

703. Mast H, Gordon PH, Mohr JP, Tatemichi TK. Central pontine myelinolysis: clinical syndrome with normal serum sodium. Eur J Med Res 1995; 1:168.

704. Norenberg MD, Papendick RE. Chronicity of hyponatremia as a factor in experimental myelinolysis. Ann Neurol 1984; 15:544.

705. Illowsky BP, Laureno R. Encephalopathy and myelinolysis after rapid correction of hyponatremia. Brain 1987; 110:855.

706. Estol CJ, Caplan LR. Reversible central pontine myelinolysis. Neurology 1990; 40 (Suppl 1):211.

707. Narins RG. Therapy of hyponatremia: does haste make waste? N Engl J Med 1986; 314:1573.

708. Ayus JC, Krothapalli RK, Arieff AI. Treatment of symptomatic hyponatremia and its relation to brain damage: a prospective study. N Engl J Med 1987; 317:1190.

709. Sterns RH. Severe symptomatic hyponatremia. Treatment and outcome: a study of 64 cases. Ann Intern Med 1987; 107:656.

710. Laureno R, Karp BI. Pontine and extrapontine myelinolysis following rapid correction of hyponatremia. Lancet 1988; I:1439.

711. Hed R, Larrson H, Fahlgren H. Acute myoglobinuria. Acta Med Scand 1955; 152:459.

712. Perkoff GI, Dioso MM, Bleisch V, et al. A spectrum of myopathy associated with alcoholism. I. Clinical and laboratory features. Ann Intern Med 1967; 67:481.

713. Haller RG, Knochel JP. Skeletal muscle disease in alcoholism. Med Clin North Am 1984; 68:91.

714. Urbano-Marquez A, Estruch R, Grau JM, et al. On alcoholic myopathy. Ann Neurol 1985; 17:418.

715. Diamond I. Alcoholic myopathy and cardiomyopathy. N Engl J Med 1989; 320:458.

716. Weber LD, Nashel DJ, Mellow MH. Pharyngeal dysphagia in alcoholic myopathy. Ann Intern Med 1981; 95:189.

717. Spector R, Choudhury A, Cancilla P, et al. Alcoholic myopathy. Diagnosis by alcohol challenge. JAMA 1979; 242:1648.

718. Rubenstein AE, Wainapel SF. Acute hypokalemic myopathy in alcoholism. Arch Neurol 1977; 34:553.

719. Estruch R, Sacanella E, Fernandez-Sola J, et al. Natural history of alcoholic myopathy: a 5 year study. Alcohol Clin Exp Res 1998; 22:2023.

720. Fernandez-Sola J, Grav Junyent JM, Urbana-Marquez A. Alcoholic myopathies. Curr Opin Neurol 1996; 9:400.

721. Urbano-Marquez A, Estruch R, Navarro-Lopez F, et al. The effects of alcoholism on skeletal and cardiac muscle. N Engl J Med 1989; 320:409.

722. Rubin E, Katz AM, Lieber CS, et al. Muscle damage produced by chronic alcohol consumption. Am J Pathol 1976; 83:499.

723. Rubin E. Alcoholic myopathy in heart and skeletal muscle. N Engl J Med 1979; 301:28.

724. Psuzkin S, Rubin E. Adenosine diphosphate effect on contractility of human actomyosin: inhibition by ethanol and acetaldehyde. Science 1975; 188:1319.

725. Louboutin JP, Nataf S, Jardel-Bousisiere J, Potiron-Josse B. Evidence for low production of lactate and pyruvate in alcoholic rhabdomyolysis. Muscle Nerve 1995; 13:784.

726. Bollaert PE, Robin-Lherbier B, Escayne JM, et al. Phosphorus nuclear magnetic resonance evidence of abnormal skeletal muscle metabolism in chronic alcoholics. Neurology 1989; 39:821.

727. Preedy VR, Patal VB, Reilly ME, et al. Oxidants, antioxidants and alcohol: implications for skeletal and cardiac muscle. Front Biosci 1999; 4:e58.

728. Ohno K, Tanaka M, Sahashi K, et al. Mitochondrial DNA deletions in inherited recurrent myogolobinuria. Ann Neurol 1991; 29:364.

729. Waldenstrom A. Alcohol and congestive heart failure. Alcohol Clin Exp Res 1998; 22 (Suppl 7):315S.

730. Peacock WF. Cardiac disease in the alcoholic patient. Emerg Med Clin North Am 1990; 8:775.

731. Preedy VR, Richardson PJ. Ethanol induced cardiovascular disease. Br Med Bull 1994; 50:152.

732. Rosenqvist M. Alcohol and cardiac arrhythmias, Alcohol Clin Exp Res 1998; 22 (Suppl 7):318S.

733. Regan TJ. Of beverages, cigarettes, and cardiac arrhythmias. N Engl J Med 1979; 301:1060.

734. Seneviratne BIB. Acute cardiomyopathy with rhabdomyolysis in chronic alcoholism. BMJ 1975; III: 378.

735. Lang RM, Borow KM, Neumann A, Feldman T. Adverse cardiac effects of acute alcohol ingestion in young adults. Ann Intern Med 1985; 103:742.

736. Abramson JL, Williams SA, Krumholz HM, Vaccarino V. Moderate alcohol consumption and risk of heart failure among older persons. JAMA 2001; 285: 1971.

737. Brion S. Marchiafava–Bignami syndrome. In: Vinken PJ, Bruyn GW, eds. Handbook of Clinical Neurology, Vol 28. Metabolic and Deficiency Diseases of the Nervous System, Part II. Amsterdam: North-Holland Publishing, 1976; 317.

738. Kohler CG, Ances BM, Coleman AR, et al. Marchiafava–Bignami disease: literature review and case report. Neuropsychiatr Neuropsychol Behav Neurol 2000; 13:67.

739. Marchiafava E, Bignami A. Sopra un alterzione del corpor calloso osservata in soggetti acoolisti. Riv Pat Nerv Ment 1903; 8:544.

740. Ironside R, Bosanquet FD, McMenemey WH. Central demyelination of the corpus callosum (Marchiafava-Bignami disease) with report of a second case in Great Britain. Brain 1961; 84:212.

741. Kosaka K, Aoki M, Kawashaki N, et al. A non-alcoholic Japanese patient with Wernicke's encephalopathy and Marchiafava-Bignami disease. Clin Neuropathol 1984; 3:231.

742. Leong ASY. Marchiafava-Bignami disease in a non-alcoholic Indian male. Pathology 1979; 11:241.

743. Lechevalier B, Andersson JC, Morin P. Hemispheric disconnection syndrome with a "crossed avoiding" reaction in a case of Marchiafava-Bignami disease. J Neurol Neurosurg Psychiatry 1977; 40:483.

744. Rosa A, Demiati M, Cartz L, et al. Marchiafava–Bignami disease, syndrome of interhemispheric disconnection, and right-handed agraphia in a left-hander. Arch Neurol 1991; 48:986.

745. Nicoli F, Vion-Dury J, Chave B, et al. Maladie de Marchiafava–Bignami: disconnexion interhémisphérique, syndrome de Balint, evolution spontanément favorable. Rev Neurol 1994; 150:157.

746. Leventhal CM, Baringer JR, Arnason BG, et al. A case of Marchiafava–Bignami disease with clinical recovery. Trans Am Neurol Assoc 1965; 90:87.

747. Helenius J, Tatlisumak T, Soinne L, et al. Marchiafava–Bignami disease: two cases with favorable outcome. Eur J Neurol 2001; 8:269.

748. Pasutharnchat N, Phanthumchinda K. Marchiafava–Bignami disease: a case report. J Med Assoc Thailand 2002; 86:742.

749. Baron R, Heuser K, Marioth G. Marchiafava–Bignami disease with recovery diagnosed by CT and MRI: demyelination affects several CNS structures. J Neurol 1989; 236:364.

750. Chang KH, Cha SH, Han MH, et al. Marchiafava–Bignami disease: serial changes in corpus callosum on MRI. Neuroradiology 1992; 34:480.

751. Yamashita K, Kobayashi S, Yamaguchi S, et al. Reversible carpus callosum lesions in a patient with Marchiafava–Bignami disease: serial changes on MRI. Eur Neurol 1997; 37:192.

752. Gass A, Birtsch C, Oster M, et al. Marchiafava–Bignami disease: reversibility of neuroimaging abnormality. J Comput Assist Tomogr 1998; 22:503.

753. Alla P, Carrere C, Dupont G, et al. Marchiafava disease: two cases with good prognosis. Presse Med 2000; 29:1170.

754. Moreaud O, Dufosse J, Pellat J. Flare-ups in Marchiafava–Bignami disease. Rev Neurol 1996: 152:560.

755. Yamamoto T, Ashikaga Y, Araki Y, et al. A case of Marchiafava–Bignami disease: MRI-findings on spin-echo and fluid-attenuated inversion recovery (FLAIR) images. Eur J Radiol 2000; 34:141.

756. Kamaki M, Kawamura M, Moriya H, et al. Callosal bleeding in a case of Marchiafava–Bignami disease. J Neurol Sci 1996; 136:86.

757. Hayashi T, Tanohata K, Kunimoto M, et al. Marchiafava–Bignami disease with resolving symmetrical putaminal lesion. J Neurol 2002; 249:227.

758. Naeije R, Franken L, Jacobivitz D, et al. Morel's laminar sclerosis. Eur Neurol 1978; 17:155.

759. Ghatak NR, Hadfield G, Rosenblum WI. Association of central pontine myelinolysis and Marchiafava–Bignami disease. Neurology 1978; 28:1295.

760. Levine S, Stypulkowski W. Experimental cyanide encephalopathy. Arch Pathol 1959; 67:306.

760a. Sage JI, VanUitert RL, Lepore FE. Alcoholic myelopathy without substantial liver disease. A syndrome of dorsal and lateral column dysfunction. Arch Neurol 1984; 41:999.

760b. Koller W, O'Hara R, Dorus W, et al. Tremor in chronic alcoholism. Neurology 1985; 35:1660.

760c. Aisen ML, Adelstein BD, Romero J, et al. Peripheral mechanical loading and the mechanism of the tremor of chronic alcoholism. Arch Neurol 1992; 49:740.

760d. Hernán MA, Chen H, Schwartzchild MA, et al. Alcohol consumption and the incidence of Parkinson's disease. Ann Neurol 2003; 54:170.

760e. Saunders-Pullman R, Shriberg J, Heiman G, et al. Myoclonus dystonia. Possible association with obsessive-compulsive disorder and alcohol dependence. Neurology 2002; 58:242.

760f. Gann H, Feige B, Fasihi S, et al. Periodic limb movements during sleep in alcohol dependent patients. Eur Arch Psychiatr Clin Neurosci 2002; 252:124.

760g. Warner GT, McAuley JH: Alcohol-induced paroxysmal nonkinesogenic dyskinesia after pallidal hypoxic insult. Mov Disord 2003; 18:455.

761. Svardsudd K. Moderate alcohol consumption and cardiovascular disease: is there evidence for a preventive effect? Alcohol Clin Exp Res 1998; 22 (Suppl 7):307S.

762. Goldberg IJ. To drink or not to drink? N Engl J Med 2003; 348:163.

763. Wannamethee SG, Shaper AG. Alcohol, coronary heart disease and stroke: an examination of the J-shaped curve. Neuroepidemiology 1998; 17:288.

764. Vogel G. Drinking studies lite? Science 1998; 279:991.

765. Hart CL, Smith GD, Hole DJ, Hawthorne VM. Alcohol consumption and mortality from all causes, coronary heart disease, and stroke: results from a prospective cohort study of Scottish men with 21 years of follow-up. BMJ 1999; 318:1725.

766. Sverdsudd K. Moderate alcohol consumption and cardiovascular disease: is there evidence for a preventive effect? Alcohol Clin Exp Res 1998; 22 (Suppl 7):307S.

767. Friedman HS. Cardiovascular effects of alcohol. Rec Dev Alcohol 1998; 14:135.

768. Figueredo VM. The effects of alcohol on the heart: detrimental or beneficial? Postgrad Med 1997; 101:171, 175.

769. Stix G. A votre santé. Should physicians tell some nondrinkers to start? Sci Am 2001; 285:24.

770. Camargo CA, Hennekens CH, Gaziano JM, et al. Prospective study of moderate alcohol consumption and mortality in U.S. male physicians. Arch Intern Med 1997; 159:79.

771. Goldberg DM, Soleas GJ, Levesque M. Moderate alcohol consumption: the gentle face of Janus. Clin Biochem 1999; 32:505.

772. Pearson TA. What to advise patients about drinking alcohol. The clinician's conundrum. JAMA 1994; 272:967.

773. Renaud S, Gueguen R. The French paradox wine drinking. Novartis Found Symp 1998; 216:208.

774. Brenner H, Rothenbacher D, Bode G, et al. Coronary heart disease risk reduction in a predominantly beer-drinking population. Epidemiology 2001; 12:390.

775. Gronbaek M, Becker U, Johanson D, et al. Type of alcohol consumed and mortality from all causes, coronary heart disease, and cancer. Ann Intern Med 2000; 133:411.

776. Mukamal KJ, Conigrave KM, Mittleman MA, et al. Roles of drinking pattern and type of alcohol consumed in coronary heart disease in men. N Engl J Med 2003; 348:109.

777. Mukamal KJ, Maclure M, Muller JE, et al. Prior alcohol consumption and mortality following acute myocardial infarction. JAMA 2001; 285:1965.

778. Caplan LR, Hier DB, DeCruz I. Cerebral embolism in the Michael Reese Stroke Registry. Stroke 1983; 14:530.

779. Hillbom M. Alcohol consumption and stroke: benefits and risks. Alcohol Clin Exp Res 1998; 22 (Suppl 7): 352S.

780. Hillbom M, Kaste M. Does ethanol intoxication promote brain infarction in young adults? Lancet 1978; II:1181.

781. Hillbom M, Kaste M. Ethanol intoxication: a risk factor for ischemic brain infarction in adolescents and young adults. Stroke 1981; 12:422.

782. Hillbom M, Kaste M. Alcohol intoxication: a risk factor for primary subarachnoid hemorrhage. Neurology 1982; 32:706.

783. Hillbom M, Kaste M. Ethanol intoxication: a risk factor for ischemic brain infarction. Stroke 1983; 14:694.

784. Syrjanen J, Valtonen VV, Ivananainen M, et al. Association between cerebral infarction and increased serum bacterial antibody levels in young adults. Acta Neurol Scand 1986; 73:273.

785. Hilton-Jones O, Warlow CP. The cause of stroke in the young. J Neurol 1985; 232:137.

786. Moorthy G, Price TR, Thurim S, et al. Relationship between recent alcohol intake and stroke type? The NINDS Stroke Data Bank. Stroke 1986; 17:141.

787. Gorelick PB, Rodin MB, Longenberg P, et al. Is acute alcohol ingestion a risk factor for ischemic stroke? Results of a controlled study in middle-aged and elderly stroke patients at three urban medical centers. Stroke 1987; 18:359.

788. Gorelick PB, Rodin MB, Langenberg P, et al. Weekly alcohol consumption, cigarette smoking, and the risk of ischemic stroke: results of a case–control study at urban medical centers in Chicago, Illinois. Neurology 1989; 39:339.

789. Haapaniemi H, Hillbom M, Jovela S. Weekend and holiday increase in the onset of ischemic stroke in young women. Stroke 1996; 27:1023.

790. Von Arbin M, Britton M, Du Faire U, Tissell A. Circulatory manifestations and risk factors in patients with acute cerebrovascular disease and in matched controls. Acta Med Scand 1985; 218:373.

791. Boysen G, Nyboe J, Appleyard M, et al. Stroke incidence and risk factors for stroke in Copenhagen, Denmark. Stroke 1988; 19:1345.

792. Taylor JR, Combs-Orme T. Alcohol and strokes in young adults. Am J Psychiatry 1985; 142:116.

793. Cullen K, Stenhouse NS, Wearne KL. Alcohol and mortality in the Busselton Study. Int J Epidemiol 1982; 11:67.

794. Stemmermann GN, Hayashi T, Resch JA, et al. Risk factors related to ischemic and hemorrhage cerebrovascular disease at autopsy: the Honolulu Heart Study. Stroke 1984; 15:23.

795. Gill JS, Zezulka AV, Shipley MJ, et al. Stroke and alcohol consumption. N Engl J Med 1986; 315:1041.

796. Gordon T, Doyle JT. Drinking and mortality: the Albany Study. Am J Epidemiol 1987; 125:263.

797. Semenciw RM, Morrison MI, Mao Y, et al. Major risk factors for cardiovascular disease mortality in adults: results from the Nutrition Canada Survey Study. Int J Epidemiol 1988; 17:317.

798. Herman B, Schmintz PIM, Leyten ACM, et al. Multivariate logistic analysis of risk factors for stroke in Tilborg, the Netherlands. Am J Epidemiol 1983; 118:514.

799. Khaw AL, Barrett-Conner E. Dietary potassium and stroke-associated mortality: a 12-year prospective study. N Engl J Med 1987; 316:235.

800. Paganini-Hill A, Ross RK, Henderson BE. Post-menopausal oestrogen treatment and stroke: a prospective study. N Engl J Med 1988; 297:519.

801. Oleckno WA. The risk of stroke in young adults: an analysis of the contribution of cigarette smoking and alcohol consumption. Public Health 1988; 102:5.

802. Klatsky AL, Friedman GD, Siegelaub AB. Alcohol and mortality: a ten-year Kaiser-Permanente experience. Ann Intern Med 1981; 95:139.

803. Lieber CS. To drink (moderately) or not to drink. N Engl J Med 1984; 310:846.

804. Henrich JB, Horwitz RI. Evidence against the association between alcohol use and ischemic stroke risk. Arch Intern Med 1989; 149:1413.

805. Editorial. Alcohol and hemorrhagic stroke. Lancet 1986; II:256.

806. Monforte R, Estruch R, Graus F, et al. High ethanol consumption as risk factor for intracerebral hemorrhage in young and middle-aged people. Stroke 1990; 21:1529.

807. Donahue RB, Abbott RD. Alcohol and hemorrhagic stroke. Lancet 1986; II:515.

808. Palomaki H, Kaste M. Does light to moderate consumption of alcohol protect against ischemic brain infarction? Stroke 1991; 22:2.

809. Ben-Shlomo Y, Markowe H, Shipley M, Marmot MG. Stroke risk from alcohol consumption using different control groups. Stroke 1992; 23:1093.

810. Korarevic DJ, Vodvodic N, Gordon T, et al. Drinking habits and death: the Yugoslavia Cardiovascular Disease Study. Int J Epidemiol 1983; 12:145.

811. Donahue RP, Abbott RD, Reed DM, Yano K. Alcohol and hemorrhagic stroke: the Honolulu Heart Study. JAMA 1986; 255:2311.

812. Kagan A, Popper JS, Rhoads GG, Yano K. Dietary and other risk factors for stroke in Hawaiian Japanese men. Stroke 1985; 16:390.

813. Tayeka Y, Popper JS, Shimizu Y, et al. Epidemiologic studies of coronary heart disease and stroke in Japanese men living in Japan, Hawaii, and California: incidence of stroke in Japan and Hawaii. Stroke 1984; 15:15.

814. Wolf PA, D'Agostino RB, Odell P, et al. Alcohol consumption as a risk factor for stroke: the Framingham Study. Ann Neurol 1988; 24:177.

815. Stamfer MJ, Coditz GA, Willett WC, et al. A prospective study of moderate alcohol consumption and the risk of coronary disease and stroke in women. N Engl J Med 1988; 319:267.

816. Bogousslavsky J, Van Melle G, Despland PA, Regli F. Alcohol consumption and carotid atherosclerosis in the Lausanne Stroke Registry. Stroke 1990; 21:715.

817. Ueda K, Hasuo Y, Kiyohara Y, et al. Hisayama: incidence, changing pattern during long-term follow-up, and related factors. Stroke 1988; 19:48.

818. Kono S, Ikeda M, Tokudome S, et al. Alcohol and mortality. A cohort study of male Japanese physicians. Int J Epidemiol 1986; 15:527.

819. Tanaka H, Ueda Y, Hayashi M, et al. Risk factors for cerebral hemorrhage and cerebral infarction in a Japanese rural community. Stroke 1992; 13:62.

820. Tanaka H, Hayashi M, Date C, et al. Epidemiologic studies of stroke in Shibata, a Japanese provincial city: preliminary report on risk factors for cerebral infarction. Stroke 1985; 16:773.

821. Iso H, Kitamara A, Shimamoto T, et al. Alcohol intake and the risk of cardiovascular disease in middle-aged Japanese men. Stroke 1995; 26:767.

822. Camargo CA. Moderate alcohol consumption and stroke. The epidemiologic evidence. Stroke 1989; 20:1611.

823. Jamrozik K, Broadhurst RJ, Anderson CS, Stewart-Wynne EG. The role of lifestyle factors in the etiology of stroke. A population-based case–control study in Perth, Western Australia. Stroke 1994; 25:51.

824. Shinton R, Sagar G, Beevers G. The relation of alcohol consumption to cardiovascular risk factors and stroke. The West Birmingham stroke project. J Neurol Neurosurg Psychiatry 1993; 56:458.

825. Beghi E, Bogliun G, Cesso P, et al. Stroke and alcohol intake in a hospital population. A case–control study. Stroke 1995; 26:1691.

826. Gronbaek M, Deis A, Sorensen TI, et al. Mortality associated with moderate intakes of wine, beer, or spirits. BMJ 1995; 310:1165.

827. Truelson T, Gronbaek M, Schnohr P, et al. Intake of beer, wine and spirits and risk of stroke. The Copenhagen City Heart Study. Stroke 1998; 29:2467.

828. Hillbom M, Numminen H, Juvela S. Recent heavy drinking of alcohol and embolic stroke. Stroke 1999; 30:2307.

829. Juvela S, Hillbom M, Palomäki H. Risk factors for spontaneous intracerebral hemorrhage. Stroke 1995; 26:1558.

830. Thrift AG, Donnan GA, McNeil JJ. Heavy drinking but not moderate or immediate drinking increases the risk of intracerebral hemorrhage. Epidemiology 1999; 10:307.

831. Longstreth WT, Nelson LM, Koepsell TD, et al. Cigarette smoking, alcohol use, and subarachnoid hemorrhage. Stroke 1992; 23:1242.

832. Teunissen LL, Rinkel GJ, Algra A, et al. Risk factors for subarachnoid hemorrhage: a systematic review. Stroke 1996; 27:544.

833. Klatsky AL, Armstrong MA, Friedman GD, et al. Alcohol drinking and the risk of hemorrhagic stroke. Neuroepidemiology 2002; 21:115.

834. Sacco RL, Elkind M, Baden-Albala B, et al. The protective effect of moderate alcohol consumption on ischemic stroke. JAMA 1999; 281:53.

835. Berger K, Ajani UA, Kase CS, et al. Light-to-moderate alcohol consumption and the risk of stroke among U.S. male physicians. N Engl J Med 1999; 341:1557.

836. Djoussé L, Ellison C, Beiser A, et al. Alcohol consumption and the risk of ischemic stroke. The Framingham Study. Stroke 2002; 33:907.

837. Dulli DA. Alcohol, ischemic stroke, and lessons from a negative study. Stroke 2002; 33:890.

838. Shaper AG, Phillips AN, Pocock SJ, et al. Risk factors for stroke in middle-aged British men. BMJ 1991; 302:1111.

839. Goldberg RJ, Burchfiel CM, Reed DM, et al. A prospective study of the health effects of alcohol consumption in middle-aged and elderly men: the Honolulu Heart Program. Circulation 1994; 89:651.

840. Hansagi H, Romelsjö A, Gerhardsson de Verfier M, et al. Alcohol consumption and stroke mortality: 20 year follow-up of 15,077 men and women. Stroke 1995; 26:1768.

841. Kiyohara Y, Kato I, Iwamoto H, et al. The impact of alcohol and hypertension on stroke incidence in a general Japanese population: the Hisayana Study. Stroke 1995; 26:368.

842. Palmer AJ, Fletcher AE, Bulpitt CJ, et al. Alcohol intake and cardiovascular mortality in hypertensive

patients: report from the Department of Health Hypertension Care Computing Project. J Hypertens 1995; 13:957.

843. Yuan JM, Ross RK, Gao YT, et al. Follow-up study of moderate alcohol intake and mortality among middle-aged men in Shanghai, China. BMJ 1997; 314:18.

844. Maskarinec G, Meng L, Kolonel L. Alcohol intake, body weight, and mortality in a multiethnic prospective cohort. Epidemiology 1998; 9:654.

845. Hart CL, Smith GD, Hole DJ, et al. Alcohol consumption and mortality from all causes, coronary heart disease, and stroke: results from a prospective cohort study of Scottish men with 71 years of follow-up. BMJ 1999; 318:1725.

846. Leppälä JM, Paunio M, Virtano J, et al. Alcohol consumption and stroke incidence in male smokers. Circulation 1999; 100:1209.

847. Romelsjö A, Leifman A. Association between alcohol consumption and mortality, myocardial infarction and stroke in 25 year follow-up of 49,618 young Swedish men. BMJ 1999; 319:821.

848. Gaziano JM, Gaziano TA, Glynn RJ, et al. Light-to-moderate alcohol consumption and mortality in the Physicians' Health Study enrollment cohort. J Am Coll Cardiol 2000; 35:96.

849. Jousilahti P, Rastenyte D, Tuomilehto J. Serum gamma-glutamyl transferase, self-reported alcohol drinking, and the risk of stroke. Stroke 2000; 31:1851.

850. Klatsky AL, Armstrong MA, Friedman GD. Alcohol use and subsequent cerebrovascular disease hospitalizations. Stroke 1989; 20:741.

851. Gill JS, Shipley MJ, Hornby RA, et al. A community case—control study of alcohol consumption in stroke. Int J Epidemiol 1988; 17:542.

852. Gill JS, Shipley MJ, Tsementzis SA, et al. Alcohol consumption: a risk factor for hemorrhagic and non-hemorrhagic stroke. Am J Med 1991; 90:489.

853. Palomäki H, Kaste M. Regular light-to-moderate intake of alcohol and the risk of ischemic stroke. Is there a beneficial effect? Stroke 1993; 24:1828.

854. Caicoya M, Rodriguez T, Corrales C, et al. Alcohol and stroke: a community case–control study in Asturias, Spain. J Clin Epidemiol 1999; 52:677.

855. Malarcher AM, Giles WH, Craft JB, et al. Alcohol intake, type of beverage, and the risk of cerebral infarction in young women. Stroke 2001; 32:77.

856. Zodpey SP, Tiwari RR, Kulkarni HR. Risk factors for hemorrhagic stroke: a case–control study. Public Health 2000; 114:177.

856a. Reynolds K, Lewis LB, Nolen JDL, et al. Alcohol consumption and risk of stroke. A meta-analysis. JAMA 2003; 289:579.

857. Palomaki H, Kaste M, Raininko R, et al. Risk factors for cervical atherosclerosis in patients with transient ischemic attack or minor ischemic stroke. Stroke 1993; 24:970.

858. Kiechl S, Willeit J, Rungger G, et al. Alcohol consumption and atherosclerosis: what is the relation: Prospective results from the Brunech Study. Stroke 1998; 29:900.

859. Bo P, Marchioni E, Bosone D, et al. Effects of moderate and high doses of alcohol on carotid atherogenesis. Eur Neurol 2001; 45:97.

860. Reed DM, Resch JA, Hayashi T, et al. A prospective study of cerebral artery atherosclerosis. Stroke 1988; 19:820.

861. Shintani S, Shiigai T, Arinami T. Silent lacunar infarction on magnetic resonance imaging (MRI): risk factors. J Neurol Sci 1998; 160:82.

862. Jorgensen HS, Nakagama H, Raaschou HO, Olsen TS. Leukoaraiosis in stroke patients. The Copenhagen Stroke Study. Stroke 1995; 26:588.

863. Yoshitake T, Kiyohara Y, Kato I, et al. Incidence and risk factors of vascular dementia and Alzheimer's disease in a defined elderly Japanese population: the Hisayama Study. Neurology 1995; 45:1161.

864. Mukamal KJ, Longstreth WT, Mittleman MA, et al. Alcohol consumption and subclinical findings on magnetic resonance imaging of the brain in older adults. The Cardiovascular Health Study. Stroke 2001; 32:1939.

865. Elias PK, Elias MF, D'Agostino RB, et al. Alcohol consumption and cognitive performance. Am J Epidemiol 1999; 150:580.

866. De Carli C, Miller BL, Swan GE, et al. Cerebrovascular and brain morphologic correlates of mild cognitive impairment in the National Heart, Lung, and Blood Institute Twin Study. Arch Neurol 2001; 58:643.

867. Herbert LE, Scherr PA, Beckett LA, et al. Relation of smoking and low-to-moderate alcohol consumption to change in cognitive function: a longitudinal study in a defined community of older persons. Am J Epidemiol 1993; 137:881.

868. Hendrie HC, Gao S, Hall KS, et al. The relationship between alcohol consumption, cognitive performance, and daily functioning in an urban sample of older black Americans. J Am Geriatr Soc 1996; 44:1158.

869. Dufouil C, Ducimetiere P, Alperovitch A. Sex differences in the association between alcohol consumption and cognitive performance: EVA Study Group. Am J Epidemiol 1997; 146:405.

870. Lemeshow S, Letenneur L, Dartigues JF, et al. Illustration of analysis taking into account complex survey considerations: the association between wine consumption and dementia in the PAQUID Study. Am J Epidemiol 1998; 148:298.

871. Ruitenberg A, van Swieten JC, Witteman JCM, et al. Alcohol consumption and the risk of dementia: the Rotterdam Study. Lancet 2002; 359:281.

872. Jousilahti P, Rastenyte D, Tuomilehto J. Serum gamma-glutamyl transferase, self-reported alcohol drinking, and risk of stroke. Stroke 2000; 31:1851.

873. Klatsky AL. Drink to your health? Sci Am 2003; 288:75.

874. Russel M, Cooper ML, Frone M, et al. Drinking patterns and blood pressure. Am J Epidemiol 1988; 128:917.

875. MacMahon SW. Alcohol consumption and hypertension. Hypertension 1987; 9:111.

876. Fuchs FD, Chambless LE, Whelton PK, et al. Alcohol consumption and the incidence of hypertension: The Atherosclerosis Risk in Communities Study. Hypertension 2001; 37:1242.

877. Cushman WC. Alcohol consumption and hypertension. J Clin Hypertens 2001; 3:166.

878. Okubo Y, Miyamoto T, Suwazano Y, et al. Alcohol consumption and blood pressure in Japanese men. Alcohol 2001; 23:149.

879. Brackett DJ, Gauvin DV, Lerner MR, et al. Dose-and time-dependent cardiovascular responses induced by ethanol. J Pharmacol Exp Ther 1994; 268:78.

880. Lip GY, Beevers DG. Alcohol, hypertension, coronary disease, and stroke. Clin Exp Pharmacol Physiol 1995; 22:189.

881. Tell GS, Rutan GH, Kronmal RA, et al. Correlates of blood pressure in community dwelling older adults. The Cardiovascular Health Study. Hypertension 1994; 23:59.

882. Gorelick PB. Alcohol and stroke. Stroke 1987; 18:268.

883. Gillman MW, Cook NR, Evans DA, et al. Relationship of alcohol intake with blood pressure in young adults. Hypertension 1995; 25:1106.

884. Randin DR, Vollenweider P, Tappy L, et al. Suppression of alcohol-induced hypertension by dexamethasone. N Engl J Med 1995; 332:1733.

885. Harper G, Casttenden CM, Potter JF. Factors affecting changes in blood pressure after acute stroke. Stroke 1994; 25:1726.

886. Keil U, Liese A, Filipiak B, et al. Alcohol, blood-pressure and hypertension. Novartis Found Symp 1998; 216:125.

887. Longstreth WT, Koepsell TD, Yerby MS, van Belle G. Risk factors for subarachnoid hemorrhage. Stroke 1985; 16:377.

888. Camargo CA, Williams PT, Vranizan KM, et al. The effect of moderate alcohol intake on serum apolipoproteins A-I and A-II: a controlled study. JAMA 1985; 253:2854.

889. Haskell WJ, Camargo C, Williams PT, et al. The effect of cessation and resumption of moderate alcohol intake on serum high-density lipoprotein subfractions. A controlled study. N Engl J Med 1984; 310:805.

890. van Tol A, Hendriks HD. Moderate alcohol consumption: effects on lipids and cardiovascular disease risk. Curr Opin Lipid 2001; 12:19.

891. Baraona E, Lieber CS. Alcohol and lipids. Rec Dev Alcohol 1998; 14:97.

892. Avogaro P, Cazzolato G, Belussi F, Bittolo Bon G. Altered apoprotein composition of HDL-2 and HDL-3 in chronic alcoholics. Artery 1982; 10:317.

893. Gorelick PB. The status of alcohol as a risk factor for stroke. Stroke 1989; 20:1607.

894. Corella D, Tucker K, Lahoz C, et al. Alcohol drinking determines the effect of the APOE locus on LDL-cholesterol concentrations in men. The Framingham Offspring Study. Am J Clin Nutr 2001; 73:736.

895. Nago N, Kayaba K, Hiraoka J, et al. Lipoprotein(a) levels in the Japanese population: influence of age and sex, and relation to atherosclerotic risk factors: the Jichi Medical School Cohort Study. Am J Epidemiol 1995; 141:815.

896. Hillbom M, Kaste M, Rasi V. Can ethanol intoxication affect hemocoagulation to increase the risk of brain infarction in young adults? Neurology 1983; 33:381.

897. Lee K, Neilsen JD, Zeeberg I, Gormasen J. Platelet aggregation and fibrinolytic activity in young alcoholics. Acta Neurol Scand 1980; 621:287.

898. Hillbom M, Kangasaho M, Kaste M, et al. Acute ethanol ingestion increases platelet reactivity. Is there a relationship to stroke? Stroke 1985; 16:19.

899. Numminen H, Syrjälä M, Benthin G, et al. The effect of acute ingestion of a large dose of alcohol on the hemostatic system and its circadian variation. Stroke 2000; 31:1269.

900. Lang WE. Ethyl alcohol enhances plasminogen activator secretion by endothelial cells. JAMA 1983; 250:772.

901. Jakubowski JA, Vailloncourt R, Deykin D. Interaction of ethanol, prostacyclin, and aspirin in determining human platelet reactivity in vitro. Arteriosclerosis 1988; 8:436.

902. Landolfi R, Steiner M. Ethanol raises prostacyclin in vivo and in vitro. Blood 1984; 64:679.

903. Fenn CG, Littleton JM. Inhibition of platelet aggregation by ethanol: the role of plasma and platelet membrane lipids. Br J Pharmacol 1981; 73:305P.

904. Haut MJ, Cowan DH. The effect of ethanol on hemostatic properties of human blood platelets. Am J Med 1974; 56:22.

905. Kangasaho M, Hillbom M, Kaste M, Vapaatolo H. Effects of ethanol intoxication and hangover on plasma levels of thromboxane B-2 formation by platelets in man. Thromb Haemost 1982; 48:232.

906. Mikhailidis DP, Barradas MA, Jeremy JY. The effect of ethanol on platelet function and vascular prostanoids. Alcohol 1990; 7:171.

907. Brust JCM. Stroke and substance abuse. In: Mohr JP, Choi D, Grotta J, Weir B, Wolf P, eds. Stroke: Pathophysiology and Management, 4th edition. New York: WB Saunders, 2004; in press.

908. Lacoste L, Hung J, Lam JY. Acute and delayed antithrombotic effects of alcohol in humans. Am J Cardiol 2001; 87:82.

909. Hendricks HF, van der Gaag MS. Alcohol, coagulation and fibrinolysis. Novartis Found Symp 1998; 26:111.

910. Torres Duarte AP, Gong QS, Young J, et al. Inhibition of platelet aggregation in whole blood by alcohol. Thromb Res 1995; 78:107.

911. DiMinno G, Mancini M. Drugs affecting plasma fibrinogen levels. Cardiovasc Drugs Ther 1992; 6:25.

912. Tsaji S, Kawano S, Michida T, et al. Ethanol stimulates immunoreactive endothelin-1 and -2 release from cultured human umbilical vein endothelial cells. Alcohol Clin Exp Res 1992; 16:347.

913. Ricker PM, Vaughan DE, Stamfer MJ, et al. Association of moderate alcohol consumption and plasma concentration of endogenous tissue-type plasminogen activator. JAMA 1994; 272:929.

914. Altura BM, Altura BT. Role of magnesium and calcium in alcohol-induced hypertension and strokes as probed by in vivo television microscopy, digital image microscopy, optical spectroscopy, ^{31}P-NMR spectroscopy and a unique magnesium ion-selective electrode. Alcohol Clin Exp Res 1994; 18:1057.

915. Fujii Y, Takeuchi S, Tanaka R, et al. Liver dysfunction in spontaneous intracerebral hemorrhage. Neurosurgery 1994; 35:392.

916. Haselager EM, Vreeken J. Rebound thrombocytosis after alcohol abuse: a possible factor in the pathogenesis of thromboembolic disease. Lancet 1977; I:774.

917. Hutton RA, Fink FR, Wilson DT, Margot DH. Platelet hyperaggregability during alcohol withdrawal. Clin Lab Haematol 1981; 3:223.

918. Ruf JC, Berger JL, Renaud S. Platelet rebound effect of alcohol withdrawal and wine drinking in rats. Relation to tannins and lipid peroxidation. Arterioscler Thromb Vasc Biol 1995; 15:140.

919. Neiman J, Rand ML, Jakowec DM, Packham MA. Platelet responses to platelet-activating factor are inhibited in alcoholics undergoing alcohol withdrawal. Thromb Res 1989; 56:399.

920. Delahousse B, Maillot F, Gabriel I, et al. Increased plasma fibrinolysis and tissue-type plasminogen activator/tissue-type plasminogen activator inhibitor ratios after ethanol withdrawal in chronic alcoholics. Blood Coagul Fibrinolysis 2001; 12:59.

921. Imhof A, Froehlich M, Brenner H, et al. Effect of ethanol consumption on systemic markers of inflammation. Lancet 2001; 357:763.

921a. Albert MA, Glynn RJ, Ridker PM. Alcohol consumption and plasma concentration of C-reactive protein. Circulation 2003; 107:443.

922. Service RF. Raising a glass to health. Science 1999; 285:2053.

923. McQueen JD, Sklar FK, Posey JB. Autoregulation of cerebral blood flow during alcohol infusion. J Stud Alcohol 1978; 39:1477.

924. Weiss MH, Craig JR. The influence of acute ethanol intoxication on intracranial physical dynamics. Bull Los Angeles Neurol Soc 1978; 43:1.

925. Persson LI, Rosengren LE, Johansson BB, Hansson HA. Blood brain barrier dysfunction to peroxidase after air embolism, aggravated by acute ethanol intoxication. J Neurol Sci 1979; 42:65.

926. Wilkins MR, Kendall MJ. Stroke affecting young men after alcoholic binges. BMJ 1985; 291:1342.

927. Berglund M. Cerebral blood flow in chronic alcoholics. Alcoholism Clin Exp Res 1981; 5:295.

928. Altura BM, Attura BT, Gebrewold A. Alcohol-induced spasms of cerebral blood vessels. Relations to cerebrovascular accidents and sudden death. Science 1983; 220:331.

929. Altura BM, Altura BT. Association of alcohol in brain injury, headaches, and stroke with brain tissue and serum levels of ionized magnesium: a review of recent findings and mechanisms of action. Alcohol 1999; 19:119.

930. Gordon EL, Nguyen TS, Ngai AC, Winn HR. Differential effects of alcohols on intracerebral arterioles. Ethanol alone causes vasoconstriction. J Cereb Blood Flow Metab 1995; 15:532.

931. Mayhan WG. Responses of cerebral arterioles during chronic ethanol exposure. Am J Physiol 1992; 262:H787.

932. Altura BM, Zhang A, Cheng TP, Altura BT. Ethanol promotes rapid depletion of intracellular free Mg in cerebral vascular smooth muscle cells: possible relation to alcohol-induced behavioral and stroke-like effects. Alcohol 1993; 10:563.

933. Altura BM, Gebrewold A, Altura BT, Gupta RK. Role of brain [Mg^{2+}] in alcohol-induced hemorrhagic stroke in a rat model: a ^{31}P-NMR in vivo study. Alcohol 1995; 12:131.

934. Crews FT, Steck JC, Chandler LJ, et al. Ethanol, stroke, brain damage, and excitotoxicity. Pharmacol Biochem Behav 1998; 59:981.

935. German JB, Walzam RL. The health benefits of wine. Annu Rev Nutr 2000; 20:561.

936. Malarcher AM, Giles WH, Croft JB, et al. Alcohol intake, type of beverage, and the risk of cerebral infarction in young women. Stroke 2001; 32:77.

937. Wollin SD, Jones PJ. Alcohol, red wine, and cardiovascular disease. J Nutr 2001; 131:1401.

938. Bell JR, Donovan JL, Wong R, et al. (+)-Catechin in human plasma after ingestion of a single serving of reconstituted red wine. Am J Clin Nutr 2000; 71:103.

939. Puddey IB, Croft KD. Alcohol, stroke and coronary heart disease. Are there anti-oxidants and pro-oxidants in alcoholic beverages that might influence the development of atherosclerotic cardiovascular disease? Neuroepidemiology 1999; 18:292.

940. Cravo ML, Camilo ME. Hyperhomocysteinemia in chronic alcoholism: relations to folic acid and vitamins B_6 and B_{12} status. Nutrition 2000; 16:296.

941. Hultberg B, Berglund M, Andersson A, Frank A. Elevated plasma homocysteine in alcoholics. Alcohol Clin Exp Res 1993; 17:687.

942. Hillbom M, Numminen H. Alcohol and stroke: pathophysiologic mechanisms. Neuroepidemiology 1998; 17:281.

943. Hines LM, Stampfer MJ, Ma J, et al. Genetic variation in alcohol dehydrogenase and the beneficial effect of

moderate alcohol consumption on myocardial infarction. N Engl J Med 2001; 344:549.

944. Swanson TH, Zinkel JL, Peterson PL. Bilateral anterior cerebral artery occlusion in an alcohol abuser with sickle-cell trait. Henry Ford Hosp Med J 1987; 35:67.

945. Nakamura M, Aoki N, Nakashima T, et al. Smoking, alcohol, sleep and risk of idiopathic sudden deafness: a case–control study using pooled controls. J Epidemiol 2001; 11:81.

946. Aronowski J, Strong R, Shirzadi A, et al. Ethanol plus caffeine (caffeinol) for treatment of ischemic stroke. Preclinical experience. Stroke 2003; 34:1246.

947. Piriyawat P, Labiche LA, Burgin WS, et al. Pilot dose-escalation study of caffeine plus ethanol (caffeinol) in acute ischemic stroke. Stroke 2003; 34:1242.

948. Joyce EM. Aetiology of alcoholic brain damage: alcoholic neurotoxicity or thiamine malnutrition? Br Med Bull 1994; 50:99.

949. Gilman S, Koeppe RA, Adams K, et al. Positron emission tomographic studies of cerebral benzodiazepine-receptor binding in chronic alcoholics. Ann Neurol 1996; 40:163.

950. Nicholas JM, Estruch R, Salamero M, et al. Brain impairment in well-nourished chronic alcoholics is related to ethanol intake. Ann Neurol 1997; 41:590.

951. Courville CB. Effects of Alcohol on the Nervous System of Man. Los Angeles: San Lucas, 1955.

952. Victor M. Persistent altered mentation due to ethanol. In: Brust JCM, ed. Neurologic Complications of Drug and Alcohol Abuse. Neurol Clin 1993; 11:639.

953. Harper C, Kril J. Patterns of neuronal loss in the cerebral cortex in chronic alcoholic patients. J Neurol Sci 1989; 92:81.

954. Harper CJ, Kril J, Daly J. Are we drinking our neurons away? BMJ 1987; 294:534.

955. Kril JJ, Harper CG. Neuronal counts from four cortical regions of alcoholic brains. Acta Neuropathol 1989; 79:200.

956. Samson Y, Baron J-C, Feline A, et al. Local cerebral glucose utilization in chronic alcoholics: a positron tomographic study. J Neurol Neurosurg Psychiatry 1986; 49:1165.

957. Freund G, Ballinger WE. Loss of muscarinic cholinergic receptors from the temporal cortex of alcohol abusers. Metab Brain Dis 1989; 4:121.

958. Kril JJ. The contribution of alcohol, thiamine deficiency and cirrhosis of the liver to cerebral cortical damage in alcoholics. Metab Brain Dis 1995; 10:9.

959. Bowden SC. Separating cognitive impairment in neurologically asymptomatic alcoholism from Wernicke–Korsakoff syndrome: is the neuropsychological distinction justified? Psychol Bull 1990; 107:355.

960. Jacobson RR, Lishman WA. Selective memory loss and global intellectual deficits in alcoholic Korsakoff's syndrome. Psychol Med 1987; 17:549.

961. Carlsson C, Claeson L-E, Karlsson K-I, Petterson L-E. Clinical, psychometric, and radiologic signs of brain damage in chronic alcoholism. Acta Neurol Scand 1979; 60:85.

962. Fox JH, Ramsey RG, Huckman MS, Proske AE. Cerebral ventricular enlargement: chronic alcoholics examined by computerized tomography. JAMA 1976; 236:365.

963. Epstein PS, Pisani VD, Fawcett JA. Alcoholism and cerebral atrophy. Clin Exp Res 1977; 1:61.

964. Lusins J, Zimberg S, Smokler H, Gurley K. Alcoholism and cerebral atrophy: a study of 50 patients with CT scan and psychological testing. Alcohol Clin Exp Res 1980; 4:406.

965. Wilkinson DA. Examination of alcoholics by computed tomographic (CT) scans: a critical review. Alcohol Clin Exp Res 1982; 6:31.

966. Carlen PL, Wortzman G, Holgate RC, et al. Reversible cerebral atrophy in recently abstinent chronic alcoholics measured by computed tomography scans. Science 1978; 200:1076.

967. Artmann H, Gall MV, Hacker H, Herrlich J. Reversible enlargement of cerebral spinal fluid spaces in chronic alcoholics. AJNR Am J Neuroradiol 1981; 2:23.

968. Ron MA, Acker W, Shaw GK, Lishman WA. Computerized tomography of the brain in chronic alcoholism. A survey and follow-up study. Brain 1982; 105:497.

969. Zipursky RB, Lim KC, Pfefferbaum A. MRI study of brain changes with short-term abstinence from alcohol. Alcoholism 1989; 13:664.

970. Muuronen A, Bergman H, Hindmarsh T, Telakivi T. Influence of improved drinking habits on brain atrophy and cognitive performance in alcoholic patients: a 5-year follow-up study. Alcoholism 1989; 13:137.

971. File SE, Mabbutt PS. Long-lasting effects on habituation and passive avoidance performance of a period of chronic ethanol administration in the rat. Behav Brain Res 1990; 36:171.

972. Walker DW, Hunter BE, Abraham WC. Neuro-anatomical and functional deficits subsequent to chronic ethanol administration in animals. Alcohol Clin Exp Res 1981; 5:267.

973. Phillips SC. The threshold concentration of dietary ethanol necessary to produce toxic effects of hippocampal cells and synapses in the mouse. Exp Neurol 1989; 104:68.

974. Durand D, St Cyr JA, Curevich N, Carlen PL. Ethanol-induced dendritic alterations in hippocampal granule cells. Brain Res 1989; 477:373.

975. Walker DW, Barnes DE, Zornetzer SF, et al. Neuronal loss in hippocampus induced by prolonged ethanol consumption in rats. Science 1980; 209:711.

976. West JR, Lind MD, Demut RM, et al. Lesion-induced sprouting in the rat dentate gyrus is inhibited by repeated ethanol administration. Science 1982; 218:808.

977. McMullen PA, St Cyr JA, Carlen PL. Morphological alterations in rat hippocampal pyramidal cell dendrites

resulting from chronic ethanol consumption and withdrawal. J Comp Neurol 1984; 225:111.

978. Bengoechea O, Gonzalo LM. Effects of alcoholization in the rat hippocampus. Neurosci Lett 1991; 123:112.

979. Arendt T, Henning D, Gray JA, Marchbanks R. Loss of neurons in the rat basal forebrain cholinergic projection system after prolonged intake of ethanol. Brain Res Bull 1988; 21:563.

980. Arendt T, Allen Y, Sinden J, et al. Cholinergic-rich brain transplants reverse alcohol-induced memory deficits. Nature 1988; 332:448.

981. Abraham WC, Rogers CJ, Hunter BE. Chronic ethanol-induced decreases in the response of dentate granule cells to perforant path input in the rat. Exp Brain Res 1984; 54:406.

982. Durand D, Carlen PL. Impairment of long-term potentiation in rat hippocampus following chronic ethanol treatment. Brain Res 1984; 308:325.

983. Rogers CJ, Hunter BE. Chronic ethanol treatment reduces inhibition in CA1 of the rat hippocampus. Brain Res Bull 1992; 28:587.

984. Cadete-Leite A, Tavares MA, Pacheco MM, et al. Hippocampal mossy fiber CA2 synapses after chronic alcohol consumption and withdrawal. Alcohol 1989; 6:303.

985. Tavares MA, Paula-Barbosa MM, Gray EG, Volk B. Dendritic inclusions in the cerebellar granular layer after long-term alcohol consumption in adult rats. Alcohol Clin Exp Res 1985; 9:45.

986. Goldstein B, Maxwell DS, Ellison G, Hammer RP. Dendritic vacuolation in the central nervous system of rats after long-term voluntary consumption of ethanol. J Neuropathol Exp Neurol 1983; 42:579.

987. Lescaudron L, Verna A. Effects of chronic ethanol consumption on pyramidal neurons of the mouse dorsal and ventral hippocampus: a quantitative histological analysis. Exp Brain Res 1985; 58:362.

988. Ferrer I, Galofre E, Fabriques I, Lopez-Tejero D. Effects of chronic ethanol consumption beginning at adolescence: increased numbers of dendritic spines on cortical pyramidal cells in adulthood. Acta Neuropathol 1989; 78:528.

989. Lundqvist C, Alling C, Knoth R, Volk B. Intermittent ethanol exposure of adult rats: hippocampal cell loss after one month of treatment. Alcohol 1995; 30: 737.

990. Zou JY, Martinez DB, Neafsey EJ, Collins MA. Binge ethanol-induced brain damage in rats: effect of inhibitors of nitric oxide synthase. Alcohol Clin Exp Res 1996; 20:1406.

991. Benthius DJ, West JR. Ethanol-induced neuronal loss in the developing rats: increased brain damage with binge exposure. Alcohol Clin Exp Res 1990; 14:107.

992. Cadete-Leite A, Tavares MA, Paula-Barbosa MM. Alcohol withdrawal does not impede hippocampal granule cell progressive loss in chronic alcohol-fed rats. Neurosci Lett 1988; 86:45.

993. Cadete-Leite A, Tavares MA, Uylings HB, Paula-Barbosa MM. Granule cell loss and dendritic regrowth in the hippocampal dentate gyrus of the rat after chronic alcohol consumption. Brain Res 1988; 473:1.

994. Phillips SC, Cragg BG. Chronic consumption of alcohol by adult mice. Effects on hippocampal cells and synapses. Exp Neurol 1983; 80:218.

995. Collins MA, Corso TD, Neafsey EJ. Neuronal degeneration in rat cerebrocortical and olfactory regions during subchronic "binge" intoxication with ethanol: possible explanation for olfactory deficits in alcoholics. Alcohol Clin Exp Res 1996; 20:284.

996. Kril JJ, Halliday GM. Brain shrinkage in alcoholics: a decade on and what have we learned? Prog Neurobiol 1999; 58:381.

997. Pfefferbaum A, Sullivan EV, Hedehus M, et al. In vivo detection and functional correlates of white matter microstructural disruption in chronic alcoholism. Alcohol Clin Exp Res 2000; 24:1214.

998. Schroth G, Naegele T, Klose U, et al. Reversible brain shrinkage in abstinent alcoholics measured by MRI. Neuroradiology 1988; 30:385.

999. Shear PK, Jernigan TL, Butters N. Volumetric magnetic resonance imaging quantification of longitudinal brain changes in abstinent alcoholics. Alcohol Clin Exp Res 1994; 18:172.

1000. Pfefferbaum A, Sullivan EV, Mathalon DH, et al. Longitudinal changes in magnetic resonance imaging brain volumes in abstinent and relapsed alcoholics. Alcohol Clin Exp Res 1995; 19:1177.

1001. deScalafani V, Ezekiel F, Meyerhoff DJ, et al. Brain atrophy and cognitive function in older abstinent alcoholic men. Alcohol Clin Exp Res 1995; 19:1121.

1002. Pfefferbaum A, Rosenbloom M, Deshmukh A, Sullivan E. Sex differences in the effects of alcohol on brain structure. Am J Psychiatry 2001; 158:188.

1003. Hommer, Momenan R, Kaiser E, Rawlings R. Evidence for a gender-related effect of alcohol on brain volumes. Am J Psychiatry 2001; 158:198.

1004. Estilaei MR, Matson GB, Payne GS, et al. Effects of chronic alcohol consumption on the broad phospholipid signal in human brain: an in vivo ^{31}P MRS study. Alcohol Clin Exp Res 2001; 25:89.

1005. Bengoechea O, Gonzalo LM. Effect of chronic alcoholism on the human hippocampus. Histol Histopathol 1990; 5:349.

1006. Mayes AR, Meudell PR, Mann D, Pickering A. Locations of the lesions in Korsakoff's syndrome. Neuropathological data on two patients. Cortex 1988; 24:367.

1007. Squire LR, Amaral DG, Press GA. Magnetic resonance imaging of the hippocampal and mammillary nuclei distinguish medial temporal lobe and diencephalic amnesia. J Neurol 1990; 10:3106.

1008. Jernigan TL, Butters N, DiTriaglia G, et al. Reduced cerebral grey matter observed in alcoholics using magnetic resonance imaging. Alcohol Clin Exp Res 1991; 15:418.

1009. Sullivan EV, Marsh L, Mathalon DH, et al. Anterior hippocampal volume deficits in nonamnesic aging chronic alcoholics. Alcohol Clin Exp Res 1995; 19:110.

1010. Harding AJ, Wong A, Svoboda M, et al. Chronic alcohol consumption does not cause hippocampal neuron loss in humans. Hippocampus 1997; 7:78.

1011. Ibanez J, Herrero MT, Insausti R, et al. Chronic alcoholism decreases neuronal nuclear size and the human entorhinal cortex. Neurosci Lett 1995; 183:71.

1012. Harding AJ, Halliday GM, Ng JLF, et al. Loss of vasopressin-immunoreactive neurons in alcoholics is dose-related and time-dependent. Neuroscience 1996; 72:699.

1013. Halliday G, Baker K, Harper C. Serotonin and alcohol-related brain damage. Metab Brain Dis 1995; 10:25.

1014. Harper C. The neurobiology of alcohol-specific brain damage, or does alcohol damage the brain? J Neuropathol Exp Neurol 1998; 57:101.

1015. Kril JJ, Halliday GM, Svoboda MD, Cartwright H. The cerebral cortex is damaged in chronic alcoholics. Neuroscience 1997; 79:983.

1015a. Mayfield RD, Lewohl JM, Dodd PR, et al. Patterns of gene expression are altered in the frontal and motor cortices of human alcoholics. J Neurochem 2002; 81:802.

1016. Schweinsburg BC, Taylor MJ, Alhassoon OM, et al. Clinical pathology in brain white matter of recently detoxified alcoholics: a ^{1}H magnetic resonance spectroscopy investigation of alcohol-associated frontal lobe injury. Alcohol Clin Exp Res 2001; 25:924.

1017. Brun A, Anderson J. Frontal dysfunction and frontal cortical synapse loss in alcoholism—the main cause of alcohol dementia? Dementia Ger Cog Disord 2001; 12:289.

1018. Monnot M, Nixon S, Lovallo W, Ross E. Altered emotional perception in alcoholics: deficits in affective prosody comprehension. Alcohol Clin Exp Res 2001; 25:362.

1019. Ambrose ML, Bowden SC, Whelan G. Working memory impairments in alcohol-dependent participants without clinical amnesia. Alcohol Clin Exp Res 2001; 25:185.

1020. Ihara H, Berrios GE, London M. Group and case study of the dysexecutive syndrome in alcoholism without amnesia. J Neurol Neurosurg Psychiatry 2000; 68:731.

1021. Maezawa Y, Yamauchi M, Searashi Y, et al. Association of restriction fragment-length polymorphisms in the alcohol dehydrogenase 2 gene with alcoholic brain atrophy. Alcohol Clin Exp Res 1996; 20:29A.

1022. Yamauchi M, Takamatsu M, Maezawa Y, et al. Polymorphism of tumor necrosis factor-beta and alcohol dehydrogenase genes and alcoholic brain atrophy in Japanese patients. Alcohol Clin Exp Res 2001; 25 (Suppl 6):7S.

1023. Muramatsu T, Kato M, Matsui F, et al. Apolipoprotein E epsilon 4 allele distribution in Wernicke–Korsakoff syndrome with and without global intellectual deficits. J Neural Trans 1997; 104:913.

1024. Tsai G, Ragan P, Chang R, et al. Increased glutamatergic neurotransmission and oxidative stress after alcohol withdrawal. Am J Psychiatry 1998; 155: 725.

1025. Tsai G, Coyle JT. The role of glutamatergic neurotransmission in the pathophysiology of alcoholism. Annu Rev Med 1998; 49:173.

1026. Chandler LJ, Newsom H, Sumners C, Crews F. Chronic ethanol exposure potentiates NMDA excitotoxicity in cerebral cortical neurons. J Neurochem 1993; 60:1578.

1027. Gotz ME, Janetzky B, Pohli S, et al. Chronic alcohol consumption and cerebral indices of oxidative stress: is there a link? Alcohol Clin Exp Res 2001; 25:717.

1028. Parsons OA, Nixon SJ. Cognitive functioning in sober social drinkers: a review of the research since 1986. J Stud Alcohol 1998; 59:180.

1029. Kubota M, Nakazaki S, Hirai S, et al. Alcohol consumption and frontal lobe shrinkage: study of 1432 non-alcoholic subjects. J Neurol Neurosurg Psychiatry 2001; 71:104.

1029a. Ding J, Eigenbrodt ML, Mosley TH, et al: Alcohol intake and cerebral abnormalities on magnetic resonance imaging in a community-based population of middle-aged adults. Stroke 2004; 35:16.

1030. Hebert LE, Scherr PA, Beckett LA, et al. Relation of smoking and alcohol consumption to incident Alzheimer's disease. Am J Epidemiol 1992; 135:347.

1031. Broe GA, Henderson AS, Creasy H, et al. A case–control study of Alzheimer's disease in Australia. Neurology 1990; 40:1698.

1032. Graves AB, van Duijn CM, Chandra V, et al. Alcohol and tobacco consumption as risk factors for Alzheimer's disease: a collaborative re-analysis of case–control studies. EURODEM Risk Factors Research Group. Int J Epidemiol 1991; 20 (Suppl 2): S48.

1033. Tsolaki M, Fountoulakis K, Chantzi E, et al. Risk factors for clinically diagnosed Alzheimer's disease: a case–control study of a Greek population. Int Psychogeriatr 1997; 9:327.

1034. Launer LJ, Feskens EJ, Kalmijn S, et al. Smoking, drinking, and thinking. The Zutphen Elderly Study. Am J Epidemiol 1996; 143:219.

1035. Galanis DJ, Joseph C, Masaki KH, et al. A longitudinal study of drinking and cognitive performance in elderly Japanese American men: the Honolulu-Asia Aging Study. Am J Public Health 2000; 90:1254.

1036. Orgogozo JM, Dartigues JF, Lafont S, et al. Wine consumption and dementia in the elderly: a prospective community study in the Bordeaux area. Rev Neurol 1997; 153:185.

1037. Lemeshow S, Letenneur L, Dartigues JF, et al. Illustration of analysis taking into account complex survey considerations: the association between wine consumption and dementia in the PAQUID Study. Am J Epidemiol 1998; 148:298.

1038. Carmelli D, Swan GE, Reed T, et al. The effect of apolipoprotein E episilon-4 in the relationships of smoking and drinking to cognitive function. Neuroepidemiology 1999; 18:125.

1039. Dufouil C, Tzourio C, Brayne C, et al. Influence of apolipoprotein E genotype on the risk of cognitive deterioration in moderate drinkers and smokers. Epidemiology 2000; 11:280.

1040. Truelson T, Thudium D, Gronbaek M. Amount and type of alcohol and risk of dementia. The Copenhagen City Heart Study. Neurology 2002; 59:1313.

1041. Mukamal KJ, Kuller LH, Fitzpatrick AL, et al. Prospective study of alcohol consumption and risk of dementia in older adults. JAMA 2003; 289:1405.

1042. Brust JCM. Wine, flavenoids, and the "water of life." Neurology 2002; 59:1300.

1042a. Hall SS. In vino vitalis? Compounds activate life-extending genes. Science 2003; 301:1165.

1043. Henn C, Loffelholz K, Klein J. Stimulatory and inhibitory effects of ethanol on hippocampal acetyl-choline release. Arch Pharmacol 1998; 357:640.

1044. Warner R, Rosett H. The effects of drinking on off-spring: an historical survey of the American and British literature. J Stud Alcohol 1975; 36:1395.

1045. Sullivan WC. A note on the influence of maternal inebriety on offspring. J Ment Sci 1888; 43:489.

1046. Lemoine P, Harousseau H, Borteyru JP, et al. Les enfants de parents alcooliques: anomalies observées. Ouest Med 1968; 25:476.

1047. Jones K, Smith DW. Recognition of the fetal alcohol syndrome in early infancy. Lancet 1973; II:999.

1048. Colangelo W, Jones DG. The fetal alcohol syndrome: a review and assessment of the syndrome and its neu-rological sequelae. Prog Neurobiol 1982; 19:271.

1049. Hanson JW, Jones KL, Smith DW. Fetal alcohol syndrome. Experience with 41 patients. JAMA 1976; 235:1458.

1050. Day NL, Jasperse D, Richardson G, et al. Prenatal exposure to alcohol: effect on infant growth and mor-phologic characteristics. Pediatrics 1989; 84:536.

1051. Hellstrom A, Svensson E, Stromland K. Eye size in healthy Swedish children and in children with fetal alcohol syndrome. Acta Ophthalmol Scand 1997; 75:423.

1052. Church MW, Abel EL. Fetal alcohol syndrome: hearing, speech, language, and vestibular disorders. Obstet Gynecol Clin North Am 1998; 25:85.

1053. Ouelette EM, Rosett HL, Rosman NP, et al. Adverse effects on offspring of maternal alcohol abuse dur-ing pregnancy. N Engl J Med 1977; 297:528.

1054. Allebeck P, Olsen J. Alcohol and fetal damage. Alcohol Clin Exp Res 1998; 22 (Suppl 7):229S.

1055. Mattson SN, Riley EP, Gramling L, et al. Neuropsychological comparison of alcohol-exposed children with or without physical features of fetal alcohol syndrome. Neuropsychology 1998; 12:146.

1056. Kaminski M, Rumeau-Rouquette C, Schwartz D. Effects of alcohol on the fetus. N Engl J Med 1978; 298:55.

1057. Coles CD, Platzman KA, Raaskind-Hood CL, et al. A comparison of children affected by prenatal alcohol exposure and attention deficit hyperactivity disorder. Alcohol Clin Exp Res 1997; 21:150.

1058. Streissguth AP, Martin DC, Barr HM, et al. Intrauterine alcohol and nicotine exposure: attention and reaction time in 4-year-old children. Dev Psychol 1984; 20:533.

1059. Streissguth AP, Barr HM, Sampson PD, et al. Attention, distraction, and reaction time at age 7 years and prenatal alcohol exposure. Neurobehav Toxicol Teratol 1986; 8:717.

1060. Bray PF. Can maternal alcoholism cause spasmus nutans in offspring? N Engl J Med 1990; 322: 554.

1061. Clarren SK, Smith DW. The fetal alcohol syndrome. N Engl J Med 1978; 298:1063.

1062. Astley SJ, Clarren SK. Measuring the facial pheno-type of individuals with prenatal alcohol exposure: correlations with brain dysfunction. Alcohol Alcohol 2001; 36:147.

1063. Pierog S, Chandavasu O, Wexler I. Withdrawal symp-toms in infants with the fetal alcohol syndrome. J Pediatr 1977; 90:630.

1064. Streissguth AP, Herman CS, Smith DW. Intelligence, behavior and dysmorphogenesis in the fetal alcohol syndrome: a report on 20 patients. J Pediatr 1978; 92:363.

1065. Streissguth AP, Clarren SK, Jones KL. Natural history of the fetal alcohol syndrome: a ten-year follow-up of eleven patients. Lancet 1985; II:85.

1066. Lemoine P, Lemoine P. Avenir des enfants de mères alcooliques (étude de 105 cas retrouvés à l'age adult) et quelques constatations d'intérêt prophylactique. Ann Pediatr 1992; 29:226.

1067. Autti-Rämö I. Twelve year follow-up of children exposed to alcohol in utero. Dev Med Child Neurol 2000; 42:406.

1068. Famy C, Streissguth AP, Unis AS. Mental illness in adults with fetal alcohol syndrome or fetal alcohol effects. Am J Psychiatry 1998; 155:552.

1069. Kelly SJ, Day N, Streissguth AP. Effects of prenatal alcohol exposure on social behavior in humans and other species. Neurotoxicol Teratol 2000; 22: 143.

1070. Jacobson SW. Specificity of neurobehavioral outcomes associated with prenatal alcohol exposure. Alcohol Clin Exp Res 1998; 22:313.

1071. Roebuck TM, Mattson SN, Riley EP. A review of the neuroanatomical findings in children with fetal alco-hol syndrome or prenatal exposure to alcohol. Alcohol Clin Exp Res 1998; 22:339.

1072. Sowell ER, Mattson SN, Thompson PM, et al. Mapping callosal morphology and cognitive correlates. Effects of heavy prenatal alcohol exposure. Neurology 2001; 57:235.

1072a. Roebuck TM, Mattson SN, Riley EP. Interhemispheric transfer in children with heavy prenatal alcohol exposure. Alcohol Clin Exp Res 2002; 26:1863.

1073. Archibald SL, Fennema-Notestine C, Riley EP, et al. A quantitative MRI study of subjects exposed to alcohol prenatally. Dev Med Child Neurol 2001; 43:148.

1074. Johnson VP, Swayze VW, Sato Y, Andreasen NC. Fetal alcohol syndrome: craniofacial and central nervous system manifestations. Am J Med Genet 1996; 61:329.

1075. Sowell ER, Jernigan TL, Mattson SN, et al. Abnormal development of the cerebellar vermis in children prenatally exposed to alcohol: size reduction in lobules I–V. Alcohol Clin Exp Res 1996; 20:31.

1076. Archibald SK, Fennema-Notestine C, Gamst A, et al. Brain dysmorphology in individuals with severe prenatal alcohol exposure. Dev Med Child Neurol 2001; 43:148.

1077. Sowell ER, Thompson PM, Mattson SN, et al. Voxel-based morphometric analyses of the brain in children and adolescents prenatally exposed to alcohol. Neuroreport 2001; 12:515.

1077a. Sowell ER, Thompson PM, Peterson BS, et al. Mapping cortical gray matter asymmetry pattern in adolescents with heavy prenatal alcohol exposure. Alcohol Clin Exp Res 2002; 26:1863.

1077b. Sowell ER, Thompson PM, Mattson SN, et al. Regional brain shape abnormalities persist into adolescence after prenatal alcohol exposure. Cereb Cortex 2002; 12:856.

1078. Chernoff GF. The fetal alcohol syndrome in mice: maternal variables. Teratology 1980; 22:71.

1079. Mukherjee AB, Hodgen GD. Maternal ethanol exposure induces transient impairment of umbilical circulation and fetal hypoxia in monkeys. Science 1982; 218:700.

1080. Ellis FW, Pick JR. An animal model of the fetal alcohol syndrome in beagles. Alcoholism Clin Exp Res 1980; 4:123.

1081. Dexter JD, Tumbleson ME, Decker JD, et al. Fetal alcohol syndrome in Sinclair (S-1) miniature swine. Alcohol Clin Exp Res 1980; 4:146.

1082. Clarren SK, Bowden DM. Fetal alcohol syndrome: a new primate model for binge drinking and its relevance to human ethanol teratogenesis. J Pediatr 1982; 101:819.

1083. Altshuler HL, Shippenberg TS. A subhuman primate model for fetal alcohol syndrome research. Neurobehav Toxicol Teratol 1981; 3:121.

1084. Tze WJ, Lee M. Adverse effects of maternal alcohol consumption on pregnancy and fetal growth in rats. Nature 1975; 257:479.

1085. Abel EL, Dintcheff BA. Effect of prenatal alcohol exposure on growth and development in rats. J Pharmacol Exp Ther 1978; 207:916.

1086. Riley EP, Lochry EA, Shapiro NR. Lack of response inhibition in rats prenatally exposed to alcohol. Psychopharmacology 1979; 62:47.

1087. Yanai J, Ginsburg BE. Audiogenic seizures in mice whose parents drank alcohol. J Stud Alcohol 1976; 37:1564.

1088. Ellis RW, Pick JR. Beagle model of the fetal alcohol syndrome, Pharmacologist 1976; 18:190.

1089. Clarren SK, Bowden DM. Measures of alcohol damage in utero in the pigtailed Macaque (*Macaca nemestrina*). In: Porter R, O'Conner M, Whelan J, eds. Mechanisms of Alcohol Damage in Utero. London: Pitman Publishing, 1984; 157.

1090. Sulik KK, Lauder JM, Dehart DB. Brain malformations in prenatal mice following acute maternal ethanol administration. Int J Dev Neurosci 1984; 2:203.

1091. Hannigan JH, Berman RF. Amelioration of fetal alcohol-related neurodevelopmental disorders in rats: exploring pharmacological and environmental treatments. Neurotoxicol Teratol 2000; 22:103.

1092. Berman RF, Hannigan JH. Effects of prenatal alcohol exposure on the hippocampus: spatial behavior, electrophysiology, and neuroanatomy. Hippocampus 2000; 10:94.

1093. Miller MW, Astley SJ, Clarren SK. Number of axons in the corpus callosum of the mature *Macaca nemestrina*: increases caused by prenatal exposure to ethanol. J Comp Neurol 1999; 412:123.

1094. Guerri C, Renau-Piqueras J. Alcohol, astroglia, and brain development. Mol Neurobiol 1997; 15:65.

1095. Shibley IA, Pennington SN. Metabolic and mitotic changes associated with the fetal alcohol syndrome. Alcohol Alcohol 1997; 32:423.

1096. McGivern RF, Clancy AN, Hill MA, Noble EP. Prenatal alcohol exposure alters adult expression of sexually dimorphic behavior in the rat. Science 1984; 224:896.

1097. Abel EL, Hazlett LS, Berk RS, Mutchnick MG. Neuro-immunotoxic effects in offspring of paternal alcohol consumption. In: Seminara D, Watson RR, Pawlowski A, eds. Alcohol, Immunomodulation, and AIDS. New York: Alan R. Liss, 1990:47.

1098. Seppala M, Raiha NC, Tamminen V. Ethanol elimination in a mother and her premature twins. Lancet 1971; II:1188.

1099. Sander LW, Snyder PA, Rosen HL, et al. Effects of alcohol intake during pregnancy in newborn state regulation: a progress report. Alcohol Clin Exp Res 1977; 1:233.

1100. Bonthuis DJ, West JR. Alcohol-induced neuronal loss in developing rats: increased brain damage with binge exposure. Alcohol Clin Exp Res 1990; 14:107.

1101. Altura BM, Altura BT, Corella A, et al. Alcohol produces spasms of human umbilical vessels: relationship to FAS. Eur J Pharmacol 1982; 86:311.

1102. Wisniewski K. A clinical neuropathological study of the fetal alcohol syndrome. Neuropediatrics 1983; 14:197.

1103. Mukherjee AB, Hodgen GD. Maternal ethanol exposure induces transient impairment of umbilical circulation and fetal hypoxia in monkeys. Science 1982; 218:700.

1104. Mann LI, Bhakthavathsalan A, Liu M, et al. Placental transport of alcohol and its effect on maternal acid–base balance. Am J Obstet Gynecol 1975; 122:837.

1105. Mann LT, Bhakkthavathsalan A, Liu M, et al. Effect of alcohol on fetal cerebral function and metabolism. Am J Obstet Gynecol 1975; 122:845.

1106. Savage DD, Montano CY, Otero MA, Paxton LL. Prenatal ethanol exposure decreases hippocampal NMDA-sensitive [^{3}H]-glutamate binding site density in 45-day-old rats. Alcohol 1991; 8:193.

1107. Noble EP, Ritchie T. Prenatal ethanol exposure reduces the effects of excitatory amino acids in the rat hippocampus. Life Sci 1989; 45:803.

1108. Queen SA, Sanchez CF, Lopez SR, et al. Dose- and age-dependent effects of prenatal ethanol exposure on hippocampal metabotropic-glutamate receptor-stimulated phosphoinositide hydrolysis. Alcohol Clin Exp Res 1993; 17:887.

1109. Kumari M, Tucku MK. Ethanol and regulation of the NMDA receptor subunits in fetal cortical neurons. J Neurochem 1998; 70:1467.

1110. Ikonomidou C, Bittigau P, Ishimaru MJ, et al. Ethanol-induced apoptotic neurodegeneration and fetal alcohol syndrome. Science 2000; 287:1056.

1111. Halmesmaki E, Valimaki M, Karonen SL, Ylikorkala O. Low somatomedin C and high growth hormone levels in newborns damaged by maternal alcohol abuse. Obstet Gynecol 1989; 74:366.

1112. Singh SP, Srivenugopal KS, Ehmann S, et al. Insulin-like growth factors (IGF-I and IGF-II), IGF-binding proteins, and IGF gene expression in the offspring of ethanol-fed rats. J Lab Clin Med 1994; 124:183.

1113. Tritt SH, Brammer GL, Taylor AN. Adrenalectomy but not adrenal demedullation during pregnancy prevents the growth-retarding effects of fetal alcohol exposure. Alcohol Clin Exp Res 1993; 17:1281.

1114. Costa LG, Guizzetti M. Muscarinic cholinergic receptor signal transduction as a potential target for the developmental neurotoxicity of ethanol. Biochem Pharmacol 1999; 57:721.

1115. Barinaga M. New experiments underscore warnings on maternal drinking. Science 1996; 273:738.

1116. Ramanathan R, Wilkenmeyer MF, Mittal B, et al. Alcohol inhibits cell–cell adhesion mediated by human L1. J Cell Biol 1996; 133:381.

1116a. Wilkemeyer MF, Chen S-Y, Menkari CE, et al. Differential effects of ethanol antagonism and neuroprotection in peptide fragment NAPVSIPQ prevention of ethanol-induced developmental toxicity. Proc Natl Acad Sci USA 2003; 100:8543.

1117. Zachman RD, Grummer MA. The interaction of ethanol and vitamin A as a potential mechanism for the pathogenesis of fetal alcohol syndrome. Alcohol Clin Exp Res 1998; 22:1544.

1118. Phillips SG, Gragg BG. Alcohol withdrawal causes a loss of cerebellar Purkinje cells in mice. J Stud Alcohol 1984; 45:475.

1119. Hemmingsen R, Jorgensen OS. Specific brain proteins during severe ethanol intoxication and withdrawal in the rat. Psychiatr Res 1980; 3:1.

1120. Samson HA, Grant KA, Coggan S, Sachs VM. Ethanol induced microcephaly in the neonatal rat: occurrence without withdrawal. Neurobehav Toxicol Teratol 1982; 4:115.

1121. O'Shea KS, Kaufman MH. The teratogenic effect of acetaldehyde: implications of the study of the fetal alcohol syndrome. J Anat 1979; 128:65.

1122. Dow KE, Riopelle RI. Ethanol neurotoxicity: effects on neurite formation and neurotrophic factor production in vitro. Science 1985; 228:591.

1123. Fisher SE, Atkinson M, Jacobson M, et al. Selective fetal malnutrition. The effect of in vivo ethanol exposure upon in vitro placental uptake of amino acids in the non-human primate. Pediatr Res 1983; 17:704.

1124. Snyder AK, Singh SP, Pullen GL. Ethanol-induced intrauterine growth retardation: correlation with placental glucose transfer. Alcoholism 1986; 10:167.

1125. Fisher SE, Duffy L, Atkinson M. Selective fetal malnutrition: effect of acute and chronic ethanol exposure upon rat placental Na,K-ATPase activity. Alcoholism 1986; 10:150.

1126. Kaufman MH. Ethanol-induced chromosomal abnormalities at conception. Nature 1983; 302:258.

1127. Gardner LI, Mitter N, Coplan J, et al. Isochromosome 9q in an infant exposed to ethanol prenatally. N Engl J Med 1985; 312:1521.

1128. Little RE, Sing CF. Association of father's drinking and infant's birth weight. N Engl J Med 1986; 314:1644.

1129. Randall CL, Anton RF. Aspirin reduced alcohol-induced prenatal mortality and malformations in mice. Alcohol Clin Exp Res 1984; 8:513.

1130. McCarver DG. ADH2 and CYPZE1 genetic polymorphisms: risk factors for alcohol-related birth defects. Drug Metab Disp 2001; 29:562.

1131. Centers for Disease Control. Sociodemographic and Behavioral characteristics associated with alcohol consumption during pregnancy. JAMA 1995; 273:1406.

1132. Sidhu JS, Floyd RS. Alcohol use among women of childbearing age—United States, 1991–1999. MMWR 2002; 51:273.

1133. Centers for Disease Control. Update: Trends in fetal alcohol syndrome—United States, 1979–1993. JAMA 1995; 273:1406.

1134. Stoler JM, Holmes LB. Under-recognition of prenatal alcohol effects in infants of known alcohol abusing women. J Pediatr 1999; 135:430.

1135. Streissguth AP, O'Malley K. Neuropsychiatric implications and long-term consequences of fetal alcohol spectrum disorders. Semin Clin Neuropsychiatry 2000; 5:177.

1136. Bearer CE, Moore C, Salvatore AE, et al. Meconium FAEE: development of a biologic marker. Alcohol Clin Exp Res 1998; 22:103A.

1137. Sampson PD, Streissguth AP, Bookstein FL, et al. Incidence of fetal alcohol syndrome and prevalence of alcohol-related neurodevelopmental disorder. Teratology 1997; 56:317.

1138. Ernhart CB, Sokol RJ, Ager JW, et al. Alcohol-related birth defects: assessing the risk. Ann N Y Acad Sci 1989; 562:159.

1139. Wright JT, Barrison IG, Waterson EJ, et al. Alcohol consumption, pregnancy, and low birthweight. Lancet 1983; I:663.

1140. Day NL, Jasperse D, Richardson G, et al. Prenatal exposure to alcohol: effect on infant growth and morphologic characteristics. Pediatrics 1989; 84:536.

1141. Graham JM, Hansen JW, Darby BL, et al. Independent dysmorphology evaluations at birth and 4 years of age for children exposed to varying amounts of alcohol in utero. Pediatrics 1988; 81:772.

1142. Ioffe S, Chernick V. Development of the EEG between 30 and 40 weeks gestation in normal and alcohol-exposed infants. Dev Med Child Neurol 1988; 30:797.

1143. Streissguth AP, Martin DC, Barr HM. Maternal alcohol use and neonatal habituation assessed with the Brazelton Scale. Child Dev 1983; 54:1109.

1144. Ernhart CH, Wolf AW, Linn PL, et al. Alcohol-related birth defects: syndromal anomalies, intrauterine growth retardation, and neonatal behavioral assessment. Alcohol Clin Exp Res 1985; 9:447.

1145. Mills JL, Graubard BI, Harley EE, et al. Maternal alcohol consumption and birthweight: how much drinking during pregnancy is safe? JAMA 1984; 252:1875.

1146. Little RE, Asker RL, Sampson PD, et al. Fetal growth and moderate drinking in early pregnancy. Am J Epidemiol 1986; 123:270.

1147. Sulik K, Johnston MS, Webb MA. Fetal alcohol syndrome: embryogenesis in a mouse model. Science 1981; 214:936.

1148. Morrow-Tlucak M, Ernhart CB, Soko RJ, et al. Underreporting of alcohol use in pregnancy: relationship to alcohol problem history. Alcoholism 1989; 13:399.

1148a. Sood B, Delaney-Black V, Covington C, et al: Prenatal alcohol exposure and childhood behavior at age 6 to 7 years: I. Dose-response effect. Peadiatrics 2001; 108: E34.

1149. Tennes K, Blackard C. Maternal alcohol consumption, birthweight, and minor physical anomalies. Am J Obstet Gynecol 1980; 138:774.

1150. Hingson R, Alpett JJ, Day N, et al. Effects of maternal drinking and marijuana use on fetal growth and development. Pediatrics 1982; 70:539.

1151. Grisso JA, Roman E, Inskip H, et al. Alcohol consumption and outcome of pregnancy. J Epidemiol Commun Health 1984; 38:232.

1152. Zuckerman B, Frank DA, Hingson R, et al. Effects of maternal marijuana and cocaine use on fetal growth. N Engl J Med 1989; 320:762.

1153. Alpert J, Zuckerman B. High blood alcohol levels in women. N Engl J Med 1990; 323:60.

1154. Mennella JA, Beauchamp GK. The transfer of alcohol to human milk—effects on flavor and the infant's behavior. N Engl J Med 1991; 325:981.

1155. Little RE, Anderson KW, Ervin CH, et al. Maternal alcohol use during breast feeding and infant mental and motor development at one year. N Engl J Med 1989; 321:425.

1156. Lindmark B. Maternal use of alcohol and breast-fed infants. N Engl J Med 1990; 322:338.

1157. Little RE. Maternal use of alcohol and breast-fed infants. N Engl J Med 1990; 322:339.

1158. Litovitz T. The alcohols: ethanol, methanol, isopropanol, ethylene glycol. Pediatr Clin North Am 33; 311:1986.

1159. Goldfrank LR, Flomenbaum NE. Toxic alcohols. In: Goldfrank LR, Flomenbaum NE, Lewin NA, et al, eds. Goldfrank's Toxicologic Emergencies, 6th edition. Stamford, CT: Appleton & Lange, 1998; 1049.

1160. Bennett IL, Cary FH, Mitchell GL. Acute methyl alcohol poisoning: review based on experiences in outbreak of 323 cases. Medicine 1953; 32:431.

1161. Swartz RD, Millman RP, Billi JE, et al. Epidemic methanol poisoning: clinical and biochemical analysis of a recent episode. Medicine 1981; 60; 373.

1162. Becker CE. Acute methanol poisoning—the blind drunk. West J Med 1981; 135:122.

1163. Klaessen CD. Nonmetallic environmental toxicants: air pollutants, solvents and vapors, and pesticides. In: Hardman JG, Limbird LE, eds. Goodman and Gilman's The Pharmacological Basis of Therapeutics, 10th edition. New York: McGraw-Hill, 2001; 1877.

1164. Sejeersted OM, Jacobsen D, Ovrebo S, et al. Formate concentrations in plasma from patients poisoned with methanol. Acta Med Scand 1983; 213:105.

1165. Burkhart KK, Kulig KW. The other alcohols. Emerg Med Clin North Am 1990; 8:913.

1166. Sharpe JA, Hostovsky M, Bilbao JM, Rewcastle NB. Methanol optic neuropathy: a histopathological study. Neurology 1982; 32:1093.

1167. Sarkola T, Eriksson CJ. Effect of 4-methylpyrazole on endogenous plasma ethanol and methanol levels in humans. Alcohol Clin Exp Res 2001; 25:513.

1168. Jacobsen D, McMartin KE. Methanol and ethylene glycol poisonings: mechanism of toxicity, clinical course, diagnosis, and treatment. Med Toxicol 1986; 1:309.

1169. Brent J, McMartin K, Phillips S, et al. Fomepizole for the treatment of methanol poisoning. N Engl J Med 2001; 344:424.

1170. Guggenheim MA, Couch JR, Weinberg W. Motor dysfunction as a permanent complication of methanol ingestion. Arch Neurol 1971; 24:550.

1171. Ley CO, Gali FG. Parkinsonian syndrome after methanol intoxication. Eur Neurol 1983; 22:405.

1172. LeWitt PA, Martin SD. Dystonia and hypokinesis with putaminal necrosis after methanol intoxication. Clin Neuropharmacol 1988; 11:161.

1173. Anderson C, Rubinstein D, Filley CM, et al. MR enhancing lesions in methanol intoxication. J Comput Assist Tomogr 1997; 21:834.

1174. McLean DR, Jacobs H, Mielke BW. Methanol poisoning: a clinical and pathological study. Ann Neurol 1980; 8:161.

1175. Jaffery JB, Aggarwal A, Ades PA, Weise WJ. A long sweet sleep with sour consequences. Lancet 2001; 358:1236.

1176. Gabow PA, Clay K, Sullivan JB, Lepoff R. Organic acids in ethylene glycol intoxication. Ann Intern Med 1986; 105:16.

1177. Piagnerelli M, Lejeune P, Vanhaeverbeek M. Diagnosis and treatment of an unusual cause of metabolic acidosis: ethylene glycol poisoning. Acta Clin Belg 1999; 54:351.

1178. Lewis LD, Smith BW, Mamourian AC. Delayed sequelae after acute overdoses or poisonings: cranial neuropathy related to ethylene glycol ingestion. Clin Pharmacol Ther 1997; 61:692

1179. Peterson CD, Collins AJ, Himes JM, et al. Ethylene glycol poisoning: pharmacokinetics during therapy with ethanol and hemodialysis. N Engl J Med 1981; 304:21.

1180. Brant J, McMartin K, Phillips S, et al. Fomepizole for the treatment of ethylene glycol poisoning. N Engl J Med 1999; 340:832.

1181. Jacobsen D. New treatment for ethylene glycol poisoning. N Engl J Med 1999; 340:879.

1182. Blakeley KR, Rinner SE, Knochel JP. Survival of ethylene glycol poisoning with profound anemia. N Engl J Med 1993: 328:515.

1183. Rich J, Scheife RT, Katz N, Caplan LR. Isopropyl alcohol intoxication. Arch Neurol 1990; 47:322.

1184. Lacouture PG, Watson S, Abrams A, et al. Acute isopropyl alcohol intoxication: diagnosis and management. Am J Med 1983; 75:680.

1185. Arnold WN. Vincent van Gogh and the thujone connection. JAMA 1988; 260:3042.

1186. Weisbord SD, Soule JB, Kimmel PL. Poison on line—acute renal failure caused by oil of wormwood purchased through the internet. N Engl J Med 1997; 337:825.

1187. Höld KM, Sirisoma NS, Casida JE, et al. Alpha-thujone (the active component of absinthe): gamma-aminobutyric acid type A receptor modulation and metabolic detoxification. Proc Natl Acad Sci USA 2000; 97:3826.

1188. Hasin DS, Grant BF, Dufour MG, Endicott J. Alcohol problems increase while physician attention declines: 1967 to 1984. Arch Intern Med 1990; 150:397.

1189. Adams WL, Barry KL, Fleming MF. Screening for problem drinking in older primary care patients. JAMA 1996; 24:1964.

1190. Pattison EM. The selection of treatment modalities for the alcoholic patient. In: Mendelson JH, Mello NK, eds. The Diagnosis and Treatment of Alcoholism. New York: McGraw-Hill, 1979:125.

1191. Klerman GL. Treatment of alcoholism. N Engl J Med 1989; 320:395.

1192. Hesselbrock MH, Eyer RE, Keener JJ. Psychopathology in hospitalized alcoholics. Arch Gen Psychiatry 1985; 42:1050.

1193. Schukit MA. The clinical implications of primary diagnostic groups among alcoholics. Arch Gen Psychiatry 1985; 42:1043.

1194. Halikas JA, Herzog MA, Mirassou MM, Lyttle MD. Psychiatric diagnoses among female alcoholics. In: Galanter M, ed. Currents in Alcoholism, Vol VIII. New York: Grune & Stratton, 1983; 283.

1195. Holden C. Is alcoholism a disease? Science 1987; 238:1647.

1196. Becker JT, Jaffe JH. Impaired memory for treatment-relevant information in in-patient men alcoholics. J Stud Alcohol 1984; 45:339.

1197. Schukit MA, Schuei MG, Gold E. Prediction of outcome in inpatient alcoholics. J Stud Alcohol 1986; 47:151.

1198. Zernig G, Fabisch K, Fabisch H. Pharmacotherapy of alcohol dependence. Trends Pharmacol Sci 1997; 18:229.

1199. Tinsley JA, Finlayson RE, Morse RM. Developments in the treatment of alcoholism. Mayo Clin Proc 1998; 73:857.

1200. Johnson BA, Ait-Daoud N. Medications to treat alcoholism. Alcohol Res Health 1999; 23:99.

1201. Agosti V. The efficacy of treatment on reducing alcohol consumption. A meta-analysis. Int J Addict 1995; 30:1067.

1202. Ciraulo DA, Sands BF, Shader RI. Critical review of liability for benzodiazepine abuse among alcoholics. Am J Psychiatry 1988; 145:1501.

1203. Linnoila MI. Benzodiazepines and alcohol. J Psychiatr Res 1990; 24 (Suppl 2):121.

1204. Hollister LE. Interactions between alcohol and benzodiazepines. Rec Dev Alcohol 1989; 7:233.

1205. Lejoyeux M, Solomon J, Ades J. Benzodiazepine treatment for alcohol-dependent patients. Alcohol Alcohol 1998; 33:563.

1206. Johnstone EC, Owens DGC, Frith DC, et al. Neurotic illness and its response to anxiolytic and antidepressant treatment. Psychol Med 1980; 10:321.

1207. Bruno F. Buspirone in the treatment of alcoholic patients. Psychopathology 1989; 22 (Suppl 1): 49.

1208. Kranzler HR, Meyer RE. An open trial of buspirone in alcoholics. J Clin Psychopharmacol 1989; 9:379.

1209. Rickels K, Chung HR, Csanalos IB, et al. Alprazolam, diazepam, imipramine, placebo in outpatients with general depression. Arch Gen Psychiatry 1987; 44:862.

1210. Barbee JG, Clark PD, Carpanzano MS, et al. Alcohol and substance abuse among schizophrenic patients presenting to an emergency psychiatric service. J Nerv Ment Dis 1989; 177:400.

1211. June HL, Greene TL, Murphy JM, et al. Effects of the benzodiazepine inverse agonist RO19-4603 alone and in combination with the benzodiazepine antagonists flumazenil, ZK 93426 and CGS 8216, on ethanol intake in alcohol-preferring (P) rats. Brain Res 1996; 734:19.

1212. June HL, Deveraju SL, Eggers MW, et al. Benzodiazepine receptor antagonists modulate the actions of ethanol in alcohol-preferring and nonpreferring rats. Eur J Pharmacol 1998; 342:139.

1212a. Johnson BA, Ait-Daoud N, Bowden CL, et al. Oral topiramate for treatment of alcohol dependence: a randomized controlled trial. Lancet 2003; 361:1677.

1213. Wright C, Moore RD. Disulfiram treatment of alcoholism. Am J Med 1990; 88:647.

1214. Fisher DM. "Catatonia" due to disulfiram toxicity. Arch Neurol 1989; 46:798.

1215. Goldfrank LR. Disulfiram and disulfiram-like reactions. In: Goldfrank LR, Fromenbaum NE, Lewin NA, et al, eds. Goldfrank's Toxicologic Emergencies, 6th edition. Norwalk, CT: Appleton & Lange, 1998; 1043.

1216. Sellers EM, Naranjo CA, Peachey JE. Drugs to decrease alcohol consumption. N Engl J Med 1981; 305:1255.

1217. Fuller RK, Roth HP. Disulfiram for the treatment of alcoholism: an evaluation of 128 men. Ann Intern Med 1979; 90:901.

1218. Fuller RK, Branchey L, Brightwell DR, et al. Disulfiram treatment of alcoholism. A Veteran's Administration Cooperative Study. JAMA 1986; 256:1449.

1219. Tennant FS. Disulfiram will reduce medical complications but not cure alcoholism. JAMA 1986; 256:1489.

1220. Schukit MA. A one-year follow-up of men given disulfiram. J Stud Alcohol 1985; 46:191.

1221. American College of Physicians. Disulfiram treatment of alcoholism. Ann Intern Med 1989; 111:943.

1222. Wilson A, Davidson WJ, Blanchard R, White J. Disulfiram implantation: trial using placebo implants and two types of controls. J Stud Alcohol 1980; 41:429.

1223. Hughes JC, Cook CC. The efficacy of disulfiram: a review of outcome studies. Addiction 1997; 92:381.

1224. Palliyath SK, Schwartz BD, Gant L. Peripheral nerve functions in chronic alcoholic patients on disulfiram: a six-month follow-up. J Neurol Neurosurg Psychiatry 1990; 53:227.

1225. Engjusen-Poulsen H, Loft S, Anderson JR, Anderson M. Disulfiram therapy: adverse drug reactions and interactions. Acta Psychiatr Scand 1992; 86 (Suppl 369): 59.

1226. Dano P, Tammam D, Brosset C, Bregigeon M. Les neuropathies périphériques dues au disulfirame. Rev Neurol 1996; 152:294.

1227. Weimer LH. Medication-induced peripheral neuropathy. Curr Neurol Neurosci Rep 2003; 3:86.

1228. Chick J. Safety issues concerning the use of disulfiram in treating alcohol dependence. Drug Saf 1999; 20:427.

1229. Rothrock JF, Johnson PC, Rothrock SM, Merkley R. Fulminant polyneuritis after overdose of disulfiram and ethanol. Neurology 1984; 34:357.

1230. Park CW, Riggio S. Disulfiram–ethanol delirium. Ann Pharmacother 2001; 35:32.

1231. Reitnauer PJ, Callanan NP, Farber RA, Aylsworth AS. Prenatal exposure to disulfiram implicated in the cause of malformations in discordant monozygotic twins. Teratology 1997; 56:358.

1232. Peachey JE, Annis HM, Bornstein ER, et al. Calcium carbimide in alcoholism treatment. 2. Medical findings of a short-term, placebo-controlled, double-blind clinical trial. Br J Addict 1989; 84:1359.

1233. Scott GE, Little FW. Disulfiram reaction to organic solvents other than ethanol. N Engl J Med 1985; 313:790.

1234. Barna P. Alcohol in anti-asthma elixirs. Lancet 1985; I:753.

1235. Kline NS, Wren JC, Cooper TB, et al. Evaluation of lithium therapy in chronic and periodic alcoholism. Am J Med Sci 1974; 268:15.

1236. Ho AK, Tsai CS. Effects of lithium on alcohol preference and withdrawal. Ann N Y Acad Sci 1976; 273:371.

1237. Dorus W, Ostow DG, Anton R, et al. Lithium treatment of depressed and non-depressed alcoholics. JAMA 1989; 262:1646.

1238. de la Fuente J-R, Morse RM, Niven RG, Ilstrup DM. A controlled study of lithium carbonate in the treatment of alcoholism. Mayo Clin Proc 1989; 64:177.

1239. Mueller TI, Stout RL, Rudden S, et al. A double-blind, placebo-controlled pilot study of carbamazepine for the treatment of alcohol dependence. Alcohol Clin Exp Res 1997; 21:86.

1240. Pettinati H. Use of serotonin selective pharmacotherapy in the treatment of alcohol dependence. Alcohol Clin Exp Res 1996; 20 (Suppl):23A.

1241. Yoshimoto K, McBride WJ, Lumeng L, Li TK. Ethanol enhances the release of dopamine and serotonin in the nucleus accumbens of HAD and

LAD lines of rats. Alcohol Clin Exp Res 1992; 16:781.

1242. McBride WJ, Bodart B, Lumeng L, Li TK. Association between low contents of dopamine and serotonin in the nucleus accumbens and high alcohol preference. Acohol Clin Exp Res 1995; 19:1420.

1243. Overstreet D, Rezvani A, Pucilowski O, Janowski D. 5-HT receptors: implications for the neuropharmacology of alcohol and alcoholism. Alcohol Alcohol 1995; 2 (Suppl):207.

1244. Higley J, Hasert M, Suomi S, Linnoila M. The serotonin reuptake inhibitor sertraline reduces alcohol consumption in nonhuman primates: effect of stress. Neuropsychopharmacology 1998; 18:431.

1245. Swift R, Davidson D, Whelihan W, Kuznetsov O. Ondansetron alters human alcohol intoxication. Biol Psychiatry 1995; 40:514.

1246. Buydens-Branchey L, Branchey MH, Nomair D, Lieber CS. Age of alcoholism onset. 2. Relationship of susceptibility to serotonin precursor availability. Arch Gen Psychiatry 1989; 46:231.

1247. Naranjo CA, Sellers EM, Sullivan JT, et al. The serotonin uptake inhibitor citalopram attenuates alcohol intake. Clin Pharmacol Ther 1987; 41:266.

1248. Naranjo CA, Sellers EM, Roach CA, et al. Zimelidine-induced variations in alcohol intake by non-depressed heavy drinkers. Clin Pharmacol Ther 1984; 35:374.

1249. Naranjo CA, Kadlec KE, Sanhueza P, et al. Fluoxetine differentially alters alcohol intake and other consummatory behaviors in problem drinkers. Clin Pharmacol Ther 1990; 47:490.

1250. Johnson BA, Ait-Daoud N. Neuropharmacological treatments for alcoholism: scientific basis and clinical findings. Psychopharmacology 2000; 149:327.

1251. Gorelick D, Pardes A. Effect of fluoxetine on alcohol consumption in male alcoholics. Alcohol Clin Exp Res 1992; 16:261.

1252. Kabel D, Petty F. A double-blind study of fluoxetine in severe alcohol dependence: adjunctive therapy during and after inpatient treatment. Alcohol Clin Exp Res 1996; 20:780.

1253. Kranzler HR, Burleson JA, Korner P, et al. Placebo-controlled trial of fluoxetine as an adjunct to relapse prevention in alcoholics. Am J Psychiatry 1995; 152:391.

1254. Janiri L, Gobbi G, Manneli P, Pozzi G. Effects of fluoxetine and antidepressant doses on short-term outcome of detoxified alcoholics. Int J Clin Psychopharmacol 1996; 11:109.

1255. Cornelius JR, Salloum IM, Ehler JG, et al. Fluoxetine in depressed alcoholics: a double-blind, placebo-controlled trial. Arch Gen Psychiatry 1997; 54:700.

1256. Tiihonen J, Ryynaenen O-P, Kauhanen J, Hakola H. Citalopram in the treatment of alcoholism: a double-blind, placebo-controlled study. Pharmacopsychiatry 1996; 29:27.

1257. Kranzler HR, Burleson JA, Brown J, Babor TF. Fluoxetine treatment seems to reduce the beneficial effects of cognitive-behavioral therapy in type B alcoholics. Alcohol Clin Exp Res 1996; 20:1534.

1258. Pettinati HM, Oslin D, Decker K. Role of serotonin and serotonin-selective pharmacotherapy in alcohol dependence. CNS Spect 2000; 5:33.

1259. Pettinati HM, Volpicelli JR, Luck G, et al. Double-blind clinical trial of sertraline treatment for alcohol dependence. J Clin Psychopharmacol 2001; 21:143.

1260. Malec TS, Malec EA, Dongier M. Efficacy of buspirone in alcohol dependence: a review. Alcohol Clin Exp Res 1996; 20:853.

1261. Tollefson G, Montague-Clouse J, Tollefson S. Treatment of comorbid generalized anxiety in a recently detoxified alcoholic population with a selective serotonergic drug (buspirone). J Clin Psychopharmacol 1992; 12:19.

1262. Kranzler HR, Burleson JA, Del Boca FK, et al. Buspirone treatment of anxious alcoholics. A placebo-controlled trial. Arch Gen Psychiatry 1994; 51:720.

1263. Malcolm R, Anton R, Randall C, et al. A placebo-controlled trial of buspirone in anxious inpatient alcoholics. Alcohol Clin Exp Res 1992; 16:1007.

1264. George D, Rawlings R, Eckardt M, et al. Buspirone treatment of alcoholism: age of onset and cerebrospinal fluid 5-hydroxyindoleacetic acid and homovanillic acid concentrations but not medication treatment predict return to drinking. Alcohol Clin Exp Res 1999; 23:272.

1265. Johnson BA, Jasinski DR, Galloway GP, et al. Ritanserin in the treatment of alcohol dependence—a multicenter clinical trial. Psychopharmacology 1996; 128:206.

1266. Wiesbeck GA, Weigers HG, Chick J, et al. Ritanserin in relapse prevention in abstinent alcoholics: results from a placebo-controlled double-blind international multicenter trial. Alcohol Clin Exp Res 1999; 23:230.

1267. Johnson BA, Campling GM, Griffiths P, Cowen PJ. Attenuation of some alcohol-induced mood changes and the desire to drink by 5HT$_3$ receptor blockade: a preliminary study in healthy male volunteers. Psychopharmacology 1993; 112:142.

1268. Sellers EM, Toneatto T, Romach MK, et al. Clinical efficacy of the 5-HT$_3$ antagonist ondansetron in alcohol abuse and dependence. Alcohol Clin Exp Res 1994; 18:879.

1269. Fadda F, Franch F, Mosca E, et al. Inhibition of voluntary ethanol intake in rats by a combination of dihydroergotoxine and thioridazine. Alcohol Drug Res 1987; 7:285.

1270. Soyka M, DeVry J. Flupenthixol as a potential pharmacotreatment of alcohol and cocaine abuse/dependence. Eur Neuropsychopharmacol 2000; 10:325.

1271. Shaw GK, Waller S, Majumdar SK, et al. Tiapride in the prevention of relapse in recently detoxified alcoholics. Br J Psychiatry 1994; 165:515.

1272. Walter H, Ramskogler K, Semler B, et al. Dopamine and alcohol relapse: D_1 and D_2 antagonists increase relapse rates in animal studies and in clinical trials. J Biomed Sci 2001; 8:83.

1273. Blum K. Suppression of alcohol craving by enkephalinase inhibition: a new opportunity in clinical treatment. Alcohol Drug Res 1987; 7:122.

1274. Herz A. Endogenous opioid systems and alcohol addiction. Psychopharmacology 1997; 129:99.

1275. Siegel S. Alcohol and opiate dependence: reevaluation of the Victorian perspective. In: Cappell HD, Glaser FB, Isreal Y, et al, eds. Research Advances in Alcohol and Drug Problems, Vol 9. New York: Plenum Press, 1986:279.

1276. Sinclair JD. The feasibility of effective psychopharmacological treatments for alcoholism. Br J Addict 1987; 82:1213.

1277. Froehlich JC, Harts J, Lumeng L, Li TK. Naloxone attenuates voluntary ethanol intake in rats selectively bred for high ethanol preference. Pharmacol Biochem Behav 1990; 35:385.

1278. Myers RD, Borg S, Mossberg R. Antagonism by naltrexone of voluntary alcohol selection in the chronically drinking macaque monkey. Alcohol 1986; 3:383.

1279. Boyle AE, Stewart RB, Macenski MJ, et al. Effects of acute and chronic doses of naltrexone on ethanol self-administration in rhesus monkeys. Alcohol Clin Exp Res 1998; 22:359.

1280. Benjamin D, Grant E, Pohorecky LA. Naltrexone reverses ethanol-induced dopamine release in the nucleus accumbens of awake, freely moving rats. Brain Res 1993; 621:137.

1281. Swift RM, Whelihan W, Kuznetsov O, et al. Naltrexone-induced alterations in human ethanol intoxication. Am J Psychiatry 1994; 151:1463.

1282. Volpicelli JR, Watson NT, King AC, et al. Effect of naltrexone on alcohol "high" in alcoholics. Am J Psychiatry 1995; 152:613.

1283. Swift RM. Drug therapy for alcohol dependence. N Engl J Med 1999; 340:1482.

1284. Volpicelli JR, Alterman AI, Hayashida M, O'Brien CP. Naltrexone in the treatment of alcohol dependence. Arch Gen Psychiatry 1992; 49:876.

1285. O'Malley SS, Jaffee AJ, Chang G, et al. Naltrexone and coping skills therapy for alcohol dependence: a controlled study. Arch Gen Psychiatry 1992; 49:881.

1286. O'Malley SS, Jaffee AJ, Chang G, et al. Six-month follow-up of naltrexone and psychotherapy for alcohol dependence. Arch Gen Psychiatry 1996; 53:217.

1287. Anton RF, Moak DH, Waid R, et al. Naltrexone and cognitive behavioral therapy for the treatment of outpatient alcoholics: results of a placebo-controlled trial. Am J Psychiatry 1999; 156:1758.

1288. Hersh D, Van Kirk JR, Kranzler HR. Naltrexone treatment of comorbid alcohol and cocaine use disorders. Psychopharmacology 1998; 139:44.

1289. Litten RZ, Allen J. Advances in the development of medications for alcoholism. Psychopharmacology 1998; 139:20.

1290. McCaul ME, Wand GE, Sullivan J, et al. Beta-naltrexol level predicts alcohol relapse. Alcohol Clin Exp Res 1997; 21:32A.

1291. Kranzler HR, Modesto-Lowe V, Van Kirk JD. Naltrexone versus nefazadone for treatment of alcohol dependence. A placebo controlled trial. Neuropsychopharmacology 2000; 22:493.

1292. Krystal JH, Cramer JA, Krol WF, et al. Naltrexone in the treatment of alcohol dependence. N Engl J Med 2001; 345:1734.

1293. Fuller RK, Gordis E. Naltrexone treatment for alcohol dependence. N Engl J Med 2001; 345:1770.

1293a. Gastpar M, Bonnet U, Böning J, et al. Lack of efficacy of naltrexone in the prevention of alcohol relapse: results from a German multicenter study. J Clin Psychopharmacol 2002; 22:592.

1294. Rubio G, Jiménez-Arriero MA, Ponce G, et al. Naltrexone versus acamprosate: one year follow-up of alcohol dependence. Alcohol Alcohol 2001; 36: 419.

1295. Heinälä P, Alho H, Kiianmaa K, et al. Targeted use of naltrexone without prior detoxification in the treatment of alcohol dependence: a factorial double-blind, placebo-controlled trial. J Clin Psychopharmacol 2001; 21:287.

1295a. Guardia J, Caso C, Arias F, et al. A double-blind, placebo-controlled study of naltrexone in the treatment of alcohol-dependence disorder: results from a multicenter clinical trial. Alcohol Clin Exp Res 2002; 26:1381.

1295b. Srisurapanont M, Jarusuraisin N. Opioid antagonists for alcohol dependence. Cochrane Database of Systematic Reviews 2002; (2):CD001867.

1295c. Ait-Daoud N, Johnson BA, Martin J, et al. Combining ondansetron and naltrexone treats biological alcoholics: corroboration of self-reported drinking by serum carbohydrate deficient transferrin, a biomarker. Alcohol Clin Exp Res 2001; 25:847.

1296. Mason BJ, Salvato FR, Williams LD, et al. A double-blind, placebo-controlled study of oral nalmephine for alcohol dependence. Arch Gen Psychiatry 1999; 56:719.

1297. Rammes G, Mahal B, Putzke J, et al. The anti-craving compound acamprosate acts as a weak NMDA-receptor antagonist, but modulates NMDA-receptor subunit expression similar to memantine and MK-801. Neuropharmacology 2001; 40:749.

1297a. Mason BJ. Acamprosate. Rec Dev Alcohol 2003; 16:203.

1298. Wilde MI, Wagstaff AJ. Acamprosate: a review of its pharmacology and clinical potential in the management of alcohol dependence after detoxification. Drugs 1997; 53:1038.

1298a. McGeehan AJ, Olive MF. The anti-relapse compound acamprosate inhibits the development of a conditioned place preference to ethanol and cocaine but not morphine. Br J Pharmacol 2003; 138:9.

1299. Mason BJ, Ownby RL. Acamprosate for the treatment of alcohol dependence: a review of double-blind, placebo-controlled trials. CNS Spectrums 2000; 5: 58.

1300. Krystal JH, Petrakis IL, Webb E, et al. Dose-related ethanol-like effects of the NMDA antagonist, ketamine, in recently detoxified alcoholics. Arch Gen Psychiatry 1998; 55:354.

1301. Krupitsky EM, Grinenko AY. Ketamine psychedelic therapy (KPT): a review of the results of ten years of research. J Psychoactive Drugs 1997; 29:165.

1302. Moncini M, Masini E, Gambassi F, Mannaioni PF. Gamma-hydroxybutyric acid and alcohol-related syndromes. Alcohol 2000; 20:285.

1303. Gessa GL, Agabio R, Carai MAM, et al. Mechanism of the antialcohol effect of gamma-hydroxybutyric acid. Alcohol 2000; 20:271.

1304. Gallimberti L, Ferri M, Ferrara SD, et al. Gamma-hydroxybutyric acid in the treatment of alcohol dependence: a double-blind study. Alcohol Clin Exp Res 1992; 16:673.

1305. Addolorato G, Caputo F, Capristo E, et al. Gamma-hydroxybutyric acid: efficacy, potential abuse, and dependence in the treatment of alcohol addiction. Alcohol 2000; 20:217.

1306. Gallimberti L, Spella MR, Soncini A, Gessa GL. Gamma-hydroxybutyric acid in the treatment of alcohol and heroin dependence. Alcohol 2000; 20: 257.

1307. Rush CR, Pazzaglia PJ. Pretreatment with isradipine, a calcium channel blocker, does not attenuate the acute behavioral effects of ethanol in humans. Alcohol Clin Exp Res 1998; 22:539.

1308. Keung W-M, Valee BL. Daidzin and daidzein suppress free-choice ethanol intake by Syrian Golden hamsters. Proc Natl Acad Sci USA 1993; 90:10008.

1309. Lin RC, Li TK. Effects of isoflavones on alcohol pharmacokinetics and alcohol-drinking behavior in rats. Am J Clin Nutr 1998; 68:1512S.

1310. Ehlers CL, Li TK Lumeng L, et al. Neuropeptide Y levels in ethanol-naïve alcohol-prefering and non-preferring rats and in Wistar rats after ethanol exposure. Alcohol Clin Exp Res 1998; 22:1778.

1311. Ehlers CL, Somes C, Cloutier D. Are some of the effects of ethanol mediated through NPY? Psychopharmacology 1998; 139:136.

1312. Hungund BK, Basavarajappa BS. Are anandamide and cannabinoid receptors involved in ethanol tolerance? A review of the evidence. Alcohol Alcohol 2000; 35:126.

1313. Arnone M, Marvani J, Chaperon F, et al. Selective inhibition of sucrose and ethanol intake by SR141716, an antagonist of central cannabinoid (CB1) receptors. Psychopharmacology 1997; 132:104.

1314. Colombo G, Agabio R, FA M, et al. Reduction of voluntary ethanol intake in ethanol-preferring sP rats by the cannabinoid antagonist SR-141716. Alcohol Alcohol 1998; 33:126.

1315. Gallate JE, McGregor IS. The motivation for beer in rats: effects of ritanserin, naloxone, and SR141716. Psychopharmacology 1999; 142:302.

1316. Mangini M. Treatment of alcoholism using psychedelic drugs: a review of the program of research. J Psychoactive Drugs 1998; 30:381.

1317. Abuzzahab FS, Anderson J. A review of LSD treatment in alcoholism. Int Pharmacopsychiatr 1971; 6:223.

1318. Zhou FC, McKinzie DL, Patel TD, et al. Additive reduction of alcohol drinking by 5HT$_{1A}$ antagonist WAY100635 and serotonin uptake blocker fluoxetine in alcohol-preferring P rats. Alcohol Clin Exp Res 1998; 22:266.

1319. Farren CK, Rezvani AH, Overstreet D, O'Malley S. Combination pharmacotherapy in alcoholism: a novel treatment approach. CNS Spectrums 2000; 5:70.

1320. Ait-Daoud N, Johnson BA, Javors M, et al. Combining ondansetron and naltrexone treats biological alcoholics: corroboration of self-reported drinking by serum carbohydrate deficient transferrin, a biomarker. Alcohol Clin Exp Res 2001; 25:847.

1321. Classics of the alcohol literature: the first American medical work on the effects of alcohol: Benjamin Rush's "An inquiry into the effects of ardent spirits upon the human body and mind" (1795). Q J Stud Alcohol 1943; 4:321.

1322. Trice HM, Staudenmeier WJ. A sociocultural history of Alcoholics Anonymous. Rec Dev Alcohol 1989; 7:11.

1323. Delbanco A, Delbanco T. A.A. at the crossroads. The New Yorker, 1995; March 20:50.

1324. Ogborne AC. Some limitations of Alcoholics Anonymous. Rec Dev Alcohol 1989; 7:55.

1325. Emrick CD. Alcoholics Anonymous: membership characteristics and effectiveness as treatment. Rec Dev Alcohol 1989; 7:37.

1326. Vaillant GE. The Natural History of Alcoholism. Cambridge, MA: Harvard University Press, 1983.

1327. Bullock ML, Culliton PD, Olander RT. Controlled trial of acupuncture for severe recidivist alcoholism. Lancet 1989; I:1435.

1328. Editorial. Many points to needle. Lancet 1990; I:20.

1329. Mayer DJ. Acupuncture: an evidence-based review of the clinical literature. Annu Rev Med 2000; 51: 49.

1330. Goodwin DW. Inpatient treatment of alcoholism—new life for the Minneapolis plan. N Engl J Med 1991; 325:804.

1331. Walsh DC, Hingson RW, Merrigan DM, et al. A randomized trial of treatment options for alcohol-abusing workers. N Engl J Med 1991; 325:775.

1332. Treatment. In: Hurley J, Horowitz J, eds. Alcohol and Health. New York: Hemisphere Publishing, 1987: 120.

1333. Sobell MB, Sobell LC. Second year treatment outcome of alcoholics treated by individualized behavior therapy: results. Behav Res Ther 1976; 14:195.

1334. Helzer JE, Robins LN, Taylor JR, et al. The extent of long-term moderate drinking among alcoholics discharged from medical and psychiatric treatment facilities. N Engl J Med 1985; 312:1678.

1335. Kissin B, Hanson M. Integrations of biological and psychological interventions in the treatment of alcoholism. In: McCrady BS, Noel NE, Nirenberg TD, eds. Future Directions in Alcohol Abuse Treatment and Research. Washington, DC: DHHS Publication No. (ADM) 85–1322, US Government Printing Office, 1988; 63.

1336. Pendery ML, Maltzman IM, West LJ. Controlled drinking by alcoholics: new findings and a reevaluation of a major affirmative study. Science 1982; 217:169.

1337. Kanaka TS, Balasubramaniam V. Stereotactic cingulotomy for drug addiction. Appl Neurophysiol 1978; 41:86.

1338. Dieckman G, Schneider H. Influence of stereotactic hypothalamotomy on alcohol and drug addiction. Appl Neurophysiol 1978; 41:93.

1339. Schottenfeld RS. Drug and alcohol testing in the workplace—objectives, pitfalls, and guidelines. Am J Drug Alcohol Abuse 1989; 15:413.

1340. Isikoff M. The nation's alcohol problem is falling through the crack. Washington Post National Weekly Edition, 1990; April 9:30.

Chapter 13
Tobacco

The use of tobacco is growing greatly and conquers men with a certain secret pleasure, so that those who have become accustomed thereto can later hardly be restrained therefrom.
—Sir Francis Bacon, Historia vitae et mortis (1623)

For thy sake, tobacco, I
Would do anything but die.
—Charles Lamb

We are in the business of selling nicotine, an addictive drug.
—Internal memo by Brown & Williamson's General Counsel (1963)

Each year, more than 400,000 Americans die as a consequence of cigarette smoking. Put another way, tobacco kills more than 1000 Americans every day. Or, put another way, tobacco accounts for 20% to 25% of all American mortality (compared with 5% for ethanol and less than 3% for all the other drugs discussed in this book).[1–6] Worldwide, tobacco causes over 3 million deaths annually. More than a third of the world's adult population smokes, and half of those who continue smoking will die prematurely from smoking related diseases.[7] Amidst such carnage, most Americans who smoke claim they would stop if they could. There is no question therefore that tobacco is addicting. It is also evident that the addictive substance in tobacco is nicotine (Figure 13–1).[8–10]

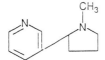

Figure 13–1. Nicotine.

Pharmacology and Animal Studies

Effects in Animals

Nicotine's pharmacological actions are biphasic: low doses stimulate nicotinic receptors, and higher doses block them. Acting both peripherally and centrally, nicotine produces complex effects. For example, heart rate may be either increased or decreased depending on actions at sympathetic and parasympathetic ganglia, carotid and aortic bodies, medullary centers, and the adrenal as well as on compensatory reflexes.[11] Central nervous system (CNS) stimulation causes tremor or seizures; CNS depression causes respiratory failure. An alerting response in the electroencephalogram may be accompanied by decreased muscle tone and reduced amplitude in the electromyogram.

In rats, dogs, and monkeys, high doses of nicotine depress locomotion, often with ataxia.[12] Low doses increase locomotion, and tolerance develops to the depressant effect of high doses but not to the stimulatory effect of low doses. Thus with chronic administration of high doses, increased locomotion emerges. In monkeys nicotine reduces aggression.[13] Nicotine improves the performance of rodents and primates on tasks involving memory, learning, and sustained attention.[14–16] In novices, nicotine causes nausea and vomiting by stimulating vagal afferents and the medullary chemoreceptor trigger zone. It also reduces appetite, mainly for sweet-tasting foods; both decreased caloric intake and increased metabolic rate and energy expenditure contribute to weight loss.[17]

Nicotine acts as a discriminative stimulus in animals, generalizing to nicotinic agonists and partially to amphetamine and cocaine.[18,19] Place preference and self-administration studies in rats, dogs, and primates confirm that nicotine is reinforcing, although less so than cocaine, and aversive effects of nicotine at high doses limits the dosage range at which it is reinforcing.[13,20–23] (Very high doses of nicotine cause vomiting, tremors, convulsions, and death.) Perhaps reflecting tolerance to nicotine's depressant effects, self-administration steadily increases during the first week of availability. Once self-administration has been established, environmental cues associated with drug delivery become powerful conditioned reinforcers—as much so as nicotine itself.[24] Nicotine's reinforcing actions are blocked by the nicotinic receptor antagonist mecamylamine. The varying degrees of tolerance to nicotine's effects appear to be more pharmacodynamic than dispositional.

Withdrawal following chronic administration in rats produces signs that peak at 18 to 22 hours and include teeth chattering, chewing, gasping, writhing, head shakes, body shakes, tremors, and ptosis; less often there is ejaculation and hind foot scratching. Increased startle response suggests heightened anxiety. Increased threshold for electrical brain-stimulation reward suggests anhedonia or a rodent equivalent of depression. These signs can be precipitated by nicotine antagonists and reversed by injection of nicotine.[19,25–27]

Nicotine, Acetylcholine Receptors, and Other Neurotransmitters/Neuromodulators

Nicotine acetylcholine receptors (nAChRs) belong to a superfamily of ligand-gated ion channels that include $GABA_A$, $5-HT_3$ serotonin, and glycine receptors. The receptor-channel complex is composed of five polypeptide subunits assembled like a rosette around a central pore. Different subunit combinations produce nAChR subtypes with different properties (e.g., speed of activation, rate of desensitization). The mammalian CNS contains nAChRs with varying combinations of $\alpha2/\alpha6$ and $\beta2/\beta4$ subunits, as well as nAChRs composed entirely of $\alpha7$ subunits. α/β nAChRs are blocked by mecamylamine; $\alpha7$ homomeric nAChRs are blocked by α-bungarotoxin.[25,28]

Physiologically released ACh is present at nAChRs for less than 2 milliseconds before being hydrolyzed by acetylcholinesterase. By contrast, nicotine, which is not broken down by acetylcholinesterase, persists in low concentration at nAChRs, causing receptor desensitization. Moreover, desensitized nAChRs have a higher affinity for agonists than resting or open nAChRs, resulting in desensitization without activation.[29] Another feature of nAChRs is that those with desensitized conformations are turned over more slowly in the cell membrane, resulting in an increase in their number. nAChR desensitization probably explains why animals have higher lever-pressing rates when nicotine is delivered intermittently rather than continuously and why tobacco addicts often report that the first cigarette smoked is the most pleasurable of the day. Increased numbers of long-lived, nonfunctional, desensitized nAChRs is of obvious relevance to nicotine tolerance, sensitization, and withdrawal.[30]

Distributed along an axis from the spinal cord to the basal telencephalon, cholinergic neurons project to nearly all brain areas. A major subsystem, projecting from the basal forebrain to the cerebral cortex and the hippocampus, probably accounts for nicotine's positive effects on memory and learning.[16] Another subsystem projects from the pedunculopontine tegmental nucleus and the laterodorsal pontine tegmental nucleus to thalamic and midbrain areas, including the ventral tegmental area (VTA) of the "reward circuit." Activation of nAChRs on presynaptic terminals causes a calcium influx that increases the release of nearly every neurotransmitter that has been studied.[30,31]

Like other addictive drugs, nicotine elevates dopamine in the nucleus accumbens (NA), and self-administration of nicotine by rats is blocked by dopamine antagonists or lesions of the NA.[32–34]

Dopamine release is facilitated by activation of nAChRs (especially those of the α2/β4 type, but also those consisting of α7 subunits) on dopaminergic neurons, as well as by activation of nAChRs on glutamatergic neurons in the VTA. The degree to which nicotine enhancement of gamma-aminobutyric acid (GABA), norepinephrine, and serotonin neurotransmission indirectly contributes to dopamine release is less certain.[31] (Nicotine injected into the serotonergic dorsal raphe nucleus in rats is anxiolytic, an effect blocked by an α4/β2 subunit receptor blocker.[35])

β2 subunit knockout mice do not self-administer nicotine, and they have a raised threshold to the effects of cocaine, including drug-seeking and NA dopaminergic release.[36,37] Conversely, previous nicotine exposure enhances the acquisition of intravenous cocaine self-administration in rats, and repeated exposure to nicotine causes not only behavioral sensitization to nicotine but also cross-sensitization to other addictive drugs. Moreover, psychostimulants, opioids, and other drugs of abuse enhance the release of ACh in the NA. Thus by increasing dopaminergic tone, nicotine influences synaptic plasticity in the reward circuit and cholinergic neurotransmission appears to play an important role in the development of sensitization to a variety of addictive agents.[38] Comparable effects in the hippocampus, moreover, might link nicotine addiction with memory and learned associates of tobacco use.[27,28,39]

nAChR subunits appear very early in embryogenesis, and stimulation of nAChRs appears to play an important role in the guidance of growth cones and the formation of synapses.[28,39]

During nicotine withdrawal in rats there is reduced dopamine release in the NA and also in the central nucleus of the amygdala, a nucleus associated with anxiety and stress responses and normally inhibited by dopamine.[40] Opioid systems probably contribute to nicotine withdrawal signs, for naloxone can precipitate them (without inducing a reduction of dopamine release in the NA) and morphine can reverse them.[26] Nitric oxide synthase (NOS) inhibitors, which attenuate morphine abstinence signs, also attenuate nicotine abstinence signs.[26] Other neurotransmitters and neuromodulators implicated in the expression of nicotine withdrawal (and of obvious relevance to the pharmacology of smoking cessation) are serotonin,

norepinephrine, glutamate, cholecystokinin-B, corticotropin releasing factor, and substance P.[25] Peripherally located nAChRs probably contribute to somatic signs of nicotine withdrawal, which can occur in the absence of affective signs and vice versa.[25]

Historical Background and Epidemiology

Origins

Nicotiana tabacum, a broad-leafed annual plant native to the Americas, was first cultivated in the Peruvian Andes between 5000 and 3000 BCE.[41,41a] Spreading throughout North and South America it was used medicinally, ritualistically (large doses induce hallucinatory trances), and recreationally by chewing, eating, drinking, and, most often, smoking, either as a cigar or in a pipe (including that symbol of friendship, the "peace pipe"). Tobacco eye drops and enemas were also available. Columbus and other New World explorers brought tobacco back to Europe, where the compulsive nature of smoking was quickly recognized. By the end of the 16th century tobacco was cultivated in Japan, China, India, Southeast Asia, Africa, and the Middle East (where it was welcomed as a drug not forbidden by the Koran).

Jean Nicot, a French envoy stationed in Lisbon, convinced of tobacco's healing powers (within the Galenic system, he identified it as "hot and dry"), sent plants and seeds to Catherine deMedici, the Queen of France, and soon afterward the "Nicotian herb" was grown in the gardens of the Vatican. It was taken as a snuff to treat an array of diseases, including kidney stones, toothache, tapeworms, dandruff, halitosis, and, in cattle, foot-and-mouth disease. Its reputation as an endurance enhancer and appetite suppressant increased its popularity as a sniffed or smoked recreational drug, as did, of course, its addictive liability. In 1735 Carolus Linnaeus named the tobacco plant *Nicotiana tabacum* in honor of Jean Nicot.

The first recorded ban on tobacco was in Lima in 1588; an ecclesiastical decree forbade priests to use tobacco during the mass. In 1604 King James I of England, associating tobacco with witchcraft, pronounced smoking "… a custom loathsome to the eye, hateful to the nose, harmful to the brain, dangerous to the lungs, and in the black, stinking fume thereof nearest resembling the horrible Stygian smoke of the pit that is bottomless." James forbade domestic production of tobacco and raised the duty on tobacco by 4000%. During the 17th century tobacco was banned in Japan, Bavaria, Switzerland, Saxony and by the Greek Orthodox Church, and its consumption was punishable by death in Russia, China, and the Ottoman Empire. (The Ottoman ruler, Murad IV, put to death more than 25,000 smokers.) During the same century, however, tobacco cultivating and trade steadily increased, including the first brand-name product, Orinoco, marketed by John Rolfe of the Jamestown Virginia Company. By 1700, Orinoco exports (inextricably linked to the slave trade) reached £38 million. George Washington was a tobacco farmer, Benjamin Franklin published advertisements for America's oldest tobacco company, P. Lorillard & Co., and a majority of the men who signed the Declaration of Independence were involved in the tobacco trade.

In 1828, Ludwig Reinmann and Wilhelm Heinrich isolated and named "nicotine," which was reported to be of benefit in treating malaria, tetanus, a variety of nervous system disorders, and, via tobacco enemas, hemorrhoids. Worldwide additions to the tobacco industry included hugely popular Cuban cigars (which stayed fresh longer than bulk tobacco) and Spanish "papelotes"— shredded tobacco wrapped in paper—which became fashionable in France as "cigarettes." In 1839 in North Carolina a new curing process produced tobacco with acidic smoke that was readily absorbed from the lungs but not from the mouth and which could be inhaled without causing undesired degrees of intoxication. Cigarettes containing this new product soon dominated the market. Between 1875 and 1880 U.S. cigarette consumption grew from 42 million to 500 million. Following the invention of a cigarette-making machine in 1880, annual consumption rose in 1889 to 2.2 billion. In 1920 it was over 100 billion.

Recent History

Under pressure from industry lobbyists, tobacco was exempted from the 1906 U.S. Food and Drugs Act, and during World Wars I and II the federal government provided cigarettes to U.S. servicemen. In 1950, however, reports began to appear statistically linking smoking and lung cancer.[42] In 1964 the U.S. Surgeon General issued a report, "Smoking and Health," which documented tobacco's causative role. The tobacco industry's response was to deny the evidence ("It's a statistical not a causal relationship"), and following its success in 1966 in watering down warning labels on cigarette packs ("cigarette smoking may be hazardous to your health") U.S. cigarette sales continued to rise.

In 1981 reports began to link passive inhalation of "environmental tobacco smoke" with lung cancer and other respiratory diseases; in 1986 a U.S. Surgeon General's Report endorsed the association; and in 1992 a U.S. Environmental Protection Agency (EPA) report identified secondhand smoke as a Group A human carcinogen.[42a] This time the tobacco industry not only denied the epidemiological evidence, but established front organizations to fund scientists who would receive highly secret "special project" awards the purpose of which was to discredit the EPA report.[43,44] (Billed as "nonprofit," these organizations bear names such as "The Advancement for Sound Science Coalition," "The Centre for Corporate Social Responsibility," "The Risk Science Institute," and "The Center for Indoor Air Research.") According to the U.S. Centers for Disease Control, of the 442,398 Americans who died in 1999 because of tobacco, 35,053 died as a consequence of exposure to secondhand smoke.[45,45a,46]

In 1988, for the first time ever, the family of a lung cancer victim won a lawsuit against a tobacco company. There followed legal action by several U.S. states against American cigarette manufacturers, which led to public release of the companies' internal documents. These revealed (1) that tobacco executives had been fully aware for decades of the addictive and carcinogenic properties of tobacco and (2) that marketing was specifically directed at children.[46,47] In a Master Settlement Agreement the industry agreed to pay US$246 billion over 25 years to cover tobacco-related medical expenses, to finance a foundation that would investigate diseases associated with tobacco, and to refrain from targeting children in advertising. Soon after this settlement the U.S. Department of Justice filed a US$289 billion lawsuit against four tobacco companies, a jury in Florida awarded a class of plaintiffs a settlement of US$145 billion, and local, state, and federal excise taxes on cigarettes rose by one-third.[48,49] (In New York City a pack of cigarettes in 2003 cost up to US$8.[50])

On the other hand, since the Master Settlement there has been no significant decrease in youth-directed magazine advertisements, and only a very small proportion of the settlement money has been used for tobacco control programs.[51–56,56a]

An attempt by the Food and Drug Administration to regulate cigarettes as "drug delivery devices" was blocked in 1996 by the U.S. Supreme Court on the grounds that Congressional approval was required. Not surprisingly, Congress, which had specifically excluded tobacco from governmental regulation under the Controlled Substances Act of 1970 and the Toxic Substances Control Act of 1976, did not grant such approval.[57,58]

Current Trends

In 2001, 22.8% of U.S. adults (46.2 million people) were current smokers, of whom 81.8% smoked daily. Prevalence of smoking was higher among men (25.2%) than women (20.7%). Prevalence was 24.0% for whites, 23.3% for blacks, 16.7% for Hispanics, 32.7% for native Americans, and 12.4% for Asians. It was 26.9% for those aged 18 to 24 years and 10.1% for those 65 years of age or older. Prevalence was 28.4% for those not completing high school, 12.3% for those with an undergraduate degree, and 8.5% for those with a graduate degree.[45] On the other hand, a 1999 survey of 14,138 U.S. college students revealed that 45.7% had used a tobacco product in the past year and 32.9% currently used tobacco. Prevalence of current cigarette smoking was 28.5%. Among males, prevalence of current cigar use was 15.7% and of smokeless tobacco 8.7%. Tobacco use was significantly more prevalent among those who also used alcohol or marijuana.[59] From 1996 to 2001 current smoking prevalence among U.S. adults remained constant in 44 states (men 25.5%, women 21.5%), fell in four, and rose in two.[59a]

During the 1990s, although increasing numbers of adult Americans continued to quit, smoking prevalence increased among children. More than 80% of smokers begin before age 18 years, and between 1992 and 1996 the proportion of eighth graders who reported smoking in the past month rose from 15.5% to 21%.[60–62] Every day in the United States 4400 children aged 12 to 17 years begin smoking (and one-third of them will die from a smoking-related disease.)[62a] Among U.S. high school students, current smoking increased from 27.5% in 1991 to 36.4% in 1997 and then fell to 22.9%.[61,62a,62b,63–65] The use of smokeless tobacco (chewing tobacco and snuff) and of non-cigarette smoking (cigar, pipe, bidi, and kretek) followed a similar pattern. White students were significantly more likely than Hispanic or black students to report current smoking.[63] Among middle school students (grades 6–8) there was a similar rise in the prevalence of tobacco use during the 1990s, but no significant change occurred during the period when tobacco use was declining among high school students. During 2002, 13.3% of middle school students used tobacco products, and 10.1% smoked cigarettes.[61b] Children can readily purchase cigarettes through Internet vendors, which seldom verify age.[65a] More than half of current cigarette smokers in middle school or high school reported that they wanted to stop smoking.[64] Factors that might have promoted cigarette use included tobacco industry expenditures on advertising and promotion (which increased during the 1990s) and the depiction of smoking in movies.[66] Factors that might have contributed to the decline in cigarette use included a 70% increase in the retail price of cigarettes during 1997–2001, increased school-based tobacco prevention programs, and increased state and national mass media anti-smoking campaigns.[67–69] (During 2003, however, states cut spending for tobacco use prevention and control programs by US$86.2 million [11.2%].[62a])

In contrast to other substance abusers, the majority of smokers take their drug continuously or frequently throughout the day, every day, craving a cigarette soon after the last is finished, while quite aware of the health consequences. The addiction liability of tobacco is aggravated by ready availability of cheap cigarettes, absence of overdose or impaired mental faculties, social acceptability, and the delay—up to decades—before the appearance of such complications as cancer, pulmonary disease, myocardial infarction, and stroke.

Globally, smoking-related mortality, which was 3 million annually in 1995 and 4.8 (uncertainty range 3.9–5.9) million in 2000, will exceed 10 million annually by 2030.[70,70a] During 2000 approximately half the deaths were in industrialized countries and half were in developing countries. Over the next few decades developing countries will claim an increasing percentage of deaths. In China, where two-thirds of men but few women are smokers, tobacco will kill 100 million of the 300 million males currently less than 30 years of age.[71,72] Multinational tobacco companies have successfully tapped into China, where cigarettes either imported or produced domestically are cheap. In 1999 representatives from more than 160 countries began meeting to negotiate a treaty on international tobacco regulation, the Framework Convention on Tobacco Control, planned for ratification in 2003. In 2001, however, a new delegation reversed earlier support of several key provisions, including obligatory taxes, restricted advertising and promotion, and passive-smoking regulations. During the 2000 U.S. elections, U.S. tobacco companies contributed US$7 million to Republicans and US$1.4 million to Democrats.[73,74]

Preparations and Acute Effects

Products

A "regular" American cigarette contains 13–20 mg nicotine and delivers 0.5–2 mg. "Low-nicotine" cigarettes contain half that amount, but smokers often titrate puffing to maintain blood levels of nicotine at around 30 ng/ml. Most pipe and cigar smokers, whose product is cured to be alkaline, absorb nicotine through the buccal mucosa and achieve lower nicotine concentrations.[75]

Increasingly popular among U.S. adolescents is the Asian practice of mixing tobacco with other products. "Kreteks" are cigarettes containing tobacco and ground clove; eugenol, the principal active ingredient in cloves, renders kreteks more addictive than plain tobacco.[76] "Bidis" are cigarettes containing tobacco wrapped in an Indian tendu or temburni leaf and available in different flavors (e.g., cherry, mango, chocolate). Bidis produce higher blood levels of nicotine, carbon monoxide, and tar than regular cigarettes.[77]

"Smokeless tobacco" includes snuff and chewing tobacco. Snuff is finely cut tobacco powder which is either inhaled through the nostrils or placed as a "quid" between the mucous membranes and the gums ("dipping"). A 20-minute dip delivers a nicotine dose of 2.0–3.5 mg. Chewing tobacco, packaged either as "twists" (ropelike leaf tobacco) or "plugs" (pressed lumps of shredded tobacco) is either chewed or placed between mucous membranes and gums, delivering a similar or slightly higher dose of nicotine. Eight to 10 dips or chews per day thus delivers a nicotine dose equivalent to 30 to 40 cigarettes per day.

Also a member of the Solanaceae family, and brought to Europe from the Americas at the same time as *Nicotiana tabacum*, *Nicotiana rusticum* contains much higher concentrations of nicotine. It is still used in "Turkish tobacco."

Acute Effects

Smoking may be either stimulating or sedating, depending on the setting and the subject's methods of titrating dosage. Smoking improves "speed and accuracy of information processing"[78] and long-term memory, reduces tension and anxiety, and increases pain threshold.[79] The usual response is arousal followed by relaxation, and smokers appear to adjust nicotine intake to favor one or the other phase. Overall, they increase or decrease their total smoking as the nicotine content of their cigarettes falls or rises.[80] Smokers do not usually describe alertness, relaxation, or euphoria as the motive for lighting a cigarette; rather the "taste of the cigarette" is perceived as the reason.[4] In fact, many smokers, while claiming inability to quit, report little or no "pleasure" in smoking.[81] On the other hand, nicotine given intravenously to smokers—but not nonsmokers—is euphorigenic, suggesting "reverse tolerance" and perhaps paralleling the locomotor effects seen in animals chronically given nicotine. In fact, among cigarette-smoking drug abusers, intravenous nicotine has been mistaken for cocaine.[21]

Burning tobacco generates more than 4000 compounds, both gaseous and particulate, including carbon monoxide, nitrogen oxides, ammonia, nitrosamines, hydrogen cyanide, sulfur-containing compounds, hydrocarbons, alcohols, aldehydes, and ketones. Nicotine, a volatile liquid, is suspended in tobacco smoke on minute particles of "tar," consisting largely of aromatic hydrocarbons, some of which are highly carcinogenic.[10] In the lung, nicotine is absorbed so quickly that it reaches the brain within 8 seconds; physiological effects are rapid and brief, increasing reinforcement potential.[10] Acute nicotine poisoning is not associated with tobacco smoking or chewing but follows accidental ingestion of tobacco by children. A small child who ingests a single cigarette or three cigarette butts has a 90% chance of becoming symptomatic.[76] Symptoms appear rapidly and include nausea, vomiting, salivation, lacrimation, abdominal pain, diarrhea, sweating, headache, miosis, agitation, delirium, fasciculations, and weakness.[11,76,82] Tachycardia and hypotension precede seizures, coma, and death from respiratory depression. Treatment consists of gastric lavage, activated charcoal, and ventilatory and blood pressure support. Atropine can be given for parasympathetic overstimulation.[76]

As in animals, tolerance develops variably to nicotine's different effects. Novices but not chronic smokers experience dizziness, nausea, and vomiting; both exhibit tremor and increased blood pressure and pulse rate. Tolerance to some of nicotine's effects seems to develop over the course of a day's smoking. For most smokers the first cigarette of the day produces the greatest subjective response, especially arousal.[10,83]

Dependence and Withdrawal

Chronic smokers experience an abstinence syndrome in which craving is strikingly out of proportion to observable signs. There is irritability, restlessness, anxiety, depression, difficulty concentrating, drowsiness, fatigue, insomnia, and headache. Performance is impaired on tests requiring attentiveness. Infrequently there is sweating, nausea, constipation, or diarrhea. Heart rate, blood pressure, and blood epinephrine levels decrease, and skin temperature and peripheral blood flow increase.[10,76,84,85] The electroencephalogram, which contains low-voltage fast activity during smoking, shows slower frequencies during abstinence.[86] Craving peaks at 24 to 48 hours and then usually diminishes gradually. In several series, irritability, anger, anxiety, and difficulty concentrating occurred in one-half to two-thirds of abstainers; by 6 months these symptoms had largely cleared, yet three-fourths of the subjects still craved cigarettes.[87] Some continue to crave for years. (Similar symptoms follow abstinence from smokeless tobacco or nicotine gum.)

Five chronic smokers in an intensive care unit (two subarachnoid hemorrhage, one intracerebral hemorrhage, one ischemic stroke, one carotid endarterectomy) developed acute delirium after 2 to 10 days of abstinence. Symptoms cleared rapidly after placement of a 21 mg nicotine patch.[88] Similar symptoms were described in terminally ill cancer patients.[89,90]

Nicotine is anorectic, probably by acting on cholinergic pathways in the lateral hypothalamus.[91] Weight gain occurs in most smokers who quit and is probably secondary both to nicotine's effects on energy expenditure and to increased eating.[92] Women are more likely than men to gain weight, but in either sex major weight gain—more than 13 kg—occurs in only a minority.[93]

Pharmacokinetics and Metabolism

The principal metabolites of nicotine, cotinine and nicotine-1N-oxide, are pharmacologically inactive. Nicotine's half-life is 1 to 4 hours and, because it induces its metabolism in the liver, shorter in chronic smokers. (Nicotine also induces the metabolism of a number of drugs, including benzodiazepines, opioids, caffeine, imipramine, propranolol, and nifedipine.) Cotinine's half-life is approximately 19 hours, and it is detectable in urine.[75,94]

Genetics

A review of 14 different studies involving 17,500 reared-together monozygotic and dizygotic twin pairs concluded that genetic factors play an important role in developing regular tobacco use. Genetic risk factors accounted for 56% of liability to tobacco use, compared with 24% for familial environmental risk factors and 20% for individual-specific environmental risk factors.[94a] A study comparing twin pairs reared either together or apart concluded that genetic effects accounted for 61% of risk and rearing/environmental effects for 20%.[95] A study from the Collaborative Study on the Genetics of Alcoholism (COGA) found an elevated risk of developing dependence on ethanol, marijuana, cocaine, or tobacco among siblings of probands dependent on these substances, and while comorbid drug dependence was common, there appeared to be independent causative factors in developing each type of substance dependence (as against a "general addictive tendency").[96]

Nicotine is oxidized to cotinine by the hepatic enzyme CYP2A6, which is highly polymorphic. Individuals carrying inactive CYP2A6 alleles have reduced nicotine metabolism, and in one report such individuals were less likely to become smokers, and if they did, they smoked fewer cigarettes per day.[97] (A proposed mechanism was that increased levels of nicotine produced noxious side effects that discouraged initiation of smoking.) Another study found no association of smoking behavior and variant alleles.[98]

Medical and Neurological Complications

Cancer, Chronic Obstructive Pulmonary Disease, and Immunosuppression

In the United States tobacco accounts for 85% of all lung cancer deaths and contributes to cancer of the oropharynx, esophagus, stomach, pancreas, kidney, breast and bladder. It accounts for 80% of all chronic obstructive pulmonary disease deaths. It is immunosuppressive.[94–101,101a] Space does not permit a detailed discussion of the mechanisms of these tobacco-related diseases, which, of course, can produce a myriad of neurological complications. (For example, patients with lung cancer develop brain and spinal cord metastases, paraneoplastic syndromes, CNS infection, and nutritional disturbance.)

Vascular Disease and Stroke

Epidemiology

A major risk factor for both coronary artery and peripheral vascular disease, tobacco accounts for about 30% of American cardiac mortality.[101,102] As regards cerebrovascular disease, although a few reports have been negative or demonstrated only insignificant trends,[103,104,104a] most case–control and cohort studies have shown that smoking also increases the risk for both occlusive and hemorrhagic

stroke.[8,104b,105–138,138a,138b] In women smokers the risk of occlusive and hemorrhagic stroke is greater in those taking oral contraceptives.[134,139–143] In a prospective cohort study of middle-aged women, smoking increased stroke risk in a dose-dependent fashion; for those smoking 25 or more cigarettes daily, the relative risk for all stroke was 3.7 and for subarachnoid hemorrhage 9.8 independent of other risk factors, including oral contraceptives, hypertension, and ethanol.[144] In another report, smoking in hypertensive men and women carried a 15-fold risk for subarachnoid hemorrhage and was a greater risk than hypertension itself.[121] In another study the treatment of hypertension reduced stroke incidence in nonsmokers but not in smokers.[145] Tobacco smoking, hypertension, and high blood cholesterol appear to act synergistically as stroke risk factors.[146] Smoking also acts synergistically with the apolipoprotein Eε4 allele in increasing the risk for ischemic stroke.[146a] Patients with ischemic stroke who smoke tend to be younger than those who do not.[147] Passive smoke exposure also increases the risk of coronary heart disease and stroke.[137,148,149]

In the Honolulu Heart Program, stroke risk was independent of coronary artery disease.[120] In a French study of women less than 45 years of age, smoking did not confer independent risk of stroke, and migraine conferred marginal risk; when both conditions were present, however, stroke risk was significantly increased.[150] Smoking is a risk factor for both central retinal artery occlusion and aortic plaque formation.[151,152] The Framingham Study found smoking to be a risk factor for subarachnoid hemorrhage.[153] Others found that among patients with aneurysmal subarachnoid hemorrhage smokers are more likely to have multiple aneurysms.[154] In one study not only was the risk for subarachnoid hemorrhage dose-dependently related to smoking, but it was greatest within 3 hours of smoking a cigarette.[155]

The Framingham Study also found that independent of age and hypertension, smoking dose-dependently increased the risk for both ischemic and hemorrhagic stroke and that this risk disappeared when smoking ceased.[156] Others confirmed reduction of risk with cessation of smoking.[110,112,157] In the Nurse's Health Study the risk of total and ischemic stroke disappeared within 2 to 4 years after cessation.[158] In a study of elderly subjects abstention from smoking was followed by improved cerebral perfusion.[159] Other workers, however, found a persistent long-term excess risk for stroke after cessation of smoking.[160] A case–control study found that an increased risk for cerebral ischemia persisted for at least 10 years in those who had stopped smoking.[127] Others reported a persistent risk for subarachnoid hemorrhage after more than 5 years of abstinence.[161,162]

Pathophysiology

Several possible mechanisms could underlie tobacco's risk for stroke.[163] Smoking aggravates atherosclerosis. In a study of identical twins discordant for smoking, carotid plaques were significantly more prominent in the smokers,[164] and in other reports smoking correlated in a dose-related fashion with severity of extracranial carotid atherosclerosis.[165–176] In the Atherosclerosis Risk in Communities (ARIC) Study, current cigarette smoking was associated with a 50% increase in the progression over 3 years of carotid artery atherosclerosis compared with never-smokers; past smoking was associated with a 25% increase and passive exposure to environmental smoke with a 20% increase.[177] Smoking one cigarette causes transient increases in arterial wall stiffness that increases the likelihood of plaque formation.[178] Smoking increases the likelihood that carotid plaques will ulcerate. In an angiographic study, intracranial carotid artery atherosclerosis correlated more with duration of smoking than with hypertension or diabetes mellitus.[179] A Japanese study found that in women a particular polymorphism of the gene for methylenetetrahydrofolate reductase (which remethylates homocysteine to methionine) was associated with increased risk for carotid atherosclerosis to a much greater degree in smokers than nonsmokers.[180]

Carbon monoxide in cigarette smoke reduces blood's oxygen-carrying capacity, and nicotine constricts coronary arteries.[181] Coronary artery constriction and increased myocardial oxygen demand induced by cocaine are exacerbated by concomitant tobacco smoking.[182] In animals nicotine damages endothelium, and increased numbers of circulating endothelial cells are found in smokers.[183,184] Neonates and children during the first year of life who were exposed to environmental tobacco smoke already demonstrated endothelial cell damage.[185] In mice chronically exposed to nicotine, aortic walls exhibited subendothelial edema and swelling of endothelial cells and mitochondria.[184] Bovine endothelial cells exposed to nicotine demonstrated giant cell formation and cellular vacuolation.[186]

Smoking acutely raises blood pressure, systole more than diastole; cerebral blood flow is reduced even after such acute effects have worn off.[187,188] Whether smoking is a risk factor for chronic hypertension is less clear,[189,190] but it accelerates the progression of chronic hypertension to malignant hypertension.[191] Smokers become tachycardic, and atrial fibrillation has followed nicotine gum chewing.[75] Demonstrating the complexity of interactions, dogs receiving ethanol followed by nicotine demonstrated synergistically increased heart rate and blood pressure, yet these excitatory effects were attenuated when ethanol followed nicotine.[192]

Smoking activates the coagulant pathway, increases platelet reactivity, and inhibits prostacyclin formation.[193–198] It also raises blood fibrinogen.[102] Elevated hemoglobin levels in smokers may also be a risk factor.[199,200] In human brain endothelial cell cultures, nicotine increased production of plasminogen activator inhibitor-1 (PAI-1).[201] Smokers have increased plasma levels of PAI-1.[202,203] In rats, nicotine-induced depletion of tissue plasminogen activator was associated with enhanced focal ischemic brain injury.[204] The increased risk of subarachnoid hemorrhage in smokers has been blamed on increased elastolytic activity in the serum.[124]

Nicotine, tars, and the gaseous components of cigarette smoke probably each contribute to cardiovascular disease.[205] Transdermal or oral nicotine produces increased plasma levels of platelet activation products (platelet factor 4 and β-thromboglobulin) and von Willebrand factor,[206,207] and stroke was reported after application of a nicotine patch.[208] However, a meta-analysis of 35 clinical trials involving transdermal nicotine patch found no excess incidence of myocardial infarction or stroke.[209] Among smokers, the risk of stroke mortality is reduced in those who smoke cigarettes with lower tar yield.[210] A Swedish study found that whereas smoking tobacco doubled the risk of stroke in men, smokeless tobacco (snuff) did not confer risk; the findings suggested that "chemical moieties produced by burning tobacco," rather than nicotine, were responsible for increased stroke risk.[210a]

Tobacco smoke and nicotine have complex effects on cerebral blood flow. Nicotine has direct and indirect effects on cerebral vessels and on neuronal nAChRs. Middle cerebral artery flow velocity increased in volunteers within a few seconds of puffing a cigarette.[211] Regional cerebral blood flow increased in the thalamus, pons, cerebellum, and visual cortex of smokers following nicotine delivered by nasal spray.[212] Exposure of rats to tobacco smoke increased cerebral blood flow and attenuated CO_2-induced vasodilation.[213] Nicotine-induced cerebral vasodilation in rats was attenuated by destroying the nucleus basalis of Meynert and abolished by blocking nAChRs in brain parenchyma.[214] In addition to direct actions of nicotine, changes in cerebral blood flow following exposure to tobacco smoke might be related to hypoxia[215] as well as to effects on thromboxane A_2, calcium and potassium channels, and nitric oxide.[216–218]

Bacterial endotoxin is an active component of cigarette smoke, and smokers have elevated plasma levels of endotoxin, which, by provoking inflammation, is an independent risk factor for atherosclerosis.[219–221]

Nicotine induces angiogenesis, and this action accelerates the growth of both neoplasms and atheroma.[222]

Progressive multifocal symptoms occurred in four young women who smoked and used oral contraceptives. Cerebral angiography demonstrated moyamoya; abnormal studies included elevated erythrocyte sedimentation rate, positive antinuclear antibodies, and elevated cerebrospinal fluid gammaglobulin (IgG). Disease progression ceased with discontinuation of oral contraceptives and reduction in smoking.[223] Tobacco and oral contraceptives were also overrepresented in another series of 39 patients with moyamoya disease.[224]

An elderly man had syncopal spells whenever he stood up after smoking a cigarette; spells ceased when he stopped smoking. Single photon emission computed tomographic (SPECT) scanning revealed reduced cerebral perfusion in "posterior circulation structures" after smoking a cigarette or chewing nicotine gum.[225]

Many brands of chewing tobacco are flavored with licorice, which contains the hypertensive, sodium-retaining, potassium-depleting glycoside glycyrrhetinic acid.[224] It is not known if this substance is an added risk factor for vascular disease.

Other Neurological Disorders

Worsening of neurological symptoms or signs has followed tobacco smoking or nicotine ingestion in patients with multiple system atrophy,[225] spinocerebellar degeneration,[226] alcoholic cerebellar degeneration,[227] and multiple sclerosis.[228] Smoking has precipitated myoclonus, ataxia, and weakness in patients with myoclonic epilepsy,[229] an effect blocked with mecamylamine; during nicotine-precipitated quadriparesis in such a patient, the soleus muscle H-reflex increased, an unexpected finding for smoking depresses the H-reflex in normal humans.[230,231]

In normal subjects, smoking induces a primary-position upbeat nystagmus that is suppressed by fixation.[232] It also impairs horizontal and vertical pursuit movements.[233] Nicotine gum produces similar alterations.[234] The effect is mediated by nAChRs of the vestibular system, perhaps peripherally as well as centrally.[235]

Smokers suffer from diminished smell, and the impairment can last for years after cessation. Anosmia has been attributed to nasal olfactory cell damage by chemicals such as acrolein, acetaldehyde, ammonia, and formaldehyde.[236]

Psychiatric Disorders

Smoking is strongly associated with mental illness. In the United States, 60% of individuals with various forms of mental illness smoke, compared with 25% in the general population. Conversely, 30% of smokers have some form of mental illness (schizophrenia, bipolar disorder, depression, post-traumatic stress disorder, attention deficit hyperactivity disorder, panic disorder, anxiety) compared with 12% in the general population. Expression of nicotinic $\alpha7$ receptor subtypes is decreased in schizophrenics, 70% of whom smoke, and nicotine normalizes the abnormal pattern of paired auditory evoked P50 waves seen in schizophrenics. (Clozapine, but not haloperidol, also normalizes the P50 abnormality.[237])

Individuals who have experienced major depression are more likely than others to be regular smokers, are less successful at quitting, and are at risk when they do quit of having recurrent depressive symptoms.[238–240] Among adolescents, depression appears to contribute to the initiation of cigarette smoking.[241] The relative roles of symptomatic relief and of underlying personality or genetic traits are uncertain.[242] A prospective cohort study found that first-incidence major depression was significantly higher in subjects with a history of nicotine dependence, whether or not they had smoked during the previous year, and that a history of major depression increased smokers' risk of progressing to nicotine dependence.[243] A twin study found that when personal smoking history was controlled, family history of smoking predicted risk for major depression and that when personal history of major depression was controlled, family history of major depression predicted smoking.[244] These findings suggest a genetic but probably non-causal link between smoking and major depression. Smoking undoubtedly contributes to the excess medical mortality associated with major depression.[245]

In a prospective study heavy cigarette smoking during adolescence increased the risk of later developing generalized anxiety disorder, agoraphobia, and panic disorder but not obsessive-compulsive disorder or social anxiety disorder. The converse was not found; adolescents with anxiety disorders were not at increased risk of becoming chronic smokers.[246]

Other Medical Complications

Exposure to tobacco smoke increases the risk of developing meningococcal disease. In a case–control study, maternal smoking was the strongest independent risk factor for invasive meningococcal disease in children less than 18 years of age (odds ratio: 3.8).[247] Cigarette smoke also is the strongest independent risk factor for invasive pneumococcal disease among immunocompetent, nonelderly adults; in a case–control study the odds ratio was 3.7 for pack-a-day current smokers and 2.4 for nonsmokers exposed to secondhand smoke for 1 to 4 hours per day.[248]

Nicotine activates $\alpha7$ nAChR subunits on lung macrophages, reducing the release of pro-inflammatory cytokines (tumor necrosis factor α, interleukins 1 and 6). As a consequence, smokers have a lower incidence of sarcoidosis and a higher incidence of active tuberculosis.[249]

Nicotine causes hyponatremia by stimulating antidiuretic hormone.[250]

Serum folate and cobalamin levels are significantly lower in current smokers than in nonsmokers. Most of the effect is attributable to differences in dietary habit. Cigarette smoke contains cyanide, however, which combines with hydroxycobalamin to form inactive cyanocobalamin.[251]

Smokers are more likely than nonsmokers to suffer from "nonspecific" back pain. Proposed mechanisms include increased coughing, diminished bone mineral content and trabecular microfractures, and reduced blood flow to vertebral bodies.[252] Postmenopausal women who smoke are at increased risk for hip fracture.[253]

Smoking is associated with a number of eye disorders. Both cataract and macular degeneration are accelerated by smoking. So-called tobacco–alcohol amblyopia is principally the result of nutritional deficiency (see Chapter 12), but toxic optic nerve damage by components of tobacco smoke (e.g., cyanide) could be contributory. Offspring of smoking mothers are at increased risk for strabismus.[254]

Smoking may aggravate rhabdomyolysis caused by ethanol, cocaine, or other drugs. Carbon monoxide in smoke produces carboxyhemoglobin, which impairs oxygen delivery to tissues.[255]

Effects on Pregnancy

Numerous studies—both case–control and prospective cohort—have addressed the effects of maternal tobacco use during pregnancy on fetal growth and development. As with other drugs, potential confounders include recall bias in retrospective studies, maternal age, socioeconomic status, education, poor prenatal care, and use of other drugs (especially ethanol). There is, however, considerable consistency across studies, leading to general agreement that maternal smoking has dose-related detrimental fetal effects.[256,257]

The evidence is especially strong for low birth weight and spontaneous abortion. A Swedish study found a statistically significant dose-related association between maternal smoking throughout pregnancy and reductions in birth weight, crown–heel length, and head circumference; quitting smoking between the first antenatal visit and the thirty-second week visit eliminated smoking-associated deficits in "brain–body weight ratio." Although this study corrected for several confounding variables, it did not consider maternal use of other drugs and ethanol.[258,259] A study from Australia found significant association between smoking throughout pregnancy and low birth weight (odds ratio: 2.52).[260] To a lesser degree exposure of nonsmokers to passive smoke also increases the likelihood of low birth weight.[261] One study found that the weight of tobacco-exposed children gradually recovered over the first 3 years of life unless ethanol exposure was also present.[262]

Maternal smoking significantly increases the risk of spontaneous abortion, abruptio placentae, and placenta previa.[263–268] Children of mothers who smoke during pregnancy had a more than threefold increased risk of sudden infant death syndrome.[269–271] Smoking during pregnancy plus lower birth weight is associated with higher childhood blood pressure.[272] Preterm infants exposed prenatally to tobacco are at increased risk for intracranial hemorrhage.[273] In utero exposure to maternal smoking increases the risk of childhood asthma independent of environmental tobacco smoke exposure.[274]

A study of 6-week-old infants found that generalized hypertonia correlated better with in utero tobacco exposure (identified by meconium and maternal urine cotinine levels) than with cocaine exposure (identified by meconium and urine benzoylecgonine levels).[275]

Neurobehavioral effects of in utero exposure to tobacco smoke become more evident as children grow older. Studies of children less than 2 years of age found impairments in motor scores, verbal comprehension, and auditory acuity.[256] Studies of children 2 to 5 years of age found significant increases in oppositional, aggressive, and hyperactive behavior.[276,277] Maternal smoking appears to be an independent risk factor for attention deficit hyperactivity disorder, conduct disorder (including criminality in adulthood), and substance abuse (especially smoking).[256,278–284]

These observations suggest that subtler intellectual impairment—undetectable by conventional epidemiological methodology—is a widespread consequence of in utero tobacco exposure. It has been pointed out that if the average IQ of such an exposed population fell by only 5 points, the proportion of those with severe retardation would triple and that of very gifted people would fall by two-thirds.[271]

Whether in utero tobacco exposure causes congenital anomalies is disputed.[257,285–287] A retrospective study—in which maternal tobacco use was probably underreported and therefore risk underestimated—found a significant association only for cardiovascular anomalies.[288] Nicotine is classified by the U.S. Food and Drug Administration as a risk level D teratogen, implying substantial fetal risk.[289]

Animal studies confirm that in utero exposure to tobacco or nicotine has adverse fetal effects. Rats or mice have reportedly had low birth weight normalizing by 1 to 2 weeks,[290] low birth weight persisting at postnatal day 29,[291] and normal birth weight but slower rate of postnatal weight gain.[292] Some studies found enhanced locomotor activity in exposed animals;[292] others did not.[256] Also reported are impaired maze tasks, avoidance responding, and appetite operant behavior.[256]

Congenital skeletal anomalies were described in mice, swine, and chicks exposed in utero to high doses of nicotine. Defects in forebrain development were described in rats.[285]

Fetal growth retardation is probably secondary in part to hypoxia and ischemia caused by nicotine and carbon monoxide.[285] In animals, nicotine reduces uterine blood flow,[293] and in pregnant humans two-pack-a-day smoking produces 10% blood carboxyhemoglobin levels, sufficient to cause an equivalent 60% reduction in fetal blood flow.[294] In addition, nicotine probably has direct toxic effects on developing brain. nAChRs are detected in the CNS early in gestation, and the density of different nAChR subtypes changes in different brain regions during development. nAChRs appear to play a role in neuronal proliferation, differentiation, and pathfinding (see above), and in animals, in utero exposure to nicotine causes reduced neuronal number, delayed neuronal maturation, and abnormal synaptogenesis.[271,295] These abnormalities involve both cholinergic and noncholinergic neurons, are lasting, and occur independently of somatic growth retardation. The second and third trimesters, rather than the first, appear to be the most vulnerable periods for these effects.[271]

Animal studies suggest that lead, thiocyanate, and cadmium contained in cigarette smoke also harms the fetus.[285,296]

Nicotine is secreted in breast milk, and case reports describe nicotine poisoning in nursing infants of mothers smoking 20 or more cigarettes a day. Symptoms include restlessness, insomnia, diarrhea, tachycardia, recurrent apnea, poor suck, flaccidity, and a grayish skin color.[285,297]

Parkinson's Disease

Numerous case–control and cohort studies confirm that cigarette smoking protects against Parkinson's disease (PD). Proposed explanations for the inverse correlation include increased mortality among smokers and a "premorbid personality type" in pre-parkinsonian patients that makes them less inclined to smoke. The effect, however, is very likely biological. In a meta-analysis of 44 case–control and four cohort studies, the relative risk of PD, compared with never smokers, was 0.59 for never smokers, 0.80 for past smokers, and 0.39 for current smokers.[298] The inverse association holds for both men and women.[299] The protective effect is less in those who develop PD later in life.[300,301] In twins discordant for PD, the twin who did not develop PD smoked more than his sibling, and this effect was more evident in monozygotic than dizygotic twins.[302] Such data support the view that the protective effect is not an artifact of shared genetic substrate. In one case–control study, the odds ratio for developing PD was 0.59 for light smokers (less than 30 pack-years) and 0.08 for heavy smokers (more than 30 pack-years); it was 0.86 for those who stopped smoking more than 20 years earlier and 0.37 for those who stopped smoking 1 to 20 years earlier.[303] Such observations support the view that the protection is both biological and lasting.

How tobacco exerts its protective effect is unclear. Cigarette smoke reduces brain monoamine oxidase (MAO) A and MAO B activity, and MAO B is involved in dopamine catabolism, with production of toxic free radicals.[304,305] Cigarette smoke reduces human striatal dopamine turnover.[306] In rats it reduces brain levels of potential neurotoxins.[307] The protective effect of smoking is modified by polymorphisms of MAO B.[308] MAO B inhibitors protect against PD caused by methylphenyltetrahydropyridine (MPTP). The protective factor in tobacco smoke might be nicotine itself.[309] Nicotine is neuroprotective in some animal models of PD, including mesencephalic hemitransection and MPTP.[310,311] It decelerates aging of nigrostriatal dopaminergic neurons.[312] Protection might involve mitochondrial

complex I (NADH-ubiquinone oxidoreductase) activity, which is deficient in PD. In a study of patients with PD and controls, cigarette smoking was protective only in men with a particular polymorphism of the mitochondrial complex I nuclear genome.[313]

Transdermal nicotine administration was ineffective in the treatment of PD.[314]

Cognitive Decline and Alzheimer's Disease

Epidemiological studies of smoking, cognitive decline and Alzheimer's disease (AD) are inconsistent. Anecdotal reports and case–control studies have claimed a decreased risk,[315–318] an increased risk,[319,320] or no correlation in either direction.[321–328,328a] Potential confounders in epidemiological studies include smoking-related diseases that select out patients and differences in education and occupation between smokers and nonsmokers.[329]

Meta-analysis of eight case–control studies revealed a significant inverse relationship between smoking and AD.[330] On the other hand, the prospective population-based Rotterdam Study found that compared with nonsmokers smokers had an *increased* risk of dementia (relative risk: 2.2) and AD (relative risk: 2.3). For smokers not carrying the apoprotein E-ε4 allele, the relative risk of AD was 4.6.[331] Similar findings were obtained in a prospective study from Northern Manhattan.[332] In the Framingham Study an apparent protective effect in women disappeared when adjusted for increased mortality in smokers; in men a trend suggested increased risk for AD.[332a] The Dutch Zutphen Elderly Study found that current smoking correlated with cognitive decline, especially in subjects with cardiovascular disease or diabetes mellitus.[332b] A CT study found that chronic smoking exaggerated age-related brain atrophy.[333] The Eurodem Study (which combined the Rotterdam cohort with those of the Danish Odense Study, the French PAQUID Study, and the U.K. MRC ALPHA Study) found accelerated cognitive decline among non-demented elderly smokers compared with never smokers.[334] The Honolulu-Asia Aging Study found that smoking in middle age increased the risk of cognitive impairment in later life.[335]

Smoking interferes with DNA repair, which declines with age.[336] Animals self-administering nicotine had markedly reduced expression of the polysialated forms of neural cell adhesion molecule (NCAM) as well as decreased neurogenesis in the dentate gyrus of the hippocampus.[336a] In adolescent rats exposure to nicotine caused CNS nAChR up-regulation with different regional patterns compared with those seen following either fetal or adult exposure. There was also neuronal damage and altered cell size in the hippocampus as well as altered synaptic activity of cholinergic, noradrenergic, dopaminergic, and serotonergic systems, which persisted for extended periods after exposure.[337] Since smoking usually begins during adolescence, these observations are obviously relevant to the apparent association between tobacco use and cognitive dysfunction.

Multiple Sclerosis

As noted above, tobacco smoking or nicotine ingestion can exacerbate symptoms or signs in patients with multiple sclerosis. In addition, several case–control and cohort studies show smoking to be a risk factor for developing multiple sclerosis, with odds ratios ranging from 1.4 to 1.9.[337a–337e] Some studies reveal a dose–response relationship.[337f] The mechanism is unclear, but nicotine and tar have immunotoxic properties,[337g] and smoking also increases the risk of developing rheumatoid arthritis.[337h]

Treatment of Nicotine Addiction

Seventy percent of smokers report that they want to quit, and one-third try to stop smoking each year, but only 20% of them seek help, and less than 10% who try to quit on their own are successful over the long-term.[338] Even with professional counseling and pharmacotherapy, however, treatment of nicotine addiction is unsatisfactory.

As of 2003, five products have been approved by the U.S. Food and Drug Administration for smoking cessation: nicotine gum, nicotine transdermal patch, nicotine nasal spray, nicotine vapor inhaler, and sustained-release bupropion. In a meta-analysis of 96 placebo-controlled studies, nicotine replacement therapy (NRT) was more effective than placebo,[338a] although some studies found it to be effective only when combined with behavioral

therapy.[339–342] Even when shown to be relatively beneficial, NRT can hardly be considered definitive. In one widely cited study, in which subjects used a 16-hour patch for 12 weeks and then tapered dosage, only 17% were still abstinent after a year compared with 4% of those receiving placebo.[343] NRT is used intermittently to prevent nicotine tolerance or sleep disruption. Long-term treatment is avoided for fear of cardiovascular and cerebrovascular complications, although such complications should be less than with smoking.[338,344–346] The same can be said for use of NRT during pregnancy.[347] A randomized controlled trial comparing the four NRT products found similar efficacy at 12 weeks of follow-up but highest compliance for the patch.[348] Gum and patch are currently available without a prescription.

A non-tobacco product that would deliver "clean" nicotine to the brain as rapidly as cigarette smoking might be more effective than gums or patches. The likelihood of such a delivery system being developed, however, is small.[348a]

Bupropion, an antidepressant with dopaminergic and noradrenergic activity, was also effective in randomized, controlled trials when combined with counseling.[349–351,351a] In one of these studies, bupropion produced significantly higher rates of abstinence than either placebo or NRT, and bupropion plus NRT was no more effective than bupropion alone.[350] In another study sustained-release bupropion plus counseling was associated with a 1-year quit rate of 33.2%.[351a] Bupropion is contraindicated in patients at risk for seizures. It attenuates the weight gain and reduces the depression associated with smoking cessation. In one study bupropion reduced other withdrawal symptoms;[350] in two other studies it did not.[349–351]

Two controlled studies demonstrated the efficacy of the antidepressant nortriptyline in smoking cessation.[352,353]

Mecamylamine, a centrally acting nicotine antagonist, reduced tobacco craving in a small group of volunteers, but smoking rates increased in subjects who were not trying to stop.[354] Both clonidine and the benzodiazepine alprazolam reduced anxiety and irritability during withdrawal; clonidine more effectively reduced craving.[355] In a controlled study clonidine produced higher abstinence rates than diazepam or placebo.[356] In another controlled study clonidine was superior to placebo but only in women.[357] In another controlled study it was not effective at all.[358] Side effects of clonidine include hypotension, tachycardia, headache, sedation, disturbed vision, and dizziness.[359]

Naloxone can trigger nicotine withdrawal symptoms in smokers,[360] and subcutaneous naloxone reportedly decreased the pleasure of cigarette smoking and helped people trying to stop.[361] Another study found it to be without effect.[362] Two trials of naltrexone failed to detect significant benefit.[363] (Heroin, methadone, and buprenorphine increase cigarette smoking, as do ethanol, amphetamine, pentobarbital, and a decrease in accustomed levels of caffeine.[364])

Pharmacological agents studied in animals and potentially useful for human nicotine addiction include dextromethorphan (which blocks α3/β4 nAChR function),[365] methyllycaconitine (which blocks α7 nAChR function),[366] the anticonvulsant γ-vinyl GABA (a GABA transaminase inhibitor, which attenuates nicotine-induced release of dopamine),[367] and acetyl-L-carnitine (an endogenous polyamine with cholinergic activity).[368] Lobeline (a herb with many nicotine-like effects: see below) appeared to offer benefit in one placebo-controlled trial.[369] Other studies were negative, however.[370,371] In rats, a nicotine conjugate vaccine attenuated nicotine's behavioral and cardiovascular effects.[372]

Meta-analysis of 22 studies of acupuncture for smoking cessation showed no benefit.[373]

The tobacco industry spends more than US$3 billion a year advertising and promoting the single most preventable cause of death in America. As noted above, much of the effort is targeted at children,[374,375] and much is devoted to forcing American-made cigarettes into foreign markets, under threat of U.S. governmental trade sanctions toward nations that resist.[376] Although momentum picked up during the 1990s, governmental antismoking efforts have been listless compared with the enthusiastic expenditures of money and energy directed against substances decreed illicit. Under the Master Settlement Agreement (MSA) of 1998 (see above), US$246 billion were to be given to the states over a 25-year period to fund a nationwide campaign of public education, and the tobacco companies promised to adopt limitations on advertising. Over the next several years, however, marketing expenditures of the cigarette industry rose dramatically and continued to target children.[54,55] Furthermore,

few of the states used the money from the settlement as intended, namely, to fund prevention and cessation programs.[53,69] In fact, during 2001 only 6% of the total MSA windfall was spent on tobacco control.[56] Well-designed prevention and cessation programs are effective; it is estimated, for example, that from 1988 to 1997 California's program (funded by an increase in cigarette taxes and focusing especially on anti-smoking media campaigns) saved more than 33,000 lives.[62,377]

Less than 20% of American smokers say their physician has advised them to stop.[53] Physicians trained to counsel patients about quitting do make a difference.[378–380] Tobacco's legality should be an incentive, not a deterrent, to such intervention. As elected officials succumb to the pressures of industry lobbyists, physicians should remind themselves that tobacco is the only product legally sold in the United States that causes disease and death when used as intended.

Lobeline

Lobelia inflata ("Indian weed," "Indian tobacco," "pukeweed," "asthma weed," "gagroot," "vomitwort," "bladderpad," "eyebright") grows throughout eastern North America. Its dried leaves were smoked for intoxicating effects by American Indians, and leaves produced for chewing were exported to England by the Shakers of New Lebanon. During the 19th century *L. inflata* was used as an emetic, expectorant, anti-asthmatic, muscle relaxant, diaphoretic, diuretic, stimulant, and to treat morphine overdose. Named after Matthias de Lobel, physician to King James I of England, *L. inflata* is still used as a tobacco substitute.[381]

Among the several pharmacologically active alkaloids of *L. inflata*, lobeline was long considered an nAChR agonist, but although it produces a number of nicotine-like effects, including anxiety reduction and improvement in learning and memory, lobeline does not support self-administration in rats, does not produce conditioned place preference, and does not generalize to nicotine in drug discrimination studies.[381,382] Lobeline actually acts as an nAChR antagonist, inhibiting nicotinic agonist-evoked dopamine release, and although high concentrations of lobeline release catecholamines from presynaptic terminals, that effect is independent of nAChRs. Despite its ineffectiveness in treating nicotine addiction (see above), lobeline's actions at presynaptic vesicular monoamine transporters, coupled with its lack of addictive liability, suggest possible use in the treatment of methamphetamine dependence[381] (see Chapter 4).

References

1. Ravenholt RT. Addiction mortality in the United States 1980: tobacco, alcohol, and other substances. Popul Dev Rev 1984; 10:697.

2. Warner KE. Health and economic implications of a tobacco-free society. JAMA 1987; 258:2080.

3. Nadelman EA. Drug prohibition in the United States: costs, consequences, and alternatives. Science 1989; 245:939.

4. Schelling TC. Addictive drugs: the cigarette experience. Science 1992; 255:430.

5. Thun MJ, Apiella LF, Henley SJ. Smoking vs other risk factors as the cause of smoking-attributable deaths: confounding in the courtroom. JAMA 2000; 284:706-712.

6. Anon. Annual smoking-attributable mortality, years of potential life lost, and economic costs—United States, 1995–1999. MMWR 2002; 51:300-303.

7. WHO. Tobacco or health, a global status report. Geneva: Switzerland, World Health Organization Publications, 1997.

8. Department of Health and Human Services. The Health Consequences of Smoking: Nicotine Addiction. A Report of the Surgeon General. Washington, DC: DHHS Publication No. (CDC) 88-8406, US Government Printing Office, 1988.

9. Benowitz NL. Pharmacologic aspects of cigarette smoking and nicotine addiction. N Engl J Med 1988; 319:1318.

10. O'Brien CP. Drug addiction and drug abuse. In: Hardman JG, Limbird LE, eds. Goodman and Gilman's The Pharmacological Basis of Therapeutics, 10th edition. New York: McGraw-Hill, 2001; 621.

11. Taylor P. Agents acting at the neuromuscular junction and autonomic ganglia. In: Hardman JG, Limbird LE, eds. Goodman and Gilman's The Pharmacological Basis of Therapeutics, 10th edition. New York: McGraw-Hill, 2001; 193.

12. Clarke PBS, Kumar R. The effects of nicotine on locomotor activity in non-tolerant and tolerant rats. Br J Pharmacol 1983; 78:329.

13. Clarke PBS. Nicotine and smoking: a perspective from animal studies. Psychopharmacology 1987; 92:135.

14. Warburton DM. Psychopharmacological aspects of nicotine. In: Wonnacott S, Russell MAH, Stolerman IP, eds. Nicotine Psychopharmacology. Molecular, Cellular, and Behavioral Aspects. Oxford: Oxford University Press, 1990; 77.

15. Stolerman IP. Behavioral pharmacology of nicotine in animals. In: Wonnacott S, Russell MAH, Stolerman IP, eds. Nicotine Psychopharmacology: Molecular, Cellular, and Behavioral Aspects. Oxford: Oxford University Press, 1990; 278.

16. Bettany JH, Levin ED. Ventral hippocampal α7 nicotinic receptor blockade and chronic nicotine effects on memory performance in the radial-arm maze. Pharmacol Biochem Behav 2001; 70:467.

17. Lupien JR, Bray GA. Nicotine increases thermogenesis in brown adipose tissue in rats. Pharmacol Biochem Behav 1988; 29:33.

18. Desai RI, Barber DJ, Terry P. Asymmetric generalization between the discriminative stimulus effects of nicotine and cocaine. Behav Pharmacol 1999; 10:647.

19. Stolerman IP, Jarvis MJ. The scientific case that nicotine is addictive. Psychopharmacology 1995; 117:2.

20. Cox BM, Goldstein A, Nelson WT. Nicotine self-administration in rats. Br J Pharmacol 1984; 83:49.

21. Henningfield JE, Mijasato K, Jasinski DR. Abuse liability and pharmacodynamic characteristics of intravenous and inhaled nicotine. J Pharmacol Exp Ther 1985; 234:1.

22. Swedberg MDB, Henningfield JE, Goldberg SR. Nicotine dependency: animal studies. In: Wonnacott S, Russell MAH, Stolerman IP, eds. Nicotine Psychopharmacology: Molecular, Cellular, and Behavioral Aspects. Oxford: Oxford University Press, 1990:38.

23. Corrigall WA. Nicotine self-administration in animals as a dependence model. Nicotine Tob Res 1999; 1:11.

24. Caggiula AR, Donny EC, White AR, et al. Cue dependency of nicotine self-administration and smoking. Pharmacol Biochem Behav 2001; 70:515.

25. Kenny PJ, Markou A. Neurobiology of the nicotine withdrawal syndrome. Pharmacol Biochem Behav 2001; 70:531.

26. Malin DH. Nicotine dependence. Studies with a laboratory model. Pharmacol Biochem Behav 2001; 70:551.

27. Dani JA, DeBiasi M. Cellular mechanisms of nicotine addiction. Pharmacol Biochem Behav 2001; 70:439.

28. Jones S, Sudweeks S, Yakel JL. Nicotinic receptors in the brain: correlating physiology with function. Trends Neurosci 1999; 22:555.

29. Mansvelder HD, McGehee DS. Cellular and synaptic mechanisms of nicotine addiction. J Neurobiol 2002; 53:606.

30. Dani JA, Ji D, Zhou FM. Synaptic plasticity and nicotine addiction. Neuron 2001; 31:349.

31. Picciotto MR, Zoli M, Rimondini R, et al. Acetylcholine receptors containing the beta-2 subunit are involved in the reinforcing properties of nicotine. Nature 1998; 391:173.

32. DiChiara G. Role of dopamine in the behavioral actions of nicotine related to addiction. Eur J Pharmacol 2000; 393:295.

33. Balfour DJ, Wright AE, Benwall ME, Birrell CE. The putative role of extrasynaptic mesolimbic dopamine in the neurobiology of nicotine dependence. Behav Brain Res 2000; 113:73.

34. Pontieeri FE, Tanda G, Ori F, et al. Effects of nicotine on the nucleus accumbens and similarity to those of addictive drugs. Nature 1996; 382:255.

35. Cheeta S, Tucci S, File SE. Antagonism of the anxiolytic effect of nicotine in the dorsal raphe nucleus by dihydro-beta-erythrodine. Pharmacol Biochem Behav 2001; 70:491-496.

36. Picciotto MR, Corrigall WA. Neuronal systems underlying behaviors related to nicotine addiction: neural circuits and molecular genetics. J Neurosci 2002; 22:3338.

37. Zachariou V, Caldarone BJ, Weathers-Lowin A, et al. Nicotine receptor activation decreases sensitivity to cocaine. Neuropsychopharmacology 2001; 24:576.

38. Schoffelmeer ANM, DeVries TJ, Wardeh G, et al. Psychostimulant-induced behavioral sensitization depends on nicotinic receptor activation. J Neurosci 2002; 22:3269.

39. Ji D, Lape R, Dani JA. Timing and location of nicotinic activity enhances or depresses hippocampal synaptic plasticity. Neuron 2001; 31:131.

40. Panagis G, Hildebrand BE, Svensson TH, et al. Selective c-fos induction and decreased dopamine release in the central nucleus of the amygdala in rats displaying a mecamylamine-precipitated nicotine withdrawal syndrome. Synapse 2000; 35:15.

41. Gately I. Tobacco: A Cultural History of How an Exotic Plant Seduced Civilization. New York: Grove Press, 2001.

41a. Brecher EM. Licit and Illicit Drugs. Boston: Little, Brown, 1972.

42. Wynder EL, Graham E. Tobacco smoking as a possible etiologic factor in bronchogenic carcinoma: a study of 684 proven cases. JAMA 1950; 143:329.

42a. U.S. Environmental Protection Agency. Respiratory Health Effects of Passive Smoking: Lung Cancer and Other Disorders. Washington, DC: U.S. Government Printing Office, 1993.

43. Ong EK, Glantz SA. Constructing "sound science" and "good epidemiology": tobacco, lawyers, and public relations firms. Am J Public Health 2001; 91:1749.

44. Yach D, Bialous SA. Junking science to promote tobacco. Am J Public Health 2001; 91:1745.

45. Cigarette smoking among adults—United States, 2001 MMWR 2003; 52:953.

45a. Mokdad AH, Marks JS, Stroup DF et al. Actual causes of death in the United States, 2000. JAMA 2004; 291:1238.

46. Pringle P. Cornered: Big Tobacco at the Bar of Justice. New York: Henry Holt, 1998.

47. Kluger R. Ashes to Ashes: America's Hundred Year Cigarette War, the Public Health, and the Unabashed Triumph of Phillip Morris. New York: Alfred A. Knopf, 1996.

48. Day S, Glater JD. Tobacco companies vow to fight $289 billion suit. NY Times, March 19, 2003.

49. Gruber J. The economics of tobacco regulation. Health Affairs 2002; 21:146.

50. O'Connell V. Bans on smoking in prison shrink a coveted market. Wall St Journal, August 27, 2003.

51. Gross CP, Soffer B, Bach PB, et al. State expenditures for tobacco control programs and the tobacco settlement. N Engl J Med 2002; 347:1080.

52. King C, Siegel M. The Master Settlement Agreement with the tobacco industry and cigarette advertising in magazines. N Engl J Med 2001; 345:504.

53. Schroeder SA. Conflicting dispatches from the tobacco wars. N Engl J Med 2002; 347:1106.

54. King C, Siegel M. The Master Settlement Agreement with the tobacco industry and cigarette advertising in magazines. N Engl J Med 2001; 345:504.

55. Chung PJ, Garfield CF, Rathouz PJ, et al. Youth targeting by tobacco manufacturers since the Master Settlement Agreement: the first study to document violations of the youth-targeting ban in magazine ads by the three top U.S. tobacco companies. Health Aff 2002; 21:254.

56. Gross CP, Soffer B, Bach PB, et al. State expenditures for tobacco-control programs and the tobacco settlement. N Engl J Med 2002; 347:1080.

56a. Schroeder SA: Tobacco conrol in wake of the 1998 Master Settlement Agreement. N Engl J Med 2004; 350:293.

57. Kessler D. A question of Intent: A Great American Battle with a Deadly Industry. New York: Public Affairs, 2001.

58. Myers ML. Tobacco, the Food and Drug Administration, and Congress. N Engl J Med 2000; 343:1802.

59. Rigotti NA, Lee JE, Wechsler H. U.S. college students' use of tobacco products: results of a national survey. JAMA 2000; 284:699.

59a. Prevalence of current cigarette smoking among adults and changes in prevalence of current and same day smoking—United States, 1996–2001. MMWR 2003; 52:303.

60. Califano JA. Substance abuse and addiction: the right to know. Am J Public Health 1998; 88:9.

61. Youth tobacco surveillance United States, 1998–1999. MMWR 2000; 49 (Suppl):1.

62. Chassin L, Presson C, Rose J, et al. The natural history of cigarette smoking from adolescence to adulthood: demographic predictors of continuity and change. Health Psychol 1996; 15:478.

62a. Tobacco use among middle and high school students—United States 2002. MMWR 2003; 52:1096.

62b. Marwick C. Increasing use of chewing tobacco, especially among younger persons, alarms surgeon general. JAMA 1993; 269:195.

63. Trends in cigarette smoking among high school students—United States, 1991–1999. MMWR 2001; 49:755.

64. Youth tobacco surveillance—United States, 2000. MMWR 2001; 50:1.

65. Trends in cigarette smoking among high school students—United States, 1991.

65a. Ribisl KM, Williams RS, Kim AE. Internet sales of cigarettes to minors. JAMA 2003; 290:1356.

66. Lyman R. In the 80's: Lights! Camera! Cigarettes! NY Times, March 12, 2002.

67. Fichtenberg CM, Glantz SA. Association of the California Tobacco Control Program with declines in cigarette consumption and mortality from heart disease. N Engl J Med 2000; 343:1772.

68. Siegel M. The effectiveness of state-level tobacco control interventions: a review of program implementation and behavioral outcomes. Annu Rev Public Health 2002; 23:45.

69. Kessler DA, Myers ML. Beyond the tobacco settlement. N Engl J Med 2001; 345:535.

70. Fagerstrom K. The epidemiology of smoking: health consequences and benefits of cessation. Drugs 2002; 62 (Suppl Z):1.

70a. Ezzati M, Lopez AD. Estimates of global mortality attributable to smoking in 2000. Lancet 2003; 362:847.

71. Liu BQ, Peto R, Chen ZM, et al. Emerging tobacco hazards in China. 1. Retrospective proportional mortality study of one million deaths. BMJ 1998; 317:1411.

72. Yang G, Fan L, Tan J, et al. Smoking in China. Findings of the 1996 National Prevalence Survey. JAMA 1999; 282:1247.

73. Waxman HA. The future of the global tobacco treaty negotiations. N Engl J Med 2002; 346:936.

74. Olson E. U.S. accused of diluting a global pact to limit use of tobacco. NY Times, May 6, 2001.

75. Benowitz NL. Pharmacologic aspects of cigarette smoking and nicotine addiction. N Engl J Med 1988; 319:1318.

76. Salomon ME. Nicotine and tobacco preparations. In: Goldfrank LR, Flomenbaum NE, Lewin NA, et al., eds. Goldfrank's Toxicologic Emergencies, 6th edition. Stamford, CT: Appleton and Lange, 1998; 1145.

77. Anon. Bidi use among urban youth—Massachusetts, March–April 1999. MMWR 1999; 48:796.

78. Pomerleau OF, Pomerleau CS. Neuroregulators and the reinforcement of smoking: towards a behavioral explanation. Neurosci Behav Rev 1984; 8:503.

79. Tripathi J, Martin B, Aceto M. Nicotine-induced antinociception in rats and mice: correlation with nicotine brain levels. J Pharmacol Exp Ther 1982; 221:91.

80. Moss RA, Prue DM. Research on nicotine regulation. Behav Ther 1982; 13:31.

81. Kozlowski LT, Wilkinson A, Skinner W, et al. Comparing tobacco cigarette dependence with other drug dependencies. JAMA 1989; 261:898.

82. Borys DJ, Setzer SC, Ling LJ. CNS depression in an infant after the ingestion of tobacco: a case report. Vet Hum Toxicol 1988; 30:20.

83. Benowitz NL. Clinical pharmacology of inhaled drugs of abuse: implications in understanding nicotine dependence. NIDA Res Monogr 1990; 99:12.

84. Pickworth WB, Fant RV, Butschky MF, et al. Effects of transdermal nicotine delivery on measures of acute nicotine withdrawal. J Pharmacol Exp Ther 1996; 279:450.

85. Jorenby DE, Hatsukami DK, Smith SS, et al. Characterization of tobacco withdrawal symptoms: transdermal nicotine reduces hunger and weight gain. Psychopharmacology 1996; 128:130.

86. Domino EF. Nicotine and tobacco dependence: Normalization or stimulation? Alcohol 2001; 24:83.

87. Hughes JR, Gust SW, Skoog K, et al. Symptoms of tobacco withdrawal. Arch Gen Psychiatry 1991; 48:52.

88. Mayer SA, Chong JY, Ridgway E, et al. Delirium from nicotine withdrawal in neuro-ICU patients. Neurology 2001; 57:551.

89. Krajnik M, Zylicz Z. Terminal restlessness and nicotine withdrawal. Lancet 1995; 346:1044.

90. Gallagher R. Nicotine withdrawal as an etiologic factor in delirium. J Pain Symp Manage 1998; 16:76.

91. Jo YH, Talmage DA, Role LW. Nicotineic receptor-mediated effects on appetite and food intake. J Neurobiol 2002; 53:618.

92. Perkins KA, Epstein LH, Marks BL, et al. The effect of nicotine on energy expenditure during light physical activity. N Engl J Med 1989; 320:898.

93. Williamson DF, Madans J, Anda RF, et al. Smoking cessation and severity of weight gain in a national cohort. N Engl J Med 1991; 324:739.

94. Wall MA, Johnson J, Jacob P, Benowitz NL. Cotinine in the serum, saliva, and urine of nonsmokers, passive smokers, and active smokers. Am J Public Health 1988; 78:699.

94a. Sullivan PF, Kendler KS. The genetic epidemiology of smoking. Nicotine Tobacco Res 1999; 1:S51.

95. Kandler KS, Thornton LM, Pedersen NL. Tobacco consumption in Swedish twins reared apart and reared together. Arch Gen Psychiatry 2000; 57:886.

96. Bierut LJ, Dinwiddie SH, Begleiter H, et al. Familial transmission of substance dependence: alcohol, marijuana, cocaine, and habitual smoking: a report from the Collaborative Study on the Genetics of Alcoholism. Arch Gen Psychiatry 1998; 55:982.

97. Tyndale R, Sellers EM. Genetic variation in CYP2A6-mediated nicotine metabolism alters smoking behavior. Ther Drug Monitor 2002; 24:163.

98. Tricker AR. Nicotine metabolism, human drug metabolism polymorphisms, and smoking behaviour. Toxicology 2003; 183:151.

99. Berger LR. Cigarette smoking and the acquired immunodeficiency syndrome. Ann Intern Med 1988; 108:638.

100. Henderson BE, Ross RK, Pike MC. Toward the primary prevention of cancer. Science 1991; 254:1131.

101. Smoking and Health. A National Status Report, 2nd edition. Rockville, MD: DHHS, Publication No. (CDC) 87-8396, 1990.

101a. Band PR, Nhu DL, Fang R, et al. Carcinogenic and endocrine disrupting effects of cigarette smoke and risk of breast cancer. Lancet 2002; 360:1044.

102. Kannel WB, D'Agostino RB, Belanger AL. Fibrinogen, cigarette smoking, and risk of cardiovascular disease: insights from the Framingham Study. Am Heart J 1987; 113:1006.

103. Herman B, Leyten ACM, van Luuk JH, et al. An evaluation of risk factors for stroke in a Dutch community. Stroke 1982; 13:334.

104. Kroger K, Buss C, Govern M, et al. Risk factors in young patients with peripheral atherosclerosis. Int Angiol 2000; 19:206.

104a. Davanipour Z, Sobel E, Alter M, et al. Stroke/transient ischemic attack in the Lehigh Valley: evaluation of smoking as a risk factor. Ann Neurol 1988; 24:130.

104b. Hammond EC. Smoking in relation to mortality and morbidity: finding in the first 34 months of followup in a prospective study started in 1959. J Natl Cancer Inst 1964; 32:1161.

105. Giroud M, Creisson E, Fayolle H, et al. Risk factors for primary cerebral hemorrhage: a population-based study—the Stroke Registry of Dijon. Neuroepidemiology 1995; 14:20.

106. Kahn HA. The Dorn study of smoking and mortality among US veterans: report on $8\frac{1}{2}$ years of observation. Natl Cancer Inst Monogr 1966; 19:1.

107. Paffenbarger RS, Wing A. Characteristics in youth predisposing to fatal stroke in later years. Lancet 1967; I:753.

108. Kurtzke JF. Epidemiology of Cerebrovascular Disease. New York: Springer-Verlag, 1969.

109. Paffenbarger RS, Williams JL. Chronic disease in former college students. XI. Early precursors of non-fatal stroke. Am J Epidemiol 1971; 94:524.

110. Rogot E. Smoking and General Mortality Among US Veterans, 1954–1969. Bethesda, MD: National Heart and Lung Institute, 1974.

111. Doll R, Peto R. Mortality in relation to smoking: 20 years' observations on male British doctors. BMJ 1976; II:1525.

112. Koch A, Reuther R, Boos R, et al. Risikofactoren bei cerebralen Durchblutungessstorungen. Verb Dtsch Ges Inn Med 1977; 83:1977.

113. Abu-Zeid HAH, Choi NW, Maini KK, et al. Relative role of factors associated with cerebral infarction and cerebral hemorrhage: a matched pair case–control study. Stroke 1977; 8:106.

114. Doll R, Gray R, Hafner B, et al. Mortality in relation to smoking: twenty-two years observations on female British doctors. BMJ 1980; I:967.

115. Salonen JT, Puska P, Tuomilehto J, et al. Relation of blood pressure, serum lipids, and smoking to the risk of cerebral stroke: a longitudinal study in Eastern Finland. Stroke 1982; 13:327.

116. Wolf PA, Kannel WB, Verter J. Current status of risk factors for stroke. Neurol Clin 1983; 1:317.

117. Candelise L, Bianchi F, Galligoni F, et al. Italian multicenter study on cerebral ischemic attacks. III. Influence of age and risk factors on cerebral atherosclerosis. Stroke 1984; 15:379.

118. Herrschaft H. Prophylaxe zerbraler Durchblutungsstorungen. Fortschr Neurol Psychiatr 1985; 53:337.

119. Bloch C, Richard JL. Risk factors for atherosclerotic diseases in the Prospective Parisian Study. I. Comparison with foreign studies. Rev Epidemiol Sante Publ 1985; 33:108.

120. Abbott RD, Reed DM, Yano K. Risk of stroke in male cigarette smokers. N Engl J Med 1986; 315:717.

121. Bonita R. Cigarette smoking, hypertension, and the risk of subarachnoid hemorrhage: a population-based case–control study. Stroke 1986; 17:831.

122. Bonita R, Scragg R, Stewart A, et al. Cigarette smoking and risk of premature stroke in men and women. BMJ 1986; 293:6.

123. Molgaard CA, Bartok A, Peddercord KM, et al. The association between cerebrovascular disease and smoking: a case control study. Neuroepidemiology 1986; 5:88.

124. Fogelholm R. Cigarette smoking and subarachnoid hemorrhage: a population-based case–control study. J Neurol Neurosurg Psychiatry 1987; 50:78.

125. Gorelick PB, Rodin MB, Langenberg P, et al. Weekly alcohol consumption, cigarette smoking, and the risk of ischemic stroke: results of a case–control study at three urban medical centers in Chicago, Illinois. Neurology 1989; 39:339.

126. Shinton R, Beevers G. Meta-analysis of relation between cigarette smoking and stroke. BMJ 1989; 298:789.

127. Donnan GA, Adena MA, O'Malley HM, et al. Smoking as a risk for cerebral ischemia. Lancet 1989; II:643.

128. Harmsen P, Rosengren A, Tsipogianni A, Wilhelmsen L. Risk factors for stroke in middle-aged men in Goteborg, Sweden. Stroke 1990; 21:223.

129. Love BB, Biller J, Jones MP, et al. Cigarette smoking. A risk factor for cerebral infarction in young adults. Arch Neurol 1990; 47:693.

130. Tuomilehto J, Bonita R, Stewart A, et al. Hypertension, cigarette smoking, and the decline in stroke incidence in Eastern Finland. Stroke 1991; 22:7.

131. Lee TK, Huang ZS, Ng SK, et al. Impact of alcohol consumption and cigarette smoking on stroke among the elderly in Taiwan. Stroke 1995; 26:790.

132. Juvela S, Hillbom M, Numminem H, et al. Cigarette smoking and alcohol consumption as risk factor for aneurysmal subarachnoid hemorrhage. Stroke 1993; 24:639.

133. Lakier JB. Smoking and cardiovascular disease. Am J Med 1992; 93:8S.

134. Milandre L, Brosset C, Habib G, et al. Cerebral infarction in patients aged 16 to 35 years. Prospective study of 52 cases. Presse Med 1994; 23:1603.

135. Benson RT, Sacco RL. Stroke prevention: hypertension, diabetes, tobacco, and lipids. Neurol Clin 2000; 18:309.

136. Kissela BM, Saverbeck L. Woo D, et al. Subarachnoid hemorrhage: a preventable disease with a heritable component. Stroke 2002; 33:1321.

137. Bonita R, Duncan J, Truelsen T, et al. Passive smoking as well as active smoking increases the risk of acute stroke. Tob Control 1999; 8:156.

138. Jamrozik K, Broadhurst RJ, Anderson CS, et al. The role of lifestyle factors in the etiology of stroke. A population-based case–control study in Perth, Western Australia. Stroke 1994; 25:51.

138a. Kurth T, Kase CS, Berger K, et al. Smoking and the risk of hemorrhagic stroke in men. Stroke 2003; 34:1151.

138b. Kurth T, Kase CS, Berger K, et al: Smoking and the risk of hemorrhagic stroke in women. Stroke 2003; 34:2792.

139. Collaborative Group for the Study of Stroke in Young Women. Oral contraception and increased risk of cerebral ischemia or thrombosis. N Engl J Med 1973; 288:871.

140. Frederiksen H, Ravenholt RT. Thromboembolism, oral contraceptives, and cigarettes. Public Health Rep 1970; 85:197.

141. Goldbaum GM, Kendrick JS, Hogelin GC, Gentry EM. The relative impact of smoking and oral contraceptive use on women in the United States. JAMA 1987; 258:1339.

142. Pettiti DB, Wingerd J. Use of oral contraceptives; cigarette smoking, and risk of subarachnoid hemorrhage. Lancet 1978; II:234.

143. Royal College of General Practitioners. Oral Contraceptives and Health. London: Pitman, 1974.

144. Colditz GA, Bonita R, Stampfer MJ, et al. Cigarette smoking and risk of stroke in middle-aged women. N Engl J Med 1988; 318:937.

145. Medical Research Council Working Party. MRC trial of treatment of mild hypertension: principal results. BMJ 1985; 291:97.

146. Pandey MR. Tobacco smoking and hypertension. J Indian Med Assoc 1999; 97:367.

146a. Pezzini A, Grassi M, Del Zotto E, et al: Synergistic effect of apolipoprotein E polymorphisms and cigarette smoking on risk of ischemic stroke in young adults. Stroke 2004; 35:438.

147. Christensen HK, Guasorra AD, Boysen G. Ischemic stroke occurs among younger smokers. Ugeskr Laeger 2001; 163:7057.

148. He J, Vupputuri S, Allen K, et al. Passive smoking and the risk of coronary heart disease—a meta-analysis of epidemiologic studies. N Engl J Med 1999; 340:920.

149. Nurminen MM, Jaakkola MS. Mortality from occupational exposure to environmental tobacco smoke in Finland. J Occup Environ Med 2001; 43:687.

150. Iglesias S, Visy JM, Hubert JB, et al. Migraine as a risk factor for ischemic stroke. A case–control study. Stroke 1993; 24:171.

151. Blackshear JL, Pearce LA, Hart RG, et al. Aortic plaque in atrial fibrillation: prevalence, predictors, and thromboembolic implications. Stroke 1999; 30:834.

152. Framme C, Spiegel D, Roider J, et al. Central retinal artery occlusion: importance of selective intra-arterial fibrinolysis. Ophthalmologe 2001; 98:725.

153. Sacco RL, Wolf PA, Bharucha NE, et al. Subarachnoid and intracerebral hemorrhage: natural history, prognosis, and precursive factors in the Framingham Study. Neurology 1984; 34:847.

154. Ellamushi HE, Grieve JP, Jager HR, et al. Risk factors for the formation of multiple intracranial aneurysms. J Neurosurg 2001; 94:728.

155. Longstreth WT, Nelson LM, Koepsell TD, van Belle G. Cigarette smoking, alcohol use, and subarachnoid hemorrhage. Stroke 1992; 23:1242.

156. Wolf PA, D'Agostino RB, Kannel WB, et al. Cigarette smoking as a risk factor for stroke. The Framingham Study. JAMA 1988; 259:1025.

157. Wannamethee SG, Shaper AG, Whincup PH, et al. Smoking cessation and the risk of stroke in middle-aged men. JAMA 1995; 274:155.

158. Kawachi I, Colditz GA, Stampfer MJ, et al. Smoking cessation and decreased risk of stroke in women. JAMA 1993; 269:232.

159. Rogers RL, Meyer JS, Judd BW, Mortel KF. Abstention from cigarette smoking improves cerebral perfusion among elderly chronic smokers. JAMA 1985; 253:2970.

160. Taylor BV, Oudit GY, Kalman PG, et al. Clinical and pathophysiological effects of active and passive smoking on the cardiovascular system. Can J Cardiol 1998; 14:1129.

161. Bell BA, Symon L. Smoking and subarachnoid hemorrhage. BMJ 1979; 1:577.

162. Taha A, Ball KP, Illingworth RD. Smoking and sub-arachnoid hemorrhage. J R Soc Med 1982; 75:332.

163. Hawkins BT, Brown RC, David TP. Smoking and ischemic stroke: A role for nicotine? Trends Pharmacol Sci 2002; 23:8.

164. Haapanen A, Koskenvuo M, Kaprio J, et al. Carotid arteriosclerosis in identical twins discordant for cigarette smoking. Circulation 1989; 80:10.

165. Bogousslavsky J, Van Melle G, Despland PA, Regli F. Alcohol consumption and carotid atherosclerosis in the Lausanne Stroke Registry. Stroke 1990; 21:715.

166. Whisnant JP, Homer D, Ingall TJ, et al. Duration of cigarette smoking is the strongest predictor of severe extracranial carotid atherosclerosis. Stroke 1990; 21:707.

167. Dempsey RJ, Diana AL, Moore RW. Thickness of carotid artery atherosclerotic plaque and ischemic risk. Neurosurgery 1990; 27:343.

168. Crouse JR, Toole JF, McKinney WM, et al. Risk factors for extracranial carotid artery atherosclerosis. Stroke 1987; 18:990.

169. Gostomzyk JG, Heller WD, Gerhardt P, et al. B-scan ultrasound examination of the carotid arteries within a representative population (MONICA Project Augsburg). Kiln Wochenschr 1988; 66 (Suppl XI):58.

170. Salonen R, Seppanen K, Rauramaa R, Salonen JT. Prevalence of carotid atherosclerosis and serum cholesterol levels in Eastern Finland. Arteriosclerosis 1988; 8:788.

171. Lassila R, Seyberth HW, Haapanen A, et al. Vasoactive and atherogenic effects of cigarette smoking: a study of monozygotic twins discordant for smoking. BMJ 1988; 297:955.

172. Tell GS, Howard G, McKinney WM, Toole JF. Cigarette smoking cessation and extracranial carotid atherosclerosis. JAMA 1989; 262:1178.

173. Dempsey RJ, Moore RW. Amount of smoking independently predicts carotid artery atherosclerosis severity. Stroke 1992; 23:693.

174. Dempsey RJ, Moore RW. A causal chain from smoking to stroke. Stroke 1992; 23:A12.

175. Mast H, Thompson JLP, Lin I-F, et al. Cigarette smoking as a determinant of high-grade carotid artery stenosis in Hispanic, black and white patients with stroke or transient ischemic attack. Stroke 1998; 29:908.

176. Kanter MC, Tegeler CH, Pearce LA, et al. Carotid stenosis in patients with atrial fibrillation. Prevalence, risk factors, and relationship to stroke in the Stroke Prevention in Atrial Fibrillation Study. Arch Intern Med 1994; 154:1372.

177. Howard G, Wagenknecht LE, Burke GL, et al. Cigarette smoking and progression of atherosclerosis. The Atherosclerosis Risk in Communities (ARIC) Study. JAMA 1998; 279:119.

178. Kool MJ, Hoeks AP, Struijker Boudier HA, et al. Short- and long-term effects of smoking on arterial wall properties in habitual smokers. J Am Coll Cardiol 1993; 22:1881.

179. Ingall TJ, Homer D, Baker HL, et al. Predictors of intracranial carotid artery atherosclerosis. Arch Neurol 1991; 48:687.

180. Inamoto N, Katsuya T, Kokubo Y, et al. Association of methylenetetrahydrofolate reductase gene polymorphism with carotid atherosclerosis depending on smoking status in a Japanese general population. Stroke 2003; 34:1628.

181. Maouad J, Fernandez F, Barrillon A, et al. Diffuse or segmental narrowing (spasm) of coronary arteries during smoking demonstrated on angiography. Am J Cardiol 1984; 53:354.

182. Moliterno DJ, Willard JE, Lange RA, et al. Coronary vasoconstriction induced by cocaine, cigarette smoking, or both. N Engl J Med 1994; 330:454.

183. Davis JW, Shelton L, Eigenberg DA, et al. Effects of tobacco and non-tobacco cigarette smoking on endothelium and platelets. Clin Pharmacol Ther 1985; 37:529.

184. Zimmerman M, McGreachie J. The effect of nicotine on aortic endothelium: a quantitative ultrastructural study. Atherosclerosis 1987; 63:33.

185. Haustein KO. Health consequences of passive smoking. Wien Med Wochenschr 2000; 150:233.

186. Talloss JH, Booyse FM. Effects of various agents and physical damage on giant cell formation in bovine aortic endothelial cell cultures. Microvasc Res 1978; 16:51.

187. Kubota K, Yamaguchi T, Abe Y. Effects of smoking on regional cerebral blood flow in neurologically normal subjects. Stroke 1983; 14:720.

188. Longstreth WT, Swanson PD. Oral contraceptives and stroke. Stroke 1984; 15:747.

189. Green MS, Jucha E, Luz Y. Blood pressure in smokers and non-smokers: epidemiologic findings. Am Heart J 1986; 111:932.

190. Pardell H, Amario P, Hernandez R. Pathogenesis and epidemiology of arterial hypertension. Drugs 1998; 56 (Suppl 2):1.

191. Isles C, Brown JJ, Cumming AM, et al. Excess smoking in malignant phase hypertension. BMJ 1979; I:579.

192. Mehta MC, Jain AC, Billie M. Combined effects of alcohol and nicotine on cardiovascular performance in a canine model. J Cardiovasc Pharmacol 1998; 31:930.

193. Seiss W, Lorenz R, Roth P, Weber PC. Plasma catecholamines, platelet aggregation and associated thromboxane formation after physical exercise, smoking, or norepinephrine infusion. Circulation 1982; 66:44.

194. Nadler JL, Velasso JS, Horton R. Cigarette smoking inhibits prostacyclin formation. Lancet 1983; I:1248.

195. Belch JJ, McArdle BM, Burns P, et al. The effects of acute smoking on platelet behavior, fibrinolysis, and haemorphology in habitual smokers. Thromb Haemost 1984; 51:6.

196. Renaud S, Blache O, Dumont E, et al. Platelet function after cigarette smoking in relation to nicotine and carbon monoxide. Clin Pharmacol Ther 1984; 36:389.

197. Nair S, Kulkarni S, Camoens HM, et al. Changes in platelet glycoprotein receptors after smoking—a flow cytometric study. Platelets 2001; 12:20.

198. Miller GJ, Bauer KA, Cooper JA, et al. Activation of the coagulant pathway in cigarette smokers. Thromb Haemost 1998; 79:549.

199. Nordenberg D, Yip R, Binkin NJ. The effect of cigarette smoking on hemoglobin levels and anemia screening. JAMA 1990; 264:1556.

200. Schwarcz TH, Hagan LA, Endean EO, et al. Thromboembolic complications of polycythemia: polycythemia vera versus smokers' polycythemia. J Vasc Surg 1993; 17:518.

201. Zidovetski R, Chen P, Fisher M, et al. Nicotine increases plasminogen activator inhibitor-1 production by human brain endothelial cells via protein kinase C-associated pathway. Stroke 1999; 30:651.

202. Simpson AJ, Gray RS, Moore NR, et al. The effects of chronic smoking on the fibrinolytic potential of plasma and platelets. Br J Haematol 1997; 97:208.

203. Margaglione M, Capucci G, d'Addedda M, et al. PAI-1 plasma levels in the general population without evidence of atherosclerosis: relation to environmental and genetic determinants. Arterioscler Thromb Vasc Biol 1998; 18:562.

204. Wang L, Kittaka M, Sun N, et al. Chronic nicotine treatment enhances focal ischemic brain injury and depletes free pool of brain microvascular tissue plasminogen activator in rats. J Cereb Blood Flow Metab 1997; 17:136.

205. Benowitz NL. The role of nicotine in smoking-related cardiovascular disease. Prev Med 1997; 26:412.

206. Benowitz NL, Fitzgerald GA, Wilson M, et al. Nicotine effects on eicosanoid formation and hemostatic function: comparison of transdermal nicotine and cigarette smoking. J Am Coll Cardiol 1993; 22:1159.

207. Blann AD, Steele C, McCollum CN. The influence of smoking and of oral and transdermal nicotine on blood pressure, and haematology and coagulation indices. Thromb Haemost 1997; 78:1093.

208. Pierce JR. Stroke following application of a nicotine patch. Ann Pharmacol 1994; 28:402.

209. Greenland S, Satterfield MH, Lanes SF. A meta-analysis to assess the incidence of adverse effects associated with the transdermal nicotine patch. Drug Saf 1998; 18:297.

210. Tang JL, Morris JK, Wald NJ, et al. Mortality in relation to tar yield of cigarettes: a prospective study of four cohorts. BMJ 1995; 311:1530.

210a. Asplund K, Nasic S, Janlert V, et al. Smokeless tobacco as a possible risk factor for stroke in men. A nested case–control study. Stroke 2003; 34:1754.

211. Boyajian RA, Otis SM. Acute effects of smoking on human cerebral blood flow: a transcranial Doppler ultrasonography study. J Neuroimag 2000; 10:204.

212. Domino EF, Minoshima S, Guthrie S, et al. Nicotine effects on regional cerebral blood flow in awake, resting tobacco smokers. Synapse 2000; 38:313.

213. Koskinen LO, Collin O, Bergh A. Cigarette smoke and hypoxia induce acute changes in testicular and cerebral microcirculation. Ups J Med Sci 2000; 105:215.

214. Uchida S, Kagitani F, Nakayama H, et al. Effect of stimulation of nicotinic cholinergic receptors on cortical cerebral blood flow and changes in the effect during aging and in anesthetized rats. Neurosci Lett 1997; 228:203.

215. Golanov EV, Ruggiero DA, Reis DJ. A brainstem area mediating cerebrovascular and EEG responses to hypoxic excitation of rostral ventrolateral medulla in rat. J Physiol (Lond) 2000; 529:413.

216. Iida M, Iida H, Dohi S, et al. Mechanisms underlying cerebrovascular effects of cigarette smoking in rats in vivo. Stroke 1998; 29:1656.

217. Gerzanich V, Zhang F, West GA, et al. Chronic nicotine alters NO signaling of Ca^{2+} channels in cerebral arterioles. Circ Res 2001; 88:359.

218. Zhang W, Edvinsson L, Lee TJ. Mechanism of nicotine-induced relaxation in the porcine basilar artery. J Pharmacol Exp Ther 1998; 284:790.

219. Hasday JD, Bascom R, Costa JJ, et al. Bacterial endotoxin is an active component of cigarette smoke. Chest 1999; 115:829.

220. Wiederman CJ, Kiechl S, Duzendorfer S, et al. Association of endotoxemia with carotid atherosclerosis and cardiovascular disease: prospective results from the Bruneck study. J Am Coll Cardiol 1999; 34:1975.

221. Risley P, Jerrard-Dunne P, Sitzer M, et al. Promoter polymorphism in the endotoxin receptor (CD14) is associated with increased carotid atherosclerosis only in smokers. The Carotid Atherosclerosis Progression Study (CAPS). Stroke 2003; 34:600.

222. Heeschen C, Jang JJ, Weis M, et al. Nicotine stimulates angiogenesis and promotes tumor growth and atherosclerosis. Nat Med 2001; 7:833.

223. Levine SR, Fagan SC, Floberg J, et al. Moyamoya, oral contraceptives, and cigarette use. Ann Neurol 1988; 24:155.

224. Morris DJ, Davis E, Latif SA. Licorice, tobacco chewing, and hypertension. N Engl J Med 1990; 322:849.

225. Johnson JA, Miller JT. Tobacco intolerance in multiple system atrophy. Neurology 1986; 36:986.

226. Spillane JD. The effect of nicotine on spinocerebellar ataxia. BMJ 1955; II:1345.

227. Schmitt J, Seelinger D, Appenzeller O, Orrison W. Nicotine and alcoholic cerebellar degeneration. Neurology 1988; 38 (Suppl 1):205.

228. Emre M, de Decker C. Nicotine and CNS. Neurology 1987; 37:1887.

229. Yoshimura I, Tabe HK, Fukushima Y, Fuyushi T. The aggravating effect of smoking on myoclonus: a case of Ramsey Hunt syndrome. Neurol Med 1988; 28:636.

230. Yokota T, Kagamihara Y, Hayashi H, et al. Nicotine-sensitive paresis. Neurology 1992; 42:382.

231. Domino EF, Von Baumgarten AM. Tobacco cigarette smoking and patellar reflex depression. Clin Pharmacol Ther 1969; 10:72.

232. Sibony PA, Evinger C, Manning KA. Tobacco-induced primary position upbeat nystagmus. Ann Neurol 1987; 21:53.

233. Sibony PA, Evinger C, Manning KA. The effects of tobacco smoking on smooth pursuit eye movements. Ann Neurol 1988; 23:238.

234. Sibony PA, Evinger C, Manning K, Pellegrini JJ. Nicotine and tobacco-induced nystagmus. Ann Neurol 1990; 28:198.

235. Pereira CB, Strupp M, Eggert T, et al. Nicotine-induced nystagmus: three-dimensional analysis and dependence on head position. Neurology 2000; 55:1563.

236. Frye RE, Schwartz BS, Dory RL. Dose-related effects of cigarette smoking on olfactory function. JAMA 1990; 263:1233.

237. Leonard S, Adler LE, Benhammou K, et al. Smoking and mental illness. Pharmacol Biochem Behav 2001; 70:561.

238. Anda RF, Williamson DF, Escobedo LG, et al. Depression and the dynamics of smoking. A national perspective. JAMA 1990; 264:1541.

239. Glassman AH, Covey LS, Stetner F, et al. Smoking cessation and the course of major depression: a follow-up study. Lancet 2001; 357:1929.

240. Niaura R, Abrams DB. Stopping smoking: a hazard for people with a history of major depression? Lancet 2001; 357:1900.

241. Kandel DB, Davies M. Adult sequelae of adolescent depressive symptoms. Arch Gen Psychiatry 1986; 43:255.

242. Glass RM. Blue mood, blackened lungs. Depression and smoking. JAMA 1990; 264:1584.

243. Kendler KS, Neale MC, MacLean CJ, et al. Smoking and major depression. A causal analysis. Arch Gen Psychiatry 1993; 50:36.

244. Breslau N, Kilbey M, Andreski P. Nicotine dependence and major depression. New evidence from a prospective investigation. Arch Gen Psychiatry 1993; 50:31.

245. Bruce ML, Leaf PJ. Psychiatric disorders and 15 month mortality in a community sample of older adults. Am J Public Health 1989; 79:727.

246. Johnson JG, Cohen P, Pine DS, et al. Association between cigarette smoking and anxiety disorders during adolescence and early adulthood. JAMA 2000; 284:2348.

247. Fischer M, Hedberg K, Cardosi P, et al. Tobacco smoke as a risk factor for meningococcal disease. Pediatr Infect Dis J 1997; 16:979.

248. Nuorti JP, Butler JC, Farley MM, et al. Cigarette smoking and invasive pneumococcal disease. N Engl J Med 2000; 342:681.

249. Floto RA, Smith KGC. The vagus nerve, macrophages, and nicotine. Lancet 2003; 361:1069-1070.

250. Adrogué HJ, Madias NE. Hyponatremia. N Engl J Med 2000; 342:1581.

251. Piyathilake CJ, Macaluso M, Hine RJ, et al. Local and systemic effects of cigarette smoking on folate and vitamin B_{12}. Am J Clin Nutr 1994; 60:559.

252. Scott SC, Goldberg MS, Mayo NE, et al. The association between cigarette smoking and back pain in adults. Spine 1999; 24:1090.

253. Baron JA, Farahmand BY, Weiderpass E, et al. Cigarette smoking, alcohol consumption, and risk of hip fracture in women. Arch Intern Med 2001; 161:983.

254. Solberg Y, Rosner M, Belkin M. The association between cigarette smoking and ocular diseases. Surv Ophthalmol 1998; 42:535.

255. Richards JR. Rhabdomyolysis and drugs of abuse. J Emerg Med 2000; 19:51.

256. Ernst M, Moolchan ET, Robinson ML. Behavioral and neural consequences of prenatal exposure to nicotine. J Am Acad Child Adolesc Psychiatry 2001; 40:630.

257. Higgins S. Smoking in pregnancy. Curr Opin Obstet Gynecol 2002; 14:145.

258. Lindley AA, Becker S, Gray RH, et al. Effect of continuing or stopping smoking during pregnancy on infant birth weight, crown–heel length, head circumference, ponderal index, and brain–body weight ratio. Am J Epidemiol 2000; 152:219.

259. Lindley AA, Gray RH, Herman AA, et al. Maternal cigarette smoking during pregnancy and infant ponderal index at birth in the Swedish Medical Birth Register, 1991–1992. Am J Public Health 2000; 90:420.

260. Chan A, Keane RJ, Robinson JS. The contribution of maternal smoking to preterm birth, small for gestational age, and low birthweight among Aboriginal and non-Aboriginal births in South Australia. Med J Aust 2001; 174:389.

261. Eskanazi B, Prehn AW, Christianson RE. Passive and active maternal smoking as measured by serum cotinine: the effect on birthweight. Am J Public Health 1995; 85:395.

262. Day N, Cornelius M, Goldschmidt L, et al. The effects of prenatal tobacco and marijuana use on offspring growth from birth through 3 years of age. Neurotoxicol Teratol 1992; 14:407.

263. Ness RB, Grisso JA, Hirschinger N, et al. Cocaine and tobacco use and the risk of spontaneous abortion. N Engl J Med 1999; 340:333.

264. Hladky K, Yankowitz J, Hansen WF. Placental abruption. Obstet Gynecol Surv 2002; 57:299.

265. Kyrklund-Blomberg NB, Gennser G, Cnattingius S. Placental abruption and perinatal death. Paediatr Perinat Epidemiol 2001; 15:290.

266. Pollack H, Lantz PM, Frohna JG. Maternal smoking and adverse birth outcomes among singletons and twins. Am J Public Health 2000; 90:395.

267. Castles A, Adams EK, Melvin CL, et al. Effects of smoking during pregnancy. Five meta-analyses. Am J Prevent Med 1999; 16:208.

268. Andres RL, Day MC. Perinatal complications associated with maternal tobacco use. Semin Neonatol 2000; 5:231.

269. Wisborg K, Kesmodel V, Henriksen TB, et al. A prospective study of smoking during pregnancy and SIDS. Arch Dis Child 2000; 83:203.

270. Pollack HA. Sudden infant death syndrome, maternal smoking during pregnancy, and the cost-effectiveness of smoking cessation intervention. Am J Public Health 2001; 91:432.

271. Slotkin TA. Fetal nicotine or cocaine exposure: which one is worse? J Pharmacol Exp Ther 1998; 285:931.

272. Blake KV, Gurrin LC, Evans SF, et al. Maternal cigarette smoking during pregnancy, low birth weight and subsequent blood pressure in early childhood. Early Hum Dev 2000; 57:137.

273. Spinello A, Ometto A, Stronati M, et al. Epidemiologic association between maternal smoking during pregnancy and intracranial hemorrhage in preterm infants. J Pediatr 1995; 127:472.

274. Gilliland FD, Li YF, Peters JM. Effects of maternal smoking during pregnancy and environmental tobacco smoke on asthma and wheezing in children. Am J Respir Crit Care Med 2001; 163:429.

275. Dempsey DA, Hajnal BL, Partridge JC, et al. Tone abnormalities are associated with maternal cigarette

smoking during pregnancy in utero cocaine-exposed infants. Pediatrics 2000; 106:79.

276. Orelebeke JF, Knol DL, Verhulst FC. Child behavior problems increased by maternal smoking during pregnancy. Arch Environ Health 1999; 54:15.

277. Wasserman RC, Kelleher KJ, Bocian A, et al. Identification of attentional and hyperactivity problems in primary care: a report from pediatric research in office settings and the ambulatory sentinel practice network. Pediatrics 1999; 103. E38.

278. Weissman MM, Warner V, Wickramaratine PJ, et al. Maternal smoking during pregnancy and psychopathology in offspring followed to adulthood. J Am Acad Child Adolesc Psychiatry 1999; 38:892.

279. Waksschlag LS, Lahey BB, Loeber R, et al. Maternal smoking during pregnancy and the risk of conduct disorder in boys. Arch Gen Psychiatry 1997; 54:670.

280. Fergusson DM, Woodward LJ, Horwood LJ. Maternal smoking during pregnancy and psychiatric adjustment in late adolescence. Arch Gen Psychiatry 1998; 55:721.

281. Milberger S, Biederman, Faraone SV, et al. Further evidence of an association between maternal smoking during pregnancy and attention deficit hyperactivity disorder: findings from a high-risk sample of siblings. J Clin Child Psychol 1998; 27:352.

282. Brennan PA, Grekin ER, Mednick SA. Maternal smoking during pregnancy and adult male criminal outcomes. Arch Gen Psychiatry 1999; 56:215.

283. Rasanen P, Hakko H, Isohanni M, et al. Maternal smoking during pregnancy and risk of criminal behavior among adult male offspring in the Northern Finland 1966 Birth Cohort. Am J Psychiatry 1999; 156:857.

284. Weitzman M, Byrd RS, Aligne CA, et al. The effects of tobacco exposure on children's behavioral and cognitive functioning: implications for clinical and public health policy and future research. Neurotoxicol Teratol 2002; 24:397.

285. Lee M-J. Marijuana and tobacco use in pregnancy. Obstet Gynecol Clin North Am 1998; 25:65-83.

286. Benowitz NL. Nicotine replacement therapy during pregnancy. JAMA 1990; 266:3174.

287. Cole H. Studying reproductive risks: smoking. JAMA 1986; 255:22.

288. Woods SRU. Maternal smoking and the risk of congenital birth defects: a cohort study. J Am Board Family Pract 2001; 14:330.

289. Drug Information for the Health Care Professional, 15th edition, Vol 1. Rockville, MD: U.S. Pharmacopeial Convention, 1995.

290. Leichter J. Decreased birth weight and attainment of postnatal catch-up growth in offspring of rats exposed to cigarette smoking during gestation. Growth Dev Aging 1995; 59:63.

291. Paulson RB, Shanfeld J, Vorhees CV, et al. Behavioral effects of prenatally administered smokeless tobacco on rat offspring. Neurotoxicol Teratol 1993; 15:183.

292. Ajarem JS, Ahmad M. Prenatal nicotine exposure modifies behavior of mice through early development. Pharmacol Biochem Behav 1998; 59:313.

293. Resnik R, Brink GW, Wilkes M. Catecholamine mediated reduction in uterine blood flow after nicotine infusion in the pregnant ewe. J Clin Invest 1979; 63:1133.

294. Bureau MA, Monette J, Shapcott D, et al. Carboxyhemoglobin concentration in fetal cord blood and in blood of mothers who smoked during labor. Pediatrics 1982; 69:371.

295. Roy TS, Sabherwal U. Effects of prenatal nicotine exposure on the morphogenesis of somatosensory cortex. Neurotoxicol Teratol 1994; 16:411.

296. Kunhert DB. Drug exposure to the fetus. The effect of smoking. NIDA Res Monogr 1991; 114:1.

297. Perraudin M, Sorin M. Intoxication probable d'un nouveau-né par la nicotine presente dans le lait de sa mère. Ann Pediatr 1978; 25:41.

297a. Louis ED, Luchsinger JA, Tang MX, et al. Parkinsonian signs in older people. Prevalence and associations with smoking and coffee. Neurology 2003; 61:24.

298. Hernán MA, Takkouche B, Caamaño F, et al. A meta-analysis of coffee drinking, cigarette smoking, and the risk of Parkinson's disease. Ann Neurol 2002; 52:276.

299. Hernán MA, Zhang SM, Rueda-deCastro AM, et al. Cigarette smoking and incidence of Parkinson's disease in two prospective studies. Ann Neurol 2001; 50:780.

300. Benedetti MD, Bower JH, Maraganore DM, et al. Smoking, alcohol, and coffee consumption preceding Parkinson's disease. A case–control study. Neurology 2000; 55:1350.

301. Marder K, Logroscino G. The ever-stimulating association of smoking and coffee and Parkinson's disease. Ann Neurol 2002; 52:261.

302. Tanner CM, Goldman SM, Aston DA, et al. Smoking and Parkinson's disease in twins. Neurology 2002; 58:581.

303. Gorell JM, Rybicki BA, Cole Johnson C, et al. Smoking and Parkinson's disease. A dose–response relationship. Neurology 1999; 52:115.

304. Hernán MA, Checkoway H, O'Brien R, et al. MAO. B intron 13 and COMT codon 158 polymorphisms, cigarette smoking, and the risk of PD. Neurology 2002; 58:1381.

305. Fowler JS, Volkow ND, Wang GJ, et al. Inhibition of monoamine oxidase B in the brains of smokers. Nature 1996; 379:733.

306. Court J, Lloyd S, Thomas N, et al. Dopamine and nicotinic receptor binding and the levels of dopamine and homovanillic acid in human brain related to tobacco use. Neuroscience 1998; 87:63.

307. Soto-Otero R, Mendez-Alvarez E, Sanchez-Sellero I, et al. Reduction of rat brain levels of the endogenous dopaminergic proneurotoxins 1,2,3,4-tetrahydroisoquinoline and 1,2,3,4-tetrahydro-beta-carboline by cigarette smoke. Neurosci Lett 2001; 298:187.

308. Checkoway H, Franklin GM, Costa-Mallen P, et al. A genetic polymorphism of MAO-B modifies the association of cigarette smoking in Parkinson's disease. Neurology 1998; 50:1458.

309. Quik M, Kulak JM. Nicotine and nicotinic receptors; relevance to Parkinson's disease. Neurotoxicology 2002; 23:581.

310. Janson A, Hedlund P, Fuxe K, et al. Chronic nicotine treatment counteracts dopamine D_2, receptor upregulation induced by a partial meso-diencephalic hemitransection in the cat. Brain Res 1994; 655:25.

311. Maggio R, Riva M, Vaglini F, et al. Nicotine prevents experimental parkinsonism in rodents and induces striatal increase of neurotrophic factors. J Neurochem 1998; 71:2439.

312. Prasad C, Ikegami H, Shimizu I, et al. Chronic nicotine intake decelerates aging of nigrostriatal dopaminergic neurons. Life Sci 1994; 54:1169.

313. Tan EK, Chai A, Zhao Y, et al. Mitochondrial complex I polymorphism and cigarette smoking in Parkinson's disease. Neurology 2002; 59:1288.

314. Vieregge A, Sieberer M, Jacobs H, et al. Transdermal nicotine in PD. A randomized, double-blind, placebo-controlled study. Neurology 2001; 57:1032.

315. Hofman A, van Duijn CM. Alzheimer's disease, Parkinson's disease, and smoking. Neurobiol Aging 1990; 11:295.

316. Ferini-Strambi L, Smirne S, Garancini P, et al. Clinical and epidemiological aspects of Alzheimer's disease with presenile onset: a case–control study. Neuroepidemiology 1990; 9:39.

317. Grossberg GT, Nakra R, Woodward V, Russell T. Smoking as a risk factor for Alzheimer's disease. J Am Geriatr Soc 1989; 37:822.

318. van Duijn CM, Hofman A. Relation between nicotine intake and Alzheimer's disease. BMJ 1991; 302:1491.

319. Shalat SL, Seltzer B, Pidcock C, Baker EL. Risk factors for Alzheimer's disease: a case–control study. Neurology 1987; 37:1630.

320. Joya CJ, Pardo CA, Londono JL. Risk factors in clinically diagnosed Alzheimer's disease: a case–control study in Colombia (South America). Neurobiol Aging 1990; 11:796.

321. French LR, Schuman LM, Mortimer JA, et al. A case–control study of dementia of the Alzheimer's type. Am J Epidemiol 1985; 121:414.

322. Jones GMM, Reith M, Philpot MP, Sahakian BJ. Smoking and dementia of Alzheimer type. J Neurol Neurosurg Psychiatry 1987; 50:1383.

323. Amaducci LA, Fratiglioni L, Rocca WA, et al. Risk factors for clinically diagnosed Alzheimer's disease: a case–control study of an Italian population. Neurology 1986; 36:922.

324. Chandra V, Philipose V, Bell PA, et al. Case–control study of late onset "probable Alzheimer's disease." Neurology 1987; 37:1295.

325. Broe GA, Henderson AS, Creasey H, et al. A case–control study of Alzheimer's disease in Australia. Neurology 1990; 40:1698.

326. Graves AB, White E, Koepsell T, et al. A case–control study of Alzheimer's disease. Ann Neurol 1990; 28:766.

327. Hebert LE, Scherr PA, Beckett LA, et al. Relation of smoking and alcohol consumption to incident Alzheimer's disease. Am J Epidemiol 1992; 135:347.

328. Elwood PC, Gallacher JE, Hopkinson CA, et al. Smoking, drinking, and other life style factors and cognitive function in men in the Caerphilly cohort. J Epidemiol Commun Health 1999; 53:9.

328a. Hebert LE, Scher PA, Beckett LA, et al. Relation of smoking and low-to-moderate alcohol consumption to change in cognitive function: a longitudinal study in a defined community of older persons. Am J Epidemiol 1993; 137:881.

329. Dartigues JF. Tobacco consumption and risk of cognitive impairment. Results of the Paquid study. Neurology 1992; 42 (Suppl 3):142.

330. Graves AB, van Duijn CM, Chandra V. Alcohol and tobacco consumption as risk factors for Alzheimer's disease: a collaborative re-analysis of case–control studies. Int J Epidemiol 1991; 20:548.

331. Ott A, Slooter AJC, Hofman A, et al. Smoking and risk of dementia and Alzheimer's disease in a population-based cohort study: the Rotterdam Study. Lancet 1998; 351:1840.

332. Merchant C, Tang M-X, Albert S, et al. The influence of smoking on the risk of Alzheimer's disease. Neurology 1999; 52:1408.

332a. Seshadri S, Wolf PA, Beiser A, et al. Smoking and the risk of Alzheimer's disease: gender, dose, and survival modify risks in the Framingham Study. Neurology 2000; 54 (Suppl 3):A396.

332b. Launer LJ, Feskens EJM, Kalmijn S, et al. Smoking, drinking, and thinking. Am J Epidemiol 1996; 143:219.

333. Kubota K, Matsuzawa T, Fujiwara T, et al. Age-related brain-atrophy enhanced by smoking: a quantitative study with computed tomography. Tohoku J Exp Med 1987; 153:303.

334. Ott A, Andersen K, Dewey ME, et al. Smoking and cognition in the elderly: prospective findings in the EURODEM Studies. Neurology, submitted.

335. Galanis DJ, Petrovitch H, Launer LJ, et al. Smoking history in middle age and subsequent cognitive performance in elderly Japanese men. The Honolulu-Asia Aging Study. Am J Epidemiol 1997; 145:507.

336. Au WW, Walker DM, Ward JB, et al. Factors contributing to chromosome damage in lymphocytes of chronic smokers. Mutat Res 1991; 260:137.

336a. Abrous DN, Adriani W, Montaron MF, et al. Nicotine self-administration impairs hippocampal plasticity. J Neurosci 2002; 22:3656-3662.

337. Slotkin TA. Nicotine and adolescent brain: insights from an animal model. Neurotoxicol Teratol 2002; 24:369.

337a. Villard-Mackintosh L, Vessey MD. Oral contraceptives and reproductive factors in multiple sclerosis incidence. Contraception 1993; 47:161.

337b. Thorogood M, Hannaford PC. The influence of oral contraceptives on the risk of multiple sclerosis. Br J Obstet Gynaecol 1998; 105:1296.

337c. Ghadirian P, Jain M, Ducic S, et al. Nutritional factors in the aetiology of multiple sclerosis: a case–control study in Montreal, Canada. Int J Epidemiol 1998; 27:845.

337d. Hernán M, Olek M, Ascherio A. Cigarette smoking and incidence of multiple sclerosis. Am J Epidemiol 2001; 154:69.

337e. Riise T, Nortvedt MW, Ascherio A. Smoking is a risk factor for multiple sclerosis. Neurology 2003; 61:1122.

337f. Franklin GM, Nelson L. Environmental risk factors in multiple sclerosis. Causes, triggers, and patient autonomy. Neurology 2003; 61:1032.

337g. Kaira R, Singh SP, Savage SM, et al. Effects of cigarette smoke on immune response: chronic exposure to cigarette smoke impairs antigen-mediated signaling in T-cells and depletes IP_3-sensitive Ca^{2+} stores. J Pharmacol Exp Ther 2000; 293:166.

337h. Silman AJ, newman J, MacGregor A. Cigarette smoking increases the risk of rheumatoid arthritis results from a nationwide study of disease discordant twins. Arthritis Rheum 1996; 39:732.

338. Rigotti NA. Treatment of tobacco use and dependence. N Engl J Med 2002; 346:506.

338a. Silagy C, Lancaster T, Stead L, et al. Nicotine replacement therapy for smoking cessation. Cochrane Database of Systematic Reviews 2002; 4:CD000146.

339. Tonnesen P, Frye V, Hansen M, et al. Effect of nicotine chewing gum in combination with group counselling on the cessation of smoking. N Engl J Med 1988; 318:15.

340. Hughes JR, Gust SW, Keenan RM, et al. Nicotine vs placebo gum in general medical practice. JAMA 1989; 261:1300.

341. Rose J, Levin ED, Behm FM, et al. Transdermal nicotine facilitates smoking cessation. Clin Pharmacol Ther 1900; 47:323.

342. Transdermal Nicotine Study Group. Transdermal nicotine for smoking cessation. JAMA 1991; 266:3134.

343. Tonnesen P, Norregaard J, Simonsen K, Sawe U. A double-blind trial of 16-hour transdermal nicotine patch in smoking cessation. N Engl J Med 1991; 325:311.

344. Benowitz NL. Pharmacodynamics of nicotine: implications for rational treatment of nicotine addiction. Br J Addict 1991; 86:495.

345. Tonnesen P, Norregaard J, Simonsen K, Sawe U. Transdermal nicotine patch for smoking cessation. N Engl J Med 1992; 326:344.

346. Sims TH, Fiore MC. Pharmacotherapy for treating tobacco dependence: what is the ideal duration of therapy? CNS Drugs 2002; 16:653.

347. Peters MJ, Morgan LC. The pharmacotherapy of smoking cessation. Med J Aust 2002; 176:486.

348. Hajek P, West R, Foulds J, et al. Randomized comparative trial of nicotine polacrilex, a transdermal patch, nasal spray, and an inhaler. Arch Intern Med 1999; 159:2033.

348a. Gray N, Boyle P. The future of the nicotine addiction market. Lancet 2003; 362:845.

349. Hurt RD, Sachs DPL, Glover ED, et al. A comparison of sustained-release bupropion and placebo for smoking cessation. N Engl J Med 1977; 337:1195.

350. Jorenby DE, Leisehow SJ, Nides MA, et al. A controlled trial of sustained-release bupropion, a nicotine patch, or both for smoking cessation. N Engl J Med 1999; 340:685.

351. Ahluwalia JS, Harris KJ, Catley D, et al. Sustained-release buprorion for smoking cessation in African Americans. A randomized controlled trial. JAMA 2002; 288:468.

351a. Swan GE, McAfee T, Curry SJ, et al. Effectiveness of bupropion sustained release for smoking cessation in a health care setting. A randomized trial. Arch Intern Med 2003; 163:2337.

352. Prochazka AV, Weaver MJ, Keller RT, et al. A randomized trial of nortriptyline for smoking cessation. Arch Intern Med 1998; 158:2035.

353. Hall SM, Reus VI, Munoz RF, et al. Nortriptyline and cognitive behavioral therapy in the treatment of cigarette smoking. Arch Gen Psychiatry 1998; 55:683.

354. Tennant FS, Tarver AL, Rawson RA. Clinical evaluation of mecamylamine for withdrawal from nicotine dependence. In: Harris LS, ed. Problems of Drug Dependence, 1983. Washington, DC: NIDA Research Monograph 49. DHHS, 1984:239.

355. Glassman AH, Jackson WK, Walsh WK, et al. Cigarette craving, smoking withdrawal, and clonidine. Science 1984; 226:864.

356. Wei H, Young D. Effect of clonidine on cigarette cessation and in the alleviation of withdrawal symptoms. Br J Addict 1988; 83:1221.

357. Glassman AH, Sterner F, Walsh BT, et al. Heavy smokers, smoking cessation, and clonidine: results of a double-blind randomized trial. JAMA 1988; 259:2863.

358. Franks R, Harp J, Bell B. Randomized controlled trial of clonidine for smoking cessation in a primary care setting. JAMA 1989; 262:3011.

359. Ornish KA, Ziscook S, McAdams LA. Effects of transferman clonidine treatment on withdrawal symptoms associated with smoking cessation. Arch Intern Med 1988; 148:2027.

360. Krishnan-Sarin S, Ropsen MI, O'Malley SS. Naloxone challenge in smokers. Preliminary evidence of an opioid component in nicotine dependence. Arch Gen Psychiatry 1999; 56:663.

361. Karras A, Kane J. Naloxone reduces cigarette smoking. Life Sci 1980; 27:1541.

362. Nemmeth-Coslett R, Griffiths RR. Naloxone does not affect cigarette smoking. Psychopharmacology 1986; 89:261.

363. David S, Lancaster T, Stead LF. Opioid antagonists for smoking cessation. Cochrane Database of Systematic Reviews. 2001; 3:CD003086.

364. Mello NK, Lukas SE, Mendelson JH. Buprenorphine effects on cigarette smoking. Psychopharmacology 1985; 86:417.

365. Hernandez SC, Bertolino M, Xiao Y, et al. Dextromethorphan and its metabolite dextrorphan block α3/β4 neuronal nicotinic receptors. J Pharmacol Exp Ther 2000; 293:962.

366. Panagis G, Kastellakis A, Spyraki C, et al. Effects of methyllycaconitine (MLA), an alpha 7 nicotineic receptor antagonist, on nicotine- and cocaine-induced potentiation of brain stimulation reward. Psychopharmacology 2000; 149:388.

367. Dewey SL, Brodie JD, Gerasinov M, et al. A pharmacologic strategy in the treatment of nicotine addiction. Synapse 1999; 31:76.

368. Persico AM, Malin DH, Wilson OB, et al. Acetyl-L-carnitine stereospecifically attenuates nicotine abstinence syndrome in the rat and facilitates smoking cessation in an open one-year follow-up trial. Soc Neurosci Abstr 1995; 21:722.

369. Schneider FH, Olsson TA. Clinical experience with lobeline as a smoking cessation agent. Med Chem Res 1996; 6:562.

370. Stead LF, Hughes JR. Lobeline for smoking cessation. The Cochrane Library, Issue 3. Oxford, Update Software, 2001.

371. Glover ED, Schneider FH, Mione PJ. A smoking cessation trial with lobeline sulfate: a pilot study. Am J Health Behav 1998; 22:62.

372. Pentel RR, Malin DH, Ennifar S, et al. A nicotine conjugate vaccine reduces nicotine distribution to brain and attenuates its behavioral and cardiovascular effects in rats. Pharmacol Biochem Behav 2000; 65:191.

373. White AR, Rampes H, Ernst E. Acupuncture for smoking cessation. Cochrane Database of Systematic Reviews 2002; 2:CD000009.

374. DiFranza JR, Richards JW, Paulman PM, et al. RJR Nabisco's cartoon camel promotes Camel cigarettes to children. JAMA 1991; 266:3149.

375. Centers for Disease Control. Comparison of the cigarette brand preferences of adult and teen-aged smokers—United States, 1989, and 10 US communities, 1988 and 1990. MMWR 1992; 41:169.

376. Vateesatokit P. The latest victim of tobacco trade sanctions. JAMA 1990; 264:1522.

377. Siegel M. The effectiveness of state-level tobacco control interventions: a review of program implementation and behavioral outcomes. Annu Rev Public Health 2002; 23:45.

378. Cummings SR, Coates TJ, Richard RJ, et al. Training physicians in counseling about smoking cessation. A randomized trial of the "Quit for Life" Program. Ann Intern Med 1989; 110:640.

379. Cohen SJ, Stookey GK, Katz BP, et al. Encouraging primary care physicians to help smokers quit. A randomized controlled trial. Ann Intern Med 1989; 110:648.

380. Manley M, Epps RP, Husten C, et al. Clinical interventions in tobacco control. A National Cancer Institute training program for physicians. JAMA 1991; 266:3172.

381. Dwoskin LP, Crooks PA. A novel mechanism of action and potential use of lobeline as a treatment for psychostimulant abuse. Biochem Pharmacol 2002; 63:89.

382. Harrod SB, Phillips SB, Green TA, et al. α-lobeline attenuates methamphetamine self-administration, but does not serve as a reinforcer in rats. Soc Neurosci Abstr 2000; 26:789.

Index

Page numbers followed by **t** and **f** stand for tables and figures, respectively.